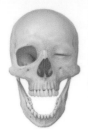

WinkingSkull.com PLUS

Test your mastery of medical physiology with this interactive online study aid.

Use the scratch-off code below to register for WinkingSkull.com *PLUS* to access:

D1569745

- **Clinical cases that correspond to the section coverage** to reinforce the physiologic concepts in that section
    - With **study questions for self-testing**, including **instantly available answers** for comparison, and **case analyses** for reinforcement
    - **Correlated with the text** making targeted review of missed concepts easy
- **More than 250 full-color images of must-know anatomy**, with "labels-on, labels-off" functionality and timed self-tests which make learning key body structures fun

Simply visit WinkingSkull.com and follow these instructions to get started today.

If you do not already have a free WinkingSkull.com account, visit WinkingSkull.com, enter the scratch off code below, and complete the registration form to create a new account.

If you already have a WinkingSkull.com account, go to the "My Account" page and click on the "Enter WinkingSkull PLUS Access Code" link. Enter the scratch-off code below.

PER COPYRIGHT,
REGISTRATION SITE UNAVAILABLE

This book cannot be returned once this panel has been scratched off.

System requirements for optimal use of WinkingSkull.com *PLUS*: * *

	WINDOWS	MAC
Recommended Browser(s)	Windows XP or Vista	MAC OS X 10.4.8 or higher
Silverlight Plug-in	Microsoft Silverlight* *After registering, follow the prompts to download Silverlight, a free plug-in required for use on the study and test pages*	
Recommended for optimal usage experience	Monitor resolutions: • A display capable of reading millions of colors • Normal (4:3) 1024 x 786 or higher	

* * *While you may find that WinkingSkull.com works with some older systems, we recommend the above as minimum requirements for using the capabilities of the site.*

Fundamentals of Medical Physiology

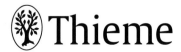

Fundamentals of Medical Physiology

Edited by
Joel Michael, PhD
Professor of Physiology
Department of Molecular Biophysics and Physiology
Rush Medical College
Chicago, Illinois

Based on the work of
Sabyasachi Sircar, MD
Professor of Physiology
University College of Medical Sciences
University of Delhi
Delhi, India

Thieme
New York • Stuttgart

Thieme Medical Publishers, Inc.
333 Seventh Ave.
New York, NY 10001

Vice President, Editorial Director, Educational Products: Anne T. Vinnicombe
Executive Editor: Kay D. Conerly
Editorial Assistant: Lauren Henry
International Production Director: Andreas Schabert
Production Editor: Kenneth L. Chumbley, Publication Services
Vice President, International Marketing and Sales: Cornelia Schulze
Chief Financial Officer: James W. Mitos
President: Brian D. Scanlan
Compositor: Manila Typesetting Company
Printer: Replika

Cover illustration drawn by Markus Voll

Library of Congress Cataloging-in-Publication Data

 Fundamentals of medical physiology/edited by Joel Michael; based on the work of Sabyasachi Sircar.
   p. ; cm.
 ISBN 978-1-60406-274-8
 1. Human physiology. I. Michael, Joel A., 1940- II. Sircar, Sabyasachi.
 [DNLM: 1. Physiological Phenomena. QT 104 F9816 2010]
 QP34.5.F863 2010
 612--dc22
                                  2010013486

Important note: Medical knowledge is ever-changing. As new research and clinical experience broaden our knowledge, changes in treatment and drug therapy may be required. The authors and editors of the material herein have consulted sources believed to be reliable in their efforts to provide information that is complete and in accord with the standards accepted at the time of publication. However, in view of the possibility of human error by the authors, editors, or publisher of the work herein or changes in medical knowledge, neither the authors, editors, nor publisher, nor any other party who has been involved in the preparation of this work, warrants that the information contained herein is in every respect accurate or complete, and they are not responsible for any errors or omissions or for the results obtained from use of such information. Readers are encouraged to confirm the information contained herein with other sources. For example, readers are advised to check the product information sheet included in the package of each drug they plan to administer to be certain that the information contained in this publication is accurate and that changes have not been made in the recommended dose or in the contraindications for administration. This recommendation is of particular importance in connection with new or infrequently used drugs.

Some of the product names, patents, and registered designs referred to in this book are in fact registered trademarks or proprietary names even though specific reference to this fact is not always made in the text. Therefore, the appearance of a name without designation as proprietary is not to be construed as a representation by the publisher that it is in the public domain.

Printed in India

5 4 3 2 1

ISBN 978-1-60406-274-8

This book is dedicated to my family: my wife Greta;

my daughters and sons-in-law, Erica Michael

and Dimitrios Donavos, and Jennifer Michael and Chris Beck;

and my grandchildren, Nicole and Allison Beck

Figure Acknowledgments

The following figures are reproduced from other Thieme sources:

Figs. 5.2, 12.1, 35.5, 35.7B, 35.8, 35.12, 78.1B-D. From *THIEME Atlas of Anatomy, General Anatomy and Musculoskeletal System*, © Thieme 2006, Illustrator: Markus Voll.

Fig. 78.1A. From *THIEME Atlas of Anatomy, General Anatomy and Musculoskeletal System*, © Thieme 2006, Illustrator: Karl Wesker.

Figs. 32.1, 33.1, 39.1, 41.1, 42.4A, 44.2, 45.1, 53.1, 67.3, 68.3, 69.1B, 77.1, 78.5B, 79.1, 81.1, 83.6, 84.4, 85.1, 85.2, 85.4, 85.9. From *THIEME Atlas of Anatomy, Neck and Internal Organs*, © Thieme 2006, Illustrator: Markus Voll.

Fig. 78.5A. From *THIEME Atlas of Anatomy, Neck and Internal Organs*, © Thieme 2006, Illustrator: Karl Wesker.

Figs. B.6, B.7B, 1.1, 3.3, 10.2, 10.3, 13.6, 13.8, 18.1, 45.17, 69.2, 69.4, 79.8. From Silbernagl S, Despopoulos A. *Color Atlas of Physiology*. Stuttgart-New York: Thieme; 2006.

Fig. 13.1. From Keuhnel W. *Color Atlas of Cytology, Histology and Microscopic Anatomy*. Stuttgart-New York: Thieme; 2003.

Fig. 23.3, 23.5, 28.1, 28.3, 29.1, 29.2. From Theml N, Diem H, Haferlach T. *Color Atlas of Hematology*. Stuttgart-New York: Thieme; 2004.

Fig. 30.2. From Burmester G-R, Pezzutto A. *Color Atlas of Immunology*. Stuttgart-New York: Thieme; 2006.

Fig. 40.7. From Mumenthaler M, Mattle H, Taub E. *Fundamentals of Neurology*. Stuttgart-New York: Thieme; 2006.

Figs. 52.3, 52.4, 52.5, 78.3. From Riede U-N, Werner M. *Color Atlas of Pathology*, Stuttgart-New York: Thieme; 2005.

Fig. 73.1. From Eastman G, Wald C, Crossin J. *Getting Started in Radiology*. 2006, Thieme Stuttgart.

Contents

Preface

This text is designed for U.S. medical school courses in physiology and is based on the original work of Dr. Sabyasachi Sircar. The goal of the text is to present the physiology that medical students need to learn in as straight forward and concise a manner as possible. I have also tried to create a text that would engage the student in learning the material ("knowing the facts") but would also provide the student with opportunities to learn to use the knowledge gained in solving real problems. American medical education is changing rapidly, with a variety of new, research-based educational paradigms being explored in the classroom. What is needed is a textbook of medical physiology that will better support student learning. I believe that this book will do that.

This book is case-based and includes a real clinical case at the beginning of each section, as well as questions related to the case throughout each chapter in the section. I have also attempted to draw student attention to recurring themes or General Models (which are described on the inside front cover of this book) that appear over and over again in every area of physiology. Both of these features are intended to help the student master the often difficult concepts and principles of physiology.

There is rich educational research literature on the benefits of the greatest possible active engagement between the learner and the material to be learned (Michael 2006). For medical students this engagement is certainly facilitated by the case-based feature of this book. Providing students with opportunities to apply the physiology they are learning to questions about a real case is engaging and encourages the learner to go beyond mere memorization to acquire the ability to apply what they know in a problem-solving context (Michael 2001). The references to General Models will help students build an integrated understanding of human physiology and will also provide tools for use in solving problems.

The organization of the book—the sequence of topics found in the ten sections—is quite conventional. Within each section the topics are covered in the order in which they are commonly taught and generally found in medical physiology courses. Nevertheless, not every course pursues these topics in the same order, and students should find that the text will assist their learning however different the sequence in their particular curriculum might be. The case and its associated questions should always be looked at first to make the most effective use of the questions included in each section.

I have been teaching physiology to medical students for forty years, and for thirty of those years I have been conducting research on learning and teaching, much of it with support from the National Science Foundation. These experiences have made it clear that learning physiology is a difficult task for anyone. Some of the problems are inherent in the discipline; physiology is a highly integrative science that is based on an understanding of physics, chemistry, and cell biology. Some of the difficulties that students encounter arise from learning resources, such as textbooks, that do not adequately support their learning. It is my hope that this text will help with both of these problems and that students using it will find it at least somewhat easier to master medical physiology.

Acknowledgments

I have learned much of what I know about teaching medical physiology from my interactions with forty classes of Rush Medical College students. Watching them learn (and sometimes not learn) has shaped my thinking about how to help the learner to learn. I also want to acknowledge two collaborators and friends, Harold Modell, PhD, and the late Allen Rovick, PhD, with whom I have debated teaching and learning for about as long as I have been at Rush. Keith Boyd, MD, of the Office of Medical Student Programs of Rush Medical College has taught me a great deal about writing cases that will help students learn.

Joel Michael, PhD
Department of Molecular Biophysics and Physiology
Rush Medical College
Chicago, Illinois

References

Michael, J. A. 2001. In pursuit of meaningful learning. *Advances in Physiology Education* 25:1145–58. Accessible on-line for free at www.advan.physiology.org.

Michael, J. 2006. Where's the evidence that active learning works? *Advances in Physiology Education* 30:159–67. Accessible on-line for free at www.advan.physiology.org.

How to Use *Fundamentals of Medical Physiology*

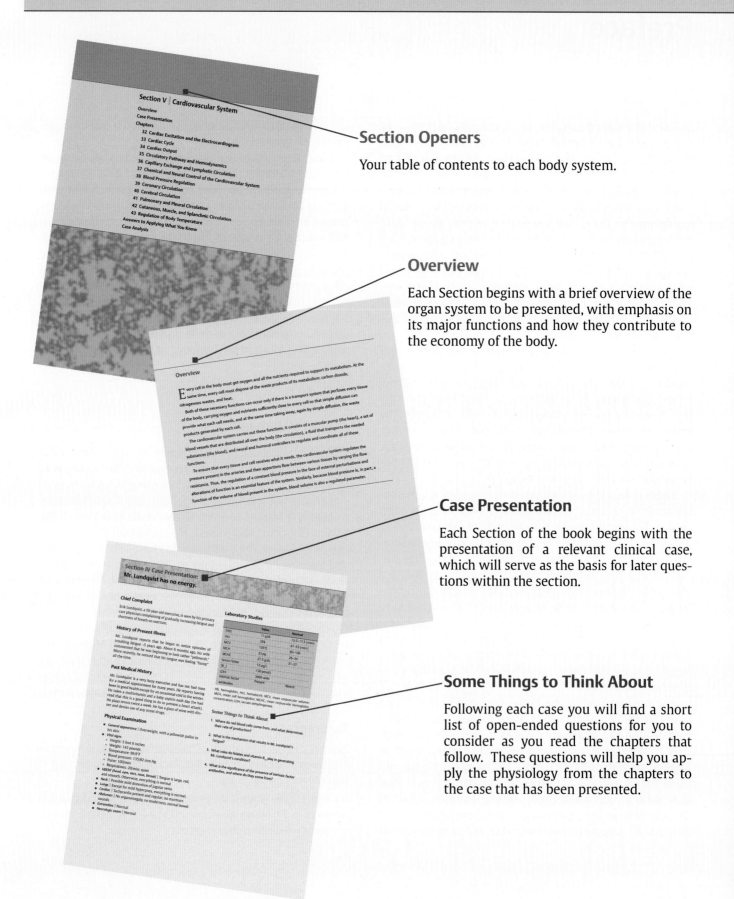

Section Openers

Your table of contents to each body system.

Overview

Each Section begins with a brief overview of the organ system to be presented, with emphasis on its major functions and how they contribute to the economy of the body.

Case Presentation

Each Section of the book begins with the presentation of a relevant clinical case, which will serve as the basis for later questions within the section.

Some Things to Think About

Following each case you will find a short list of open-ended questions for you to consider as you read the chapters that follow. These questions will help you apply the physiology from the chapters to the case that has been presented.

General Models

There are a number of phenomena that are present in many different places in the body and we have referred to these as "general models." These general models are described in the table located on the inside of the front cover. Throughout the text we have drawn your attention to the applicability of these models to physiologic phenomena wherever they occur.

Summary

At the end of each chapter you will find a Summary of the important points that have been presented.

Applying What You Know

At the end of each chapter you will find questions relating the case presented at the beginning of the section to the physiology discussed in the chapter you have just read. You can confirm that you have understood the chapter by correctly answering these questions.

Answers to Applying What You Know

At the end of each Section of the book, you will find brief answers to the Applying What You Know questions from each chapter.

Case Analysis

At the end of each section a brief analysis of the opening case is presented. This analysis will provide some information about the case from a clinical perspective and will also explain the (patho-) physiological mechanisms that give rise to the patient's condition.

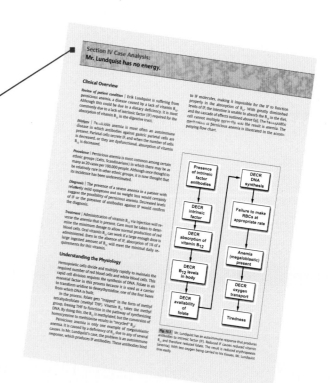

Section I | Foundations of Physiology

Overview

Chapters

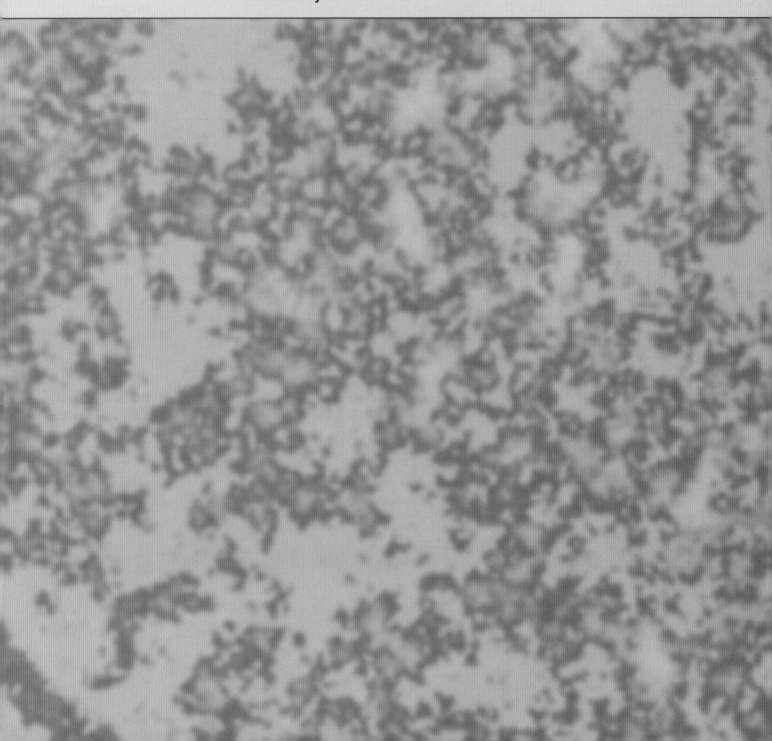

Overview

Physiology is a biological science. The questions it asks about the organism, and the answers that it generates, are informed by what we know about cells, the constituent parts of the organism. Thus, physiology builds on a knowledge base arising from such fields as biochemistry and molecular biology. The first three chapters of this section provide an overview of the structures and functions of the cell, the cell membrane, and the processes by which genetic information is used to make the cell.

One of the central concepts in physiology is homeostasis, the constancy of the *milieu interieur*, an idea set forth by Claude Bernard in 1865. In the fourth chapter the concept of homeostasis and its relationship to control systems is discussed.

The cell is the smallest unit of life, and all organisms are made up of one or more cells. Every animal cell uses nutrients that it obtains from the external world in some manner to generate the energy that is required to power all of its functions. Every cell arises from a parent cell.

The cell is bounded by a membrane (see Chapter 2) with special properties and many important functions. One function of the membrane is to contain the contents of the cell, its constituent parts (the organelles), and the solutes that are essential for the life of the cell. In this chapter we will describe the organelles whose various functions contribute to the life and health of the cell.

Cell Organelles

An *organelle* is a membrane-limited subcellular entity that can be isolated by centrifugation at high speeds. It includes the nucleus, mitochondria, endoplasmic reticulum, Golgi apparatus, peroxisome, lysosome, and plasma membrane (**Fig. 1.1**). The nucleolus, ribosomes, and cytoskeleton proteins are not organelles because they are not membrane-bound. However, they are considered here, along with the nucleus, because of their important functions in the cell.

The various subcellular fractions can be separated by differential centrifugation. *Low-speed* centrifugation precipitates the nuclei. *Intermediate-speed* centrifugation separates out the mitochondria, lysosomes, and peroxisomes. *High-speed* centrifugation precipitates the free ribosomes and endoplasmic reticulum (ER), both smooth and rough. These precipitates are collectively called *microsomes*. For example, the commonly used clinical term *hepatic microsomal enzymes* refers to the enzymes contained in smooth endoplasmic reticulum in liver cells. These enzymes play a key role in several important physiologic reactions and in the detoxification of drugs and poisons.

Apparatus for Protein Synthesis

The **nucleus** consists mainly of the chromosomes. Except in germ cells, the chromosomes occur in pairs, one from each parent. Each chromosome consists of a long strand of deoxyribonucleic acid (DNA). It is wrapped at intervals around a core of histone proteins to form a *nucleosome* (**Fig. 1.2A**). Thus, a chromosome is like a string of beads. The whole complex of DNA and proteins is called *chromatin*. When the cell is not dividing, only clumps of chromatin can be seen in the nucleus. During cell division, the coiling around histones is loosened, probably by acetylation of the histones, and the chromosomes become distinct.

The nucleus is enclosed in a double membrane containing pores (nuclear pores) through which messenger ribonucleic acid (mRNA) can pass out, and some of the proteins synthesized in the cytosol (the intracellular fluid and all the solutes contained in it) can enter back into the nucleus. The nuclear

pores are guarded with two rings that open and close to regulate the passage of large molecules. The transport through the nuclear pore requires proteins called *importins* and *exportins*.

Nucleolus | The nucleus of most cells, especially the growing cells, contains one or more nucleoli (**Fig. 1.1**). The nucleolus is the site of ribosome synthesis. It contains the genes for ribosome synthesis, along with a considerable amount of RNA and proteins representing ribosomes in various stages of production. Cells that are actively synthesizing proteins have prominent nucleoli.

Ribosomes are the sites of protein synthesis (**Figs. 1.1** and **1.2B**). They are small granules of RNA. Ribosomes may be present free in the cytosol or on the surface of the rough endoplasmic reticulum. The *free ribosomes* synthesize cytoskeletal proteins and other cytoplasmic proteins, such as hemoglobin. The proteins synthesized by them also find their way into the nucleus, mitochondria, and peroxisomes. The *bound ribosomes* are located on the rough ER. They synthesize all membrane proteins and most of the proteins destined for secretion. The proteins synthesized are extruded into the rough ER. Bound and free ribosomes are structurally identical and interchangeable, and the cell can adjust the relative number of each as its metabolism changes. Both types of ribosomes usually occur in clusters called *polyribosomes* attached to one mRNA molecule, an arrangement that increases the rate of polypeptide synthesis. The ribosomes of eukaryotes and prokaryotes are entirely dissimilar. Hence, in bacterial infections, antibiotics such as tetracycline and streptomycin are able to selectively inhibit the prokaryotic ribosomes of the bacteria, but not of the human cells.

Secretory (Exocytic) Apparatus

Rough endoplasmic reticulum | The endoplasmic reticulum, whether rough or smooth, is made of a series of membranous tubules in the cytoplasm of the cell (**Figs. 1.1** and **1.2B**). The rough ER has ribosomes attached to its cytoplasmic side. It is concerned with protein synthesis and the initial folding of polypeptide chains. After the polypeptide chain is formed, it is modified (posttranslational modification) to the final protein by chemical modifications of the amino acid residues, cleavage

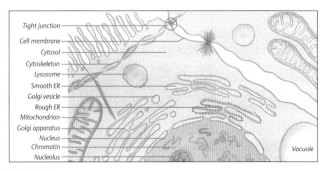

Tight junction
Cell membrane
Cytosol
Cytoskeleton
Lysosome
Smooth ER
Golgi vesicle
Rough ER
Mitochondrion
Golgi apparatus
Nucleus
Chromatin
Nucleolus
Vacuole

Fig. 1.1 An epithelial cell and some of its organelles. ER, endoplasmic reticulum.

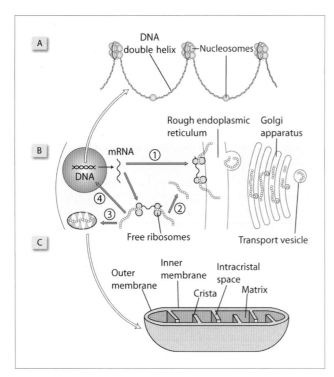

Fig. 1.2 **(A)** The double helix of DNA is magnified, showing it as a "string of beads". DNA forms the strings, while nucleosomes (histone proteins) form the beads. **(B)** Peptides synthesized on the rough endoplasmic reticulum mostly end up in the Golgi apparatus (1), while those synthesized by the free ribosomes either end up as cytoplasmic proteins (2) or find their way into the mitochondria (3) or the nucleus (4). **(C)** The mitochondrion is magnified, showing the outer and inner membranes, the matrix, and the intracristal spaces. mRNA, messenger ribonucleic acid.

of the polypeptide chain, and folding and packaging of the protein into its ultimate, often complex configuration.

Most proteins synthesized in the ribosomes have at their amino terminal a special sequence of 15 to 30 amino acids called the *signal peptide*. As the protein enters the rough ER, the signal peptide remains at the leading end; hence, it is also called the *leader sequence*. The signal peptide, and with it, the rest of the peptide, is guided into the ER by the signal recognition particle (SRP) present in the cytosol. The process is analogous to a needle guiding a thread. The SRP binds to receptors present on the surface of the ER and thereby anchors the signal peptide to the ER. Thereafter, the signal peptide dissociates from the SRP and binds to the protein (translocon) that forms the pores of the endoplasmic reticulum. The signal peptide is then cleaved from the rest of the peptide by a signal peptidase. In the case of hormones, removal of the signal peptide results in the conversion of preprohormone to prohormone (precursor forms of the hormone). Before secretion, additional amino acid residues are removed in the Golgi apparatus, resulting in the formation of the hormone.

The final step in posttranslational modification is protein folding. The way the protein gets folded is determined by the sequence of the amino acids in the polypeptide chain. Special protein molecules called *molecular chaperones* are sometimes

required for ensuring a proper protein folding. If a fully formed polypeptide chain folds too soon, it will not be able to enter the ER. Such failure usually does not occur because the polypeptide chain enters the ER well before it is completely synthesized. Thus, while the signal protein is entering the ER, the other end of the polypeptide is still lengthening due to continuing translation. The process is called *cotranslational insertion*. The polypeptide chain anchors the ribosome on which it is synthesized to the ER. The ER is called a rough ER when a large number of ribosomes are anchored to it.

The **Golgi apparatus (Figs. 1.1** and **1.2B)** is a stack of six or more membrane-enclosed sacs (cisterns). The cell contains one or more Golgi apparatuses, usually near the nucleus. Each Golgi apparatus is a polarized structure with a *cis* (convex) side and a *trans* (concave) side. Membranous vesicles containing newly synthesized proteins bud off from the rough ER and fuse with the *cis* side of the Golgi apparatus. The proteins are then passed from cistern to cistern, finally reaching the *trans* side, from which vesicles bud off into the cytoplasm and are finally exocytosed (**Fig. 1.2B**).

Secretory vesicles budding off from the trans-Golgi are released to the cell exterior through exocytosis. The passage of the vesicle from the Golgi body to the exterior can be along nonconstitutive or constitutive pathways. In the *constitutive* or *unregulated pathway,* the contents of the secretory vesicles are exocytosed immediately. The exocytosis results not only in secretion, but also in the incorporation of bits of new membrane into the existing cell membrane. Vesicles are also pinched off from the cell membrane by endocytosis. These vesicles, called *endosomes,* eventually become lysosomes (see below). In the *nonconstitutive* or *regulated pathway,* the secretory vesicles are released in a regulated fashion only on appropriate external stimulation, as in glandular cells and neuronal endings.

Apparatus for Metabolic Reactions

Mitochondria (Figs. 1.1 and **1.2C)** are sausage-shaped structures made of an outer membrane and an inner membrane that is folded to form shelves (*cristae*). The space between the two membranes is called the *intracristal* (or *intermembrane*) *space*, and the space inside the inner membrane is called the *matrix space*. The *outer membrane* of each mitochondrion is studded with the enzymes concerned with biologic oxidations, providing raw materials for the reactions occurring in the matrix space. The *matrix space* contains enzymes of the citric acid cycle and enzymes required for β-oxidation of fatty acids. The *inner membrane* contains succinate dehydrogenase and adenosine triphosphatase (ATP) synthetase. The *intracristal space* contains adenyl kinase and creatine kinase. The enzymes in the matrix, inner membrane, and intermembrane space are *marker enzymes* for mitochondriae; that is, they are found nowhere else.

Mitochondria have their own genome, which suggests that mitochondria were once autonomous organisms that came to develop a symbiotic relation with eukaryotic cells. Compared with the nuclear genome, the mitochondrial genome contains much less DNA. The mitochondrial DNA codes certain key enzymes of oxidative phosphorylation.

All the mitochondria in the zygote come from the ovum; therefore, the inheritance of mitochondrial DNA is entirely maternal. Mitochondrial DNA mutates far more frequently than nuclear DNA. Mutations in mitochondrial DNA cause a large number of relatively rare diseases.

Peroxisomes are cellular storehouses of metabolic enzymes. The peroxisome matrix contains nearly 50 enzymes that catalyze a variety of metabolic reactions. Peroxisomes in the liver detoxify alcohol and other harmful compounds. The marker enzymes for peroxisomes are catalase and urate oxidase.

Peroxisome membrane also has an elaborate mechanism for importing several enzymes into its matrix. An autosomal mutation that produces a defect in peroxisome membrane transport is the cause of Zellweger syndrome, which is fatal in infancy. Conversely, clofibrate, the drug used for lowering blood lipids, causes an increase in the number of peroxisomes. It is only one of the *several peroxisome proliferators* that are known to increase the number of peroxisomes.

The **smooth endoplasmic reticulum (Fig. 1.1)** is the site of steroid synthesis. Steroid-secreting cells are rich in smooth ER. The enzymes responsible for the synthesis of membrane phospholipids reside in the cytoplasmic surface of the cisterns of the ER. As phospholipids are synthesized at that site, they self-assemble into bimolecular layers, thereby expanding the membrane and promoting the detachment of *lipid vesicles* from it. These vesicles then travel to other sites, donating their lipids to other membranes.

Smooth ER is also the site of detoxification of drugs and poisons in other cells, especially liver cells. Hepatic detoxification has important implications in pharmacology and medicine. Liver cell ER is also the site where glucose-6-phosphate is stripped of its phosphate radical before releasing glucose into the blood. Glucose-6-phosphatase is the marker enzyme for smooth ER. In striated (skeletal and cardiac) muscle, the smooth ER is called the *sarcoplasmic reticulum*. It stores Ca^{2+} in high concentration and plays an important role in muscle contraction.

Digestive Apparatus

Lysosomes (Fig. 1.1) are membranous bags containing hydrolytic enzymes. The cell employs lysosomal enzymes for digesting large molecules of proteins, polysaccharides, fats, and nucleic acids. Lysosomes bud off from the *trans* face of the Golgi apparatus. Lysosomal enzymes are synthesized in the rough ER and then processed by the Golgi apparatus. The marker enzyme for lysosome is acid phosphatase.

The lysosomal membrane has a hydrogen-ion pump that pumps in H^+ from the cytosol and lowers the lysosomal pH to 5.0, which is the optimum pH for the lysosomal enzymes. The characteristic granules of the granulocytic leukocytes are actually lysosomes. Phagocytic vacuoles fuse with the lysosome, whose enzymes digest the phagocytosed matter. The products of enzymatic digestion are absorbed into the cytosol, while the rest is exocytosed. The lysosomes also engulf worn-out components of the cell in which they are located, forming autophagic vacuoles, and return the digested products for reuse by the cell. When a cell dies, lysosomal enzymes cause autoly-

sis of the remnants. Apoptosis by lysosomal enzymes is often important in the process of development. For example, in the embryonic stage, the hands are webbed until lysosomes digest the tissues between the fingers.

Small amounts of enzymes that leak out of lysosomes into the cytosol normally get inactivated due to the absence of acidic pH. However, large leakages cause destruction of the cell. In gout, phagocytes ingest uric acid crystals, and such ingestion triggers the extracellular release of lysosomal enzymes that contribute to the inflammatory response in the joints.

When a lysosomal enzyme is congenitally absent, it results in a rare but well-known group of disorders called the *lysosomal storage disorders*. In this, the lysosomes become engorged with indigestible substrates. For example, in Tay-Sachs disease, a lipid-digesting enzyme is missing. It leads to brain dysfunction due to engorgement of brain cells with lipids.

Cytoskeletal Apparatus

The cytoskeleton (**Fig. 1.1**) comprises three types of filaments: microtubules, microfilaments, and intermediate filaments. All three are made of protein subunits. They not only maintain the structure of the cell, but also permit it to change shape and move.

Microtubules and microfilaments are long polymers that move about by depolymerization at one end (the minus end) and polymerization at the other (the plus end). Both serve as "railroads" on which certain proteins called *molecular motors* can "walk" (**Fig. 1.3B**). Both lend some amount of structural solidity to the cell. However, there are differences too.

Microtubules are tubular structures, ~15 to 20 nm in diameter. A microtubule is made of α-tubulin and β-tubulin subunits that form stacks of rings containing 13 subunits (**Fig. 1.3A**). The molecular motors for a microtubule are *kinesin* and *dynein*. Microtubules are generally involved in the movement of cellular components, transporting secretory granules, vesicles, and mitochondria from one part of the cell to another. One end of its molecular motor binds to the transport vesicle, while the other end "walks" on the microtubule. They also form mitotic spindles, which move the chromosomes in mitosis. The anticancer drug paclitaxel binds to microtubules and makes them so stable that organelles cannot move, and mitotic spindles cannot form, leading to cell death. Microtubule assembly is prevented by colchicine and vinblastine.

Microfilaments are filamentous structures, ~35 nm in diameter. They are made of two F-actin (filamentous actin) strands that are coiled helically (**Fig. 1.3D**). Each F-actin strand is a polymer of G-actin (globular actin) subunits. The molecular motor of microfilaments is myosin. Microfilaments are concerned with motility of the cell itself. The most well-known function of microfilaments is their role in muscle contraction: the actin filaments in muscle are microfilaments. Microfilaments are anchored to the plasma membrane by anchoring proteins. Microfilaments and the anchoring proteins together form a dense matrix beneath the cell membrane, which is particularly abundant at the *zonulae adherentes* (intercellular junctions). Microfilaments are abundant in lamellipodia, the processes that cells put out when they crawl along surfaces. Bundles

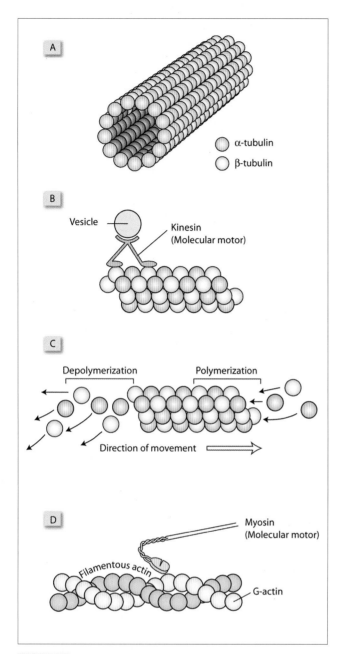

Fig. 1.3 Microtubules and microfilaments. **(A)** A microtubule is made of α-tubulin and β-tubulin. Thirteen of these subunits form rings that stack up to form a hollow tubule. **(B)** A kinesin molecule carrying a vesicle is moving on a microtubule. **(C)** The microtubules themselves can move about in the cytoplasm by depolymerizing at one end and polymerizing at the other. **(D)** Two strands of F-actin are intertwined and are moved by the myosin molecule.

of microfilaments are also present in the core of microvilli, where they lend structural support. Also, when a cell divides, it is pinched in two by a constricting band of microfilaments.

Intermediate filaments have a diameter (8–10 nm) that is between that of a microtubule and a microfilament. They are made of cytokeratin. Unlike microtubules or microfilaments, these proteins are very stable and remain mostly polymerized. They are also more abundant than either of the other

two structures. They serve as the "bones" of the cell, giving structural strength to it. For example, the nucleus sits in a cage made of intermediate filaments. In axons, the intermediate filaments are called *neurofilaments*: they maintain the axonal diameter. Intermediate filaments are also present in desmosomes (intercellular junctions).

The **centrosome** is located near the nucleus. It is made of two centrioles, which are short cylinders arranged at right angles to each other (**Fig. 1.4**). Microtubules in groups of three run longitudinally in the walls of each centriole. There are nine of these triplets spaced at regular intervals around the circumference.

The centrioles are surrounded by a small amount of γ-tubulin. Microtubules grow out of this γ-tubulin in the pericentriolar material; hence, the centrosome is also called the *microtubule-organizing center*. When a cell divides, the centrosomes duplicate themselves, and the pairs move apart to form the poles of the mitotic spindles, which are made of microtubules.

Cilia and flagella are motile processes of cells. Cilia usually occur in large numbers on the cell surface, whereas flagella are usually limited to one or a few per cell. Both have the same diameter, but flagella are about 10 times longer. They also differ in their pattern of beating. Dynein is the molecular motor responsible for the beating of flagella and cilia. The propulsion of a sperm is an example of flagellar action. The mucokinesis in the respiratory tract is brought about by ciliary action.

Both flagella and cilia resemble the centriole in having an array of nine tubular structures in their wall, but they have an additional pair of microtubules in the center (**Fig. 1.4**). Also, there are two rather than three microtubules in each of the nine circumferential structures. The microtubule assembly of a cilium or flagellum is anchored in the cell by a *basal body*, which is structurally identical to the centriole. It is from the basal body that the cilium or the flagellum starts to grow.

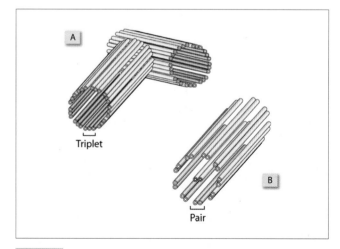

Fig. 1.4 **(A)** A pair of centrioles lying at right angles to each other. Each centriole is made of nine circumferential triplets of microtubules. **(B)** A cilium or a flagellum is made of nine circumferential pairs and one central pair of microtubules.

Intercellular Junctions

Intercellular junctions (**Fig. 1.5**) fasten cells to each other and to the basement membrane. They are of four types: zona occludens, zona adherens, desmosomes, and gap junction. Gap junctions not only fasten cells together, but, more importantly, permit passage of water, electrolytes, and ionic currents through them.

The **zona occludens or tight junction** is a bandlike ridge just below the apex of a cell. The membranes of the adjacent ridges are apposed tightly, leaving little space in between. Some are so tight that they do not allow water and ions to pass through them; therefore, they are called *tight* tight junctions. Others that are more permeable are called *leaky* tight junctions. These have important functions in the renal tubules. Tight junctions also help to maintain polarity of the cells. Membrane proteins in the apical region of the cell cannot float across the band of zona occludens.

The **zona adherens** is another band immediately below the zona occludens. However, the band is formed not by a ridge, but by microfilaments running under the surface of the membrane. The membranes of adjacent cells are apposed less tightly here, leaving a gap of ~20 nm. Like zona occludens, they strongly bind adjacent cells and also lend polarity to the cell by preventing the drift of integral membrane proteins. However, they are quite permeable to water and ions.

The **desmosome or macula adherens** is not a band, but a row of junctional patches below zona adherens (*macula = spot*). Like zona adherens, these spot-junctions leave 20 nm clefts between adjacent membranes. Intermediate filaments of the two adjacent cells converge on their respective side of the junction. The desmosome therefore not only attaches adjacent cells, but also lends structural stability to the entire epithelium by anchoring together the cytoskeleton of the adjacent cells. A *hemidesmosome* (one-half of a desmosome) attaches a cell to the basement membrane.

The **gap junction** consists of a pair of *hemichannels* or *connexons* inserted into the membrane of adjacent cells (**Fig. 1.6**). Each connexon is made of six identical protein subunits called *connexins,* which enclose a central channel. When the corresponding connexons of the adjacent cell link up end to end, they form a continuous channel that permits substances to pass through from cell to cell. Each connexin is made of four transmembrane peptide segments. Mutant connexons produce Charcot-Marie-Tooth disease, a form of peripheral neuropathy.

At gap junctions, the intercellular space narrows down to 3 nm, thereby helping in binding the cells together. However, their real physiologic significance lies in allowing ions to

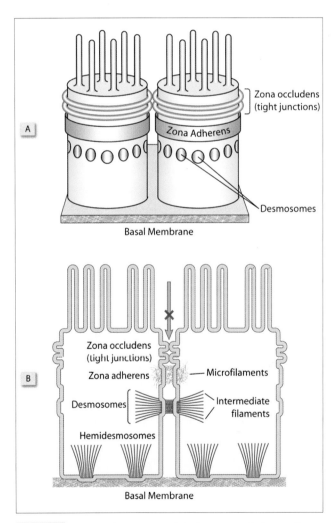

Fig. 1.5 Intercellular junctions. **(A)** The zona occludens and zona adherens form a continuous ring around the cell. The desmosomes form an interrupted ring around the cell. **(B)** Longitudinal section of two cells showing intercellular junctions. The zona occludens forms the tightest junctions and usually does not permit movement of electrolytes across them.

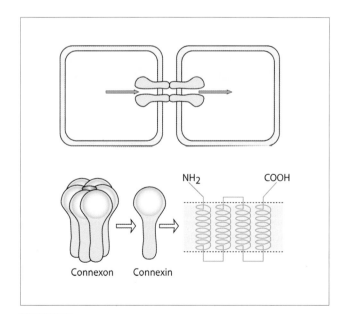

Fig. 1.6 Gap junctions connecting adjacent cells are designed to permit free communication through them. A gap junction is made of two connexons, one in the membrane of each of the adjacent cells (*top*). Each connexon is made up of six connexins (*bottom left*). Each connexin (*bottom, middle*) is made of a long peptide chain that traverses the membrane four times (*bottom, right*).

flow through them—they conduct ionic current. This enables electrical excitation to spread from cell to cell, as in smooth and cardiac muscles. The pore size of a gap junction decreases when intracellular Ca^{2+} is high or pH is low, both of which are commonly associated with cell damage. Closure of gap junctions in response to these stimuli isolates damaged cells, so that the Ca^{2+} and H^+ do not spread from the damaged to the normal cells.

Cell Adhesion Molecules

Cell adhesion molecules (CAMs) are surface glycoproteins present on the cell membrane surface. They are important for binding to other cells as well as to the extracellular matrix, where they bind to laminins. Apart from holding the tissues together, CAMs have important roles in inflammation and wound healing, embryonic development, axonal growth, and tumor metastasis. The four important groups of CAMs are selectins, integrins, cadherins, and the immunoglobulin G (IgG) superfamily of immunoglobulins. *Selectins* are required for capturing the free-flowing neutrophils and making them roll along the endothelial wall. Integrins and IgG superfamily immunoglobulins are present on the endothelium. They bring about a firm adhesion of the neutrophil with the endothelium. Neutrophilic migration through the endothelial wall (diapedesis) requires dissociation of intercellular cadherin contacts.

Summary

- Cell organelles are intracellular, membrane-limited structures that serve many different functions within the cell.

- Protein synthesis involves the nucleus, the nucleolus, the ribosomes, and the rough endoplasmic reticulum.

- Secretion of proteins and other products of cell synthesis to the exterior of the cell involves the rough endoplasmic reticulum working together with the Golgi apparatus.

- The cell's metabolic reactions take place in the mitochondria, peroxisomes, and smooth endoplasmic reticulum.

- Unwanted molecules in the cell interior are digested by enzymes found in the lysomes.

- The cell contains a cytoskeleton made up of microtubules and micro- and intermediate filaments.

- Intracellular junctions (the zona occludens, zona adherens, desmosomes, and gap functions) fasten cells to each other and to the basement membrane.

The cell's organelles and its intracellular solutes (some inorganic and some organic) are contained within the cell by its membrane. The membrane has limited and selective permeability; it maintains the intracellular concentration of electrolytes and biologic compounds that is distinctly different from that of the extracellular fluid. Cell membrane function is thus an essential one for the health and survival of the cell.

Membrane Composition

Membranes are complex structures composed of lipids, proteins, and carbohydrates. The cell membrane contains proteins and lipids in a *mass ratio* of 50:50. An average membrane protein is several times larger than the average lipid molecule, but lipid molecules are ~50 times more numerous than protein molecules. The ratio is not absolute and varies from membrane to membrane. The exact ratio between the two varies with the function of the cell. For example, the myelin sheath of nerves has ~75% lipids and 25% proteins, whereas membranes involved in energy transduction, such as the inner mitochondrial membrane, have 75% proteins and 25% lipids.

The major membrane lipids are phospholipids, glycosphingolipids, and cholesterol. Membrane phospholipids are of two types: the phosphoglycerides (**Fig. 2.1A**), which are more abundant, and the sphingomyelins (**Fig. 2.1B**), which are prominent in the myelin sheath. Glycosphingolipids present in the membrane include cerebrosides and gangliosides (**Figs. 2.1C and 2.1D**). Both are derivatives of sphingosine. Cholesterol is also present in the cell membrane, where it plays an important role in determining membrane fluidity (see below).

The plasma membrane contains over 100 different proteins: enzymes, transport proteins, structural proteins, antigens (e.g., for histocompatibility), and receptors for various molecules. The external side of membrane proteins has oligosaccharide chains (carbohydrates) attached to them.

Membrane Structure

Lipid Bilayer

Membrane lipids are amphipathic; that is they contain both hydrophobic and hydrophilic regions. The hydrophilic (polar) region is their globular head; the hydrophobic (nonpolar) regions are their fatty acid tails. The membrane lipids are organized into a continuous bilayer (as seen in **Fig. 2.2A**) in which the hydrophobic regions of the phospholipids are shielded from the aqueous environment, while the hydrophilic regions are immersed in water. Proteins are found inserted into this lipid bilayer and are classified into integral proteins and peripheral proteins.

Integral proteins are anchored to membranes through a direct interaction with the lipid bilayer. Some of them span the entire thickness of the membrane, often traversing the membrane several times (**Fig. 2.2B**). Others are located more on the outside or inside of the membrane.

Integral proteins are amphipathic, consisting of two hydrophilic ends separated by an intervening hydrophobic region that traverses the hydrophobic core of the bilayer. The hydrophilic ends of the integral protein are found outside the membrane, on either its external or internal surface. Integral

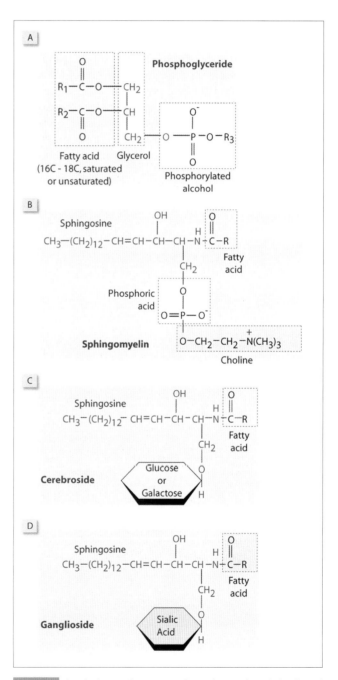

Fig. 2.1 (A,B) Chemical structure of membrane phospholipids and (C,D) glycosphingolipids.

proteins serve as (1) *channels,* which permit the passage of selected ions through the membrane; (2) *carriers* (or transporters), which translocate substances across the membrane by binding to them; (3) *pumps,* which are carriers that split adenosine triphosphate (ATP) and use the energy derived for membrane transport of substrates; (4) *receptors* (located on the outside), which bind to specific molecules and generate a chemical signal initiating intracellular reactions; and (5) *enzymes* catalyzing reactions at the membrane surfaces, both outer and inner.

Peripheral proteins do not interact directly with the phospholipids in the bilayer. They are associated with integral proteins via electrostatic interactions. They are located on both surfaces of the membrane. Peripheral proteins serve as cell adhesion molecules (CAMs) that anchor cells to neighboring cells and to the basal lamina. They also contribute to the cytoskeleton when present on the cytoplasmic side of the membrane. For example, ankyrin, a peripheral protein located on the inside of the membrane, anchors spectrin (a cytoskeletal protein in the erythrocyte) to band-3 (an integral protein of erythrocyte membrane). Ankyrin plays an important role in the maintenance of the biconcave shape of the erythrocyte (**Fig. 2.2C**).

Fluid Mosaic

The fluid mosaic model of membrane structure has been likened to icebergs (membrane proteins) floating in a sea of predominantly phospholipid molecules (**Fig. 2.3A**). Phospholipids also float about in the plane of the membrane. This diffusion, termed *translational diffusion,* can be as rapid as

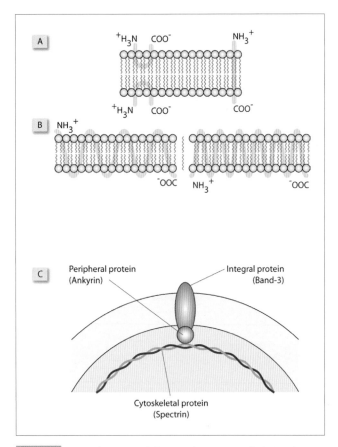

Fig. 2.2 Integral proteins. **(A)** Integral proteins with their polar residues projecting out. **(B)** A molecule of G-protein spanning the membrane seven times, and a glucose transporter molecule, spanning the membrane 12 times. **(C)** A peripheral protein anchoring the integral protein to the cytoskeletal protein of an erythrocyte.

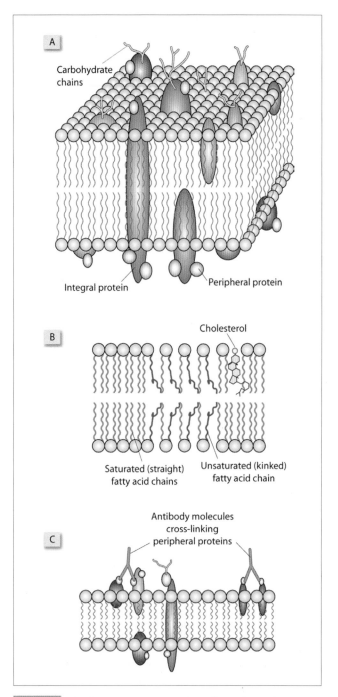

Fig. 2.3 Membrane structure. **(A)** The cell membrane showing integral and peripheral proteins. **(B)** Intercalation of kinked unsaturated fatty acid chains and cholesterol molecules spaces out the phospholipid molecules and affects membrane fluidity. **(C)** Antibody molecules cross-linking peripheral proteins. This reduces the mobility of integral proteins and reduces membrane fluidity.

several micrometers per second. Several membrane transport processes and enzyme activities depend on the optimum fluidity of the cellular membrane. As membrane fluidity increases, there is a rise in membrane permeability to water and small hydrophilic solutes. The fluidity of a cell membrane depends on the lipid composition of the membrane, the density of integral proteins, and the temperature.

Role of fatty acids | A lipid bilayer made up of only one type of phospholipid changes from a liquid state to a rigid crystalline state (gel state) at a characteristic freezing point. This change in state is known as a phase transition, and the temperature at which it occurs is called the phase transition temperature (T_m). The T_m is higher (fluidity is low) when the constituent fatty acid chains are long and mostly saturated (without double bonds). Long chains have greater interactions among themselves, making the membrane stiffer. Saturated fatty acids have straight tails, whereas unsaturated fatty acids have kinked tails. As more kinks are inserted in the tails, the membrane becomes less tightly packed, and therefore its fluidity increases (**Fig. 2.3B**), a change with consequences for membrane function.

Role of cholesterol | The presence of cholesterol in the membrane makes it possible for the cell membrane to maintain its fluidity across a wide range of temperatures. The number of cholesterol molecules in the membrane can be as high as the number of phospholipids. At high cholesterol:phospholipid ratios, the transition temperature is abolished altogether; that is, the membrane always remains fluid. Cholesterol is found among the phospholipids of the membrane, with its hydroxyl group at the aqueous interface and the remainder of the molecule among the fatty acid tails of phospholipids (**Fig. 2.3B**). At temperatures above the T_m, cholesterol partially immobilizes those portions of the fatty acid chains that lie adjacent to it and thus makes the membrane stiffer. At temperatures below the T_m, it minimizes the mutual interaction of the hydrocarbon tails of fatty acids and thereby increases membrane fluidity.

Membrane areas having a high density of integral proteins have low membrane fluidity due to protein–protein interaction. Some of the protein–protein interactions taking place within the plane of the membrane may be mediated by interconnecting peripheral proteins, such as cross-linking antibodies (**Fig. 2.3C**). These peripheral proteins may then restrict the mobility of integral proteins within the membrane.

Membrane Asymmetry

Membranes are asymmetric structures. This asymmetry is of two types: regional asymmetry and inside–outside asymmetry.

Regional asymmetry refers to the specialization of the cell membrane at different sites on the cell. For example, in renal tubules (see Chapter 53) and intestinal mucosal cells (see Chapter 70), only the membrane facing the lumen (tubular or intestinal) is thrown into folds, forming microvilli. Similarly, only the membranes that are contiguous with adjacent cells show specializations for intercellular tight junctions.

Inside–outside (transverse) asymmetry refers to the structural differences through the thickness of the cell membrane. For example, the phospholipids are not symmetrically disposed across the membrane thickness. The choline-containing phospholipids (lecithin and sphingomyelin) are located mainly in the outer molecular layer; the aminophospholipids (phosphatidylserine and cephalin) are preferentially located in the inner layer. Cholesterol is generally present in larger amounts on the outside than on the inside. Glycolipids lie exclusively on the outside of the membrane. Proteins too are differentially located in the outer, inner, or middle parts of the membrane. The carbohydrates are attached only to the membrane proteins on the outer surface. In addition, specific enzymes are located exclusively on the outside or inside of membranes, as in the mitochondrial and plasma membranes.

Membrane Disorders

Mutation of membrane proteins affects their function as receptors, transporters, ion channels, enzymes, and structural components. For example, in *hereditary spherocytosis,* there is mutation in the genes encoding spectrin, resulting in the tendency of the red blood cell (RBC) to become spherical rather than biconcave (see Chapter 21). Membrane proteins can trigger the production of antibodies by the immune system; when the antibody binds to the membrane protein, it alters its function. Autoantibodies to the acetylcholine receptor in skeletal muscle cause *myasthenia gravis.* Ischemia can quickly affect the integrity of various ion channels in membranes. The fragility of red cells is critically dependent on the protein:cholesterol ratio in the RBC membrane.

Membrane Transport

Simple Diffusion

Because simple diffusion involves no expenditure of biologic energy, it can occur only from a region of high solute concentration to a region of low solute concentration. Simple diffusion is the result of the random motion of molecules, and it occurs in both directions across the membrane. However, the diffusion down the concentration gradient is much greater than the diffusion against the gradient. Hence, the **net diffusion** is always down the concentration gradient. The rate of simple diffusion is directly proportional to the concentration gradient across the membrane (**Fig. 2.4**) and the permeability of the membrane to the solute. The membrane permeability to a substance depends on the molecule's size, lipid solubility, and electrical charge.

Gases such as oxygen (O_2), carbon dioxide (CO_2), and nitrogen (N_2) and hydrophobic molecules such as steroid hormones and weak organic acids and bases readily diffuse through the cell membrane.

Small uncharged polar molecules like water and urea can diffuse across the lipid bilayer, but not in physiologically sufficient amounts. Much larger amounts of water pass through membrane channels called *aquaporins*, which are present on all cells. Aquaporins do not allow ions to pass through them. The aquaporin molecules are stored in endosomes inside the cells. When suitably stimulated, they are rapidly translocated to the cell membrane. Similarly, urea employs specific transporters for crossing the membrane in larger amounts.

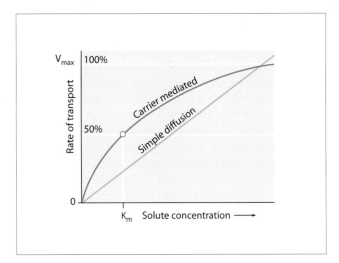

Fig. 2.4 Chemical kinetics of simple diffusion (*blue line*) and carrier-mediated membrane transport (*red line*). Note that although the rate of carrier-mediated transport plateaus at high solute concentration, there is no such limit to simple diffusion.

Large uncharged hydrophilic molecules such as glucose cannot diffuse through the lipid bilayer. Biologic membranes employ carrier-mediated transport for glucose.

Charged particles, whether large (amino acids) or small (Na^+, K^+, Cl^-, and Ca^{2+} ions), cannot diffuse across the lipid bilayer. Amino acids employ membrane transporters to cross the membrane. Ions cross the membranes, often in large amounts, through membrane channels. Ion channels do not allow water to pass through them.

Carrier-mediated Transport

Membrane transport can also occur through carrier-mediated transport, which employs certain integral membrane proteins as carriers or transporters for specific substrates. It may occur without any energy expenditure (facilitated diffusion) or may involve energy expenditure (active transport). When a carrier transports only a single substance, it is called a *uniporter*. When it transports more than one substance in the same direction, it is called a *cotransporter* or *symporter*. When it transports two substances in opposite directions, it is called a *countertransporter* or *antiporter*.

The rate of carrier-mediated transport depends on the concentration gradient across the membrane (**Fig. 2.4**), the number of carriers available (which is the rate-limiting parameter), and the rapidity of bonding and dissociation of the carrier with its substrate. The rate of transport cannot exceed a certain maximum, called the V_{max}. At V_{max}, all substrate-binding sites on the carrier are saturated. The substrate concentration at which the transport is 50% of the maximum is called the binding constant (K_m) of the carrier.

Carrier-mediated transport can be blocked by inhibitors that bear structural similarity to the physiologic substrate and compete with the physiologic substrate for a place on the carrier. Once they bind to the carrier, these inhibitors may not dissociate easily, thereby blocking the transport mechanism. For example, the carrier-mediated transport of glucose is blocked by phloridzin.

The inhibitors are often classified as competitive and noncompetitive. If an inhibitor binds irreversibly to the carrier, leaving no chance for the substrate to compete for a place on the carrier, the inhibition is called *noncompetitive*. The carrier in effect gets inactivated. If, however, the inhibitor binds reversibly, the physiologic substrate has a reasonable probability of competing and dislodging the inhibitor from the binding site. The inhibition is then said to be *competitive*.

It is unlikely that the carriers, which are integral membrane proteins, actually move through the thickness of the membrane, carrying their substrate with them. The inside-outside asymmetry of membrane proteins is too stable to permit such movements. Rather, a *ping-pong mechanism* has been proposed (**Fig. 2.5A**). In this model, the carrier protein exists in two principal conformations: ping and pong. In the pong state, it is exposed to high concentrations of solute, and the molecules of the solute bind to specific sites on the carrier protein. Transport occurs when a conformational change to the ping state exposes the carrier to a lower concentration of solute. The transition between the ping and pong states is powered by the bond energy released when the carrier binds to the solute. This is true for all carrier-mediated transport. In active transport (**Fig. 2.5B**), the binding of ATP to the carrier provides the energy needed to move the solute against its electrochemical gradient.

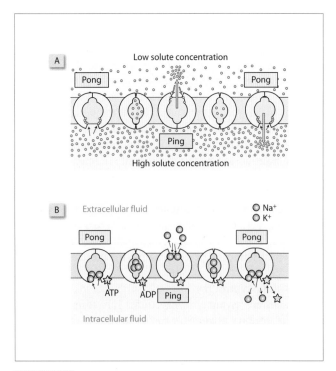

Fig. 2.5 The ping-pong model of carrier-mediated transport. **(A)** Facilitated diffusion. Note that transport of solute occurs in both directions. However, transport is greater from higher to lower solute concentration. **(B)** Active transport. Binding sites for sodium ions (Na^+) are present only at the inner side, whereas binding sites for potassium ions (K^+) are present only at the outer side of the membrane carrier. This ensures that Na^+ can only move out, whereas K^+ can only move in. ADP, adenosine diphosphate; ATP, adenosine triphosphate.

While integral membrane proteins employ the ping-pong mechanism for transporting ions, certain microbes synthesize small organic molecules called *ionophores* that transport ions by actually traveling across the membrane. These ionophores contain hydrophilic centers that bind specific ions and a hydrophobic exterior that allows them to dissolve in the membrane and diffuse across it.

Passive carrier-mediated transport, also called *facilitated diffusion*, can transport substrates only from a region of high concentration to a region of low concentration. Like simple diffusion, it is bidirectional—it occurs in both directions. However, when the concentration on one side is higher than the other, the difference in the kinetics of solute–carrier interaction ensures that there is a **net flux** of solute movement from high to low concentration.

Glucose and other large uncharged hydrophilic molecules have extremely slow rates of simple diffusion across the lipid bilayer. They cross the membrane much faster through facilitated diffusion. Examples of facilitated diffusion are the cotransport of Na^+ with monosaccharides or amino acids in renal tubular cells (see Chapter 55) and intestinal mucosal cells (see Chapter 70). An example of facilitated countertransport is the Cl^--HCO_3^- antiporter found in renal tubular cells and gastric parietal cells.

Facilitated diffusion is faster than simple diffusion, but the amount transported by facilitated diffusion is limited by the availability of the carrier. Hormones can regulate facilitated diffusion by changing the number of carriers available. For example, insulin increases glucose transport into cells by moving glucose transporters from an intracellular reservoir into the membrane.

Primary-active carrier-mediated transport involves energy expenditure. The energy comes mostly from ATP that is hydrolyzed by the carrier protein itself, which also acts as an ATPase. Unlike passive transport, active transport can transport substrates against a concentration gradient. The best-known example of a carrier ATPase is the Na^+-K^+ ATPase. It has binding sites for both ATP and Na^+ on the cytoplasmic side of the membrane, but the K^+ binding site is located on the extracellular side of the membrane (**Fig. 2.5B**). This asymmetry of location of the binding sites explains why, unlike facilitated diffusion, primary-active transport can occur only in one direction. Ouabain or digitalis inhibits this ATPase by binding to the extracellular site on the transporter.

Secondary-active carrier-mediated transport represents a combination of primary-active transport and facilitated diffusion. It is exemplified by glucose transport across renal tubular cells and intestinal mucosal cells (**Fig. 2.6**). The basolateral border of the cell lowers the intracellular Na^+ concentration through primary active transport of Na^+ ions to the exterior. The low intracellular Na^+ concentration provides the necessary concentration gradient for Na^+ to diffuse in passively at the luminal border through facilitated cotransport with glucose. Thus, the Na^+-K^+ ATPase indirectly powers the movement of glucose into the cell, and glucose can move in against a concentration gradient so long as Na^+ diffuses in along a concentration gradient.

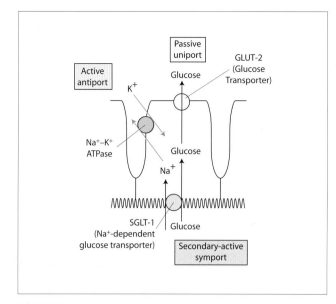

Fig. 2.6 Passive, active, and secondary-active transport. Sodium-dependent glucose transporter-1 (SGLT-1) transports glucose against its concentration gradient. The energy for this uphill transport is derived from the favorable concentration gradient for sodium ion (Na^+) with which it is cotransported. The Na^+ concentration gradient is created by the Na^+–K^+ adenosine triphosphatase (ATPase).

Endocytosis

Endocytosis is the process by which cells take up macromolecules and large particles from the extracellular environment. The process requires ATPase, Ca^{2+}, and microfilaments. Endocytosis occurs by invagination of the plasma membrane so as to enclose a small droplet of extracellular fluid and its contents. The invagination gets pinched off at its neck to form an endocytotic vesicle. The vesicle then transports its contents to other organelles by fusing with their membranes.

Alternatively, it can fuse back with the plasma membrane. Depending on what is endocytosed, endocytosis is called phagocytosis or pinocytosis. Endocytosis of cells, bacteria, viruses, or debris is called *phagocytosis*. Endocytic vesicles containing these particles fuse with primary lysosomes to form secondary lysosomes, where the ingested particles are digested. Endocytosis of water, nutrient molecules, and parts of the cell membrane is called *pinocytosis*.

Fluid-phase pinocytosis is a nonselective process in which the cell takes up fluid and all its solutes indiscriminately. Vigorous fluid-phase pinocytosis is associated with internalization of considerable amounts of the plasma membrane. To avoid reduction in the surface area of the membrane, the membrane is replaced simultaneously by exocytosis of vesicles. In this way, the plasma membrane is constantly recycled.

Absorptive pinocytosis is also called *receptor-mediated pinocytosis*. It is responsible for the uptake of selected macromolecules for which the cell membrane bears specific receptors. Such uptake minimizes the indiscriminate uptake of fluid or other soluble macromolecules. The vesicles formed during absorptive pinocytosis are derived from invaginations (pits) that are coated on the cytoplasmic side with a filamentous material called *clathrin*, a peripheral membrane protein. Such pits are called *coated pits.*

An example of absorptive pinocytosis is provided by the endocytosis of low-density lipoprotein (LDL) molecules. The molecules bind with their receptor on the plasma membrane, and the receptor-LDL complexes are internalized by means of coated pits. The endocytotic vesicles fuse with lysosomes in the cell. The receptor is released and recycled back to the cell surface membrane, but the LDL is metabolized.

Endocytosed hormone receptors can trigger intracellular events after being endocytosed. Following pinocytosis, these hormone receptors form *receptosomes,* vesicles that avoid lysosomes and deliver their contents to other intracellular sites, such as the Golgi body.

Receptor-mediated endocytosis can at times be self-defeating. Viruses causing hepatitis, poliomyelitis, and acquired immunodeficiency syndrome (AIDS) gain access into the cell through this mechanism. Iron toxicity also begins with excessive uptake of iron through endocytosis.

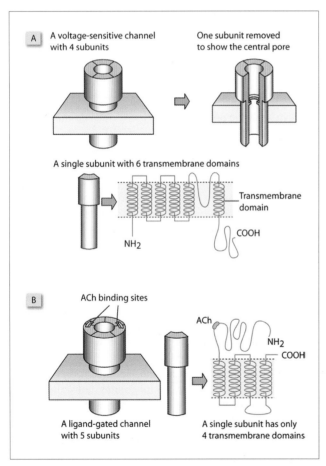

Fig. 2.7 **(A)** Structure of a voltage-gated channel. It is made of four subunits, with each subunit made of six transmembrane domains. The subunits enclose a central pore. **(B)** Structure of a ligand-gated cation channel. It is made of five subunits, each with four transmembrane domains. The subunits enclose a central pore. The binding sites for acetylcholine (ACh) are present on the exterior at the junctions between two adjacent subunits.

Exocytosis

Exocytosis is the process for release of macromolecules formed in the cell to the exterior. Exocytosis is associated with an increase in the area of the plasma membrane. Working in tandem with fluid-filled endocytosis, this process is involved in remodeling of the membrane. Exocytosed molecules are of three types. Some attach to the cell surface and become peripheral proteins, for example, antigens. Some become part of the extracellular matrix, such as collagen and glycosaminoglycans. Some enter the extracellular fluid and serve as hormones or neurotransmitters. These are exocytosed only when the cell is stimulated.

Membrane Channels

Ion channels are integral membrane proteins that enclose a central pore. They traverse the entire thickness of the cell membrane, projecting a little at both the outer and inner membrane surfaces.

The structural characteristics of some ionic channels are shown in **Fig. 2.7** and are summarized in **Table 2.1**. A voltage-sensitive Na^+ ion channel, for example, is made of four subunits designated as α, β, γ, and δ. Each subunit in turn is made of six coiled transmembrane segments designated S1–S6. In general, channels have variable numbers of subunits and transmembrane domains having different designations.

Ion Channel Specificity

Ion channels are highly specific for certain ions. Although it is understandable that a larger ion cannot pass through a smaller channel, it requires some explanation as to why smaller ions do not pass through larger channels. This is explained by the *closest-fit hypothesis.* The hydration of ions is an important consideration in this hypothesis.

The smaller an ion, the more highly localized is its charge, and the stronger is its electric field. Smaller ions, such as Na^+ (crystal radius of 0.095 nm), have stronger effective electric fields than larger ions, such as K^+ (crystal radius of 0.133 nm). As a result, smaller ions attract water more strongly. Thus, the strong electrostatic attraction for water causes Na^+ to have a larger water shell.

Table 2.1 Structural Characteristics of Ionic Channels

	Number of Subunits	Number of Transmembrane Domains per Subunit
Voltage-gated Na^+ and K^+ channels	4 subunits. All are α-type and are designated I, II, III, and IV	6 (S1, S2, S3, S4, S5, and S6)
Ligand-gated cation channel	5 subunits. 2 are α-type, 1 each are β, γ, and δ	4 (M1, M2, M3, and M4)

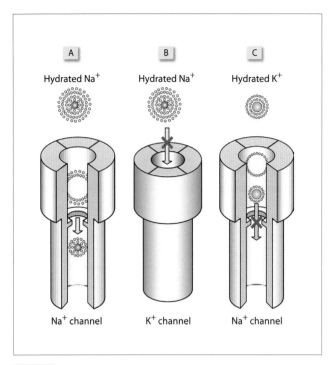

Fig. 2.8 The closest-fit theory of ion channel specificity. **(A)** A sodium ion (Na$^+$) passes through the outer and inner pores. **(B)** A hydrated sodium ion is unable to pass through the outer pore of a potassium ion (K$^{+)}$ channel. **(C)** A hydrated K$^+$ is unable to pass through the inner pore.

For passing completely through a channel, an ion has to negotiate two barriers: an *outer pore* and another pore called the *selectivity filter* located midway inside the channel (**Fig. 2.8**). The ion enters the outer pore with its complete water of hydration. Once it arrives at the inner selectivity filter, the ion sheds most of its water shell and forms a weak electrostatic bond with the polar (carboxyl) residues of the amino acids that line the channel wall. This electrostatic bond must release adequate energy for stripping the ion of its water shell. The energy released is maximum when the unhydrated ion fits closely in the channel and is less if it floats loosely within the channel.

The hydrated Na$^+$ ion is larger than the hydrated K$^+$ ion, and as would be expected, a Na$^+$ channel has a larger diameter than a K$^+$ channel. A hydrated Na$^+$ ion is a little too large to pass through the outer pore of a K$^+$ channel. The hydrated K$^+$ ion is slightly less in diameter than the Na$^+$ channel, yet it is unable to pass through the Na$^+$ channel because the selectivity filter of the Na$^+$ channel is oversized for a K$^+$ ion bereft of its water shell. Hence, the energy released due to the electrostatic attraction between the K$^+$ ion and the wall of the Na$^+$ selectivity filter is inadequate for stripping the K$^+$ ion of its water shell. With its shell intact, the K$^+$ is unable to negotiate the selectivity filter of the Na$^+$ channel.

Types of Channels

What makes channels unique as compared with other mechanisms of membrane transport is that they can be gated (opened or closed) precisely. Depending on the factors that produce

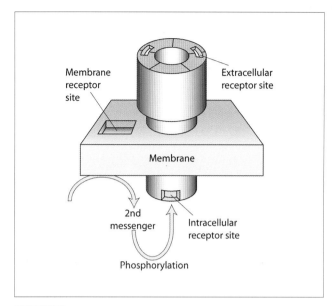

Fig. 2.9 Ligand-binding sites may be located on the outer membrane surface, or they may be present on the outer or inner parts of a membrane channel.

their opening and closing (gating), ion channels are classified into four types.

Voltage-gated channels are gated by changes in membrane potential. Examples are voltage-gated Na$^+$, K$^+$, and Ca^{2+} channels.

Ligand-gated channels are regulated by chemicals that bind to them (ligands). The ligand affects channel permeability in different ways (**Fig. 2.9**). (1) It can bind to the receptor channel protein at an extracellular site (e.g., in acetylcholine receptors). (2) It can bind to the channel at an intracellular site (e.g., pronase, local anesthetics). (3) It can bind to membrane receptors and activate a second messenger cascade, leading to phosphorylation of channel protein.

Mechanically gated channels have pores that respond to mechanical stimuli like the stretch of the membrane.

Resting channels are not gated at all. Resting channels make a substantial contribution to the membrane potential.

Apart from these physiologic channels, membrane pores may be created in pathologic situations. Diphtheria toxin and activated serum complement components like the C5b-C6-C7-C8-C9 fragment can produce large pores in cellular membranes and thereby provide macromolecules with direct access to the cell interior.

Summary

- The cell membrane controls the movement of solutes into and out of the cell.

- The cell membrane is a lipid bilayer in which are embedded a large number of different proteins that serve different functions.

- Transport of solutes across the membrane occurs by four different processes: passive diffusion (down a gradient), carrier-mediated transport (also down a gradient), primary-active transport (against a gradient), and secondary-active transport (also against a gradient).

- Channels are membrane-spanning proteins (some always open, others gated by different stimuli) through which solutes can diffuse down a gradient.

The characteristics of a cell are determined by its structural proteins and the proteinaceous enzymes that control its metabolic functions. The structure and hence the functions of proteins are determined by their amino acid sequence, which in turn is determined by the information coded into the nucleic acids in the cell's nucleus. That is to say, the structure and functions of a cell are determined by its genes. A change in the composition of the nucleic acid, a change in the genes, alters the protein synthesized, sometimes with deleterious consequences.

The genetic information in the nucleus is coded into the structure of deoxyribonucleic acid (DNA). DNA can replicate itself so that every daughter cell that results from cell division has exactly the same genetic information. DNA can also produce messenger and transfer ribonucleic acid (RNA), which leaves the nucleus and when in the cytoplasm gives rise to the synthesis of proteins. This process of information transfer from DNA to RNA to proteins is often referred to as the central dogma of molecular biology.

Nucleic Acids

DNA is made up of a set of basic subunits called nucleotides (**Fig. 3.1A**). A nucleotide is made of a nitrogenous base, a pentose sugar molecule, and up to three phosphate groups. The pentose sugar may be deoxyribose or ribose. Accordingly, the

nucleic acid is either DNA or RNA. DNA is found in the chromosomes, but it is present in the mitochondria too. RNA, though synthesized in the nucleus, is present mostly in the cytosol. In both DNA and RNA, the nucleotides are linked to each other by phosphodiester bonds, forming long chains of nucleotides. The codes for the synthesis of different types of amino acids reside in the sequence of the different nucleotides in the DNA. There are four types of nucleotides in DNA depending on the type of their nitrogenous base, which are adenine (A), guanine (G), cytosine (C), and thymine (T). Similarly, the nucleotides in RNA contain adenine, guanine, cytosine, or uracil (U). The nucleotide chain has two free ends, a 5′ (read five prime) end and a 3′ end. The sequence of nucleotides in a segment of DNA or RNA is conventionally stated from the 5′ end to the 3′ end.

DNA has a double helical structure (**Fig. 3.1B**), with its two strands interconnected by hydrogen bonds. RNA usually does not assume a double helical structure, but folds upon itself 10 times to form various shapes. There are three major types of RNA: ribosomal RNA (rRNA), transfer RNA (tRNA), and messenger RNA (mRNA). The rRNA, along with several proteins, forms the ribosomes upon which protein synthesis takes place. The tRNA transports specific amino acids from the cellular amino acid pool to the ribosomes, which are the sites of protein synthesis. The mRNA acts as a template of the genetic code contained in the DNA, and it contains the information needed to build the proteins coded for by a particular gene.

Genetic Code

The genetic code is made of three-lettered words (triplets or codons), each letter representing a particular nucleotide. Each triplet codon always codes for the synthesis of a specific amino acid. It is possible to arrange four nucleotides into 64 ($4^3 = 64$) different triplets. Of these, 61 code for amino acids, and the remaining 3 (UAG, UGA, UAA) are called *stop codons*. Because the number of codons (61) exceed the number of amino acids to be coded for (20), several amino acids have more than one codon coding for them (**Table 3.1**). The reverse is not true: one codon never represents more than one amino acid.

Not all stretches of DNA in the chromosome code for proteins. For example, if the nucleotide sequence in a stretch of RNA is 5′-AUG-CCA-UUG-GAU-UAA-3′, then the polypeptide coded by it is methionine-proline-leucine-aspartic acid. UAA does not code for any amino acid; rather, it signals that the chain should stop growing further. UAA is therefore a stop codon. Long stretches of DNA in eukaryotic cells do not code for protein. These noncoding regions are known as introns. The intervening stretches that code for proteins are known as exons.

Mutation refers to a permanent change in the genetic code. Such changes can have lethal effects (although this is not always the case) on an organism due to alterations in the protein encoded by the mutated segment of the DNA.

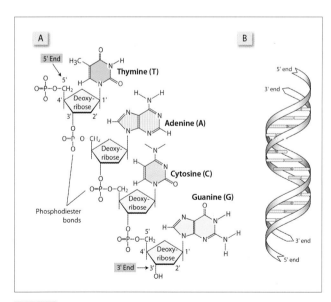

Fig. 3.1 **(A)** Nucleotides of deoxyribonucleic acid (DNA). Each of the four nucleotides (T, A, C, and G) consists of a common pentose sugar and different nitrogenous base. **(B)** The double helix structure of DNA. The nucleotides of each DNA strand form hydrogen bonds with their complementary nucleotide on the other strand.

Table 3.1 Codons for Amino Acids and Stop Codons

Glycine	GGU, GGC, GGA, GGG
Alanine	GCU, GCC, GCA, GCG
Valine	GUU, GUC, GUA, GUG
Leucine	UUA, UUG, CUU, CUC, CUA, CUG
Isoleucine	AUU, AUC, AUA
Serine	UCU, UGC, UCA, UCG, AGU, AGC
Threonine	ACU, ACC, ACA, ACG
Cysteine	UGU, UGC
Methionine	AUG
Aspartic acid	GAU, GAC
Aspartine	AAU, AAC
Glutamic acid	GAA, GAG
Glutamine	CAA, CAG
Arginine	CGU, CGC, CGA, CGG, AGA, AGG
Lysine	AAA, AAG
Histidine	CAU, CAC
Phenylalanine	UUU, UUC
Tyrosine	UAU, UAC
Tryptophan	UGG
Proline	CCU, CCC, CCA, CCG
Stop codons	UAA, UAG, UGA

DNA Replication

During cell division, each strand of the double-stranded DNA creates an identical copy of itself. This is known as *DNA replication*. In eukaryotes (like bacteria), DNA replication begins at multiple sites along the DNA helix, but in prokaryotes (like humans), the replication begins at a single site. The site(s) must contain a unique nucleotide sequence. At the site(s) of replication, the two strands of DNA unwind, forming a replication fork. Unwinding requires the enzyme DNA helicase. A complementary nucleotide sequence is assembled on each of the separated DNA strands. Because a DNA strand is read out only in the 3′ to 5′ direction, the complementary DNA strands grow in opposite directions, as shown in **Fig. 3.2A**. Replication requires the enzyme DNA polymerase. The initiation of replication requires an RNA primer, a short RNA segment attached to the 3′ end of the DNA strands.

Transcription

Transcription is the process by which messenger RNA is synthesized using one of the DNA strands as the template (**Figs. 3.2B** and **3.3**). The part of the template bearing the nucleotide sequence TATAAA (the TATA box), read in the 5′ to 3′ direction, signals the initiation of transcription. These sequences are called the promoter regions of the DNA.

The enzyme RNA polymerase binds to the DNA at the promoter region. Transcription begins a few nucleotides downstream from the promoter site. This produces a growing chain of RNA bearing complementary nucleotides. Transcription stops

when the RNA polymerase reaches an area on the DNA known as the termination region.

Translation

Translation is the process of mRNA-guided protein synthesis (**Fig. 3.3**). The mRNA is formed in the nucleus. It leaves the nucleus to enter the cytosol and reaches the ribosome. Protein synthesis takes place on the ribosomal surface. Translation requires the availability of amino acids that are to be incorporated into the peptide, the mRNA bearing the codons, the tRNA bearing the anticodons and having a binding site for one amino acid, and ribosomes on which the protein assembly can take place. Also required are guanosine triphosphate (GTP) and adenosine triphosphate (ATP) as energy sources and several protein factors that are necessary for the initiation, elongation, and termination of the peptide chain.

Initiation of translation begins with the binding of the mRNA with the ribosome so that the initiation codon of the mRNA (the first codon that is to be translated) is located at

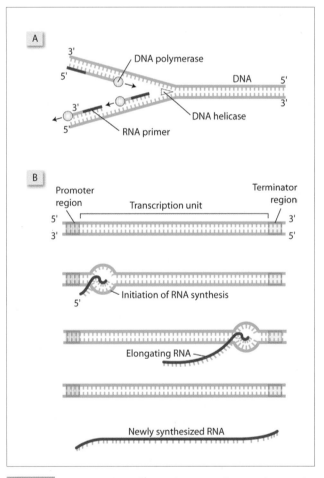

Fig. 3.2 **(A)** Deoxyribonucleic acid (DNA) replication showing the replication fork. Two enzymes are required, one to "unzip" the DNA helix as replication proceeds, the other to add the successive nucleotides required to build the complementary strand of DNA. **(B)** Transcription (ribonucleic acid [RNA] synthesis) is a process in which the DNA is read, and a strand of RNA containing that code is constructed. The RNA will be used to build the protein specified by the DNA codon.

the P-site (*P* for peptide) of the ribosome, and its second codon is located at the A-site (*A* for amino acid) of the ribosome. Next, a tRNA carrying methionine binds to the initiation codon AUG in the mRNA. Protein molecules called initiation factors bind to the complex, lending it stability.

Elongation of the peptide chain occurs when a second tRNA carrying the corresponding amino acid (say, tryptophan) binds to the next codon (UGG) on the mRNA at the A-site of the ribosome. This binding requires GTP and an elongation factor. Next, the methionine molecule binds to the tryptophan molecule to form a dipeptide. The reaction is catalyzed by the enzyme peptidyltransferase and an rRNA molecule. The tRNA left behind by methionine dissociates from the P-site. The tRNA now moves to the vacant P-site, carrying its dipeptide and the second codon (UGC) with it. A fresh tRNA carrying a third amino acid now binds to the A-site, and the cycle repeats all over again, resulting in a growing peptide chain.

Termination of translation occurs when a stop codon (say, UAA) on the mRNA comes to occupy the A-site. There are no tRNAs for stop codons; therefore, the peptide chain cannot grow further. Instead, the peptide chain is released from the tRNA carrying it through hydrolysis. The hydrolysis requires peptidyltransferase, releasing factors, and GTP.

Cell Proteins: The Results of Transcription and Translation

The proteins that result from the processes of transcription and translation serve many functions in the cell: (1) some proteins serve as essential structural components for the cell; (2) a great many of the proteins function as enzymes, catalyzing all of the cell metabolic activities; and (3) some proteins are "exported" from the cell and function as hormones or other signaling molecules.

There are, however, two issues that must be addressed. First, every cell in an organism has exactly the same DNA, but cells obviously differ from one another in a great many different ways. Not every cell produces every possible protein. How does this diversity, the differentiation of cells, come to be? Second, cells are not static, unchanging systems; cell function is constantly changing to contribute to the maintenance of homeostasis. How does modulation of cell function occur when the basic information coded into its DNA is unchanging?

The answer to both questions lies in the fact that the transcription of genes *is not* an automatic, obligatory process. Transcription requires the presence of proteins (themselves the product of transcription and translation of genes) called *transcription factors* (**Fig. 3.3A**). Some transcription factors promote transcription of a particular gene, whereas others can inhibit it. Thus, which genes are expressed (undergo transcription) and which are not expressed depends on the presence of transcription factors.

Cell Differentiation and Development
A fertilized egg will undergo repeated cell division, ultimately resulting in the embryo and then the fetus. Each of those cells

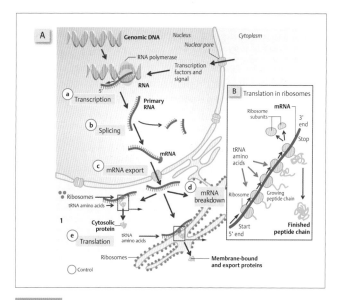

Fig. 3.3 **(A)** Transcription of the deoxyribonucleic acid (DNA) code into messenger ribonucleic acid (mRNA). mRNA leaves the nucleus and is then used to build the various kinds of proteins that determine cell structure and function (translation). **(B)** The building of a protein (a peptide chain) by a ribosome. Transfer RNA (tRNA) carries the required amino acids to the ribosome for assembling into the peptide being built.

has exactly the same genetic information encoded in its DNA, but cells rapidly differentiate in a wide variety of cell types, each doing different things. This must mean that they are expressing different sets of genes.

This process of differentiation and development is driven by the fact that the egg contains not only DNA from the mother, but also proteins and mRNA. And the distribution of these substances is not uniform. Therefore, as the fertilized egg divides, and those cells divide repeatedly, each daughter cell receives a different set of proteins and mRNA molecules that serve as transcription factors. It takes ~12 cell divisions before transcription and translation begins in the cells of the zygote (and the maternal proteins and mRNA are degraded). At this point, then, which genes are expressed and which are not is determined by the presence of a specific set of transcription factors.

The result is liver cells that make and secrete albumin, something that muscle cells cannot do, and pancreatic islet cells that synthesize insulin, which other cells cannot do.

Modulation of Cell Function
Hormones are chemical messengers released by endocrine cells (see Chapter 75) that are able to alter the functions of all cells that possess receptors for those hormones. There are two classes of hormones, both lipophilic, that are able to enter the nucleus and bind to receptors. The hormone + receptor complex is then able to function as a transcription factor, either increasing or decreasing the re-encryption of a particular protein.

For example, when the concentration of sodium falls, a reflex is initiated that eventually results in the release of the hormone aldosterone (a lipophilic, steroid hormone) from the adrenal cortex. Collecting duct cells in the kidneys have receptors for aldosterone in their nucleus. The result is increased transcription of genes required for the collecting duct cells to synthesize more sodium transport proteins required for greater reabsorption of sodium (thus conserving sodium in a situation where sodium concentration is too low).

Summary

- An organism's genetic information, the blueprint from which it is constructed, is contained in the molecules of DNA found in the nucleus.

- The DNA in the nucleus is replicated each time a cell divides.

- The genetic code in DNA is read out in the process of transcription; the result is a set of messenger RNA molecules that code for the synthesis of proteins.

- Translation is the building of proteins (many of which serve as the enzymes that direct the cell's metabolism) by the messenger RNA.

- Cell differentiation and development, and the modulation of cell functions, result from changes in the cell proteins (enzymes) that are produced by the cell.

We are all familiar with a great many different man-made devices that function as control systems. These devices are designed to hold some particular condition at a constant level or magnitude despite disturbances (whether from outside the device or from within it) that would change the value of that parameter. For example, the cruise control on an automobile holds the speed of the car constant despite the uphill and downhill terrain that is being driven across. The heating/cooling plant in a building is designed to hold the temperature in the building constant in the face of changing temperatures outside. Finally, the level of water in a toilet tank is controlled by a simple system that involves a float and a valve that opens and closes to keep the water at the desired level.

Each of these devices is a negative feedback control system. In the body, we will see that there are a great many such control systems that contribute to a state referred to as *homeostasis.*

Control Systems

Every control system contains a set of components that have functions necessary for the system to do its job of holding something constant.

First, a decision must be made about which variable is to be *regulated* (held constant). An essential aspect of this decision is that the variable must be measurable if it is to be regulated.

Thus, there must be a *sensor* in the system whose output (whatever its nature) is proportional to the magnitude of the regulated variable. There must also be a device with which the desired value of the regulated variable can be set; this is often referred to as the *set-point* or *reference value*. In a heating/cooling system, the *regulated* variable is the building temperature, the sensor is a thermometer (which produces an electrical output proportional to temperature), and the set point is determined by a device for indicating what temperature is desired. In many temperature-control systems, the sensor and the set point are built into a single unit placed wherever the temperature is to be regulated.

The control system must also be able to compare the desired, set-point value to the actual value of the variable as measured by the sensor. This component is, not surprisingly, called the *comparator*. The output of the comparator is an *error signal* that defines the relationship between the desired and actual values ("temperature is too high" or "temperature is too low") and quantitates that difference ("room temperature needs to increase by 2 degrees").

The error signal is then used to alter the function of those *effectors* that are capable of changing the value of the regulated variable. In a heating system, this is typically a furnace, which can be turned on or turned up to increase the flow of heat into the building.

Such systems are said to incorporate negative feedback because the change in effector function that is generated is always the opposite of the change that has occurred to the regulated variable.

Table 4.1 lists the standard components of a negative feedback control system. **Fig. 4.1A** illustrates the arrangement of the components of a generic negative feedback control system, and **Fig. 4.1B** illustrates one example of such a system (a heating system in a building).

There is another way in which a control system might contribute to maintaining the value of some variable more or less constant. This is called *anticipatory control*, and it is dependent on the ability to predict changes in the regulated variable that will occur in the future. For example, if the temperature regulating system for a building has a thermometer outside the building, it can use information about the change in outdoor temperature (a disturbance) to signal the need for the furnace to begin running before the building temperature actually begins to change. The combination of negative feedback control and anticipatory control can hold a regulated variable within tighter limits.

Homeostasis

One of the great insights of 19th-century physiologist Claude Bernard was that the body attempts to maintain the state of its internal environment (*milieu interieur*) constant. That is to say, the body *regulates* the values of a great many physiologic variables, attempting to hold them constant in the face of disturbances in the external environment and disturbances in the organism (changing functions, damage to physiologic systems). These variables are said to be homeostatic regulated. **Table 4.2** is a list of some of the most important homeostatic systems that will be discussed in this book.

The systems that accomplish homeostatic regulation are negative feedback control systems. Just like the man-made system previously described, physiologic negative feedback

Table 4.1   The Components of a Negative Feedback Control System

Component	Function
Sensor	Measures the value of the variable to be regulated
Set-point or reference value	Establishes the value at which the regulated variable is to be held
Comparator	Compares the set-point value and the actual measured value
Error signal	The difference between the set-point value and the actual value
Effector(s)	System component(s) that determine(s) the value of the regulated variable

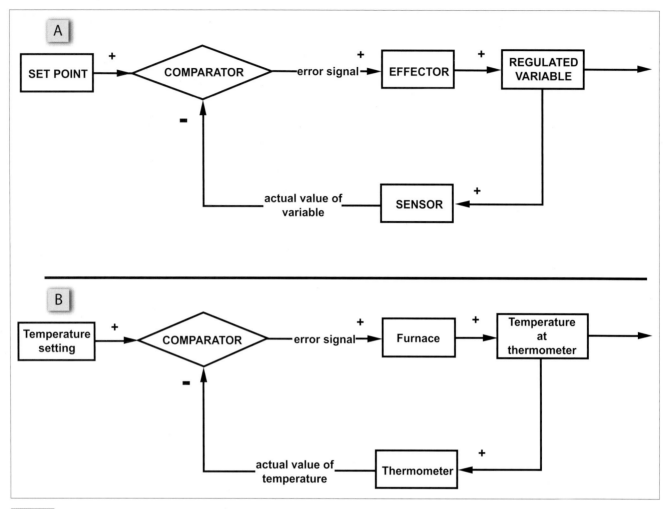

Fig. 4.1 **(A)** A generic negative feedback system, showing its components and the organization of these components. **(B)** A home heating system, showing its components; such a system is one example of a negative feedback system. The plus sign (+) at the head of an arrow indicates that the relationship between the variables is a direct one; as the input increases, the output increases. The minus sign (–) indicates that the relationship between the variables is inverse; as the input increases, the output decreases and conversely.

systems are made up of a set of standard components. All homeostatic systems have a sensor, a *receptor*, which can measure the value of the variable to be regulated. There is some mechanism for determining the set point, the value of the regulated variable that the system will attempt to hold constant. The set-point value and the actual value of the variable that is present are compared, and the output of the comparator is an error signal that represents the magnitude of the change that has to be produced to restore the regulated variable to its set-point value. The error signal then alters the behavior of the effector(s) that determine the value of the regulated variable. A change to the regulated variable results in changes in physiologic functions that cause the regulated variable to return to its set-point value.

Table 4.2 A List of Some Important Homeostatic Systems

Regulated Variable	Sensor	Effector(s)	
Arterial blood pressure	Carotid baroreceptors	Heart, blood vessels	Chapter 38
Body core temperature	Thermoreceptors in hypothalamus and skin	Muscle, sweat glands, cutaneous circulation	Chapter 43
Arterial PO_2 and PCO_2	Chemoreceptors in carotid sinus and brainstem	Respiratory muscles	Chapter 50
Osmolarity of body fluids	Hypothalamic osmoreceptors	Collecting ducts of the renal tubules	Chapter 56
Plasma potassium concentration	Cells of the adrenal cortex	Kidney tubule cells	Chapter 59
Plasma glucose concentration	Beta cells in the pancreas	Liver, muscle, and adipose cells	Chapter 81

Abbreviations: PCO_2, partial pressure of carbon dioxide; PO_2, partial pressure of oxygen.

In studying a physiologic system, it is not always easy to identify the components of the negative feedback system regulating a particular system or the mechanisms that serve those functions. For example, plasma glucose concentration is homeostatically regulated. The sensor in the system is the β-cell in the pancreas, which effectively measures glucose concentration by, in effect, determining the rate of entry of glucose into the cell. This same cell, however, also determines the set point and uses the difference between the set point and the actual plasma glucose concentration to determine the release of the hormone insulin. It is insulin that alters the function of liver, muscle, and adipose cells to change their uptake of glucose, thus altering the plasma glucose concentration.

In some cases, we simply do not know the mechanism by which the set point is determined, or even where in the system it is determined, although the behavior of the system clearly reveals that there is such a component somewhere.

Not All Physiologic Parameters Are Regulated

It is important to keep in mind the fact that not all physiologic variables are homeostatically regulated. For example, to regulate blood pressure (Chapter 38), the cardiovascular system alters the function of the heart and the blood vessels. Thus, blood pressure is the *regulated* variable, but heart rate, stroke volume, and peripheral resistance are *controlled* variables. In a real sense, the body does not care what value the heart rate assumes, as long as changes in heart rate contribute to regulating blood pressure.

Remember, too, that only a variable that can be measured can be regulated. Although one might argue that blood flow to the peripheral tissues is the most important cardiovascular variable, the body has no flow meters and therefore cannot regulate flow directly.

Failures of Homeostasis

The body's ability to regulate the internal environment is not perfect. External disturbances and normal changes in the activity of the body can result in deviations of regulated variables from their set-point levels. For example, blood glucose is regulated at a concentration of ~100 mg/dL (Chapter 81). However, following a meal, blood glucose climbs much above this level as the meal is digested, and the productions of digestion are absorbed into the blood. The blood glucose regulatory mechanisms are working normally (**Fig. 4.2**), and blood glucose will eventually return to its regulated level, but the system is not capable of maintaining a perfectly constant value for blood glucose under all conditions.

Homeostatic regulation can also fail when one particular system is involved in regulating two different variables. For example, the cutaneous circulation is controlled by two different systems, one that regulates blood pressure (see Chapter 38) and one that regulates body temperature (Chapter 43).

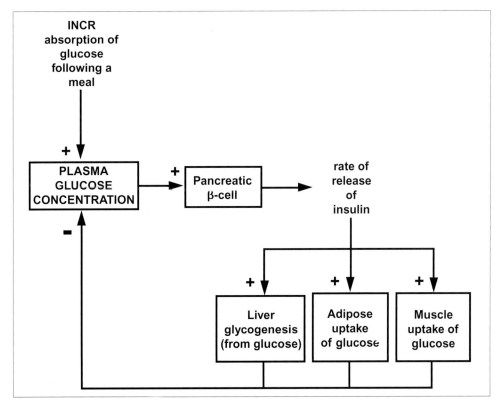

Fig. 4.2 The negative feedback system that contributes to the regulation of plasma glucose concentration. The β-cell is the glucose sensor, set point, and comparator. Insulin released by the β-cells alters the function of three different types of cells (the effectors in the system) to determine the plasma glucose concentration that is present. In the face of a disturbance that increases plasma glucose (the consequences of eating a meal), the system acts to lower the plasma glucose concentration.

During severe exercise, the need to maintain blood pressure takes priority over the need for a constant body temperature, and the cutaneous blood changes in a way that can result in hyperthermia.

Homeostasis can also fail when pathology (disease) is present in the organism. When such disturbances remain small, the body can often compensate, and little or no change occurs in the internal environment. However, larger disturbances, or chronic disturbances, can lead to failure to hold one or more physiologic parameter constant. Death is a consequence of widespread failure to maintain homeostasis.

Summary

● A negative feedback system can be employed to regulate (hold more or less constant in the face of disturbances) the value of some system variable.

● A negative feedback system is made up of elements that can measure the magnitude of the regulated variable, a set point that establishes the desired value of the variable, a comparator to generate an error signal, and a set of components whose function can be controlled to determine the value of the regulated variable.

● In the body, the state of the internal environment (the values of many physiologic variables) is held more or less constant in the face of disturbances from the external world and from within the body itself. This state of constancy is referred to as homeostasis.

● Homeostasis is maintained by a large number of negative feedback systems.

Section II | Physiology of Nerves and the Autonomic Nervous System

Overview

The nervous system is one of two information-processing and transmitting systems in the body (the other being the endocrine system). The nervous system employs electrical signals to conduct information-bearing signals over individual neurons, with these signals often traveling long distances. Neurons transmit information to other neurons or to effector cells (muscles or glands) using chemical transmitters.

The nervous system conveys information rapidly between specific neurons and between specific neurons and specific effector cells. It operates in a similar manner to a telephone system.

The nervous system mediates all of our interactions with the external environment (sensory and motor). It also controls our internal organs and organ systems to maintain homeostasis.

Section II Case Presentation:
Ann Adams is getting weak.

Chief Complaint

Ann Adams, a 19-year old secretary, presents with increasingly severe muscle weakness, eyelid and mouth droop, and slurred speech.

History of Present Illness

Ms. Adams awoke yesterday with weakness of her right hand and arm. When she looked in the mirror, she noticed that she had a droopy right eyelid and a droop to her mouth on the right side when she tried to grin. She also noted that her speech was slightly slurred.

As the day went on, her symptoms gradually progressed, including a deterioration of her speech to the point of being unintelligible. She found that, with rest, her problems would transiently improve only to recur when she exerted herself again.

This morning she came to see you because her problems had not resolved. In addition, she has developed a weak neck, requiring hand support to maintain it in an upright position.

Past Medical History

Ann has no past history of major illness or neurologic problem. She has experienced no recent trauma. She denies fever or chills. She uses no medication. She has not traveled recently, been exposed to any chemicals or fumes, or been around people who are ill.

Physical Examination

- *General appearance* | Ann Adams is a depressed-looking white woman who cried on several occasions during the evaluation.
- *Vital signs*
  - Temperature: 98.8°F
  - Blood pressure: 102/70 mm Hg
  - Pulse: 94/minute
  - Respirations: 16/minute
- *HEENT (head, eyes, ears, nose, throat)* | Bilateral ptosis and widening of the nasolabial folds, with the right greater than the left.
- *Neurologic exam* | Normal mental status. Ms. Adams is right-handed. Speech was fluent but slurred, and it decreased in volume as the exam progressed. Motor exam revealed 4+/5+ strength throughout. However, it was noted that all muscle groups could be fatigued over time against resistance. Deep tendon reflexes were normal, and no pathologic reflexes were present. Sensory exam was normal. Cerebellar function and gait were normal.

Hospitalization

You admit her to the hospital for further evaluation.

Laboratory Studies

Complete blood count (CBC), electrolytes (Ca, Cl, PO_4, Mg, K, Na), a panel of 12 blood chemistry values (albumin, alkaline phosphatase, bilirubin total, blood urea nitrogen, total protein, uric acid, Ca, cholesterol, creatinine, glucose, PO_4, serum glutamic oxaloacetic transaminase [SGOT]), urinalysis, electrocardiogram (ECG), and chest x-ray were all normal.

Motor Nerve Conduction Studies

The right ulnar nerve was electrically stimulated with surface electrodes placed on the skin over the nerve. The resulting muscle electrical activity recorded with surface electrodes was normal in amplitude and latency.

Sensory Nerve Conduction Study

The right ulnar nerve was electrically stimulated distally, and the compound action potential was measured over the nerve proximally. The amplitude and latency of the response were normal.

Electromyography

A percutaneous needle electrode was inserted into the muscle, and the muscle electrical activity in response to motor nerve stimulation was measured.

Recording from the abductor digiti minimi muscle (little finger) revealed an initially normal response amplitude. After five repetitive nerve stimulations (at 2/second), the response amplitude had decreased by 8% (normal is a decrement of < 10%).

Recording from the right deltoid muscle (shoulder) in the same way resulted in a 38% decrement in the response (normal is a decrement of < 10%).

Tensilon Test

The patient was given 2 mg of Tensilon (edrophonium chloride, a drug that inhibits the action of the cholinesterase enzyme) intravenously. Within 30 seconds her speech became stronger and clearer, she felt stronger, and her ptosis disappeared. About 10 minutes later, however, her problems gradually reappeared.

Antibody Study

A serum study for acetylcholine receptor antibodies revealed 23 nmol/L (normal is < 0.5).

Treatment

The patient was begun on treatment with Mestinon (pyridostigmine bromide; Valeant Pharmaceuticals International, Aliso Viejo, CA). The initial dose was 60 mg every 4 hours. Initially, the patient noted a marked improvement in muscle strength. However, after several days she began experiencing diarrhea, anxiety, and a recurrence of weakness.

Her dose was adjusted over the next several days with improvement in her symptoms and a near total return to normal.

At the time of discharge, her regimen was Mestinon 45 mg orally at 7:30 AM and 11:30 AM, and 30 mg at 2:30 PM and 9:30 PM.

Some Things to Think About

1. Ms. Adams is experiencing muscle weakness. Where in the neuromuscular system might pathologic changes give rise to weakness?

2. In nerve conduction studies, electrical stimulation is used to elicit neural activity. What is the mechanism by which this occurs?

3. Nerve conduction studies performed in an attempt to determine the cause of Ms. Adams' problem yielded normal values. What parameters determine the conduction velocity of nerves?

4. Ms. Adams' problem seems to be located at the neuromuscular junction. Where at this structure might there be a functional problem?

5. How might the physiology of the neuromuscular junction be manipulated to help alleviate Ms. Adams' symptoms?

The Structure of Neurons

The neuron or nerve cell (**Fig. 5.1**) is called an excitable cell because it can conduct electric impulses, called action potentials, which encode various types of motor and sensory information. A neuron has a cell body called the soma and two kinds of processes, namely, the axon and the dendrites.

It must be noted that muscles cells (see Section III) are also excitable cells, as are many gland cells (see Section IX).

The neuron contains most of the organelles present in a typical cell. However, the centriole, which is necessary for mitosis, is absent in the mature neuron, which does not undergo mitosis. The cisternae of the rough endoplasmic reticulum are disposed in parallel arrays called *Nissl bodies.* Due to their ribosomic RNA content, Nissl bodies stain intensely with chromophilic dyes and are very conspicuous. Polyribosomes are also found free in the cytoplasm. Nissl bodies are present in the soma and dendrites but are usually absent from the axon hillock and the axon. Smooth endoplasmic reticulum is present in all parts of the neuron.

The *cytoskeleton* of the neuron is made of microtubules, microfilaments, and intermediate filaments. In neurons, intermediate filaments are called *neurofilaments.* Under the light microscope, a network of *neurofibrils* (~2 μm in diameter) is seen around the nucleus, extending into the dendrites and the axon. Neurofibrils are actually bundles of neurofilaments and microtubules. In certain degenerative diseases like Alzheimer's disease, the neurofilament protein gets altered, resulting in the formation of characteristic lesions called *neurofibrillary tangles.*

The **axon** arises as a single long process from the *axon hillock,* which is a conical extension of the cell body. The axon is thicker and much longer than dendrites of the same cell. In some neurons, the axon may be myelinated. In certain very small local-circuit neurons, for example, the amacrine cells of the retina, there may be no axon at all. The part of the axon between the axon hillock and the beginning of the myelin sheath is called the *initial segment.* In response to the various synaptic inputs on the dendrites, the axon hillock and initial segment give rise to an action potential and hence are together called the *spike trigger zone.* The axon conducts the action potential over long distances.

The axon is sometimes defined as the process that carries signals away from the soma. Similarly, dendrites are sometimes defined as the processes that carry impulses toward the soma. However, these definitions are too limited in their scope. In a pseudounipolar cell or a bipolar cell, the axon carries information both toward and away from the cell.

Dendrites are the multiple cell processes that branch extensively immediately after arising from the soma. The dendritic tree so formed provides most of the surface for receiving signals from other neurons via their synapses with axon terminals. Dendrites often look "thorny" due to numerous minute projections called *spines* present on their surface. The spines are the sites of synaptic contact, connected to the main shaft by a thin neck and ending in a more bulbous head. Each spine forms at least one synapse. During synaptic transmission, calcium (Ca^{2+}) concentration rises in the spine. The thin neck of the spine prevents the rise in Ca^{2+} concentration in the spine from spreading to the main shaft and results in an increased duration of postsynaptic potentials in the dendrites.

Spines decrease in number after neuronal deafferentiation or nutritional deprivation and exhibit structural changes in older people and in individuals with certain chromosomal abnormalities (trisomies 13 and 21). The synaptic inputs produce local potentials that get algebraically summated on the surface of dendrites. Short dendrites usually do not produce action potentials, but conduct graded potentials that can be summated. Dendrites that are very long may conduct action potentials.

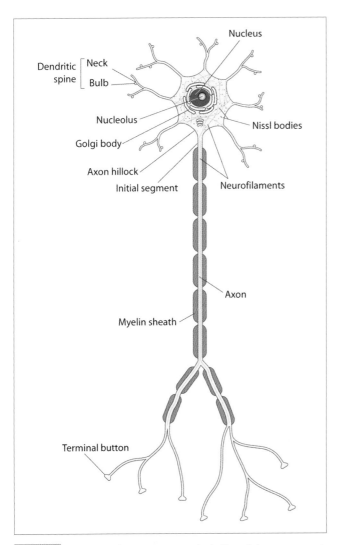

Fig. 5.1   Structure of a neuron. Note the bulb and the narrow neck of the dendritic spines. Not all neurons have myelinated axons like this one does.

Myelination of Neurons

Myelination of axons (the presence of high-resistance tissue surrounding the axon) increases their speed of conduction but greatly increases their diameter. In motor nerves, speed is important. Hence, motor neurons to muscles and sensory fibers from muscles (proprioceptive fibers) are heavily myelinated. Inside the brain, neurons span short distances, and hence speed of conduction is less important. Rather, the space available inside the cranium is limited, and it is advantageous to have thinly myelinated or unmyelinated neurons that occupy less space, allowing more neurons to be accommodated inside the cranium.

Myelination begins at ~4 months in utero and is complete by ~5 years. Motor nerve roots are largely myelinated at birth, but the optic nerve and sensory roots lag behind by 3 to 4 months. The corticospinal tracts require a year for full myelination, and commissural axons of the cerebral hemispheres take 7 years or more. It is only after the completion of myelination that a neuron becomes fully functional. In the infant, functions like vision, walking, and performance of directed movements are possible only after the completion of myelination.

Peripheral myelination | The myelin sheath is produced by glial cells called *Schwann cells* that encircle the axon, forming around it a thin sleeve called the *sheath of Schwann*. The myelin sheath is composed of several layers of cell membrane wrapped spirally around the axon (**Fig. 5.2A**). The myelin gets compacted by the elimination of the intervening cytoplasm. The so-called unmyelinated axons are also covered by a single layer of membrane and the cytoplasm of the enveloping Schwann cell. However, the myelin is not prominent.

Externally, the Schwann cell is covered by a basal lamina and the endoneurium. The myelin sheath is interrupted at the *nodes of Ranvier*, where the axon is covered by a thin sleeve of basal lamina. Persistence of the sleeve after nerve injury serves to guide the regenerating axons along the right path.

Central myelination | Schwann cells are found only in peripheral nerves. Myelination of neurons in the central nervous system is produced by a type of neuroglial cell called the *oligodendrocyte* (**Fig. 5.2B**). A single oligodendrocyte can myelinate as many as 60 axons.

Morphologic Classification of Neurons

Golgi type I and type II neurons | Large cells with long axons are called *Golgi type I neurons* or *projection neurons.* They include the neurons that form peripheral nerves and long tracts of the brain and spinal cord. Small neurons with relatively short axons are called *Golgi type II* neurons or *local circuit neurons.* The total number of cells in the human nervous system is ~1 trillion, most of which are local circuit neurons that have proliferated markedly in the course of evolution. The evolutionary increase in the number of sensory neurons has been much less. The number of motor neurons has remained relatively small at ~2 million.

Pseudopolar, bipolar, and multipolar neurons | Except in early embryonic stages, *true unipolar neurons* are not found in vertebrates. However, the primary sensory neurons (neurons conveying impulses from the sensory receptors to the spinal cord) are *pseudounipolar* (**Fig. 5.3A**). During early development, these neurons are bipolar, but later, the roots of the two processes shift around the perikaryon and fuse into a single stem. The

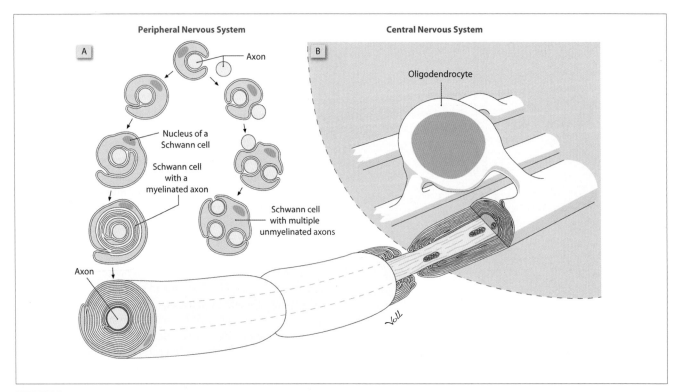

Fig. 5.2 **(A)** Myelination of peripheral neurons by Schwann cells. **(B)** Myelination of central neurons by oligodendrocytes.

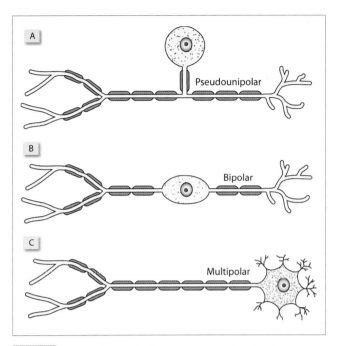

Fig. 5.3 **(A)** Pseudounipolar, **(B)** bipolar, and **(C)** multipolar neurons. In all three of these types of neurons, information propagates from right (where stimuli act on the neurons) to left (where information is passed on to other neurons).

stem and both its branches are myelinated axons. There may be short dendritic processes at the end of the distal branch, often in association with some kind of receptor structure. In *bipolar neurons* (**Fig. 5.3B**), an axon projects from each end of a fusiform cell body. Cells of this type are found in the vestibular and cochlear ganglia and in the nasal olfactory epithelium. Most vertebrate neurons, especially in the central nervous system, are *multipolar* (**Fig. 5.3C**). The dendrites branch profusely to form the dendritic tree. There is usually a single axon.

Organization of Neurons

The nervous system is divided into the *central nervous system* (CNS), constituted by the brain and the spinal cord, and the *peripheral nervous system* (PNS), constituted by neurons lying outside the CNS. The *autonomic nervous system* (ANS) is a motor, or efferent, system that encompasses both the CNS and PNS. An aggregation of neuronal cell bodies located inside the CNS is called a *nucleus*. An aggregation of neuronal cell bodies located outside the CNS is called a *ganglion*. A compact bundle of axons located inside the CNS is called a *tract*. A compact bundle of axons located outside the CNS is called a *nerve*.

Axoplasmic Transport

Axoplasmic transport, the movement of substances between the cell soma and the axon terminals, is vital to nerve cell functions. There are two forms of axonal transport: fast and slow. Fast axoplasmic transport has a velocity of 20 to 400 mm per day and may be anterograde or retrograde in direction. Slow axoplasmic transport occurs at 0.2 to 0.4 mm per day and is always anterograde.

Fast Axoplasmic Transport

Fast anterograde transport occurs along microtubules. It occurs from the soma to axon terminal and is driven by the molecular motor *kinesin*. It transports membrane-bounded organelles like short segments of the endoplasmic reticulum, mitochondria, small vesicles, actin, myosin, and the clathrin used in recycling of synaptic vesicle membrane.

Fast retrograde transport occurs from the nerve terminals to the cell body, returning materials for degradation or reuse. These materials include proteins and small molecules picked up by the axon terminal. It employs the molecular motor *dynein* and has one-third the velocity of anterograde transport. Retrograde transport is responsible for carrying tetanus toxin and neurotropic viruses such as herpes simplex and rabies directly to cell bodies in the CNS. It has been employed by neuroanatomists for charting out neural pathways.

Slow Axoplasmic Transport

Slow transport carries protein subunits of neurofilaments, tubulins of the microtubules, and soluble enzymes. It also moves some cytosol with it. The mechanism of slow axonal transport is not clear: probably the cytoskeleton moves as a whole due to the continual polymerization at the leading end and depolymerization at the trailing end, and the axoplasmic matrix moves with it.

Neuroglia

Neuroglia, meaning nerve glue, is the connective tissue of the brain. In the CNS, neuroglial cells are 10 times more numerous than neurons. These cells provide structural and trophic support to neurons and depending on their type, serve other important functions. Although they are interconnected through gap junctions, glial cells do not conduct action potentials. The major neuroglial cells are astrocytes, oligodendroglia, and microglia (**Fig. 5.4**). The Schwann cells of peripheral nerves

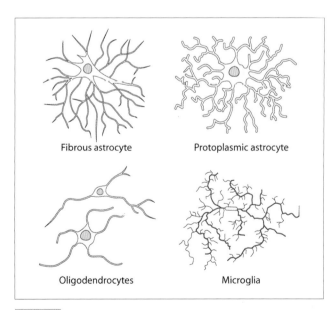

Fig. 5.4 Four different neuroglial cells found in the central nervous system.

and the ependymal cells of cerebral ventricles are also considered to be neuroglial cells.

Astrocytes are star-shaped glial cells. They form the skeleton of the CNS. In the developing nervous tissue, astrocytes provide the framework along which young neuronal cells migrate to their final positions. They form an insulation around synapses to prevent chaotic spread of nerve impulses. These astrocytes around synapses have an important role in reestablishing synaptic contact following disruption of synapses. Astrocytes proliferate and form scars after neuronal damage. They clear the neural tissues of potassium (K^+) and excess neurotransmitters that accumulate extracellularly following neural activity. Through their processes and footplates on the walls of blood vessels, astrocytes contribute to the formation of the blood–brain barrier. Astrocytes also store glycogen. When stimulated by neurotransmitters like norepinephrine, they convert the glycogen into glucose and release it for the consumption of the neurons.

Oligodendrocytes resemble astrocytes, but as their name indicates, they have fewer dendrites. They myelinate neurons of the CNS.

Microglial cells resemble oligodendrocytes, but as the name suggests, they are much smaller in size. They are phagocytic cells that clear up myelin and cellular debris in injured areas.

Summary

- Neurons have a cell body (soma) and two kinds of processes arising from the soma: an axon and a set of dendrites.

- The axons of motor neurons (and some sensory neurons) are myelinated and therefore have a higher conduction velocity.

- The nervous system has three major subdivisions: the central nervous system (CNS), the peripheral nervous system (PNS), and the autonomic nervous system (ANS).

Applying What You Know

5.1. Ms. Adams had two nerve conduction studies done on her ulnar nerve (which runs down the outside of the forearm and is easily accessed for such studies). Both studies yielded normal responses. If you could look at this nerve under a microscope, what would you see? And how would what you see help you to interpret the results of the nerve conduction study?

The conduction of a nerve impulse or action potential is an electrical phenomenon. The inner surface of the "resting" nerve membrane is negatively charged with respect to its outer surface, giving the nerve membrane an electrical polarity. This potential is called the *resting membrane potential (RMP)*. When this polarity is briefly reversed, it serves as a signal that is conducted over long distances along the nerve membrane. This signal is called the *action potential (AP)*. However, before discussing the action potential (Chapter 7) or its conduction over the nerve membrane (Chapter 13), it is necessary to understand the origin of the resting membrane potential. This is discussed below in detail.

It is important to point out that muscle cells, too, have a resting membrane potential, and that it originates from the same mechanisms as are seen in nerve cells and described below. Furthermore, changes to the resting membrane potential in muscle serve the same function as they do in nerve cells.

Finally, it should be remembered that all cells, even those for which information processing is not an important function, exhibit a resting potential.

Diffusion Potential

The inner surface of a cell membrane is usually charged negative with respect to its outer surface (**Fig. 6.1**). The potential of the inner surface of the membrane with respect to its outer surface is called the *membrane potential*. The potential is called a membrane potential because it exists essentially on the membrane. The cations and anions form layers on the outer and inner membrane surfaces, respectively. The membrane potential is produced by the passive diffusion of ions across the membrane. Hence, it is also called a *diffusion potential*.

The membrane potential changes markedly when the membrane is electrically stimulated (when an electrical current is made to flow across the membrane, whether artificially in the laboratory or by a physiologic process). The potential recorded

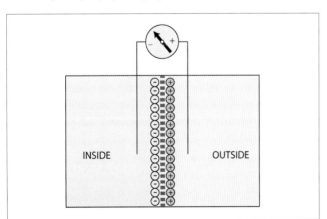

Fig. 6.1   A potential of approximately –80 mV is measurable across the cell membrane (the actual value varies somewhat in different cell types). The potential exists essentially at the membrane, with anions and cations layered on the opposite surfaces of the cell membrane.

intracellularly when a cell is not stimulated is called the *resting membrane potential* (RMP), and the membrane is said to be *polarized*. The unmyelinated axonal membrane has an RMP of –70 mV. The membrane potential is more negative (–90 mV) in striated muscles and less negative (–50 mV) in certain smooth muscles. The general principles of membrane potential, however, are the same in all excitable tissues. Most of the discussion on membrane potential in the following passages assumes a membrane potential of –80 mV. When the inside of the membrane becomes more negative, it is said to be *hyperpolarized*. When the inside of the membrane becomes less negative, it is said to be *depolarized*. When following depolarization, the membrane returns to the polarized state, it is said to be *repolarized*.

Origin of Diffusion Potential

The activity of the Na^+–K^+ pump in the cell membrane builds up a large concentration of Na^+ outside the cell (in the extracellular fluid [ECF]) and a large concentration of K^+ inside the

---

General Models: Energy and Flow

It is worth noting at this point that there are two features of the diffusion potential that you will see again and again in many different contexts while learning physiology.

The action of the Na+–K+ pump in creating a concentration gradient across the cell membrane for Na+ and K+ is a crucial feature of all cells. It also must be noted that the Na+–K+ pump utilizes biologic energy in the form of adenosine triphosphate (ATP) to transport solutes against their concentration gradients. Pumping ions requires that work be done and that ATP be available to provide the energy to do that work. Essentially every function of the body requires that work be done; therefore, provisions to continuously supply ATP to every cell are essential.

We can think of this phenomenon as being one example of a **general model**, one that we will have to deal with repeatedly. For example, we will see (Chapter 14) that contraction of muscle requires the availability of ATP. We will refer to this model as the formation and transformation of the energy model (the **energy model** for short).

There is another **general model** here that is also worth noting. Na⁺ and K⁺ move down their concentration gradients and in doing so create a diffusion potential. For anything to move, heat or matter of any kind (any solutes, water, blood, air), an energy gradient must be present, and there must be a pathway through which the flow can occur. But any such pathway will present some opposition to flow. We can thus state that flow is determined by the magnitude of the gradient that is present and inversely determined by the resistance to flow that is present. We will see many other examples of this as the **flow model** as we describe other physiologic systems (flow of blood in the circulation, flow of air in the airways).

cell (intracellular fluid [ICF]). It also indirectly contributes to the buildup of a large Cl⁻ concentration in the ECF. It is important to note that the concentration of an ion can be expressed as mM/L (millimoles per liter) or as mEq/L (milliequivalents/liter). A millimole is a measure of the number of particles of a substance that is present; a milliequivalent is a measure of the number of charges that are present. For monovalent ions such as Na^+, K^+, or Cl^-, a mM/L is exactly the same as a mEq/L.

The membrane potential develops when these ions leak back along their respective concentration gradients (i.e., when Na^+ leaks back from ECF into the cell, and K^+ leaks out from the cell to the ECF). The streams of ions that leak back from high to low concentration are called *leak currents* or *channel currents* to differentiate them from the *pump current* produced by the Na^+–K^+ pump. In its resting state, the membrane has a high permeability to K^+ (it is very leaky for K^+), but its permeability to Na^+ is much less (it is less leaky for Na^+). Hence, the amount of K^+ that leaks out in a given time is much more than the amount of Na^+ that leaks in through the membrane in the same time. As a result, an excess of K^+ accumulates in the cells, the amount of which is too small to change the ECF or ICF concentrations of K^+, but large enough to make the exterior of the membrane positive with respect to its interior by many millivolts.

Diffusion potential of a single ion | Before trying to understand the diffusion potential of an ion, it is important to recall that whenever an ion is distributed asymmetrically across a membrane, there exists a unique potential E_{ion} that will prevent its diffusion. This potential is called the Nernst potential of the ion. It can be calculated using the Nernst equation:

$$E_X = -61\log_{10}\frac{[X]_i}{[X]_o} \qquad (6.1)$$

If the ions are allowed to diffuse, they produce a diffusion potential. The following passages explain why the diffusion potential produced by an ion is exactly equal to its Nernst potential.

General Model: Balance of Forces

One useful way to think about the diffusion potential is that it is an electrical potential gradient that exactly balances the flux of an ion produced by a concentration gradient. It is thus an example of another general model, the balance of forces model. It follows, then, that a change in either the concentration or electrical potential gradient will result in a flux of ions (a current).

Take the case illustrated in **Fig. 6.2**. Assume that the membrane is permeable only to K^+ and impermeable to Na^+ and Cl^-. Assume also that the membrane potential E_m is 0 mV to start with. The following sequence of events will occur: (1) K^+ diffuses out of the cell along its concentration gradient. The resultant decrease in intracellular K^+ concentration is so small (< 10 picoEq/dL) that it hardly produces any change in the K^+ concentration gradient or its rate of outward diffusion. (2) Because the membrane is impermeable to both Na^+ and Cl^-, the diffusion of K^+ produces an intracellular negativity, which is not nullified by the diffusion of Na^+ in the opposite direction, or by

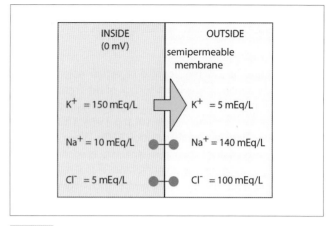

Fig. 6.2 Distribution of ions across a semipermeable membrane that is permeable only to potassium ions. Potassium (K^+) ions will diffuse out, resulting in a diffusion potential that will be equal to the Nernst potential of K^+.

the diffusion of Cl^- in the same direction. (3) The intracellular negativity reduces the rate of subsequent outward diffusion of K^+ because opposite electrical charges attract one another. (4) As the outward diffusion of K^+ continues, the membrane becomes increasingly negative inside, and the outward diffusion of K^+ keeps decreasing. (5) When the membrane potential reaches about –90 mV (which is the Nernst potential for K^+), the outward net K^+ diffusion stops (although there is still random movement of the ions in both directions across the membrane). Hence, the diffusion potential produced by a single ion will always equal its own Nernst potential (**Fig. 6.3**).

The intracellular negativity pulls back the extracellular cations to the external surface of the membrane. Similarly, the external positivity attracts the intracellular anions to the internal surface of the membrane. Hence, opposite charges line up on opposite surfaces of the membrane. Together, the membrane and the opposite charges on its opposite surfaces form a parallel-plate capacitor in which the membrane is the dielectric. The capacitance of a parallel-plate capacitor is inversely proportional to the thickness of the dielectric. Because the membrane is very thin, the capacitance of the membrane is quite high. It is important to consider membrane capacitance in thinking about the conduction of nerve impulses (Chapter 9).

Diffusion potential of multiple ions | When multiple ions are diffusing across the membrane, each ion tries to drive the membrane potential toward its own Nernst potential. The resultant diffusion potential (E_m) is called the *equilibrium potential of the membrane*. It is given by the Goldman equation:

$$V_m = 61 \ \log\frac{P_K[K_0]+P_{Na}[Na_0]+P_{Cl}[Cl_i]}{P_K[K_i]+P_{Na}[Na_i]+P_{Cl}[Cl_0]} \qquad (6.2)$$

where P_K, P_{Na}, and P_{Cl} are the conductances (permeability) of K^+, Na^+, and Cl^-, respectively.

When only one ion is permeable, the equation reduces to the Nernst equation.

In other words, when the permeability of one ion far exceeds that of the others, the equilibrium potential of the

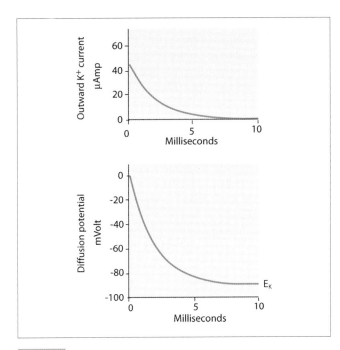

Fig. 6.3 Consequences of the ionic distribution shown in **Fig. 6.2**. The outward diffusion of potassium (K$^+$) ions declines with the build-up of a diffusion potential (which opposes the movement of positively charged K$^+$ ions). The diffusion stops when the diffusion potential equals the Nernst potential of K$^+$.

membrane will approach the Nernst potential of the most permeable ion. The implications are as follows: (1) There is a balance of currents, with each diffusing ion trying to drive the equilibrium potential toward its own Nernst potential. For example, Na$^+$ tries to drive the RMP toward +70 mV, K$^+$ tries to drive the RMP toward –90 mV, and Cl$^-$ tries to drive the RMP toward –80 mV. (2) The ion that is more permeable and more distant from the equilibrium potential is more effective in driving the equilibrium potential toward its own Nernst potential. (3) The equilibrium potential, or the RMP, assumes a value of –80 mV. At this RMP, both Na$^+$ and K$^+$ are moderately effective and balance each other. The effectiveness of the Na$^+$ ion comes from the distance of its Nernst potential from the RMP. On the other hand, the effectiveness of the K$^+$ ion comes from its moderate permeability. The Nernst potential of Cl$^-$ is equal to the RMP; hence, it is unable to influence the RMP.

Membrane Currents

In the case illustrated in **Fig. 6.4**, the outward diffusion of the positively charged K$^+$ ions will tend to hyperpolarize the membrane. In other words, K$^+$ carries a hyperpolarizing current. Because K$^+$ is flowing out, it constitutes an outward hyperpolarizing current. Similarly, Na$^+$ carries an inward depolarizing current, and Cl$^-$ carries an inward hyperpolarizing current.

The number of ions flowing out per second per square centimeter of the membrane (current density) can be calculated from Ohm's law. Because the reciprocal of resistance is conductance, Ohm's law can be rewritten as

$$\text{Current (I)} = \text{Potential (E)} \times \text{Conductance (g)} \quad (6.3)$$

Outward current per unit membrane area (μA/cm^2)

$$= \left[\begin{array}{cc} \text{Membrane} & \text{Nernst potential} \\ \text{potential} & \text{of an ion} \\ \text{(mV)} & \text{(mV)} \end{array} \right] \times \begin{array}{c} \text{Ionic conductance} \\ \text{per unit membrane area} \\ \text{(mmho/cm}^2) \end{array}$$

$$(6.4)$$

Thus,

$$\begin{aligned} I_{Na} &= (E_m - E_{Na}) \times g_{Na} \\ I_K &= (E_m - E_K) \times g_K \\ I_{Cl} &= (E_m - E_{Cl}) \times g_{Cl} \end{aligned} \quad (6.5)$$

where I_{Na}, I_K, and I_{Cl} are the membrane currents, E_{Na}, E_K, and E_{Cl}, are the Nernst potentials, and g_{Na}, g_K, and g_{Cl} are the membrane conductances for Na$^+$, K$^+$, and Cl$^-$ ions, respectively. These formulas explain why the membrane current of an ion is directly proportional to the difference between the membrane potential and the Nernst potential of the ion. This point is illustrated through the following example.

Figure 6.4 shows the intracellular and extracellular concentrations of Na$^+$, K$^+$, and Cl$^-$ and their membrane conductances. Based on these data, the membrane currents of these ions at two different membrane potentials, 0 mV and –80 mV, have been calculated (assuming that the membrane con-

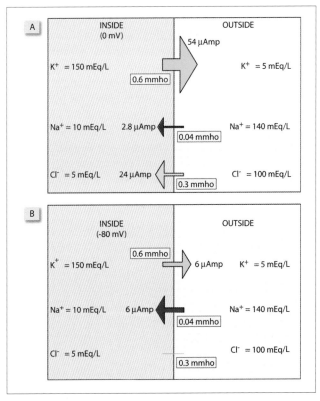

Fig. 6.4 **(A)** The membrane potential is 0 mV. The total hyperpolarizing current (78 μAmp) carried by potassium (K$^+$) and chloride (Cl$^-$) diffusing down their concentration gradients far exceeds the depolarizing sodium (Na$^+$) current (2.8 μAmp) caused by Na$^+$ diffusing down its concentration gradient. **(B)** The membrane potential is –80 mV. Now, the outward hyperpolarizing K$^+$ current exactly balances the inward depolarizing Na$^+$ current.

Table 6.1 Calculation of Ionic Currents (I_{ion}) at Two Different Membrane Potentials, 0 mV and –80 mV, Using the Formula $I_{ion} = (E_m – E_{ion}) \times g_{ion}$

Membrane Potential (E_m)	Nernst Potential of (E_{ion} in mV)	Membrane Conductance of (g_{ion} in mmho)	Membrane Current of Ion (I_{ion} in µAmp)
0 mV	$E_K = -90$	$g_K = 0.6$	$I_K = 54$
0 mV	$E_{Na} = +70$	$g_{Na} = 0.04$	$I_{Na} = 2.8$
0 mV	$E_{Cl} = -80$	$g_{Cl} = 0.3$	$I_{Cl} = 24$
–80 mV	$E_K = -90$	$g_K = 0.6$	$I_K = 6$
–80 mV	$E_{Na} = +70$	$g_{Na} = 0.04$	$I_{Na} = 6$
–80 mV	$E_{Cl} = -80$	$g_{Cl} = 0.3$	$I_{Cl} = 0$

ductances of the ions do not change with changes in membrane potential, which is not literally correct, as explained later) and tabulated (**Table 6.1**).

When membrane potential is at 0 mV, K^+ will carry a strong outward hyperpolarizing current (54 µA), Na^+ will carry a weak inward depolarizing current (2.8 µA), and Cl^- will carry a strong inward hyperpolarizing current (24 µA). Thus, the total hyperpolarizing current (78 µA) carried by K^+ and Cl^- far exceeds the depolarizing Na^+ current (2.8 µA). The intracellular potential therefore becomes negative.

With increasing negativity, the depolarizing Na^+ current increases and the hyperpolarizing currents of K^+ and Cl^- decrease. When membrane potential reaches –80 mV, K^+ will carry a moderate outward hyperpolarizing current, Na^+ will carry a moderate inward depolarizing current, and Cl^- current stops because –80 mV equals E_{Cl}. At this stage, the hyperpolarizing and depolarizing currents are equal, and the membrane potential does not change any further. The potential at which an equilibrium is established between the depolarizing and hyperpolarizing membrane currents denotes the resting membrane potential of the membrane. Expressed mathematically,

$$I_{Na} + I_K + I_{Cl} = 0 \qquad (6.6)$$

$$\therefore \{(V_m - E_{Na}) \times g_{Na}\} + \{(V_m - E_K) \times g_K\} + \{(V_m - E_{Cl}) \times g_{Cl}\} = 0 \qquad (6.7)$$

By expanding and rearranging, we get

$$V_m = \frac{(E_K \times g_K) + (E_{Na} \times g_{Na}) + (E_{Cl} \times g_{Cl})}{g_K + g_{Na} + g_{Cl}} \qquad (6.8)$$

This is the Hodgkin-Huxley equation for calculation of membrane potential. More accurate values are given by the Goldman equation, the derivation of which is beyond the scope of this book. Simply note that for the same set of ionic concentrations and conductances, the Hodgkin-Huxley equation and the Goldman equation give slightly different values.

Chloride current | It should be clear from the foregoing discussions that Na^+ always carries an inward depolarizing current, and K^+ always carries an outward hyperpolarizing current. The Cl^- current is somewhat different. Unlike Na^+ or K^+ ions, Cl^- ions do not have a pump transporting them. Hence, the Cl^- gradient is created entirely by the RMP, which pushes out Cl^- ions from the cell. Thus, the Nernst potential of Cl^- equals the RMP. Consequently, there is no significant Cl^- current across the resting membrane. Several types of nerve cells, however, do pump out Cl^- through secondary active transport using K^+–Cl^- cotransport. In these cells, the E_{Cl} is slightly more negative than the RMP, and Cl^- carries a weak, inward hyperpolarizing current.

Another situation in which the E_{Cl} and RMP are different is when the g_{Na} increases massively, as during an action potential. In this situation, the Cl^- sets up a moderately strong inward hyperpolarizing current.

Effect of Changes in Extracellular Fluid Ionic Concentrations

Extracellular ionic concentrations are much more prone to perturbations as compared with intracellular concentrations. Any variation in ECF ionic concentration alters the Nernst potential of the ion. However, the change in Nernst potential is less for ions that have high concentration in the ECF (Na^+, Cl^-) and more for K^+, which has a low ECF concentration. **Table 6.2** shows that for a given amount of change in ECF concentration (e.g., 5 mEq/L), the percentage change in $[C_o] / [C_i]$ is much greater for K^+ (100%) than for Na^+ (3.6%) or for Cl^- (5%). The changes in the Nernst potentials are correspondingly larger. Hence, perturbations in extracellular K^+ concentration have large effects on membrane potential. As shown in the above example, a 5 mEq/L increase in the ECF concentration of Cl^- will hyperpolarize the membrane slightly as its Nernst potential changes from –79.4 mV to –80.7 mV. However, a similar increase in ECF K^+ will depolarize the membrane markedly as its Nernst po-

Table 6.2 Effect of Increasing the Extracellular Fluid (ECF) Concentration of Ions on the Nernst Potential

Nernst Potential for Ions when ECF Concentration Is Normal			
Ion	ICF Conc. (mEq/L)	ECF Conc. (mEq/L)	Nernst Potential (mV)
Na^+	10	140	69.9
K^+	150	5	–90.1
Cl^-	5	100	–79.4
Nernst Potential for Ions when ECF Concentrations Are Increased by 5 mEq/L			
Ion	ICF Conc. (mEq/L)	ECF Conc. (mEq/L)	Nernst Potential (mV)
Na^+	10	145	70.8
K^+	150	10	–71.7
Cl^-	5	105	–80.7

Abbreviations: ICF, intracellular fluid; ECF, extracellular fluid.

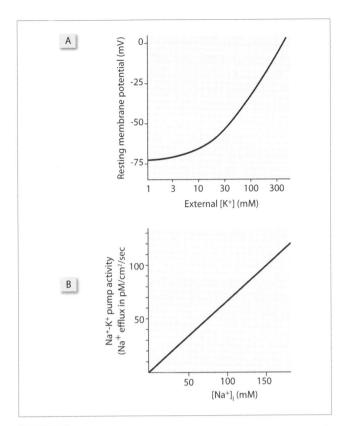

Fig. 6.5 **(A)** Effect of increasing the extracellular potassium (K^+) concentration of the membrane potential. **(B)** Dependence of sodium (Na^+)–K^+ pump activity on the intracellular Na^+ concentration. (**[A]** Adapted from Curtis HJ, Cole KS. Membrane resting and action potentials from the squid giant axon. J Cell Comp Physiol 1942;19:139.)

tential changes from –90.1 mV to –71.7 mV. Hence, addition of KCl to the bathing solution of an excitable tissue depolarizes the cells (**Fig. 6.5A**).

Pump Current

The role of the Na^+–K^+ pump in the development of membrane potentials is easily misunderstood. This is unfortunate because the membrane potential is one of the best understood areas of physiology. Before considering the role of the Na^+-K^+ pump in membrane potential, two facts that are discussed below must be understood.

A strong pump that is working slowly | The first thing that must be realized is that the Na^+-K^+ pump works very feebly in the cells. It serves to pump out the Na^+ that diffuses back into the cell and pumps in the K^+ that diffuses out of the cell. In the resting membrane, these ion fluxes are small. However, during an action potential, large amounts of Na^+ diffuse in, and equally large amounts of K^+ diffuse out. These are pumped back to the extracellular and intracellular compartments, respectively, for the maintenance of cell homeostasis.

Let us imagine the original situation when the ECF and ICF concentrations were equal, and the Na^+-K^+ pump just got into action. The pump activity must have been very high ini-

tially because the intracellular Na^+ concentration was high. However, as more and more Na^+ was pumped to the exterior, the pump current got reduced. This is because the activity of the Na^+–K^+ pump is directly proportional to the intracellular Na^+ concentration (**Fig. 6.5B**). At the usual intracellular Na^+ concentration of 10 mEq/L, the pump current is feeble and adds only about –3 mV to the diffusion potential.

An electrogenic pump rendered electroneutral | The second important thing that must be realized is that, although the Na^+–K^+ pump is potentially electrogenic (because it pumps out three Na^+ ions for every two K^+ ions that are pumped in), at no stage is the pump able to build up a significant membrane potential. This is because as soon as the pump creates a negative potential inside the cell, chloride ions rush out of the cell and restore electroneutrality. Thus, in effect, the Na^+–K^+ pump pumps out three Na^+ ions and one Cl^- ion for every two K^+ ions it pumps in. The real role of the Na^+–K^+ pump is that it builds up a high K^+ concentration within the cell and a high Na^+ concentration outside the cell, setting the stage for the development of a diffusion potential.

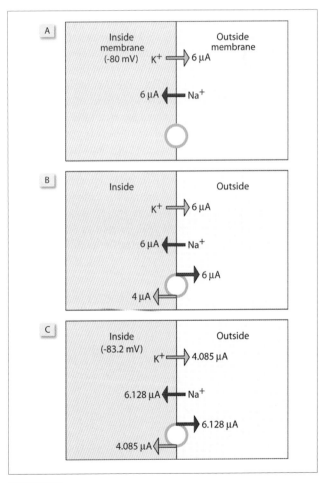

Fig. 6.6 Effect of pump current on cell homeostasis and membrane potential. **(A)** Membrane potential is –80 mV. Pump is not operational. The leak currents balance each other. **(B)** Pump is operational, resulting in an unbalanced outward potassium (K^+) current of 2 μA. **(C)** Membrane potential is –83.2 mV. Leak currents and pump currents get readjusted accordingly.

Restoration of the Concentration Gradients across the Membrane

During the resting state, a cell with a polarized membrane continuously loses K$^+$ to the exterior and gains Na$^+$ through their respective channels. The membrane potential does not change because the outward K$^+$ current balances the inward Na$^+$ current. However, due to these continuous channel currents, the intracellular and extracellular concentrations of these ions tend to equalize, and the membrane potential disappears over time. However, that does not happen due to the Na$^+$–K$^+$ pump, which pumps out three Na$^+$ ions for every two K$^+$ ions transported inside.

Balancing pump current with channel current | Suppose that in a resting nerve cell, the channel currents produce Na$^+$ influx and K$^+$ efflux in a ratio of 1:1. Yet the Na$^+$–K$^+$ pump, which produces Na$^+$ efflux and K$^+$ influx in a ratio of 3:2, is able to restore cell homeostasis. Before understanding how the same is possible, it is important to recall that the activity of the Na$^+$–K$^+$ pump (and the resultant pump current) increases when the intracellular concentration of Na$^+$ rises.

Let us take the example shown in **Fig. 6.6**. When the pump is inactive, the leak currents of Na$^+$ and K$^+$ balance each other (both are 6 µA), so that the membrane potential does not change. However, cell homeostasis is threatened as the intracellular concentration of K$^+$ and extracellular concentration of Na$^+$ decrease continuously. To prevent these losses, the Na$^+$–K$^+$ pump becomes operational, generating an outward Na current of 6 µA and an inward K$^+$ current of 4 µA. (Recall that the Na$^+$ and K$^+$ pump currents are in a ratio of 3:2.) The pump current, of Na$^+$ exactly balances the leak current of Na$^+$. However, the K$^+$ leak current is not fully balanced by the K$^+$ pump current, and there remains an unbalanced K$^+$ leak current of 2 µA. This outward K$^+$ current hyperpolarizes the membrane slightly, taking the membrane potential to –83.2 mV. The hyperpolarization reduces the K$^+$ leak current to 4.085 µA and increases the Na$^+$ leak current to 6.128 µA. The increase in Na$^+$ leak current stimulates the pump activity, so

that the pump currents for K$^+$ and Na$^+$ become 4.085 µA and 6128 µA, respectively. The pump currents now completely balance the leak currents, and cell homeostasis is no longer threatened.

In the new equilibrium, the following may be noted: (1) The Na$^+$ current (6.128 µA) and K$^+$ current (4.085 µA) are in a ratio of 3:2. This is true for both leak currents and pump currents. (2) The activity of the Na$^+$-K$^+$ pump has made a difference of only 3.2 mV.

Summary

- The membranes of all cells are electrically polarized, with the interior of the cell electrically negative to the outside of the cell.

- This resting membrane potential (RMP) is a consequence of the nonuniform distribution of Na$^+$ and K$^+$ across the membrane.

- This ion distribution is the result of the operation of the Na$^+$–K$^+$ pump, which utilizes biochemical energy to transport these ions against their concentration gradient.

- Diffusion of these two ions down the concentration gradient (leak currents) results in an RMP of –70 mV in unmyelinated axons and –90 mV in striated muscle cells.

Applying What You Know

6.1. Ms. Adams' electrolyte concentrations were all normal. However, if her potassium concentration was abnormally high, what effect would that have on the resting potential of her cells? What would happen if her potassium concentration was abnormally low? Explain.

Action Potential

The action potential (AP), the nerve impulse, is the signal that is conducted along the axon over long distances (or over a muscle cell) without a reduction in amplitude. Any transient change in the resting membrane potential, a depolarization or hyperpolarization, small or large in magnitude, can constitute a signal. However, except for the AP, all other membrane electrical signals decrease in amplitude after traveling short distances along a membrane. The AP consists of a brief reversal of membrane polarity followed by a quick restoration of the normal polarity. In neurons, the whole process lasts a few milliseconds. In skeletal muscle cells, the AP is similarly short, but in cardiac and smooth muscle cells, it is very much longer (see **Figs. 18.4** and **19.1**).

All-or-none law | An AP is usually full-sized with a fixed amplitude of ~110 mV (from –70 mV to +40 mV). Subthreshold stimuli cannot trigger APs. Once triggered, an AP runs its entire course, producing a fully fledged spike. This is known as the *all-or-none law.*

The all-or-none law does not rule out a change in AP amplitude, if the prevailing conditions of membrane potential and excitability, ionic concentrations, and temperature are changed. It only emphasizes that the magnitude of the spike (which depends on concentrations) does not increase or decrease in a *graded* manner with changes in the stimulus strength: it is either maximum (all), or it is not triggered at all (none). However, a change in stimulus strength alters the frequency with which APs are generated.

Phases of action potential | The AP, which is recorded using an intracellular electrode (**Fig. 7.1A**), has five phases: prepotential, depolarization, repolarization, after-depolarization, and hyperpolarization (**Fig. 7.1B**). (1) The *prepotential,* also called the "foot" of the AP, is a local membrane potential that drifts slowly toward –55 mV, which is called the *firing level or threshold.* Strictly speaking, it is not a part of the AP. (2) During *depolarization,* the potential shoots up to +40 mV in less than a millisecond. (3) During *repolarization,* the potential drops to near resting levels, about –40 mV. This phase also lasts less than a millisecond. The depolarization and repolarization phases of the AP together constitute the *spike potential.* Although the total duration of the nerve AP (the time it takes for the membrane potential to return to its resting level) can be many milliseconds, the spike lasts for no more than 2 to 3 msec. It is the spike potential rather than the entire AP that can truly be termed the nerve impulse. (4) During *after-depolarization,* the rate of repolarization slows down and gradually reaches the resting potential of –70 mV. This slow phase of repolarization lasts ~2 msec. (5) During *after-hyperpolarization,* the intracellular negativity overshoots the normal resting value of –70 mV to reach a more negative value of about –75 mV. It lasts for nearly 40 msec before slowly returning to the normal resting potential of –70 mV.

The duration of the AP generated in other excitable cells can be quite a bit longer than in the nerve cell; in heart muscle, the AP can be 400 msec long.

Membrane excitability during action potential | An AP is triggered only if the stimulus raises the membrane potential above the firing level of –55 mV. The minimum strength of a stimulus that can trigger an AP is called a *threshold stimulus.*

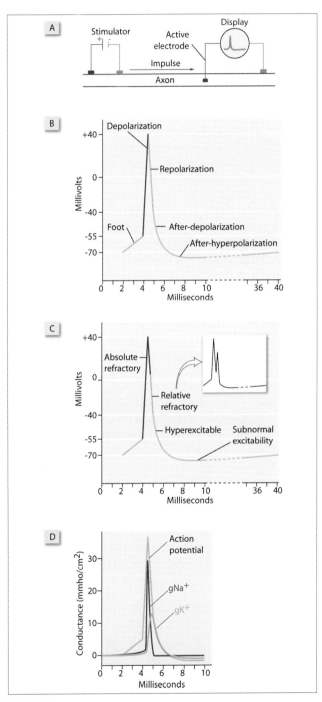

Fig. 7.1 **(A)** Set up for the recording of an action potential (AP). **(B)** Phases of an AP. **(C)** Refractory periods of an AP. Inset shows a second, smaller AP triggered during the relative refractory period. **(D)** Ionic conductances during an AP.

The membrane is *refractory* (i.e., not responsive) to a second stimulus during most of the spike (**Fig. 7.1C**). From the spike onset until repolarization is approximately one-third complete, the membrane is *absolutely refractory*; that is, no stimulus howsoever strong can elicit a response. Thereafter, until the onset of after-depolarization, the membrane is *relatively refractory*; that is, a sufficiently high stimulus can elicit a response. During after-depolarization, the membrane is hyperexcitable. Having just come out of the refractory period, the membrane is excitable, and being closer to the firing level makes it *hyperexcitable*. During hyperpolarization, the membrane excitability is low, but it slowly returns to normal. The *effective refractory period* (ERP) includes the absolute refractory period and the early part of the relative refractory period. At the end of ERP, the membrane is able to conduct physiologically produced APs. If the membrane is in the relative refractory period, the action potentials are smaller and are conducted slowly.

The presence of a refractory period limits the frequency with which a neuron (or a muscle cell) can generate and propagate APs.

Origin and spread of action potential | During the depolarization phase of AP, ionic currents flow between the depolarized membrane and the adjacent polarized areas, which then get depolarized, too. When the depolarization of the adjacent area exceeds 15 mV, a fresh AP is triggered in the adjacent area. In this way, the AP travels along the membrane as a wave of depolarization.

If every AP is triggered by another in its immediate vicinity, how is the first AP stimulated? It stands to reason that ultimately an AP must be triggered by other types of physiologically generated electrical signals. These electrical signals are of different types. The excitatory postsynaptic potential (EPSP) and end plate potential (EPP) are produced by chemical transmission at synapses (see Chapter 11). The receptor potential is generated by the transduction of light, sound, heat, chemical, or mechanical stimuli into electrical signals (see Chapter 10). APs can also be triggered experimentally by a pair of stimulating electrodes: the AP gets triggered at the cathode.

Ionic conductances during action potential | All phases of the AP except the prepotential are the direct consequence of the permeability (conductance) changes of sodium (Na^+) and potassium (K^+), which are due to channel activation and inactivation. An increase in Na^+ conductance depolarizes the membrane, and an increase in K^+ permeability repolarizes (or hyperpolarizes) the membrane. The actual membrane potential at any instant is determined by the relative magnitudes of Na^+ and K^+ permeability (**Fig. 7.1D**).

General Model: Flow

The flow of Na^+ and K^+ ions across the membrane is always determined by the electrochemical (concentration and electrical potential) gradient across the membrane and the ease with which these ions can move across it—the conductance for each ion (conductance = 1/resistance). This general model describes ion flow in all cells, as well as the flow of blood in the circulation and air in the respiratory tree.

The prepotential is induced by some external source of negative potential. The source may be an external electrode (a cathode) or a depolarized area on the membrane in the immediate vicinity. Depolarization occurs due to a steep rise in Na^+ conductance. Repolarization occurs due to two reasons: the rapid rise of K^+ conductance shortly after the surge in Na^+ conductance, and the spontaneous inactivation of the Na^+ channels, which open during the depolarization phase. During after-depolarization, the K^+ conductance is considerably more than the Na^+ conductance. Hence, the potential drifts back slowly toward the resting value. Hyperpolarization occurs because K^+ conductance is still high, although the Na^+ conductance has returned to normal.

Effect of temperature on the action potential | Temperature affects the rate at which membrane channels open and close. With a fall in temperature, the depolarization phase becomes less steep due to slower opening of Na^+ channels (**Fig. 7.2**). Also, the overshoot goes higher due to a slower onset of Na^+ channel inactivation and a delayed rise in K^+ conductance.

Membrane Stimulation

In clinical situations, both the positive and negative electrodes are placed extracellularly, usually on the surface of the skin. When current is passed through the electrodes, the part of the nerve below the cathode gets excited, and the part of the nerve below the anode gets hyperpolarized. In the electrodes, the current is carried by electrons; in the tissues, the current is carried by ions, both positive and negative. The direction of the current is conventionally the direction of flow of positive ions.

Cathodal stimulation | When the stimulating electrodes are turned on, the anions and cations start flowing along the electric field set up between the electrodes. Initially, the ions are unable to flow across the membrane at sites where the field intersects the membrane. Hence, at these sites, the ions pile up on both surfaces of the membrane. These ionic currents are called *capacitive currents*. Immediately below the cath-

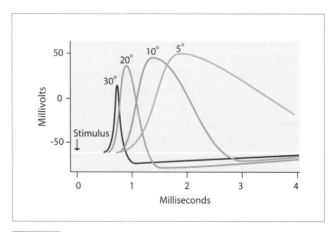

Fig. 7.2 Effect of temperature on the AP. As the temperature falls, both the duration and the amplitude of the AP increase. (Adapted from Hodkin AL, Katz B. The electrical activity of the giant axon of the squid. J Physiol (Lond) 1949; 109:245.)

ode, the extracellular anions flowing away from the cathode line up on the outer membrane surface, whereas the axoplasmic cations flowing toward the cathode adhere to the inner membrane surface (**Fig. 7.3A**). These events result in a change in membrane potential, which is called an *electrotonic potential*. The potential that develops under the cathode is called *catelectrotonic potential*, whereas the potential that develops under the anode is called *anelectrotonic potential*. When the electrodes are removed, the electrotonic potentials disappear very quickly.

The catelectrotonic potential is the direct effect of the cathodal electric field. Another potential, called the local potential, develops simultaneously at the same site under the effect of the catelectrotonic potential. The local potential develops due to the opening of the membrane Na^+ channels, and it lasts a little longer after the electrodes are removed. If the local potential is strong enough, it triggers the AP.

Anode-break excitation | Sometimes the membrane gets excited at the anode when the stimulus is switched off. This is called anode-break excitation. If the stimulus is applied for a sufficient length of time, the ions start crossing the membrane, setting up a *resistive current*. Thus, under the anode there is a large increase in the inward diffusion of Na^+ into the axon and a large decrease in the outward efflux of K^+. However, these ionic fluxes are unable to change the membrane potential so long as the anodal current is passing through it, and the membrane remains hyperpolarized due to the potential drop

occurring along the path of the anodal current. The moment the anode is switched off, the combination of high Na^+ influx and low K^+ efflux depolarizes the membrane and triggers an AP.

Membrane accommodation | When a catelectrotonic potential depolarizes the membrane rapidly to the firing level, an AP is triggered. However, when the catelectrotonic potential depolarizes the membrane slowly to the firing level, the AP often fails to be triggered. This phenomenon is called membrane accommodation and is due to Na^+ channel inactivation. When the membrane depolarizes, both Na^+ and K^+ channels open up. If the depolarization occurs very slowly, more and more Na^+ channels open up, only to get quickly inactivated. The K^+ channels remain open and tend to restore the membrane potential. By the time the potential reaches the firing level, most of the Na^+ channels have become inactivated, whereas the K^+ channels remain open as long as the membrane remains depolarized. Therefore, the explosive depolarization fails to occur. If, however, the membrane depolarizes rapidly to the firing level, a large number of Na^+ channels open all at once. Before they become inactivated, they are able to trigger off the AP by overcoming the effect of K^+ channels. For the same reason, the square pulse is more effective than the sawtooth pulse in stimulating the membrane (**Fig. 7.3B**).

Graded Potentials

Unlike APs, local potentials do not obey the all-or-none law. They are proportional to the stimulus strength and hence are also called *graded potentials*. Other examples of graded potentials are the receptor potential and the end plate potential. Some of the differences between graded potentials and APs are listed in **Table 7.1**.

Table 7.1 Differences between Graded Potential and Action Potential

Graded Potential	Action Potential
Amplitude proportionate to stimulus strength and can get summated	Amplitude constant for all suprathreshold stimuli and cannot be summated
Can be a depolarization or hyperpolarization	Always a depolarization
Conduction is associated with reduction in magnitude	Conducted without reduction in magnitude
Can be generated spontaneously in response to physical or chemical stimuli	Generated only in response to membrane depolarization

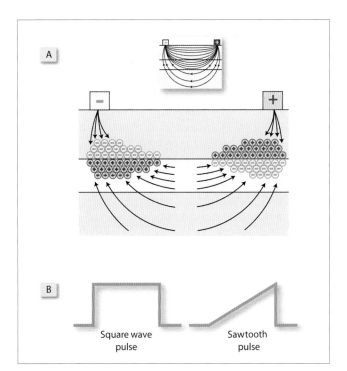

Fig. 7.3 **(A)** Current flowing from anode to cathode, intersecting the axonal membrane in its path. Beneath the cathode, anions accumulate outside, and cations accumulate inside the membrane. Beneath the anode, there is accumulation of cations outside and anions inside the membrane. **(B)** A square-pulse stimulus rises sharply to its peak level and effectively triggers an AP, whereas a sawtooth pulse, which rises to its peak slowly, often fails to trigger an AP.

Summary

- The AP is an all-or-none electrical signal generated in an excitable membrane by a threshold depolarization.

- When the membrane has generated an AP, it becomes refractory for a time and cannot generate a second AP until the refractory period is over.

- The AP is triggered by a sudden opening of voltage-gated Na^+ channels through which an inward current passes. This is followed somewhat later by the opening of a voltage-gated K^+ channel and an outward current.

Applying What You Know

7.1. Ms. Adams undergoes several nerve conduction studies in which electrical stimuli are applied to the nerve. What must the stimulus do to the nerve membrane to excite an AP? Explain.

Channel Dynamics

Effect of Membrane Potential on Channel Permeability

The excitability properties of nerve and muscle cells—their ability to generate action potentials — is a consequence of the presence of two special ion channels in their membrane. These are a voltage-dependent Na^+ channel and a voltage-dependent K^+ channel. These channels open (activate) and close (deactivate) with changes in the membrane potential. Individual channels obey the all-or-none law: they are either fully open or fully closed. When the membrane depolarizes, the probability of a channel being open increases. Stated simply, as the membrane depolarizes, more and more channels change from the fully closed to the fully open state.

When the membrane depolarizes, both Na^+ and K^+ channels open up, resulting in significant increases in their conductances (i.e., membrane permeability). The increase in conductance is essentially proportional to the change in membrane potential.

Sodium channel inactivation | Though both Na^+ and K^+ conductances increase with membrane depolarization, the increase in Na^+ conductance does not last long. In other words, if the membrane is kept depolarized long enough, the Na^+ channels that are initially activated start closing down spontaneously after a few milliseconds (**Fig. 8.1A**). This process is called *Na+ channel inactivation.* Na^+ channels recover from inactivation only after the membrane returns to the normal resting membrane potential (RMP). Na^+ channel activation has two important consequences: the *refractory period* and *membrane accommodation.*

The conductance of Na^+ channels is determined by two gates: the activation and inactivation gates (**Fig. 8.1B**). The activation and inactivation gates are also called the m gates and h gates, respectively. The origins of the names "m" and "h" are to be found in the empirical equations developed in the 1950s by Hodgkin and Huxley to describe the time course of voltage changes during an action potential. During depolarization, the activation gate opens quickly, followed slowly by the closure of the inactivation gate. This results in a brief interval during which the channel remains open. During repolarization, the activation gate closes first, followed by the opening of the inactivation gate, so that the channel remains closed throughout repolarization.

Effect of Channel Permeability on Membrane Potential

Stabilizing effect of potassium channels | When the membrane potential becomes less negative, the K^+ channels open up (**Fig. 8.2A**). Opening of the K^+ channels increases the outward hyperpolarizing current and thereby makes the membrane more negative. Conversely, if the membrane potential becomes more negative, a large number of K^+ channels close down, and the membrane potential drifts to a less negative value. Thus, whenever there is a change in membrane potential, the

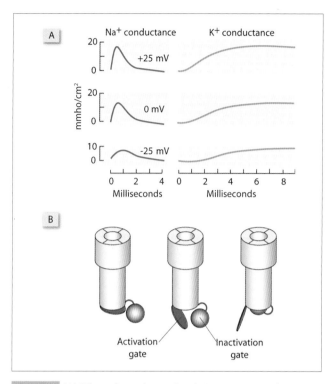

Fig. 8.1 **(A)** Effect of membrane depolarization on membrane permeability to potassium (K^+) and sodium (Na^+) ions over a period of 4 to 8 milliseconds. The effects of three different grades of depolarization are shown here, as the membrane is depolarized to +25 mV (*above*), 0 mV (*middle*), and –25 mV (*bottom*). Note that the changes in membrane permeability of Na^+ are transient, whereas those of K^+ are sustained as long as the membrane remains depolarized. **(B)** Activation (m) and inactivation (h) gates of a sodium channel.

activated K^+ channels tend to restore the membrane potential to the original level. Hence, K^+ channels are said to have a stabilizing effect on the membrane potential: they tend to prevent any change in membrane potential.

Destabilizing effect of sodium channels | When the membrane depolarizes, the Na^+ channels start opening up (**Fig. 8.2B**). The opening of the Na^+ channels increases the inward depolarizing current and thereby depolarizes the membrane further, leading to the opening of greater numbers of Na^+ channels. Thus, there is a positive feedback spiral (the *Hodgkin cycle*), resulting in a very rapid change in membrane potential and opening of nearly all the Na^+ channels. Because the opening of even a few Na^+ channels can trigger off this vicious cycle, resulting in large changes in membrane potential, Na^+ channels are said to have a destabilizing effect on membrane potential.

Firing level | It is clear from **Fig. 8.1A** that when the membrane depolarizes, the rise in Na^+ conductance is much quicker than the rise in K^+ conductance. Hence, even a small depolarization should destabilize the membrane potential and set off

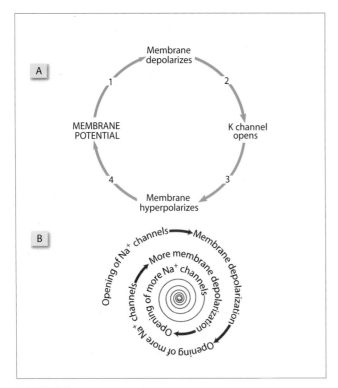

Fig. 8.2 Effect of channel permeability on membrane potential. **(A)** Stabilizing effect of potassium (K^+) ions on membrane potential. When the membrane is depolarized (becomes less negative), K^+ channels open, the flux of K^+ out of the cell increases, and the membrane potential becomes more negative. **(B)** The Hodgkin cycle, explaining the destabilizing effect of sodium (Na^+) ions on membrane potential. When Na^+ channels open, the influx of Na^+ increases, and more Na^+ enters the cell; the membrane potential becomes more positive, opening more Na^+ channels.

the Hodgkin cycle. What actually happens is that the membrane quickly repolarizes following a small depolarization. Why is this so?

The question is best answered by the following argument, which explains why the slightest depolarization of the membrane is immediately opposed by g_K and g_{Cl} even when these conductances remain unchanged. If, additionally, the K^+ channels open up, the g_K increases, and the opposition to membrane depolarization is even greater. Thus, a fairly large increase in g_{Na} is required before the Hodgkin cycle can be set off. The membrane potential at which this occurs is called the *firing level* or *threshold*.

Agents Altering Channel Function

Several naturally occurring substances affect the permeability of Na^+ or K^+ channels. These compounds have been used extensively in research for studying channel properties using the voltage clamp technique.

Specific channel blockers | The activation of Na^+ channels is blocked by *tetrodotoxin* (TTX) and *saxitoxin* (STX). These bind to the extracellular sites on the Na^+ channel and prevent the activation of Na^+ channels, thereby rendering the membrane inexcitable. The inactivation of Na^+ channels is blocked by *pro-*

nase, which binds to intracellular sites on the Na^+ channel. The inactivation of the K^+ channel is blocked by *tetraethylammonium* (TEA). It prolongs the action potential.

Local anesthetics are lipid-soluble substances that bind to intracellular sites on the Na^+ channels. Some of them, such as lidocaine and procainamide, tend to produce a frequency-dependent block; that is, they produce a conduction block only after the membrane conducts a train of action potentials. This is probably because the local anesthetic molecule binds to an intracellular site on the channel. In its charged form, the local anesthetic molecule gains access to its binding site within the pore only when the channel is in an open state. Moreover, the local anesthetic seems to bind more tightly to the inactivated form of the Na^+ channel.

Nonspecific channel modulators | Calcium (Ca^{2+}) ions bind to the negatively charged groups in the membrane phospholipids. Because the concentration of Ca^{2+} ions is much higher outside the cell than inside the cell, Ca^{2+} ions bind mainly on the outer surface of the membrane. This does not affect the overall membrane potential, which is determined only by the Nernst potentials of the diffusible ions. However, it does produce small, local areas of hyperpolarization and thereby reduces the excitability of the Na^+ channels located in the vicinity.

Lowering the concentrations of extracellular Ca^{2+} can cause spontaneous impulse generation, which can be reversed by the addition of Ca^{2+} or other bivalent ions, probably because of their stabilizing effects on the channel. Spontaneous impulse generation in nerves due to low serum Ca^{2+} can result in widespread muscle spasms and paresthesias (false sensations). When muscle contraction is present, this is called *tetany* and is commonly seen when an individual hyperventilates or in patients with hypoparathyroidism.

Channel Characterization

Voltage Clamp Technique

Measuring the electrical conductance of a membrane involves measuring membrane currents at different voltages. A major hurdle in these efforts is the explosive change in membrane potential that occurs once the voltage touches the threshold. This led to the search for a technique that would "clamp" the membrane potential at any desired value despite the surge in current.

In the voltage clamp technique (**Fig. 8.3**), the membrane potential can be stepped rapidly to a predetermined level of depolarization (called the *command potential*) by passing current across the cell membrane. Every time the membrane potential tends to change from the command potential, the clamp circuit opposes the change in potential by injecting a precisely calculated feedback current.

Patch Clamp Technique

Before the advent of the patch clamp technique, the voltage clamp technique was used to determine conductance of a whole membrane with a mixed population of different types of channels. The conductance characteristics of a single type of

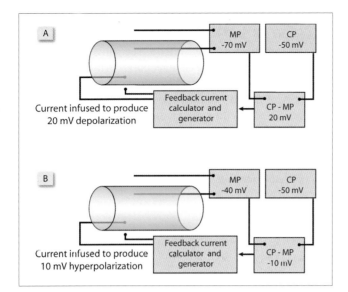

Fig. 8.3 **(A)** Membrane potential (MP = –70 mV) is made equal to the command potential (CP = –50 mV) by injecting a calculated amount of current. **(B)** If the membrane potential tries to change from –50 to –40 mV, it is immediately corrected by injecting a current calculated to produce 10 mV hyperpolarization.

channel were deduced by blocking the other known channels present in the membrane. For example, **Fig. 8.4** shows the records of membrane conductance before and after application of TTX. The conductance measured after applying TTX gives the K^+ conductance provided the membrane has only Na^+ and K^+ channels.

With the patch clamp technique, it is possible to record the conductance of a single channel. A small, fine, polished glass micropipette with a tip diameter of ~1 μm is pressed against the membrane. The pipette is filled with a solution having a

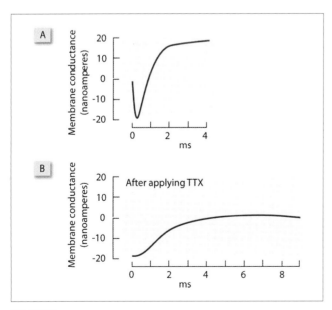

Fig. 8.4 **(A)** Conductance of a membrane that contains only sodium (Na^+) and potassium (K^+) channels. **(B)** Conductance of the same membrane after blocking the Na^+ channels with tetrodotoxin (TTX).

composition like the extracellular fluid. A metal electrode in contact with the electrolyte in the micropipette connects the pipette to a special electric circuit that measures the current flowing through channels in the membrane under the pipette tip. A small amount of suction to the patch pipette greatly increases the tightness of the seal between the pipette and the membrane. The result is a seal with extremely high resistance (the gigaohm seal) between the inside and outside of the pipette.

Patch clamping (**Fig. 8.5A**) offers three types of experimental possibilities: (1) The experimenter can apply various stimuli from within the pipette and measure the behavior of the trapped channels. (2) The experimenter can detach the membrane from the cell, thereby exposing the cytoplasmic side of the channels. (3) The membrane patch can be ruptured

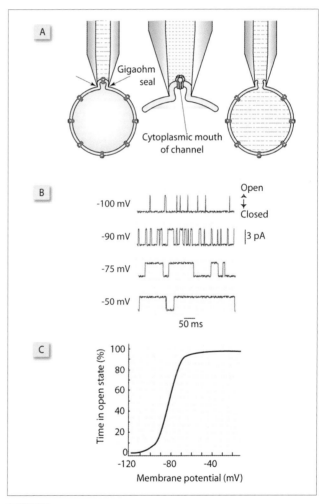

Fig. 8.5 **(A)** Three methods of the patch clamp technique. **(B)** Channel current of a single channel recorded through a patch clamp. The channel current obeys the all-or-none law: it is either 3 pA (maximum) or 0 pA (minimum). As the membrane is depolarized in steps (–100 mV, –90 mV, –75 mV, and –50 mV), the channel remains open for longer durations. **(C)** Graph showing the relation between membrane potential and the time spent by the channel in the open state. (Adapted from Ackerman MJ, Clapham DE. Ion channels: basic science and clinical disease. N Eng J Med 1997;337:1575.)

without breaking the gigaohm seal so that the experimenter can alter the constituents of the living cell's cytoplasm.

Channel currents recorded by patch clamp | One striking observation made possible through patch clamp studies of single channels is that channels obey the all-or-none law: they are either fully open (conducting a maximum current of ~3 pA) or are fully closed (**Figs. 8.5B** and **8.5C**). Also, channels are usually not continuously open, but switch frequently between the open and closed states. The probability of a channel being open at any instant increases as the membrane depolarizes.

Channel Structure

The molecular structures of several channels have been characterized, and the sites responsible for specific channel characteristics have been identified. The structure of an ion channel has been described in Chapter 2. Some of the details of a voltage-sensitive Na$^+$ channel are shown in **Fig. 8.6**. The S-4 transmembrane segments in each homologous domain of the α-subunit contain the voltage sensors. The positively charged

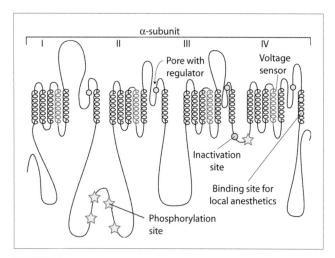

Fig. 8.6 The ultrastructure of the α-subunit of the sodium channel showing its functionally important sites.

amino acid in the third position within S-4 is the actual voltage sensor. S-5 and S-6 transmembrane segments and the short membrane-associated P loop (segments SS1 and SS2) enclose between them the channel pore. Certain amino acids in the P loop are critical for determining conductance and ion selectivity of the Na$^+$ channel and its ability to bind TTX and saxitoxin. The short intracellular loop connecting homologous domains III and IV serves as an inactivation gate. The loops between I and II and between III and IV are susceptible to phosphorylation. Phosphorylation at these two sites impairs channel activation and inactivation, respectively.

Summary

- The activation gate of the voltage-gated Na$^+$ channel opens quickly when depolarized to threshold and just as quickly spontaneously closes. The inactivation gate then closes and cannot be opened for a time.

- When open, the voltage-gated Na$^+$ channel produces a positive-feedback effect because the inward Na$^+$ current further depolarizes the membrane, thus opening more Na$^+$ channels.

- The voltage-gated K$^+$ channel opens more slowly when depolarized to threshold and spontaneously closes.

- The voltage-gated Na$^+$ channel is a membrane-spanning protein with three functional domains: the voltage sensor, the gated pore, and the inactivation gate.

Applying What You Know

8.1. If we could pharmacologically alter Ms. Adams' voltage-dependent Na$^+$ channels so that they stayed open 50% longer than normally, what effect would this have on the amplitude of her action potentials? Would this change or alleviate her symptoms? Explain.

Action potentials in neurons and muscle cells propagate (are conducted) over the entire cell rapidly and with no reduction in their amplitude (action potentials are an all-or-none phenomenon). The mechanism of this conduction is basically the same in nerve and muscle, but we will discuss the mechanism as it operates in neurons. However, remember that this description applies to muscle action potentials as well.

Mechanism of Nerve Conduction

Electrotonic Conduction

Local currents | When an action potential is in its depolarization phase, local currents flow from the depolarized membrane to the adjacent polarized areas and depolarize them, too. In the axoplasm, the current flows away from the depolarized area. The current then flows out through the axonal membrane and returns through the extracellular fluid. This passive flow of local currents to adjacent membrane areas is called *electrotonic conduction*. The local current circuit has three components: (1) the internal longitudinal current or axoplasmic current, which flows through the axoplasm; (2) the radial or membrane current, which flows out through the membrane; and (3) the external longitudinal current, which flows through the extracellular fluid. The effect of local currents becomes smaller with distance (**Fig. 9.1A**). In an unmyelinated neuron, a fully fledged action potential (peak-to-peak) of 110 mV can produce a depolarization of 15 mV at a distance of 1.0 mm, but a depolarization of only 2.0 mV at a distance of 2.0 mm.

General Model: Flow

Local currents flow because of the presence of an electrical potential gradient. The resistance along each piece of the circuit determines the magnitude of the current that flows. The equation that describes this phenomenon, Ohm's law, is identical in form to the equation describing blood flow in the circulation.

Factors affecting electrotonic conduction | Electrotonic conduction is determined by four physical factors: (1) The axoplasmic resistance (Ri) offered by the axoplasm to the flow of axoplasmic current. The thinner the axon, the higher is the axoplasmic resistance, and the weaker is the electrotonic conduction. (2) The resistance (Ro) offered by the extracellular fluid to the outer longitudinal current. The greater this resistance, the weaker is the electrotonic conduction. Ro usually remains constant. (3) The resistance (Rm) offered by the membrane to the transmembrane current. When Rm is high (compare **Fig. 9.1B** *left* and *right*), the membrane current falls, resulting in higher axoplasmic current and stronger electrotonic conduction. Rm is high when the membrane is thick, as in the myelinated segment of the neuron. (4) The electrical capacitance (Cm) of the membrane. The greater the membrane

capacitance, the poorer is the electrotonic conduction. An electrical impulse is conducted by inducing a potential change in its adjacent area. The greater the capacitance of a structure, the more it resists any change in its potential. Hence, if the capacitance of the adjacent area is higher, it takes longer to induce a potential change in that area; therefore, electrotonic conduction slows down. Cm is low when the membrane is thick, as in the myelinated segment of the neuron.

Propagation of Action Potential

Local currents from one action potential spread to the adjacent membrane area and depolarize it to the threshold level, triggering another action potential, and the process continues. Thus, there are two essential components of action potential propagation: (1) The flow of local currents, which depolarize the adjacent membrane, is called the *conductive component* of impulse propagation. This electrotonic conduction of membrane depolarization is associated with progressive decrease in the magnitude of depolarization. (2) The triggering of a fresh action potential in the adjacent membrane is called the *regenerative component* of impulse propagation. The new action potential depolarizes the membrane maximally and thereby restores the depolarization to its original peak-to-peak magnitude of 110 mV.

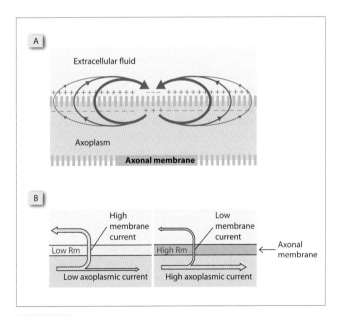

Fig. 9.1   **(A)** In an unmyelinated membrane, local currents get smaller with distance (thickness of line is proportional to magnitude of current) because of high axoplasmic resistance (Ri), low membrane resistance (Rm), and high membrane capacitance (Cm). High Cm is shown as a dense distribution of membrane charge. **(B)** Membrane resistance and currents. (*Left*) When membrane resistance, Rm, is low, the membrane current is high. When membrane resistance is high (*right*), membrane current decreases, and axoplasmic current rises (currents are proportional to the thickness of the arrows).

Without the conductive component, an action potential cannot be conducted at all. Without the regenerative component, an action potential can be conducted only up to a limited distance beyond which it will fade out. Before the local currents fade out completely, a fresh action potential must be generated for its continued propagation. The conductive component is very fast and depends on the electrical characteristics (the cable properties) of the membrane. The regenerative component is much slower.

Nerve Conduction Velocity

Nerve conduction velocity can be affected by factors influencing electrotonic conduction (conductive component), the action potential (regenerative component), or both.

Axon diameter | An axon with a larger diameter allows easier passage to axoplasmic current because the resistance of a conductor is inversely related to its cross-sectional area. When the electrotonic conduction is stronger, and the adjacent membrane is depolarized to the firing level more quickly, conduction velocity increases. In an unmyelinated fiber, the speed of propagation is directly proportional to the square root of the fiber diameter (D).

$$\text{Conduction velocity} \propto \sqrt{D}$$

Temperature | When temperature decreases, the duration of the action potential (especially the spike) increases markedly. This increases the delay in conduction caused by the action potential and thereby slows down conduction velocity.

Resting membrane potential (RMP) | When the membrane is hyperpolarized, it has two effects: it speeds up electrotonic conduction but slows down the generation of action potential because of the greater time required for the membrane to depolarize to threshold potential. The resultant effect on conduction velocity is variable but usually causes a decrease. The following example should make it clear.

Suppose a membrane has an RMP of –80 mV, and a part of it depolarizes to +40 mV during an action potential. The potential difference between the depolarized and repolarized areas will be 120 mV. If, however, the RMP is –100 mV, and it depolarizes to +40 mV, the potential difference between depolarized and repolarized areas will be 140 mV. This higher potential difference will set up stronger local currents, resulting in faster electrotonic conduction. However, hyperpolarization is usually associated with a reduction in peak depolarization. In that case, there will be no increase in electrotonic conduction. Moreover, a hyperpolarized membrane takes longer to reach the firing level and therefore slows down the regeneration component.

On the other hand, when the RMP is less negative, it slows down both electrotonic conduction and the generation of action potential. The latter occurs because persistent depolarization causes inactivation of a large number of sodium (Na$^+$) channels. As a result, the spike generated is stunted and wider.

Firing level (threshold potential) | If the threshold potential is low, then an action potential can trigger another action potential a longer distance away, where the local currents are small. Thus, the conduction velocity increases. The threshold potential effectively decreases when the concentration of divalent ions (particularly Ca^{2+}) in the extracellular fluid decreases.

Myelination and Saltatory Conduction

Myelination speeds up conduction by influencing both conductive and regenerative components.

Effect on conductive component | Myelination increases the membrane resistance and decreases the membrane capacitance (**Fig. 9.2**). The increase in membrane resistance reduces the transmembrane current and increases the axoplasmic current; therefore, the membrane space constant increases (see below). The decrease in membrane capacitance decreases the membrane time constant (see below). Together these properties ensure that the depolarization produced in one node is electrotonically conducted quickly and adequately through the myelinated segments and triggers action potentials several nodes away. This is called *saltatory conduction* (Latin: *saltere* means "to jump"). In a myelinated neuron, the conduction velocity is directly proportional to the fiber diameter (**Fig. 9.3**).

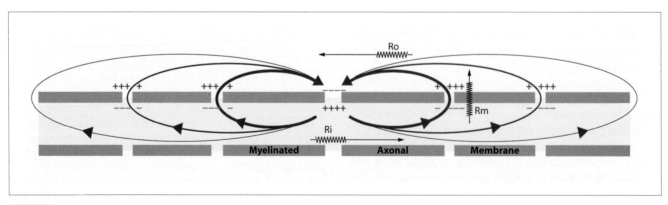

Fig. 9.2 In the myelinated axon, local currents travel long distances. Myelinated membrane does not permit passage of current through it due to its high low membrane resistance (Rm). Also, myelination decreases membrane capacitance (Cm), which is shown here as the sparsely distributed charges on the membrane.

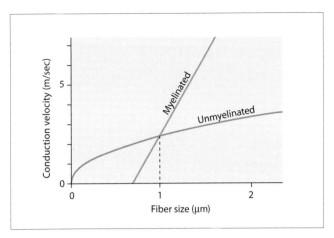

Fig. 9.3 Relationship of fiber diameter to conduction velocity. For the same fiber diameter, myelinated neurons conduct faster only when the fiber size is > 1 µm. (Adapted from Rushton WAH. A theory of the effects of fiber size in medullated nerve. J Physiol (Lond) 1951;115:116.)

Conduction velocity ∝ Axonal diameter

Effect on regenerative component | Due to poor permeability to potassium (K^+), the resting potential in the myelinated segment is only –3 to –6 mV, and no action potential is generated in the membrane in the myelinated segment of the axon. Action potentials are generated only in the unmyelinated nodes, which are 0.2 to 1.0 mm apart. Fewer action potentials mean less delay in conduction: there is a higher conduction velocity.

However, unmyelinated axons with a diameter < 1 µm have conduction velocities that are greater than myelinated axons of the same size (see left-hand side of **Fig. 9.3**). One reason for this is the following. The total diameter of a myelinated axon is the sum of the diameter of the axon and the thickness of the myelin sheath. For a given total diameter of myelinated axon, the greater the thickness of the myelin sheath, the smaller is the diameter of the axon. Although a thick myelin sheath would speed up conduction, a thin axon would slow down conduction. For diameters < 1 µm, even a thin myelin sheath would reduce the axonal diameter to the point where axoplasmic resistance increases tremendously, and conduction slows down markedly.

Nerve Conduction Failure

In a myelinated neuron, an action potential is conducted over long distances electrotonically before triggering a fresh action potential. Although this mechanism increases the speed of propagation, it is also fraught with the risk of conduction failure. Conduction failure will occur if (1) the electrotonic conduction is so weak that it fades out completely before traveling to the next node, or (2) the electrotonic conduction is so slow that the original action potential completes itself (returns to the RMP) before the local currents can reach the next node. Normally, this risk is negligible because in a myelinated neuron, the electrotonic conduction from one action potential

(1) is strong enough to trigger a fresh action potential more than 10 nodes away (not just in the next node) and (2) is fast enough that the impulse travels 10 nodes by the time the original action potential reaches its peak.

Space and time constants | For a quick and assured nerve conduction, a strong electrotonic conduction is necessary. Strong electrotonic conduction occurs when (1) axoplasmic resistance (Ri) is low, (2) external longitudinal resistance (Ro) is low, (3) membrane resistance (Rm) is high, and (4) membrane capacitance (Cm) is low. From the above-mentioned cable properties, two indicators of electrotonic conduction can be calculated: the space constant and the time constant of the nerve membrane.

The *space constant* (λ) of a membrane tells us how far a change in membrane potential will be conducted electrotonically. It is the distance a potential is conducted along the membrane before it reduces to 37% of its original strength. The space constant is 0.5 mm for unmyelinated nerves and 3.0 mm for myelinated neurons. The greater the space constant, the farther the currents will flow (**Fig. 9.4A**). It is given by the formula

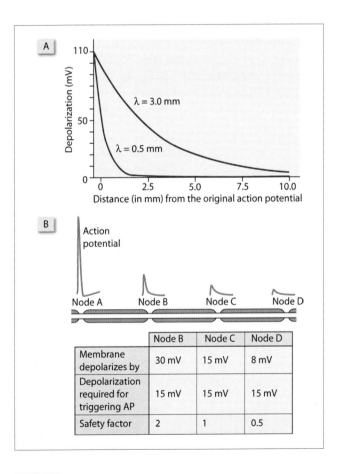

Fig. 9.4 **(A)** Effect of membrane space constant on the spread of an action potential (AP). On a membrane with a low space constant, any depolarization potential will fade away within a short distance. **(B)** The safety factor in nerve conduction. The action potential at node A will trigger action potentials at nodes B and C, but not at node D.

$$\lambda = \sqrt{\frac{Rm}{Ro+Ri}} \qquad (9.1)$$

A large axon has a low Ri, and its myelination increases the Rm. Thus, a large myelinated axon has a high space constant.

The *time constant* τ of a membrane tells us how quickly the electrotonic conduction will occur. It is the time taken by a stimulus potential to raise the membrane potential to 63% of its own strength. The greater the time constant, the slower the currents will flow. It is given by the formula

$$\tau = Rm \times Cm \qquad (9.2)$$

A myelinated axon has low capacitance. Hence, its time constant is low and conduction velocity is high. Conversely, the muscle membrane has high capacitance. Hence, its time constant is high and conduction velocity is low.

Safety factor | For triggering an action potential, the membrane needs to be depolarized by 15 mV, from –70 mV (the RMP) to –55 mV (the firing level). Thus, an electrotonic depolarization of 15 mV is the minimum required for propagation of a nerve impulse. **Fig. 9.4B** shows an action potential in node A and the depolarization it produces at nodes B (30 mV), C (15 mV), and D (8 mV). Hence, an action potential will be triggered in nodes B and C, but not in node D.

The ratio of membrane depolarization that actually occurs at a node to the membrane depolarization required for triggering an action potential is called the *safety factor of nerve conduction*.

$$\text{Safety factor} = \frac{\text{Membrane depolarization ocurring at a node}}{\text{Depolarization required for triggering action potential}} \qquad (9.3)$$

Conduction across a node occurs only if the safety factor is > 1. If the safety factor is < 1, conduction failure occurs. The higher the safety factor, the more certain (or safe) is the conduction of a nerve impulse across a node. In the given example, the safety factors in nodes B, C, and D are 2.0, 1.0, and 0.5, respectively.

Factors Causing Conduction Failure

There are several factors that block nerve conduction. Some of these are implicated in diseases of nerve conduction, whereas

Table 9.1 Susceptibility of Fibers of Different Diameters (A, B, C; see Table 9.2) to Local Anesthetics, Pressure, and Hypoxia

Susceptibility to	Most Susceptible	Less Susceptible	Least Susceptible
Local anesthetics	C	B	A
Pressure	A	B	C
Hypoxia	B	A	C

Table 9.2 Classification of Nerve Fibers Based on Their Diameter and Conduction Velocity

	Function	Fiber Diameter (μ)	Conduction Velocity* (m/s)	Spike Duration (ms)
Aα	Somatic motor proprioception	12–20	100	0.5
Aβ	Touch, pressure	5–12	60	0.5
Aγ	Fusimotor	3–6	40	0.5
Aδ	Pain, temperature crude touch	2–5	20	0.5
B	Preganglionic autonomic (thinly myelinated)	< 2	10	1.0
C	Postganglionic autonomic, pain, temperature (all are unmyelinated)	< 1	2	2.0

*Range: ± 20%.

others have been employed therapeutically as anesthetics. Nerve fibers of different diameters differ in their susceptibility to conduction block by different factors (**Table 9.1**). The classification of nerve fibers into types A, B, and C based on their diameters is given in **Table 9.2**.

Local anesthetics bind to Na+ channels and block them. Blockade of Na+ channels abolishes the action potentials. Myelinated axons have a high density of Na+ channels at the nodes (**Table 9.3**). At therapeutic concentrations, local anesthetics are unable to block all the Na+ channels in a node; hence, myelinated nerves are relatively less sensitive to local anesthetics. Unmyelinated axons, on the other hand, have a much lower density of Na+ channels and are therefore much more susceptible to local anesthetics.

Pressure compresses axons, reducing the axonal diameter with a consequent increase in the axoplasmic resistance. Pressure on the axons therefore impairs electrotonic conduction. The effect of pressure on nerve conduction explains neuropraxia (the temporary failure of nerve function or conduction due to pressure or structural damage of the affected cell). Large, myelinated neurons (type A), which rely heavily on the efficient electrotonic conduction through axoplasm, are the worst

Table 9.3 Channel Density in Different Parts of the Neuron

Site	Channels/μ³
Soma	50–75
Initial segment	250–500
Myelinated segment of axon	< 25
Node of Ranvier	2000–12,000
Unmyelinated axon	100
Axon terminal	25–75

affected by pressure, followed by the smaller neurons (types B and C).

Hypoxia | Smaller cells require less oxygen. Hence, the smallest C fibers are least susceptible to hypoxic damage. However, the largest A neurons are not very susceptible to hypoxia. Hypoxia reduces the activity of the Na$^+$–K$^+$ ATPase, which is required for restoring the intracellular ionic concentrations after a neuron has conducted several action potentials. This restorative oxygen requirement is low in large myelinated neurons where action potentials are generated only at the nodes. It turns out to be, therefore, that the B fibers are the most susceptible to hypoxia, followed by A and C fibers.

Demyelination | A demyelinated axon (as is present in many different neurologic conditions) is not the same as an unmyelinated axon. Like the unmyelinated axon, the demyelinated axon has poor electrotonic conduction. However, unlike the unmyelinated axon, the demyelinated axon does not have a sufficient number of sodium channels on its internodal segment and is therefore incapable of generating closely spaced action potentials for ensuring safe propagation of impulses. Thus, in a demy-

elinated neuron, an action potential often fails to get electrotonically conducted from one node to the next. In short, the safety factor of nerve conduction in a demyelinated axon is low.

A rise in temperature, as occurs in fever, predisposes to conduction failure in a demyelinated axon. The rise in temperature decreases both the duration of the spike and its amplitude (see **Fig. 7.2**). The decrease in spike duration speeds up conduction, but the reduction in spike amplitude reduces the safety factor of conduction. In a normal axon, the safety factor is quite high. Therefore, the reduction in safety factor does not cause conduction failure; rather, the conduction becomes faster due to the shorter duration of the action potential. In a demyelinated axon, the safety factor is very low, and any further reduction causes conduction failure.

Ephaptic Conduction

Ephapse means "false synapse," and it refers to nerve-to-nerve interactions that occur due to electrical coupling between adjacent neurons or axons. Ephaptic conduction is unusual in

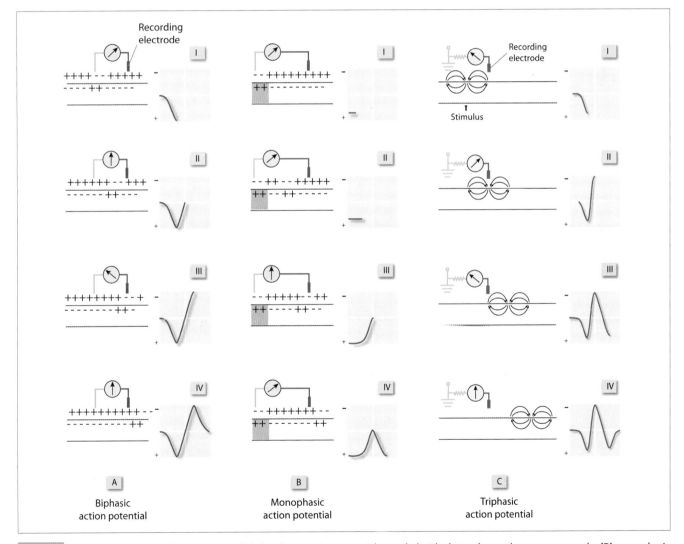

Fig. 9.5 Extracellularly recorded action potential. **(A)** Biphasic action potential recorded with electrodes on the nerve or muscle, **(B)** monophasic action potential recorded when one electrode is placed on a crushed region of the tissue, **(C)** triphasic action potential recorded with electrodes in the extracellular fluid, not on the tissue.

the normal nervous system, although there are some data to suggest that electrical coupling occurs in damaged nervous systems.

Ephaptic interaction, however, is the rule between cardiac muscle cells and single-unit smooth muscle cells, which have gap junctions between adjacent cells. For electrical excitation to spread from one cell to another, the local current must be able to complete its circuit through the adjacent cell. This requires a low-resistance bridge that would permit the inner longitudinal current to flow easily from one neuron to another. Such low-resistance bridges are provided by gap junctions (also called *electrical synapses*) between adjacent neurons.

General Model: Communications

Electrical coupling between cells provides another mechanism by which information can spread through a tissue or organ. Because electrical signals propagate with a high velocity, they make possible the coordinated response of a large number of cells.

Conduction of the Action Potential in Muscle Cells

Conduction of the action potential in muscle cells occurs by the same mechanism as was described for unmyelinated axons. Although the velocity of conduction is lower in muscle cells than in myelinated axons, it is fast enough to ensure that all parts of the muscle cell contract at the same time (see Chapter 14).

Electroneurography

Measurement of Nerve Conduction Velocity

Compound action potential | A peripheral nerve is made of many axons with different conduction velocities. When a nerve trunk is excited with a large enough stimulus, all the axons in it get excited. A monophasic record obtained from the nerve surface some distance away (an extracellular recording) shows multiple peaks, each peak corresponding to the action potentials of a group of axons having similar conduction velocities **(Fig. 9.5)**. The record so obtained is called the *compound action potential* **(Fig. 9.6)**.

Suppose the time interval between the stimulus and the appearance of the first peak (i.e., Aα) is t_1. If the distance between the stimulating and recording electrodes is d_1, the conduction velocity (V_1) of the nerve fiber represented by that peak (i.e., Aα) is given by the formula

$$V_1 = d_1 / t_1 \qquad (9.4)$$

Similarly, the conduction velocity (V_2) of Aβ; will be d_2/t_2, and so on. Conduction velocities in infants are roughly half of the adult values, reaching the adult range by 5 to 8 years. They decline by 1 m/sec per decade between 20 and 55 years and thereafter, at the rate of 3 m/sec per decade. Nerve fibers

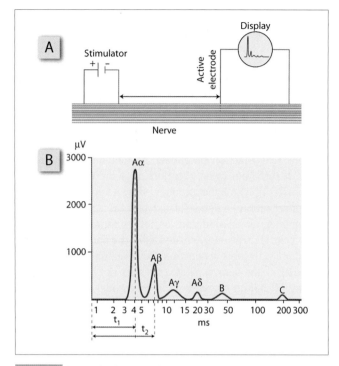

Fig. 9.6 **(A)** Method of recording a compound action potential. **(B)** A compound action potential in a mixed nerve. The sequence of peaks proceeding from left to right reflects a spectrum of axon diameters (and myelination) and hence conduction velocities CRO.

have been classified on the basis of their conduction velocities **(Table 9.2)**.

Electromyography

Electromyography (EMG) is the recording of the electrical activity of the muscle using surface electrodes placed on the muscle or, more commonly, needle electrodes inserted into the muscle. The needle electrode consists of a pointed steel cannula through which runs a fine silver, steel, or platinum wire that is insulated except at its tip. The potential difference between the outer cannula and inner wire is recorded, and the patient is grounded by a separate surface electrode. The ground lead is attached to the same limb as the muscle to be examined.

The standard protocol for EMG recording is as follows. (1) The electrode is inserted into the muscle while it is relaxed, and the *insertion activity* is noted. (2) The muscle is then explored systematically with the electrode for the presence of any spontaneous activity. Normally, there is no spontaneous activity. (3) Thereafter, the subject is asked to contract the muscles voluntarily, and the motor unit potentials are recorded from different sites on the muscle at different grades of contraction. (4) Finally, the subject is asked to contract the muscle maximally (against resistance), and the interference pattern is recorded.

Summary

- The action potential propagates by electrotonic spread of current and the regeneration of the action potential at every piece of membrane that is depolarized to threshold. One result is that the amplitude of the action potential is the same everywhere on an excitable cell.

- The velocity of conduction is determined by the diameter of the axon (or muscle cell) and the presence of myelin.

- The compound action potential is a surface recording of the electrical activity in a tissue (nerve or muscle).

Applying What You Know

9.1. I Ms. Adams' nerve conduction velocities are normal. What does this finding tell you about possible causes of her problem? Explain.

9.2. The EMG studies of Ms. Adams' deltoid muscle showed a marked decrease in the amplitude of the response on repetitive stimulation. What does this tell you about the muscle action potential? Explain.

Action potentials can be elicited by direct electrical stimulation of a neuron or muscle cell. As will be discussed in Chapter 11, one neuron generating an action potential can elicit an action potential in another electrically excitable cell by chemical transmission. How, under normal circumstances, are action potentials *initiated* in the body?

One answer to this question is that sensory receptors (see below) monitoring the external and the internal environments generate electrical signals that give rise to action potentials that are then conducted to the nervous system, where they give rise to a variety of responses.

Sensory Transduction

The term *receptor* refers to two different kinds of structures in the body, and it is important that they not be confused. A *sensory receptor* is a modified neuron or nerve endings that encodes information and conveys it to the nervous system. A *ligand-binding receptor* is a large molecule present on the cell membrane or inside the cell that binds a certain specific molecule and thus initiates a cascade of biochemical reactions.

A sensory receptor responds only to a specific stimulus, which is called the *adequate stimulus*, and most sensory receptors have only one adequate stimulus (**Fig. 10.1**). Stimuli other than the adequate stimulus usually do not stimulate the receptor. However, if a stimulus is strong enough, it can cause several kinds of sensory receptors to respond. For example, photoreceptors respond to a blow to the head or the eye, producing a perceptible flash of light called a *phosphene.*

There are two broad classes of sensory receptors. Exteroreceptors respond to stimuli from the external world, such as light, heat, sound, and touch. The special senses (sight, hearing, taste, smell, etc.) provide us with information about the external environment. Interoreceptors respond to stimuli generated within the body, and these visceral sensory systems enable the body to maintain a state of homeostatic balance. We will be focusing exclusively on such visceral afferent systems.

Generator Potential

On application of the adequate stimulus, the receptor membrane, typically depolarizes (although there are a few receptors that hyperpolarize). The magnitude of the depolarization is proportional to the strength of the stimulus and is usually several millivolts (**Fig. 10.2**). This potential is known as the *generator potential.* The generator potential is a local potential that does not actively propagate but can trigger an action potential in another part of the receptor cell or in the neuron that innervates the receptor cell if it (the generator potential) is large enough.

Mechanoreceptors are stimulated when their membrane is deformed by pressure or is stretched, opening up the stretch-sensitive cation channels present on the membrane; one particular type of mechanoreceptor is the *baroreceptor*, which responds to changes in pressure. In *thermoreceptors,* the Na^+–K^+ pump activity is highly sensitive to temperature changes. A fall in the temperature of a *cold receptor* is associated with reduced Na^+–K^+ ATPase activity, with resultant depolarization of the membrane. A rise in the temperature of a *warm receptor*, on the other hand, activates temperature-sensitive Na^+ channels, resulting in membrane depolarization. *Chemoreceptors*, which respond to certain molecules ("chemicals"), and *photoreceptors* (which respond to quanta of light) are coupled to G proteins and initiate an intracellular cascade of reactions. *Nociceptors* (that signal pain) contain in their membrane certain proteins that convert thermal, mechanical, or chemical energy into a depolarizing potential. One such protein is the capsaicin or vanilloid receptor.

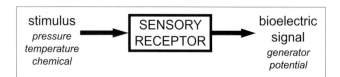

Fig. 10.1   Sensory receptors are specialized neurons that convert some stimulus (pressure, temperature, the presence of some molecule) into a bioelectric signal, the generator potential. Receptors are most sensitive to some particular stimulus (often referred to as the adequate stimulus), although many of them can respond to any stimulus if it is large enough.

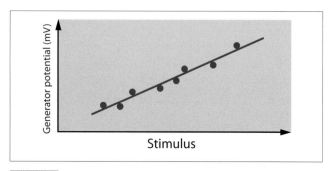

Fig. 10.2   Sensory receptors most commonly depolarize when stimulated, giving rise to a generator potential. The amplitude of the generator potential is proportional to the amplitude of the stimulus.

Table 10.1 Sensory Receptors Monitoring the Internal Environment

Stimulus	Sensory Receptor Type	What Is Being Measured
Mechanical pressure	Baroreceptors	Blood pressure (see Chapter 38)
Volume	Volume receptors	Atrial volume (see Chapter 38)
Length	Stretch receptors	Airway size (see Chapter 49)
Temperature	Thermoreceptors	Hypothalamic temperature (see Chapter 43)
		Skin temperature (see Chapter 43)
Osmotic pressure	Osmoreceptors	Body fluid osmolarity (see Chapter 57)
Chemicals	Chemoreceptors	Partial pressure of oxygen (see Chapter 50) Partial pressure of carbon dioxide (see Chapter 50)

The generator potential spreads electrotonically and thus decrements quickly with distance. However, if the generator potential reaches a region of the receptor cell with normal electrical excitability, an action potential will be generated.

Coding the Information in the Stimulus

Action potentials are all-or-none phenomena, and coding of information about the stimulus cannot occur by varying the amplitude of the action potential. There are three questions that must be asked about the stimulus and must be coded somehow by the receptor: (1) What is the adequate stimulus? (2) Where is the adequate stimulus impinging on the body? and (3) How strong is the stimulus?

Coding the Nature of the Stimulus
Sensory receptors respond to one particular form of stimulus. Each receptor is connected to a neural pathway that connects to neural circuitry in a particular place in the nervous system. Thus, an action potential pulse train reaching the visual cortex is responded to as signaling a visual stimulus, even if the initial excitation of the receptors was the result of mechanical energy affecting the receptors. Thus, it is the specificity of the wiring of the nervous system that identifies the stimulus. The sensory pathway is thus referred to as a *labeled line*.

Coding the Location of the Stimulus
Some receptors are located on a surface structure (the skin, the retina of the eye), and the location of a stimulus on this surface is a vitally important piece of information. Here, too, the wiring of the nervous system provides a specification of

the receptors being stimulated. The location of a stimulus applied to the right thumb is signaled by the particular neural pathway that is activated.

In the same way, receptors located in the visceral organs are wired into particular neural pathways. Thus, the carotid baroreceptors (which signal the blood pressure present in the carotid sinus) send a neural signal to the medullary cardiovascular control center, and neural activity along that pathway is processed as coming from that location.

Thus, the location of a stimulus is coded by the particular labeled line that carries the neural signals from the receptor to the central nervous system.

Coding of Stimulus Intensity
There are two different ways in which the intensity of the stimulus is coded: frequency coding and population coding. Both coding schemes are in use at all times.

In *frequency coding,* the frequency of the action potentials generated is proportional to the magnitude of the generator potential, which, in turn, is proportional to the magnitude of the stimulus affecting the receptor (**Fig. 10.3**). Some receptors also signal the rate of change of the stimulus magnitude, so that the same stimulus magnitude yields a different firing frequency depending on whether the stimulus at that moment is increasing or decreasing.

In *population coding,* the strength of a stimulus also determines the number of sensory receptors stimulated. A strong stimulus stimulates multiple receptors, whereas a threshold stimulus might excite only a single receptor. Sensory receptors with the lowest thresholds are recruited first. The number of sensory units stimulated provides the brain with information about the stimulus strength.

Receptor Adaptation
When a steady stimulus is applied to a receptor, the frequency of the action potentials generated may decline gradually (**Fig. 10.4**). This gradual decline in receptor response to a stimulus is called *receptor adaptation*, and it explains why many stimuli, when present continuously, tend to be perceived with decreasing intensity. Some receptors, notably nociceptors, vestibular receptors, and muscle spindle, do not show adaptation.

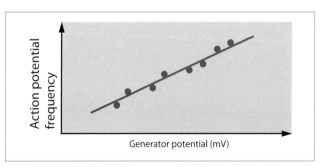

Fig. 10.3 If the generator potential depolarizes the electrically excitable membrane to threshold the receptor will fire an action potential. The larger the generator potential, the faster the frequency of firing action potentials.

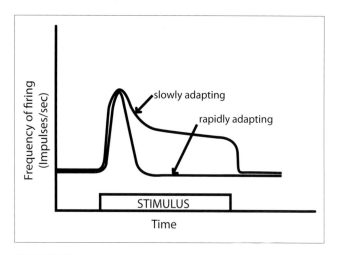

Fig. 10.4 Rapidly and slowly adapting sensory receptors. With a maintained stimulus, the response of the receptor (its frequency of firing) decreases, possibly to zero (it stops firing).

Adaptation may be slow or rapid. *Slow adaptation* is brought about by the inactivation of Na^+ and calcium (Ca^{2+}) channels or through the activation of Ca^+-dependent K^+ channels. In either case, the alteration in membrane potential makes it more difficult for action potentials to be generated. *Rapid adaptation* occurs when, as in the case of the Pacinian corpuscle (a kind of touch receptor in the skin), the receptor structure filters out the steady component. When pressure is applied to a Pacinian corpuscle, it initially causes deformation of all its concentric layers and deforms the nerve ending in its core. However, the inner layers slowly regain their original position, relieving the pressure on the nerve ending, although the outer layers remain deformed.

Summary

- Transduction is the conversion of a physical or chemical stimulus into an electrical signal that can give rise to a train of action potentials.

- Because the action potential is an all-or-none phenomenon, the magnitude of a stimulus can only be coded by the frequency of firing of the sensory pathway.

- In many sensory systems, maintained stimulation of a receptor causes a decrease in the magnitude of the response, a phenomenon called *adaptation*.

Applying What You Know

10.1. Conduction in Ms. Adams' sensory nerves in the ulnar nerve appears to be normal when stimulated electrically. Can you conclude that the function of the related sensory receptors is also normal? Explain.

An action potential does not get conducted from one cell to another unless there are low resistance electrical pathways connecting the two cells. Although gap junctions do occur between cardiac muscle cells and some smooth muscle cells (see Chapters 18 and 19), they are not present in skeletal muscle or in neurons. Thus, special mechanisms are required for the impulse to travel from one neuron to another (synaptic transmission) or from a neuron to a skeletal muscle cell (neuromuscular transmission). The mechanisms of synaptic transmission and neuromuscular transmission are quite similar, although transmission at the neuromuscular junction is somewhat simpler. The structure of the neuromuscular junction is illustrated in Fig. 13.8.

Neuromuscular Transmission

The steps of neuromuscular transmission (**Fig. 11.1A**) can be summed up as follows: (1) An action potential is conducted down the motor axon to the prejunctional axon terminal. (2) Depolarization of the terminal buttons opens up voltage-gated calcium (Ca^{2+}) channels in its membrane. Ca^{2+} moves into the terminal along an electrochemical gradient. (3) Elevated Ca^{2+}

concentration in the terminal button causes exocytosis of synaptic vesicles filled with the transmitter acetylcholine (ACh) into the myoneural cleft. (4) The ACh released from synaptic vesicles diffuses across the myoneural cleft and binds to specific acetylcholine receptors on the motor end plate. (5) The binding of ACh to the ACh receptor increases the conductance of the postjunctional membrane to Na^+ and K^+, resulting in a transient depolarization of the postjunctional membrane. This depolarization is called the *end-plate potential* (EPP). (6) The EPP is transient because acetylcholine is quickly hydrolyzed by the enzyme acetylcholinesterase (AChE) into choline and acetate. AChE is present in high concentration in the junctional cleft. (7) The postjunctional membrane cannot generate action potentials. However, the EPP depolarizes the adjacent muscle membrane by electrotonic conduction. When the depolarization exceeds the threshold, an action potential is triggered in the adjacent muscle membrane.

General Model: Communications

The chemical transmission mechanism employed at the neuromuscular junction and synapse is one example of how cells communicate with one another. It has some important similarities to one of the mechanisms used by the endocrine system to communicate with distant target cells; a specific chemical substance (a transmitter or hormone) binds to a specific membrane receptor, initiating a response in the cell. The intracellular signaling pathways used in neural pathways are essentially the same as those used in endocrine mechanisms.

Acetylcholine as a Neurotransmitter
Synthesis of acetylcholine | ACh is synthesized in the cytosol of the motor nerve terminal in the presence of the enzyme choline O-acetyltransferase.

$$Acetyl\text{-}CoA + Choline \xrightarrow{\text{Choline O-acetyltransferase}} Acetylcholine + CoA$$

Neurons cannot synthesize choline, which is obtained from the diet. Significant amounts of choline are taken up from the junctional cleft into the nerve terminal through Na^+-coupled secondary-active transport. After synthesis, ACh is incorporated into the synaptic vesicles. Empty synaptic vesicles originate in the soma and are transported distally by axoplasmic flow. Some are formed in the axon, and some are formed in the terminal button itself.

Release of acetylcholine | ACh is released into the myoneural cleft by exocytosis of synaptic vesicles. The exocytosis is triggered by the rise of Ca^{2+} in the terminal button. The release of acetylcholine occurs in quanta or packets. Each quantum corresponds to the content of one synaptic vesicle—10,000 molecules of ACh.

Inactivation of acetylcholine | ACh diffuses from its site of release by diffusion. More importantly, it is hydrolyzed into

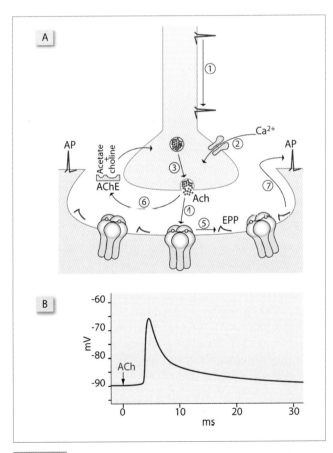

Fig. 11.1 **(A)** Major steps in neuromuscular transmission (see text for details). **(B)** An end-plate potential (EPP with an amplitude—a depolarization—of 25 mV).

acetate and choline by the enzyme AChE present in the basal lamina. Choline is taken up from the synaptic cleft and reused for the synthesis of acetylcholine.

Acetylcholine receptors | ACh has to diffuse 1 µm to reach the end plate, which it does in less than a millisecond. ACh binds to ACh receptors located on the ACh-gated cation channels present on the postjunctional membrane. The binding is short lasting because as the ACh concentration in the cleft falls, ACh quickly dissociates from its receptor, in accordance with the laws of chemical kinetics. Unbound ACh is enzymatically degraded by acetylcholinesterase. Formation of an ACh-receptor complex opens up the channels to both Na^+ and K^+, and as a result, the postjunctional membrane gets depolarized. According to the Goldman equation, the membrane potential (V_m) is given by

$$V_m = 61 \log \frac{P_K[K_0] + P_{Na}[Na_0] + P_{Cl}[Cl_i]}{P_K[K_i] + P_{Na}[Na_i] + P_{Cl}[Cl_0]} \quad (11.1)$$

Assuming $P_K = P_{Na}$, and ignoring P_{Cl} (because both P_K and P_{Na} increase markedly in comparison to P_{Cl}), the above formula reduces to

$$V_m = 61 \log \frac{[K_0] + [Na_0]}{[K_i] + [Na_i]} \quad (11.2)$$

Or (see **Table 6.2** for the concentrations of the ions involved)

$$V_m = 61 \log \frac{5 + 140}{150 + 10} \quad (11.3)$$

$$= -2.6 \text{ mV}$$

Thus, the simultaneous increase in Na^+ and K^+ permeability drives the membrane potential toward 0 mV. However, the presence of ACh in the cleft is normally extremely short-lived. Hence, the ligand-gated cation channels remain open for a very short time, permitting only a very small local depolarization (0.5 mV) of the membrane. Larger depolarization is possible if ACh remains attached to the channels for longer durations. This knowledge is used in the treatment of myasthenia gravis (see below) in which the channels are kept open for longer periods.

Postjunctional Potentials

Miniature end-plate potential (MEPP) | Each quantum of ACh released into the synaptic cleft produces a small depolarization called a *miniature end-plate potential* (MEPP), which is 0.5 mV in amplitude and not large enough to trigger an action potential in the adjacent muscle plasma membrane. MEPPs occur spontaneously even when the neuron is not stimulated, with an average frequency of ~1/sec. Such sporadic MEPPs have no physiologic effect. A large number of MEPPs must be produced synchronously to bring about a substantial change in the potential of the motor end plate.

End-plate potential (EPP) | Each action potential reaching the axonal ending results in the release of ~60 vesicles or quanta of ACh, with each quantum containing 10,000 ACh molecules. The 600,000 ACh molecules (more than enough despite the simultaneous degradation of ACH by AChE in the myoneural cleft) bind to 300,000 ACh receptors (2 ACh molecules must bind to a receptor for it to open) and produce 300,000 MEPPs, each having an amplitude of 0.5 mV. These MEPPs summate spatially, taking the membrane potential from –90 mV to –65 mV (**Fig. 11.1B**). This 25 mV change in membrane potential is called the *end-plate potential* (EPP). The EPP gets conducted electrotonically from the end plate to the adjacent muscle fiber membrane, which then gets depolarized to its firing level and generates an action potential. No action potential is generated in the end plate itself.

Only 6 quanta of ACh are necessary for the transmission of the action potential across the neuromuscular junction, but as many as 60 are released. This provides a 10-fold safety factor for neuromuscular transmission. As a result, transmission at the neuromuscular junction is said to be one-to-one; one action potential in the motor nerve innervating a muscle cell causes one action potential in the muscle cell.

Drugs Affecting Neuromuscular Transmission

Drugs Affecting Acetylcholine Release

Aminopyridines increase the duration of the action potential in the nerve terminal, probably by blocking the voltage-gated K^+ channels on the nerve terminals. Prolongation of action potential results in greater Ca^{2+} influx and release of more quanta of ACh. These drugs have found some limited use in treating Lambert-Eaton myasthenic syndrome (see below).

Botulinum toxin produces muscular paralysis by inhibiting the exocytosis of synaptic vesicles. Although best known for causing food poisoning, in recent years botulinum toxin (Botox) has found therapeutic use as a long-acting muscle relaxant whose effect lasts 3 to 4 months. Botox has been used in the treatment of squint, facial wrinkles, achalasia (to relax the lower esophageal sphincter), anal fissure (to relax the anal sphincter), and skeletal deformities that occur due to muscle spasm.

Alpha-latrotoxin is the toxin of the black widow spider *Lactrodectus mactans*. It binds to receptors on the presynaptic membrane. The binding results in massive Ca^{2+} influx into the presynaptic terminal with consequent release of large amounts of ACh, leading to muscle spasm. The spider is commonly found in North America, where it causes the greatest number of deaths from arthropod bites.

Hemicholiniums are drugs that block the choline transport system and inhibit choline uptake. Prolonged treatment with hemicholiniums depletes the neuronal store of transmitter and ultimately decreases the ACh content of the quanta.

Drugs Inhibiting Acetylcholinesterase

Anticholinesterases (anti-ChE) are drugs that bind to AChE, thereby preventing it from hydrolyzing ACh (**Fig. 11.2A**). The AChE is freed only after it hydrolyzes the anti-ChE bound to it.

By inactivating AChE, anti-ChE drugs permit large amounts of ACh to accumulate in the myoneural cleft. As a result, the EPP is larger (more depolarization) and dramatically prolonged. The initial response is a depolarization that results in persistent muscle contraction (spasm). However, after a few seconds, the motor end plate becomes inexcitable due to channel desensitization. Channel desensitization is not the same as channel inactivation. Desensitization occurs in a ligand-gated channel when the ligand remains attached to the channel receptor for several milliseconds. The molecular mechanism of channel desensitization is not well understood. Anti-ChE drugs are of two types: reversible and irreversible.

Reversible inhibitors | Reversible anti-ChE drugs such as neostigmine are readily hydrolyzed by AChE. Therefore, in a few hours, the AChE becomes available once again for inactivating ACh. Reversible inhibitors are used in the treatment of myasthenia gravis and in curare poisoning.

Irreversible inhibitors | Organophosphate compounds such as malathion and Baygon (S.C. Johnson & Son, Racine, WI) (insecticides), diisopropyl phosphofluoridate (DFP, Dyflos), and nerve gas used in chemical warfare are poorly hydrolyzed by AChE and remain attached to the AChE molecule for several weeks. AChE is therefore unable to bind and hydrolyze ACh. The persistence of ACh in the myoneural cleft causes desensitization of the channels in the motor end plate. Hence, irreversible anti-ChE produces deadly paralysis.

Drugs Blocking Acetylcholine Receptors

Drugs that bind to acetylcholine receptors are of two types: those that do not have any intrinsic activity (nondepolarizing blocker) and those that mimic the action of acetylcholine (depolarizing blocker). Drugs that have an affinity for acetylcholine receptors but do not have any intrinsic activity produce nondepolarizing neuromuscular block. They do not depolarize the end plate, but keep the ACh receptors blocked so that ACh is unable to bind to them. Drugs that mimic the action of acetylcholine produce depolarizing neuromuscular blocker.

Nondepolarizing neuromuscular blocker | An example of a nondepolarizing neuromuscular blocker is d-tubocurarine. It has no effect of its own, but by binding to the ACh receptor, it prevents ACh from producing neuromuscular transmission. This results in muscle paralysis that can be fatal due to the paralysis of respiratory muscles. An ACh receptor will bind more of the agonist that is present in the highest concentration. If the concentration of ACh in the cleft is increased by administering anti-AChE, the ACh molecules are able to dislodge d-tubocurarine from the ACh receptors, making them functional again. Hence, the neuromuscular block produced by tubocurare is said to be reversible. d-Tubocurarine is obtained from curare, a toxin extracted from certain plants, which was used on poison arrows by South American natives to paralyze their prey. α-Bungarotoxin found in the venom of the krait also produces nondepolarizing blocker.

Depolarizing neuromuscular blocker | An example of a depolarizing neuromuscular blocker is succinylcholine. It is poorly inactivated by AChE; therefore, its action is much more prolonged than that of ACh. It binds to ACh receptors in the motor end plate and causes muscle spasm when administered in a moderate dosage. In a high dosage, however, it induces desensitization of the ACh-gated channels with consequent paralysis. It is commonly used as a muscle relaxant during abdominal surgery (to provide the surgeon with easier access into the viscera). The block produced by succinylcholine is called irreversible because even if the succinylcholine molecules are dislodged from the ACh receptors, the channels remain desensitized for a longer period.

Diseases of Neuromuscular Transmission

Myasthenia gravis is characterized by severe skeletal muscular weakness and rapid onset of fatigue. It is associated with the destruction of ACh receptors on the motor end plate. Fewer ACh receptors result in fewer MEPPs and smaller EPP.

Myasthenia gravis is caused by autoantibodies to ACh receptors on the motor end plate. The antibodies block the ACh-receptors so that ACh cannot bind to them. The antibodies also cross-link the ACh-receptors, triggering their removal by endocytosis (**Fig. 11.2B**). Alternatively, it has been suggested that the disease is associated with benign tumor of the thymus (thymoma) and a hypersecretion of thymopoietin, which binds to the ACh receptors to inactivate them.

Neostigmine, an anti-ChE drug, produces striking symptomatic improvement, each dose acting for several hours. When AChE is administered, ACh persists in the myoneural cleft for a longer period, resulting in larger MEPPs that add up to produce an EPP large enough to trigger an action potential. It is so because the presence of ACh in the cleft is normally extremely short-lived. Hence, the ligand-gated cation channels remain open for a very short time, permitting a very small MEPP. Larger MEPPs are possible if ACh remains attached to the channels for longer duration. If the channels are reduced in number, a larger MEPP at every channel can compensate to produce a normal end-plate potential.

Treatment also includes suppression of autoimmunity by immunosuppressants, thymectomy, and plasmapheresis.

In **Lambert-Eaton myasthenic syndrome (LEMS)**, autoantibodies damage the voltage-gated Ca^{2+} channels present in the nerve endings at the neuromuscular junction (**Fig. 11.2B**). This decreases the Ca^{2+} influx that causes acetylcholine release during neuromuscular transmission and results in muscle weakness. Symptoms of LEMS are alleviated with continued muscular activity due to the progressive accumulation of Ca^{2+} in the terminal buttons, with consequent improvement of ACh release from the nerve ending. This is in contrast to the symptoms of myasthenia gravis, which get aggravated with continued muscular activity due to the progressive reduction of ACh release from the nerve endings.

Transmission at the Synapse

A synapse is the site where the information carried by a train of action potentials travels across the 20 to 40 nm-wide gap (called the *synaptic cleft*) separating one neuron (the presynaptic neuron) from another (the postsynaptic neuron). Most commonly, the axon terminal forms the presynaptic element

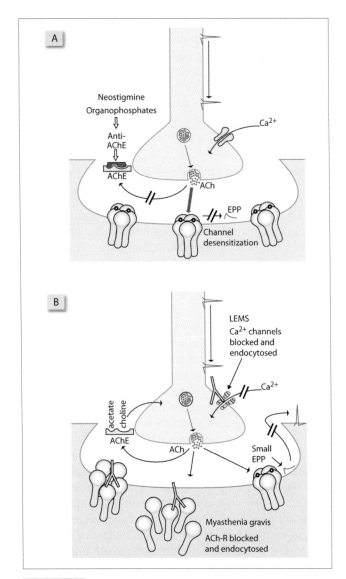

Fig. 11.2 **(A)** Effect of anti-acetylcholinesterase (AChE) drugs. **(B)** Pathophysiology of myasthenia gravis and Lambert-Eaton myasthenic syndrome (LEMS). Antibody binding to the acetylcholine receptor blocks their ability to respond to acetylcholine (ACh). ACh-R, receptor; EPP, end-plate potential.

present in the synaptic vesicles are released into the synaptic cleft. (5) The neurotransmitter binds to ionic channels present on the postsynaptic neuron. (6) The binding of neurotransmitter to the ion channels opens up the channel, allowing ions to flow across the postsynaptic membrane. If the ionic current is a depolarizing current, the postsynaptic neuron depolarizes, triggering an action potential in it (if the membrane potential reaches threshold) and thereby completing the process of synaptic transmission. (8) The neurotransmitter released is cleared from the synaptic cleft quickly through reuptake into the presynaptic terminal or nearby glial cells (the most common mechanism), rapid enzymatic degradation, or quick diffusion away from the synaptic cleft. The neurotransmitter glutamate has its own specific transporter for reuptake, whereas other small-molecule transmitters share a common transporter.

The process of synaptic transmission involves several steps; therefore, it takes ~0.5 msec to cross the 20 nm-wide synaptic cleft. In comparison, an impulse traveling the same distance along an uninterrupted nerve membrane takes only 0.2 to 40 nsec. Synaptic transmission is thus a much slower process than nerve conduction, and the time taken to cross the synapse is called the *synaptic delay*. The greater the number of synapses in a neural path, the slower is the speed with which an impulse travels along it. Thus, the conduction velocity along a pathway provides an estimate of the number of synapses in the path.

Differences between the Neuromuscular Function and Synapses

Although the basic steps involved in synaptic transmission are identical to those that occur at the neuromuscular junction, there are several important differences. (1) Transmission at the synapse is never one-to-one, and spatial and temporal summation is required to generate a postsynaptic action potential. (2) Although the EPP is always excitatory, postsynaptic potentials can be either excitatory or inhibitory. (3) Transmission at the synapse can be modulated by mechanisms that alter the release of transmitter from the presynaptic neuron. (4) Although the only transmitter employed at the neuromuscular junction is ACh, there are a large number of different transmitters employed at synapses.

Postsynaptic Potentials

Excitatory postsynaptic potential (EPSP) | The binding of the neurotransmitter to receptors on the postsynaptic membrane triggers the opening of the ligand-gated Na^+ channels on the postsynaptic membrane. The resultant rise in the Na^+ conductance depolarizes the postsynaptic membrane. The depolarization thus produced is called the excitatory postsynaptic potential (EPSP) (**Fig. 11.3**). The magnitude of the EPSP is 8 mV. The depolarization starts with a latency of 0.5 msec, rises to its peak in 2.0 msec, then declines with a half-life of 4.0 msec.

Inhibitory Postsynaptic Potentials

The soma and dendrites of a neuron usually have synaptic connections with a large number of axon terminals. Not all of them produce an EPSP. Any number of them can produce an

of the synapse, and the dendrites form the postsynaptic element. Accordingly, the most common type of synapse is the axodendritic synapse, though axosomatic and axoaxonic synapses are also quite common. The transmission at the synapse is mediated by chemicals called neurotransmitters released from the presynaptic neuron terminal.

The sequence of events that occur at a synapse is essentially identical to those that occur at the neuromuscular junction. (1) An action potential arrives at the presynaptic nerve terminal and depolarizes the presynaptic membrane. (2) When the membrane depolarizes to –40 to –20 mV, the voltage-gated Ca^{2+} channels in the presynaptic terminal open up, resulting in an influx of free Ca^{2+} into the nerve terminal. (3) The rise in intracellular Ca^{2+} stimulates the exocytosis of synaptic vesicles from the presynaptic terminal. (4) The neurotransmitters

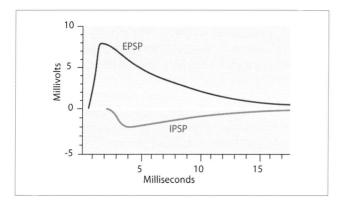

Fig. 11.3 Excitatory postsynaptic potential (EPSP) and inhibitory postsynaptic potential (IPSP).

inhibitory postsynaptic potential (IPSP). The IPSP is produced when the neurotransmitter increases the conductance of the postsynaptic membrane to K^+ ions, producing hyperpolarization of the membrane. Its magnitude is 2 mV. The hyperpolarization has a latency of 2 msec, attaining its maximum at 4 milliseconds, then returning to the resting potential with a half-life of 3 msec (**Fig. 11.3**).

Table 11.1 summarizes the differences between the EPSP and the IPSP.

Synaptic integration | The soma-dendritic tree acts as an integrator that summates all the EPSPs and IPSPs. Depending on the summated postsynaptic potential, synaptic transmission may or may not occur. Suppose there are five presynaptic neurons synapsing on one postsynaptic neuron. If two of the presynaptic neurons produce an EPSP (8 mV each), and the other three produce IPSPs (–2 mV each), the summated potential will be +10 mV, and synaptic transmission will occur. On the other hand, if only one of them produces an EPSP, and the other four produce IPSPs, then the summated potential will equal zero, and no synaptic transmission will occur.

The type of summation described above is called *spatial summation* because the postsynaptic potentials are "separated in space"; that is, they are produced simultaneously at different sites on the soma or dendrite of the postsynaptic neuron (**Fig. 11.4**). Another type of summation called *temporal summation* occurs when the postsynaptic potentials are "separated

Table 11.1 A Comparison of Excitatory Postsynaptic Potential (EPSP) and Inhibitory Postsynaptic Potential (IPSP)

EPSP	IPSP
Produced when excitatory neurotransmitters (e.g., glutamate) are released	Produced when inhibitory neurotransmitters (e.g., GABA and glycine) are released
Associated with the opening of ligand-gated Na^+ channels	Associated with the opening of ligand-gated K+ channels
Has a potential of +8 mV	Has a potential of –2 mV

Abbreviation: GABA, γ-aminobutyric acid.

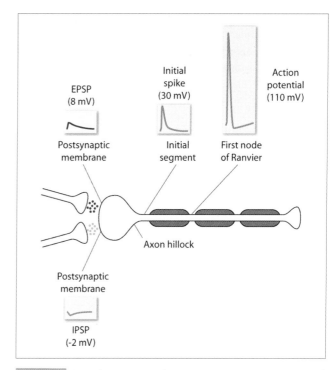

Fig. 11.4 Spatial summation of an excitatory postsynaptic potential (EPSP) and inhibitory postsynaptic potential (IPSP), and the generation of initial spike and action potential.

in time." For example, if an inhibitory presynaptic neuron fires off three action potentials in quick succession before the decay of the previous ones, each time producing an IPSP of –2 mV at the same site, then the summated potential will be about –6 mV.

Summation of postsynaptic potentials is made easier by the membrane characteristics of the dendrites: the EPSPs and IPSPs produced on the dendrites do not decay quickly, a property called the *holding capacity* of dendrites. Temporal summation is more complete when the time constant of the membrane is high. Spatial summation is more complete when the space constant of the membrane is high. (Time and space constants are explained in Chapter 9.) The holding capacity is greater in the axodendritic synapses on the dendritic spines. The thin neck of the spine prevents the high Ca^{2+} concentration in the spine (during synaptic transmission) from spreading to the main shaft, increasing the holding capacity of the dendrites.

Initial spike and action potential | If the summated postsynaptic potential is an excitatory potential, it depolarizes the *initial segment* (the axon hillock and the proximal unmyelinated part of the unmyelinated axon) by ~30 mV. This depolarization, which is called the *initial spike,* is more than adequate for triggering a fully fledged action potential at the first node of Ranvier. The initial segment has the lowest threshold of excitation as compared with the other parts of the soma because it has a higher density of voltage-dependent Na^+ channels.

The action potential triggered by the initial spike travels not only anterogradely along the axon, but also retrogradely to the soma and dendrites. This retrogradely conducted potential, although identical to the action potential, is called by a different name, the *soma-dendritic (SD) spike*. It serves to restore the soma and dendrites to the resting potential, allowing fresh summation of subsequently generated EPSPs and IPSPs. It is like making calculations on a slate, then wiping the slate clean for a fresh set of calculations.

Presynaptic Inhibition and Facilitation

The facilitatory neuron stimulates the release of excitatory neurotransmitters. The facilitatory neuron usually releases serotonin, which acts through serotonergic receptors to activate cyclic adenosine monophosphate (cAMP)–dependent phosphokinase A (as in group IIA hormones) and phosphokinase C (as in group IIC hormones). Together, phosphokinase A and phosphokinase C open up the L-type Ca^{2+} channels, thereby enhancing neurotransmitter release. Phosphokinase A additionally shuts down K^+ channels, resulting in prolongation of the depolarization, which keeps the Ca^{2+} channels open for a longer period.

In **presynaptic inhibition (Fig. 11.5)**, the inhibitory neuron releases γ-aminobutyric acid (GABA), which binds to $GABA_A$ or $GABA_B$ receptors on the presynaptic neuron terminals. Stimulation of the ionotropic $GABA_A$ receptors increases the membrane permeability to chloride (Cl^-) ions. Because the Nernst potential of Cl^- is close to the resting membrane potential, the rise in Cl^- permeability does not change the membrane potential. However, the high Cl^- conductance tends to stabilize the membrane potential near E_{Cl} (i.e., the membrane potential does not change easily), in accordance with the general rule that the membrane potential tends to stay near the Nernst potential of the highly permeable ion. Thus, when an action potential arrives at the presynaptic axon terminal, the depolarization of the presynaptic membrane is less than usual, and the presynaptic action potential is dwarfed. The smaller action potential is associated with the release of less neurotransmitter from the presynaptic axon terminal.

Stimulation of the metabotropic $GABA_B$ receptors increases the membrane permeability to K^+ ions and decreases the membrane permeability to Ca^{2+} ions. The rise in K^+ permeability hyperpolarizes the membrane, dwarfing the presynaptic action potentials and reducing Ca^{2+} influx. The reduction in Ca^{2+} permeability further reduces the Ca^{2+} influx and with it, the neurotransmitter release.

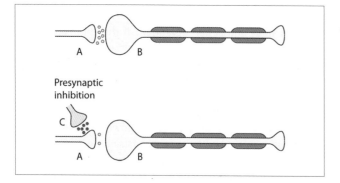

Presynaptic inhibition

Fig. 11.5 The mechanism of presynaptic inhibition involves reducing the release of excitatory transmitter from the presynaptic neuron.

Synaptic Transmitters

Chemical transmission at all neuromuscular junctions utilizes acetylcholine. At synapses, there are a large number of different transmitters employed. Some of these are excitatory (glutamate, ACh in same synapses, norepinephrine at some synapses), and others are inhibitory (GABA, glycine, ACh at some synapses, norepinephrine at some synapses).

For each of these transmitters, there is a synthetic pathway in the presynaptic neuron to make the transmitter. There are generally enzymes that are responsible for degrading the enzymes to terminate their action.

Summary

- Transmission from a motor neuron to a skeletal muscle occurs through the release of acetylcholine at the neuromuscular junction.

- Acetylcholine binds to receptors on the muscle membrane that open, allowing an inward Na^+ current, which depolarizes the muscle membrane (produces an end-plate potential); an action potential in the muscle membrane results.

- Transmission at the neuromuscular junction is normally one-to-one.

- Transmission from neuron to neuron occurs at a synapse. Transmitter is released by the presynaptic neuron and binds to receptors on the postsynaptic membrane. The receptor then opens, allowing an inward current that alters postsynaptic membrane potential.

- Transmission at the synapse is never one-to-one; spatial and temporal summation is always required.

- The postsynaptic potentials can be either depolarizing (the EPSP) or inhibitory (the IPSP).

Applying What You Know

11.1. Why did the improvement of Ms. Adams' symptoms following the administration of Tensilon last only a short time?

11.2. Failure of transmission at the neuromuscular junction can occur for many different reasons: (1) failure to release acetylcholine, (2) failure of acetylcholine to bind to the postjunctional receptor, or (3) failure of the muscle membrane to generate an action potential. Which data about Ms. Adams' signs and symptoms can be used to distinguish between these possibilities? Explain.

11.3. Mestinon is an anticholinesterase that allows ACh to occupy the ACh-receptor for a longer time. This results in a larger EPP, which increases the safety factor for transmission at the neuromuscular junction. What other manipulation of the system would improve Ms. Adams' symptoms? Explain.

The autonomic nervous system (ANS) is essentially a visceral *efferent* system that controls (excites or inhibits) the contraction of cardiac and smooth muscles, as well as certain secretory and metabolic processes. Visceral *afferents* are sometimes called autonomic afferents. However, many disagree and consider the ANS to be only an efferent system. In this chapter, we will consider the ANS to be strictly an efferent neural pathway.

The hypothalamus plays an important role in the regulation of autonomic activity and has been called the head ganglion of the ANS. Information from all regions of the central nervous system (CNS) reach the hypothalamus, and this can influence autonomic responses. Although it was earlier believed that the ANS is not under voluntary control, there is a growing body of evidence that individuals skilled in the arts of yoga, meditation, and relaxation can exert at least some voluntary control over their blood pressure and heart rate that are normally regulated by the ANS.

The ANS is made up of two components: the sympathetic and the parasympathetic (**Fig. 12.1** and **Table 12.1**). The two

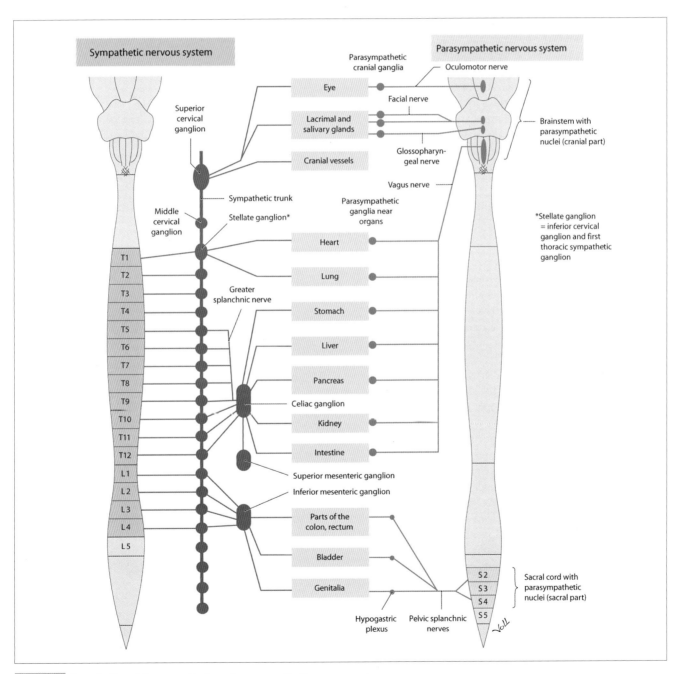

Fig. 12.1 Organization of the sympathetic and parasympathetic nervous system.

components have important similarities and differences in both anatomic and functional characteristics. *Anatomically,* the sympathetic fibers originate from the thoracic and lumbar segments of the spinal cord (the thoracolumbar outflow), whereas the parasympathetic fibers originate from the brainstem and the sacral segments of the spinal cord (the craniosacral outflow). *Functionally,* the sympathetic system is involved with controlling many individual catabolic processes (increasing the expenditure of energy) and can also be activated in "fight-or-flight" situations. The parasympathetic system is concerned with the vegetative aspects of day-to-day living and supports the anabolic processes of the body.

Although a motor nerve travels all the way from the spinal cord to the muscle it innervates, the autonomic pathway from the spinal cord to the target organ is made of two neurons that synapse in an autonomic ganglion. The neuron originating from the spinal cord is the preganglionic neuron; the one that reaches the target organ is the postganglionic neuron. In general, sympathetic ganglia are located close to the spinal cord, whereas parasympathetic ganglia are located close to the target organ. However, there are exceptions to this rule, as discussed below. It is important to stress here that no nerve is entirely made of autonomic fibers. The vagus nerve, which carries most of the parasympathetic fibers to the viscera, also carries sensory fibers and nerve fibers supplying skeletal muscles.

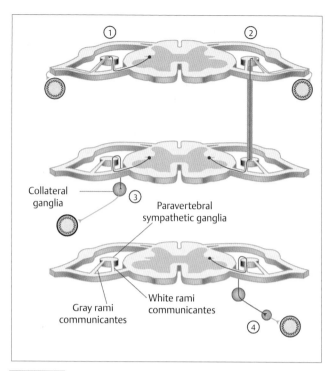

Fig. 12.2 Sympathetic preganglionic and postganglionic neurons. The preganglionic fiber may relay in (1) the segmental sympathetic ganglion, (2) the sympathetic ganglion of a higher or lower spinal segment, (3) a collateral ganglion, or (4) a ganglion near the target organ.

General Models: Communication and Homeostasis

The ANS is one of the information-processing systems of the body that make a major contribution to coordinating the activity of all of the organ systems. As a neural system, it transmits information from cell to cell using action potentials and synaptic transmission. The ANS plays a major role in controlling the visceral organs to maintain homeostasis.

Sympathetic Nervous System

Preganglionic sympathetic neurons originate from cells located in the intermediolateral horn of the thoracolumbar (T1–L3) spinal gray matter. The preganglionic fibers leave the spinal cord through its ventral root along with the somatic nerves (**Fig. 12.2**). However, they soon exit the ventral root through the *white rami communicantes* to enter the paravertebral sympathetic ganglion. The white ramus communicans is white because it is formed entirely of preganglionic sympathetic fibers that are thinly myelinated B fibers. Postganglionic neurons originating in the sympathetic chain leave the ganglion through the *gray rami communicantes* and reenter the ventral root to enter the spinal nerve. The gray ramus communicans is gray in color because the postganglionic sympathetic fibers are unmyelinated C fibers. Some fibers ascend or descend along the sympathetic trunk to a variable extent and make synapses with the cells of the upper or lower sympathetic ganglia.

Some preganglionic sympathetic fibers pass uninterrupted through the paravertebral sympathetic ganglia. They emerge from the paravertebral ganglia as splanchnic nerves and synapse in the collateral ganglia (e.g., celiac, otic, mesenteric).

Some preganglionic fibers pass uninterrupted even through the collateral ganglion to synapse in ganglia in or near the target organ (e.g., in the genital tract). The postganglionic neurons innervating these organs are very short. Finally, some preganglionic fibers synapse directly with the chromaffin cells of the adrenal medulla. The chromaffin cells secrete enipinephrine when stimulated.

Parasympathetic Nervous System

Preganglionic parasympathetic neurons are present in the craniosacral outflow from the CNS. Parasympathetic nerves are present in the *cranial nerves* (CNs) III, VII, IX, and X and originate in the nuclei of the corresponding CNs. *In the sacral part* of the spinal cord, the parasympathetic fibers originate in the intermediolateral gray horn of S1–S4 and pass out through the ventral spinal root of the corresponding nerves. In both cases, the parasympathetic preganglionic fibers travel all the way to the target organ and synapse with the cells of the postganglionic parasympathetic neurons present in the parasympathetic ganglia located near or in the organ.

Autonomic Neurotransmission

Postganglionic parasympathetic fibers release mostly acetylcholine (ACh) as their neurotransmitter. ACh has two types of receptors: muscarinic and nicotinic. Muscarinic receptors are found on target organs. They are blocked by atropine.

Postganglionic sympathetic fibers release mostly norepinephrine. However, there are exceptions to this general rule:

Table 12.1 Responses of Effector Organs to Autonomic Nerve Impulses and Circulating Catecholamines

Effector Organs	Cholinergic Response	Noradrenergic Impulses	
		Receptor	Response
Eyes			
Radial muscle of iris		α	Contraction (mydriasis)
Sphincter muscle of iris	Contraction (miosis)		
Ciliary muscle	Contraction for near vision	β	Relaxation for far vision
Heart			
Sinoatrial node	Decrease in heart rate, vagal arrest	β	Increase in heart rate
Atria	Decrease in contractility and increase in conduction velocity	β	Increase in contractility and conduction velocity
Atrioventricular node	Decrease in conduction velocity	β	Increase in conduction velocity
His-Purkinje system	Decrease in conduction velocity	β	Increase in conduction velocity
Ventricles	Decrease in contractility	β	Increase in contractility
Arterioles			
Coronary	Constriction	α	Constriction
		β	Dilation
Skin and mucosa	Dilation	α	Constriction
Skeletal muscle	Dilation	α	Constriction
		β	Dilation
Cerebral	Dilation	α	Constriction
Pulmonary	Dilation	α	Constriction
		β	Dilation
Abdominal viscera		α	Constriction
		β	Dilation
Salivary glands	Dilation	α	Constriction
Renal		α	Constriction
		β	Dilation
Systemic veins		α	Constriction
		β	Dilation
Lungs			
Bronchial muscle	Contraction	β	Relaxation
Bronchial glands	Stimulation	α	Inhibition
		β	Stimulation
Stomach			
Motility and tone	Increase	α, β	Decrease
Sphincters	Relaxation	α	Contraction
Secretion	Stimulation	α	Inhibition
Intestine			
Motility and tone	Increase	α, β	Decrease
Sphincters	Relaxation	α	Contraction
Secretion	Stimulation	α	Inhibition

(Continued on page 66)

Table 12.1 *(Continued)* **Responses of Effector Organs to Autonomic Nerve Impulses and Circulating Catecholamines**

Effector Organs	Cholinergic Response	Noradrenergic Impulses	
		Receptor	Response
Gallbladder and ducts	Contraction	β	Relaxation
Urinary bladder			
Detrusor	Contraction	β	Relaxation
Trigone and sphincter	Relaxation	α	Contraction
Ureters			
Motility and tone	Increase	α	Increase
Uterus	Variable	α	Contraction
		β	Relaxation
Male sex organs	Erection	α	Ejaculation
Skin			
Pilomotor muscles		α	Contraction
Sweat glands	Generalized secretion	α	Slight, localized secretion
Spleen capsule		α	Contraction
		β	Relaxation
Adrenal medulla	Secretion of epinephrine and norepinephrine		
Liver		α, β	Glycogenolysis
Pancreas			
Acini	Increased secretion	α	Decreased secretion
Islets	Increased insulin and glucagon secretion	α	Decreased insulin and glucagon secretion
		β	Increased insulin and glucagon secretion
Salivary glands	Profuse, watery secretion	α	Thick, viscous secretion
		β	Amylase secretion
Lacrimal glands	Secretion	α	Secretion
Nasopharyngeal glands	Secretion		
Adipose tissue		α, β	Lipolysis
Juxtaglomerular cells			Increased renin secretion
Pineal gland			Increased melatonin synthesis and secretion

sympathetic vasodilator fibers and sympathetic fibers innervating sweat glands have acetylcholine as their neurotransmitter.

The adrenergic receptors on target organs are of three types: α_1, β_1, and β_2. Norepinephrine acts mainly on α_1 receptors and, to a lesser degree, on β receptors. In general, α receptors mediate excitation of smooth muscles, β_1 receptors mediate excitation of cardiac muscle, and β_2 receptors mediate inhibition of smooth muscles. The autonomic effects on different organs are summarized in **Table 12.1**.

Ganglionic transmission | At the synapse between the preganglionic and postganglionic neurons, the neurotransmitter is ACh, which acts on nicotinic cholinergic receptors located on the postganglionic neuron. These nicotinic receptors are blocked by ganglion blockers such as hexamethonium. Some cholinergic receptors in the ganglia are of the muscarinic type.

Activation of the postsynaptic receptors in the ganglion leads to the generation of an excitatory postsynaptic potential (EPSP) in the postganglionic cell and occasionally produces an inhibitory postsynaptic potential (IPSP). The various neurotransmitters, the receptor they activate, and the type of postsynaptic potentials they produce are summarized in **Table 12.2**.

Autonomic Function Tests

Several autonomic function tests are available for diagnosing underactivity of the ANS. The heart rate responses to the Valsalva maneuver (Valsalva ratio) and a change of posture from standing to lying (S/L ratio) have been used to assess parasympathetic function. The galvanic skin resistance (GSR) has been used to assess sympathetic function. The resistance offered by skin to a galvanic current is low when it is moist; therefore, GSR gives a measure of sweating. Because sweating increases during anxiety, GSR has been used in the lie detector. For the same reason, GSR has been used with patients dealing with anxiety for providing biofeedback on the amount of nervous sweating.

Table 12.2 Major Neurotransmitters of the Autonomic Nervous System

Neurotransmitter	Receptor	Postsynaptic Potential
Acetylcholine	Nicotinic	Fast EPSP (30 ms)
Acetylcholine	Muscarinic	Slow EPSP (30 s)
Dopamine	D_2	Slow IPSP (2 s)
GnRH	GnRH receptor	Late slow EPSP (4 s)

Abbreviations: EPSP, excitatory postsynaptic potential; GnRH, gonadotropin-releasing hormone; IPSP, inhibitory postsynaptic potential.

Summary

- The autonomic nervous system is made up of two branches: the sympathetic and the parasympathetic.

- Each ANS pathway is a made up of two neurons, a preganglionic neuron located at the thoracolumbar spinal cord (sympathetic) or central nervous system and sacral cord

parasympathetic, and a postganglionic neuron that innervates visceral effectors.

- The transmitter at the ANS ganglia is acetylcholine acting on nicotinic receptors.

- The transmitter at the effectors is acetylcholine (parasympathetic) acting on muscarinic receptors and norepinephrine acting at α-adrenergic receptors and β-adrenergic receptors.

Applying What You Know

12.1. Mestinon affects ACh receptors on skeletal muscle, thus alleviating Ms. Adams' symptoms. What does Mestinon do to the ACh receptors in autonomic ganglia? Explain.

Answers to Applying What You Know

Chapter 5

1 Ms. Adams had two nerve conduction studies done on her ulnar nerve (which runs down the outside of the forearm and is easily accessed for such studies). Both studies yielded normal responses. If you could look at this nerve under a microscope, what would you see? And how would what you see help you to interpret the results of the nerve conduction study?

The ulnar nerve is a bundle of axons, some originating from cell bodies in the spinal cord (motor neurons) and others originating from cell bodies in the periphery (sensory neurons). If you were to examine the ulnar nerve under a microscope, you would see axons of varying size, some myelinated and others unmyelinated. You could presumably count the number of each kind of axon and tabulate the distribution of sizes. Such a count would not, however, tell you much about the function of these axons.

The fact that conduction along these axons is normal (normal conduction velocities, normal latencies) tells you that the axons are functioning normally, suggesting that their distribution of sizes and state of myelination are all normal. However, you cannot tell whether the cell bodies and their inputs (sensory stimuli or synaptic) are normal.

Chapter 6

1 Ms. Adams' electrolyte concentrations were all normal. However, if her potassium concentration were abnormally high, what effect would that have on the resting potential of her cells? What would happen if her potassium concentration were abnormally low? Explain.

The Na$^+$–K$^+$ pump in the cell membrane maintains a high extracellular concentration of Na$^+$ and a high intracellular concentration of K$^+$ by pumping potassium into the cell and sodium out of the cell. The resting membrane potential (RMP) is largely the creation of the "leak" of K$^+$ down its concentration gradient out of the cell and the smaller leak of Na$^+$ down its concentration gradient into the cell. Thus, abnormally high extracellular [K$^+$] (hyperkalemia) would reduce the K$^+$ leak and therefore result in a less negative RMP; the membrane would be depolarized. On the other hand, if the extracellular [K$^+$] became abnormally low (hypokalemia), the "leak" would get larger, and the RMP would become more negative; the membrane would hyperpolarize. Either change will affect the excitability of every excitable cell in the body (nerve and muscle).

Chapter 7

1 Ms. Adams undergoes several nerve conduction studies in which electrical stimuli are applied to the nerve. What must the stimulus do to the nerve membrane to excite an action potential? Explain.

An action potential occurs when the excitable membrane (remember, that means either a nerve or a muscle cell) is depolarized (becomes less negative). The state of voltage-dependent Na$^+$ and K$^+$ channels in the membrane, whether or not they are open (activated), depends on the potential across the membrane. Thus, an electrical stimulus must depolarize the membrane to its threshold (the membrane potential at which the number of voltage-dependent Na$^+$ channels that are activated is great enough to start to depolarize the membrane further) to trigger an action potential.

Chapter 8

1 If we could pharmacologically alter Ms. Adams' voltage-dependent Na+ channels so that they stayed open 50% longer than normally, what effect would this have on the amplitude of her action potentials? Would this change or alleviate her symptoms? Explain.

If the voltage-dependent Na$^+$ channels remained open for a longer time when activated (before spontaneously inactivating), more Na$^+$ would enter the cell, making the membrane more positive during the spike of the action potential (AP). That is to say, the membrane potential would move closer to the Na$^+$ Nernst potential, and the amplitude of the action potential would increase. Note that this does not violate the all-or-none principle, which says that under the existing conditions (whatever they may be), the action potential is always the same size; clearly, with the conditions changed by the drug, the amplitude of the AP will change.

However, this pharmacologic change would not directly help Ms. Adams. Both her motor nerves and her muscle cells are able to generate normal APs. Making those APs larger would not address her problem, which is that her end-plate potentials (EPPs) are too small because of the binding of antibodies to the postjunctional ACh receptors.

Chapter 9

1 Ms. Adams' nerve conduction velocities are normal. What does this finding tell you about possible causes of her problem? Explain.

Normal conduction velocity of the compound action potential in a nerve suggests that the number of myelinated and unmyelinated axons is normal and that the size of these axons is unchanged. Thus, one can conclude that Ms. Adams' problem is not the result of an axonal conduction defect (such as is present in demyelinating diseases like multiple sclerosis). However, such a study provides no information about either the function of her neuromuscular junctions or the functional state of her muscles.

2 The EMG studies of Ms. Adams' deltoid muscle showed a marked decrease in the amplitude of the response on repetitive stimulation. What does this tell you about the muscle action potential? Explain.

The EMG recorded from a muscle is the "sum" of the action potentials generated by all of the muscle cells making up the whole muscle. Thus, the EMG is a kind of compound action potential. The decrease in the magnitude of the EMG most likely results from the failure of some muscle cells to fire APs. This would occur if there is a problem at the neuromuscular junction that blocks transmission. This failure of transmission would functionally result in muscle weakness.

Chapter 10

1 Conduction in Ms. Adams' sensory nerves in the ulnar nerve appears to be normal when stimulated electrically. Can you conclude that the function of the related sensory receptors is also normal? Explain.

The nerve conduction test only examines the function of the axon in response to external electrical stimulation. Such a test does not stimulate the sensory endings of those axons, so one can conclude nothing about the ability of the sensory endings to generate an appropriate neural signal carrying information about the nature, location, and magnitude of the adequate stimulus.

Chapter 11

1 Why did the improvement of Ms. Adams' symptoms following the administration of Tensilon last only a short time?

Tensilon is an inhibitor of the cholinesterase enzyme that breaks down acetylcholine. Thus, while Tensilon is active, it will result in larger EPPs (the channels stay open longer), and thus more muscle cells will contract. However, Tensilon itself will diffuse away from the neuromuscular junction and also is subject to metabolic degradation. Both of these will terminate its action and leave Ms. Adams with her muscle weakness unaltered.

2 Failure of transmission at the neuromuscular junction can occur for many different reasons: (1) failure to release acetylcholine, (2) failure of acetylcholine to bind to the postjunctional receptor, or (3) failure of the muscle membrane to generate an action potential. Which data about Ms. Adams' signs and symptoms can be used to distinguish between these possibilities? Explain.

Transmission at the neuromuscular junction requires release of adequate amounts of transmitter, binding of the transmitter to postjunctional receptors, opening of the receptor cation channels, and generation of an action potential in the muscle fiber.

Nerve conduction studies have established that the motor nerves are probably functioning normally. The normal EMG on initial stimulation suggests that the muscle cells are able to generate action potentials. The fact that blocking the action of acetylcholinesterase improves transmission is strong evidence that Ms. Adams' symptoms arise from a problem with the ACh receptors at her neuromuscular junctions. Ms. Adams has antibodies that bind to the ACh receptor, preventing them from functioning.

3 Mestinon is an anticholinesterase that allows ACh to occupy the ACh receptor for a longer time. This results in a larger EPP, which increases the safety factor for transmission at the neuromuscular junction. What other manipulation of the system would improve Ms. Adams' symptoms? Explain.

To improve Ms. Adams' symptom, muscle weakness, particularly on repetitive use, we have to increase the probability of transmission occurring at her neuromuscular junctions. Increasing the duration of action of ACh is one approach to accomplishing this.

Another approach would be to alter the voltage-dependent Na^+ channels in her muscle cell membranes. If these channels became more sensitive to depolarization so that at any membrane potential they were more likely to be activated, then the probability of a muscle action potential would be increased, and more muscle cells would contract.

Chapter 12

1 Mestinon affects ACh receptors on skeletal muscle, thus alleviating Ms. Adams' symptoms. What does Mestinon do to the ACh receptors in autonomic ganglia? Explain.

Mestinon affects transmission at the muscarinic receptors on skeletal muscle. There are, however, other muscarinic receptors on effectors innervated by the parasympathetic system. The occurrence of diarrhea on the initial dose of Mestinon suggests that smooth muscle in her intestine was being affected by the drug.

The receptors in autonomic ganglia, on the postganglionic cell, are nicotinic, so Mestinon will have minimal affect on transmission at the autonomic ganglia because the receptors are different.

Clinical Overview

Review of patient's condition | Ann Adams is suffering from myasthenia gravis, a disease in which muscle weakness is present. In many cases, repeated use of a muscle leads to profound fatigue and increasing weakness in that muscle.

Etiology | Myasthenia gravis (MG) is an autoimmune disease in which the body's host defense system mistakenly creates antibodies against a normal constituent of the body. In MG, antibodies are produced that bind to the acetylcholine receptors at the motor end plate. This both inactivates these receptors and brings about their destruction. With fewer ACh receptors available at the end plate, the end-plate potential (EPP) is smaller than normal, and transmission can fail. The innervated motor unit (all the muscle fibers innervated by a particular motor neuron) then cannot be made to contract, and muscle weakness is experienced.

Prevalence | Myasthenia gravis is an uncommon disease.

Diagnosis | There are three symptoms that when present lead to the diagnosis of myasthenia gravis. One is muscle weakness, which may be accentuated by repetitive use, although the latter is not always present. Electrophysiologic studies of nerve conduction showing normal sensory nerve activity, normal conduction in motor nerves, but failure of electrical activity in the affected muscles on repeated stimulation are also diagnostic. Finally, antibodies to the acetylcholine receptor are present in more than 70% of patients with generalized (involving many muscles) MG.

Treatment | Administration of anticholinesterase drugs dramatically improves the patient's condition. Such drugs increase the size of the end-plate potential, so that even with fewer ACh receptors available, the EPP is large enough to trigger an action potential in the muscle cell membrane.

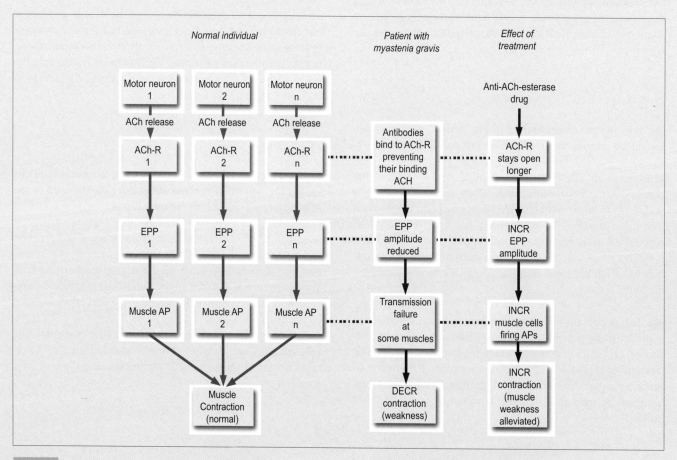

Fig. II.1 (*Left*) Mechanisms triggering muscle contraction in a normal individual. (*Middle*) In a patient with myasthenia gravis such as Ms. Adams', the consequence of binding of antibodies to AChR is to inhibit muscle contraction. (*Right*) The mechanism by which treatment alleviates Ms. Adams' symptoms. ACh, acetylcholine receptor; AP, action potential; EPP, end-plate potential.

Understanding the Physiology

Skeletal muscle cells are stimulated to contract by the motor neuron that innervates them. Acetylcholine, the transmitter at all skeletal muscles, is released from the endings of the motor neuron axon in vesicles and diffuses across the gap. When two ACh molecules bind to a receptor, the channel opens, and both Na^+ and K^+ can diffuse across the membrane under the influence of their electrochemical gradients. Each vesicle contains 10,000 molecules of ACh and results in a miniature endplate potential (MEPP) of ~0.5 mV. However, a large number of vesicles are released simultaneously, and the result is a postjunctional membrane depolarization (an EPP) that summates to an amplitude of 25 mV. The EPP is more than large enough to trigger an action potential in the innervated muscle fibers. Thus, in a normal muscle, transmission between the motor nerve and the muscle cell it innervates is one-to-one.

At a normal motor end plate, the safety factor, the ratio of the amplitude of the EPP produced to the threshold depolarization required to trigger an action potential in the muscle cell, is very large. This means that random fluctuations in the MEPP and the small decrease in the MEPP that results from repetitive stimulation of the end plate still leave the EPP more than large enough to always fire the muscle action potential.

In the patient with myasthenia gravis, the presence of antibodies that bind to ACh receptors results in the destruction of receptors and a decrease in the size of the EPP. The safety factor becomes much smaller, and the decrement with repetitive firing can now result in failure of transmission and thus a reduced contraction. The result is muscle weakness.

The normal processes of triggering a muscle contraction, the changes produced by the disease process, and the mechanism by which treatment works are illustrated in **Fig. II.1**.

Section III | Physiology of Muscle

Overview

Case Presentation

Chapters

Answers to Applying What You Know

Case Analysis

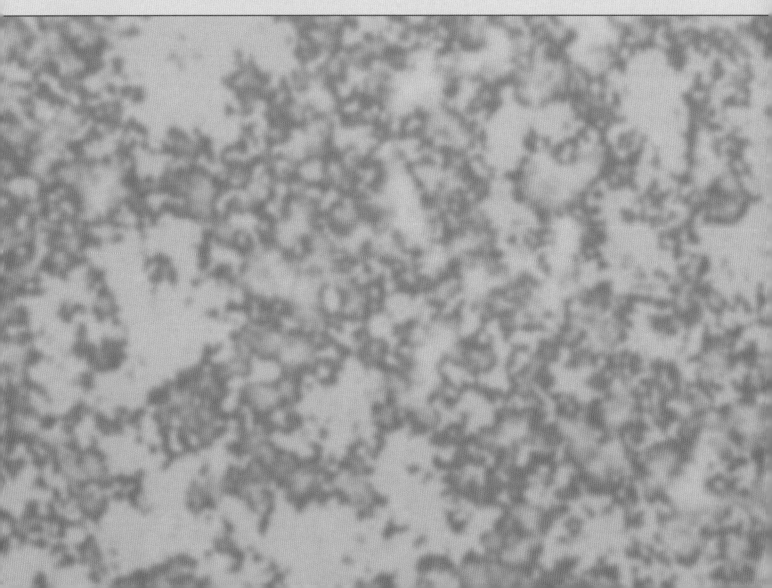

Overview

Muscle cells are of three types: skeletal, smooth, and cardiac; they are electrically excitable cells. As neurons are specialized for the conduction and transmission of information using action potentials, muscle cells are specialized to contract (shorten) and generate force when stimulated. Muscle cells transform the energy stored in adenosine triphosphate (ATP) molecules into mechanical work; this transformation results in either force generation (if the cell length is kept constant) or contraction (shortening).

In all three types of muscle, contraction or force generation is accomplished by an ordered array of two proteins: actin (the thin filament) and myosin (the thick filament). The movement of these proteins along each other results from release of energy by the myosin-ATPase.

The trigger for muscle contraction is an electrical signal on the cell membrane. For skeletal and cardiac muscle, this signal is an action potential; some smooth muscle cells generate action potentials, whereas others respond to other electrical signals.

When electrically excited, muscle cells exhibit a rapid increase in the concentration of calcium (Ca^{2+}) in their cytoplasm. In skeletal muscle, this increase results from the release of Ca^{2+} from intracellular stores. In cardiac and smooth muscle, the Ca^{2+} comes both from intracellular stores and from the extracellular fluid compartment. The Ca^{2+} released then disinhibits the myosin-ATPase, the enzyme releases energy from ATP, and actin and myosin move by one another. The result is work done by the muscle.

Muscle cells are effectors that determine various functions in every organ system of the body.

Section III Case Presentation:
Jeremy Wright's surgery goes wrong.

Reason for Admission

Jeremy Wright is a 47-year-old man scheduled to undergo a cholecystectomy (removal of his gallbladder) for relief of cholelithiasis (gallstones).

Preadmission Work-up

- *Vital signs*
  - Temperature: 36.5°C
  - Blood pressure: 135/82 mm Hg
  - Pulse: 75/min
  - Respirations: 16/min
- *Laboratory studies*
  - Complete blood count: normal
  - Blood chemistries: normal
  - Urinalysis: normal
  - Chest x-ray: normal
  - Electrocardiogram (ECG): normal

Preparation for Surgery

Succinylcholine (which binds to nicotinic acetylcholine receptors at the motor end plate and is degraded only very slowly; it acts as a muscle relaxant) and halothane (a general anesthetic) were administered.

Shortly after the administration of the anesthetic (but before the start of the surgery), the anesthesiologist noticed that the patient began to exhibit fasciculations (spontaneous skeletal muscle contractions). This was rapidly followed by muscle rigidity (skeletal muscle contractures characterized by hard muscles and stiff joints). In addition, the patient's body temperature began to rise rapidly, increasing from 36.5°C prior to the administration of anesthesia up to 39°C within a half hour following general anesthesia. It was also noted that end-tidal PCO_2 (the partial pressure of CO_2) was increasing. The ECG showed a sinus tachycardia developing.

At this time, administration of halothane and succinylcholine were halted, and the surgery was canceled. The patient was hyperventilated to lower end-tidal PCO_2. The patient's temperature continued to climb, reaching 41°C in slightly less than 1 hour.

Ice packs were applied to the patient to help reduce his now dangerous core temperature. The results of a quick blood screening are

$$[K^+]_p = 6.0 \text{ mEq/L}$$
$$pH = 7.30$$
$$\text{Anion gap} = 15 \text{ mEq/L}$$
$$\text{Creatine kinase} = 12,000 \text{ U/L}$$

The slightly elevated plasma $[K^+]$ was initially dismissed as unimportant.

Attempts to bring the patient's temperature down continued. A second blood test confirmed the presence of a lactic acidosis (the anion gap was increased to 17 mEq/L, and pH had fallen to 7.28), and a now distinct hyperkalemia (elevated extracellular K^+) was present. The muscle rigidity was slightly reduced, and the rate of increase of temperature declined significantly. However, the patient began to show cardiac arrhythmias (an irregular heartbeat). The patient's rigidity was reduced somewhat, and the need for ice packs continued to decrease significantly. However, the heartbeat became erratic, and the patient's blood pressure began to fall significantly.

To reverse this developing condition, dantrolene (a drug that blocks release of Ca^{2+} from the sarcoplasmic reticulum) was administered intravenously. The muscle rigidity began to disappear, and body temperature no longer increased. The application of ice packs brought down body temperature. Over time extracellular $[K^+]$ and pH returned to normal. Cardiac function also returned to normal.

Mr. Wright was moved to the intensive care unit (ICU), where he was closely monitored for the next 48 hours.

Some Things to Think About

1. Why was succinylcholine administered to Mr. Wright in preparation for undergoing abdominal surgery?

2. Why do Mr. Wright's muscles become rigid?

3. Why does Mr. Wright become hyperkalemic? What role does K^+ play in muscle function?

4. Why does Mr. Wright's body temperature begin to increase?

13　Functional Anatomy of Muscle

Muscle cells of all types are cells whose special function in the body is to convert biologic energy (ATP) into the generation of force or shortening (contraction). Muscles are the "motors" of the body, allowing us to move about in the world (skeletal muscle), to pump blood (cardiac muscle), and to move the food we eat through the gastrointestinal tract (smooth muscle). Our understanding of the mechanisms by which muscle functions is based on an appreciation for the structure of muscle.

Muscle Fibers

Muscles are contractile tissues whose cells are traditionally called *fibers*. Histologically, some muscle fibers show cross-striations; others do not. Functionally, some muscles conduct electrical excitation ephaptically, with the action potential spreading from cell to cell. Such muscle fibers can contract spontaneously. In other muscles, ephaptic conduction is absent. These muscle cells contract only when stimulated through the nerve fibers that innervate them. Accordingly, there are four types of muscle fibers based on their histologic and functional characteristics (**Table 13.1**).

Skeletal muscle fibers are striated in appearance, cylindrical, and multinucleate (**Fig. 13.1A**). They are 10 to 30 cm in length—long enough to justify the term *fiber*. They are formed by fusion of several smaller cells into a multinucleate syncytium. Skeletal muscles are so named because they are attached to bones by tendons and move the bones and the loads borne by them. They are the only muscles under voluntary control.

Smooth muscle cells are nonstriated in appearance, fusiform (spindle-shaped), and uninucleate (**Fig. 13.1B**). They are 0.02 to 0.5 mm in length. *Single-unit* (or *visceral*) *smooth muscles* are present in the walls of the gastrointestinal and genitourinary tract. All the fibers in a single-unit smooth muscle contract together, near simultaneously or sequentially, due to the presence of cell-to-cell conduction of electrical excitation. *Multiunit* (or *motor-unit*) *smooth muscles* are found in the intrinsic muscles of the eye, piloerector muscles, and vas deferens and in the walls of large elastic arteries. Fibers of multiunit smooth muscles contract in response to nerve stimulation in much the same way as skeletal muscle fibers. However, they are innervated by autonomic fibers that are not under voluntary control.

Cardiac muscle cells are striated, ~0.1 mm-long cylindrical fibers, some of which are branched (**Fig. 13.1C**). The cells

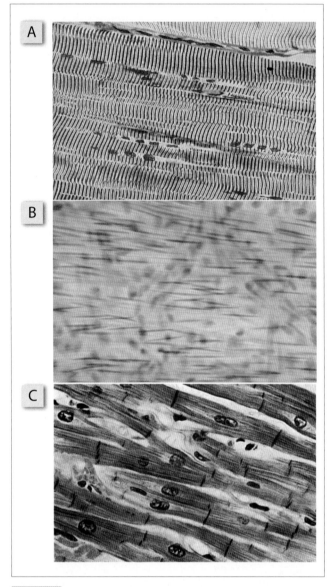

Fig. 13.1 Muscle cells: **(A)** Skeletal muscle fibers, **(B)** smooth muscle fibers, and **(C)** cardiac muscle cells.

are joined end to end, forming *intercalated disks* that provide low-resistance bridges for passage of electrical excitation from cell to cell. Cardiac muscle is found only in the heart; hence its name.

Cardiac muscle has functional resemblances with both smooth muscle and skeletal muscle. Cardiac muscle resembles visceral smooth muscle in that it exhibits automaticity and emphatic conduction, and its contractility is affected by hormones. Cardiac muscle resembles skeletal muscle in that it contains regular sarcomeres delimited by Z-disks, exhibits a similar length–tension relationship, and its contraction is regulated by the troponin–tropomyosin complex.

Table 13.1 Classification of Muscle Fibers

	Striated	Nonstriated
Ephaptic conduction present	Cardiac muscle	Single-unit smooth muscle
Ephaptic conduction absent	Skeletal muscle	Multiunit smooth muscle

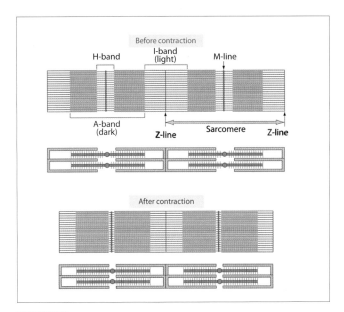

Fig. 13.2 Dark and light bands in striated muscle. Contraction reduces the widths of the I-band and H-band, but the width of the A-band remains unchanged.

Contractile Apparatus of a Striated (Skeletal and Cardiac) Muscle

Like all other cells, the striated muscle fiber has a cell membrane (called the sarcolemma), smooth endoplasmic reticulum (called sarcoplasmic reticulum), cytoplasm (called sarcoplasm), and cytoskeletal proteins The *cytoskeletal proteins* are of three types: contractile, regulatory, and anchoring proteins. The *contractile proteins* are myosin and actin. These two proteins interact to generate the contractile force in a muscle. The *regulatory proteins* are tropomyosin and troponin, and they regulate the interaction between actin and myosin. The *anchoring proteins* are α-actinin, titin, nebulin, and dystrophin. These proteins anchor the cytoskeletal proteins to each other, as well as to the sarcolemma and the extracellular matrix.

The cytoskeletal proteins are disposed in a remarkably orderly way because of which the muscle fiber shows transverse *striations* when viewed under the light microscope. With special techniques, the striations are seen to correspond with dark and light bands (see **Fig. 13.2**). The line called the Z-line extends through the middle of the light band. The part of the muscle fiber that extends between two consecutive Z-lines is called a *sarcomere,* which is the contractile unit of muscle. During muscle contraction, the Z-lines come closer together, and the sarcomeres shorten.

Sarcoplasmic reticulum | In a muscle cell, the sarcoplasmic reticulum (SR) is arranged in a highly geometric way (**Fig. 13.3**) with tubules (the *longitudinal* or *L-tubules*) running parallel to the length of the fiber. These tubules are disposed along the entire length of the A- and I-bands. They end in dilated sacs called *terminal cisterns.*

T-tubules (*traverse tubules*) are disposed radially, coursing from the surface toward the center of the fiber. The transverse tubules are invaginations of the sarcolemma into the cell (**Fig. 13.3**). They typically occur at the A–I junctions in mammals and at the Z-disk in amphibians. Being extensions of the sarcolemma, the T-tubules conduct the action potentials from the sarcolemma into the interior of the cell along its membranes.

Myosin filaments are thick and disposed longitudinally at the center of a sarcomere (**Fig. 13.3**). A myosin filament is made of two intertwined heavy H-chains (**Fig. 13.4A**). The heavy chain has a globular head and a long tail. The tails are helically intertwined; the heads remain separate. Each globular head contains two additional light L-chains. In the sarcomere, the myosin tails are grouped into a bundle from which the globular heads called myosin heads project out (**Fig. 13.4B**).

Digestion with trypsin (**Fig. 13.4A**) generates two fragments of the myosin molecule: the heavy meromyosin (HMM) and the light meromyosin (LMM). The HMM contains the globular head as well as part of its fibrous tail. It can be split further by papain into two parts: the globular HMM S1, which has all the adenosine triphosphatase (ATPase) activity and actin-binding ability, and the fibrous HMM S2, which has none of it. The LMM

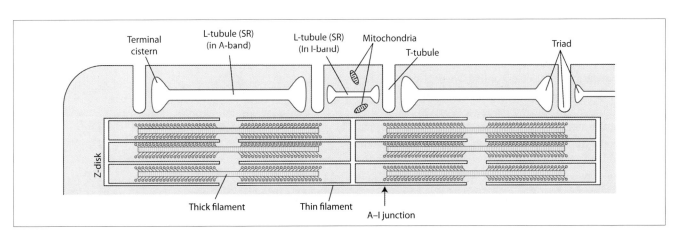

Fig. 13.3 The transverse and longitudinal tubules. The T-tubule and two lateral cisterns on its sides constitute a triad. Note that the L-tubules (the sarcoplasmic reticulum [SR]) in the I-band are shorter and less regular than the L-tubules in the A-band. This is because the I-band region is crowded with mitochondria. Moreover, the width of the I-band changes during muscle contraction, subjecting the L-tubule to compression. The T-tubule and two terminal cisterns on their sides constitute a triad.

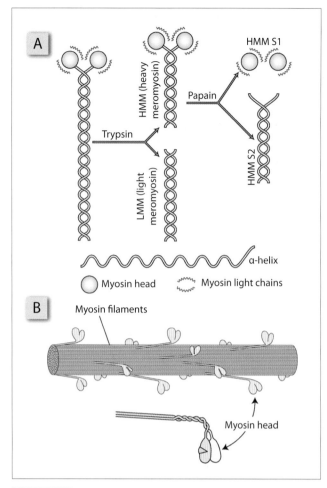

Fig. 13.4 Myosin filaments are made up of repeating subunits. **(A)** Structure of myosin filaments. **(B)** Organization of myosin filaments.

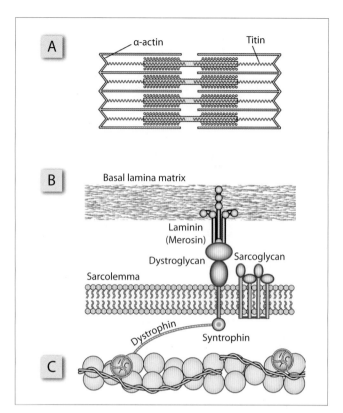

Fig. 13.5 Anchoring proteins in muscle. **(A)** α-Actinin anchors the thin filaments to the Z-disk, and titin filaments anchor the thick filaments to the Z-disk. **(B)** Dystrophin-associated glycoproteins anchor the contractile machinery of each sarcomere to the muscle fiber and the whole muscle. **(C)** Actin is a chain of globular proteins with active sites along the molecule that play a key role in contraction. The control proteins tropomyosin (the thread wrapped around the actin filament) and troponin (the bead attached to the tropomyosin) can also be seen.

comes entirely from the fibrous tail of the myosin molecule. It does not have any ATPase activity or actin-binding ability.

Actin filament is a double helical filament (F-actin) (**Fig. 13.5C**). It is made of globular subunits called G-actin. There are specific sites on the actin filament that bind to the myosin head during muscle contraction. These sites are called *active sites.*

Tropomyosin is a filamentous molecule (**Fig. 13.6**) that consists of two chains, α and β. The tropomyosin filament lies in the groove between the two filaments of actin, and each tropomyosin filament spans seven G-actin subunits. Tropomyosin keeps the active sites of the actin molecules covered when the muscle is not contracting. For contraction to be initiated, the tropomyosin filament must slide off and uncover the active sites (see Chapter 14).

Troponin is attached to tropomyosin (see **Fig. 13.6**). It has three subunits: troponin-T that binds to tropomyosin, troponin-C that binds to four ions of Ca^{2+}, and troponin-I that holds the tropomyosin filament over the active sites on actin so long as troponin-C is not bound to Ca^{2+}.

Anchoring Proteins of a Striated Muscle

The α-*actinin* is located in the Z-band. It cross-links the actin filaments anchoring them to the Z-band (**Fig. 13.5A**). *Titin* (earlier called connectin or gap filament) is a large elastic filament that interconnects the Z-disks (**Fig. 13.5A**). The sarcomere

resists stretching because of the titin filaments that provide what is called the series elastic component (see Chapter 16) of the muscle. When the sarcomere is stretched so there is no overlap between actin and myosin filaments, the titin filaments become more apparent in the gap between the actin and myosin

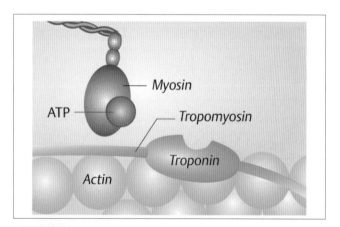

Fig. 13.6 The control protein tropomyosin is wrapped around the actin molecule. Attached to the tropomyosin molecule are troponin molecules. These control proteins play a role in triggering muscle contraction. ATP, adenosine triphosphate.

filaments. *Nebulin* is an inextensible filament connected at one end to the α-actinin in the Z-disk and to the tropomyosin-troponin complex at regular intervals.

Dystrophin-associated glycoproteins include some proteins that are extracellular (dystroglycan and laminin), some located on the inner side of sarcolemma (dystrophin, syntrophin, and utrophin), and some that span the membrane thickness (sarcoglycan, sarcospan). Dystrophin, the best known of these, anchors actin to the membrane through syntrophin, and also to the basal lamina matrix through dystroglycan and laminin (**Fig. 13.5B**). Genetic defects in the dystrophin molecule produce Duchenne muscular dystrophy.

Smooth Muscles

Smooth muscles have functionally important anatomic differences with skeletal muscles (**Fig. 13.7**). (1) The sarcolemma shows short invaginations into the cytoplasm called caveoli, which are analogous to the T-tubules in skeletal fibers. (2) There are several fusiform densities present in the cytoplasm (cytoplasm dense bodies) and along the inner surface of the sarcolemma (subsarcolemmal dense plaque). The cytoplasmic dense bodies contain the protein α-actinin and are the equivalent of the Z-disks in skeletal muscle fibers. Subplasmalemmal dense plaques contain vinculin and talin. Extending between cytoplasmic dense bodies are three types of filaments: actin, myosin, and intermediate filaments. Intermediate filaments are made of desmin (in vascular smooth muscle, it is made of vimentin) that provides a cytoskeletal framework. (3) The ratio of actin and myosin filaments is ~12:1 in smooth muscles compared with ~2:1 in skeletal muscles. The myosin filaments

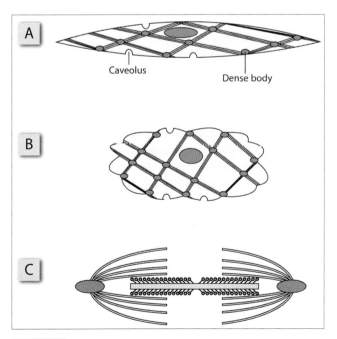

Fig. 13.7 Smooth muscle fiber. **(A)** Structure of a smooth muscle fiber. **(B)** A smooth muscle fiber in the contracted state. **(C)** Actin fibers radiate from the dense bodies, with several actin filaments surrounding a single myosin filament.

are different in skeletal and smooth muscles. In smooth muscles, the projecting heads of the myosin molecules form cross-bridges with the actin filaments along their entire length, whereas the thick filaments of skeletal muscle have a bare central segment that is devoid of cross-bridges. (4) The regulatory proteins tropomyosin and troponin that are present in skeletal muscle are absent in smooth muscle. Instead, smooth muscles contain calmodulin, which is analogous to troponin.

Neuromuscular Junction

A junction between two neurons that permits the passage of an electrical impulse across it is called a synapse (see Chapter 11). The neuromuscular junction (**Fig. 13.8**) is essentially a synapse that exists between an axonal ending and a muscle fiber. As the axon innervating a skeletal muscle fiber approaches its termination, it loses its myelin sheath. The axis cylinder then branches into several bulb-shaped endings called *terminal buttons*, each of which innervates a muscle fiber. The terminal buttons contain many small *synaptic vesicles* that contain acetylcholine, which is the neurotransmitter at neuromuscular junctions. The sites of the prejunctional membrane that are specialized for vesicular release of neurotransmitter are called the *active zones*.

The terminal buttons come in close proximity with a thickened trough on the muscle membrane called the *motor end plate* that bears receptors for acetylcholine (ACh). The motor end plate is thrown into folds called the *junctional folds*. The acetylcholine receptors are clustered at the crest of each junctional fold, which are positioned opposite the active zones of the prejunctional membrane. The 100 nm-wide space between the terminal button and the motor end plate is called the *myoneural cleft*. The cleft is not uniformly wide. It is less than 1 nm in width at the tips of the junctional folds. Within the cleft is a basement membrane or the *basal lamina* made of collagen and other matrix proteins. The enzyme *acetylcholinesterase* (AChE) is anchored to the collagen fibrils of the basement membrane.

Synapse en passant in Smooth Muscle

Unlike the motor end plate of a skeletal muscle fiber, smooth muscles do not show any specialization at their site of contact with the axon. Moreover, the axon innervating smooth muscle does not end at the site of innervation. Rather, it shows multiple swellings or varicosities along its course that liberate neurotransmitters. Each axon forms multiple junctions with muscle cells along its path. Such synapses are called *synapse en passant* (**Fig. 13.9**). This is unlike in skeletal muscle, where the neuron must branch and terminate to innervate multiple fibers. Finally, the neurotransmitters released from the varicosities (the *junctional neurotransmitters*) can be either ACh or norepinephrine. This is unlike the axonal ending in skeletal muscle that releases only acetylcholine.

Contact junctions | In multiunit smooth muscles, the varicosities come in close contact with individual cells, forming contact junctions (**Fig. 13.9A**). Here, the muscle membrane is separated from the varicosity by a gap of roughly the same width as in a neuromuscular junction. Hence, the junctional delay (i.e., time taken for the impulse to travel from the neuron

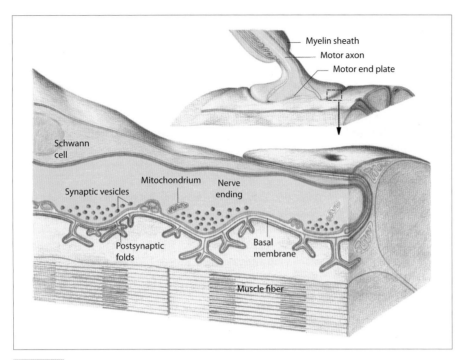

Fig. 13.8 The structure of the neuromuscular junction in skeletal muscle.

to the muscle membrane) is comparable to that in a neuromuscular junction of a skeletal muscle.

Diffuse junction | In single-unit smooth muscle, the varicosities do not come in close contact with any cell. Neurotransmitters from the varicosities diffuse to reach all the muscle cells. This arrangement has been called a diffuse junction (**Fig. 13.9B**). The junction delay is considerably more in diffuse junctions.

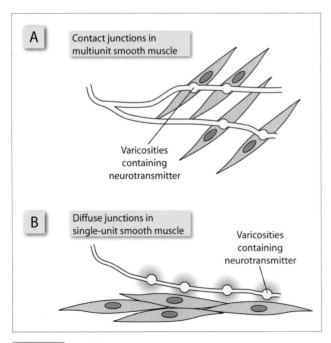

Fig. 13.9 Synapse en passant on smooth muscle. **(A)** Contact junctions. **(B)** Diffuse junctions.

Summary

- There are three different muscle types: skeletal, cardiac, and smooth. They share many properties, but they also exhibit important differences in structure and function.

- In all three muscle types, contraction results from the interaction of two contractile proteins, actin (the thin filament) and myosin (the thick filament).

- Associated with the contractile proteins are other proteins whose function is to control the activity of myosin-ATPase.

- Skeletal muscle is innervated by motor neurons, and the site of innervation is the neuromuscular junction. Smooth muscle is innervated by the autonomic nervous system at a variety of types of neuromuscular junctions.

Applying What You Know

13.1. When succinylcholine is administered to Mr. Wright, he develops a flaccid paralysis. When halothane anesthesia is started, he quickly develops skeletal muscle contractures. Contrast these two quite different states of his muscles in terms of the state of his sarcomeres.

13.2. Describe the sequence of events that occur at the skeletal muscles when succinylcholine is administered to Mr. Wright. What happens to his muscles, and why does it happen?

Contractile Mechanism

The shortening of a muscle fiber occurs due to the sliding of actin filaments on myosin filaments. The process that causes this shortening is called *cross-bridge cycling*; it is briefly summarized in **Fig. 14.1A**. This process is triggered by the increase in cytosolic calcium (Ca^{2+}) and its binding to troponin (**Fig. 14.1B**).

Cross-bridge Cycling

Adenosine triphosphate (ATP) binds to myosin ATPase present on the myosin head and splits into adenosine diphosphate (ADP) and an inorganic phosphate (P_i). The energy released activates the myosin head, which is now ready to bind to actin. The activated myosin head binds with the active sites of actin filaments, forming actomyosin. Simultaneously, the myosin head flexes at its hinge. As a result, the actin filament slides on the myosin filament, bringing the Z-disks closer together and thereby shortening the sarcomere. As the myosin head flexes, the ADP and P_i present on it are released, making room for a fresh molecule of ATP. When ATP binds to myosin ATPase, the myosin head detaches from actin, and the cross-bridge cycle is repeated.

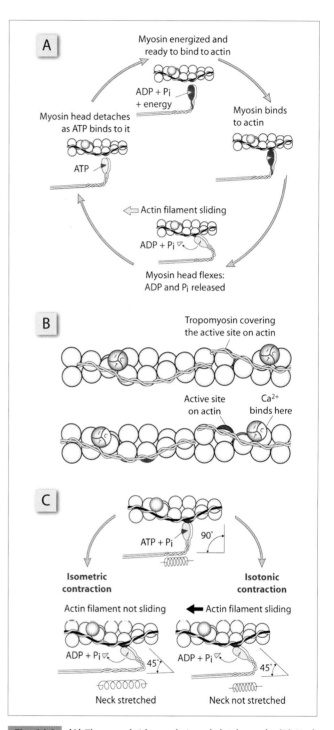

Fig. 14.1 **(A)** The cross-bridge cycle in a skeletal muscle. **(B)** Binding of calcium ions to troponin-C shifts the tropomyosin molecule, uncovering the active sites on actin that bind to myosin heads. **(C)** The power stroke in isometric and isotonic contraction. In isometric contraction, the actin filament cannot slide, resulting in the stretching of the neck of the actin filament. ADP, adenosine diphosphate; ATP, adenosine triphosphate; P_i, inorganic phosphate.

General Model: Energy

The use of the energy in ATP by muscle cells to shorten is only one example of a general model that can be used to understand many physiologic processes. It is a particularly obvious example because we can directly experience the work (for which energy must be expended) of the muscle cells as we move our limbs.

Power stroke | When the muscle is in a relaxed state, the myosin head is in the high-energy 90-degree conformation. The high-energy state is brought about by the energy released when an ATP molecule binds to myosin ATPase (present on the S-1 head) and is hydrolyzed into ADP and P_i. The activated myosin head binds to one of the several active sites on the actin filament to form the actin–myosin–ADP–P_i complex. Formation of the complex triggers two near-simultaneous events: (1) the flexion of the myosin head, which now changes to the low-energy 45-degree conformation; and (2) the release of the P_i and ADP from the complex.

The *flexion of the myosin head* from the high-energy 90-degree conformation to the low-energy 45-degree conformation generates mechanical force and is called the *power stroke*. It has either or both of the following effects (**Fig. 14.1C**). If the load on the muscle is small, then the actin filament slides over the myosin filament, producing muscle shortening (isotonic contraction). If the load on the muscle is large, then the actin and ADP + P_i myosin filaments are unable to slide over each other (isometric contraction). Flexion of the myosin head will instead stretch the elastic neck of the myosin molecule (see Chapter 16 and the description of the series elastic component).

The *release of ADP and P_i* allows a fresh ATP molecule to bind to the myosin head. The myosin–ATP complex has a low affinity for actin; therefore, it results in the dissociation of the myosin head from the actin filament. The freshly bound ATP molecule is split, the myosin head is reactivated, and the cycle is repeated.

Dark and light bands | Long before the mechanism of muscle contraction was understood, it was observed that the skeletal muscle showed cross-striations that appeared as alternate light and dark bands under the light microscope (**Fig. 14.2**). These light and dark bands are barely visible when the muscle fiber is perfectly focused, but they become prominent when the fiber is defocused slightly by lowering or raising the objective of the microscope. The band that appears to be dark on lowering the objective will appear to be light when the objective is raised, and vice versa. By convention, all references to the dark and light bands are those observed when the objective of the microscope is lowered.

The dark band contains highly refractile material and is birefringent or anisotropic; hence, it is called the anisotropic or A-band. The A-bands are coextensive with the myosin filaments. The A-band is birefringent because the actin and myosin fibers overlap in this zone. The light bands are called isotropic or I-bands; they are present in the region containing only actin filaments. The I-band is bisected by the transverse Z-line. The A-band is bisected by the H-band and the M-line. During contraction, the width of the A-band remains constant, and the widths of the I-band and H-band decrease.

The above observations served as a lodestar for a century of research on the mechanism of muscle contraction. Any theory of muscle contraction had to account for the above observations. The sliding filament theory satisfactorily explains them all.

Initiation and Termination of Cross-bridge Cycling

Tropomyosin | The cross-bridge cycling is switched off or on by the tropomyosin molecule, which slides on the actin molecule to cover or uncover the active sites on it. Tropomyosin covers the active sites on actin when the sarcoplasmic calcium (Ca^{2+}) concentration is low and uncovers them when it rises.

Troponin | The regulatory action of Ca^{2+} on tropomyosin is mediated by troponin (Tp), a protein made up of three subunits, TpC to which Ca^{2+}-binding occurs, and TpI and TpT. When the sarcoplasmic Ca^{2+} concentration rises, four ions of Ca^{2+} bind to TpC. The TpC–$4Ca^{2+}$ complex induces changes in TpI and TpT, which, in turn, bring about a shift of tropomyosin away from the active sites on actin. When the sarcoplasmic Ca^{2+} falls, Ca^{2+} dissociates from TpC, and tropomyosin slides back on the actin filament to cover the active sites.

Sarcoplasmic calcium concentration | The Ca^{2+} concentration in the sarcoplasm is quite low. The concentration in the L-tubule is about a thousand times higher because Ca^{2+} is continuously pumped from the sarcoplasm into the L-tubule by Ca^{2+}-ATPase. These calcium pumps are located on the membranes along the entire length of the L-tubule. Most of the Ca^{2+} that enters the L-tubule moves to the terminal cisterns, where it is bound in large amounts to a calcium-binding protein called *calsequestrin*.

When the sarcolemma depolarizes, the depolarization spreads to the T-tubules, too. When the T-tubule depolarizes, the Ca^{2+} present in the lateral cisterns diffuses out into the sarcoplasm through special Ca^{2+} channels called the *ryanodine receptor* (RYR) channels. The released Ca^{2+} is taken up almost immediately and pumped back into the L-tubules by Ca^{2+}-ATPase. Hence, the Ca^{2+} concentration rises in the sarcoplasm for a very brief period and has been aptly called the *Ca2+ pulse*. During the Ca^{2+} pulse, the sarcoplasmic Ca^{2+} concentration rises a thousandfold, from $\sim 10^{-7}$ to 10^{-4} moles/L.

The sarcoplasmic Ca^{2+} concentration is determined by a dynamic balance between (1) the rate at which Ca^{2+} enters it from the lateral cisterns and (2) the rate at which Ca^{2+} is pumped back into the L-tubules. When the frequency of action potentials increases, the sarcoplasmic Ca^{2+} also increases. Conversely, a decrease in the frequency of action potentials results in a fall in sarcoplasmic Ca^{2+}.

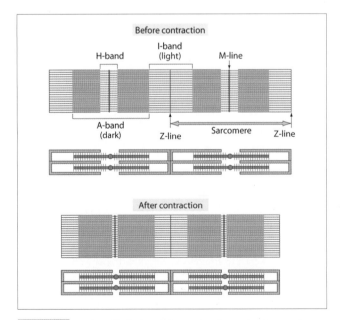

Fig. 14.2 Dark and light bands in a striated muscle. Contraction reduces the widths of the I-band and H-band, but the width of the A-band remains unchanged.

General Models: Reservoir and Balance of Forces

The cytoplasm of muscle cells is a reservoir in which the concentration of calcium that is present is determined by the rate at which calcium enters from the extracellular space, the rate at which calcium is pumped out of the cell, the rate at which calcium enters from the sarcoplasmic reticulum (SR), and the rate at which calcium is pumped back into the SR. Changes to any of these processes will change the balance determining calcium concentration; hence, muscle function will change.

Role of ATP | ATP has three roles in muscle contraction and relaxation. (1) It provides the energy for the power stroke of the myosin head. (2) It brings about a dissociation of the myosin head from the actin filament. (3) It brings about muscle relaxation by pumping out Ca^{2+} from the sarcoplasm into the L-tubules.

Muscle relaxation occurs when the cross-bridge cycle is interrupted. It is a common misconception that ATP causes muscle relaxation by disengaging the actin and myosin filaments. Disengagement of actin and myosin by ATP does not stop the cross-bridge cycle; rather, it keeps the cycle going. Disengagement of actin and myosin by ATP is followed immediately by a fresh interaction between actin and myosin and results in another power stroke. Hence, for the cycle to stop, the dissociation of myosin heads from actin must be accompanied by a lowering of sarcoplasmic Ca^{2+} and the consequent covering of the active sites on actin. When a muscle becomes fatigued, its ATP content decreases. Depletion of ATP slows down the pumping of Ca^{2+} into sarcoplasmic tubules and therefore increases the sarcoplasmic Ca^{2+} concentration. The active sites on actin remain uncovered (due to high sarcoplasmic Ca^{2+}) and bound to the myosin heads (because ATP is also required for the dissociation of myosin heads from actin). The muscle therefore fails to relax completely and remains in a partially contracted state called *contraction remainder*. For identical reasons (i.e., depletion of ATPs), the muscles become rigid after death, a state known as *rigor mortis*.

Excitation–Contraction Coupling

The term *excitation–contraction coupling* refers to the events between the generation of sarcolemmal action potential and the outpouring of Ca^{2+} from L-tubule cisterns into the sarcoplasm. For years, researchers have tried to understand how the depolarization of the T-tubules results in an outpouring of Ca^{2+} from the lateral cisterns, although there is no continuity between them. Presently, the favored theory is that of mechanically interlocked receptors of the T-tubule and lateral cistern, as explained below.

General Model: Flow

For molecules or ions such as Ca^{2+} to move from one location to another, energy must be expended. This energy can come from a concentration gradient, as is the case here (calcium leaving the lateral cisterns), or from the expenditure of biologic energy by a "pump." In addition, there must be an open pathway through which the ions can move. Thus, to understand muscle function, it is essential to understand the mechanism by which Ca^{2+} gets into the sarcoplasm.

The resting membrane potential (RMP) of skeletal muscle is about −90 mV. The action potential runs along the T-tubule to enter deep into the muscle fiber (**Fig. 14.3**). When the action potential reaches up to the tip of the T-tubule, it activates certain voltage-gated receptors called *dihydropyridine receptors*

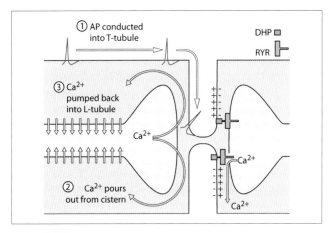

Fig. 14.3 Excitation–contraction coupling. The T-tubule above is shown as polarized, while below, it is shown as depolarized. Depolarization of the T-tubule results in outpouring of Ca^{2+} from the lateral cistern. When Ca^{2+} binds to its binding site on troponin, contraction occurs. AP, action potential; DHP, dihydropyridine receptor; RYR, ryanodine receptor.

(DHPs) located on the T-tubule membrane. Activated DHPs trigger the opening of the RYR Ca^{2+} release channels located on the lateral cisterns. This is possible because the lateral cisterns are located very close to the tips of the transverse tubules, and the protein chains of DHP and RYR are mechanically interlocked. When the DHP is activated by the depolarization of the T-tubule, it undergoes a conformational change, which results in the RYR being pulled open mechanically.

Muscle Energetics

Energy Source for Muscle Contraction
The ATP store of a muscle cell is exhausted in the first 3 seconds of exercise. Thereafter, the ATP stores are replenished continuously by the dephosphorylation of creatine phosphate reserves of the muscle fiber.

In another 5 seconds, the creatine phosphate reserves also get depleted, and a further supply of energy for ATP replenishment comes from glycolysis. However, the lactic acid accumulation associated with glycolysis makes it difficult for muscle contraction to continue beyond 1 minute. Continuous exercise for several hours is possible only when the ATP is replenished continuously through the Krebs cycle. The efficiency of the muscles under aerobic conditions is ~20%.

Despite being an inefficient and short-term process of ATP generation, the value of glycolysis lies in that, unlike the Krebs cycle, its peak rate is not limited by the oxygen supply to the muscle. It is therefore ideal for short but severe exercise, such as a 100-meter sprint. The Krebs cycle, on the other hand, provides a steady supply of ATP at a rate limited by the oxygen uptake of the tissues and is indispensable for a marathon.

Muscle Heat
Early researchers carefully recorded the heat produced in muscle to understand the mechanism of muscle contraction. These

details corroborate the current concepts of the contractile and elastic properties of the muscle and also indicate the timings of the physical and chemical processes that underlie muscle contraction.

Resting heat is the heat produced in the unstimulated muscle. It is the energy released due to the basic cellular metabolism and activity of the Na^+–K^+ pump.

Activation heat is produced at the onset of muscle contraction, before any generation of tension and/or shortening. Activation heat is associated with the release of Ca^{2+} from SR and the activity of myosin ATPase activity during cross-bridge cycling. Repeated activation of the muscle fiber, as occurs during muscle tetanus, results in the summation of activation heat. The total activation heat released during the course of a sustained muscle contraction is called the *maintenance heat.*

Shortening heat occurs during the actual process of shortening. It is absent in isometric contraction. Shortening heat is the energy released in overcoming the viscous forces inside the muscle while shortening. The sum of activation (or maintenance) heat and shortening heat is called the *initial heat.*

Recovery heat is the heat liberated due to the activity of Ca^{2+}–ATPase as it pumps Ca^{2+} back into the SR and due to the regeneration of ATP as well as other energy substrates. Recovery heat begins almost immediately after the onset of contraction and continues for several minutes after the cessation of contraction, indicating that increased Ca^{2+}–ATPase activity and ATP regeneration begin soon after contraction starts.

Relaxation heat is the amount of heat produced in addition to the recovery heat. It is released when an isotonically contracted muscle is stretched back by the load to its original length and is attributable to the viscous resistance to isotonic muscle relaxation.

Summary

- Shortening or force generation of muscle is the result of the sliding of actin filaments on myosin filaments.

- Actin and myosin interact with one another at cross-bridges, which are the sites of myosin–ATPase activity.

- The activity of cross-bridges is controlled by the local concentration of Ca^{2+}, which interacts with control proteins to disinhibit myosin–ATPase.

- Function requires the availability of ATP, which comes from a variety of metabolic pathways.

Applying What You Know

14.1. Dantrolene is administered to Mr. Wright to stop the continuous cycling of his skeletal muscle cross-bridges and the consequent hyperthermia and hyperkalemia. Explain how dantrolene accomplishes this. Why are Mr. Wright's heart and vascular smooth muscle not affected?

14.2. Mr. Wright develops a marked hyperkalemia at the height of his abnormal response to being prepared for surgery. By what mechanism is Mr. Wright's plasma [K^+] increased?

14.3. Mr. Wright also develops a marked lactic acidosis. What is the mechanism by which this occurs? Is this response related to the hyperkalemia that is present? Explain.

15 Characteristics of Muscle Contraction

The structural unit of a skeletal muscle is a muscle fiber, but its functional unit is the motor unit (see below). Although most of the properties of the whole muscle are also present in each muscle fiber, some of its properties can be related only to the behavior of its motor unit. Hence, the gross characteristics of muscle contraction are discussed under two headings: the single-fiber characteristics and the motor-unit characteristics.

Single Muscle Fiber

Although discussed as the characteristics of a single muscle fiber, most of the experiments discussed in the following text can also be performed with the whole muscle. How can we be sure that the experimentally observed properties of a whole muscle are also valid for the muscle fiber? For example, we know that when a train of stimuli is applied, the muscle generates more tension than it does in response to a single stimulus. There could be two reasons for this increase in muscle tension. One possibility is that multiple stimuli activate more muscle fibers. The other possibility is that multiple stimuli increase the contractility of each muscle fiber. In practice, we rule out the first possibility by employing a maximal stimulus for stimulating the muscle. When a maximal stimulus is applied to a muscle, all the muscle fibers contract. Hence, the increase in muscle tension cannot be attributed to stimulation of a greater number of fibers. Rather, it must be the response of individual muscle fibers. Most experiments on whole muscle employ maximal stimulus for stimulating the muscle.

The all-or-none law | A single muscle fiber obeys the all-or-none law: it either contracts maximally or not at all, depending on whether the stimulus is of threshold intensity or subthreshold. Although muscle fibers obey the all-or-none law, the whole muscle does not. As the stimulus strength increases, more and more fibers in the muscle are stimulated, and the muscle shows a graded response to the stimuli.

The actin–myosin filaments themselves do not obey the all-or-none law. This can be shown in skinned fibers in which the sarcolemma of the muscle fiber is removed. The filaments show graded contraction proportional to the calcium (Ca^{2+}) concentration of the bathing fluid. Why then does the whole fiber obey the all-or-none law? It is because the sarcolemma depolarizes in an all-or-none fashion. If it were possible to produce graded depolarization of the sarcolemma, the muscle fiber, too, would show graded contractions.

Single Muscle Twitch

The single muscle twitch (commonly called the simple muscle twitch) may be recorded in the isotonic or isometric condition. In isotonic recording, the muscle is made to contract against minimal load, and the shortening is recorded using a system of levers. In isometric recording, the contracting muscle is not allowed to shorten, and the tension (force) developed is recorded using a tension transducer.

Recording a perfectly isotonic contraction requires that the load on the muscle is zero. Recording of a perfectly isometric contraction requires that the load is completely immovable. Both are technically impossible. For recording isotonic muscle shortening, the muscle has to move a writing lever. The recording lever itself has a finite weight, which acts as a load on the muscle. Hence, it is not possible to record a perfectly isotonic muscle contraction.

On the other hand, for recording an isometric increase in muscle tension, the muscle is made to produce a very small displacement of a very heavy load. The displacement, which is measured after magnification, gives an indirect measure of the degree of muscle tension. If no displacement is produced in the recording device, then the muscle tension cannot be assessed. Hence, no recording can be perfectly isometric.

As a practical approximation, isotonic recording is made using a very light isotonic lever that is moved easily by the muscle. Isometric recording is made using a tension transducer, which serves two purposes. (1) It acts like a heavy load, allowing only minimal muscle shortening in response to large contractile forces. (2) It produces a measurable current that is proportional to the muscle shortening. The current produced is therefore proportional to the rise in muscle tension.

Phases of a muscle twitch | A typical isotonic twitch recorded from a frog's sartorius muscle takes ~0.6 second and shows three phases (**Fig. 15.1A**). (1) The *latent phase* is the

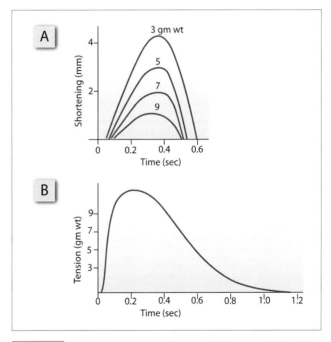

Fig. 15.1 **(A)** Single muscle twitches recorded *isotonically* from frog sartorius muscle. The heavier the load, the less the muscle shortens and the briefer the twitch. **(B)** Single muscle twitch recorded *isometrically* from frog sartorius muscle. (Adapted from Jewell BR, Wilkie DR. The mechanical properties of relaxing muscle. J Physiol (Lond), 1960, 152:30.)

time taken by the impulse to travel along the nerve to the neuromuscular junction, and through neuromuscular transmission, excitation–contraction coupling, the initial isometric phase of contraction, and the inertia of the recording lever. The latent period is longer when the distance between the point of nerve stimulation and the neuromuscular junction is more, or when a heavier load prolongs the initial isometric contraction phase. (2) *Isotonic contraction* is the phase in which the muscle shortens by up to 20% of its resting length. The greater the load, the shorter is the isotonic contraction phase, and the less is the shortening. (3) *Isotonic relaxation* is the phase in which the muscle gets stretched back to its original length by the dead weight suspended from the recording lever. The relaxation period is prolonged when the dead weight is lighter. If the load on the muscle is zero, the muscle will not regain its original length: a muscle that has contracted isotonically remains shortened until it is restored to its original length by stretching.

Isotonic versus isometric twitch | There are salient differences between the time courses of isotonic and isometric twitches (**Fig. 15.1**). Isotonic contraction has a longer latent period. This is because no contraction is entirely isotonic: all isotonic contractions begin with a brief phase of isometric contraction, which accounts for a part of the latent period of isotonic contractions. For the same reason, the total duration of isotonic shortening is less than the duration of rise in isometric tension. The peak isotonic shortening occurs after peak isometric tension.

Slow and fast twitch muscles | Depending on the duration of a single twitch, muscle fibers are categorized into slow twitch and fast twitch muscle fibers (**Fig. 15.2A**). Slow twitch fibers rely on oxidative metabolism and are red due to their myoglobin content. Fast twitch fibers are pale in color because they lack myoglobin. Most muscles contain a varying admixture of both types of fibers and are called pale muscles, examples of which are the gastrocnemius muscle, the extraocular muscles, and the dorsal interossei. They contract quickly but are easily fatigable. Muscles that contain only red fibers are called red muscles, examples of which are the coleus and the lumbricals. Their contractions are slow and sustained and are not easily fatigued.

Summation of twitches and muscle tetanus | When two stimuli are so timed that the second twitch starts before the completion of the first, the second twitch records a greater shortening (or tension) than the first. This is called *summation of twitches* (**Fig. 15.2B**). As the interval between the two stimuli is decreased, individual peaks of the two twitches become less discernible until only a single large twitch is observed. When multiple stimuli are delivered in quick succession to produce summation of twitches, the muscle gets *tetanized*—it remains contracted and does not relax. If the stimuli are spaced sufficiently close, the individual peaks fuse to produce a complete tetanus, and the contraction reaches a near-perfect plateau. If the peaks of the individual twitches are discernible, it indicates the presence of brief relaxation between peaks, and the tetanus is said to be incomplete.

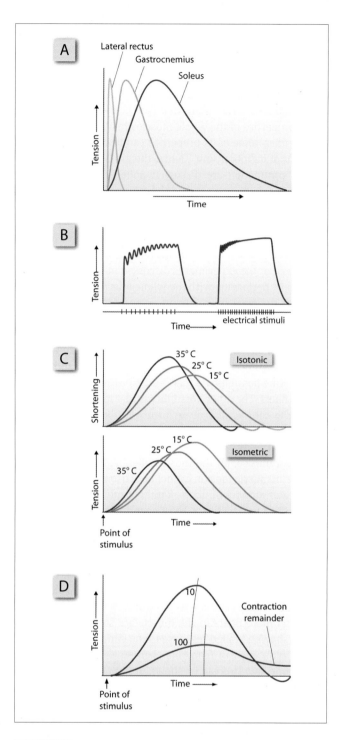

Fig. 15.2 **(A)** Isometric twitches of inferior rectus, gastrocnemius, and coleus. **(B)** Subtetanic and tetanic contractions. **(C)** Effect of temperature on isotonic contractions and isometric contractions. **(D)** Muscle fatigue. The figure shows the 10th twitch and the 100th twitch obtained when the muscle is repeatedly stimulated in rapid succession.

Tetanic tension is about four times the twitch tension. There are two theories for this higher tension generated during muscle tetanus: one theory assumes that during a single twitch, the amount of Ca^{2+} released into the sarcoplasm is not enough to produce tetanic tension. When the muscle is stimulated in rapid succession, Ca^{2+} is released into the sarcoplasm with each stimulus, and there is a progressive accumulation of Ca²⁺ in the sarcoplasm. Tetanic tension is reached when sarcoplasmic Ca²⁺ levels reach their maximum. Studies with the Ca²⁺-sensitive photoprotein aequorin show that sarcoplasmic Ca²⁺ does increase on stimulation in rapid succession. On the other hand, there are experiments to suggest that even during a single twitch, enough Ca²⁺ is released into the sarcoplasm to cause complete shortening of its sarcomeres. However, the Ca²⁺ starts moving back into the sarcoplasmic reticulum well before the muscle tension is able to rise to tetanic levels. During tetanus, Ca²⁺ is continuously present in the sarcoplasm; therefore, the muscle gets adequate time to reach tetanic tension.

Effect of temperature on muscle contraction | A rise in temperature reduces the isometric twitch tension of muscles (**Fig. 15.2C**). A rise in temperature (within physiologic limits) promotes the activity of Ca²⁺– ATPase, which pumps Ca²⁺ back faster into the sarcoplasmic reticulum and hastens relaxation. Contraction is quicker, too, due to faster diffusion of Ca²⁺ from the reticulum to the sarcoplasm. Because the duration of the Ca²⁺ pulse decreases with the rise in temperature, less time is available for the rise of twitch tension. Hence, the strength of an isometric muscle twitch falls at a higher temperature. For the same reason, temperature does not have much effect on tetanic tension.

Isotonic shortening of muscles increases with a rise in temperature. This is due to the decrease in the internal viscoelastic resistance to shortening, which more than compensates for the reduction in muscle tension.

Muscle fatigue is associated with a fall in muscle tension and an increase in relaxation time (**Fig. 15.2D**). The fatigue occurs at least partly due to ATP depletion in the muscle itself and is most prominently revealed by its incomplete relaxation. In a large motor unit, fatigue can also occur at the neuromuscular junction.

However, the depletion of acetylcholine occurs only at prolonged, high-frequency (> 50 Hz) stimulation. In real life, psychological fatigue occurs in the central synapses of the brain earlier than in the muscle itself. This fatigue can, however, be overcome by adequate encouragement and motivation.

Length–tension relationship | The length of a muscle, when it is detached from its bony attachments, is called its *equilibrium length*. If the muscle is stimulated after stretching it passively, the contractile force developed by it will vary depending on the amount of passive stretch. In other words, the contractile force developed by a muscle depends on its initial length. The force of muscle contraction recorded at various initial lengths of the muscle is shown in **Fig. 15.3A**. The force recorded is the total force: it is the sum of the active contractile force and the passive recoil of the muscle in response to stretching. If the muscle is stretched but not stimulated, the force recorded will give the passive recoil force. The active contractile force generated by the muscle can be obtained by subtracting the passive recoil force from the total tension. It is seen that as the muscle is stretched from its equilibrium length, the active tension first increases to a maximum and then decreases. The length at which the muscle generates the maximum contractile force is called its *resting length*. The

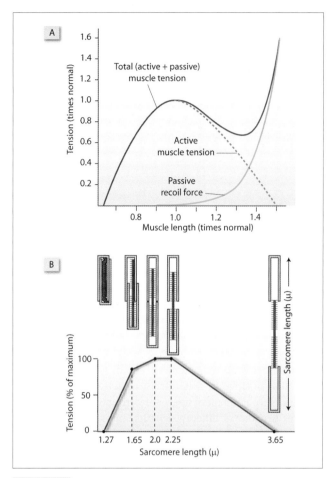

Fig. 15.3 Length–tension relationship in a skeletal muscle fiber. **(A)** Active, passive, and total tension in a muscle, which is stimulated at different preloaded conditions. **(B)** Cross-bridge overlap at different sarcomere lengths. (Adapted from Gordon AM, Huxley AF, Julian FJ. The variation in isometric tension with sarcomere length in vertebrate muscle fibers. J Physiol (Lond), 1960, 152:30.)

resting length of a sarcomere is 2.0 to 2.25 μ. The rise and fall of active tension occur due to the varying degrees of cross-bridge overlap (**Fig. 15.3B**).

Muscle contractility | Because the strength of muscle contraction varies with muscle length, it is important that studies on muscle contractility are made on isometric contraction. An increase in muscle contractility is associated with a rise in peak tension, an increase in the rate of rise and fall in tension, and a shortening of the duration of contraction. Thus, the rise in peak tension that occurs with a fall in temperature (**Fig. 15.2C**) does not signify a rise in contractility because the contraction and relaxation periods are prolonged. Muscle contractility is an important consideration in cardiac muscle physiology.

Preload versus afterload | *Preload* is the load placed on a muscle before the muscle contracts. It serves to stretch the muscle sarcomeres, thus producing a passive tension in the muscle. This passive tension increases muscle contraction in two ways: (1) It adds an elastic recoil force to the muscle during its contraction. (2) It stretches the muscle to its resting length, producing the optimum length–tension relationship (described

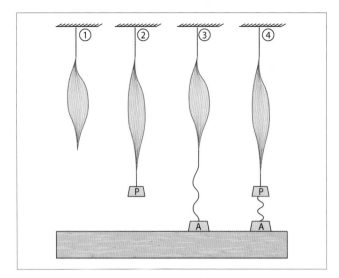

Fig. 15.4 Different types of muscle loading. (1) Unloaded muscle (ignoring the weight of the muscle itself). (2) Preloaded muscle. (3) After-loaded muscle. (4) Preloaded and after-loaded muscle.

below) for active force generation. In real-life situations, it is a common practice to prestretch a muscle using antagonist muscles. Through experience, we learn how much force our muscles generate at different lengths, and unconsciously, we adjust the muscle length before initiating a movement to develop the power we want.

Afterload is the load that the muscle encounters after it starts shortening. The contraction of an afterloaded muscle is comparatively less. In real-life situations, after-loaded contractions tend to occur in novel situations when there are unexpected perturbations in load.

A muscle can also be partly preloaded and partly after-loaded (**Fig. 15.4**). The concept of preload and afterload is also applicable to the heart, which is made of striated muscle. A heart can withstand a greater preload than afterload without going into cardiac failure.

Motor Unit

A solitary motor neuron with all its peripheral branches and innervated extrafusal muscle fibers is called a *motor unit*. The term *motor unit* is sometimes extended to multiunit smooth muscles, too. The motor unit is the functional unit of muscle contraction in vivo.

The motor unit obeys the all-or-none law: when the nerve fiber of the motor unit is stimulated, all the fibers of the motor unit will either contract maximally or not contract at all, depending upon whether the stimulus is of threshold or subthreshold intensity.

Innervation ratio | The number of muscle fibers innervated by a single neuron is called the innervation ratio of the motor unit. The ratio is low in muscles concerned with precision movement and high in those requiring power rather than precision. For example, the extraocular muscles have the lowest innervation ratio of less than 6 per axon, whereas the

gastrocnemius muscle has an innervation ratio of up to 2000 per axon.

Motor unit territory | In the transverse section of a muscle, the area occupied by a single motor unit is called the motor unit territory. For example, the territory of a motor unit in biceps ranges from 2 to 15 mm in diameter. There are extensive overlaps of the motor unit territories of different motor units, and muscle fibers belonging to different motor units intermingle singly (**Fig. 15.5A**). It is uncommon to find two or more motor fibers of the same motor unit lying adjacent to each other. The extensive intermingling of motor fibers from different motor units results in smoothing of the muscle contraction.

End-plate zone | The motor end plates of all the muscle fibers in a motor unit are aligned in a narrow band called the *end-plate zone* or *innervation zone*. It is located midway between the ends of the muscle fibers (**Fig. 15.5B**). However, the end-plate zones of different motor units are not always aligned.

Motor Recruitment

When a muscle begins to contract, a few units contract first. If the power generated is inadequate, more units are "recruited."

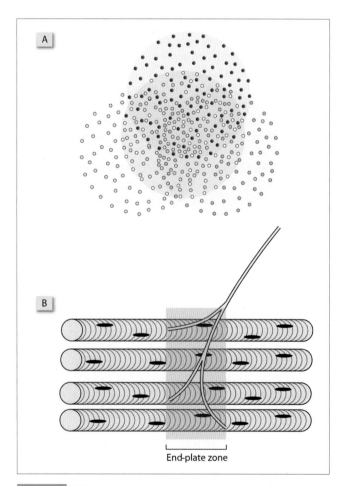

Fig. 15.5 **(A)** Motor unit territories of four motor units (shown in different colors) seen in cross section. Fibers intermingle singly, as shown in the central overlapping area. **(B)** End-plate zone of a muscle.

This process of employing a progressively greater number of motor units for muscle contraction is called *motor recruitment.*

Henneman (size) principle | When a muscle contracts against a load, the smallest motor units (which have only a few muscle fibers in them) are recruited first. If the force generated is insufficient, then the larger motor units are recruited. This order of recruitment from the smaller to the larger motor units is described by the Henneman principle or the *size principle.* In fact, the largest motor units in a muscle are idle most of the time because such large muscle forces are rarely required. On stimulation, the larger motor units are found to be more excitable than the smaller ones. Hence, the orderly recruitment from smaller to larger units occurs due to the way the motor system is organized and not because of their intrinsic excitability.

One strength of the Henneman principle is that it accounts for muscles' fine gradation of low-intensity movements, as well as their bursts of power for moving heavy loads. The Henneman principle brings out an interesting similarity between the motor and the sensory system. Because progressively larger motor units are recruited, it means that as the load increases, the number of motor fibers recruited increases exponentially. This exponential rise in motor strength in response to a linear rise in motor neuron discharge is reminiscent of the Weber-Fechner law, which states that the stimulus intensity must rise exponentially to produce a linear rise in sensory neuronal discharge (**Fig. 15.6**).

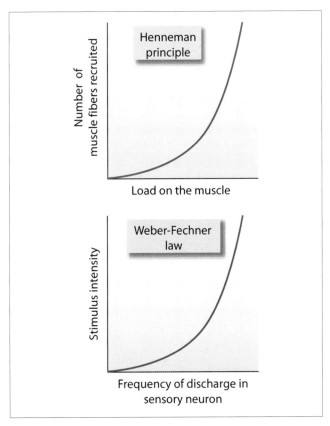

Fig. 15.6 Similarity between Henneman (motor) principle and Weber-Fechner (sensory) law.

Type I and Type II Motor Units

A motor unit contains only one type of muscle fiber: either all the fibers are red, or all are white. Accordingly, motor units are called type I (red) and type II (white) motor units (**Table 15.1**).

Type I (red) motor units are adapted for slow and sustained (tonic) contractions without fatigue. They are smaller and are the first to be recruited whenever a muscle contracts. These units are therefore almost continuously (i.e., tonically) active during routine activity. This is also the reason why all muscles must have at least a few type I motor units in them. Because type I units contract continuously for prolonged

Table 15.1 Comparison between Type I and Type II Motor Units

Motor Unit	Type I	Type II
Names	Slow oxidative	Fast glycolytic
	Red fibers	White fibers
	Tonic fibers	Phasic fibers
	S (slow)	F (fast)
Metabolism	Aerobic	Anaerobic
Glycolytic capacity	Low	High
Oxidative capacity	High	Low
Fatigability	Little or none	Rapid
Fiber length	Small	Large
Fiber diameter	Small	Large
Glycogen content	Low	High
Mitochondria	High	Low
Sarcoplasmic reticulum (SR)	Normal	Extensive
Ca^{2+} pumping into SR	Moderate	High
Capillary density	High	Low
Blood supply	High	Normal
Myoglobin content	High	Low
Myosin ATPase activity	Low	High
Phosphorylase	Low	High
Succinic dehydrogenase	High	Low
NADH dehydrogenase	High	Low
Number of units in a muscle	Many	Few
Number of terminals per axon	Few	Many
Axon diameter	Small	Large
Conduction velocity	Slow	Fast
Order of recruitment	Early	Later
Twitch duration	Long	Brief
Tetanic tension	Small	Large

Abbreviations: ATPase, adenosine triphosphatase; NADH, nicotinamide adenine dinucleotide.

periods without fatigue, they have to be dependent on aerobic metabolism, and are endowed with a high capillary density for ensuring an adequate oxygen supply. However, the capillaries get squeezed between contracting muscle fibers, and blood flows through the capillaries only during intermittent muscle relaxation. Hence, red fibers contain myoglobin for storing oxygen and ensuring adequate oxygen supply during tonic contractions. Myoglobin gets rapidly oxygenated during the brief phases of relaxation that occur in between contractions. Type I units are present mostly in postural muscles, which do not require speedy contractions. In keeping with the requirements, axons of these units have smaller diameter and slow conduction velocity.

Type II (white) motor units are adapted for brief (phasic) bursts of powerful contractions. They are inactive most of the time and are recruited much later when the type I motor units fail to move the load. They contract only in short bursts (i.e., phasically) when a brief but powerful contraction is needed. In keeping with their function, axons of type II units have larger diameter with greater conduction velocity.

For contracting and relaxing quickly, white muscle fibers have more extensive sarcoplasmic reticulum with a higher capacity for pumping Ca^{2+}. They also have a faster isoenzyme of myosin–ATPase. Because these muscles are fast muscles, they have little time for taking up O_2 and glucose from blood. Hence, white fibers depend on anaerobic metabolism and store adequate glycogen in them. However, the lactic acidosis resulting from anaerobic metabolism makes the white fibers fatigue-prone.

Summary

- The contraction of single muscle fibers is all-or-none; the contraction either occurs or does not occur depending on the stimulus strength.

- There are important differences between isometric contractions or twitches (muscle length does not change) and isotonic twitches (length does change).

- The strength of skeletal muscle contraction can be altered by recruiting additional muscle fibers to contract, by increasing the frequency of stimulation to produce tetanic summation, and by altering the length of the muscle when it contracts.

- There are two types of muscle fibers, type I (red) and type II (white), with different functional properties.

Applying What You Know

15.1. Predict what pattern of neural activity you would observe in Mr. Wright's motor nerves during his contractures. Explain.

15.2. During Mr. Wright's contractures, what muscle fiber types are active? Explain.

Physical Models of Muscle

The contractile properties of the muscle explain how the muscle shortens actively in response to a stimulus. However, it does not explain (1) how the muscle regains its original length after it is stretched passively and (2) how the muscle is able to contract even when its external length does not change. These characteristics of muscle are attributable to its elasticity. To explain how the elastic and contractile components are arranged in the muscle, the two-compartment model and the three-compartment model of muscle were proposed. Later models have incorporated several more compartments to explain all the observed characteristics of gross muscle contraction. However, for most purposes, the three-compartment model suffices.

General Model: Elasticity

All biologic structures, from cells to tissues to organs, are elastic structures. That is to say, changes in length or size require the presence of an energy gradient. The elastic properties of muscle are integral to their function and the function of the tissues and organs in which they are found.

The Two-Compartment Model

The two-compartment model assumes that the muscle has a contractile component (CC) and an elastic component (EC). The CC represents the actin and myosin filaments. The CC is considered to be plastic; that is, when stretched, it produces no elastic recoil. The CC is therefore unable to return to its original length after it has been stretched. The EC represents the elastic element, which resists stretch and restores a contracted muscle to its resting length.

In the two-compartment model (see **Figs. 16.1A** and **16.1B**), there is only one elastic component that may be located either in series with the comtractile component (as a *series elastic component* [SEC]) or in parallel with it (as a *parallel elastic component* [PEC]). In either case, such a model is unable to explain all the observed phenomena related to muscle elasticity.

If an elastic element is inserted in series with the contractile component (**Fig. 16.1A**), the CC would continue to elongate when the muscle is stretched and would ultimately snap, while the SEC would remain unstretched. However, the SEC does explain how the muscle is able to contract without a change in length and why the muscle reverts to its resting tension at the end of an isometric contraction. This is because during isometric contraction, the SEC gets stretched, and during relaxation, it recoils and stretches out the CC.

To resist muscle stretching, an elastic component must be present in parallel with the CC (**Fig. 16.1B**). However, a parallel elastic component cannot explain how a muscle regains its original length after isometric contraction. A parallel elastic

element will simply fold up during active shortening of the CC; therefore, it will be unable to provide the necessary elastic recoil for restoration of the original muscle length. Nonetheless, it does explain why the muscle resists passive stretching.

The Three-Compartment Model

The inadequacy of the two-compartment model led to the proposing of the three-compartment model of muscle elasticity (**Fig. 16.1C**), in which the presence of two elastic components was posited, one in series with the CC of the muscle (SEC) and the other in parallel (PEC). In this model, the SEC explains how the muscle is able to contract even when its external length does not change. It also explains how it regains its original length after contracting isometrically. The PEC is the reason why the muscle regains its original length after it is passively stretched. The SEC resides in the elastic neck of myosin filaments, and in the case of a whole muscle, in the tendon. The PEC resides in the sarcolemma and the gap filaments.

Effect of Load

Phases of Muscle Contraction

A muscle that contracts tetanically against a load shows three phases that differ in the extent of shortening and the amount of tension generated (**Fig. 16.2A**).

Initial isometric contraction phase | All muscle contractions begin with this phase in which the shortening of the CC merely stretches the SEC. The load does not move, and there is no change in the external length of the muscle (hence the name *isometric*). Stretching of the SEC is associated with a rise in muscle tension. As the shortening of the CC continues, the SEC gets stretched more and more. Stretching of the SEC results in a rise of muscle tension until the tension equals the load. This point marks the end of the initial isometric phase.

Intermediate phase of isotonic contraction | This phase commences when the muscle tension exceeds the load, and the load starts moving. There is no further stretching of the SEC and no further increase in muscle tension (tone) during this phase.

Terminal phase of the ineffective contraction | As the muscle shortens, the force generated by its CC changes in accordance with the length–tension relationship. Once the muscle becomes shorter than the resting length, any further shortening is associated with a decrease in tension. When the tension generated decreases and equals the load, the contraction becomes ineffective; that is, there is no further change in muscle length or tension despite the continuation of muscle stimulation and continuous cross-bridge cycling.

Force–Velocity Relationship

When the load is immovable, there is no isotonic contraction, and the contraction becomes entirely isometric. Conversely, when the load is zero, the initial isometric phase disappears,

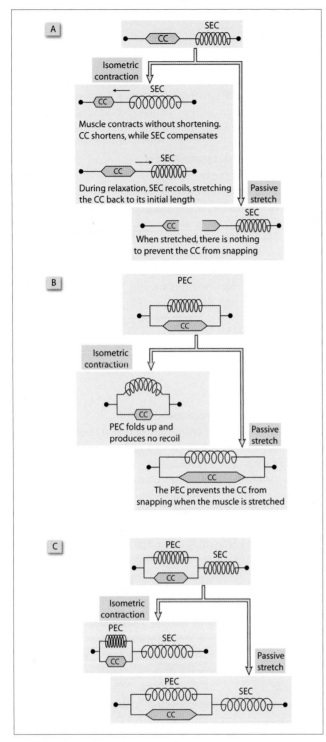

Fig. 16.1 **(A)** Two-compartment model with the elastic component in series (SEC). The model explains the mechanism of isometric contraction but fails to explain the effect of passive stretch. **(B)** Two-compartment model with the elastic component in parallel (PEC). The model explains the mechanism of recoil of muscles following passive stretch but fails to explain the mechanism of isometric contraction. **(C)** The three-compartment model of the muscle showing the contractile component (CC), PEC, and SEC. When the muscle contracts without external shortening, the shortening of CC is compensated by the stretching of SEC. When the muscle is passively stretched, all the components are stretched. The recoil of the PEC restores the CC to its original length.

and the contraction begins with the isotonic phase. The muscle initially shortens at its maximum velocity (V_{max}) and shortens to ~60% of its resting length. Thereafter, the force generated by its CC is zero (in accordance with the length–tension relationship), and the contraction enters its terminal isometric phase (**Fig. 16.2B**). Between these two extremes (zero load and immovable load), all contractions have variable durations of isotonic and isometric contraction. With increasing load, the duration of the initial and terminal isometric contraction increases, and the velocity of isotonic shortening keeps decreasing. The extent of shortening also decreases.

Isotonic and Isometric Contractions

The terms *isometric* and *isotonic contraction* usually refer to the extreme ends of the force–velocity graph. Isometric contractions occur while trying to move the immovable. Isotonic contraction is rarely seen in its pure form: the weight of the

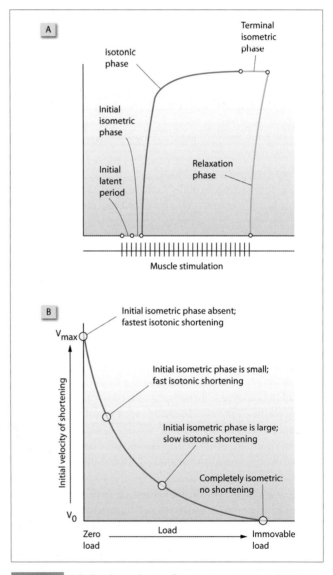

Fig. 16.2 **(A)** The three phases of a tetanic contraction. **(B)** Force–velocity relationship in a skeletal muscle.

muscle itself constitutes a load on the muscle. The differences are summarized in **Table 16.1**.

Energy expenditure in isometric contraction | In isometric contraction, there is no external shortening of the muscle; therefore, the external work done (force × distance moved) is zero. Yet sustained isometric contraction is associated with fatigue, indicating that the contraction requires continuous energy expenditure. The energy is utilized for doing "internal" work—for stretching the SEC. It may be argued that the SEC needs to be stretched but once, and thereafter no further energy expenditure should be required. That is not correct. The SEC continuously tends to recoil back each time the myosin head dissociates from the actin filament, and it requires continuous energy-intensive cross-bridge cycling to keep the SEC stretched. The situation is analogous to a car kept stationary on an incline with its engine running, by adjusting the clutch and the accelerator pedals. The car continuously burns fuel and yet does no external work. The car can also be kept stationary by switching off the engine and applying the brakes. The situation then becomes analogous to the latch phenomenon of smooth muscles discussed in Chapter 18.

Summary

- The full range of muscle responses requires the presence of elastic elements in muscle.

- To understand all phases of isometric (muscle length is fixed) and isotonic (muscle is allowed to shorten) contractions requires consideration of the behavior of the elastic elements in muscle.

Applying What You Know

16.1. Mr. Wright exhibits stiff joints while being anesthetized. Describe the contractions occurring at a joint under these conditions.

Table 16.1 Comparison of Isotonic and Isometric Contraction

Isometric Contraction	Isotonic Contraction
Shortening of the CC is compensated by stretching of the SEC.	Shortening of the CC results in shortening of muscle. The SEC is not stretched.
Tension rises due to stretching of SEC.	Because the SEC is not stretched, tension remains unchanged.
No shortening occurs; therefore, no external work is done.	Shortening occurs, and external work is done.
Occurs at the beginning and end of all contractions	Occurs in the middle of a contraction
Isometric phase increases when load increases.	Isotonic phase decreases when load increases.
Heat released is less and therefore more energy-efficient.	Heat released is more (due to the release of heat of shortening) and therefore is less energy-efficient.
An isometric twitch has a shorter latent period, shorter contraction period, and longer relaxation period.	An isotonic twitch has a longer latent period, longer contraction period, and shorter relaxation period.
A rise in temperature decreases isometric twitch tension.	A rise in temperature increases isotonic twitch shortening.

Abbreviations: CC, contractile component; SEC, series elastic component.

Muscle Tension versus Shortening

The external work done by a muscle is observable as the change in either its length (*muscle shortening*) or its stiffness (*muscle tension*). The shortening of a muscle depends on the length of the muscle—the number of sarcomeres in series. The tension developed by the muscle is proportional to the physiologic (not anatomic) cross-sectional area of the muscle — the number of sarcomeres disposed in parallel. The anatomic *cross-sectional area* is the cross-sectional area of the muscle at its thickest parts. The *physiologic cross-sectional area* is the sum of the cross-sectional areas of all the muscle fibers at their thickest part. Based on the relative amounts of tension and excursion, muscle contraction has been classified into three types: isometric, eccentric, and concentric. Eccentric contractions generate the maximum amounts of tension, followed by isometric and isotonic contractions.

In **isometric contraction**, there is a rise in muscle tension, but there is no muscle shortening. The shortening is zero if the load is immovable or if an antagonistic muscle contracts with equal force. Also called static or holding contractions, the functional role of isometric contractions is mostly to stabilize the joints.

In **eccentric contraction**, there is a simultaneous increase in muscle length and tension. This occurs when a contracting muscle is subjected to an external force greater than the active tension generated. It is also called *lengthening contraction.* Eccentric contractions decelerate body segments and provide shock absorption, for example, when walking or landing from a jump. Elbow flexors contract eccentrically when the glass of water is lowered to the table. Another example of eccentric contraction is the quadriceps muscle when the body is being lowered to sit on a chair. The tension of an eccentric contraction increases as the speed of active lengthening increases.

In **concentric contraction**, the muscle shortens, while the muscle tension may increase (auxotonic), decrease (meiotonic), or remain unchanged (isotonic). *Auxotonic contraction* is associated with a continuous rise in muscle tension and is seen while pulling a spring. *Meiotonic contraction* is associated with a fall in tension. It is seen when the muscle acts on a device like the clasp knife, which offers resistance that is initially high, but drops suddenly. *Isotonic contraction* is not associated with any change in muscle tension and is seen when the load remains unchanged throughout contraction. It is seen when a load is lifted by flexing the elbow. The speed of shortening in a concentric contraction is inversely proportional to the tension produced.

Internal Architecture of Muscle

The body requires a wide range of excursion and tension, and muscles tend to specialize in one or the other. The relative amounts of muscle tension and excursion produced by a muscle are determined by its internal architecture (**Fig. 17.1**, **Table 17.1**).

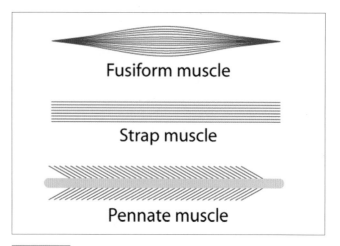

Fig. 17.1　Internal structure of muscle. There are three types of muscles based on the orientation of individual muscle fibers within the whole muscle.

In **strap and fusiform muscles**, the fibers run through the entire length of the muscle. Each fiber, therefore, must be at least as long as the muscle itself. Hence, for a given volume of muscle, only a limited number of fibers can be accommodated in parallel. Fusiform muscles have a larger physiologic cross-sectional area than strap muscles, which are generally thin and long. Accordingly, strap muscles (e.g., sartorius, gracilis, and semitendinosus) can quickly contract through a large range of excursion but develop relatively weaker tension as compared with fusiform muscles.

In **pennate muscles**, the length of the fibers is much smaller than the length of the muscle. Hence, a very large number of fibers can be accommodated in a relatively small volume of muscle. This reduces the excursion (the extent to which the muscle can contract) but greatly augments the tension generated. Most of the muscles in the body are of pennate structure (e.g., the vasti of the quadriceps, soleus, and gastrocnemius). In pennate muscles, both the excursion and the tension contributed by individual fibers to the whole muscle are reduced due to the oblique disposition of fibers.

Muscle Action

Laws of muscle action | The outcome of muscle contraction in terms of the movements in the skeletal lever system is known as muscle action. Muscles rarely contract alone; rather,

Table 17.1　Muscle Excursion and Tension of Different Types of Muscles

	Excursion	Tension
Straplike	High	Low
Fusiform	Moderate	Moderate
Pennate	Low	High

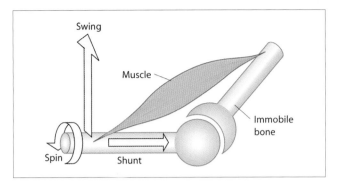

Fig. 17.2 Components of muscle action at the joint.

several muscles contribute to produce the desired force and resulting motion. Although the resultant effect is often quite complex, muscles abide by certain elementary principles known as the *laws of muscle action*. The *law of approximation* states that a contracting muscle tends to bring its origin and insertion together. The *law of detorsion* states that a contracting muscle tends to bring its origin and insertion into the same plane.

Components of muscle action | The muscle action at the joint can be resolved into three components (**Fig. 17.2**). The *swing component* tends to change the angulation of the joint. The *shunt component* tends to compress the articular surfaces. The *spin component* tends to rotate the bone about its long axis. The swing component is discussed further with the skeletal lever system (see below).

Integrated Muscle Action

The functional role of a muscle in any movement can be classified into three different types: agonist, antagonist, and synergist. The synergist in its turn may act as an assistant mover, neutralizer, or stabilizer.

An **agonist** is a contracting muscle or a muscle group that is the principal muscle producing a joint motion. The agonist always contracts actively to produce a concentric, isometric, or eccentric contraction. An agonist is also called a *prime mover*, indicating that the muscle provides the most important force creating a particular torque.

An **antagonist** is a muscle (or muscle group) that possesses the opposite anatomic action of the agonist. The antagonist is usually a noncontracting muscle that neither assists nor resists motion, but that passively elongates or shortens to permit the motion to occur. For example, during elbow flexion, the biceps brachii muscle is an agonist, and the triceps brachii is an antagonist. When the agonist and antagonist contract simultaneously, the result is isometric contraction of both, with consequent stiffening of the muscle and immobilization of the joint. The antagonist then functions as a stabilizer (see below). Body builders show off their biceps by simultaneously contracting the triceps.

A **synergist** contracts at the same time as the agonist. The action of the synergist may be nearly identical to that of the agonist, partially antagonistic to the agonist, or neither. Accordingly, a synergist may serve three different roles as an assistant mover, neutralizer, or stabilizer. An *assistant mover* is a servile synergist muscle that can aid the prime mover to act as an emergency muscle either when great force is required or when paralysis has occurred. For example, during elbow flexion, the brachioradialis acts as the assistant mover, with the brachialis serving as the prime mover. The *neutralizer* is a partially antagonistic synergist muscle that opposes an unwanted action of the prime mover. For example, the pronator teres prevents the supination action of the biceps brachii during elbow flexion. Another example is the wrist extensors preventing wrist flexion when long flexors of the fingers contract to close the fist. A *stabilizer* is a synergist muscle that steadies or supports a proximal joint so that another muscle may act effectively at a distal joint. This contraction is generally isometric. For example, the wrist extensors often act as stabilizers so that the hand can be used effectively. To reach out with the hand, the scapula must be stabilized against the thorax. This is done by the rhomboids.

The relationships of muscles as agonists, antagonists, and synergists are situational and not absolute. When a person in a sitting position flexes his elbow to lift a load in hand, the flexors contract concentrically and are called agonists. The extensors are the antagonists, and they are relatively relaxed and elongate to permit the elbow flexion motion. To lower the load, the elbow is extended. In this situation, the flexors perform an eccentric contraction and are still called agonists, whereas the extensors remain relatively inactive and are still called antagonists. But when the person is placed in the supine position with the shoulder in 90 degrees flexion and is asked to perform the same motion of elbow flexion and extension, the agonist–antagonist relation is reversed. Now the elbow extensors are the agonists for elbow extension (concentric contraction) and for elbow flexion (eccentric contraction), whereas the flexors are the antagonists for both these motions.

Actions of Two-Joint Muscles

Many muscles in the human body cross two or more joints. Examples are the biceps brachii, the long head of the triceps brachii, the hamstrings, the rectus femoris, and several muscles crossing the wrist and finger joints. These muscles affect motion simultaneously at both or all of the joints over which they pass.

Active insufficiency | During joint movements, the passive tensions in two-joint muscles change much more than that in one-joint muscles. During certain joint movements, two-joint muscles become excessively slack, thereby failing to produce active tension (*active insufficiency*). An example of active insufficiency is seen in the finger flexors, which cannot produce a tight fist when the wrist is in flexion. A tight fist is possible only when the wrist is in a neutral position.

Passive insufficiency | During certain other movements, two joint muscles get stretched excessively, thereby restricting the range of joint movements (*passive insufficiency*). An example of passive insufficiency is seen in the gastrocnemius, which restricts ankle dorsiflexion when the knee is flexed. A larger range of ankle dorsiflexion is possible when the knee is in flexion due to the change in the tightness of the gastrocnemius.

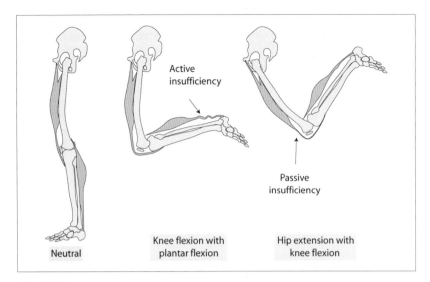

Neutral	Knee flexion with plantar flexion	Hip extension with knee flexion

Fig. 17.3 Action at a two-joint muscle. Active insufficiency of the gastrocnemius muscle occurs due to excessive slackness when there is knee flexion with plantar flexion. Passive insufficiency of the rectus femoris muscle occurs due to excessive stretching when there is knee flexion with hip extension.

Both active and passive insufficiency can occur at the same time in a pair of antagonists. A good example is the combined movement of hip extension and knee flexion (**Fig. 17.3**). This movement produces active insufficiency of the hamstrings and passive insufficiency of the rectus femoris. Conversely, simultaneous hip flexion and knee extension cause passive insufficiency of the hamstrings and active insufficiency of the rectus femoris.

Skeletal Lever System

A joint represents the fulcrum (F) of a lever system (see **Fig. 17.4**), in which the swing component of muscle action provides the effort (E) for moving the external load (L). Most body levers are of class III. They magnify the swing component. The skeletal lever system delivers muscle power to the load. The lever does not magnify power, which remains unchanged. It merely alters the ratio of force transmitted to the load and the excursion of the load. In all three classes of lever, what is gained in excursion is lost in force, and what is gained in force is lost in excursion. Class II levers always produce force gains (high mechanical advantage), whereas class III levers always produce excursion gains (low velocity ratio).

Class I lever ⏐ Examples of a class I lever include the atlantooccipital joint, where the weight of the head is balanced by neck extensor muscle force. A head that tips forward in sleep is extended by the neck extensors when the person wakes up (**Fig. 17.5A**). Conversely, in full extension, the center of gravity of the head lies behind the axis, so that the flexor muscles now act to pull the head forward. The same leverage system works to balance the trunk at the hip joints in standing.

Class II lever ⏐ There are fewer examples of class II levers in our body. The anterior fibers of the masseter muscle usually pass in front of the back molar teeth. Therefore, as the mandible is elevated, the food crushed between these teeth lies closer to the axis of the temporomandibular joint than the anterior part of the muscle. Class II levers provide a force advantage such that large weights can be supported or moved by a smaller force (**Fig. 17.5B**).

Class III lever ⏐ The vast majority of lever systems within the body are class III levers, with the joint closer to the muscle attachment than to the load. Contraction of the brachialis, an elbow flexor, causes motion at the fulcrum of the elbow joint, which results in elbow flexion, raising the object in the hand as well as the weight of the forearm. Class III levers give the advantage of higher speed and larger excursion. They are ideal for most muscles that contract through a small range with great force (**Fig. 17.5C**).

Lever systems, though, can be considered in several ways, depending on the points of reference chosen and the axis about which movement occurs. For example, during plantarflexion of the foot against resistance by contracting the triceps surae, the whole foot acts as a class I lever if the ankle joint is

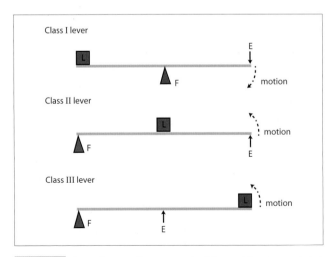

Fig. 17.4 Three classes of levers. F is the fulcrum (the pivot point), L is the load, and E is the effort applied.

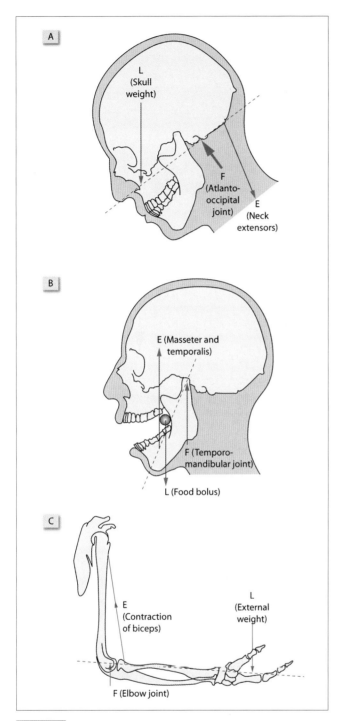

Fig. 17.5 Examples of levers in the musculoskeletal system. **(A)** Class I lever. **(B)** Class II lever. **(C)** Class III lever. F, L, and E are explained in **Fig. 17.4**.

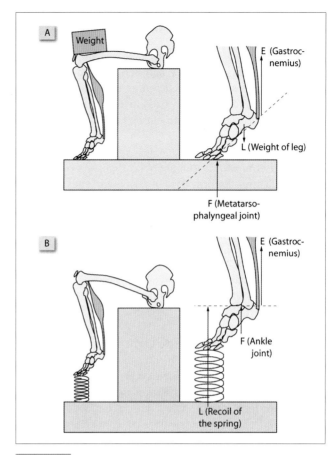

Fig. 17.6 **(A)** Plantar-flexion against resistance can be viewed as a Class I lever. **(B)** Plantar-flexing to raise the heel can be viewed as a Class II lever.

considered as the axis (**Fig. 17.6A**). However, if the foot is on the ground with the subject sitting with a weight on the bent knees, then contraction of the same muscles can be seen to cause rotation about the metatarsophalangeal joints, raising the load (weight of the leg) acting at the ankle joint. This is a class II lever system (**Fig. 17.6B**).

Summary

- Skeletal muscle use in vitro always involves some combination of isometric (no shortening, but tension is developed) and isotonic (shortening does occur) contraction.

- The two or more muscles that connect to the skeleton around a joint can act as agonists, antagonists, or synergistically in producing movement at that joint.

Applying What You Know

17.1. Following the induction of anesthesia, Mr Wright is observed to develop "muscle rigidity" with "hard muscles and stiff joints." What kind of muscle contraction is occurring? Why do his joints appear "stiff"?

There are several differences between smooth and skeletal muscles. The structural differences have been discussed in Chapter 13 and are briefly listed in **Table 18.1**. The functional characteristics of smooth muscles are discussed in this chapter.

Compared with skeletal muscles, smooth muscles have delayed onset of contraction and relaxation: the contraction begins ~200 msec after the peak of a spike and ends 500 msec after excitation is over. Smooth muscles have lower energy requirements for contraction and can maintain a high tension without actively contracting (latching). Smooth muscles have a higher percentage of shortening. A smooth muscle fiber can contract (shorten) to almost 30% of its initial length. Finally, smooth muscles are able to readjust their resting length, that is, the length at which they generate maximum active tension (plasticity).

Mechanism of Smooth Muscle Contraction

The cross-bridge cycling in smooth and skeletal muscles is identical, and each cross-bridge cycling of a myosin head generates the same amount of shortening (1 nm) and tension. However, the regulation of smooth muscle contraction is different (**Fig. 18.1**). Smooth muscle does not contain tropomyosin or troponin. One of the light chains of the myosin filament located in the neck region, called the *regulatory chain of myosin,* serves the function of tropomyosin. Similarly, a calcium-binding protein called *calmodulin* serves the role of troponin.

Phosphorylation of myosin cross-bridges ‖ When sarcoplasmic Ca^{2+} rises (**Fig. 18.1A**), the Ca^{2+} binds to calmodulin (**Fig. 18.1B**). The Ca^{2+}–calmodulin complex activates the enzyme *myosin light chain kinase* (MLCK), which in turn phosphorylates the myosin regulatory chain (**Figs. 18.1C** and **18.1D**). Phosphorylation of the regulatory chain (often called *cross-bridge phosphorylation*) permits actin–myosin interaction, and the cross-bridge cycling starts (**Fig. 18.1E**). The

Table 18.1 Structural Differences between Skeletal and Smooth Muscle Fibers

Skeletal Muscle Fiber	Smooth Muscle Fiber
Large, cylindrical, and multinucleate	Small, spindle-shaped, and uninucleate
Well-developed T-tubules	Caveoli, which are rudimentary T-tubules
HZ-disks	Dense bodies that are analogous to Z-disks
Actin and myosin filaments are roughly equal in number.	Actin filaments far outnumber the myosin filaments.
Actin filaments are parallel.	Actin filaments radiate from the dense bodies.

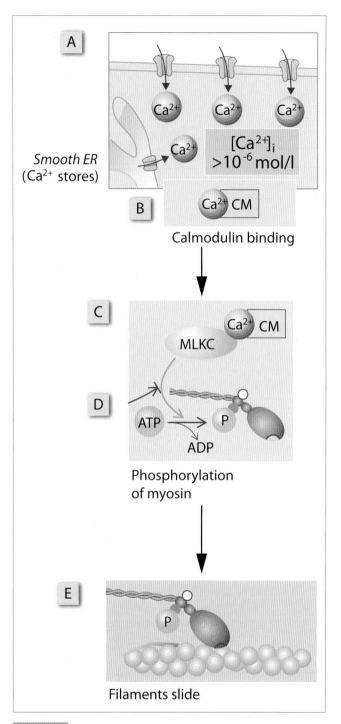

Fig. 18.1 Control of cross-bridge cycling in smooth muscle. ADP, adenosine diphosphate; ATP, adenosine triphosphate; CM, calmodulin; MLCK, myosin light chain kinase.

cycling stops when another enzyme, called *myosin phosphatase,* dephosphorylates the regulatory chain.

Variability of the average cycling rate ‖ Cross-bridge cycling occurs only when the myosin cross-bridge is phosphorylated. Dephosphorylation prevents the attachment as well as the detachment of cross-bridges. In a smooth muscle cell, some cross-bridges may be cycling, whereas others are halted at any one instant, depending on whether or not the cross-bridge is phosphorylated. Hence, the average cycling rate of all the cross-bridges in a sarcomere at any instant can be anything from zero (when none of the cross-bridges are phosphorylated) to maximum (when all the cross-bridges are phosphorylated).

Latch mechanism | When the cycling rate is high, the work done is high, too. The shortening speed and the contractile force rise. When the average cycling rate is low, work done is also low. The shortening speed is low, and so is the active tension generated. However, the resistance to passive tension in the muscle increases. This is because as the cycling rate decreases, more and more myosin heads remain *latched* to the actin filament.

When the rate of cross-bridge cycling nears zero, the energy consumption is minimal, and the muscle goes into a state that is analogous to the contraction remainder of a fatigued skeletal muscle: such a muscle cannot generate active tension but can effectively resist passive stretching. This suits the smooth muscle well because in most instances, it has to resist stretch rather than actively move a load. Smooth muscles are mostly found in the walls of hollow viscera that must resist excessive stretching, such as the arterial walls. Rarely is smooth muscle required to move a heavy load.

Plasticity | The smooth muscle defies the usual length–tension relationship that is valid for striated muscles. Unlike a striated muscle fiber that can contract to roughly 60% of its initial length, a smooth muscle fiber can contract to almost 30% of its initial length. Similarly, when stretched passively, the passive tension it develops gradually reduces to the prestretch level. In other words, whether actively contracted or passively stretched, the smooth muscle fiber tends to behave as if it is always at its resting length. This phenomenon is called plasticity and is possible due to a process in which the thick filaments dissolve and reorganize themselves so that at longer fiber lengths, the thick filaments are shorter but more numerous and are disposed in series. Conversely, at shorter lengths, the thick filaments are longer and are disposed in parallel (**Fig. 18.2**).

Excitation and Inhibition of Smooth Muscle

Based on how smooth muscles are stimulated or inhibited, smooth muscle cells are classified into single-unit and multiunit types. *Multiunit smooth muscles* are stimulated only

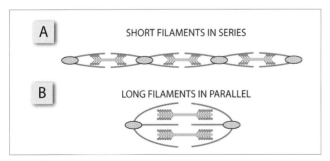

Fig. 18.2 Forty-eight cross-bridges disposed in series (A) and parallel (B).

through nerves, quite like skeletal muscle fibers. *Single-unit smooth muscles* show ephaptic conduction; that is, the excitation spreads from cell to cell via gap-junctions, resulting in the contraction of all the fibers in a unit. Single-unit smooth muscles are excited in several ways that include (1) spontaneous excitation through a pacemaker, (2) ephaptic excitation from adjacent cells, (3) stimulation through autonomic nerves—by neurotransmitters, (4) stimulation by hormones, (5) stimulation by stretch, and (6) stimulation by cold temperature.

Some hormones and neurotransmitters even inhibit smooth muscle contraction. For inhibition to occur, the muscle must already be contracting in response to some other excitatory stimulus. For example, a smooth muscle excited through a pacemaker is inhibited by a nerve secreting inhibitory neurotransmitter. Smooth muscles that remain contracted most of the time and relax only in response to inhibitory stimuli are called *tonic smooth muscles.* Examples of tonic smooth muscles are the smooth muscles of gastrointestinal and urogenital sphincters. Smooth muscles located in the walls of blood vessels and airways also remain partially contracted. On the other hand, muscles forming the walls of gastrointestinal and urogenital tracts remain mostly relaxed and contract only in response to excitatory stimuli. These are called *phasic smooth muscles.*

General Model: Communications

Smooth muscle is responsive to information reaching it from a variety of sources, including cell–cell communications via circulating humoral agents and via neural transmission.

Mechanisms of Excitation–Contraction Coupling

With so many types of stimuli exciting a smooth muscle, the excitation–contraction coupling in smooth muscle is not unexpectedly a diverse phenomenon. There are at least three different ways in which the smooth muscle excitation can be coupled to its contraction and two sources from which Ca^{2+} can be mobilized: extracellular and intracellular (**Fig. 18.3**).

In **electromechanical coupling**, the smooth muscle is excited through sarcolemmal depolarization. When the membrane depolarizes, voltage-gated Ca^{2+} channels present on the sarcolemma open up, and Ca^{2+} moves into the sarcoplasm from the extracellular fluid. This Ca^{2+} stimulates the release of more Ca^{2+} from the sarcoplasmic reticulum (SR). This is called *Ca^{2+}-induced Ca^{2+} release* (CICR). A fully fledged action potential (AP) is not always required for electromechanical coupling. In a multiunit smooth muscle fiber, even subthreshold electrotonic depolarizations can raise the sarcoplasmic Ca^{2+} sufficiently to bring about excitation–contraction coupling.

A fall in temperature also excites the smooth muscles. It does so by inhibiting the Na^+–K^+ pump, thereby depolarizing the sarcolemma. This is possible because, unlike in striated muscles, the Na^+–K^+ pump makes a substantial direct contribution to membrane potential in smooth muscle.

In **pharmacomechanical coupling**, the muscle is excited by chemical agents in the absence of any membrane depolariza-

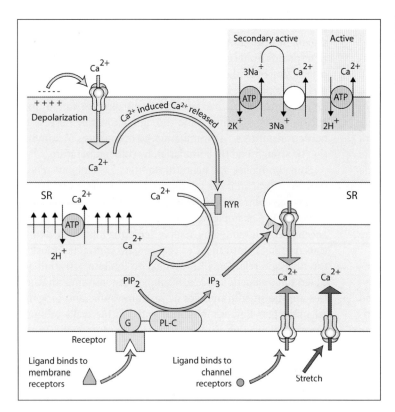

Fig. 18.3 Excitation–contraction coupling in smooth muscle. Note that calcium enters the sarcoplasm from the extracellular space through several different mechanisms (most important) *and* from the sarcoplasmic reticulum (less important because the sarcoplasmic reticulum is poorly developed in smooth muscle). ATP, adenosine triphosphate; G, G protein; IP, PIP, PL-C, phospholipase C; RYR, ryanodine receptor; SR, sarcoplasmic reticulum.

tion. There are two mechanisms of pharmacomechanical coupling: (1) Neurotransmitters and hormones bind to membrane receptors to activate group II hormonal mechanisms (see Chapter 75) to release Ca^{2+} from the SR. (2) Neurotransmitters and hormones bind directly to ligand-gated Ca^{2+} channels on the sarcolemma and open them up, letting in extracellular Ca^{2+}.

In **mechanomechanical coupling**, smooth muscles are excited by stretch, which opens up stretch-sensitive Ca^{2+} channels on the sarcolemma, letting in extracellular Ca^{2+}.

General Model: Flow

The entry (flow) of Ca^{2+} into the sarcoplasm, whether from the SR or the extracellular space, is driven by the concentration gradient for calcium.

Resting Membrane Potential

Unlike in the skeletal muscle, the resting membrane potential (RMP) of the smooth muscle cell is less, approximately –50 mV. In single-unit smooth muscles, the RMP is often unstable, oscillating between –55 and –35 mV. These oscillations are called *pacemaker potentials*. They occur due to rhythmic changes in either Ca^{2+} channel permeability or the activity of the Na^+–K^+ pump. In skeletal muscle, the electrogenicity of the Na^+–K^+ pump contributes directly very little to the RMP. In smooth muscle, the Na^+–K^+ pump makes a more significant contribution (–20 mV) to the RMP.

Action Potentials

In multiunit smooth muscle, even a subthreshold depolarization without an AP is associated with some amount of contrac-

tion. APs are, however, essential for single-unit smooth muscle to contract because only an AP can excite several smooth muscle fibers through ephaptic conduction. A subthreshold depolarization will fade out after traveling a short distance. In single-unit smooth muscle, the excitation needs to spread from cell to cell. Not unexpectedly, subthreshold depolarizations have no role in the contraction of single-unit smooth muscle.

The APs in single-unit smooth muscles (**Fig. 18.4**) are of three types: (1) spike potentials, which are similar to the AP in a skeletal muscle fiber; (2) APs with plateaus, which are similar to cardiac APs; and (3) spikes on oscillatory pacemaker potentials, which are observed only in smooth muscles.

There is a slow and rhythmic oscillation of the resting membrane potential between –55 and –35 mV. Spike potentials are triggered, in singles or in bursts, only at the peak of the oscillations when the potential touches the firing level. The pacemaker potentials themselves are not associated with contractions. Contractions occur only after the spikes.

Effect of Autonomic Neurotransmitters

Smooth muscles are innervated only by autonomic nerves. The potentials generated in smooth muscle when they are stimulated through autonomic nerves are called *junctional potentials*. They may be excitatory junctional potentials (EJPs) or inhibitory junctional potentials (IJPs), depending on whether the neurotransmitter secreted at the junction depolarizes or hyperpolarizes the smooth muscle membrane.

Acetylcholine | ACh binds to ligand-gated ACh receptors present on smooth muscles and depolarizes the membrane. The ACh receptors present on smooth muscles are of the muscarinic type. In multiunit smooth muscles, the depolarization triggers APs. In single-unit smooth muscles with spontaneous

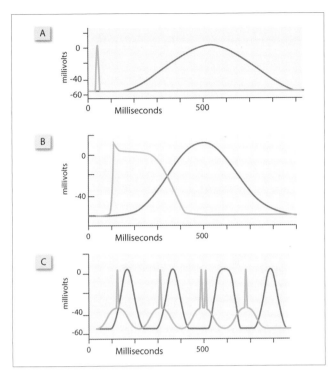

Fig. 18.4 Action potentials (green) and the resulting contractions (yellow) in smooth muscles. **(A)** A single spike potential producing a single muscle twitch. **(B)** Action potential with a plateau. It is associated with a prolonged contraction. **(C)** Pacemaker potential with superimposed spikes.

APs, the depolarization results in a higher frequency of APs. The APs themselves become slightly smaller and wider. The contractions become stronger and more frequent.

The effect of **catecholamines** on smooth muscle depends on the type of receptor stimulated. Adrenergic receptors are of two types, α and β. In general, β-adrenoceptors are inhibitory, causing relaxation, whereas α-adrenoceptors may be either excitatory or inhibitory. Inhibitory α- and β-adrenoceptors are widely distributed in gastrointestinal smooth muscles. *Excitatory α-adrenoceptors* are present mainly in vascular and urogenital smooth muscles and gastrointestinal sphincters. They produce membrane depolarization by increasing Na^+ permeability. *Inhibitory α-adrenoceptors* induce relaxation mainly through membrane hyperpolarization caused by an increase in K^+ permeability. The inhibition is quicker and short-lasting. *Inhibitory β-adrenoceptors* induce relaxation mainly by suppressing spontaneous pacemaker activity, with or without hyperpolarization of the membrane. The spike characteristics are not affected much.

Effects of Ovarian Hormones

The effects of ovarian hormones on uterine smooth muscle are complicated by the type of excitation–contraction coupling, hormonal interactions, and differences in the circular and longitudinal uterine smooth muscles. In general, estrogens stimulate and progesterone relaxes uterine smooth muscles. Stimulation generally occurs when the muscle depolarizes,

and its spike-frequency increases. Conversely, inhibition occurs when the muscle hyperpolarizes, and the spike frequency decreases.

Occasionally, both estrogen and progesterone violate this general rule, possibly because they affect both electromechanical and pharmacomechanical coupling. For example, they may stimulate contractions through pharmacomechanical coupling while inhibiting the spike discharges.

Summary

- The contractile mechanism of smooth muscle is the same as that of skeletal muscle.

- Intracellular Ca^{2+} interacts with different control proteins; smooth muscle has no troponin/tropomyosin, but uses calmodulin and myosin light chain kinase to activate myosin ATPase.

- Multiunit smooth muscle and single-unit smooth muscle are stimulated and inhibited by different mechanisms.

- Electrical stimulation of smooth muscle can involve a variety of different membrane electrical phenomena (APs and/or slow depolarizations).

- Smooth muscle is innervated by the autonomic nervous system, which can stimulate or inhibit its contraction.

Applying What You Know

18.1. If dantrolene blocks the release of Ca^{2+} in smooth muscle (and it is not known whether this occurs or not), how would that effect manifest itself in the course of Mr. Wright's stay in the operating room? What would you expect to observe that does not, in fact, seem to be present?

Cardiac muscle fibers are of two types: nonautomatic and automatic. The nonautomatic fibers of the atria and ventricles generate contractile force. The automatic fibers are spontaneously excitable and constitute the conducting system of the heart. They contribute relatively little to force generation, as they have fewer myofibrils and mitochondria and have poorly developed sarcoplasmic reticulum.

Cardiac muscle has functional resemblances with both smooth muscle and skeletal muscle. Cardiac muscle resembles visceral smooth muscle in that it shows automaticity and ephaptic conduction, and its contractility is affected by hormones. Cardiac muscle resembles skeletal muscle in that it contains regular sarcomeres delimited by Z-disks and shows similar length–tension relationship; additionally, its contraction is regulated by the troponin–tropomyosin complex.

Cardiac Action Potentials

Cardiac action potentials (APs) are more like those of the smooth muscle than those of neurons or skeletal muscle. The APs of automatic cardiac fibers comprise single spikes on the peaks of an oscillating membrane potential. APs of nonautomatic cardiac fibers have a characteristic plateau. This prolonged plateau increases the duration of the cardiac AP.

Action Potential in Nonautomatic Cardiac Fibers

The AP in a nonautomatic cardiac fiber shows a characteristic plateau. In all, it has five phases (**Fig. 19.1**). The absolute refractory period of cardiac AP includes phases 0, 1, and 2; in phase 3, the cardiac muscle is in the relative refractory period. The cardiac AP is thus refractory for most of its duration.

Phase 0 is the phase of depolarization that occurs due to the opening of Na^+ channels, resulting in a *fast inward depolarizing current*.

Phase 1 is the partial repolarization that occurs due to sodium (Na^+) channel inactivation and a transient increase in potassium (K^+) permeability (the *transient outward K^+ current*).

Phase 2 is the plateau during which the membrane repolarizes either very slowly or not at all. It occurs due to (1) the opening of sarcolemmal *L-type calcium (Ca^{2+}) channels* (L for long-lasting) that lets in a slow, inward depolarizing current and (2) the closure of a distinct set of K^+ channels called the *inward rectifying K^+ channels*.

The K^+ channels normally open up when the membrane depolarizes. In cardiac muscles, some K^+ channels (the inward-rectifying K^+ channels) do exactly the opposite; that is, they remain open when the membrane is polarized and close down with depolarization. Hence, at the resting membrane potential, they make a substantial contribution to the total K^+ current. Conversely, during the sustained depolarization of the plateau phase, they close down. If they remained open during depolarization, large amounts of K^+ would flow out of the cell throughout the plateau phase, a loss that would be difficult to replenish.

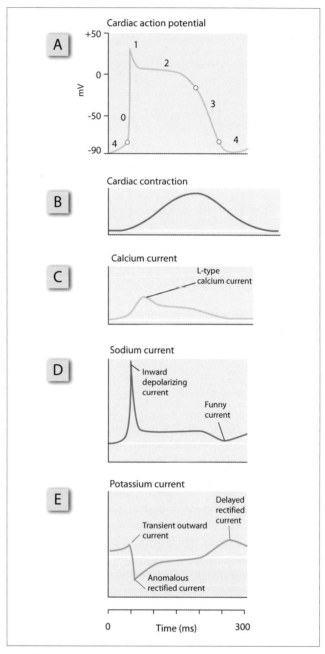

Fig. 19.1 **(A)** Cardiac action potential and **(B)** the resulting cardiac contraction. Also shown are **(C)** calcium (Ca^{2+}), **(D)** sodium (Na^+), and **(E)** potassium (K^+) currents associated with the action potential.

Phase 3 is the phase of complete repolarization. It occurs due to two outward K^+ currents through two different types of K^+ channels: (1) The *delayed outward rectified K^+ current* flows through voltage-gated channels that are activated slowly. (2) The *Ca^{2+}-activated K^+ current* flows through K^+ channels that are activated by the elevated sarcoplasmic Ca^{2+} levels.

Phase 4 is the resting phase with a potential of about –90 mV. It is maintained by a *resting K^+ current*, the largest contributor to which is the inward rectifying K^+ current mentioned above.

Action Potential in Automatic Cardiac Fibers

Phases of action potential | The AP of an automatic cardiac fiber shows salient differences from that of a nonautomatic fiber (**Fig. 19.2A**). (1) The RMP is less negative (–70 mV) than in nonautomatic cardiac fibers (–90 mV). (2) Phase 0 is less steep, and its peak is less sharp (more rounded) than phase 0 in nonautomatic fibers. This is because the depolarization in phase 0 occurs due to an increase in Ca^{2+} permeability. This is unlike phase 0 of nonautomatic cells, which is produced by an increase in Na^+ permeability. (3) In the absence of the plateau (phase 2), phases 1 and 3 blend into a single phase of repolarization called phase 3. (4) Phase 4 of the AP shows a slow drift toward the threshold potential until phase 0 is triggered. This characteristic phase 4 is also called the *pacemaker potential* or the *diastolic depolarization.*

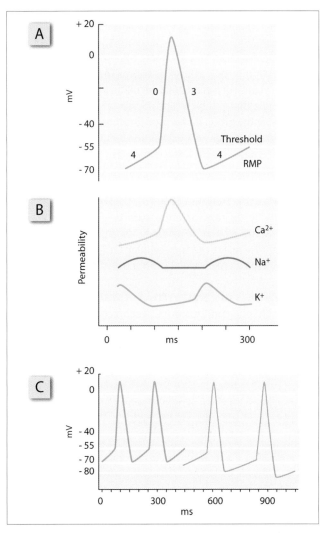

Fig. 19.2 **(A)** Cardiac pacemaker potential and **(B)** the associated permeability changes to calcium (Ca^{2+}; top), sodium (Na^+; middle), and potassium (K^+; bottom). **(C)** Effect of acetylcholine on cardiac pacemaker. RMP, resting membrane potential.

Ionic basis of pacemaker potential | Permeability changes in all three ions, that is, Na^+, K^+, and Ca^{2+} (**Fig. 19.2B**), are responsible for the slow diastolic depolarization. (1) The "funny" *Na^+ current* is carried by a population of funny Na^+ channels that open up when the membrane hyperpolarizes beyond –50 mV (instead of closing down like the regular Na^+ channels). The resulting Na^+ influx depolarizes the membrane toward threshold. (2) The *outward (delayed) rectifier K^+ current* is carried by channels that open up with depolarization and close down as the membrane repolarizes (just like ordinary channels). However, the opening and closing of channels are somewhat slow or delayed; therefore, there is a slight phase lag between the membrane potential and the K^+ permeability changes. As a result, when the membrane is fully depolarized, the K^+ permeability is still increasing. Conversely, when the membrane is fully repolarized, the K^+ permeability is still decreasing. This delayed decrease in outward K^+ current following full repolarization contributes to the subsequent diastolic depolarization. (3) An *inward Ca^{2+} current* contributes to phase 4 depolarization.

Autonomic effects | Epinephrine stimulates the β receptors of sinoatrial (SA) node cells, thus increasing the rate of phase 4 depolarization and decreasing the threshold for firing. This, of course, results in an increase of heart rate.

Acetylcholine (ACh) stimulates the muscarinic receptors of the SA node cells, hyperpolarizing the pacemaker cells, reducing the steepness of the phase 4 depolarization, and finally making the threshold for firing more positive (**Fig. 19.2C**). All of these changes result in a slower heart rate.

Abnormal Potassium Currents

Certain types of K^+ channels assume importance in cardiac disorders (**Table 19.1**). Arachidonic acid and other fatty acids that are liberated from ischemic cardiac cells activate *arachidonic acid-activated K^+ channels,* thereby shortening the duration of the cardiac AP and with it, the duration of cardiac systole. The effect is more pronounced at the acidic pH that is often present during ischemia.

In addition, there are the *Na^+-activated potassium channels* that get activated in a heart overloaded with Na^+ ions, following digitalis administration, for example. Hence, the Q-T interval of the electrocardiogram (ECG) is shortened in a patient receiving digitalis.

Cardiac Contraction

Excitation–Contraction Coupling

As in smooth muscle, the sarcoplasmic Ca^{2+} concentration in the cardiac muscle is kept low by two types of Ca^{2+} transport across the muscle cell membrane. One is a primary active transport in which a Ca^{2+}-$2H^+$ antiport occurs using Ca^{2+}-ATPase for splitting ATP. The other is a secondary active transport in which a passive Ca^{2+}-$3Na^+$ antiport is coupled to an active Na^+–K^+ antiport (**Fig. 19.3**).

The sarcoplasmic Ca^{2+} pulse is produced predominantly by mobilization of intracellular Ca^{2+} from the sarcoplasmic reticulum when the ryanodine channels on lateral cisterns open

Table 19.1 Normal and Abnormal Cardiac Potassium (K^+) Currents of Clinical Importance

Normal K^+ Currents	Role
Transient outward K^+ current	Opens briefly immediately after depolarization; contributes to early repolarization
Anomalous (inward) rectifier K^+ current	Responsible for the resting potential; closes with repolarization; thus, opposes depolarization and prolongs the plateau
Delayed (outward) rectified K^+ current	Opens at the end of plateau
	Initiates repolarization.
Ca^{2+}-activated K^+ current	Activated by the rise in sarcoplasmic Ca^{2+} concentration that occurs at the onset of contraction; accelerates repolarization and thereby shortens the action potential
ACh-activated K^+ current	Activated in response to vagal stimulation; hyperpolarizes the resting cell, thereby slowing the sinoatrial node and shortening the atrial action potential
Abnormal K^+ currents	Role
Na^+-activated K^+ current	Activated by high sarcoplasmic Na^+ concentrations; accelerates repolarization in a Na^+-overloaded heart
ATP-sensitive K^+ current	Normally inhibited by adenosine triphosphate (ATP); opens in energy-starved heart
Arachidonic acid-activated K^+ current	Activated by arachidonic acid and other fatty acids, especially at acidic pH

up. This mobilization is triggered by a smaller amount of extracellular Ca^{2+} that enters through the sarcolemma when the membrane is excited, and binds to the ryanodine receptors. This process is called *calcium-induced calcium release* (CICR). Although cardiac fibers show T-tubules as in skeletal muscle fibers, these T-tubules do little else other than to let in extracellular Ca^{2+} like the rest of the sarcolemma. The influx of Ca^{2+} into the cardiac muscle cell is essential for contraction of cardiac muscle; the intracellular stores are not sufficient to maintain contact for many beats. The contraction starts just after depolarization and lasts until ~50 msec after repolarization is completed (**Fig. 19.1**).

Cross-bridge Cycling and Sliding of Filaments

The cross-bridge cycling in cardiac muscle is no different from that of skeletal or smooth muscle. However, its regulation shares the features of both. Like the skeletal muscle, its onset and termination are controlled by the troponin–tropomyosin complex. Like the smooth muscle, the contractility of cardiac muscle is sensitive to phosphorylation.

Modulation of Cardiac Muscle Contractility

Phosphorylation | At least three components of the cardiac excitation–contraction coupling machinery are susceptible to phosphorylation (**Fig. 19.3**). (1) Phosphorylation of sarcoplasmic Ca^{2+} channels results in their remaining open for longer durations. Sarcoplasmic Ca^{2+} concentration therefore rises and results in quicker and stronger contraction. (2) Phosphorylation of troponin-I inhibits binding of Ca^{2+} to troponin-C, thereby facilitating relaxation. (3) *Phospholamban* is a regulatory protein present only in cardiac muscles. It controls the activity of the sarcoplasmic Ca^{2+} pump. When phosphorylated, phospholamban stimulates the Ca^{2+} pump in the L-tubules and lowers sarcoplasmic Ca^{2+} concentration, thereby accelerating relaxation. The overall effect of activation of the intracellular phosphorylation system is to increase the strength of contraction (positive inotropic effect), and speed of contraction (positive chronotropic effect), as well as to quicken relaxation. Phosphorylation of intracellular regulatory proteins is induced by catecholamines, which bind to sarcolemmal β_1 receptors and activate the group IIa hormonal mechanism.

Membrane pump and exchanger | The Na^+–K^+ pump on the sarcolemma lowers intracellular Na^+. This promotes the entry of extracellular Na^+ into the cell in exchange for Ca^{2+} efflux. In other words, the sarcolemma pumps out Ca^{2+} through secondary active transport (**Fig. 19.3**). Inhibition of this active transport—by digitalis or other cardiac glycosides (a group of structurally similar to compounds that increase cardiac contractility)—raises the intracellular Ca^{2+} concentration and thereby increases myocardial contractility.

Characteristics of Cardiac Muscle Contraction

Due to ephaptic conduction between cardiac myocytes, the contraction of cardiac muscle obeys the all-or-none law: it either contracts completely or does not contract at all, depending on whether the strength of the stimulus is threshold or subthreshold.

General Model: Communications

This type of cell–cell communications is an essential feature of cardiac muscle and contributes to the coordinated contraction of the entire heart so that pumping of blood results.

Cardiac muscle also shows summation of contraction. When a quiescent cardiac muscle starts contracting spontaneously (as occurs at the onset of idioventricular rhythm), its first few contractions show a progressive increase in height. The phenomenon is known as the positive staircase effect

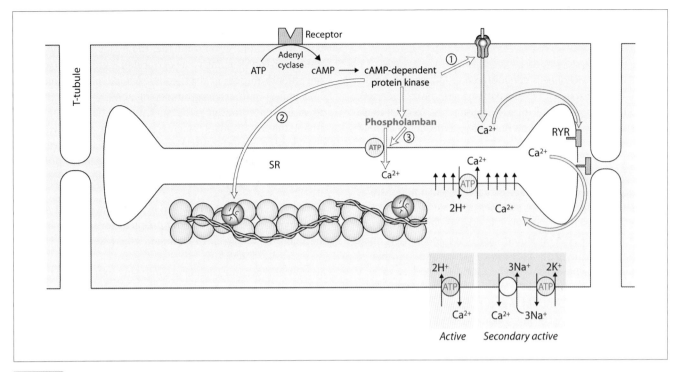

Fig. 19.3 Excitation–contraction coupling in cardiac muscle and the modulation of cardiac contractility. ATP, adenosine triphosphate; cAMP, cyclic adenosine monophosphate; RYR, ryanodine receptor; SR, sarcoplasmic reticulum.

(**Fig. 19.4**) and occurs due to the cumulative increase in sarcoplasmic calcium concentration. A similar *positive staircase effect* is seen over a few beats immediately after an increase in heart rate. Conversely, a *negative staircase effect* (progressive reduction in strength of contraction) is observed for a few seconds immediately after a decrease in heart rate.

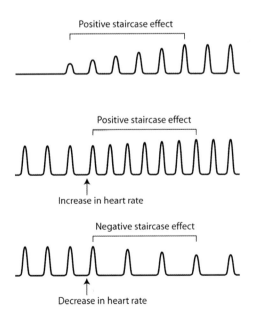

Fig. 19.4 Summation of cardiac contraction. Positive staircase effect occurs when a quiescent heart starts beating or when there is a sudden increase in heart rate. Negative staircase effect occurs following a sudden decrease in heart rate.

Although cardiac contractions show the staircase effect, they never fuse together because the cardiac muscle cannot be stimulated in quick succession due to its long refractory period. Thus, unlike skeletal muscle, cardiac muscle cannot be tetanized.

Summary

- Cardiac muscle shares some properties with skeletal muscle (an ordered array of actin and myosin, use of troponin and tropomyosin as control proteins) and some properties with smooth muscle (automaticity, electrical coupling of cells).

- The ventricle muscle cell (force generating) has an AP that is due to the interaction of several different voltage-dependent membrane channels.

- The AP of SA node and conducting system cells exhibit automaticity (spontaneous firing); its rate of firing is controlled by the autonomic nervous system.

- Unlike skeletal muscle, contraction of cardiac muscle is dependent on the entry of Ca^{2+} from the external cellular fluid.

Applying What You Know

19.1. If dantrolene blocks the release of Ca^{2+} in cardiac muscle (and it is not clear that this actually occurs), how would that effect manifest in the course of Mr. Wright's experience in the operating room? What would you expect to observe that does not, in fact, seem to be present?

Answers to Applying What You Know

Chapter 13

1 When succinylcholine is administered to Mr. Wright, he develops a flaccid paralysis. When halothane anesthesia is started, he quickly develops skeletal muscle contractures. Contrast these two quite different states of his muscles in terms of the state of his sarcomeres.

When Mr. Wright is in a state of flaccid paralysis, no force is being generated by his muscles, and the sarcomeres are at their resting length, with little or no overlap between actin and myosin. When the muscles are maximally contracted (contractures present), the sarcomeres are short, and there is maximal overlap of the actin and myosin (maximum number of cross-bridges are possible).

2 Describe the sequence of events that occur at the skeletal muscles when succinylcholine is administered to Mr. Wright. What happens to his muscles, and why does it happen?

When succinylcholine is administered to Mr. Wright, the drug binds to ACh receptors at his motor end plates. These receptors open, an inward Na^+ current is generated, and an end-plate potential results. The muscle cells are depolarized, and fire action potentials (APs) and contraction occur. However, the succinylcholine molecule is resistant to degradation by AChesterase, and the receptor therefore remains open. The muscle membrane is subjected to a sustained depolarization. This causes the voltage-dependent Na^+ channels in the muscle membrane to enter the inactive state, and thus the muscle membrane becomes electrically inexcitable. With no APs being generated, there is no release of Ca^{2+} from the sarcoplasmic reticulum (SR). The Ca^{2+} pump in the SR membrane sequesters calcium in the SR, reducing the Ca^{2+} concentration around the cross-bridges. This results in a flaccid paralysis.

Chapter 14

1 Dantrolene is administered to Mr. Wright to stop the continuous cycling of his skeletal muscle cross-bridges and the consequent hyperthermia and hyperkalemia. Explain how dantrolene accomplishes this. Why are Mr. Wright's heart and vascular smooth muscle not affected?

The Ca^{2+} that triggers contraction of skeletal muscle comes from the SR. The amount of Ca^{2+} stored in the SR and released is more than enough to raise the intracellular concentration of Ca^{2+} to the level required to produce contraction in skeletal muscle. This means that skeletal muscle contraction is independent of the extracellular concentration of Ca^{2+}.

Dantrolene prevents the exit of Ca^{2+} from the SR. The continued action of the inward Ca pump in the SR membrane then sequesters the Ca^{2+} back in the SR, reducing the concentration in the sarcoplasm. Muscle contraction ceases.

In cardiac and smooth muscle, there is a source of Ca^{2+} in addition to the SR, namely, the extracellular fluid. When cardiac and smooth muscle is electrically excited, voltage-dependent Ca channels in the sarcolemma open, and Ca^{2+} enters the cells down its concentration gradient. Thus, the Ca^{2+} concentration around the cross-bridges is increased by Ca^{2+} from the SR (poorly developed in smooth muscle) and from outside the cell. Dantrolene therefore has little effect on these two forms of muscle because it does not block the entry of extracellular calcium.

2 Mr. Wright develops a marked hyperkalemia at the height of his abnormal response to being prepared for surgery. By what mechanism is Mr. Wright's plasma $[K^+]$ increased?

Mr. Wright becomes hyperkalemic (his extracellular potassium concentration increases above normal) when the ATP in his muscle is depleted by the continuous cross-bridge cycling that is occurring. With decreased ATP availability, the Na^+–K^+ pump in the sarcolemma slows down, and the rate of K^+ influx also slows; therefore, the extracellular concentration rises. It is also likely that the sarcolemma is damaged by these changes, thus resulting in the intracellular K^+ being "dumped" into the extracellular fluid.

3 Mr. Wright also develops a marked lactic acidosis. What is the mechanism by which this occurs? Is this response related to the hyperkalemia that is present? Explain.

The continuous cycling of cross-bridges causes a depletion of ATP in the muscle cell. At the same time, the rigidly contracted muscle compresses the blood vessels perfusing it, and the supply of oxygen to the muscle is compromised. The result of both these processes is that glycolysis (the metabolism of glycogen, a storage form of glucose) is promoted in an effort to continue the production of ATP. Lactic acid is a by-product of the glycolysis metabolic pathway.

Chapter 15

1 Predict what pattern of neural activity you would observe in Mr. Wright's motor nerves during his contractures. Explain.

Mr. Wright's muscle contractures are the result of the release of Ca^{2+} from his muscle SR trigger by the interaction of the halothane anesthesia and a genetic defect involving his SR calcium channels. The contractures occur independently of activity in his motor nerves and chemical transmission at the neuromuscular junction. The halothane has certainly rendered Mr. Wright unconscious, and it is therefore unlikely that there is any neural activity in his motor nerves.

2 During Mr. Wright's contractures, what muscle fiber types are active? Explain.

Because Mr. Wright's contractures are *not* the result of neural inputs to the muscles, but are the result of dumping calcium into the myoplasm, all types of muscle fibers will be affected.

Chapter 16

1 Mr. Wright exhibits stiff joints while being anesthetized. Describe the contractions occurring at a joint under these conditions.

Mr. Wright's stiff joints are a consequence of the simultaneous contraction of all of the muscles around a joint. Under these conditions, when muscles with opposing actions are contracting at the same time, there is little or no movement of the joint. This means that the muscles are contracting isometrically because no shortening is occurring.

Chapter 18

1 If dantrolene blocks the release of Ca^{2+} in smooth muscle (and it is not known whether this occurs or not), how would that effect manifest itself in the course of Mr. Wright's stay in the operating room? What would you expect to observe that does not, in fact, seem to be present?

If dantrolene blocked the release of Ca^{2+} in smooth muscle, one consequence would be reduced contraction of vascular smooth muscle, vasodilatation (blood vessels would get larger), and a fall in blood pressure. Mr. Wright does experience a fall in blood pressure, but only when his cardiac arrhythmia (irregular heartbeat) reduces cardiac pumping, which then reduces the flow of blood out of the heart.

Chapter 19

1 If dantrolene blocks the release of Ca^{2+} in cardiac muscle (and it is not clear that this actually occurs), how would that effect manifest in the course of Mr. Wright's experience in the operating room? What would you expect to observe that does not, in fact, seem to be present?

If dantrolene blocked the release of Ca^{2+} from cardiac muscle SR, the disinhibition of myosin–ATPase would be reduced, there would be less cross-bridge cycling, and less force would be generated. The ability of the heart to pump blood would be compromised, and blood pressure would fall. There is no evidence that this has occurred in Mr. Wright's case; the fall in pressure that eventually occurs is due to the arrhythmia that occurs.

Furthermore, there is no unequivocal evidence that dantrolene affects the calcium release channel in cardiac muscle. There are many calcium channel subtypes, and it does not appear that the subtypes present in cardiac muscle are altered in patients who experience malignant hyperthermia.

Section III Case Analysis:
Jeremy Wright's surgery goes wrong.

Clinical Overview

Review of patient condition | Jeremy Wright is prepped for routine gallbladder surgery with succinylcholine and then administered halothane anesthesia. He immediately develops malignant hyperthermia, and the surgery is halted.

Etiology | Certain individuals respond to general anesthetic agents, particularly gaseous ones, with a response in which skeletal muscle sarcoplasmic reticulum (SR) releases all of its stored calcium, continuously activating the contractile machinery, with several physiologic consequences following.

Malignant hyperthermia in response to anesthesia appears to be the result of any of a large number of single gene mutations affecting the synthesis of calcium (Ca^{2+}) release channels in muscle SR. Thus, there is a distinct tendency for this problem to occur in several members of a family.

Prevalence | The prevalence of the occurrence of this phenomenon is difficult to determine, with estimates ranging from 1 in 3000 to 1 in 50,000 surgical procedures. The prevalence of the gene mutations is even more difficult to determine because many individuals with such mutations may never be subjected to anesthesia in a way that would trigger malignant hyperthermia.

Diagnosis | The immediate presence of increased end-tidal PCO_2 (reflecting the greatly increased muscle metabolism), muscle rigidity, and rising temperature is diagnostic for this condition and should alert the surgical staff to take immediate measures to terminate the procedure and reverse the problem.

Treatment | Dantrolene is a drug that blocks the Ca^{2+} release channels in muscle SR. The Ca pumps present in the SR membrane then take up the Ca^{2+} in the muscle cytoplasm, sequestering it in the SR. This terminates the cross-bridge cycling that is generating heat (hyperthermia), causing the sodium–potassium (Na^+–K^+) pump to slow and $[K^+]_p$ to increase, causing a lactic acidosis, and resulting in tachycardia (elevated heart rate) and cardiac arrhythmias.

Understanding the Physiology

A skeletal muscle contracts when stimulated by the motor nerves that innervate it. This requires signal transmission at the motor end plate (neuromuscular junction). Succinylcholine blocks transmission by essentially binding to the acetylcholine (Ach) receptor in a nonreversible manner. Thus, the initial excitation that occurs following succinylcholine binding and the opening of the cation channel is followed by a flaccid paralysis of the muscles that can no longer respond to neural activity in the motor nerves. This flaccid paralysis makes surgical procedures through the wall of the abdomen much easier to accomplish.

However, certain individuals with any of several possible gene mutations respond to general anesthesia in an unusual way. The Ca^{2+} channels in their skeletal muscle SR open and stay open. The result is that the Ca^{2+} sequestered in the SR floods into the myoplasm, raising the $[Ca^{2+}]$ there. This disinhibits the myosin–adenosine triphosphatase (ATPase), causing sustained muscle contraction. Heat is an unavoidable by-product of the energy-yielding steps involved. With heat production dramatically increased and heat disposal mechanisms unable to keep up, body temperature must climb steeply.

The continuous cycling of the cross-bridges (sustained muscle contraction) begins to use up the adenosine triphosphate (ATP) available in the muscle and creates a hypermetabolic state in which oxygen (O_2) consumption increases, as does the generation of carbon dioxide (CO_2). One consequence is that the Na^+–K^+ pump begins to slow, and the accumulation of K^+ inside the cells decreases. The result is an increase in extracellular $[K^+]$ (hyperkalemia). At the same time, the decreased ATP availability, coupled with decreased muscle perfusion (in part because the contracted muscles compress the blood vessels perfusing the muscles), promotes anaerobic mechanism and the production of lactic acid. This causes a lactic acidosis (and the anion gap widens).

The effects of all these insults on the heart are to increase the firing rate of the sinoatrial node, the cardiac pacemaker, resulting in a tachycardia. Eventually, the heart rate can become erratic (an arrhythmia is present).

The treatment of a potentially lethal condition requires closing the SR Ca^{2+} channels so that the Ca^{2+} in the myoplasm can be pumped back into the SR, stopping the cross-bridge cycling and heat generation. Dantrolene is a drug that does exactly this in skeletal muscle. It is not clear whether dantrolene has the same effect on smooth muscle or cardiac muscle.

It is also essential that all of the effects resulting from the pathologic increase in muscle intracellular Ca^{2+} be brought under control: body temperature must be reduced, end-tidal CO_2 brought back to normal, pH restored to normal, $[K^+]$ reduced, the arrhythmia eliminated, and the tachycardia reversed. The seriousness of these conditions explains why continued monitoring of the patient in the intensive care unit is necessary.

The accompanying flow chart (**Fig. III.1**) illustrates the mechanisms that generate Mr. Wright's condition.

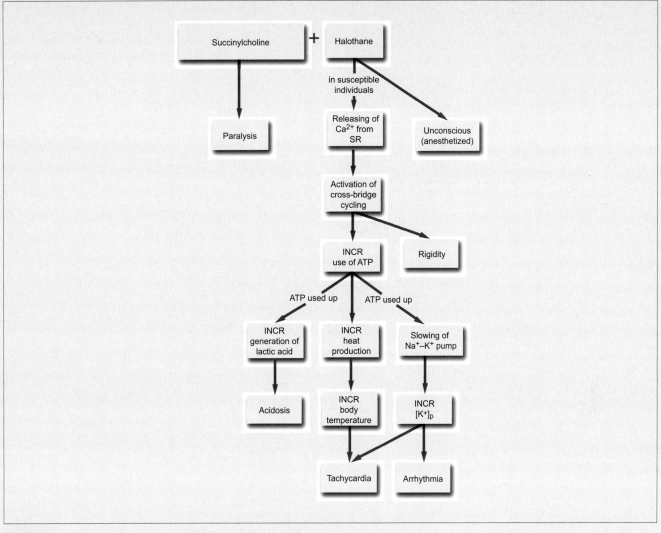

Fig. III.1 Mr. Wright's response to halothane anesthesia is abnormal and unexpected. It is the consequence of a genetic defect that results in an SR membrane that reacts to the anesthetic by opening calcium channels.

Section IV | Blood and Immune System

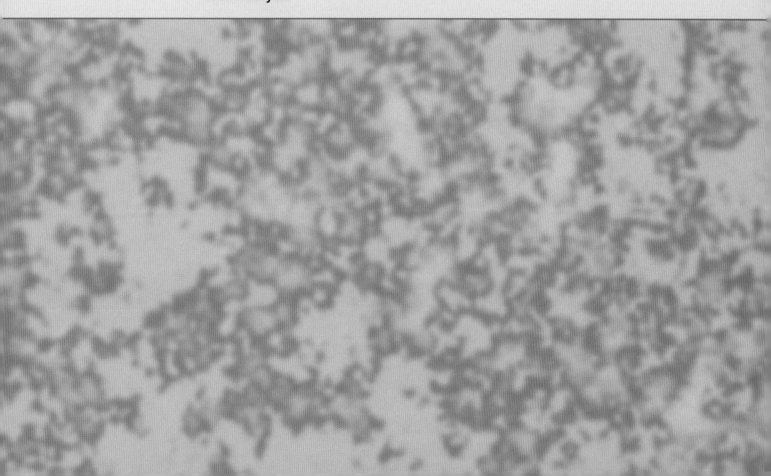

Overview

Blood is a fluid (plasma) in which are suspended several kinds of cells. Blood has several important functions. (1) It transports oxygen, carbon dioxide, nutrients, hormones, and so on, around the body as it is pumped through the circulation. Some of these substances are present in solution, and others are carried by red blood cells. (2) Damage to the integrity of the circulatory system is maintained by the clotting mechanisms, a complex system of cells, the platelets, and proteins in solution. (3) The blood is a major locus for the body's immune system.

Red blood cells (RBCs) are produced in bone marrow and are filled with hemoglobin, a protein that reversibly binds oxygen. The production of RBCs is regulated by the hormone erythropoietin. Hematinic factors that promote the production of RBCs and hemoglobin include iron (an essential component of hemoglobin), folic acid, and vitamin B_{12}.

Blood clotting results from the interaction of plasma proteins and a large number of clotting factors, which activate one another to produce a blood clot. The clotting process must be carefully controlled to stop bleeding where and when it occurs but not cause clots to form, because they can damage the circulation by blocking blood flow.

The immune system is made up of five different white blood cells and other cells. The system destroys foreign invaders (bacteria, viruses, proteins), as well as damaged endogenous cells (e.g., tumor cells).

Chief Complaint

Erik Lundquist, a 50-year-old executive, is seen by his primary care physician complaining of gradually increasing fatigue and shortness of breath on exertion.

History of Present Illness

Mr. Lundquist reports that he began to notice episodes of troubling fatigue ~5 years ago. About 6 months ago, his wife commented that he was beginning to look rather "yellowish." More recently, he noticed that his tongue was feeling "funny" all the time.

Past Medical History

Mr. Lundquist is a very busy executive and has not had time for a medical appointment for many years. He reports having been in good health except for an occasional cold in the winter. He takes a multivitamin and a baby aspirin each day (he had read that this is a good thing to do to prevent a heart attack). He plays tennis twice a week. He has a glass of wine with dinner and denies use of any street drugs.

Physical Examination

- *General appearance* | Overweight, with a yellowish pallor to his skin
- *Vital signs*
  - Height: 5 foot 6 inches
  - Weight: 143 pounds
  - Temperature: 99.9°F
  - Blood pressure: 135/82 mm Hg
  - Pulse: 100/min
  - Respirations: 20/min; quiet
- *HEENT (head, eyes, ears, nose, throat)* | Tongue is large, red, and smooth. Otherwise, everything is normal
- *Neck* | Possible mild distention of jugular veins
- *Lungs* | Except for mild hyperpnea, everything is normal.
- *Cardiac* | Tachycardia present and regular; no murmurs
- *Abdomen* | No organomegaly, no tenderness, normal bowel sounds
- *Extremities* | Normal
- *Neurologic exam* | Normal

Laboratory Studies

	Value	Normal
[Hb]	11 g/dL	13.5–17.5 (men)
Hct	33%	41–53 (men)
MCV	120 fL	80–100
MCH	33 pg	26–34
MCHC	27.5 g/dL	31–37
Serum folate	12 µg/L	
[B$_{12}$]	130 pmol/L	
LDH	3400 units	
Intrinsic factor antibodies	Present	Absent

Hb, hemoglobin; Hct, hematocrit; MCV, mean corpuscular volume; MCH, mean cell hemoglobin; MCHC, mean corpuscular hemoglobin concentration; LDH, lactate dehydrogenase.

Some Things to Think About

1. Where do red blood cells come from, and what determines their rate of production?

2. What is the mechanism that results in Mr. Lundquist's fatigue?

3. What roles do folates and vitamin B$_{12}$ play in generating Mr. Lundquist's condition?

4. What is the significance of the presence of intrinsic factor antibodies, and where do they come from?

Body Fluids

The percentage of body weight that is accounted for by water is ~60% in men, 50% in women, and 65 to 75% in infants. Women have the least proportion of body water because they have more adipose tissue than men. In both genders, water constitutes ~72% of the lean (adipose-free) body mass. In a man weighing 60 kg, the volume of total body water (TBW) is ~36 L. This water is divided into various compartments, as shown in **Fig. 20.1**. Approximately 66.6% of TBW is present in the intracellular compartment (ICF), and 33.3% is present in the extracellular compartment (ECF).

Extracellular fluid (ECF) is present outside the cells. Of the 12 L of ECF, 3 L is present inside the blood vessels as intravascular fluid or plasma, whereas the remainder is present around the cells as interstitial fluid and is separated from the intravascular fluid only by the walls of the blood vessels. Some of the ECF is present in specialized compartments and is called transcellular fluid. Examples include cerebrospinal fluid, synovial fluid, pleural fluid, pericardial fluid, peritoneal fluid, intraocular fluid, gastrointestinal secretions, and urine.

The volume of the various body compartments can be measured by injecting into them an indicator substance and then estimating its volume of distribution from the degree of its dilution. The indicator substance used must fulfill certain criteria. For measurement of body fluid compartments, the most relevant consideration is that the indicator should remain confined to the compartment whose volume is to be measured and should get uniformly diluted by the fluid in the compartment (**Table 20.1**). Other considerations are that the indicator should be nontoxic; should not change (pharmacologically or otherwise) the fluid volume; should not be metabolized, al-

Table 20.1	Indicators for Measuring Body Fluid Compartments
Total body water (TBW) volume	Deuterium oxide (heavy water), tritium oxide, aminopyrine
Extracellular fluid (ECF) volume	Sodium thiosulfate, sucrose, inulin, mannitol
Intravascular space	Evans blue (T–1824), $^{131}I_2$ (These bind to plasma albumin, and therefore cannot escape from the blood vessels.)

tered, or excreted in significant amounts in a short time; and should be easy to estimate in the laboratory.

Two compartments whose volumes can only be calculated indirectly are the intracellular fluid (TBW volume – ECF volume) and the extravascular fluid (ECF volume – plasma volume).

Example

One hundred mg of inulin (a sugar that cannot enter cells) was injected intravenously into a 60 kg man. After 30 minutes, the inulin concentration was found to be 0.75 mg/dL. Also, 25 mg was excreted in urine during that period. Calculate the extracellular volume.

Solution

The ECF will be given by the volume of distribution of inulin, which is equal to

$$\text{vol} = \frac{\text{amt}}{\text{conc}} \qquad (20.1)$$

$$\text{vol} = \frac{100-25}{0.75} \times 100$$

$$\text{vol} = 10,000 \text{ mL} \, (10 \text{ L})$$

Body fluid osmolarity | The normal osmolarity of body fluids is ~290 mOsm/L (this is a measure of the solute particles present in the fluid and an indirect measure of the hydrostatic pressure that the solution would generate). Some ions, like potassium, magnesium, and phosphate (K^+, Mg^{2+}, and PO_4^{3-}), are predominantly intracellular. Others, like sodium, chloride, and calcium (Na^+, Cl^-, and Ca^+), are predominantly extracellular and are important contributors to ECF osmolarity.

It should be clear from **Table 20.2** that the major contributors to the body osmolarity are Na^+ and Cl^-. The total body osmolarity can be calculated by adding up the millimolar concentrations of Na^+ (140), K^+ (5), Cl^- (100), bicarbonate (HCO_3^-; 25), glucose (5), and urea (5), and adding another 10 for other less-abundant ions. Alternatively, it can be quickly calculated by the formula

$2 \times Na^+$ concentration + glucose osmolar concentration + urea osmolar concentration

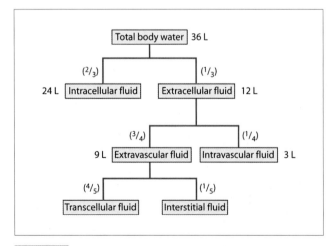

Fig. 20.1 Body fluid compartments. The calculation of total body water assumes a 60 kg man and is only an approximation because the percentage of body fat in any individual will affect the percentage of body weight that is water.

Table 20.2 Important Contributors to Body Osmolarity

Constituent	Concentrate
Na^+	135–155 mmol/L
Cl^-	90–110 mmol/L
HCO_3^-	25 mmol/L
K^+	3.5–5.0 mmol/L
Glucose	60–100 mg/dL (3.4–5.6 mmol/L)
Blood urea nitrogen	10–20 mg/dL (3.6–7.1 mmol/L)

This formula is convenient for quickly calculating body fluid osmolarity when it rises alarmingly in hyperglycemia or uremia. Proteins do not contribute significantly to body fluid osmolarity because their molar concentration is low. However, the *oncotic pressure* (the osmotic pressure due to solutes that cannot cross the membrane) of the plasma proteins does play an important role in determining the movement of water across the cell membrane and across the walls of capillaries.

Blood

The body contains ~5 L of blood, of which approximately half is water. The functions of blood are transport of respiratory gases (O_2 and CO_2), nutrients, metabolites, and hormones to and from all the cells of the body. It provides defense against infection and has a role in the maintenance of body temperature, acid–base balance, and fluid–electrolyte balance. It has an inbuilt mechanism (hemostasis) for preventing its own loss from the body.

Composition of blood | Blood is made of formed (cellular) elements (45%) and plasma (55%). The two can be separated by centrifuging whole blood at ~1000 G (usually equivalent to ~3000 rpm in a small centrifuge). The bulk of the cellular elements of blood is made of RBCs or erythrocytes. Others include the white blood cells (WBCs) or leukocytes and the platelets or thrombocytes (**Table 20.3**).

The plasma contains innumerable substances in solution, of which proteins (the plasma proteins) are an important con-

Table 20.3 Normal Values for the Cellular Elements in Human Blood

Red blood cells	Men	5.5 (± 1.0) million/µL
	Women	4.8 (± 1.0) million/µL
White blood cells		
Total leukocytic count		4000–11,000/µL
Differential leukocytic count	Neutrophils	3000–6000 (50–70%)
	Eosinophils	150–300 (1–4%)
	Basophils	0–100 (0–1%)
	Lymphocytes	1500–4000 (20–40%)
	Monocytes	300–600 (2–8%)
Platelets		200,000–500,000/mL

stituent. The major constituents of plasma are summarized in **Table 20.4**. Plasma contains, among other substances, coagulation proteins. Hence, like blood, plasma clots on standing. Plasma without the coagulation proteins is called *serum*. It is obtained by allowing whole blood to clot. As the clot hardens, it shrinks and extrudes the serum. Serum has essentially the same composition as plasma except that its clotting factors have been consumed, and it has a higher serotonin content due to the breakdown of platelets during clotting.

Erythrocytic sedimentation | When anticoagulated blood is allowed to stand in a long vertical tube, its erythrocytes settle down, leaving clear plasma at the top of the tube. The rate at which the erythrocytes settle down in a tube of standard dimensions (2.5 mm inner diameter, 200 mm height) is called the *erythrocytic sedimentation rate* (ESR) and is one of the oldest hematologic tests that is still in use.

The most important factor that determines ESR is the extent of rouleaux formation by erythrocytes (see **Fig. 21.1**). Rouleaux formation is determined mainly by the nature of plasma. Increased rouleaux formation occurs when plasma contains increased amounts of fibrinogen (as in pregnancy) and serum globulin (as in inflammatory diseases). RBC characteristics also affect rouleaux formation and therefore affect the ESR, too. RBCs with higher MCHC (mean corpuscular hemoglobin concentration) tend to fall more slowly in plasma than those with normal or low MCHC. Excessive nonuniformity of shape (poikilocytosis) or size (anisocytosis) of the RBCs reduces ESR.

Two well-known pathologic causes of elevated ESR are tuberculosis and rheumatoid arthritis. However, ESR is elevated in so many diseases that it has little diagnostic utility. It is elevated in almost all inflammatory disorders and collagen diseases. Its main utility is in prognosis, that is the prediction of the probable course of a disease in an individual and the chances of recovery. Thus, during a 6-month course of tuberculosis treatment, serial measurements of ESR can indicate whether the patient is improving. It has similar use in certain malignancies, especially Hodgkin disease.

Plasma Proteins

Properties of plasma proteins | Plasma proteins are large molecules with molecular weights ranging mostly from 50,000 to 300,000 daltons. With the exception of albumin, nearly all plasma proteins are glycoproteins containing oligosaccharides. The oligosaccharide chains are responsible for certain properties of plasma proteins, such as solubility, viscosity, charge,

Table 20.4 Constituents of Plasma

Constituents	Examples
Electrolytes	Na^+, K^+, Cl^-, HCO_3^+
Proteins	Albumin, globulin, amino acids
Carbohydrates	Glucose
Lipids	Cholesterol, fatty acids
Minerals	Ca^{2+}, PO_4^{3-}
Enzymes	Alkaline phosphatase, amylase
Metabolites	Bilirubin, urea, uric acid, creatinine

and denaturation. Like most other proteins, their charged residues tend to be located on the surface of the molecule.

Certain properties of plasma protein molecules are attributable to their large size and high molecular weight. For example, unlike electrolytes or other smaller molecules, they can be separated from the plasma by ultracentrifugation. They are unable to pass across the capillary membrane and consequently exert an oncotic pressure of ~25 mm Hg. Owing to their size and particularly their shape, they greatly contribute to blood viscosity. The plasma protein fibrinogen is also a significant contributor to blood viscosity.

Another set of properties of plasma proteins is attributable to the presence of polar residues like NH_3^+ and COO^- on their molecular surface. Thus, plasma protein molecules are soluble in water and show electrophoretic mobility. They are amphoteric in nature because the polar residues comprise both positive amino (NH_3^+) and negative carboxyl (COO^-) groups. The plasma proteins act as efficient buffers by virtue of their amphoteric nature. Their polar residues bind easily with, and therefore serve as good carriers for, metallic ions and steroids.

Functions of plasma proteins | The two important functions of plasma proteins are (1) retaining the fluid portion of blood in the capillaries by virtue of the oncotic pressure they exert and (2) buffering body fluids. Besides these general functions, different plasma proteins have specific functions: they can act variously as nutrients, enzymes, hormones, antibodies, clotting and fibrinolytic factors, carrier molecules, and scavengers (**Table 20.5**).

The carrier function of plasma proteins aids in the transportation of hormones with very low solubility in plasma. Hormones bound to carriers have a longer half-life in blood. Binding the hormones to plasma proteins prevents the rapid filtration of hormones through the glomeruli. The protein-bound hormone also acts as a reservoir of the hormone. When the free hormone level falls, the bound hormone readily dissociates from the carrier protein and restores the free hormone level.

The scavenger function of plasma proteins comes into play after cell necrosis, which is associated with the release of large amounts of actin (present in the cytoskeleton of cells) into the circulation. These are scavenged by gelsolin that depolymerizes F-actin, and Gc protein (also called the vitamin D-binding protein) that binds to G-actin.

Table 20.5 Some Examples of Plasma Proteins and Their Functions

Plasma Protein	Function
Lipoproteins	Nutrients
Amylase, alkaline phosphatase	Enzymes
Anterior pituitary hormones, angiotensin	Hormones
γ-Globulin	Antibodies
Fibrinogen, prothrombin, fibrinolysin	Clotting and fibrinolytic factors
Albumin, ceruloplasmin, transferrin	Carriers
Gelsolin, Gc protein	Scavengers

Types of plasma proteins | Only two types of plasma proteins, albumin and globulin, were originally separated using the salting out technique. More advanced techniques later showed the globulin fraction to be highly heterogeneous. The term *globulin* now signifies a large group of plasma proteins (designated as α_1, α_2, β, and γ). The albumin fraction is more homogeneous. The term *albumin* has therefore been retained to denote the largest single protein in the albumin fraction; the remaining proteins in that fraction have been given other names, such as prealbumin.

The plasma concentration of total proteins in adults is ~7 g/dL, of which albumin accounts for more than half—4 g/dL. Albumin molecules far outnumber globulin molecules; therefore, albumin is the principal contributor to plasma oncotic pressure. When plasma albumin falls, the plasma oncotic pressure decreases and results in edema.

Synthesis of plasma proteins | The γ-globulins (immunoglobulins) are produced by plasma cells. Most other plasma proteins are synthesized in the liver. However, contributions to plasma proteins also come from macrophages (complement), intestinal cells (apoproteins), and endothelial cells (coagulation factors).

The relation of plasma proteins to diet has been studied in dogs rendered hypoproteinemic by repeated plasmapheresis. It was noted that the 10 essential amino acids have to be provided in the diet for the satisfactory synthesis of plasma proteins. Usually, dietary proteins of animal origin favor albumin synthesis, whereas those of plant origin favor globulin synthesis.

Hypoproteinemia due to increased protein losses occurs in nephrotic syndrome and in protein-losing enteropathy. Hypoproteinemia due to reduced protein synthesis occurs in liver diseases, malabsorption, malnutrition, prolonged starvation, and chronic inflammation (due to inhibition of hepatic synthesis of albumin by inflammatory mediators). The midpregnancy fall in total plasma protein concentration is largely due to hemodilution and occurs despite the increase in hepatic synthesis of globulin.

Hyperproteinemia is seen in acute inflammation and in multiple myeloma. Globulins increase sharply during any acute inflammation. These are called *acute-phase proteins*. They include C-reactive proteins (CRP), so called because they react with C-polysaccharide of pneumococci. Other acute-phase proteins are α_1-antitrypsin, haptoglobin, von Willebrand factor, and fibrinogen. C-reactive proteins increase in chronic inflammation and malignancy, too. These acute-phase proteins are important for nonspecific immunity of the body. In multiple myeloma, plasma cells secrete large amounts of immunoglobulins, resulting in hypergammaglobulinemia.

General Model: Reservoir

The blood, the contents of the vascular compartment, serves as a reservoir for a great many substances with essential roles in the economy of the body. We will be describing a great many physiologic processes that put substances into the blood and a great many processes that take these same things out of the blood.

Summary

- The body contains a high percentage of water (~60% in men and 50% in women).

- Total body water is distributed between the intracellular compartment and the extracellular compartment.

- Body fluid osmolarity is ~290 mOsm/L, and water moves quickly between compartments to maintain the same osmolarity everywhere.

- The blood is 55% plasma (water and solutes) and 45% cells.

- Plasma proteins are particularly important solutes, carrying out many different functions.

Applying What You Know

20.1. Calculate Mr. Lundquist's total body water and his intracellular fluid (ICF) and extracellular fluid (ECF) volumes.

20.2. Mr. Lundquist's hematocrit (Hct) is low. What parameters might be altered from their normal values to give rise to this state?

The red blood cells (RBCs), or *erythrocytes*, are biconcave, circular, disk-shaped cells without a nucleus, mitochondria, or ribosomes. The average life span of an RBC in the circulation is 120 days. The RBC count is highest on the first day of life. The changes in RBC count with age parallel the changes in hemoglobin concentration (see **Fig. 22.1**). The RBC counts in men and women are given in **Table 20.3**.

An abnormally high RBC count is called *polycythemia* and is seen in chronic hypoxic conditions (living at high altitude). The malignant form of polycythemia is called *polycythemia vera*. Whether benign or malignant, polycythemia is associated with high blood viscosity and increased resistance to blood flow, resulting in stagnant hypoxia and peripheral cyanosis (see Chapter 50).

Of major importance is the hemoglobin content in RBC cytoplasm. The advantages of carrying hemoglobin within a cell versus free form in the plasma are threefold: (1) It prevents the rapid degradation and elimination of the hemoglobin. (2) It prevents the marked increase in the plasma viscosity that would occur if hemoglobin were present as a plasma protein. (3) It prevents blood from exerting a high osmotic pressure across the capillary wall.

The biconcave shape of the RBC gives it a large surface-to-volume ratio—the most efficient shape for rapid gas exchange. The RBC is flexible and readily distorted during its passage in the circulation; as it passes through capillaries, it assumes a parachute-like configuration (**Fig. 21.1A**). Erythrocytes are mostly round, but a few of them are slightly oval. The term *poikilocytosis* refers to an excessive variation in RBC shape. The mean diameter of RBCs as measured directly is 7.2 μm. The disk thickness is 2 μm. Excessive variation in RBC size is called *anisocytosis*. It may be due to an increase in the number of small or large cells or both.

Rouleaux formation | Within a blood vessel, in the absence of significant flow, the RBCs tend to form rouleaux; that is, they tend to align themselves to form stacks (**Fig. 21.1B**). This is a reversible phenomenon. Plasma proteins like fibrinogen interact with the protein coating of RBCs to promote rouleaux formation. Albumin and globulins also induce rouleaux formation, but only at concentrations much higher than normal.

Chromicity | RBC staining is deeper at the periphery of the cell and fades at the center (the central pallor). Cells that stain normally are assumed to have a normal concentration of hemoglobin and are called *normochromic*. The term *hypochromia* is used to describe a decrease in the intensity of staining. Hypochromia is usually associated with a decrease in the mean cell hemoglobin concentration (MCHC)—a decrease in the concentration of hemoglobin in the RBCs (see below). However, cells that are thinner than normal (as in thalassemia) may appear slightly hypochromic even though the MCHC is normal. The term *hyperchromia* is used to describe an increase in the intensity of staining of the RBC, in which the cell stains

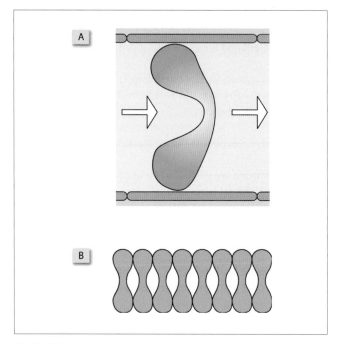

Fig. 21.1 **(A)** A red blood cell assumes a parachute-like shape for squeezing through a capillary. **(B)** Rouleaux formation.

more deeply, and the central pallor is not apparent. Such an appearance is usually due to an increase in the thickness of the cell, and not to an increase in MCHC.

Spherocytes (spherical erythrocytes) show both an increase in thickness and an elevated MCHC. They certainly are hyperchromic. In megaloblastic anemia, the RBC diameter is increased, but MCHC remains normal. Whether or not the cells should be called hyperchromic depends on what is meant by the term *hyperchromia*. Considering the ambiguity of the term *hyperchromia*, it is best abandoned in favor of the more objective MCHC.

Volume of packed red cells (VPRC) is total volume of packed RBCs (preferable to the term *packed cell volume* (PCV) that was used earlier) in 100 mL of blood. It is determined by centrifuging the blood at a high speed in a graduated centrifuge tube. The centrifugation results in the separation of three layers: a supernatant layer of plasma, a sediment layer of RBCs, and a thin buffy coat separating the two. The *buffy coat* is made of leukocytes and platelets. The volume of RBC sediment gives the VPRC. The VPRC is a useful clinical test that is used for detecting anemia and polycythemia. However, a normal RBC count or VPRC does not rule out an absolute deficiency or excess of RBCs in the body: it might be a case of hemodilution (as in pregnancy) or hemoconcentration (as in dehydration).

When hematologic measurements are made electronically, VPRC is computed from the product of RBC count and the mean RBC volume. When thus computed, the term *VPRC* becomes a misnomer because no "packing" of RBC is involved. The term *hematocrit* (Hct) is therefore currently preferred over VPRC.

Red Cell Indices

The RBC indices refer to the mean corpuscular volume (MCV), the mean corpuscular hemoglobin (MCH), and the mean corpuscular hemoglobin concentration (MCHC). These indices are calculated from VPRC, the hemoglobin concentration, and the RBC count. The three indices are related by the formula

$$MCHC = \frac{MCH}{MCV} \tag{21.1}$$

The **mean cell volume** (MCV) is the average volume of the RBCs. It is calculated by dividing the packed cell volume (VPRC) by the RBC count. The result is expressed in femtoliters (fL) or cubic micrometers (μ^3).

$$MCV = \frac{VPRC}{RBC\ count} \tag{21.2}$$
$$VPRC = 0.45$$
$$RBC\ count = 5 \times 10^{12}/L$$

$$MCV = \frac{0.45}{5 \times 10^{12}/L}$$
$$= 0.09 \times 10^{-12}/L$$
$$= 90 \times 10^{-15}/L = 90\ fL$$

Normal MCV = 85 ± 8 fL

The **mean cell hemoglobin** (MCH) is the average mass of hemoglobin (in picograms [pg]) contained in each RBC. It is increased in spherocytosis and megaloblastic anemia. The MCH is calculated by dividing the amount of hemoglobin in 1 L of blood by the number of RBCs present in 1 L of blood (the RBC count).

Example:

$$MCH = \frac{Hb\ concentration}{RBC\ count} \tag{21.3}$$
$$Hb\ concentration = 15\ g/dL = 150\ g/L$$
$$RBC\ count = 5 \times 10^{12}/L$$

$$MCH = \frac{150\ g/L}{5 \times 10^{12}/L}$$
$$= 30 \times 10^{-12}g = 30\ pg$$

Normal MCH = 30 ± 2 pg

The **mean cell hemoglobin concentration** (MCHC) is the average concentration of hemoglobin in an erythrocyte. MCHC is increased in spherocytosis and sickle cell anemia. MCHC is calculated by dividing the amount of hemoglobin in 1 L of blood by the volume of packed cells in 1 L of blood (VPRC).

$$MCHC = \frac{Hb\ concentration}{VPRC} \tag{21.4}$$
$$Hb\ concentration = 15\ g/dL$$
$$VPRC = 0.45$$

$$MCHC = \frac{15\ g/dL}{0.45}$$
$$= 33.33\ g/dL$$

Normal MCHC = 33 ± 2 g/dL

Red Blood Cell Metabolism

The mature RBC has a low metabolic activity and consumes very little oxygen. Its energy requirements are met through glycolysis. Ninety percent of the glycolysis occurs through the *Embden-Meyerhof pathway* (see **Fig. 74.2**), but with a difference: in erythrocytes, the glycolytic step catalyzed by phosphoglycerate kinase is bypassed (**Fig. 21.2**). The significance of this modified pathway is the production of 2,3 DPG (diphosphoglycerate) that influences the affinity of hemoglobin for oxygen and thereby has important physiologic consequences. Acidemia decreases DPG in the RBC by hindering glycolysis, and hypoxia increases DPG by inhibiting the Krebs cycle. Hormones that increase DPG formation include the thyroid hormone, growth hormone, and androgens.

Another important advantage of the Embden-Meyerhof pathway is that it generates nicotinamide adenine dinucleotide and hydrogen (NADH + H$^+$). Normally, methemoglobin is formed continually by the auto-oxidation of hemoglobin. Simultaneous reduction of methemoglobin by NADH + H$^+$

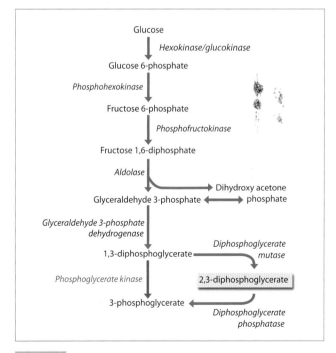

Fig. 21.2 The Embden-Meyerhof pathway in erythrocytes. Compare it with **Fig. 74.2**.

keeps the proportion of methemoglobin below 1% of the hemoglobin content.

Ten percent of glycolysis occurs through the *pentose phosphate pathway,* also called the hexose monophosphate (HMP) shunt. The significance of this pathway is that it generates nicotinamide adenine dinucleotide phosphate and hydrogen (NADPH + H$^+$), which is required for the reduction of glutathione. Reduced glutathione protects the sulfhydryl groups of hemoglobin against oxidation. NADPH + H$^+$ is also needed for the maintenance of normal RBC fragility.

Red Blood Cell Turnover

Erythropoiesis

In the adult, the erythrocytes are produced in the bone marrow. The erythrocytic precursor cells are the proerythroblasts, erythroblasts (early, intermediate, and late), and reticulocytes.

Erythropoietin | The production of erythrocytes is regulated by a hormone called *erythropoietin.* Erythropoietin is a glycoprotein secreted mainly by the kidney (85%) and liver (15%). In the kidney, erythropoietin-secreting cells are found in the interstitium of the inner cortex and outer medulla, lying just outside the tubular basement membrane.

Erythropoietin increases erythropoiesis by acting on the bone marrow as well as the fetal yolk sac, liver, and spleen, where it promotes (1) proliferation of committed stem cells, (2) differentiation of erythropoietic stem cells to proerythroblasts, (3) hemoglobin synthesis, by increasing globulin synthesis and potentiating δ-amino levulinic acid synthetase, and (4) release of erythrocytes from bone marrow.

The factors that promote erythropoietin secretion are (1) hypoxia; (2) alkalosis; (3) hormones, such as growth hormone, prolactin, thyroid hormones, catecholamines, corticosteroids, and androgens; and (4) hemolysates (products, mainly nucleotides, released following RBC destruction), such as cyclic adenosine monophosphate (cAMP), NAD$^+$, and NADP$^+$. Stimulation of erythropoietin by hypoxia (whether from prolonged exposure to high altitude or pathology that results in decreased O$_2$ uptake) is a physiologic feedback mechanism through which the number of erythrocytes is increased whenever there is increased destruction of RBCs resulting in the release of hemolysates and causing O$_2$ deficiency in the tissues. The increase in RBC count tends to improve tissue oxygenation.

General Model: Homeostasis

The cells that produce and release erythropoietin are functioning like sensors in a homeostatic mechanism. It is only possible to regulate a variable that you can measure, and in this case it appears that the stimulus being measured is actually PO$_2$ rather than number or concentration of RBCs.

Nutritional requirements for erythropoiesis | Vitamin B$_{12}$ and folate are essential for DNA synthesis. Deficiency of either of them results in, among other things, megaloblastic anemia.

Iron is essential for hemoglobin synthesis. Deficiency of iron, occurring mostly due to inadequate intake, is one of the most common causes of anemia. An adequate supply of high-quality protein in the diet is essential for supplying amino acids for the synthesis of the globin component of hemoglobin. Available protein is prioritized for hemoglobin synthesis; hence, the protein deficiency must be very marked before hemoglobin synthesis is impaired.

Red Blood Cell Destruction

About 1% of the RBCs, generally the older and the abnormal ones, are removed daily from circulation by macrophages lining the walls of sinusoids, where the blood flow is slow, as in the liver, spleen, and bone marrow. Inside the macrophage, hemoglobin is degraded into bilirubin after removing the iron from it. The iron and bilirubin are released into circulation.

Red blood cell fragility | Due to certain pathologic changes in its membrane or in its contents, the RBC sometimes becomes mechanically more fragile—more vulnerable to deforming stresses than normal RBCs. Such cells are removed from circulation by macrophages in larger numbers than normal cells. A convenient method for testing RBC fragility is to test for its *osmotic fragility.* Erythrocytes are suspended in a series of saline solutions with strengths ranging from 0.9 to 0.3%. RBCs with normal osmotic fragility start showing hemolysis (RBC rupture with loss of hemoglobin) in 0.5% saline and are completely hemolyzed in 0.35% saline (**Fig. 21.3**). However, a normal or low osmotic fragility does not rule out the possibility of a high mechanical fragility. In sickle cell anemia, the sickle-shaped erythrocytes have a high mechanical fragility. However, the osmotic fragility of the sickle cells is normal or even low.

In **hereditary spherocytosis,** the spherocytes (spherical erythrocytes) hemolyze more readily: they start hemolyzing at higher saline concentration. This is because spherocytes, as the name suggests, are rather more spherical than discoid, which leaves them with little margin for swelling in hypotonic solutions. Spherocytes are removed by the spleen in large numbers, resulting in hemolytic anemia (see below). Spherocytosis is caused by abnormalities of the protein network that maintains the shape and flexibility of the RBC membrane (see

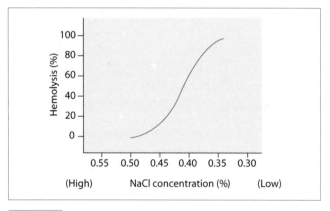

Fig. 21.3 Osmotic fragility curve. The curve shifts to the left when the osmotic fragility of red blood cells increases.

Fig. 2.2B). Ankyrin, a peripheral protein located on the inside of the membrane, anchors spectrin (a cytoskeletal protein in the RBC) to band-3, an integral protein of the erythrocyte membrane. Defects in band-3, spectrin, and ankyrin have all been observed in the spherocytes.

G6PD deficiency | The deficiency of the enzyme glucose 6-phosphate dehydrogenase (G6PD), a key enzyme in the pentose phosphate pathway, reduces the production of NADPH + H^+. In the absence of adequate NADPH + H^+, the susceptibility of RBCs to hemolysis increases. Severe G6PD deficiency also inhibits the ability of granulocytes to kill bacteria and thereby predisposes to severe infections.

Anemias

Anemia is variously defined as a reduction in hemoglobin concentration or RBC count in the peripheral blood, or the total RBC mass in the body, below the norm for the age and sex of the patient. The total RBC mass is not affected by hemodilution or hemoconcentration.

A man is usually said to be anemic when his hemoglobin falls below 13.0 g/dL, and a woman, when her hemoglobin falls below 11.5 g/dL. Somewhat arbitrarily, anemia is called moderate when it falls below 9 g/dL and severe when it falls below 6 g/dL. The fall of the hemoglobin concentration below normal values is usually, but not always, accompanied by a fall in the RBC count. Thus, occasionally, especially in the hypochromic microcytic anemia of iron deficiency, the RBC count is normal, although the hemoglobin is significantly reduced due to the low hemoglobin content of individual cells.

There are two main classifications of anemia: the laboratory classification, based on the characteristics of the RBC, and the etiological classification, based on the cause of the anemia.

The **laboratory classification** is based on the values of MCV and MCHC. In normocytic anemias, the MCV is within the normal range. Most *normocytic anemias* are also normochromic with a normal MCHC, but mild hypochromia may occur occasionally. If the erythrocytes are normocytic and normochromic, why should there be anemia at all? The anemia in these cases results from a low RBC count, which reduces the hemoglobin concentration in the blood. In *microcytic anemias*, the MCV is reduced. Microcytic anemias are mostly hypochromic with the MCHC reduced. In *macrocytic anemias*, the MCV is increased. Most macrocytic anemias are normochromic, but a mild hypochromia (reduced MCHC) may occur in some cases.

The **etiological classification** of anemias is based on the cause of anemia (**Fig. 21.4**). Broadly, the cause can be due to a deficiency of hemopoietic factors (deficiency anemia), excessive breakdown of erythrocytes (hemolytic anemia), or excessive blood loss (hemorrhagic anemia). *Deficiency anemias* occur due to reduced hemoglobin synthesis or impaired RBC formation, which can occur when there is a deficiency of iron (iron-deficiency anemia), or due to vitamin B_{12} or folate deficiency (megaloblastic anemia). *Hemolytic anemias* are relatively uncommon. RBCs are destroyed in large numbers either due to some defect in the RBC itself (intracorpuscular defect), or due to some defect in its immediate environment (extra-

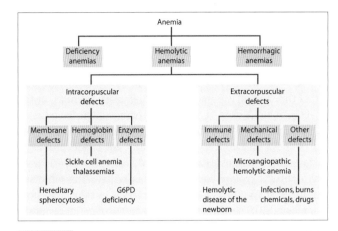

Fig. 21.4 Classification of anemias based on the root cause of the problem: deficiency anemias result from a lack of substrates to make hemoglobin; hemolytic anemias are a consequence of destruction of red blood cells; hemorrhagic anemias result from blood loss. G6PD, glucose 6-phosphate dehydrogenase.

corpuscular defect). *Hemorrhagic anemia* is a common form of anemia and can be due to acute or chronic blood loss. Anemia following acute blood loss (acute posthemorrhagic anemia) results in hemodilution. This is because the plasma is restored much faster than the cellular elements. The result is a normocytic, normochromic anemia. Anemia due to chronic blood loss (chronic posthemorrhagic anemia) tends to show features of iron deficiency, a microcytic, hypochromic anemia. *Hemodilutional anemia* occurs when there is hypervolemia due to fluid retention. The physiologic anemia of pregnancy occurs due to the hemodilution caused by aldosterone.

Signs and symptoms | Anemia results in reduced oxygen-carrying capacity of blood, resulting in tissue hypoxia. The hypoxia causes symptoms such as easy fatigability (due to muscle hypoxia) and faintness (due to cerebral hypoxia), especially on exertion. The hypoxia brings about several compensatory responses. Although these responses alleviate tissue hypoxia, they also produce symptoms such as *breathlessness* due to compensatory stimulation of the respiratory center and *palpitation* due to compensatory increase in cardiac output. The raised cardiac output creates turbulence of blood during its passage through the cardiac valves, resulting in clinical signs such as *cardiac murmurs*. The reduction in RBC count reduces blood viscosity and thereby contributes to the likelihood of turbulence and the resultant murmurs (see Appendix A, Turbulent versus Laminar Flow section, Reynolds number).

Blood picture | In *megaloblastic anemia*, there is marked macrocytosis, anisocytosis, and poikilocytosis. There is neutropenia with aged, hypersegmented neutrophils, and thrombocytopenia. This is because the production of other blood cells is also affected due to impaired DNA synthesis.

In *iron deficiency anemia*, the erythrocytes are typically microcytic and appear hypochromic in blood film. Both MCH and MCHC are reduced. The RBC count is also reduced.

In *hemolytic anemias*, the reticulocyte count is increased due to the appearance of larger reticulocytes that are less mature. These are released prematurely from bone marrow into circulation under the stimulation of erythropoietin in response to increased demand. Hence, these reticulocytes are called *shift reticulocytes.* A few nucleated RBCs (erythroblasts released prematurely into circulation) may also be seen.

Bone marrow picture | The state of bone marrow reflects either the cause of the anemia (as in deficiency anemias) or the effect of anemia (as in hemolytic and hemorrhagic anemias).

In *megaloblastic anemia,* the proerythroblasts and erythroblasts show megaloblastic changes and are called promegaloblasts and megaloblasts, respectively. Compared with their erythroblastic counterparts, megaloblasts have the following features: (1) The cell is larger with a larger nucleus and more cytoplasm. (2) The chromatin is more reticular (loose mesh) than the erythroblast, which has a more clumped chromatin. Clumping of chromatin is a sign of cell maturity. (3) Hemoglobinization of the cytoplasm proceeds normally. Thus, nuclear maturation (indicated by the state of chromatin) can be said to be lagging behind cytoplasmic maturation (indicated by hemoglobinization). (4) Due to maturation arrest, the primitive precursor cells (e.g., promegaloblast) are more numerous than usual.

In *iron deficiency anemia,* the bone marrow shows proliferation of the precursor cells (erythroid hyperplasia) with a larger proportion of the mature forms. Some of the precursor cells show scanty, polychromatic cytoplasm (a sign of cytoplasmic immaturity) with a pyknotic nucleus (a sign of nuclear maturity). It indicates that cytoplasmic maturation lags behind nuclear maturation.

In *hemolytic anemias,* the RBC precursors show excessive proliferation (erythroid hyperplasia). Normally, white cell precursors are three to five times more numerous than RBC precursors: the myeloid to erythroid ratio is from 3 to 5:1. In erythroid hyperplasia, their numbers become roughly equal (1:1). The marrow space in the bone widens, resulting in detectable bone changes in radiographs.

Summary

- RBCs contain hemoglobin, which is necessary for the transport of oxygen and carbon dioxide in the circulation.

- RBCs are produced in the bone marrow, and this process is controlled by the hormone erythropoietin.

- RBCs have an average life span of 120 days and are removed from the circulation by macrophages.

- An abnormally low concentration of hemoglobin is called anemia, and there are many different causes of such a condition.

Applying What You Know

21.1. Mr. Lundquist has a hematocrit (Hct) that is significantly lower than normal. How does this relate to his chief complaint of fatigue and shortness of breath?

22 Hemoglobin

Hemoglobin is an oxygen-binding protein present in the cytoplasm of red blood cells (RBCs). It transports oxygen from the lungs to the tissues and also transports carbon dioxide from the tissues to the lungs. Hemoglobin is also a particularly important contributor to the acid–base buffering capacity of blood (see Chapter 63).

Hemoglobin in the newborn | The hemoglobin concentration of blood from the umbilical cord averages 16.5 g/dL. The cord blood is representative of the infant's blood before birth. Shortly after birth, the hemoglobin value of normal infants increases rapidly, the hemoglobin on the first day of life being 18.5 g/dL. This is due to the result of two processes. (1) There is a transfusion of RBCs from the placenta to the infant. Hemoglobin values are significantly higher in infants in whom the cord is not tied for a few minutes after delivery, allowing extra placental blood to pass into the infant. (2) There is a rapid reduction of plasma volume in the neonate, resulting in hemoconcentration. The reduction in plasma volume allows the infant to accommodate the extra maternal blood cells obtained through transfusion. After the first 2 days, there is a marked fall in hemoglobin concentration for 2 weeks, stabilizing by the third month at 12.0 g/dL. At the end of the first year, it starts rising toward the adult level. The adult values of hemoglobin are 15.5 ± 2.5 g/dL for men and 14.0 ± 2.5 g/dL for women (**Fig. 22.1**).

Estimation of hemoglobin | As a colored substance, the hemoglobin concentration of a blood sample can be easily estimated by comparing its color to that of a reference hemoglobin solution. However, difficulty in colorimetry is posed by the fact that the color of hemoglobin is not constant; it is bright red when fully oxygenated and bluish red when deoxygenated. Hence, before colorimetry, it is important to oxygenate the hemoglobin completely (the oxyhemoglobin method) or to denature it using acid (acid-hematin method), alkali (alkali-hematin method), or cyanide (cyanmethemoglobin method).

Structure of hemoglobin | Hemoglobin, molecular weight 64,450 daltons, is a globular molecule comprising four sub-

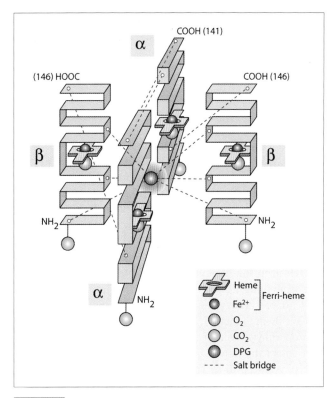

Fig. 22.2 Structure of hemoglobin shown schematically.

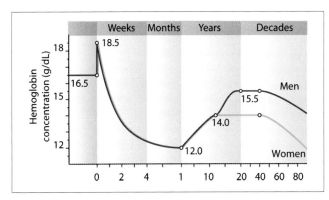

Fig. 22.1 Hemoglobin concentration at different ages.

units, each subunit consisting of a polypeptide chain and *heme*, an iron-containing porphyrin (**Fig. 22.2**). The four polypeptide chains present in a hemoglobin molecule together constitute the protein called *globin*. One gram of hemoglobin contains 3.4 mg of iron and can carry up to 1.34 mL of oxygen.

Different forms of hemoglobin have different polypeptide chains in them. Hemoglobin A, which comprises 97% of the hemoglobin in adults, is made up of two α chains, each containing 141 amino acid residues, and two β chains, each containing 146 amino acid residues. It is symbolically written as HbA $(\alpha_2\beta_2)$. There are salt links (noncovalent, electrostatic bonds) between the terminal carboxyl residues (COO⁻) and the intermediate amino residues (NH₃⁺) of the four polypeptide chains. The iron atom of heme is attached between the histidine residues of the α chain at positions 58 and 87 (also called His-E7 and His-F8, respectively). In the β chain, the iron atom is attached between histidine residues at positions 63 and 92. In the deoxygenated state, the iron atom is located a little outside the plane of the ring in the direction of His-F8.

Fetal hemoglobin or HbF $(\alpha_2\beta_2)$ is the main form of hemoglobin in the fetus. It has greater affinity for oxygen. It is more resistant to alkali denaturation; therefore, the routine alkali-hematin method fails to estimate HbF unless the solution is heated in a water bath for 4 minutes. HbF disappears from the RBCs of normal infants by the age of 6 months,

123

although very small amounts (< 2%) can be detected in the RBCs of most children and adults.

HbA$_2$ ($\alpha_2\beta_2$) is present in small amounts (< 3% in normal adults). Hb-Bart's (γ_4) is present in the fetus in small amounts. Hb-Gower 1($\zeta_2\epsilon_2$), Hb-Gower 2($\alpha_2\epsilon_2$), and Hb-Portland ($\zeta_2\epsilon_2$) are embryonic forms of hemoglobin.

Hemoglobin Synthesis

Heme is formed by the condensation of succinyl-coenzyme A (succinyl-CoA; derived from the citric acid cycle in mitochondria) and glycine to form α-amino-β-ketoadipic acid (**Fig. 22.3**). The condensation requires pyridoxal phosphate for the activation of glycine. α-Amino-β-ketoadipic acid gets rapidly decarboxylated to δ-amino levulinate (ALA). It is the rate-controlling step in heme synthesis and occurs in the mitochondria in the presence of ALA synthetase.

Two molecules of ALA condense in the cytosol to form porphobilinogen in the presence of ALA dehydratase. Four molecules of porphobilinogen condense to form uroporphyrinogen-III in the presence of uroporphyrinogen synthetase. Uroporphyrinogen-III is converted to coproporphyrinogen-III by the decarboxylation of the acetate groups (A), which changes them to methyl (M) groups. The reaction is catalyzed by uroporphyrinogen decarboxylase. Coproporphyrinogen-III then enters the mitochondria, where it is converted to protoporphyrinogen-III by the mitochondrial enzyme coproporphyrinogen oxidase, which catalyzes the decarboxylation and oxidation of two propionic acid chains into vinyl groups. Another mitochondrial enzyme, porphyrinogen oxidase, converts protoporphyrinogen-III to protoporphyrin-III. Protoporphyrin is a component of several cellular enzymes (e.g., cytochromes, catalase, and P-450 microsomal enzymes). The final step in heme synthesis involves the incorporation of ferrous iron into protoporphyrin in a reaction catalyzed by heme synthetase or ferrochelatase, another mitochondrial enzyme.

Reactions of Hemoglobin

Oxygenation | Oxygen binds reversibly with hemoglobin to form oxyhemoglobin. The oxygen molecule occupies the sixth coordinate position of the iron atom, which remains in the ferrous state. The insertion of the O$_2$ molecule has the following effects. The iron atom moves into the plane of the heme molecule. As the iron atom moves, it pulls the His-F8 along it, distorting the polypeptide chains. The distortion of the polypeptide chains results in the rupture of the salt links between the chains and the release of H$^+$ ions. (Thus, oxygenated hemoglobin has a different buffering capacity than does nonoxygenated hemoglobin.) The quaternary structure of hemoglobin changes from the taut (T) state to the relaxed (R) state.

Four O$_2$ molecules bind to a molecule of hemoglobin, one each to a heme molecule. The insertion of the first molecule of O$_2$ increases the affinity of sites 2 and 3 for O$_2$. After sites 2 and 3 are filled, the affinity of site 4 is increased further. This phenomenon is called *cooperative binding kinetics*. It re-

sults in the sigmoid O$_2$-dissociation curve of hemoglobin (see **Fig. 48.1B**).

Buffering of hydrogen ions | H$^+$ ions bind to the NH$_2$ of the intermediate histidine residues to form NH$_3^+$. These NH$_3^+$

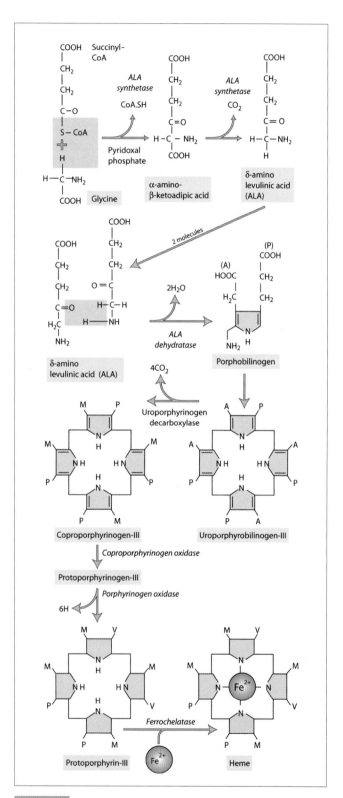

Fig. 22.3 Steps in hemoglobin synthesis. A, acetate; H, hydrogen; M, methyl; N, nitrogen; P, propionate; V, vinyl.

groups interact with the terminal COO^- groups to form salt links. Formation of salt links reduces the binding of O_2 to hemoglobin. Conversely, binding of O_2 to hemoglobin breaks the salt links and releases the H^+ ions. Thus, oxygenation of hemoglobin reduces the buffering capacity of hemoglobin. Conversely, the buffering of H^+ by hemoglobin decreases its oxygenation. The buffering of H^+ ions is also important for the transport of carbon dioxide (CO_2) in plasma as bicarbonates.

Formation of carbamino hemoglobin | CO_2 binds avidly to the terminal αNH_2 groups of valine in the β polypeptide chain and less avidly to the ones in the α polypeptide chain.

$$R-N-H+CO_2 = R-N-COO^- + H^+$$
$$\quad\ \ |\qquad\qquad\qquad |$$
$$\quad\ \ H\qquad\qquad\qquad H$$

The reaction produces a carbamate and releases H^+, which is buffered by the intermediate histidine residues of hemoglobin. These reactions favor the formation of salt links that make oxygenation more difficult. Thus, whenever CO_2 is transported in blood, whether as carbamino hemoglobin or as bicarbonates, it is associated with a reduction in the oxygenation capacity of hemoglobin. This phenomenon is called the *Bohr effect*.

Reaction with 2,3-diphosphoglycerate (DPG) | Only a single molecule of DPG binds to a molecule of hemoglobin. The DPG molecule occupies the central cavity enclosed by the four polypeptide chains of hemoglobin. It is held in place by salt bridges with three NH_3^+ groups on each p polypeptide chain. One is the NH_3^+ group of the terminal valine residue; the two others belong to the intermediate lysine and histidine residues. Formation of the salt links makes it difficult for O_2 to bind to hemoglobin and shifts the O_2 dissociation curve to the right (see **Fig. 52.2**).

Formation of carboxyhemoglobin | Carbon monoxide (CO) reacts with hemoglobin to form carboxyhemoglobin. The affinity of hemoglobin for CO is 200 times higher than its affinity for O_2. It binds exactly where O_2 binds to heme. The result is a reduction in the transport of O_2 in the blood.

Formation of methemoglobin | The ferrous iron (Fe) of hemoglobin is susceptible to oxidation by superoxides and other oxidizing agents, forming methemoglobin (hemoglobin with its iron in ferric form), which cannot carry oxygen. The red cell possesses an effective *methemoglobin reductase system* for reducing Fe^{3+} back to Fe^{2+}. The system comprises NADH + H^+, cytochrome b5, and cytochrome b5 reductase.

$$Hb\text{-}Fe^{3+} + Cyt\ b5\ red \rightarrow Hb-Fe^{2+} + Cyt\ b5\ ox$$

$$Cyt\ b5\ ox + NADH + H^+ \xrightarrow{Cyt\ b5\ reductase} Cyt\ b5\ red + NAD^+$$

Methemoglobinemia can occur due to genetic deficiency of methemoglobin reductase. It is also caused by the ingestion of certain drugs, such as sulphonamides. When more than 10% of the normal hemoglobin changes to methemoglobin, it causes a dusky discoloration of the skin resembling cyanosis.

Glycosylation of hemoglobin | Hemoglobin is non-enzymatically glycosylated by the glucose that enters the erythrocytes. The amount of glycosylated hemoglobin (HbA_{1c}) is proportionate to the blood glucose concentration and is normally ~5%. The HbA_{1c} level reflects the average blood glucose concentration over the preceding 6 to 8 weeks and serves as an index of long-term control of diabetes mellitus. Thus, a patient who is not very careful about controlling his hyperglycemia and takes an insulin injection only before visiting the physician would have a normal blood glucose, but his HbA_{1c} would remain elevated.

Hemoglobin Disorders

Hemoglobinopathies

Hemoglobinopathies refer to abnormalities in the amino acid sequence of the polypeptide chains of hemoglobin. Examples of hemoglobinopathies are HbS, HbC, and HbE. They occur due to a defect in the gene that directs the synthesis of these polypeptide chains. Several abnormal hemoglobins have no harmful effects, but HbS results in sickle cell anemia, a potentially fatal disorder.

Sickle cell anemia | In HbS, the α chains are normal, but the β chains are abnormal, with a valine residue at position 6 instead of the usual glutamic acid. This substitution results in the formation of certain reactive sites called *sticky patches* on the β chain, which bind to *sticky receptors* on the α chains of HbS. This binding causes polymerization of HbS (**Fig. 22.4**), forming long, fibrous precipitates. The precipitates distort the erythrocyte, making it sickle shaped. Because polymerization results in fewer molecules of hemoglobin, the osmotic pressure exerted by hemoglobin decreases, and the sickle cell becomes dehydrated. For the same reason, the sickle cell can imbibe more water without bursting, and its osmotic fragility is lower than normal cells. The mechanical fragility of sickle cells is, however, higher because polymerization of hemoglobin deforms the membrane and makes it rigid. The membrane also gets altered chemically, favoring the deposition of IgG and complement on its surface.

Sickling occurs only in deoxygenated hemoglobin. The conformational change that occurs with oxygenation hides the sticky receptors in the deeper regions of the molecules so that they are not present on the surface, and no sickling can occur. Sickling is also reduced in cells that have more HbF because HbF has sticky receptors but no sticky patches. Hence, in effect, HbF blocks the sticky patches of HbS. As a result, they prevent the formation of long polymers of HbS (**Fig. 22.4C**).

Sickling of red cells causes two types of problems:

1. Sickle cells are hemolyzed in large numbers, resulting in hemolytic anemia. The hemolysis is both intravascular and extravascular. *Intravascular hemolysis* occurs due to cell lysis caused by complement activation. It also occurs because of the fragmentation of the rigid cells due to mechanical stress as they pass through narrow capillaries. *Extravascular hemolysis* occurs due to excessive phagocy-

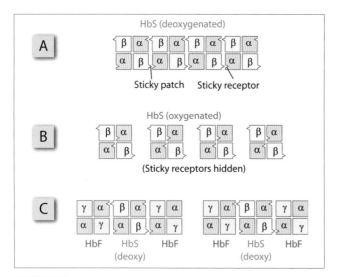

Fig. 22.4 Sticky receptors and sticky patches in sickle cell anemia. **(A)** Polymerization of deoxygenated HbS. **(B)** Lack of polymerization in oxygenated HbS. **(C)** Lack of polymerization of deoxygenated HbS in the presence of HbF. Only trimers are formed.

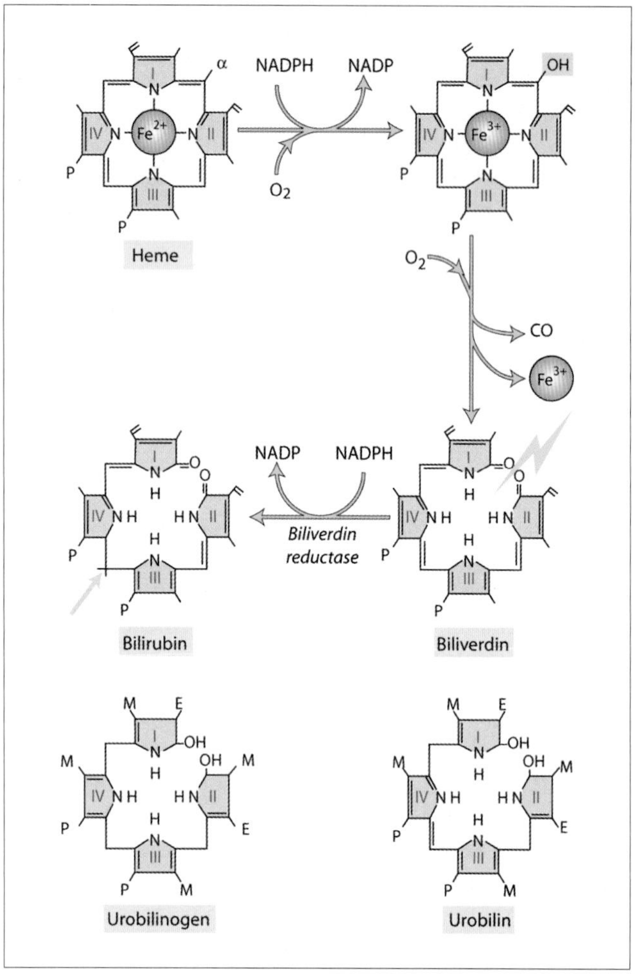

Fig. 22.5 Steps in hemoglobin degradation.

tosis of the immunoglobulin G- (IgG-) coated sickle cells by macrophages in splenic sinusoids.

2. Sickle cells also obstruct the capillary microcirculation. The reasons include increased rigidity of the cell, increased tendency of sickle cells to adhere to the endothelium, and a general increase in blood viscosity. The occlusion causes stagnant hypoxia and severe ischemic pain (vasoocclusive crisis). The hypoxia causes sickling of more cells and sets off a vicious cycle.

Thalassemias

Thalassemias refer to the reduced synthesis or absence of one of the pair of polypeptide chains of hemoglobin. When one of the chains is present in a reduced concentration, the affected polypeptide nevertheless has a normal sequence of amino acids. This condition occurs due to defects in the regulatory portion of the globin genes. Decreased or absent α and β polypeptides are called α and β thalassemia, respectively. Decreased polypeptide synthesis has two effects: (1) a general reduction in the amount of hemoglobin synthesized, resulting in anemia, and (2) an imbalance between the amounts of different α and β chains. In α thalassemia, for example, in the absence of α chains, four β chains aggregate to form β_4, called *HbH*. These aggregates precipitate in the cytoplasm and cause membrane damage. Red cells with these aggregates are removed in large numbers by splenic macrophages, causing hemolytic anemia.

Hemoglobin Breakdown

Formation of bilirubin | Aged erythrocytes are phagocytosed by macrophages in the lining of the sinusoids in the liver, bone marrow, and spleen. Inside the macrophage, the

heme molecule is cleaved off globin (**Fig. 22.5**). Globin is degraded into amino acids and reused. The Fe^{2+} in the porphyrin is converted into Fe^{3+}. The ring is broken to release the iron and carbon monoxide, resulting in the formation of *biliverdin*, a green pigment. These reactions are catalyzed by heme oxygenase, an enzyme complex present in the microsomes of macrophages. The fate of the released iron is discussed in Chapter 24. The biliverdin is converted into *bilirubin*, a yellow pigment, by biliverdin reductase, which reduces the methyl bridge between pyrrole III and pyrrole IV to a methylene group.

Excretion of bilirubin | Bilirubin is poorly soluble in water and is transported in plasma bound to albumin. In the hepatic sinusoids, bilirubin dissociates from albumin to enter the liver cells through facilitated diffusion. Bilirubin is lipid soluble and tends to persist inside the cell. The hepatocytes conjugate bilirubin with *uridine diphosphate (UDP) glucuronic acid,* making it water soluble so that it can be excreted in bile. The reaction is catalyzed by the enzyme *glucuronyl transferase* present in hepatic microsomes (i.e., the smooth endoplasmic reticulum of the liver cells). The reaction occurs in two stages as shown below. The conjugated bilirubin is excreted into the hepatic canaliculi through active transport. This active transport is the rate-limiting step in the entire process of bilirubin excretion.

$$\underset{\substack{+\\ \text{Bilirubin}}}{\overset{\text{UDP}}{\text{Glucuronic acid}}} \xrightarrow{\underset{\text{transferase}}{\text{UDP glucuronyl}}} \underset{\substack{+\\ \text{UDP}}}{\overset{\text{Bilirubin}}{\text{monoglucuronide}}}$$

$$\underset{\substack{+\\ \text{Bilirubin}\\ \text{monoglucoronide}}}{\overset{\text{UDP}}{\text{Glucuronic acid}}} \xrightarrow{\underset{\text{transferase}}{\text{UDP glucuronyl}}} \underset{\substack{+\\ \text{UDP}}}{\overset{\text{Bilirubin}}{\text{diglucuronide}}}$$

Formation and excretion of urobilinogen | The conjugated bilirubin excreted in bile is acted upon by intestinal bacteria in the terminal ileum and the colon. The bacterial enzyme β-glucuronidase splits off the glucuronide and converts bilirubin into *urobilinogen* (also called stercobilinogen), a colorless compound. About 20% of the urobilinogen formed is reabsorbed from the intestine and reexcreted by the liver into the intestine through bile. This constitutes the *enterohepatic cycle* of urobilinogen. A relatively small amount of urobilinogen that is absorbed from the intestine is excreted in urine. Most of the urobilinogens (colorless) formed in the intestine are further oxidized to *urobilins* (colored compounds) and excreted in feces. The darkening of feces on standing in air is due to conversion of the fecal urobilinogens to urobilins.

Hyperbilirubinemia

The normal serum bilirubin level ranges from 0.3 mg to 1.0 mg/dL. Most of this bilirubin is in the unconjugated form (0.2–0.7 mg/dL). The serum level of conjugated bilirubin is 0.1 to 0.3 mg/dL.

The term *jaundice* or *icterus* refers to the yellowish discoloration of the skin and mucous membranes caused by hyperbilirubinemia. Clinical jaundice is apparent when serum bilirubin exceeds 2 mg/dL. The excess bilirubin in blood may be mostly conjugated or mostly unconjugated. If more than 50% of the bilirubin is conjugated, it is called *predominantly conjugated* hyperbilirubinemia. If less than 15% is conjugated, it is called *predominantly unconjugated* hyperbilirubinemia (**Table 22.1**).

Unconjugated Bilirubinemia

Unconjugated bilirubinemia occurs when bilirubin is produced in excess of what can be conjugated in the liver. It is also called *retention hyperbilirubinemia*. Unconjugated bilirubin is insoluble in water: it is transported in plasma in bound form with albumin. Because albumin is not filtered into urine, unconjugated bilirubin does not appear in the urine (**Fig. 22.6A**). Hence, in unconjugated bilirubinemia, the jaundice is acholuric (no bile in urine).

Albumin has two binding sites for bilirubin: a high-affinity site and a low-affinity site. The high-affinity sites on albumin molecules can bind unconjugated bilirubin up to a concentration of 20 mg/dL. Unconjugated bilirubin in excess of this

Table 22.1 Conjugated versus Unconjugated Bilirubinemia

Conjugated Bilirubinemia	Unconjugated Bilirubinemia
Jaundice is choluric.	Jaundice is acholuric.
Jaundice is mostly due to posthepatic causes. Hepatic causes include infective hepatitis.	Jaundice is mostly due to prehepatic causes. Hepatic causes include neonatal jaundice.
Kernicterus can never occur.	Kernicterus can occur.
Stool may be clay colored.	Stool is never clay colored.
Van den Berg reaction is direct.	Van den Berg reaction is indirect.

amount is bound to the low-affinity site on albumin and dissociates readily. Being lipid soluble, unconjugated bilirubin can cross the blood–brain barrier. It is unable to penetrate the adult brain in large amounts, but in infants, hyperbilirubinemia in excess of 20 mg/dL results in a neurologic disorder called *kernicterus* due to deposition of bilirubin in the lipid-rich basal ganglia.

Unconjugated bilirubinemia can occur due to *prehepatic causes*, such as excessive hemolysis, or due to *hepatic causes*, such as decreased hepatic conjugation of bilirubin. Gilbert syndrome (mild reduction in UDP glucuronyl transferase), Crigler-Najjar syndrome type II (moderate reduction in UDP glucuronyl transferase), and Crigler-Najjar syndrome type I (UDP glucuronyl transferase absent) are hepatic causes of unconjugated bilirubinemia that have genetic etiology. A more common cause is neonatal jaundice.

In **neonatal jaundice,** also called *physiologic jaundice of the newborn,* up to 5 mg/dL of hyperbilirubinemia may be present normally. It appears within 2 to 5 days of birth and lasts for about a week. In the fetus, bilirubin is removed from the circulation by the placenta. At birth, the newborn has to excrete its own bilirubin suddenly, but its hepatic conjugation of bilirubin is still inadequate due to reduced UDP-glucuronyl transferase activity. As a result, hyperbilirubinemia occurs. The hyperbilirubinemia subsides when the newborn's liver matures. The jaundice can be prevented by administration of *phenobarbital* to the pregnant mother or to the newborn. Phenobarbital belongs to a group of drugs called hepatic microsomal enzyme inducers. Microsomal inducers increase the activity of glucuronyl transferase. Neonatal jaundice can be reduced by *phototherapy*. Exposure of the skin to white or blue lights causes photoisomerization of bilirubin to water-soluble lumirubin, which is rapidly excreted in bile without requiring any conjugation.

Conjugated Bilirubinemia

Conjugated bilirubinemia occurs when there is impaired hepatic excretion of bilirubin, and the conjugated bilirubin is returned to the circulation. It is also called *regurgitation hyperbilirubinemia*. Conjugated bilirubin is water soluble and is present in plasma in dissolved form. It gets easily filtered into

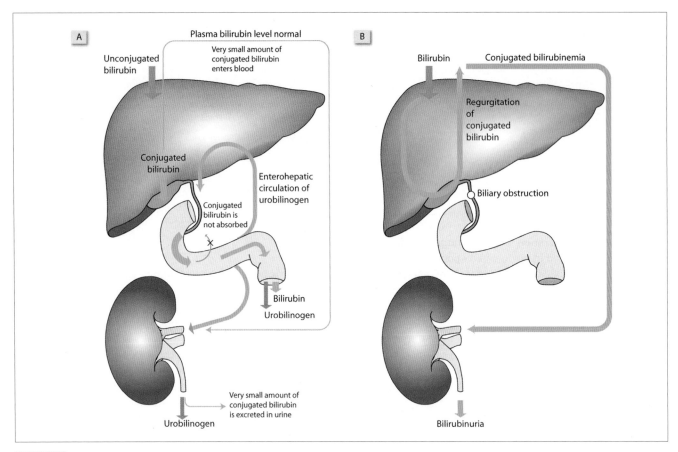

Fig. 22.6 Hyperbilirubinemia. **(A)** Unconjugated bilirubinemia. **(B)** Conjugated bilirubinemia.

urine (**Fig. 22.6B**). Hence, in conjugated bilirubinemia, the jaundice is *choluric* (bile pigment present in urine). Conjugated bilirubinemia can occur due to posthepatic or hepatic impairment of bilirubin excretion.

Posthepatic causes of hyperbilirubinemia (obstructive jaundice) include obstruction of bile ducts and intrahepatic biliary canaliculi. In these conditions, the conjugated bilirubin formed in the liver cells cannot flow out of the biliary canaliculi easily and therefore regurgitates into the hepatic sinusoids, resulting in conjugated hyperbilirubinemia. Because the bile does not enter the intestine, the stool is pale (clay-colored). No urobilinogen is formed either; therefore, none is excreted in the urine.

Hepatic causes include hepatocellular diseases and certain genetic defects in bilirubin excretion, such as Dubin-Johnson syndrome and rotor syndrome. In hepatocellular diseases, all three functions of the liver cells are impaired: uptake of bilirubin, conjugation of bilirubin, and excretion of bilirubin. However, it is the excretion that is most affected, leading to conjugated rather than unconjugated bilirubinemia. Hepatocellular jaundice is therefore choluric and is associated with pale stools. The urine urobilinogen levels first increase and then decrease with increasing severity of hepatocellular jaundice. The *initial rise* in urine urobilinogen is due to a reduction in hepatic reuptake of the urobilinogen absorbed from the intestine into blood. Hence, the urobilinogen is eli-

minated in larger amounts in urine. The *subsequent fall* in urine urobilinogen is due to the reduced excretion of bilirubin into the intestine with consequent reduction in the intestinal urobilinogen synthesis. For the same reason, a rising urinary urobilinogen level in a patient with jaundice under treatment is a good sign.

Hemoglobinemia

When there is excessive removal of erythrocytes by macrophages, it is called *extravascular hemolysis*: it is associated with the release of bilirubin in blood. When there is excessive breakdown of erythrocytes inside the blood vessels, it is called *intravascular hemolysis:* it is associated with the release of free hemoglobin into circulation.

When hemoglobin is released into circulation in large amounts, plasma proteins bind to it so that iron is not lost from the body into the urine. The complexes formed are taken up by hepatocytes, and the iron is recycled. Free hemoglobin released into circulation first combines with *haptoglobin*. When the binding capacity of haptoglobin is exceeded, the hemoglobin gets converted into methemoglobin. The ferriheme (heme containing Fe^{3+}) dissociates from globin and binds to *hemopexin*. When the binding capacity of hemopexin too is exceeded, the ferriheme is bound to plasma *albumin* to form methemalbumin. Low plasma haptoglobin level is an early indicator of excessive hemoglobin breakdown. Low plasma hemopexin or the appearance of methemalbumin in plasma indicates severe increase in hemoglobin breakdown. When the binding capacities of all three plasma proteins are exceeded, hemoglobin starts circulating in blood in free form (hemoglobinemia).

Freely circulating hemoglobin is taken up by macrophages and broken down, resulting in hyperbilirubinemia. Hemoglobin is also filtered into the renal tubules. Small amounts of hemoglobin are removed from the tubules through endocytosis by tubular cells. The iron is stored in renal tubular cells as *hemosiderin*. Hemosiderinuria occurs when these tubular cells are desquamated into tubules. When a large amount of hemoglobin is filtered into the tubules, it is passed into the urine (hemoglobinuria). If the urine is alkaline, the hemoglobin is oxygenated to oxyhemoglobin (pink) in the urinary tract. If the urine is acidic, the hemoglobin is oxidized to methemoglobin (dark brown). The urine color varies accordingly.

Summary

- Hemoglobin is composed of four polypeptide chains and heme, an iron-containing porphyrin.

- The synthesis of hemoglobin begins with the reduction of succinyl-CoA and glycine and successive steps requiring the presence of appropriate enzymes.

- Hemoglobin reversibly binds oxygen and buffers hydrogen ions.

- Both the globin component of hemoglobin and the Fe^{2+} are salvaged from RBCs removed from the circulation and reused to make new RBCs.

Applying What You Know

22.1. Mr. Lundquist's [Hb] = 11 g/dL, and he is clearly anemic. How does this relate his presenting symptom of fatigue?

22.2. Calculate an approximate value for the oxygen content of Mr. Lundquist's arterial blood.

Hemopoiesis

In the fetus, all blood cells originate in the mesenchyme. During the first 2 months of fetal life, blood formation takes place in the yolk sac (**Fig. 23.1A**). Thereafter, the liver becomes the main site of hemopoiesis until about the seventh month, with the spleen making a small contribution. Hemopoiesis commences inside the bone marrow in the third month, and by the seventh month, it is the major site of hemopoiesis (**Fig. 23.1B**).

After birth, red blood cells (RBCs), granulocytes, and platelets are formed in the bone marrow. The marrow makes only a small contribution to lymphocyte production, which occurs mainly in other lymphoid tissues. Monocytes are formed in the bone marrow and partly in the spleen and lymphoid tissues. The spleen, liver, and lymph nodes resume their hemopoietic activity only when there is an excess demand for blood cell formation that cannot be met with bone marrow hyperactivity alone. Such hemopoiesis that occurs outside the bone marrow is called *extramedullary hemopoiesis* and is most common in infants and young children in whom the entire marrow cavity is occupied by red (hemopoietic) marrow, leaving little space for expansion of the marrow cavity.

Stem cells | There are three functionally different stem cells: the *pluripotent stem cell,* which can give rise to any blood cell; the *myeloid stem cell,* giving rise to erythrocytes, granulocytes of all types, monocytes, and platelets; and the *lymphocyte stem cell,* which gives rise only to lymphocytes. All stem cells possess two fundamental properties: self-renewal—pro-

ducing more stem cells through mitosis—and differentiation and commitment, which is the ability to differentiate into any of the mature specialized blood cells.

Progenitor cells | With time, the capability of a stem cell for self-renewal diminishes, and its commitment to a particular line of differentiation increases. When the self-renewal capability is lost, the cell is no longer called a stem cell, but is termed a *progenitor cell*. Progenitor cells are committed to one or at the most two lines of development. Progenitor cells are more numerous than stem cells and like stem cells, are present in both bone marrow and circulating blood. Stem cells and progenitor cells cannot be differentiated morphologically. They both look like a large lymphocyte. However, they can be separated by immunologic techniques, taking advantage of the different types of molecules present on their cell membrane. Progenitor cells are recognized by their ability to give rise to clones (colonies or a group of cells) of differentiated cells in the presence of growth factors. Hence, progenitor cells are also called colony-forming cells (CFC) or colony-forming units (CFU).

Progenitor cells may be multipotent or unipotent (**Figs. 23.2, 23.3**). An example of multipotent progenitor cells is the CFU-

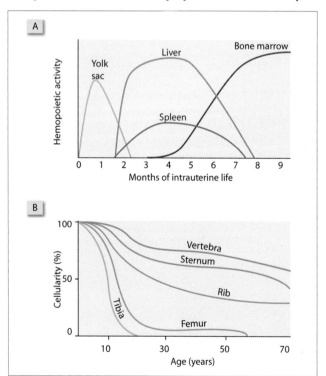

Fig. 23.1 **(A)** Sites of extramedullary erythropoiesis. **(B)** Percentage of red marrow in different bones.

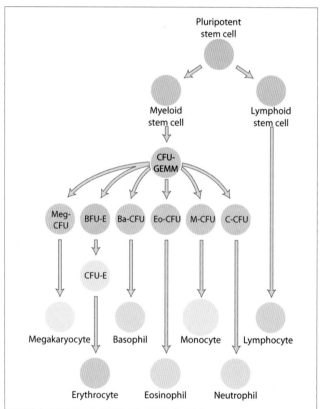

Fig. 23.2 Hemopoietic pathways for the production of red blood cells and white blood cells. CFU-GEMM, colony-forming unit: granulocyte, erythroid, megakaryocyte, macrophage; Meg-CFU, megakaryocytes-colony-forming unit; BFU-E, burst-forming units-erythrocyte; Ba-CFU, Ba-CFU basophil colony-forming unit; Eo-CFU, Eo-CFU eosinophil colony-forming unit; M-CFU, M-CFU macrophage colony-forming unit; G-CFU, G-CFU neutrophil colony-forming unit.

GEMM (colony-forming unit: granulocyte, erythroid, mega-karyocyte, macrophage). Examples of unipotent progenitor cells are CFU-E (erythroid) and Meg-CFU (megakaryocytes). The erythroid series has two types of erythroid progenitor cells: burst-forming units-erythrocyte (BFU-E) and colony-forming units-erythrocyte (CFU-E). BFU-E forms large colonies, whereas CFUE forms much smaller colonies.

Progenitor cells undergo both multiplication and maturation before they are released into the bloodstream. The growth and differentiation of hemopoietic cells are controlled by cytokines. Cytokines that control the granulocytic and thrombocytic series are called *colony-stimulating factors* (CSF). G-CSF stimulates granulocytic precursors, M-CSF stimulates monocytic precursors, and GM-CSF stimulates both. Cytokines that stimulate the lymphocytic series are called *interleukins*. The cytokine stimulating the erythroid series is called *erythropoietin*.

Erythropoiesis

The regulation of erythropoiesis is discussed in Chapter 21. The first cell of the erythroid series is the pronormoblast, which matures successively into the normoblasts, the reticulocyte, and finally an erythrocyte in ~7 days.

The *pronormoblast* (12–20 μm) has a large nucleus that occupies most of the cell. The nucleus contains several nucleoli. The chromatin is finely reticular. The cytoplasm is intensely basophilic (dark blue) because of its high RNA content.

The *normoblasts* are classified into the early (basophilic) normoblast, intermediate (polychromatic) normoblast, late (orthochromatic) normoblast, and reticulocyte (**Fig. 23.4**). Mitotic division occurs up to the stage of the intermediate normoblast, and mitosis is most active at this stage. The late normoblast is not capable of mitotic division. As it proceeds through these stages, the cell and its nucleus become smaller, chromatin becomes thicker and coarser, and the cytoplasm

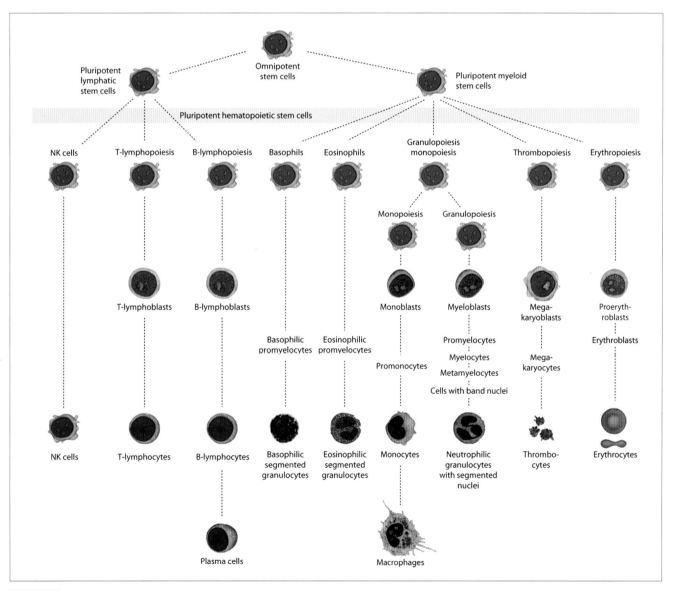

Fig. 23.3 Hemopoietic cells.

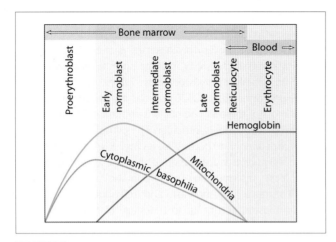

Fig. 23.4 Cytoplasmic changes during erythropoiesis.

becomes less basophilic. The nucleoli disappear in the early normoblast stage. Hemoglobin appears in the intermediate normoblast stage. The acidophilic tint of hemoglobin makes the cytoplasm polychromatic (blue-gray violet). The nucleus becomes pyknotic (a deeply staining, structureless mass) and is extruded in the late normoblast stage. With the loss of the nucleus, formation of new ribosomes in the cytoplasm ceases. The cytoplasm still has a faint polychromatic tint.

The *reticulocyte* is a disk-shaped, nonnucleated cell, of slightly larger volume and diameter than the mature erythrocyte. The hemoglobin content is about the same as that of the mature cell. The cytoplasm still contains small amounts of ribosomic RNA, which results in a faint polychromatic tint with Romanowsky stains. With supravital stain such as brilliant cresyl blue, the RNA appears in the form of a fine reticulum; hence the name reticulocyte. As the reticulocyte matures, the RNA is catabolized, and ribosomes disintegrate. The reticulocyte takes ~2 days to mature to an erythrocyte. Reticulocytes are present in the circulation, where they comprise 0.2 to 2.0% of the RBC count. Their number increases in hemolytic anemia and following treatment of deficiency anemias.

The formation of microcytes in iron deficiency and macrocytes in vitamin B$_{12}$ is linked to the mitotic activity of erythrocytic precursors. When hemoglobin reaches the critical concentration of ~20 g/dL, it enters the nucleus through nuclear pores and reacts with nuclear histone. The reaction inhibits DNA replication and thereby disables mitosis. In iron deficiency, the critical hemoglobin concentration is reached later, allowing mitosis to continue longer and resulting in the formation of smaller RBCs. Conversely, vitamin B$_{12}$ is essential for DNA synthesis; therefore, its deficiency inhibits mitosis, resulting in the formation of megaloblasts and macrocytes.

Leukopoiesis

Granulocytic (myeloid) series | The first recognizable cell of the granulocytic series is the myeloblast (15–20 µm), from which the mature granulocytes develop through a series of cells: the promyelocyte, myelocyte, metamyelocyte, and band cell. Apart from the difference in granules, the myelo-

cyte, metamyelocyte, and band form have similar morphologic characteristics. The maturation of the granulocytes is characterized by the development of azurophilic granules (in the promyelocyte stage), disappearance of nucleoli, appearance of specific granules (in the myelocyte stage), and cessation of mitosis (in the metamyelocyte stage). There is a progressive loss of cytoplasmic basophilia, ripening of the nucleus, which ultimately becomes segmented, and the development of motility and ability to act as a phagocyte.

Lymphocytic series | The lymphoblast resembles the myeloblast except that its nucleus contains fewer nucleoli and coarser chromatin. Lymphoblasts give rise successively to the large and small lymphocytes, both of which are found in the circulation.

Monocytic series | Monocytes are formed mainly in the bone marrow and migrate to the spleen and lymphoid tissues. The earliest cell is the monoblast, which gives rise to the promonocyte and the mature monocyte. The monoblast is a large cell that cannot be distinguished from the myeloblast on morphologic grounds alone. The promonocyte (20 µm) has a large kidney-shaped nucleus. The chromatin is reticular. The cytoplasm is a dull gray-blue and may contain fine azurophilic granules.

Thrombopoiesis

The megakaryoblast (20–30 µm) is the first cell in the platelet series. It develops into a larger promegakaryocyte and a still larger megakaryocyte (30–90 µm). The megakaryocyte (**Fig. 23.5**) has a single multilobed nucleus with coarse clumps of chromatin. The cytoplasm is light blue and contains fine azurophilic granules. The cell margin is irregular and may show pseudopodia. Platelets are formed by the breaking off of small fragments of these megakaryocytes.

Bone Marrow

Bone marrow is liquid in consistency. Its color is either red or yellow. Hemopoiesis occurs in the red marrow. Yellow marrow is composed mainly of fat cells. An adult has ~3 to 4 L of bone marrow, nearly half of which is red marrow. Besides hemopoietic cells, mature blood cells, and fat cells, bone marrow contains reticulum cells and reticulin fibers, blood vessels, and nerves. The reticulin fibers form a supporting network for the hemopoietic cells that lie outside the blood vessels. The reticulum cells are potentially hemopoietic and form part of the functional reserve of the marrow (see below). The ratio of white blood cells (WBCs) to nucleated RBCs is normally ~3 to 5:1. Megakaryocytes and lymphoid follicles are also present, though in smaller numbers.

The marrow sinusoids connect the arterial capillaries with the venules. Developing blood cells lie outside the sinusoids. Unlike the spleen, the marrow sinusoids form a closed system with no openings into the extravascular spaces. Hence, the newly formed cells have to cross the sinusoid walls before entering the circulation. The sinusoids are innervated by sensory nerve fibers. These nerves explain the pain produced when marrow is aspirated.

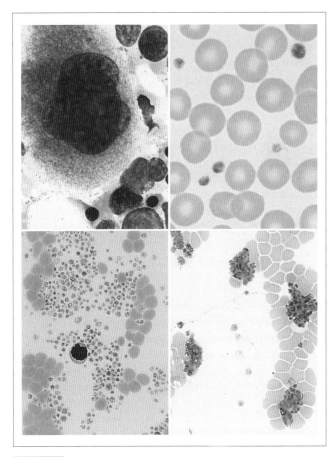

Fig. 23.5 Megakaryocytes (*above, left*) and thrombocytes.

At birth, the marrow in all the bones of the body appears red and contains no fat. By the age of 5 years, fat cells begin to appear, and the red marrow in the long bones gradually is replaced by yellow fatty marrow. The replacement occurs first in the bones of the hands and feet and then in the bones of the arms and legs from the distal to the proximal ends. By the age of 20 years, red marrow is found only in the bones of the thorax (ribs, clavicles, scapula, and sternum), vertebra, skull, pelvis, and the upper one-third of the femur and humerus shafts (**Fig. 23.1B**).

Bone marrow reserve | The bone marrow has a large reserve capacity that enables it to increase its output to as much as 13 times normal. The reserve capacity of the marrow is comprised of two components. The *functional reserve* is attributable to stem cells in the marrow that start proliferating and differentiating. Initially, only the intermediate normoblasts and myelocytes start proliferating. Later, even the more primitive early normoblasts and promyelocytes start proliferating. The *anatomical reserve* is in the form of the fat cells that can be readily replaced by active hemopoietic cells. The replacement of fat cells occurs initially in the red marrow itself, which becomes redder in color. Later, yellow marrow is transformed into red marrow, either by activation of the dormant stem cells or by migration of stem cells from red marrow. Still later, the bone is eroded by the expanding marrow cavity.

Bone Marrow Biopsy

Bone marrow biopsy is an important method of investigation in blood disorders. There are two main methods of biopsy. In *aspiration biopsy,* bone marrow is aspirated through a specially constructed wide-bore needle. The aspirate consists of marrow diluted with a variable amount of blood. Films of the aspirated marrow are made on glass slides; they are stained as blood films using a Romanowsky stain. The sternum and the posterior iliac crest are the sites of choice for marrow aspiration. The anterior iliac crest and spinous processes of the lumbar vertebrae are also suitable for marrow aspiration. In *trephine biopsy,* a specially constructed trephine (hollow tube with serrated cutting edge) is used to obtain the biopsy specimen. Trephine biopsy gives a histologic section in which bony trabeculae, hemopoietic tissue, fat cells, and blood vessels are seen—the architecture of the marrow is preserved.

The following features are systematically noted in bone marrow biopsy: (1) the cellularity of the marrow, indicating whether it is hyperactive or hypoactive; (2) the type and activity of erythropoiesis, which can indicate megaloblastic anemia; (3) the number and type of developing WBCs, which can indicate leukemias; (4) the number and type of megakaryocytes; (5) the myeloid–erythroid ratio, which is normally ~3 to 5:1 (reduction of the ratio to 1:1 suggests erythroid hyperplasia); (6) the iron content of the marrow (seen as hemosiderin granules or ferritin); and (7) the presence of foreign or tumor cells, parasites, or organisms.

Summary

- Hemopoiesis is the production of blood cells of all types. In the adult, it occurs in bone marrow.

- Hemopoiesis begins with pluripotent stem cells that differentiate into pluripotent lymphatic stem cells (the progenitors of all lymphocytes) and pluripotent myeloid stem cells (the progenitors of all of the other WBCs and erythrocytes).

Applying What You Know

23.1. Is Mr. Lundquist's anemia due to a decreased rate of production of red blood cells or an increased rate of destruction of red blood cells? How do you know?

24 Hematinic Factors

The production of red blood cells (RBCs) and the hemoglobin that they contain is determined by many physiologic factors. Agents or processes that result in increased hemoglobin concentration or increased production of RBCs are said to be hematinic. Three such factors to be considered here are iron (an essential component in hemoglobin), folic acid (needed for DNA synthesis), and vitamin B_{12} (needed to maintain an appropriate level of folate).

Iron

It is important to note that iron balance is achieved solely by control of absorption rather than by control of excretion. Iron is not directly excreted; it is lost from the body only when iron-laden cells are lost, especially epithelial cells from the gastrointestinal tract.

Mechanism of Iron Absorption

Iron absorption occurs almost entirely in the duodenum (**Table 24.1**). Only 5% of the ingested iron is normally absorbed. A non-vegetarian diet contains iron mostly in the heme form; a vegetarian diet contains iron in the nonheme form. The absorption of nonheme and heme iron occurs by different mechanisms.

Dietary nonheme iron is ingested mainly in the form of insoluble salts, such as $Fe(OH)_3$ and $FePO_4$, and insoluble complexes with dietary substances, such as phytates (present in grains and bran), polyphenols (present in legumes, tea, coffee, and wine), egg white, and bovine milk protein. In its insoluble form, iron is unable to diffuse in adequate amounts to the intestinal brush border (see Chapter 70).

Gastric acid is necessary for iron absorption because it dissolves the insoluble ferric (Fe^{3+}) salts and complexes. The dissolved Fe^{3+} forms complexes with reducing substances in the diet, such as ascorbic acid and cysteine (present in meats), and is reduced to Fe^{2+} (ferrous). The intestinal brush border can absorb only Fe^{2+}. Hence, iron absorption is impaired in subjects with gastrectomy or achlorhydria (inability to secrete HCl in the stomach).

The enzyme *ferric reductase,* present on the intestinal brush border, reduces any remaining Fe^{3+} to Fe^{2+}. Ferrous iron is taken up into the intestinal mucosal cells (enterocytes) through facilitated diffusion across the luminal border. Once inside, the Fe^{2+} is oxidized to Fe^{3+} by the enzyme *ferroxidase* and bound to apoferritin to form *ferritin.* At the basolateral border of the enterocyte, the ferritin dissociates to release Fe^{3+}, which diffuses out into the blood through facilitated diffusion.

Dietary heme iron is freed from its apoprotein (globin) by exposure to gastric acid and proteases. The free heme, containing iron in the Fe^{2+} form, is transported into the enterocyte intact by a specific *heme transporter.* Inside the enterocyte, the enzyme *heme oxygenase* releases Fe^{2+} from heme and adds it to the free Fe^{2+} pool in the enterocyte. The subsequent fate of heme and nonheme Fe^{2+} is the same. Absorption of heme iron is relatively unaffected by the presence of other foods in the diet.

Regulation of Iron Absorption

The intestinal mucosal cell absorbs iron in proportion to the body's need for iron to maintain the rate of erythropoiesis. As mentioned above, the iron absorbed into the mucosal cell binds to apoferritin to form ferritin. The ferritin then releases

Table 24.1 Nutritional Aspects of Iron

Dietary form	Ferric (Fe^{3+})
Daily requirements	10–20 mg in diet (Only 10% of the dietary intake is absorbed.)
Sources	Meat, liver, egg, leafy vegetables, whole wheat, and jaggery (a type of sugar)
Absorption	Fe^{3+} is reduced to Fe^{2+} by ferric reductase present on enterocytes. Reducing substances such as vitamin C enhance absorption. Phosphates and phytates (present in cereals) decrease absorption by forming insoluble complexes with iron.
Site of absorption	Duodenum and upper jejunum
Body resources	5 g (in the liver, spleen, bone marrow, lymph nodes, and the RES cells)
Storage forms	⅔ as ferritin and ⅓ as hemosiderin
Transport form	As Fe^{2+} bound to transferrin; as ferritin (ferric hydrophosphate) bound to apoferritin
Role	Synthesis of hemoglobin, myoglobin, and cytochromes (intracellular enzymes)
Causes of deficiency	Decrease in dietary intake or absorption; increased demand (pregnancy) or losses (hemorrhage)
Effects of deficiency	Iron deficiency anemia
Effects of excess	Hemosiderosis and hemochromatosis
Diagnosis of deficiency	Serum iron level (normal =120 µg/dL) and total iron-binding capacity (normal = 250–450 µg/dL)
Therapeutic form	Ferrous sulfate

Abbreviation: RES, reticuloendothelial system.

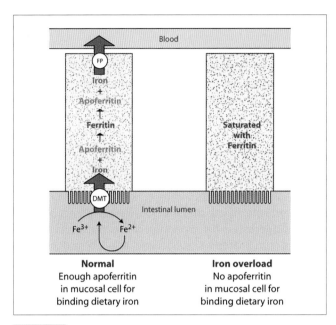

Fig. 24.1 Regulation of iron absorption. DMT, dimethyltryptamine; FP, ferroportin.

iron into the bloodstream and reverts back to apoferritin. The *mucosal block theory* (**Fig. 24.1**) says that when the body iron stores are high, mucosal ferritin does not release iron into the bloodstream (in accordance with the dynamics of chemical equilibrium). Consequently, the mucosal cells remain loaded with ferritin. With all the apoferritin converted into ferritin, the mucosal cell is not able to take up any more luminal iron. Mucosal cells have a life span of 3 to 4 days, at the end of which they get sloughed off into the intestine. Mucosal ferritin iron is also lost with them, ridding the body of its unwanted iron.

Iron Cycle

The term *iron cycle* (**Fig. 24.2A**) refers to the uptake of iron from plasma into erythrocytes and its eventual return to the plasma after the death of the erythrocytes. Each day ~30 mg of iron goes through this cycle. Iron travels from plasma to the bone marrow, where it is incorporated into hemoglobin. At the end of their life span, erythrocytes are engulfed by macrophages lining the sinuses of the liver, spleen, and bone marrow. After phagocytosis, the RBC membrane is lysed, heme is released from hemoglobin, and iron is liberated by the enzyme heme oxygenase, completing the cycle.

Not all of the iron in blood is recycled. For example, the pulmonary alveolar macrophages (PAM) lack the ability to return the iron to the circulation; they store the iron. These iron-laden macrophages may remain in the tissues, or they may enter the circulation only to leave the body subsequently through the intestine. Similarly, iron is taken up each day by many tissues for the synthesis of nonhemoglobin, iron-containing enzymes, and proteins such as cytochromes, catalases, and myoglobin. The amount of iron lost to these tissues daily is ~2 mg, which must be replenished in the diet. These tissues include (1) the liver, which takes up the largest amount of iron next only to the RBCs; (2) the placenta, which transfers the iron to the fe-

tus; (3) intestinal mucosal cells, which store iron as ferritin, thereby regulating iron absorption; (4) skeletal muscles, which produce myoglobin; and (5) proliferating cells that require excess cytochromes and catalases.

Iron Transport in Plasma

The plasma protein that transports iron is called *transferrin*. It is a glycoprotein, and it binds up to two atoms of Fe^{3+}. Transferrin is synthesized chiefly in the liver. Its rate of synthesis is inversely related to the amount of iron stored in the body. Hence, in iron deficiency, plasma transferrin increases. Clinically, the amount of transferrin is expressed in terms of the amount of iron it will bind, that is, the *total iron-binding capacity* (TIBC). Transferrin-mediated transport ensures delivery of iron only to those cells that need iron, that is, the RBC precursors. Unbound iron becomes distributed to all cells equally, irrespective of their iron requirement. The importance of transferrin is apparent in *congenital atransferrinemia*, where erythrocytes show signs of iron deficiency, but tissues are loaded with iron.

Regulation of Cellular Uptake of Iron

Transferrin delivers its iron to the RBCs and other tissues by binding to specific *transferrin receptors*. The rate of iron uptake by a cell is related to the number of transferrin receptors on its surface. During erythropoiesis, the number of transferrin receptors reaches its peak in intermediate normoblasts when hemoglobin first makes its appearance. Cells shed their receptors as their iron requirement decreases. The shed receptors can be found in plasma in a concentration that correlates with the rate of erythropoiesis.

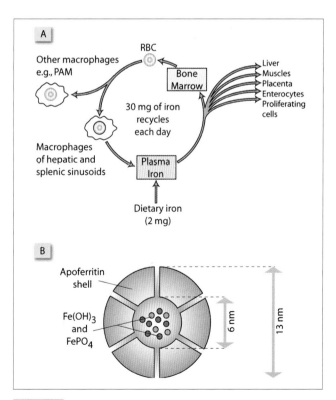

Fig. 24.2 **(A)** The iron cycle. **(B)** Structure of ferritin. RBC, red blood cell; PAM, pulmonary alveolar macrophage.

When plasma iron concentration is high, the cells inhibit the synthesis of transferrin receptors and increase the synthesis of apoferritin, thereby limiting further acquisition of iron and facilitating storage of any excess. In contrast, when plasma iron concentration is low, the cells increase the synthesis of transferrin receptors and reduce the synthesis of apoferritin, maximizing iron entry and utilization while minimizing the diversion of iron into stores.

Iron Storage Proteins

The two iron storage compounds are ferritin and hemosiderin. Iron exchanges mostly with ferritin. The exchange with the hemosiderin is much slower.

Ferritin (**Fig. 24.2B**) is made of an iron-free apoferritin (protein) shell with a hollow central cavity containing a complex of $Fe(OH)_3$ and $FePO_4$. The cavity communicates with the surface by six channels, through which iron can enter and leave. A fully saturated ferritin molecule can hold up to ~4500 iron atoms.

Hemosiderin represents a more stable form of storage iron than ferritin. It is formed in the macrophages and hepatocytes when a large amount of iron accumulates in them. Hemosiderin is a dense aggregate of ferritin crystals. It is formed inside the lysosome and is therefore usually membrane-bound. The lysosomal enzymes digest the proteins of the ferritin. As a result, the iron increases in concentration and polymerizes. Lipids and other substances are added to the aggregate, making the composition of hemosiderin quite variable. The iron in hemosiderin is mostly in the form of Fe_2O_3 (**Table 24.2**).

General Model: Reservoir

In attempting to understand the complex processes involved in maintaining an appropriate level of iron in the body, it is useful to keep in mind the reservoir model. To maintain a constant and appropriate iron level requires keeping track of the inputs of iron to the system (diet and absorption) as well as the sources of loss of iron from the system.

Table 24.2 Comparison of Ferritin and Hemosiderin

Ferritin	Hemosiderin
Composition fairly consistent	Composition highly variable
Not enclosed by membrane	Usually enclosed by membrane
Less iron content (~20%)	More iron content (~30%)
Protein content higher	Protein content lower
Iron in the form of $Fe(OH)_3$ and $FePO_4$	Iron in the form of Fe_2O_3
Water-soluble	Water-insoluble
Stains with Prussian blue	Does not stain with Prussian blue

Iron Storage Disorders

Siderotic granules are granules of nonheme iron in the RBC. The granules represent the iron present in excess of requirements for hemoglobin synthesis. *Siderocytes* are RBCs containing siderotic granules; precursor cells (normoblasts and reticulocytes) containing siderotic granules are called *sideroblasts*. Sideroblasts are normally present in bone marrow. Siderocytes appear in the blood in significant numbers after splenectomy. This is because normally the spleen temporarily sequesters reticulocytes released from bone marrow until they complete heme synthesis, using up all their iron (siderotic) stores. Following splenectomy, reticulocyte maturation occurs in the peripheral blood; thus, siderocytes appear in blood.

Hemosiderosis is the deposition of hemosiderin in the tissues. The term *siderosis* is broader and includes the deposition of other forms of iron too, such as ferritin. *Hemochromatosis* is a hereditary condition in which the iron overload occurs due to increased iron absorption from the gut. However, the term is also used synonymously with hemosiderosis. To avoid confusion, the hereditary form of hemosiderosis is called primary hemochromatosis; the other forms are called secondary hemochromatosis.

Hemosiderosis is of four types: local hemosiderosis, hemolytic or transfusional hemosiderosis, nutritional hemosiderosis, and primary hemochromatosis. In local hemosiderosis, the iron deposition is localized to a small part of the body. In others, the hemosiderin deposits are found throughout the body.

Local hemosiderosis develops when there is hemorrhage into the tissues. Macrophages phagocytose the RBCs and store their iron as ferritin and hemosiderin. If the hemorrhage is small, the macrophages migrate away from the site, but if the hemorrhage is large, the hemosiderin-laden macrophages remain at the site.

Hemolytic hemosiderosis is seen in hemolytic anemias. It is also called transfusional hemosiderosis because it occurs following repeated blood transfusion. Initially, the hemosiderin accumulates in the mononuclear phagocytic system (MPS) cells, but in prolonged and severe cases, the parenchymal cells, like those of the liver and myocardium, are also overloaded with hemosiderin.

Nutritional hemosiderosis occurs due to an increased intake of iron. It is sometimes caused by excessive consumption of red wine, which has a high iron content. Alcohol also increases the absorption of iron.

Primary hemochromatosis is a genetic disease that results in increased absorption of iron from the gut. Its exact mechanism is not known.

Folic Acid

Folic acid is another essential factor contributing to hemoglobin and RBC production. Folic acid, or *pteroylglutamic acid*, consists of the base pteridine attached to one molecule each of *p-aminobenzoic acid* (PABA) and *glutamic acid* (**Fig. 24.3A**). Animals cannot synthesize folates; therefore, they require folate in their diet. In plants, folic acid is present as a *polyglutamate conjugate* consisting of a polypeptide chain of seven

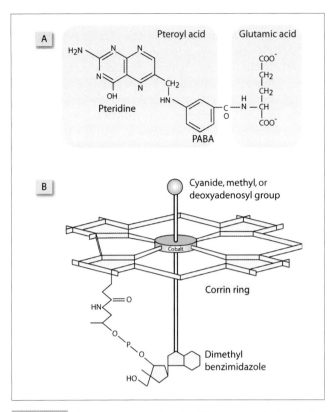

Fig. 24.3 (A) Structure of folic acid. (B) Structure of vitamin B₁₂. PABA, *p*-aminobenzoic acid; THF, tetrahydrofolate.

glutamate residues. In liver (consumed as food), the major folate is a *pentaglutamyl conjugate.* These *polyglutamyl folates* in the diet are broken down by intestinal enzymes to *monoglutamyl folates* for absorption. Most of this is reduced to *tetrahydrofolate* (THF) in the intestinal cell by the enzyme *folate reductase.* THF is the active form of folic acid (**Table 24.3**).

Action of Folic Acid

Folic acid is important for DNA synthesis, an essential step in the daily production of new RBCs. *THF* acts as a carrier for activated one-carbon units such as *methyl, methylene, methenyl, formyl,* and *formimino.* By transferring a methyl group, it helps in DNA synthesis (**Fig. 26.4**), which requires methylation of uridine to thymidine. Serine provides the methyl group required. THF transfers the methyl group from serine to uridine in two steps. (1) Serine transfers the methylene group to THF to form glycine and methylene-THF. (2) Methylene-THF transfers the methyl group to uridine and, in the process, gets converted to *dihydrofolate* (DHF).

The regeneration of THF from DHF occurs in the presence of *folate reductase.* If the THF is not regenerated, it results in folate deficiency, which can be overcome only by excess dietary intake. *Methotrexate,* an anticancer drug, is an inhibitor of folate reductase. By preventing the regeneration of THF, it impairs DNA synthesis. Hence, it especially impairs the function of vigorously multiplying cells that have to synthesize a lot of DNA.

Table 24.3 Nutritional Aspects of Vitamin B₁₂ and Folic Acid

	Folic Acid	**Cobalamin**
Dietary form	Polyglutamates	Deoxyadenosyl-cobalamin
Daily requirements	200 µg	2 µg
Sources	Liver, leafy vegetables, yeast, and legumes	Animal products (meat, liver, fish, eggs, and milk)
Absorption	Pancreatic carboxypeptidases reduce poly- to mono-glutamates. Jejunal mucosal cells convert monoglutamates to absorbable methyl-THF	Intrinsic factor secreted by the parietal cells binds to B₁₂ as well as to the ileal receptors, thereby facilitating diffusion
Site of absorption	Ileum	Ileum
Body resources	500 mg (in liver, erythrocytes, and leukocytes)	5 mg (in liver)
Storage forms	5-methyl THF	Deoxyadenosyl-cobalamin
Transport form	5-methyl THF	As methylcobalamin bound to transcobalamin
Role	DNA synthesis in blood cells	DNA synthesis in blood cells
Causes of deficiency	Decreased dietary intake or absorption; increased demand (pregnancy)	Low intake/absorption; high demand pregnancy) or losses (fish tapeworm infestation)
Active form	Tetrahydrofolate	Methylcobalamin and deoxyadenosylcobalamin
Effects of deficiency	Megaloblastic anemia	Megaloblastic anemia
Effects of excess	Water-soluble. Excess is excreted.	Water-soluble. Excess is excreted.
Diagnosis of deficiency	Serum folic acid level (normal = 200 ng/dL); FIGLU test (increased urinary excretion of formiminoglutamic acid)	Serum B₁₂ level (normal = 50 µg/dL); methyl-malonic acid test (increased urinary excretion in deficiency)
Therapeutic form	Pteroylglutamic acid	Hydroxycobalamin

Abbreviations: FIGLU, formiminoglutamic acid; THF, tetrahydrofolate.

Some of the methylene-THF formed gets converted (trapped) into *methyl-THF*. It is called the *methyl trap* or the *folate trap.* Recovery of THF from methyl-THF requires vitamin B$_{12}$.

Folate Deficiency

The common causes of folate deficiency are (1) *inadequate intake,* mostly due to an unbalanced diet (common in alcoholics; teenagers, who are affected by food fads/consume too much junk food); (2) *increased requirements,* as in pregnancy, infancy, malignancy, and increased hematopoiesis (chronic hemolytic anemias); (3) *malabsorption due to celiac sprue;* and (4) *folate inhibitors* such as methotrexate.

Because folic acid is important for DNA synthesis and cell division, the cells that multiply rapidly, such as the hemopoietic cells, are especially affected. Erythropoiesis, leukopoiesis, and thrombopoiesis all are affected. Defective erythropoiesis results in anemia. The RBC precursors such as the normoblasts grow in size but fail to divide in time, resulting in large cells called *megaloblasts.* The anemia that is associated with the presence of megaloblasts in bone marrow is called *megaloblastic anemia.* The erythrocytes that appear in the circulation are also large (macrocytes).

Vitamin B$_{12}$

Vitamin B$_{12}$ is essential for RBC production. Vitamin B$_{12}$ (*cobalamin*) is a corrin ring (similar to a porphyrin ring) with a cobalt ion at its center (**Fig. 24.3B**). The vitamin is synthesized entirely by bacteria and certain fungi. It is absent from plants unless they are contaminated by bacteria or fungi. Although colonic bacteria synthesize cobalamin, the colonic cobalamins are unabsorbable in humans. Animals, especially ruminants, are, however, able to absorb colonic cobalamins. Humans derive their cobalamins from the meat, milk, and especially the liver of these animals. The commercial preparation is *cyanocobalamin.* The stability of this compound and therefore its shelf life are much higher than other forms of cobalamin (**Table 24.3**).

Absorption and Storage

The intestinal absorption of vitamin B$_{12}$ is possible only if the vitamin B$_{12}$ is bound to the *intrinsic factor,* a glycoprotein secreted by parietal cells of the gastric mucosa. Dietary vitamin B$_{12}$ is bound to proteins.

In the acidic pH of the stomach, vitamin B$_{12}$ dissociates from dietary proteins and binds to haptocorrin, also called R-binder, which is present in swallowed saliva. In the alkaline pH of the duodenum, pancreatic trypsin releases vitamin B$_{12}$ from R-binder and allows it to bind to the intrinsic factor. The intrinsic factor–methylcobalamin complex binds to specific receptors in the ileum and is absorbed by endocytosis. Inside the mucosal cells, cobalamin is transferred from intrinsic factor to transcobalamin II, another cyanocobalamin-binding protein. Transcobalamin II transports cobalamin in blood (**Fig. 24.4**). Cobalamin is stored in the liver, bound to transcobalamin.

The absorption of vitamin B$_{12}$ is impaired in achlorhydria because it is not released from dietary proteins. It is also

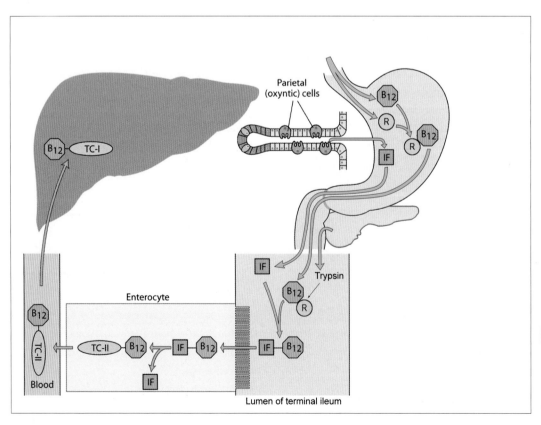

Fig. 24.4 The role of intrinsic factor (IF) and R-binder in the absorption of vitamin B$_{12}$. FIGLU, formiminoglutamic acid; THF, tetrahydrofolute.

impaired in pancreatic insufficiency because it is not released from R-binder.

The **Schilling test** is used for estimating vitamin B_{12} absorption. In this test, a small dose of radiolabeled vitamin B_{12} is administered orally, and the amount of B_{12} absorbed is assessed by measuring the radioactivity in urine. If the absorption of vitamin B_{12} appears to be reduced, the test is repeated after supplementing intrinsic factor along with oral radioactive vitamin B_{12}.

Actions of Vitamin B_{12}

Inside the cells, cobalamin is converted into its active forms: methylcobalamin and deoxyadenosylcobalamin. *Methylcobalamin* is required for THF recovery from methyl trap and S-adenyl methionine (SAM) production. *Deoxyadenosylcobalamin* is a coenzyme for an important gluconeogenetic reaction.

THF recovery and SAM production | The recovery of THF from the methyl trap and SAM production are interlinked (**Fig. 24.5**). Cobalamin removes the methyl group from methyl-THF and in the process gets converted into methylcobalamin. Methylcobalamin then transfers the methyl group to homocysteine,

which gets converted into methionine. Cobalamin gets regenerated in the process. One of the products of methionine is SAM, which is important for maintenance of myelin in neurons.

The above reactions explain an observation of great clinical importance. Vitamin B_{12} deficiency produces megaloblastic anemia and neurologic symptoms. Megaloblastic anemia occurs because the folate that gets trapped in the methyl trap is not recovered, resulting in folate deficiency. Hence, an increase in dietary folate improves the megaloblastic anemia caused by vitamin B_{12} deficiency. The neurologic deficiencies, however, are not improved by folate administration. It is therefore important not to administer folate supplements indiscriminately. If there is a deficiency of vitamin B_{12}, the folate supplements prevent the occurrence of megaloblastic anemia. In the absence of megaloblastic anemia, the vitamin B_{12} deficiency tends to go undiagnosed, although the neurologic changes associated with it continue unabated. The above reaction also explains the occurrence of *homocystinuria* in vitamin B_{12} deficiency.

Gluconeogenesis | Deoxyadenosylcobalamin is the coenzyme for conversion of methylmalonyl-coenzyme A (CoA) to succinyl-CoA. This is a key reaction in the pathway of conversion of propionate (an amino acid) to succinyl-CoA (a member of the citric acid cycle); it is therefore of significance in the process of gluconeogenesis. The urinary excretion of methylmalonyl-CoA is increased (methylmalonic aciduria) in vitamin B_{12} deficiency and has been used as a test for vitamin B_{12} deficiency.

Vitamin B_{12} Deficiency

Dietary deficiency of vitamin B_{12} is uncommon even in vegetarians who obtain adequate vitamin B_{12} in milk. Most cases of vitamin B_{12} deficiency are due to a reduction in intestinal absorption of vitamin B_{12}, the causes of which can be (1) *inadequate intrinsic factor* (IF), as in pernicious anemia and gastrectomy; (2) *disorders* (*sprue, enteritis*) or *resection of terminal ileum;* and (3) *competition for cobalamin* by fish tapeworm and bacteria (in the blind loop syndrome), which consume most of the cobalamin in the intestine, leaving little for absorption.

The main effects of vitamin B_{12} deficiency are (1) megaloblastic anemia, (2) glossitis (sore tongue), (3) *neurologic manifestations* due to demyelination and axonal degeneration of peripheral nerves and posterolateral columns of the spinal cord, and (4) biochemical consequences, such as homocystinuria and methylmalonic aciduria.

Pernicious anemia is an autoimmune disease that destroys most of the gastric mucosa, abolishing almost completely the secretion of not only IF, but also gastric HCl (*achlorhydria*) and pepsin. The abolition of IF secretion impairs vitamin B_{12} absorption, producing all the signs of vitamin B_{12} deficiency, notably megaloblastic anemia.

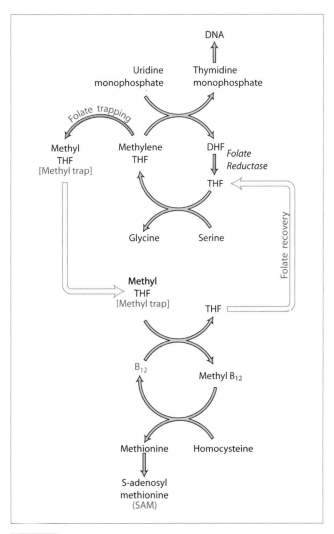

Fig. 24.5 The role of folate in DNA synthesis, the folate trap, and the role of vitamin B_{12} in folate recovery. DHF, dihydrofolate; IF, intrinsic factor; THF, tetrahydrofolate.

Summary

● Factors that increase the production of hemoglobin or RBCs are called *hematinic factors.*

● The three principal hematinic factors are iron, folate, and vitamin B_{12}.

- Absorption of iron in the gastrointestinal tract is regulated at the intestinal mucosal cells via an iron-transporting protein, apoferritin.

- Folate is essential for DNA synthesis; with reduced levels of folate, the rapidly reproducing hematopoietic cells in bone marrow cannot make RBCs.

- Vitamin B_{12} plays an essential role in the recovery of folate in the metabolic pathways that produce DNA.

Applying What You Know

24.1. A test has revealed that Mr. Lundquist is producing antibodies against intrinsic factor. Describe the consequences that would be expected.

The outcome of indiscriminate transfusion of blood from one individual (the donor) to another (the recipient) can be fatal. This happens when certain immunoglobulins (called *agglutinins*) present in the recipient's plasma react with certain antigenic proteins (called *agglutinogens*) on the donor's erythrocytes. The reaction results in the lysis of the donor's erythrocytes with lethal consequences. Both agglutinogens and agglutinins are of several different types, and each agglutinogen has a specific agglutinin with which it reacts. By ensuring that the recipient's plasma does not have the agglutinins that are specific for the agglutinogens on the donor erythrocytes, fatal outcomes from transfusions can be avoided. Establishment of a system of blood groupings has made it possible to minimize the occurrence of this problem.

Blood Group Systems

Blood is grouped based on the type of agglutinogen present on the erythrocytes. Thus, blood group A has A agglutinogen on its erythrocytes; blood group M has M agglutinogen on its erythrocytes. All blood groups obey, in whole or in part, *Landsteiner's law,* which states that (1) when the red blood cells (RBCs) contain a particular agglutinogen, the corresponding agglutinin is always absent in the plasma of that blood; and (2) when a particular agglutinogen is not present on the RBCs, the corresponding agglutinin is always present in the plasma. The first clause of the law is always true, but the second clause is valid only for the ABO blood groups.

Although innumerable agglutinogens have been identified in the blood, the important ones are those that are widely prevalent in the population and that cause the worst transfusion reactions. These are called the *major blood group systems:* the ABO and the rhesus (CDE) systems. Some blood groups are found only in a small proportion of the population and occasionally produce mild transfusion reactions. These are called the *minor blood group systems:* MN, P, and so on. In addition to the major and minor blood groups, there are *familial blood groups,* which are prevalent only in a few families.

The **ABO system** comprises two agglutinogens, A and B, whose corresponding agglutinins are α and β. Accordingly, there are four blood groups in the ABO system: *group A,* which has A agglutinogen; *group B,* which has B agglutinogen; *group AB,* which has both; and *group O,* which has neither. Group A has β agglutinin, group B has α agglutinin, group AB has neither, and *group O* has both (**Table 25.1**). Both α and β agglutinins are immunoglobulin M (IgM), which is very effective in causing agglutination (clumping) of the RBCs.

In the United States, ~40% of the population has A group, 11% has B group, and 45% has O group blood. Only 4% has AB group blood. These proportions vary in different countries and ethnic groups.

The **rhesus blood group** agglutinogens were first discovered in the erythrocytes of rhesus monkeys. Rhesus blood

Table 25.1 ABO and Rhesus Blood Groups

Group		Agglutinogen	Agglutinin
ABO system	A	A	β
	B	B	α
	AB	A and B	–
	O	–	α and β
Rhesus system	Rh+	D	–
	Rh–	–	–

group comprises a system of three agglutinogens: C, D, and E. However, for practical purposes, the term *rhesus agglutinogen* refers to the D agglutinogen, which produces the worst transfusion reactions. Accordingly, the rhesus system comprises only two blood groups, rhesus positive (Rh-positive or D+) and rhesus negative (Rh-negative or D–), depending on the presence or absence of D agglutinogen (**Table 25.1**).

Unlike in the ABO system, there are no natural antibodies to rhesus agglutinogens. Anti-D antibodies develop only when a D– person is transfused with D+ blood. Once produced, these antibodies persist in blood for years and can produce serious reactions during a second transfusion.

Anti-D agglutinins are predominantly immunoglobulin G (IgG) and partly immunoglobulin M (IgM). Unlike IgM, which is very effective in agglutinating agglutinogen-bearing RBCs, IgG does not agglutinate RBCs, although they do react with the agglutinin. Such immunoglobulins that do not cause agglutination are called *incomplete antibodies*. Although they do not agglutinate RBCs, IgG-coated RBCs still get lysed due to the activation of complement on their surface (see Humoral Immunity section, the complement system, Chapter 31).

Blood Grouping

For *ABO blood grouping,* the test sample of blood or erythrocyte suspension is reacted with sera containing α and β (called antiserum A and antiserum B). The sample is grouped according to the serum that agglutinates its RBCs (**Fig. 25.1**).

Rhesus blood grouping can be done in the same way as ABO grouping if the anti-D agglutinin used is of the IgM type. If the anti-D agglutinin used is IgG, the D+ RBCs will get coated with anti-D agglutinin, but there will be no agglutination of the cells. The coated RBCs will agglutinate only on subsequent addition of Coombs (anti-immunoglobulin) serum (**Fig. 25.2**). Agglutination will also occur if the IgG anti-D is potentiated by adding albumin to it.

Genotypes and Inheritance

The *ABO phenotypes* are controlled by a pair of codominant alleles A and B. An individual who has inherited A agglutinogen from one parent and B agglutinogen from the other parent

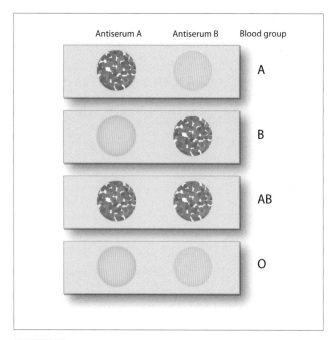

Fig. 25.1 The agglutination test for blood grouping.

will have the AB blood group. Similarly, an individual whose phenotypic blood group is B may have either the genotype BB (homozygous) or BO (heterozygous), as shown in **Table 25.2**.

The *Rh phenotypes* are controlled by three sets (C, D, and E) of two alternative alleles (dominant and recessive). Each

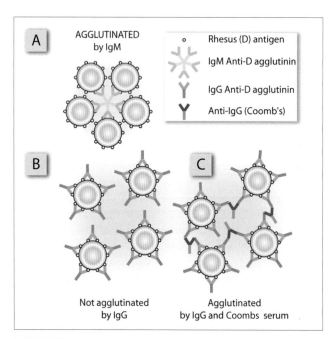

Fig. 25.2 Rhesus agglutinogens and agglutinins. **(A)** Rhesus-(D-) positive red blood cells (RBCs) agglutinated by immunoglobulin M (IgM) anti-D agglutinins. **(B)** D+, RBCs coated but not agglutinated by immunoglobulin G (IgG) anti-D agglutinins. **(C)** IgG anti-D coated RBCs agglutinated by anti-IgG, which bind to IgG molecules by their stem (Fc).

Table 25.2 Genotypes of ABO Blood Groups

Blood Group	Possible Genotype(s)
A	AA, AO
B	BB, BO
AB	AB
O	OO

phenotype has a variable number of possible genotypes. For example, cde has only one possible genotype, ccddee. CDE, on the other hand, can have eight possible genotypes: CCDDEE, CCDDEe, CCDdEE, CCDdEe, CcDDEE, CcDDEe, CcDdEE, and CcDdEe.

Agglutinogens and Agglutinins

The **ABO agglutinogens** represent only a few of the approximately one million agglutinogens present on an erythrocyte. The ABO agglutinogens are glycosphingolipids (oligosaccharide plus sphingolipid). The antigenicity of the agglutinogens resides in the oligosaccharide moiety. The ABO agglutinogens are present on the RBC membrane as external proteins. O group cells contain a nonantigenic H substance from which both A and B agglutinogens are derived. The genes for A and B agglutinogens are located on chromosome 9. They code the synthesis of transferase A and transferase B, the two enzymes that are responsible for conversion of substance H into A and B agglutinogens.

ABO agglutinogens are not confined to erythrocytes alone; they are widely found in the secretory glands of gastrointestinal, respiratory, and genitourinary tracts. The secreted agglutinogens are, however, not glycosphingolipids, but glycoproteins (oligosaccharide plus protein).

Rhesus agglutinogens | Unlike the ABO agglutinogens, rhesus agglutinogens are integral membrane proteins. They are not found anywhere other than on RBCs.

ABO agglutinins | The agglutinins α and β are absent at birth but develop over the first 3 to 6 months of life. They are produced as a result of exposure to ABO-like polysaccharides that are abundant in microbes, seeds, and plants. These natural antibodies are immunoglobulins of the IgM type. Subsequent exposures to ABO agglutinogens, as in the course of mismatched transfusion, also produce agglutinins. Such immune agglutinins are often of the IgG type.

Rhesus agglutinins | There are no natural antibodies to rhesus agglutinogens. Agglutinins formed against them are of the IgG type.

Importance of Blood Groups

Transfusion of blood | The main importance of blood groups lies in ensuring compatible blood transfusion. This is discussed in detail below.

Association with diseases | The incidence of certain diseases is related to the blood group. For example, duodenal ulcers are twice as common in group O nonsecretors than in group A or B secretors; tumors of the salivary glands, stomach, and pancreas are more common in group A than in group O individuals.

Blood Transfusion

Autologous Blood Transfusion

Autotransfusion is completely free from the risks of transfusion reactions and transfusion-transmitted diseases. In this, the patient's own blood is withdrawn in advance of elective surgery and then transfused back if needed during the surgery. Up to 1.5 L of blood is withdrawn over a 3-week period while the person receives iron supplements.

Blood Grouping and Cross-matching

Autotransfusion is only occasionally possible. More commonly, the patient needs a blood donor. Preferably, the blood groups of the donor and the recipient should be the same. In an emergency, there may be no time to find out the blood group of the patient, and even when known, the blood of the same group may not be available. In such situations, blood group O– may be transfused indiscriminately to all patients in dire need of transfusion. This is because O– group blood has no agglutinogens, and the chances of fatal reactions occurring following a mismatched transfusion (O– group blood donated to persons with A+, B+, or AB+ blood groups) are the lowest. Persons with O– blood group are therefore called *universal donors*. In the same way, persons with AB blood group are *universal recipients*. In an emergency, they can be transfused with any of the ABO blood groups. This is because AB group blood has neither α nor β agglutinins.

The idea of a universal donor is not always safe. Normally, the α and β agglutinins present in the transfused O group blood are greatly diluted by the recipient's plasma and therefore are unable to lyse the recipient's erythrocytes. It may be argued that the donor's agglutinogens also get diluted. That, however, is not true. The effective concentration of agglutinogens is determined by their concentration on the surface of the erythrocyte, which remains unchanged even after the dilution of erythrocytes in the recipient's plasma. However, the O group donor may have very high titers of α and β agglutinins: these may cause hemolysis of the recipient's erythrocytes. Such O group donors are called *dangerous universal donors*.

Transfusion of blood of the same group does not guarantee a reaction-free transfusion. The donor's and recipient's blood may be ABO and rhesus compatible, but the donor might have P agglutinogens, and the recipient might have anti-P agglutinins. Because there are innumerable minor and familial blood groups that are never ascertained, the donor's and recipient's blood have to be directly tested (cross-matched) against each other. Cross-matching may be major or minor. *Major cross-matching* involves testing the donor's erythrocytes against the recipient's serum. *Minor cross-matching* involves testing the recipient's erythrocytes against the donor's serum.

Blood grouping, however, does help in narrowing down the search for compatible blood. For example, if the recipient is B+, the blood bank technician needs to test only a few samples of B+ blood for the perfect compatibility. Without blood grouping, a much larger number of random blood samples would have to be cross-matched.

Complications of Transfusion

Fatal *hemolytic reactions* can occur in a mismatched transfusion. Rapid hemolysis results in liberation of free hemoglobin into the plasma, often resulting in severe jaundice and renal tubular damage. When reactions occur, transfusion must be stopped immediately and the patient intravenously injected with rapid-acting corticosteroids. Febrile reactions occur due to destruction of leukocytes and platelets by antibodies against them.

Circulatory overload can develop if transfusion is too rapid. The rate of transfusion should not exceed 1 mL per kilogram body weight per hour.

Hemosiderosis is caused by repeated blood transfusions, as in thalassemic patients. There is iron deposition in, and consequent damage to, several organs, such as the liver, heart, and endocrine organs.

Electrolyte disturbances, especially hyperkalemia and hypocalcemia, are not uncommon. *Hyperkalemia* occurs because in stored blood the erythrocytes leak out intracellular K^+ into the plasma. *Hypocalcemia* occurs because stored blood contains citrates as an anticoagulant. When transfused into a recipient, the citrates are metabolized. However, if the rate of transfusion exceeds the rate of citrate metabolism, the citrates chelate calcium (Ca^{2+}) in the recipient's blood, causing hypocalcemia.

Anemia hypoxia (Chapter 50) can be a problem in patients receiving a large transfusion of stored blood. RBCs in stored blood have very low amounts of 2,3-diphosphoglycerate (DPG) in them. Hence, stored blood has a high affinity for O_2; consequently, it tends to give off less O_2 to the tissues.

Transmission of diseases like hepatitis B or C and acquired immunodeficiency syndrome (AIDS) constitutes a serious risk.

Hemolytic Disease of the Newborn

Erythroblastosis Fetalis

If an Rh– mother bears an Rh+ baby in two consecutive pregnancies, the second baby is prone to develop hemolytic disease. The hemolytic disease can also occur in the first baby if the Rh– mother is sensitized to rhesus agglutinogens by a prior Rh+ blood transfusion.

During the first pregnancy, the mother is sensitized to Rh agglutinogens of the fetus due to leakage of fetal erythrocytes into the maternal circulation. The leak occurs late in the third trimester or during parturition when the maternal and fetal bloods come in contact for the first time. However, agglutinins are not formed quickly or in significant titers on first exposure, and the first D+ fetus usually is born unharmed. A second D+ fetus, however, evokes rapid formation of anti-D agglutinins in the third trimester.

The anti-D formed is almost entirely of the IgG type, which can cross the placental barrier. The agglutinins therefore cross over to the fetal circulation, hemolyzing the fetal RBCs. The hemolysis triggers compensatory hyperactivity of the fetal erythropoietic organs, resulting in the appearance of immature erythroblasts in the fetal circulation, which gives this disorder its name.

Depending on its severity, erythroblastosis fetalis takes one of the following forms. In severe cases, the fetus experiences severe edema formation and often dies in utero. The condition is called *hydrops fetalis*. Less severe cases result in jaundice of the newborn, and the condition is called *icterus neonatorum gravis*. The jaundice is much less severe before birth because the mother conjugates and excretes most of the fetal bilirubin load. However, the problem is exacerbated immediately after birth. The mildest cases result only in an anemia called the *congenital anemia of the newborn*.

Kernicterus is a complication of icterus neonatorum gravis. It is a neurologic syndrome in which unconjugated bilirubin is deposited in the basal ganglia. The condition is uncommon in adults, but infants are vulnerable to it because their blood–brain barrier is more permeable. Moreover, because the liver is not mature enough in infancy, there is a greater rise in the plasma concentration of unconjugated bilirubin, which is lipid soluble and crosses the blood–brain barrier more easily.

The diagnosis of erythroblastosis fetalis is confirmed only if anti-D agglutinins are detected in fetal RBCs or in maternal blood. Anti-D-coated fetal RBCs agglutinate on adding Coombs serum. The test is called the *direct Coombs test*. For detecting anti-D agglutinin in maternal blood, the agglutinin must first be adsorbed in "carrier" RBCs. Subsequent addition of Coombs serum will cause the RBCs to agglutinate. The test is called the *indirect Coombs test*.

Prevention of the condition is possible by not allowing the mother to get sensitized to Rh agglutinogens during the first pregnancy. This is done by administering a single dose of anti-Rh serum during the first 72 hours postpartum. The anti-Rh antibodies promptly destroy any Rh agglutinogens that might gain access to maternal circulation and prevent the mother from developing active immunity against the Rh agglutinogen.

Treatment of the newborn consists of exchange transfusion in which the hemolyzed blood of the newborn is withdrawn from a suitable peripheral artery, and fresh Rh– blood is transfused simultaneously into a convenient peripheral vein.

Fetal ABO Hemolytic Disease

Fetal ABO hemolytic disease, which has a similar mechanism to that described above, is surprisingly mild. There are at least four reasons for this: (1) Fetal erythrocyte membrane possesses fewer A and B agglutinogenic sites. (2) Anti-A and anti-.B agglutinins do not bind complement on the fetal erythrocyte. (They do so in adults, causing severe hemolysis in ABO incompatibility.) (3) Anti-A and anti-B are mostly IgM, which does not cross the placenta. (4) The small amounts of IgG anti-A and anti-B that do cross the placenta bind to several types of cells other than RBCs. Consequently, their effect on erythrocytes is diluted.

Summary

- Blood is grouped by the type of agglutinogens present on the RBCs.

- The two major groups are the ABO and the rhesus (Rh).

- Safe transfusion requires the matching of the ABO group of the donor with that of the recipient.

Applying What You Know

25.1. If Mr. Lundquist were to need a transfusion, which blood group could he safely receive? Explain.

26 Blood Platelets and Hemostasis

Blood Platelets

Blood platelets, or *thrombocytes*, are thin, biconvex, anucleate disks 2 to 4 µm in diameter. They are produced in bone marrow by fragmentation of very large nucleated cells called *megakaryocytes*. They are released into the blood, where they have a life span of ~10 days.

Blood platelets have at least four functions. (1) When the endothelium is disrupted, the breach is closed by a mass of platelets called the *platelet thrombus* or the *platelet plug*. (2) Phospholipids present on the surface of platelets have an essential role in blood coagulation. Some of the key reactions take place only on the surface of platelets. (3) Platelet granules release several prohemostatic and antihemostatic substances, as well as factors that are important in tissue healing. (4) Platelets have a weak phagocytic activity.

Platelet Structure

In stained blood smears, platelets exhibit two concentric zones: a peripheral zone called the hyalomere and a central zone called the granulomere (**Fig. 26.1**). The *hyalomere* has a circumferential bundle of microtubules that maintain the shape of the platelet. It also has actin and myosin proteins. When the intracellular calcium concentration rises, the myosin light chain kinase is activated, and the myosin interacts with actin filaments, resulting in platelet contraction. The *granulomere* contains a canalicular system, secretory granules, one or two mitochondria, and scattered particles of glycogen. However, the platelet lacks a nucleus and is therefore unable to synthesize proteins.

The **platelet canalicular system** is of two types. The *surface-connected canalicular system* is analogous to the T-tubules of a skeletal muscle cell. It is open on the platelet surface at several sites and is the major pathway for the discharge of secretory products upon activation of the platelets. The *dense tubular system* is analogous to the L-tubule of a skeletal muscle cell.

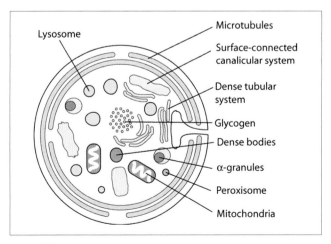

Fig. 26.1 Structure of a thrombocyte.

It maintains a high concentration of calcium (Ca^{2+}) inside it. This Ca^{2+} is released into the platelet cytosol when the platelet is activated.

The **platelet granules** are of three types: α-granules, dense granules, and lysosomal granules. The contents of α-granules and dense granules are secreted on platelet activation; the lysosomal granules are secreted when the platelet begins to disintegrate.

α-Platelet granules secrete numerous substances, most of which are already present in plasma and therefore do not have any physiologic role. An example is the *von Willebrand factor* (vWF), which is important for platelet adhesion. Adequate amounts of vWF come from endothelial secretions; therefore, the presence or absence of vWF in platelets does not affect platelet adhesion. The important α-granule proteins are those that are absent from plasma until secreted by activated platelets and are as follows. (1) *Platelet factor 4* inhibits the antithrombin III–heparin system. (2) *Thrombospondin* binds to the glycoprotein receptors on the platelet surface and brings about platelet aggregation. (3) *Platelet-derived growth factor* (PDGF) and *transforming growth factor-β* (TGF-β) are chemoattractants for leukocytes, smooth muscle cells, and fibroblasts. They also stimulate mitosis of these cells. Thus, they help in inflammation and wound healing. (The term *platelet-derived growth factor* is inappropriate because these factors are secreted not only by platelets, but also by monocytes, macrophages, and endothelin cells.) (4) *Fibronectin* helps in the adhesion of platelets to the site of injury.

Dense platelet granules secrete *adenosine diphosphate (ADP)*, which amplifies platelet activation. Patients with hereditary disorders that prevent the storage of adequate quantities of ADP in the dense granules have moderate bleeding disorders. Dense granules also secrete *serotonin,* which constricts arterioles, thereby helping in hemostasis.

Platelet integrins | The platelet bears on its surface *integrins,* which are cell adhesion molecules. Chemically, these molecules are glycoproteins (GP) and have various subtypes. GP Ib is present on all platelets. GP IIb–IIIa is formed only after platelet activation. GP I is important for platelet adhesion, whereas GP IIb–IIIa is important for platelet aggregation.

Platelet Count

The normal platelet count is 150,000 to 400,000/cc of blood. **Thrombocytopenia** is the condition in which there is a fall in platelet count below 150,000/cc of blood. It results in *purpura,* a bleeding disorder. When the purpura occurs without any obvious cause, it is called primary thrombocytopenic purpura. Secondary thrombocytopenic purpura (where the cause is identifiable) occurs following drug administration (e.g., aspirin), in malignancies (e.g., leukemias, aplastic anemia, and bone marrow infiltration), and in hypersplenism, in which an abnormally hyperactive spleen destroys platelets and other blood cells in larger than usual numbers. Life-threatening

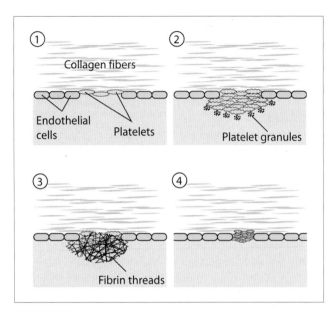

Fig. 26.2 Formation of a platelet plug. (1) A few platelets adhere to the collagen fibers below the disrupted endothelium. (2) Several more platelets aggregate at the site, forming a platelet plug. (3) Fibrin threads are deposited in the plug, making it firm. (4) Platelet plug contracts, pulling together the edges of the disrupted endothelium.

thrombocytopenia occurs in hemorrhagic dengue fever, a viral disease.

Thrombocytosis is the condition in which there is a rise of the platelet count above 400,000/cc of blood. Individuals with thrombocytosis are predisposed to thrombotic events. The common causes of thrombocytosis are acute hemorrhage, surgery, and trauma, particularly bone fractures. Splenectomy causes thrombocytosis by reducing the number of platelets that are removed from circulation.

Hemostasis

The term *hemostasis* refers to the stoppage of bleeding. It occurs in three major steps: constriction of the damaged blood vessels, formation of a hemostatic plug (**Fig. 26.2**), and clot retraction and dissolution.

Constriction of the damaged vessel slows down the bleeding. Unless the blood flow slows down, any clot formed is washed away. The immediate constriction occurs mainly due to the direct response of vascular smooth muscle to injury. A little later, further constriction is induced by the serotonin released from platelets that adhere to the site of injury.

Formation of a platelet plug arrests the bleeding by plugging the breach in the endothelium. The platelet plug is formed by a large number of tightly packed platelets.

Consolidation of the platelet plug occurs through the formation of fibrin threads that run criss-cross through it. This involves the enzymatic conversion of the plasma protein fibrinogen into fibrin through an elaborate process called coagulation or clotting. The fibrin threads bind to the integrins on platelets and anchor the platelets tightly together into a thrombus or clot.

Clot retraction (shrinking of the clot) pulls the edges of the wound together, making wound healing easier. Clot retraction occurs due to the contraction of platelets. Integrins are also required for clot retraction because they anchor platelets to fibrin threads.

Fibrinolysis (dissolution of the clot) is necessary for the restoration of normal blood flow to the healed tissue. Fibrinolysis is produced by a substance called *plasmin,* which splits fibrin enzymatically. Plasmin is formed from plasminogen by *tissue plasminogen activator* (t-PA) secreted by endothelial cells. Newly formed clots, which are rich in platelets, are less susceptible to fibrinolysis than older clots. This is because platelets release *plasminogen activator inhibitor.* This ensures that clots are lysed only after sufficient time has elapsed during which tissue healing can occur.

Platelet Plug Formation

The formation of a platelet plug begins when platelets come in contact with the subendothelial collagen fibers (collagen fibers lying under the endothelium of blood vessels) that get exposed as a result of injury (**Fig. 26.3**). The platelet plug is formed in four stages: platelet adhesion, platelet activation, platelet aggregation, and platelet contraction.

Platelet adhesion requires the presence of the von Willebrand factor (vWF), a glycoprotein secreted by the vascular endothelial cells and present in plasma (**Fig. 26.3A**). When the endothelium is disrupted (**Fig. 26.3B**), the circulating vWF binds to the exposed subendothelial collagen fibers. On binding with collagen, vWF gets altered so that it is now able to bind with GP lb present on the platelet surface. The vWF thereby anchors the platelet to subendothelial collagen.

Platelet activation refers to the rise in intracellular Ca^{2+} concentration that occurs in the platelet after it gets anchored to collagen through vWF (**Fig. 26.3B**). The contact with collagen activates group II-C hormonal mechanisms (see Chapter 75) in the platelet. The IP_3 (the second messenger of group II-C hormones) formed triggers the release of Ca^{2+} from the dense tubular system of platelets into the platelet cytosol. Activated platelets contract (due to activation of actin–myosin interaction), develop pseudopodia (due to reorganization of microtubules), discharge their granules (due to Ca^{2+}-mediated exocytosis), and develop another type of integrin on its surface called GP IIb–IIIa (**Fig. 26.3C**).

The rise in Ca^{2+} during platelet activation also leads to the formation of thromboxane A_2 inside the platelet (**Fig. 26.4**). Thromboxane A_2 leads to further rise in cytosolic Ca^{2+}. Thus, there is a positive feedback cycle of platelet activation. The ADP secreted by the dense granules contributes to platelet activation by inducing thromboxane A_2.

Platelet aggregation | The GP IIb–IIIa on the platelet surface binds to *thrombospondin* (**Fig. 26.3D**), an adhesive protein secreted by the platelet itself. GP IIb–IIIa also binds to fibrinogen present in plasma. Aggregation of platelets occurs due to the cross-linking of thrombospondin with fibrinogen (**Fig. 26.3E**).

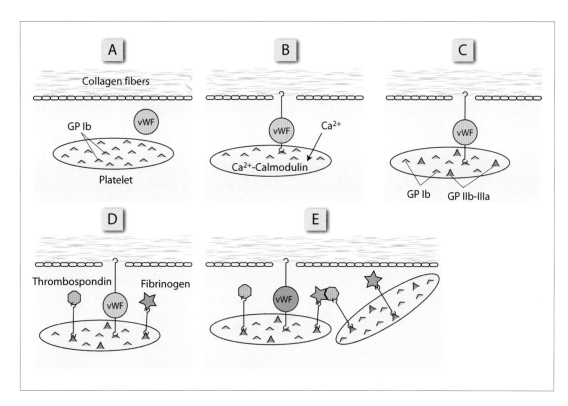

Fig. 26.3 Schematic illustration of platelet adhesion and aggregation (see text for details). GP, platelet glycoprotein; vWF, von Willebrand factor.

Blood Coagulation

Blood coagulation is brought about through a cascade system in which one activated factor activates another factor. The cascade ends with the formation of fibrin. The coagulation factors are listed in **Table 26.1**.

The coagulation process is initiated by two different mechanisms, the extrinsic and the intrinsic (**Fig. 26.5**). The two pathways soon converge on a common pathway that begins with the activation of factor IX and ends with the formation of fibrin threads.

The extrinsic pathway is initiated by the *tissue factor*, a glycoprotein released by the injured tissues. The intrinsic pathway is initiated by contact of blood platelets with negatively charged surfaces, such as glass. It is called "intrinsic" because all the necessary factors required in this pathway are present in the plasma itself. It is through the intrinsic pathway that blood clots when allowed to stand in a glass test tube. Injured blood vessels, too, can trigger the intrinsic pathway because injury exposes the collagen fibers in the vessel wall. Collagen provides the negative surface that triggers the intrinsic pathway.

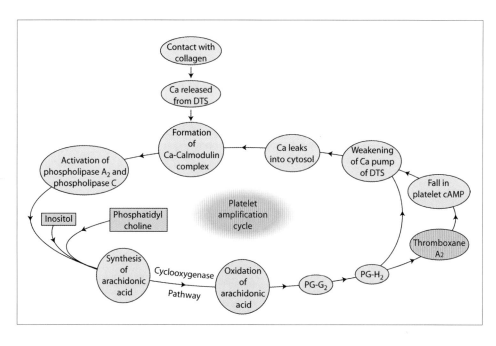

Fig. 26.4 The amplification cycle for platelet activation. See also **Fig. 26.2**. DTS, dense tubular system; PG, prostaglandin; cAMP, cyclic adenosine monophosphate.

Table 26.1 Coagulation Factors

I	Fibrinogen
II	Prothrombin
III	Thromboplastin
IV	Calcium ions
V	Labile factor
VI	Has been dropped; earlier called accelerin
VII	Stable factor; earlier called preaccelerin
VIII	Antihemophilic globulin
IX	Christmas factor
X	Stuart–Prower factor
XI	Plasma thromboplastin antecedent
XII	Hagman-factor
XIII	Fibrin stabilizing factor (Laki-Lorand factor)
HMWK	High-molecular-weight Kininogen
Pre-K	Prekallikrein
Ka	Kallikrein
PPL	Platelet phospholipids

Initiation of the intrinsic pathway requires four contact activation factors: factor XII, factor XI, prekallikrein, and high-molecular-weight kininogen (HMWK). Factor XII is activated to XIIa when it comes in contact with a negatively charged surface. Factor XIIa in its turn activates XI to XIa. The formation of XIIa is greatly enhanced through feedback activation by pre-

kallikrein (**Fig. 26.6**): XIIa activates prekallikrein to kallikrein, which, in turn, activates more XII to XIIa.

HMWK is responsible for attracting prekallikrein and factor XI (both are bound to HMWK in plasma) to the site of reaction with factor XII. This is possible because HMWK, like factor XII, is attracted toward negatively charged surfaces, which provide the site of reaction.

Initiation of the extrinsic pathway occurs when tissue factor (TF), a glycoprotein, is released from fibroblasts and smooth muscle cells of the vessel wall. TF is the cofactor of both factors VII and VIIa. The binding of TF with factor VII or VIIa has to occur in the presence of membrane phospholipids. Hence, the reaction occurs mainly on the fibroblasts of the vessel wall, with the fibroblast cell membrane providing the phospholipids necessary for the reaction.

When TF binds to factor VII, it promotes its activation to VIIa. When TF binds to factor VIIa, the TF–VIIa complex catalyzes the activation of factor IX (**Fig. 26.5**), and though somewhat weakly, the activation of factor X.

Activation of factors VII, VIII, and V (**Fig. 26.6**) does not occur in the regular course of the cascade. Factor VII is activated by several factors, the most important ones being TF and factor IXa. It is also activated by VIIa (autoactivation). Factor V and factor VIII are activated only through feedback activation. In the coagulation cascade, activation of factor VIII and factor V occurs before activation of factor X and much before the formation of thrombin. However, the activation of factors V and VIII requires Xa and thrombin. Initially, only traces of Xa

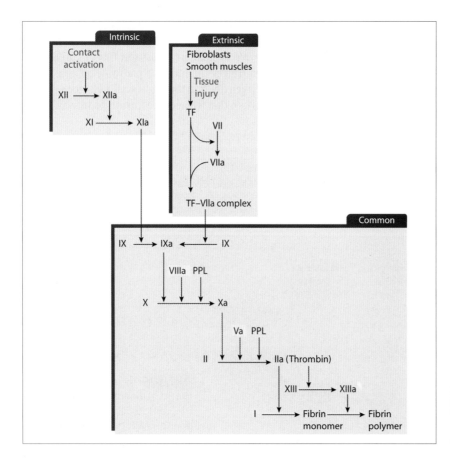

Fig. 26.5 The coagulation cascade. All steps require calcium ions (not shown). TF, tissue factor; PPL, platelet phospholipids (present on platelet surface).

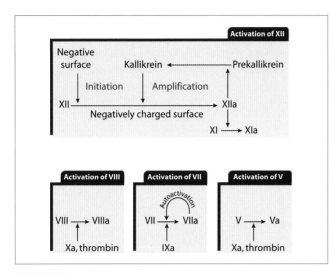

Fig. 26.6 Activation of factors XII, VIII, VII, and V.

and thrombin may be available for the activation of factors V and VIII. However, as coagulation proceeds, more and more factor Xa and thrombin are generated and are available for activation of factors V and VIII.

Activation of factor X requires platelet phospholipids; therefore, it occurs on the platelet surface. A complex of factors X, IXa, VIIIa, platelet phospholipids, and calcium ions (X–IXa–VIIIa–PPL–Ca^{2+} complex), called *tenase,* forms on the platelet surface (**Fig. 26.7A**) and results in the activation of factor X to Xa.

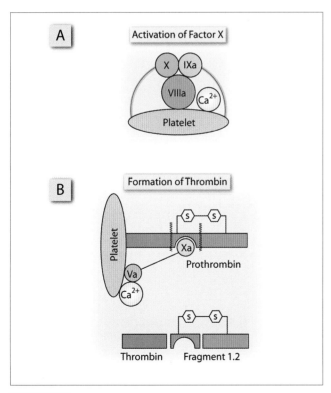

Fig. 26.7 **(A)** The IXa–VIIIa–PPL–Ca^{2+} complex (tenase) that activates factor X into Xa. **(B)** The Xa–Va–PPL–Ca^{2+} complex that splits prothrombin into thrombin. PPL, platelet phospholipids.

Formation of thrombin, too, requires platelet phospholipids and therefore occurs on the platelet surface. Thrombin is cleaved off from the prothrombin molecule by the Xa–Va–PPL–Ca^{2+} complex that binds to prothrombin (**Fig. 26.7B**). Factor Xa splits the prothrombin molecule at two sites, forming thrombin and a residual fragment called *fragment 1.2.* In hypercoagulable states, fragment 1.2 serves as a useful marker for excessive thrombin formation.

Formation of fibrin monomers | Fibrin monomers are formed from fibrinogen by the action of thrombin. The fibrinogen molecule is made of three pairs of nonidentical chains: the Aα, Bβ, and γ chains (**Fig. 26.8**). The three chains are disposed symmetrically with their NH$_2$ groups linked together by disulfide bonds into a central nodule (or the disulfide knot). Thrombin cleaves off short segments from the NH$_2$ terminals of Aα and Bβ chains to form fibrin monomer.

Polymerization of fibrin monomers | The fibrin monomers initially polymerize through weak noncovalent bonds to form fibrin strands. The bonds are formed both end to end (between the distal nodules) as well as side to side (between the central nodule and the distal nodule). In the central nodule, the bonds are formed at the active sites formed by the detachment of the NH$_2$ groups from Aα and Bβ chains (**Fig. 26.9**).

Stabilization of fibrin polymers | The fibrin polymers are formed through noncovalent bonding of fibrin monomers and are therefore mechanically weak. It is made stronger and more resistant to fibrinolysis by factor XIIIa, which polymerizes fibrin by catalyzing the formation of peptide bonds between fibrin monomers (**Fig. 26.9**).

Factor XIII is cleaved by thrombin into its active form XIIIa. Following activation, factor XIII undergoes a conformational change so that its cysteine molecules get exposed at the sur-

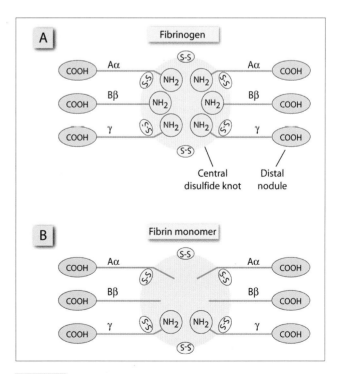

Fig. 26.8 Structure of **(A)** fibrinogen and **(B)** fibrin monomer.

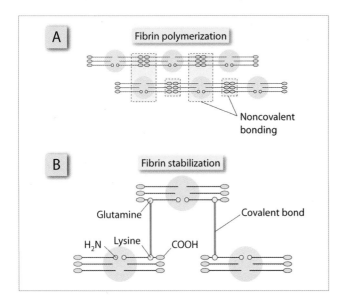

Fig. 26.9 **(A)** Polymerization of fibrin molecules through noncovalent bonding. **(B)** Fibrin stabilization by factor XIII. Shown here are the peptide bonds formed between the glutamine and lysine residues on the γ-chains of the fibrin monomers.

face. It is these cysteine molecules that catalyze the formation of peptide bonds between fibrin monomers.

Role of factor IV | Calcium is required for all the steps of the coagulation cascade. Clinical hypocalcemia does not impair coagulation for which Ca^{2+} has to fall to very low levels. Death due to hypocalcemic tetany occurs well before plasma Ca^{2+} can fall to such levels.

Summary

- Platelets are small blood cells produced in bone marrow that play an important role in blood clotting.

- Hemostasis involves several responses of the damaged vessel, platelets, and the formation of fibrin.

- The coagulation cascade involves the interaction of a large number of clotting factors in the blood.

Applying What You Know

26.1. Patients like Mr. Lundquist with pernicious anemia commonly also exhibit thrombocytopenia (a reduced number of platelets). How would this condition affect the clotting of Mr. Lundquist's blood? What would be the mechanism of this effect?

Antihemostatic Mechanisms

The coagulating tendency of blood is balanced in vivo by endogenous antihemostatic mechanisms (**Fig. 27.1**) that prevent clotting inside the blood vessels and dissolve any clots that do form. In addition, there are exogenous antihemostatic mechanisms that have been exploited for therapeutic purposes.

General Models: Balance of Forces

Most physiologic phenomena exhibit this sort of balance of forces in which multiple factors facilitate or inhibit a particular process. It is usually easy to determine the consequence of a single factor changing, but it is much more difficult to predict the outcome of several factors changing.

Factors Inhibiting Platelet Aggregation

Normally, a delicate balance exists between thromboxane A_2, which promotes platelet aggregation, and prostacyclin (PGI_2), which inhibits platelet aggregation. Thromboxane A_2 is produced by platelets; PGI_2 is produced by endothelial cells. Both are produced by the cyclooxygenase pathway of arachidonic acid oxidation (**Fig. 27.2**). Prostacyclin stimulates membrane adenyl cyclase and raises cyclic adenosine monophosphate (cAMP) levels in platelets. cAMP stimulates Ca–ATPase (adenosinetriphosphatase) and thereby increases the pumping of Ca^{2+} into the dense tubular system of the platelet with consequent lowering of cytosolic Ca^{2+}. Prostacyclin thus prevents platelet activation; thromboxane A_2 reduces the cAMP levels in platelets, resulting in the opposite effect.

Aspirin irreversibly (for the remaining life of the platelet) inhibits the cyclooxygenase pathway of arachidonic acid oxidation. By interrupting the amplification cycle for platelet activation (see **Fig. 26.4**), aspirin minimizes platelet activation and aggregation. This makes aspirin a valuable drug for the prevention of thrombosis. Aspirin also inhibits arachidonic acid oxidation in endothelial cells, thereby reducing prostacyclin secretion. However, the effect is comparatively weaker. Ingestion of certain fish oils prolongs the bleeding time: certain fatty acids found in fish oils decrease arachidonic acid release from platelet membrane phospholipids and thus limit the synthesis of thromboxane A_2.

Factors Inhibiting Coagulation

Protein C pathway | Three protein factors, protein C, thrombomodulin, and protein S, constitute an important negative feedback pathway that keeps blood coagulation under control (**Fig. 27.3**). *Protein* C is activated by factors Xa and thrombin. The activated protein C inactivates factors VIIIa and Va, the two key factors responsible for the formation of thrombin and Xa. The inactivation requires the presence of two cofactors, *protein S* and *thrombomodulin*. Protein S and protein C are plasma proteins. Thrombomodulin is a protein present on vascular endothelium.

Antithrombin–heparin system | *Antithrombin III* is present in plasma as well as in vascular endothelium. It inactivates several coagulation factors, including thrombin. *Heparin sulfate* is present only in the vascular endothelium. It inhibits both the production of thrombin (from prothrombin) and the action of thrombin (on fibrinogen). Heparin potentiates antithrombin III.

Exogenous anticoagulants | In vivo, a plasma Ca^{2+} level low enough to impair blood clotting is incompatible with life. However, clotting can be prevented in vitro if Ca^{2+} is removed from

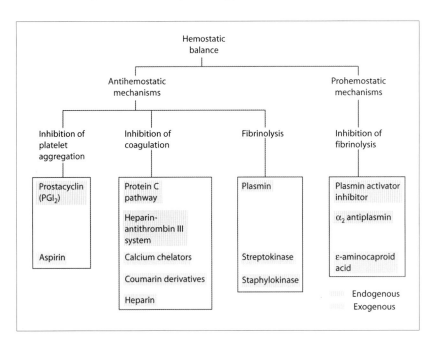

Fig. 27.1 Antihemostatic and prohemostatic mechanisms.

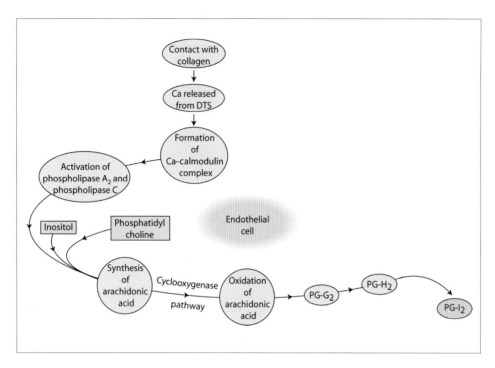

Fig. 27.2 Prostacyclin synthesis in endothelial cells. Compare with **Fig. 26.4**. DTS, dense tubular system; PG, prostaglandin.

blood by the addition of substances such as oxalates, which form insoluble salts with Ca^{2+} or by the addition of chelating agents that bind Ca^{2+}.

Coumarin derivatives such as *dicumarol* and *warfarin* are effective anticoagulants. These compounds inhibit the reduc-

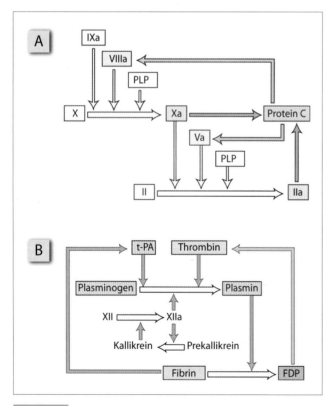

Fig. 27.3 (A) The protein C pathway for inhibition of coagulation. (B) Plasminogen activation. FDP, fibrin degradation products; PLP, pyridoxal phosphate; t-PA, tissue plasminogen activator. Red = stimulation; blue = inhibition.

tion of vitamin K to its active form vitamin KH_2, resulting in the impaired synthesis of factors II, VII, IX, and X (VKDP, see below). However, coumarin derivatives are not administered when the anticoagulant effect needs to be reversed quickly. Such a situation arises, for example, during dialysis of blood, when the blood drawn from the patient's vein must be treated with an anticoagulant before passing it through the dialysis machine, and the anticoagulant must be quickly neutralized before reinfusing the blood into the patient's vein. Heparin is the anticoagulant of choice in such situations because its effect is quickly neutralized by *protamine,* a highly basic protein that forms an irreversible complex with heparin.

Factors Causing Fibrinolysis

Plasmin (fibrinolysin) is the principal fibrinolytic factor. It is formed from a circulating glycoprotein called plasminogen. Plasmin lyses both fibrin and fibrinogen. Exogenous plasmin activators include the bacterial enzymes *streptokinase* and *staphylokinase.* These are used in the treatment of early myocardial infarction for lysing clots in coronary arteries.

The main endogenous activator of plasmin is the *tissue plasminogen activator* (t-PA), which is present in the endothelial cells. In its absence, there is extensive spontaneous fibrin deposition. There are also defects in growth and fertility because plasmin not only lyses clots but also plays a role in cell motility and in ovulation.

Epinephrine stimulates endothelial cells to secrete t-PA. In violent deaths, a large amount of adrenaline is released into the blood. The adrenaline causes rapid release of t-PA from endothelial cells, causing massive fibrinolysis. Hence, the blood remains fluid and incoagulable even after death, an observation of forensic importance. The catalytic efficiency of t-PA increases several hundred-fold when it binds to fibrin. This is an example of autoinactivation, wherein fibrin indirectly brings about its own degradation. Human t-PA is now produced by recombinant DNA techniques and is available for clinical use. It lyses clots in the coronary arteries if given to patients soon after the onset of myocardial infarction.

Another activator of plasmin is thrombin. However, the products of fibrinogen breakdown (called fibrinogen *degradation products*) inhibit the activity of thrombin. Thus, there is a negative feedback that controls plasmin generation. Plasmin is also activated by kallikrein and factor XIIa (**Fig. 27.3**). It is interesting to note that fibrinolysis is initiated by the same factors that initiate coagulation (kallikrein and factor XIIa) or are involved in the final stages of coagulation (thrombin, fibrinogen).

Prohemostatic Mechanisms

Fibrinolysis Inhibitors

Exogenous inhibitors of fibrinolysis include drugs like ε-*aminocaproic acid.* Dentists sometimes apply it locally during tooth extraction.

Endogenous inhibitors of fibrinolysis include *plasminogen activator inhibitors* (PAI), which inhibit the activation of plasmin, and $α_2$-antiplasmin that inhibits plasmin directly. During clotting, the fibrin threads bind to both plasminogen activators like t-PA and plasminogen activator inhibitors like $α_2$-antiplasmin. Hence, both fibrinolytic and antifibrinolytic substances are present inside the thrombus.

Hemorrhagic Disorders

Hemorrhagic disorders are of three types: vascular disorders due to increased capillary fragility, platelet disorders that result in inadequate formation of platelet plugs, and coagulation disorders (**Fig. 27.4**) that result from weakness of the platelet plug.

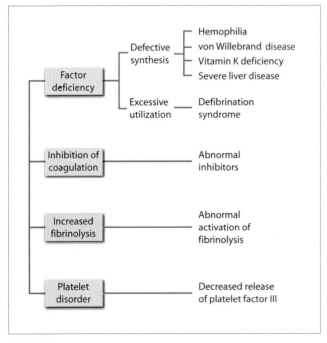

Fig. 27.4 Types of coagulation disorders.

The characteristics of bleeding due to vascular and platelet disorders are similar. They tend to cause spontaneous bleeding, resulting in purplish patches on the skin or mucous membranes. The condition is called *purpura.* The term purpura comes from the word *purple*, which denotes the color of the bleeding patches. Coagulation disorders do not cause purpura. Spontaneous bleeding, when it does occur in severe coagulation disorders, occurs in joints and muscle. Bleeding mostly occurs following injury and does not stop easily. Although the bleeding characteristics give some clue regarding their cause (vascular/platelet or coagulation disorders), the final diagnosis requires confirmatory tests.

Tests for Vascular and Platelet Disorders

The **tourniquet test** is positive in most cases of thrombocytopenia. It is performed by placing the sphygmomanometer cuff around the upper arm and raising the pressure to halfway between the arterial and venous blood pressures. The idea is to permit arterial flow but occlude the venous return to increase severely the capillary hydrostatic pressure distal to the cuff. The pressure is kept elevated for 5 minutes. After the cuff is deflated and the congestion disappears, the number of petechiae in the cubital fossa is counted. If more than 20 petechiae are present in an area of 3 cm diameter, the test is positive and suggests thrombocytopenia.

The **bleeding time** is estimated by pricking the finger or the earlobe to a measured depth and mopping the blood that flows out at regular intervals. The normal bleeding time is 2 to 6 minutes. Bleeding time increases in thrombocytopenia.

Clot retraction | Fresh blood is taken in a test tube and incubated in a water bath at 37°C. Clot retraction is indicated by the pulling away of the clot from the sides of the tube. Normally, clot retraction should begin in 1 hour and be complete in 24 hours. Also, the volume of serum left behind after complete clot retraction is about half the volume of blood. The clot retraction time is prolonged in thrombasthenia.

Tests for Coagulation Disorders

Although platelet phospholipid is required for clotting, the coagulation time is not affected by moderate thrombocytopenia. This is the reason why a platelet count is not considered to be a test for coagulation disorder. However, the coagulation time may be affected in severe thrombocytopenia.

Whole blood clotting time tests the intrinsic and common pathways. It is the time taken for blood to clot spontaneously in a glass tube. Normal clotting time is 5 to 11 minutes. The test is not sensitive: clotting time is prolonged only in severe coagulation disorders. However, it remains a useful and simple test for controlling the dose of heparin during anticoagulant therapy.

Partial thromboplastin time (PTT) assesses the intrinsic and common pathways of coagulation. In this test, the intrinsic coagulation pathway is activated by incubating the plasma with kaolin (a contact factor) in the presence of Ca^{2+} and platelet lipid substitute. Normally, the plasma clots within 45 seconds. If the clotting time is prolonged by more than 10 seconds, the result is considered abnormal.

Prothrombin time (PT) assesses the extrinsic and common pathways of coagulation. In this test, the extrinsic coagulation pathway is activated by incubating the plasma with tissue factor (factor III) and Ca^{2+}. Because the time taken varies with the type of tissue factor used, the test is always performed simultaneously on the patient's plasma and a sample of normal plasma. Because tissue factor from different sources varies, the international standardized ratio (INR) is often calculated. The INR = $(PTpatient/PTnormal)^X$, where X is a measurement of the activity of the tissue factor used in the test. INR values near 1 are normal.

Thrombin time estimates the fibrinogen concentration in plasma and therefore tests the common pathway. It is the time taken by plasma to clot after addition of thrombin to it. With a standardized thrombin solution, plasma clots in 15 seconds. Prolongation to 18 seconds or more is regarded as abnormal.

Thromboplastin generation test (TGT) is a test for the intrinsic pathway. It is done in two stages. In stage I, thromboplastin is produced by reacting together factors XII, XI, IX, VIII, V, platelet phospholipids, and Ca^{2+}. Stage II estimates the amount of thromboplastin formed in stage I by adding it to normal plasma (containing prothrombin and fibrinogen) and noting the time taken for fibrin formation.

Platelet Disorders

Bleeding due to a reduction in platelet count is called *thrombocytopenic purpura.* Bleeding disorders can also be due to defects in platelet adhesion or aggregation. Platelet adhesion is impaired in von Willebrand disease, in which there is deficiency of von Willebrand factor. von Willebrand disease is also associated with defective coagulation. Platelet aggregation is impaired in *thrombasthenia,* a rare hereditary disorder in which the GP IIb–IIIa receptors are not formed following platelet activation. (see **Table 27.1.**)

Vascular Disorders

Bleeding disorders from vascular causes are often called *athrombocytopenic purpura.* Strictly speaking, the term *athrombocytopenic* should also include functional disorders of platelets such as thrombasthenia. However, because these are rare conditions, the term usually refers to vascular disorders. Two well-known vascular causes of bleeding are *scurvy* (see **Table 66.2**), which causes failure of collagen formation associated with impaired hydroxyproline synthesis, and *Cushing syndrome,* which causes loss of perivascular supporting tissues. Other causes are severe infections, drugs, and senile purpura (due to atrophy of collagen in old age).

Coagulation Disorders

Hemophilia is caused by a genetic deficiency of factor VIII (hemophilia A or classical hemophilia) or of factor IX (hemophilia B or Christmas disease). Hemophilia A is three times more common than hemophilia B, occurring in 1 in 10,000 male births. Hemophilia is inherited as a sex-linked (on X chromosome) disorder mostly transmitted by women who themselves have no symptoms. To have frank hemophilia, a woman has to be homozygous for the hemophilic gene. Female carriers of hemophilia, who are heterozygotes, usually produce sufficient factor VIII for normal hemostasis.

Hemophilia is characterized by bleeding into soft tissues, muscles, and weight-bearing joints. Hematuria and nose bleeds are common. Hemophilic bleeding can result in large collections of partially clotted blood putting pressure on adjacent tissues. Despite frequent bleeding, severe iron-deficiency anemia is uncommon in hemophiliacs because most of the bleeding is internal, and the iron released is recycled.

A prolonged PTT is considered diagnostic for hemophilia. Hemophilia is treated with factor VIII concentrate. ε-Aminocaproic acid (EACA) has been used in hemophilia, especially during dental extractions. It is a potent antifibrinolytic agent that inhibits plasminogen activators present in oral secretions and stabilizes clot formation in oral tissue.

In **von Willebrand disease,** patients bleed excessively due to a congenital deficiency of vWF. Its incidence is ~1 in 1000, and if one considers subclinical cases, too, it is as high as 1 in 100. In addition to promoting platelet adherence, vWF serves as a carrier protein for factor VIII in plasma and increases its plasma half-life. In the absence of vWF, factor VIII cannot be maintained at adequate levels in the plasma. An analogue of vasopressin, *desamino-arginine-vasopressin,* is often given to these patients just before surgery to induce endothelial cells to release their stores of vWF.

Vitamin K deficiency | Vitamin K is obtained partly from food, especially green leafy vegetables (as vitamin K_1 or *phylloquinone*), and partly from the bacterial flora in the intestine, which synthesizes the vitamin (as *menaquinone*). When one source is deficient, the other compensates. Dietary vitamin K_1 is fat-soluble and requires bile salts for its absorption. Bacterial vitamin menaquinone is water-soluble and is absorbed even in the absence of bile.

The physiologically active form of vitamin K is vitamin KH_2 (reduced hydroquinone). In the liver, vitamin K is reduced to vitamin KH_2. Liver cells store enough vitamin K to last a month; therefore, inadequate dietary intake is not a common cause of vitamin K disorder. There are three major causes of vitamin K deficiency. (1) *Antibiotics* eliminate intestinal bacteria and reduce the synthesis of menaquinone. (2) *Intestinal malabsorption* of vitamin K can occur in obstructive jaundice. Due to the absence of bile, absorption of fats and fat-soluble vitamins is impaired. (3) *Hepatocellular diseases* cause vitamin K deficiency by impairing its conversion to the active form.

Vitamin K deficiency results in low plasma levels of both procoagulants and some anticoagulants. These proteins are called *vitamin K-dependent proteins* (VKDP). The procoagulants are factors II, VII, IX, and X. The anticoagulants are protein C and protein S. The plasma level of factor VII is the first to decrease when vitamin K deficiency is present.

The vitamin K-dependent proteins undergo some posttranslational processing before they are secreted. This involves carboxylation of about 10 of their terminal glutamic acid residues. Vitamin KH_2 serves as a cofactor in the carboxylation reaction. In the process, vitamin KH_2 gets oxidized to vitamin K oxide. Vitamin KH_2 is subsequently regenerated from vitamin K oxide by the enzyme epoxide reductase. This is called the

Table 27.1 Clinical Differences between Vascular or Platelet Disorders and Coagulation Disorders

Vascular/Platelet Disorders	Coagulation Disorders
Bleeding usually confined to the skin.	Bleeding usually in deeper tissues.
Bleeding usually takes the form of confluent petechiae and small ecchymosis.	Bleeding usually takes the form of large ecchymoses.
Spontaneous bleeding is common.	Spontaneous bleeding is uncommon.
Wound bleeding	Wound bleeding
a. is excessive	a. is less profuse
b. is immediate	b. is delayed for several hours
c. stops quickly on application of local pressure	c. does not stop quickly on application of local pressure
d. lasts < 48 hours	d. continues > 48 hours
e. rarely recurs	e. tends to recur

vitamin K cycle (**Fig. 27.5**). The commonly used anticoagulants warfarin and dicumarol are inhibitors of the enzyme epoxide reductase and prevent the regeneration of the physiologically useful vitamin KH_2.

Thrombotic Disorders

Formation of clots inside blood vessels is called *thrombosis* to distinguish it from the normal extravascular clotting of blood. Thrombi can occlude the arterial supply to the organs in which they form. Bits of thrombus (emboli) sometimes break off and travel in the bloodstream to distant sites, blocking the blood supply to other organs.

Three factors predispose to thrombosis. (1) *Hemodynamic factors:* Thrombosis is prone to occur where blood flow is sluggish, for example, in the veins of the legs after surgery, following delivery of a baby, or during long air flights because the slow flow permits activated clotting factors to accumulate instead of being washed away. (2) *Vascular factors:* Thrombosis tends to occur where the arterial intima is damaged by atherosclerotic plaques. (3) *Blood factors:* A congenital absence of protein C leads to massive intravascular coagulation and usually death in infancy. A genetic abnormality in factor V, making it resistant to inactivation by protein C, is a more common cause of thrombosis. Hypercoagulability of blood can occur due to a rise in plasma levels of vWF. It is an acute-phase protein, and its plasma level rises in inflammatory states. Plasma vWF level also rises during the third trimester of pregnancy.

Disseminated Intravascular Coagulation

Disseminated intravascular coagulation (DIC) has two phases, the thrombotic phase and the fibrinolytic phase.

In the **thrombotic phase,** there is formation of numerous small thrombi and emboli throughout the microvasculature, causing blockage of circulation and ischemic organ damage. The clots also use up most of the coagulation factors and platelets, resulting in bleeding tendencies. Hence, the condition is also called *defibrination syndrome* or *consumption coagulopathy.*

In the **fibrinolytic phase,** there is fibrinolysis of the clots. The fibrin degradation products that are formed have an antihemostatic effect and aggravate bleeding.

DIC usually occurs in *metastatic malignancies* (malignancies that spread to various parts of the body) and massive trauma because malignant or necrotic tissues release tissue factor into the circulation, triggering coagulation.

DIC also occurs in gram-negative septicemia because the endotoxin from *gram-negative bacteria* activates factor XII and stimulates the secretion of tissue factor. DIC is more common during pregnancy because pregnancy is associated with a rise in plasma fibrinogen level and vWF. DIC also occurs following snakebite: the venom of the Malaysian pit viper has a direct effect on fibrinogen, converting it to fibrin.

Summary

- There must be a balance between mechanisms that promote blood clotting and those that oppose it.

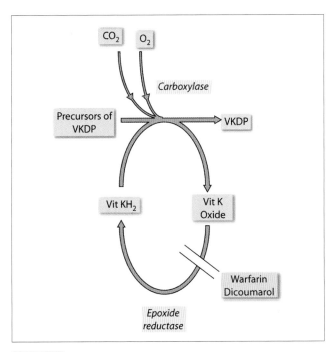

Fig. 27.5 Vitamin K cycle. VKDP, vitamin K-dependent proteins.

- Antihemostatic mechanisms include inhibition of platelet aggregation, inhibition of coagulation, and fibrinolysis.

- Prohemostatic mechanisms inhibit fibrinolysis.

Applying What You Know

27.1. Predict the results of subjecting Mr. Lundquist's blood to the following tests: (1) partial thromboplastin time, (2) prothrombin time, and (3) thrombin time. Explain your predictions.

Leukocytes (white blood cells) are classified into granulocytes (neutrophils, eosinophils, and basophils) and agranulocytes (monocytes and lymphocytes). The cytoplasm of granulocytes contains secretory granules that readily take up Romanowsky-type stains. Monocytes and lymphocytes do not have granules in their cytoplasm and are therefore called agranulocytes. The granules that distinguish the different types of granulocytes are called *specific* or *secondary granules*. They make their appearance only in the myelocyte stage. Another set of granules called the *primary* or *azurophilic granules* are common to all granulocytes. They appear in the promyelocyte stage but become obscured by the appearance of the specific granules in the myelocyte stage. All cytoplasmic granules, primary or secondary, contain biologically active substances that are involved in inflammatory and allergic reactions.

Neutrophils approach, ingest, and kill bacteria. Eosinophils attack parasites that are too large to be engulfed by phagocytosis. They enter tissues and are especially abundant in the mucosa of the respiratory, lower urinary, and gastrointestinal tracts. They increase in number in allergic diseases. Basophils, which resemble mast cells, release histamine and other inflammatory mediators. They are important in immediate-type hypersensitivity reactions. The relative and absolute counts of leukocytes are given in **Table 20.3**.

Neutrophils

The neutrophil (**Fig. 28.1**) is 10 to 14 μm in diameter. It is circular in shape, but the shape keeps changing due to ameboid movements. Its nucleus is multilobed with up to six lobes; hence, the neutrophil is also called a *polymorphonuclear leuko-*

cyte. The number of lobes is related to the age of the neutrophils, with the younger ones having a single-lobed horseshoe-shaped nucleus, and the older ones having a multilobed nucleus. The frequency distribution of neutrophils with different numbers of lobes is called the *Arneth count* and is done to assess the average age of neutrophils in circulation. Nearly 45% of the neutrophils are trilobed and in the right stage of maturity for optimum functioning, 20% are overaged with four or five lobes, and 35% are underaged with fewer than three lobes. A preponderance of immature cells is called a "shift to the left," whereas a preponderance of the older cells is called a "shift to the right."

Of the total number of neutrophils present in blood, only 50% are circulating in the blood at any moment, while another 50% remain marginated (sidelined) on vessel walls or sequestered (isolated) in closed capillaries. Margination of neutrophils is the first step in their migration to the tissues, which is their ultimate destination. After migration into tissues, they never return to the bloodstream and survive in tissues only for a few days. The average half-life of neutrophils in the circulation is only 6 hours. Up to 100 mL of packed neutrophils is eliminated daily, mainly in the intestine and in respiratory secretions. Neutrophils that die in tissues are taken up by macrophages.

For every neutrophil in the circulation, there are ~100 mature neutrophils held in bone marrow as a reserve. These stored neutrophils enter the bloodstream when they are stimulated by cortisol or by a granulocyte-inducing factor derived from dead leukocytes. Thus, an increase in the blood neutrophilic count can occur in three ways. (1) Mobilization of marginated or sequestered neutrophils from blood vessels. Epinephrine, exercise, and corticosteroids produce transient neutrophilia in

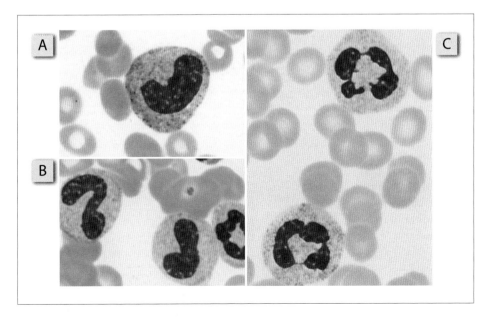

Fig. 28.1 Neutrophils. **(A)** Transitional form between a metamyelocyte and a band cell. **(B)** Two band cells. **(C)** Segmented neutrophilic granulocytes.

this way. (2) Release of stored neutrophils from bone marrow. This, too, produces a transient neutrophilia. (3) Stimulation of neutrophil production in bone marrow.

Neutrophilic granules | Like all granulocytes, neutrophils have two types of granules: the azurophilic granules that are also present in other granulocytes, and the specific granules that are peculiar to neutrophils alone and give them their name.

Azurophilic granules are released into phagocytic vacuoles containing ingested microbes. The contents of the azurophilic granule include myeloperoxidase and defensins. *Myeloperoxidase* is a protein that catalyzes the production of hypochlorite (OCl^-) from chloride and hydrogen peroxide produced by the oxygen burst. It imparts a greenish color to the pus. *Defensins* are cationic proteins that kill a variety of bacteria, fungi, and viruses.

Although the contents of the azurophilic granules are mostly secreted into phagocytic vacuoles, some enzymes may escape into surrounding tissues. This happens when the ingested organism is large, and the phagocytic vacuole cannot be completely sealed off. The enzymes, particularly elastase, cause considerable damage to the surrounding tissues. Such damage underlies several disorders, including rheumatoid arthritis and pulmonary emphysema.

Specific granules are largely released into the extracellular space. They are released early, when the neutrophil moves toward the site of inflammation. The major constituent of specific granules is an iron-binding protein called *apolactoferrin*. By binding iron, lactoferrin exerts a bactericidal effect by depriving bacteria of their necessary iron. It also contains *collagenase*, which facilitates neutrophilic mobility by hydrolyzing the extracellular matrix. The membrane of specific granules bears integrin molecules. When the granules fuse with the cell membrane, these integrin molecules appear on the cell membrane, where they perform an important role in chemotaxis.

Neutrophil count | An increase in neutrophil count is called *neutrophilia*, and a decrease is called *neutropenia*. Because neutrophils, comprise the bulk of leukocytes, neutrophilia is associated with leukocytosis (an increase in the total leukocytic count), and neutropenia is associated with leukopenia (a decrease in the total leukocytic count). Conversely, most cases of leukocytosis are due to neutrophilia, and most cases of leukopenia are due to neutropenia.

At birth, neutrophilic leukocytosis (25,000/cc) is present. The neutrophil count returns to normal after 1 week. In adults, the neutrophilic count can show a transient increase due to mobilization of neutrophils from the marginal pool. The phenomenon is called the *shift-leukocytosis* and is mostly due to the stimulation by glucocorticoid secretion. Marked shift-leukocytosis with neutrophilia occurs after strenuous exercise. During pregnancy, the leukocytosis increases until term and peaks at parturition, with the count sometimes doubling. Leukocytosis also occurs when an individual has anxiety or stress of any kind. Finally, there is a diurnal factor, with the leukocytic count increasing slightly in the afternoon (the afternoon tide).

Neutrophilia occurs in (1) infections and septicemia, especially with pyogenic cocci (e.g., *Staphylococci*) and bacilli (e.g., *Escherichia coli*), as well as with nonpyogenic organisms (e.g., diphtheria and cholera bacilli); (2) hemorrhage and trauma, as in surgery, fractures, crush injuries, and burns; (3) malignancies such as myeloid leukemia; (4) cardiac disorders, such as myocardial infarction; (5) metabolic disturbances, such as renal failure and diabetic coma; and (6) with use of medications, such as epinephrine.

Neutropenia commonly occurs in (1) viral infections, such as influenza, measles, and infective hepatitis; (2) bacterial infections, such as typhoid fever; (3) aplastic anemia; and (4) hypersplenism.

Neutrophilic Functions

The major role of neutrophils is to protect the host against infectious agents. To fulfill this role, neutrophils are endowed with the capability to sense infection, migrate to the site of the infecting organism, and then destroy the infectious agent.

Chemotaxis | Neutrophils are attracted toward the site of infection by chemoattractant molecules, which are detected by specific receptors on the neutrophilic membrane. These chemoattractants are either molecules released by the degradation of bacteria and damaged tissue cells or molecules formed through the interaction of bacteria with the host defense system. Notable among the latter are complement C5 (see **Table 31.1**), leukotriene B4 (which is the most potent chemoattractant molecule known yet), secretions of platelet α-granules (platelet factor 4, platelet-derived growth factor), and secretions of mast cell granules (see below).

Margination | When a neutrophil flowing inside a capillary approaches an area of inflammation, it becomes marginated—it is attracted to the capillary endothelium and starts rolling along its surface (**Fig. 28.2**). Margination usually occurs in a postcapillary venule. The margination is caused by the binding of selectins (cell adhesion molecules) present on the

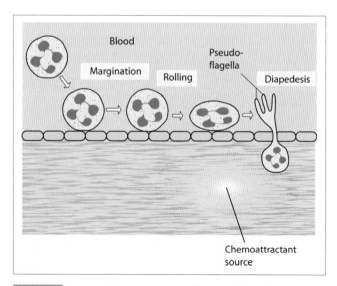

Fig. 28.2 Neutrophilic margination, rolling, and diapedesis are parts of the body's response to the presence of infection.

endothelial cells, with the carbohydrate molecules present on the surface of neutrophils. Endothelial selectins are more numerous in areas where there is inflammation. However, they are present normally, too, which is the reason why nearly half the circulating neutrophils remain marginated.

Activation | While rolling along the endothelial surface, if the neutrophil comes in contact with chemoattractant molecules, it becomes activated. The activation is mediated by G-protein. Activation of neutrophils is associated with degranulation of the specific granules to the neutrophil cell surface and a marked increase in neutrophilic adhesion to endothelial cells, resulting in the cessation of rolling. This occurs due to the appearance of integrins (cell adhesion molecules) on the surface of the neutrophil, which bind with its receptors on endothelial cells.

Diapedesis | Neutrophils next insinuate themselves through the walls of the capillaries between endothelial cells by a process called diapedesis. The neutrophils then migrate to the tissue along the chemoattractant gradient. During diapedesis, the neutrophil elongates and develops a broad "head" called a lamellipodium, which contains the bulk of the cytoplasm, and a thin forked "tail" called the pseudoflagellum. There is degranulation of specific granules from the lamellipodium.

Phagocytosis | Neutrophils have on their surface receptors for the Fc fragment of immunoglobulin molecules. When these Fc receptors bind to the IgG and complement proteins present on bacterial surface (see Chapter 31, Effector Phase of Immune Response section, opsonization), it triggers increased neutrophilic motility, exocytosis, and respiratory burst, thereby facilitating phagocytosis. These responses are mediated by G-protein.

During phagocytosis, the granulocyte membrane extends pseudopodia around the particle. The pseudopodia fuse to form a phagocytic vacuole and enclose the particle in it. The primary (lysosomal) and secondary (specific) granules fuse with the phagocytic vacuole and discharge into it enzymes such as lysozyme, myeloperoxidase, cathepsin G, elastase, lactoferrin, and cationic proteins called defensins. Following the respiratory burst, superoxide anion and its metabolites H_2O_2 and hypohalites diffuse into the phagocytic vacuole and initiate oxygen-dependent microbial killing.

Respiratory burst | Within seconds of stimulation, neutrophils sharply increase their oxygen uptake, a phenomenon known as the respiratory burst. The increased oxygen uptake is utilized for oxidation of glucose via the hexose monophosphate shunt, resulting in the production of nicotinamide adenine dinucleotide phosphate (NADPH) and reduced glutathione (GSH). NADPH reduces molecular oxygen to superoxide ion (O_2^-) and then to H_2O_2. GSH helps in detoxifying the extra H_2O_2 produced.

The reduction of O_2^- to H_2O_2 inside the neutrophil is catalyzed by the enzyme superoxide dismutase (SOD). The O_2^- that escapes from neutrophils into extracellular space is reduced to H_2O_2 by ceruloplasmin, an acute-phase protein. Neither O_2^- nor H_2O_2 has significant bactericidal activity, though the H_2O_2 formed in the tissues damages cells and the connective tissue matrix. However, in the presence of the azurophilic granule

enzyme myeloperoxidase, H_2O_2 oxidizes halide ions (Cl^-, Br^-, I^-) to form hypohalites (HOCl, HOBr, HOI), which are powerful microbicidal agents.

$$2O_2 + NADPH = 2O_2^- + NADP^+ + H^+$$
(weak bactericidal)

$$2O_2^- + 2H^+ \xrightarrow{\underset{\text{Ceruloplasmin (extracellular)}}{\text{Superoxide dismutase (intracellular)}}} H_2O_2 + O_2$$

$$H_2O_2 + 2Cl^- \xrightarrow{\text{Myeloperoxidase}} 2HClO$$
(strong bactericidal)

Disorders of Neutrophilic Functions

Abnormal polymerization of actin filaments in neutrophils or a congenital deficiency of leukocytic integrins results in *neutrophil hypomotility.* In a group of rare hereditary disorders known collectively as *chronic granulomatous disease,* the inability of neutrophils and monocytes to generate O_2^- leads to recurrent bacterial infections. Severe *congenital glucose 6-phosphate dehydrogenase (G6PD) deficiency* causes susceptibility to multiple infections due to failure to generate the NADPH necessary for O_2^- production. In *congenital myeloperoxidase deficiency,* microbial killing power is reduced because hypohalite ions are not formed.

Eosinophils

Eosinophils (**Fig. 28.3**) contain a bilobed nucleus and large, coarse granules that stain orange-red with Wright stain. Like neutrophils, eosinophils are distributed in an intravascular compartment made up of a marginal pool and a circulating pool of equal size. Its half-life in circulation is ~8 hours. For each circulating eosinophil, ~100 eosinophils are present in the tissues, primarily in the skin and in the submucosa of the respiratory, gastrointestinal, and genitourinary tracts.

Eosinophils are attracted to tissue sites of allergic reactions by chemotactic factors secreted by mast cells. At the site of the allergic reaction, eosinophils degrade mast cell products and thereby decrease the clinical manifestations of allergic responses.

Eosinophilic granules | The predominant constituent of eosinophilic granules is a material called *major basic protein* (MBP), which plays a key role in the eosinophil's ability to damage the helminthic larvae. Also present in the large granules is a potent bactericidal called *eosinophilic cationic protein,* a neurotoxic protein, and an *eosinophil peroxidase* with properties different from the myeloperoxidase of neutrophils. The smaller eosinophilic granules contain *aryl sulfatase B,* an enzyme that can inactivate the sulfur-containing leukotrienes liberated by mast cells in immediate hypersensitivity reactions. Eosinophils secrete *lysophospholipase,* which forms crystals called Charcot-Leyden crystals in the pulmonary secretions of patients with asthma.

Eosinophilic count | Glucocorticoids cause margination and sequestration of circulating eosinophils, lowering the eosinophilic count. The eosinophilic count shows a diurnal variation that varies inversely with the diurnal fluctuations in glucocorticoid levels (see **Fig. 79.6**). It is lowest at 8 AM and highest at midnight. Emotional stress decreases it. The eosinophil count decreases progressively during the intermenstrual period.

Eosinophilia occurs in (1) allergic disorders such as asthma, drug allergy, and food sensitivity; (2) parasitic infestations, such as hookworm, tapeworm, hydatid, and filaria. In general, eosinophilia is more pronounced with parasites causing tissue infection than with those causing intestinal infestations; (3) skin diseases such as eczema, dermatitis, and scabies; and (4) pulmonary eosinophilia, a group of diseases associated with pulmonary infiltration. Their cause is unknown, but it could be related to filarial infestation.

Eosinopenia occurs in (1) endocrine disorders, such as Cushing disease, and (2) stress, as in acute infection, traumatic shock, surgical operation, severe exercise, burns, acute emotional stress, or exposure to cold.

Basophils and Mast Cells

Basophils

The mature basophil (**Fig. 28.3**) has a lighter staining nucleus than the neutrophil. It seldom contains more than two lobes. The cytoplasm is pink and contains a varying number of large, deeply staining basophilic granules. The granules are usually not very numerous, and although they do not pack the cytoplasm, as do eosinophil granules, they overlie the nucleus and tend to obscure its detail.

Basophils remain in the blood only for a few hours, after which they move into tissues. Their fate in the tissues is uncertain. Contrary to earlier belief, basophils do not transform into mast cells in tissues. The basophil surface membrane contains receptors for the Fc fragment of immunoglobulin E (IgE) molecules. Basophil degranulates when an antigen reacts with IgE bound to basophils and thereby interconnects the IgE molecules on the basophil surface (see **Fig. 30.2**, Immediate hypersensitivity). Basophilic granules contain histamine, which mediates allergic reactions. Basophils also contain the proteoglycan chondroitin sulfate, whose function in the basophil is not known.

Basophilia occurs in chronic myeloid leukemia and hypersensitivity states. *Basopenia* occurs in Cushing disease and in the case of prolonged corticosteroid therapy. It also occurs when there is neutrophilic leukocytosis, as in infections.

Mast Cells

Mast cells are cells similar to basophils. They are found wandering in connective tissues, especially beneath epithelial surfaces. Mast cells are most abundant at those places where the body comes in direct contact with the environment, for example, in the lung, skin, lymphoid tissues, and submucosal layers of the digestive tract. The similarities and differences between basophils and mast cells are summarized in **Table 28.1**.

Mast cells contain inflammatory mediators, such as histamine, leukotrienes, prostaglandins, and chemotactic factors. Excessive mast cell degranulation produces clinical manifestations of allergy and even anaphylaxis. Leukotrienes released by the mast cell trigger the bronchospasm and the mucosal edema of bronchial asthma. The slow-reacting substance of anaphylaxis or SRS-A is a mixture of leukotrienes C4, D4, and E4 (see Chapter 37, Paracrine Control section, Prostaglandins). Mast cells also participate in immune response and tissue repair. They release tumor necrosis factor in response to bacterial products by an antibody-independent mechanism, thus contributing to the nonspecific natural immunity. Mast cells also contain the Charcot-Leyden crystal protein and small amounts of major basic protein.

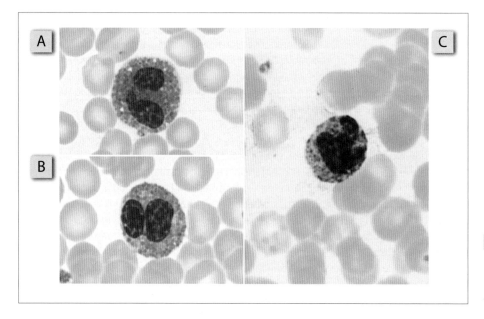

Fig. 28.3 Eosinophils and basophils. **(A,B)** Eosinophils with corpuscular, orange-stained granules; **(C)** basophils with corpuscular granules that stain deep blue to violet.

Table 28.1 Comparison of Basophil and Mast Cell

Both Basophil and Mast Cell	
Are derived from marrow stem cells	
Are stimulated to grow by the same interleukins	
Have surface receptors for IgE and degranulate when an antigen interlinks the IgE on their surfaces	
Basophil	**Mast Cell**
Is present in the bloodstream	Is present in tissues
Has a multilobed nucleus	Has a round nucleus
Granules contain chondroitin sulfate	Granules contain heparin

Abbreviation: IgE, immunoglobulin E.

Summary

- There are three types of granulocytes: neutrophils, eosinophils, and basophils.

- Neutrophils have several functions that contribute to host defense against infectious agents.

- Eosinophils play a role in allergic responses.

- Basophils play a role in immune responses.

Applying What You Know

28.1. Patients with pernicious anemia often exhibit leukopenia (a reduced white cell count). What roles do leukocytes play in host defense?

Monocytes

Monocytes (**Fig. 29.1**) are spherical cells. When suspended in isotonic fluid, their diameter is 9 to 12 µm, but when flattened in dried blood smears, they measure up to 14 to 18 µm in diameter. They have a relatively abundant dull blue cytoplasm with a few azurophilic granules. The nucleus is round or kidney-shaped and is eccentric in position. Its chromatin stains less intensely than that of lymphocytes, and there are one or two nucleoli.

Monocytes originate in bone marrow and circulate in blood for 3 days before migrating through the walls of postcapillary venules into the connective tissue of various organs, where they differentiate into tissue macrophages. Tissue macrophages do not reenter circulation, but persist in the tissues for another 3 months. Circulating monocytes perform no important function and are only a mobile reserve of cells capable of migrating into tissues and developing into macrophages.

Monocytosis (an increase in monocyte count, see **Table 20.3**) occurs in (1) bacterial infections, such as tuberculosis and typhoid; (2) protozoal infections, such as malaria; (3) rickettsial infections; (4) neoplastic diseases, such as infectious mononucleosis, Hodgkin disease, and monocytic leukemia; and (5) chronic inflammatory diseases, such as rheumatoid arthritis, collagen diseases, ulcerative colitis, and regional enteritis.

Mononuclear Phagocytic System

Tissue macrophages settle at several strategic locations in the body and constitute the tissue–macrophage system. Monocytes and macrophages together constitute the mononuclear phagocytic system. The mononuclear macrophage system was earlier called the reticuloendothelial system (RES), a term that encompassed a large collection of phagocytic cells. Any cell capable of taking up a vital dye such as trypan blue and particulate materials like colloidal carbon was called an RES cell. The RES therefore included (1) reticulum cells of the spleen and the lymph nodes; (2) cells lining the lymphatic and blood sinuses of the lymph nodes, spleen, and liver (Kupffer cells); (3) monocytes of blood; and (4) tissue macrophages. The reticuloendothelial system was so named because it included the reticulum cells of the spleen and lymph nodes and also the cells lining the splenic and hepatic sinusoids, which were thought to be endothelial cells. It was later discovered that the true endothelial cells and fibroblasts were also capable of taking up the dye, and although they were weakly phagocytic, they were for some time included under the RES.

The RES was later renamed the mononuclear phagocytic system (MPS). It includes (1) precursor cells from bone marrow; (2) promonocytes from bone marrow; (3) monocytes from bone marrow and blood; and (4) macrophages in the liver (Kupffer cells), spleen, lymph node, bone marrow, lung (pulmonary alveolar macrophages, also called dust cells), connective tissue (histiocytes), pleura and peritoneum, bones (osteoclasts), and central nervous system (microglial cells). The criteria for identifying a cell of the MPS are vigorous phagocytosis and pinocytosis and its ability to attach firmly to a glass surface. Reticulum cells of the spleen and lymph nodes, endothelial cells, and fibroblasts are not included in the MPS.

The functions of the MPS are as follows. (1) Macrophages ingest cell debris, broken erythrocytes, fibrin, and bacteria; therefore, they are important in inflammation and healing. (2) Bacteria entering the tissues through blood or lymph are sequestered and destroyed by the macrophages. (3) Macrophages process antigens and thereby play an important part

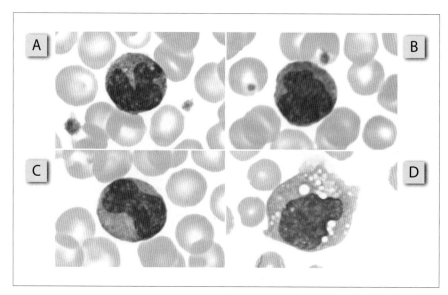

Fig. 29.1 (A–C) Range of appearances of typical monocytes with lobed nucleus, gray-blue stained cytoplasm, and fine granulation. (D) Phagocytic monocyte with vacuoles.

in the immune response. Macrophages are also very efficient in phagocytosing antigen-antibody-complement complexes because they have receptors for immunoglobulins and complement. (4) Macrophages, especially those in the spleen, remove aged erythrocytes. The heme moiety is divested of its iron, which is stored in the macrophages. (5) Macrophages store excess lipids and mucoprotein and become swollen to form "foam cells." (6) Twenty or more macrophages can fuse to form a multinucleate "giant cell," up to 50 μm in diameter, that engulfs a bacillus, especially the tubercle bacillus.

Lymphocyte

Lymphocytes (7–11 μm) have a deeply staining, slightly indented nucleus with a thin rim of clear blue cytoplasm (**Fig. 29.2**). They contain no specific granules, but may have a few small azurophilic granules.

Large and small lymphocytes | About 10 to 20% of the lymphocytes in peripheral blood are *large lymphocytes* (11–15 μm). These were believed to be in an early stage of development from the lymphoblast, which is larger than the lymphocyte. However, it is now known that these large lymphocytes are actually natural killer (NK) cells. They nonspecifically kill any cell that is coated with immunoglobulin IgG. This phenomenon is called antigen-dependent cell-mediated cytotoxicity (ADCC). Large lymphocytes require neither any prior sensitization nor major histocompatibility (MHC) molecules (see Chapter 31, Initial Phase of Immune Response section) for antigen recognition. They are therefore responsible for innate immunity rather than acquired immunity. They are particularly effective against tumor cells and virus-infected cells.

Small lymphocytes produce acquired immune response. They are classified as B lymphocytes, which mediate humoral immunity, and T lymphocytes, which mediate cellular immunity. These subtypes are not morphologically distinguishable, but have distinctive molecules on their cell membranes (surface markers) that are identifiable by immunocytochemical methods.

Lymphocytic count | The normal lymphocytic count is given in **Table 20.3**. *Lymphocytosis* occurs in (1) viral infections (e.g., mumps, measles, chicken pox, influenza, and viral hepatitis), (2) bacterial infections (e.g., typhoid, tuberculosis, and whooping cough), (3) parasitic infections (e.g., toxoplasmosis), (4) malignancies (e.g., lymphocytic leukemia and lymphocytic lymphoma), and (5) autoimmune diseases (e.g., myasthenia gravis and thyrotoxicosis).

Lymphopenia occurs in (1) acquired immunodeficiency syndrome (AIDS), (2) pancytopenia from any cause (e.g., aplastic anemia, bone marrow infiltration, and hypersplenism), and (3) corticosteroid administration.

Lymphocytic Processing

The committed lymphocytic stem cells soon differentiate into the committed B and T cells. The committed B lymphocytic stem cells are processed (rendered mature and immunocompetent) in the bone marrow (B for bursa of Fabricius, the site of B cell processing in birds). The committed T lymphocytic stem cells are processed in the thymus. The processing involves brisk proliferation with frequent mutations during cell divisions. These mutations may have a role in the development of antibody specificity. In the thymus, a factor called thymosin plays an important role in the processing of T lymphocytes.

Following processing, the mature T and B cells enter the circulation, where they are present in a 70:30 ratio. Many of them leak out through the postcapillary venules to settle in the peripheral lymphoid tissues (see below). Some of the lymphocytes return again to the circulation through the lymphatics draining these lymphoid tissues. At any given time, only ~2% of the lymphocytes are in the peripheral blood; the rest remains in the lymphoid organs. Within the peripheral lymphoid tissues, the T and B lymphocytes are found in distinct zones, as shown in **Table 29.1**. After birth, some lymphocytes are still formed in the bone marrow, but most are formed in the lymph nodes, thymus, and spleen from precursor cells that originally came from bone marrow.

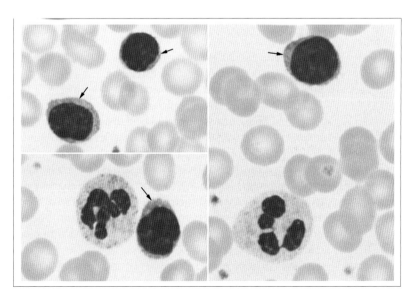

Fig. 29.2 Lymphocytes (*arrows*).

Table 29.1 Distribution of B and T Lymphocytes in Peripheral Lymphoid Tissues

Peripheral Lymphoid Tissue	B-Lymphocyte	T Lymphocyte
Lymph node	Subcapsular cortex, germinal centers, and medullary cord	Diffuse cortex
Spleen	Germinal centers and red pulp	Periarteriolar sheath
Alimentary and respiratory tracts	Submucous follicles	Interfollicular areas in submucosa

Lymphoid Tissues

Lymphocytes occur individually in blood, lymph, and connective tissues. They also occur in densely packed aggregates. The term *lymphoid tissue* includes all aggregations of lymphocytes and lymphocyte-rich organs, such as the thymus, lymph nodes, and spleen.

The lymphoid tissues in which lymphocytes are processed, the thymus and bone marrow, are called *central* or *primary lymphoid tissues.* The lymphoid organs in which processed lymphocytes are seeded are called *peripheral* or *secondary lymphoid tissues.* They include lymph nodes, the spleen, the lymphoid tissues associated with the alimentary tract (including the tonsils in the oral cavity and the Peyer's patches in the terminal ileum), respiratory and urinary tracts, and a portion of lymphocytes in bone marrow.

Thymus

The thymus is located anterior to the heart. In a small child, it may extend up to the neck, almost to the level of the thyroid gland. The thymus reaches its greatest size during puberty. After puberty, the thymus regresses (thymic involution), during which the thymic lymphocytes and epithelial cells are increasingly replaced by adipose tissue, though some thymic tissue persists throughout life.

The thymus consists of a cortex and a medulla. The cortex contains lymphocytes and thymocytes (precursors to the lymphocytes). The medulla contains mostly epithelial cells. The thymus is the first organ to become lymphoid in the fetus, as it gets seeded by blood-borne lymphocytes from the yolk sac and the fetal liver. The seeding is aided by thymotaxin, a chemotactic factor secreted by the thymus. Lymphocytes processed in the thymus are called T lymphocytes. During their processing in the thymus, the T lymphocytes develop surface molecules (also called surface markers) called CD-4 and CD-8, which form the basis for categorizing T cells into the T4 and T8 cells. The lymphocytes also develop MHC molecules and antigenic receptors. Lymphocytes that develop receptors against self-antigens undergo apoptosis, which explains why more than 90% of the lymphocytes die in the cortex of the thymus.

Lymph Node

The lymph node (**Fig. 29.3A**) has an outer cortex, where the lymphocytes are tightly packed, and an inner cortex, where the lymphocytes are diffusely distributed. The lymph node also contains the medullary cords, which are dense aggregations of lymphocytes around small blood vessels. Present inside the outer cortex are the germinal centers, which are circular zones with sparsely distributed lymphocytes at their center.

The lymph node is an effective filter located in the path of lymphatics that removes most of the microbes, malignant cells, and macromolecules from the lymph. After entering the lymph node, the lymph vessels open into the larger lymph sinuses. The lumens of these lymph sinuses are crisscrossed by a mesh formed by the modified epithelial cells called reticular cells. Macrophages are attached to this reticular mesh and also line the walls of the sinuses.

As the lymph flows through the lymph sinus, the bacteria are phagocytosed by the macrophages in the sinuses. Most of the bacteria, however, are filtered out of the lymph vessels and are deposited in the node, where they are phagocytosed by the macrophages and initiate an immune response. Viruses enter the lymphocytes but are not destroyed; rather, they persist in the lymphocytes and are distributed throughout the body. The lymph node is not an efficient barrier to malignant cells, which tend to accumulate in the lymph node and overflow into other nodes. Hence, when removing a malignant tumor, the surgeon also removes the draining lymph nodes to arrest the further metastasis of the malignant cells.

The lymphocytes in the germinal centers of the lymph node proliferate to form more lymphocytes. However, most of the lymphocytes present in the lymph node are seeded from blood flowing through the node. The macrophages in the lymph node are derived from monocytes in blood. Granulocytes do not enter the lymph node in significant numbers.

Spleen

The spleen (**Fig. 29.3B**) is divided into small compartments by connective tissue trabeculae extending inside from its fibrous capsule. Between the trabeculae is a meshwork of fine reticular connective tissue called the *splenic pulp.* Splenic arteries and veins travel in the trabeculae before entering the pulp. As they traverse the pulp, the arteries are surrounded by aggregations of immunocompetent lymphocytes, forming a periarterial sheath. At places, the periarterial sheath contains germinal centers, which are circular zones with sparsely distributed lymphocytes at their center. The periarterial sheath and the germinal centers constitute the white pulp. The red pulp consists of splenic sinuses that are engorged with blood and therefore red in color.

The circulation of the spleen has fast and slow components. The fast component is represented by the nutritive blood

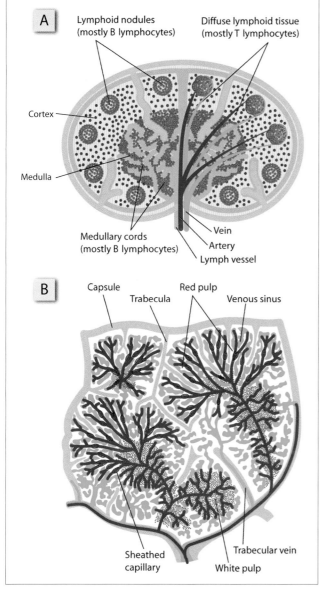

Fig. 29.3 (A) Structure of a lymph node. (B) Structure of the spleen. (Adapted from Faucett DW. A Textbook of Histology. 12th ed. New York: Chapman & Hall, Springer Science and Business Media; 1994.)

that are not as flexible as normal RBCs and consequently are unable to squeeze through the intercellular gaps between the endothelial cells that line the splenic sinuses. The process is called culling. Hence, splenectomy is helpful in elevating the RBC count in conditions like spherocytosis and autoimmune hemolytic anemias that are associated with excessive removal of RBCs. (3) The spleen acts as a reservoir for lymphocytes, plasma cells, monocytes, and platelets. It does so by preferentially sequestering newly released cells from the bone marrow, forming a reservoir inside it. In lower animals, it acts as a reservoir for whole blood, too. (4) The spleen is important for defense against blood-borne infections. Splenectomy renders the body vulnerable to fatal septicemia. (5) The macrophages in the spleen perform their usual functions of storage and immunity.

Certain patients of chronic splenomegaly develop neutropenia, anemia, and thrombocytopenia. The blood picture becomes almost normal after splenectomy. The condition is called hypersplenism and occurs probably due to increased sequestration and destruction of blood cells in the splenic pulp.

Summary

- Monocytes are the precursor cells of tissue macrophages, which play an important role in host defense.

- Lymphocytes play an essential role in immunologic host defense.

- Lymphoid tissues are found in the thymus, lymph nodes, and spleen and contain large numbers of lymphocytes.

Applying What You Know

29.1. Both Miss Adams, the patient with myasthenia gravis, and Mr. Lundquist, who has pernicious anemia, are likely to exhibit an increase in the number of lymphocytes. Explain why this is likely to be so.

supply in which blood stays within blood vessels. The slow component represents the nonnutritive blood supply that leaves arterioles and percolates through large numbers of phagocytes and lymphocytes before entering the splenic sinuses and passing back into the general circulation.

The functions of the spleen are as follows. (1) The spleen produces erythrocytes in the second half of fetal life. It can resume erythrocyte production in adult life if the bone marrow gets destroyed. (2) The spleen is the most effective lymphoid organ for the removal of aged erythrocytes from the circulation. The macrophages lining splenic sinusoids remove mildly damaged red blood cells (RBCs) that have reacted with antibodies or drugs. It also removes abnormal RBCs, such as spherocytes, sickle cells, and cells containing malarial parasite,

Immunity

Immunity refers to the body's ability to resist foreign substances (recognized as non-self) such as microbes or toxins that are potentially damaging to the body. Immunity may be natural or acquired. Acquired is further classified as actively acquired (active immunity) or passively acquired (passive immunity).

Natural (Innate) Immunity

Natural (innate) immunity refers to the nonspecific defense mechanisms of the body, which include the following: (1) phagocytosis by leukocytes and the monocyte–macrophage system cells; (2) destruction of ingested microbes by gastric acid; (3) resistance of the skin to microbial infection; (4) plasma enzymes, such as lysozymes that lyse bacteria, basic polypeptides that inactivate certain gram-positive bacteria, and complement, which destroys foreign substances; and (5) natural killer (NK) cells, which nonspecifically destroy foreign cells, tumor cells, and infected cells.

Inflammation is a form of natural immunity. It is associated with warmth (calor), redness (rubor), pain (dolor), and swelling (tumor). Thus, if any external or internal part of the body becomes swollen, red, painful, and warm, it is called an *inflammation*. The suffix *itis* is added to the name of the part to signify its inflammation, for example, gastritis, enteritis, hepatitis, myocarditis, meningitis, and encephalitis. The warmth, redness, and swelling of inflammation are due to the vasodilatation associated with inflammation. The vasodilatation, along with the increased capillary permeability associated with inflammation, results in exudation of plasma into interstitial spaces. The exudate contains large numbers of inflammatory cells, mainly neutrophils.

Immune surveillance is another form of natural immunity. It is the continuous recognition and destruction of tumor cells that keep appearing in the body throughout life. Immune cells identify tumor cells by the tumor-specific antigens. Although all types of immune cells are involved in the surveillance, the natural killer cells are especially dedicated to the surveillance. NK cells do not need to be stimulated by the tumor antigens. The mere contact with NK cells kills the tumor cells.

Tumor cells have several mechanisms for evading immunologic surveillance. They include the following: (1) A few isolated tumor cells express too little antigen to stimulate the immune system, and by the time the host's tumor immunity is adequate, the tumor burden is overwhelmingly large. The mechanism is called "sneaking through." (2) Tumor cells can shed or internalize their antigens and thereby evade detection. (3) Tumor cells decrease the expression of their class I molecules and thereby evade the associated recognition of the tumor antigens. (4) Tumor antigens generally do not express class II molecules and therefore do not stimulate the helper T cells. This makes tumor cells poorly immunogenic. (5) Certain molecules, such as sialomucin, tend to cover and mask the tumor antigens, disabling immune cells from detecting them. This has been called "antigenic blindfolding." (6) A subpopulation of T8 cells called *suppressor T cells* (T_s) is tumor-friendly. They suppress the development of the usual immune response to tumor antigens by inhibiting the differentiation of T_c cells and inhibiting the activity of macrophages. (7) Tumor cells can synthesize substances that reduce host immunity that is targeted at them.

Acquired (Adaptive) Immunity

Acquired (adaptive) immunity is a highly specific defense mechanism of the body that is targeted specifically at foreign materials introduced into the body. The foreign material may be an antigen or a hapten.

An *antigen* is usually a high-molecular-weight protein, but it may also be a low-molecular-weight protein (e.g., insulin) or a high-molecular-weight polysaccharide (e.g., dextran). Immunogenic molecules require some degree of chemical complexity. Large substances lacking chemical complexity, such as nylon, polyacrylamide, and Teflon (DuPont Pharma, Wilmington, DE), are not immunogens. The specificity of an antigen is due to specific areas of its molecule called determinant sites or epitopes. One protein can have several epitopes, and these may differ from each other not only in their specificity, but also in their antigenic potency.

A *hapten* is usually a nonprotein substance that has little or no antigenic property by itself, but which combines with a protein to form a new antigen capable of stimulating production of specific immunoglobulins, the specificity of which depends upon the hapten fraction rather than the carrier protein. A secondary response can be elicited by a subsequent challenge by the same carrier–hapten complex, but not by the hapten combined with a different carrier. The hapten, however, does not require the protein carrier to react with the antibody produced. Lipids and simple carbohydrates that are not antigenic, as well as the more complex polysaccharides that are poorly antigenic, are often powerful haptens.

Active immunity involves a direct encounter with the antigen. An essential aspect of active-acquired immune response is the development of *immunologic memory* of the antigen so that on subsequent encounters, the response to the same antigen is more vigorous.

When an antigen is introduced into an animal for the first time, there is an interval varying from 4 days to 4 weeks before any antibody can be detected in the serum. Then, a rise in the antibody titer, which reaches its maximum by 6 days to 3 months, follows. This response is called the *primary response* (**Fig. 30.1, Table 30.1**). When the same antigen is injected into the body again, there is an immediate drop in the circulating antibody titer due to its neutralization by the injected antigen. However, after 2 to 3 days, there is a rapid rise in titer that reaches its peak after 7 to 14 days. The antibody titer is much higher than in the primary response. This response is called

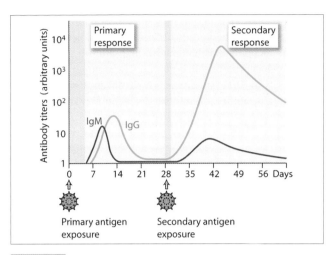

Fig. 30.1 Primary and secondary immune responses. Note also the class switch: in the primary response, the rise in immunoglobulin M (IgM) occurs before the rise in immunoglobulin G (IgG) and is produced in a comparable amount. In the secondary response, IgG appears earlier, and its amount far exceeds the amount of IgM produced.

the *secondary response.* Even after the antibody titer falls off, it remains higher than the titer achieved during the primary response. The main features of the secondary response are therefore threefold: a smaller dose of antigen required to produce it, a shorter lag, and greater antibody production.

Active immunization against a microbe can be achieved by injecting its antigens into the body. When the microbe invades the body, a secondary response is elicited by its antigens, and it is quickly destroyed before it can multiply and infect the body. Subsequent attacks by the same microbe only help in boosting the secondary response and prolonging the immunity.

Passive immunity is acquired without an encounter with the antigen, as when the mother passes her antibodies to the fetus through the placenta or colostrum, or when antibodies are injected therapeutically. Passively acquired immunity does not confer immunologic memory.

Passive immunization can be achieved by injecting preformed antibodies (produced in animals or in another person) against specific microbial antigens. When the microbe subsequently invades the body, it is quickly eliminated by the

injected antibodies, which, too, are consumed in the process. Such prompt elimination, however, preempts the development of active immunity.

Immunotherapy

Immunotherapy is the therapeutic use of immunologic methods for eliminating tumor cells. **Nonspecific immunotherapy** relies on the activation of immune responses that are not tumor-specific, but nonetheless inhibit tumor growth. This is done by injecting cytokines, such as tumor necrosis factor.

Specific immunotherapy involves injecting the patient with tumor cells or tumor antigens to induce immunity against tumor antigens. It is often supplemented by injection of cytokines for stimulating the differentiation of helper T cells, which are usually not formed in large numbers in the natural antitumor immune responses. *Monoclonal antibodies* (originating from a single clone of cells and therefore highly immune-specific) directed against tumor antigens have been used in immunotherapy to treat cancer. However, most cancer cells undergo antigenic modulation, rendering the antibodies ineffective. An agent called an *immunotoxin* or the "magic bullet" combines the selectivity of monoclonal antibodies with the killing power of anticancer drugs. It consists of antitumor toxins linked to monoclonal antibodies specific for tumor cells only. Once the antibody binds to the tumor cell, the tumor cell internalizes the antibody, along with the toxin that ultimately kills it.

Immunomodulation

Immunoenhancement

Immunoenhancement means enhancing the humoral or cell-mediated immune response against antigens. *Adjuvants* (Latin *adjuvere,* to help) are substances that, when mixed with an antigen before injection, nonspecifically enhance the immune response to the antigen. An adjuvant may be a cell-wall constituent (e.g., muramyl dipeptide) from tubercle bacilli or gram-negative bacteria, such as diphtheria or whooping cough bacilli. Other adjuvants are alum, mineral oil, lanolin, and detergents. The first adjuvant to be discovered was Freund adjuvant. It contains heat-killed *Mycobacterium tuberculosis,* mineral oil, and

Table 30.1 Differences between Primary and Secondary Immune Response

	Primary Response	Secondary Response
Responding B cells	Unsensitized B cells	Memory B cells
Latent period	5–10 days	1–3 days
Peak antibody titer	Smaller	Larger
Persistence of antibody titer	Short	Long
Predominating antibody class	IgM appears earlier	IgG appears earlier
Induced by	All immunogens, including TI antigens	Only T-cell-dependent protein antigens
Dose of antigen required	High	Low

Abbreviations: IgG, immunoglobulin G; IgM, immunoglobulin M.

lanolin. A similar adjuvant that is in wide use is the bacillus Calmette-Guérin (BCG). Named after its originators, BCG is an attenuated strain of *M. tuberculosis*.

Adjuvants enhance immunogenicity of soluble protein antigens by converting them into particulate forms. This promotes increased phagocytic uptake and, subsequently, a delayed and sustained release of the antigen (the depot effect). Injection of adjuvants often causes granuloma formation at the site of injection after several days. A granuloma is an aggregation of macrophages, lymphocytes, giant cells, and fibroblasts, formed within a meshwork of connective tissue fibers.

Immunosuppression

Immunosuppression is used therapeutically in inflammations, organ transplantation, autoimmune disorders, Rh blood antigen sensitization, and cancers of the hemopoietic system.

Nonspecific immunosuppression can be induced by physical and chemical methods. *Physical methods* of immunosuppression include the removal of lymphoid tissue by surgical means or by irradiation. Surgical removal of the thymus has been performed for the alleviation of myasthenia gravis. Removal of other lymphoid organs changes the immune response only slightly. *Chemical immunosuppressants* include corticosteroids.

Specific immunosuppression is the abolition of the response to a particular antigen, leaving the response to all other antigens intact. *Antigen-induced suppression* is used for allergen desensitization. However, the suppression is transient. The rationale is that if several small doses of an antigen are given over time, the body stops reacting to that antigen. An example of *antibody-mediated suppression* is the prevention of Rh blood antigen sensitization in susceptible pregnant women. *Antilymphocytic serum reacts* selectively with lymphocytes, inactivating their antigenic receptors. Because of several side effects, it has limited use in humans.

Immunodeficiency

Immunodeficiency can be caused by genetic or environmental factors, or both. Immunodeficiency diseases can affect humoral immunity, cell-mediated immunity, phagocytosis, or the complement system. Most immunodeficiency diseases involve only B cells. Examples are the X-linked agammaglobulinemia and X-linked hyper-IgM syndrome.

Acquired immunodeficiency syndrome | (AIDS) was first identified in 1981. It is characterized by dramatic weight loss, night sweats, swollen lymph nodes, and high susceptibility to opportunistic infections. It is also associated with neuropsychiatric abnormalities. The definition of AIDS is explicit in its name. It is "acquired" because it is not inherited. It is an "immunodeficiency" because the immune system breaks down. It is a "syndrome" because it is associated with several diseases that take advantage of the body's collapsed defenses.

AIDS spreads by intimate homosexual or heterosexual contact, by exposure to infected blood or blood products, or from mother to child during pregnancy. It is caused by an RNA retrovirus that has been named the human immunodeficien-

cy virus type 1 (HIV-1). AIDS patients have lymphopenia involving primarily the T_4 cells because the T_4 molecule acts as a specific receptor that binds with high affinity to the HIV's envelope glycoprotein called gp 120. The number of circulating NK cells in AIDS patients is not significantly reduced, but their cytotoxic ability is diminished. The humoral dysfunction associated with AIDS is an inability to produce an adequate IgM response. HIV virus does not kill the infected T_4 cells—clever viruses do not. Rather, they activate them to T_H1 cells. This leads to a widespread activation of the immune system, which causes immunologic destruction.

Monocytes also express the antigens of T_4 cells and therefore get infected with HIV virus. Monocytes are more refractory to the cytopathic effects of the virus: the virus can survive in these cells and get transported to different parts of the body, such as the brain and lung. Thus, monocytes serve as a major reservoir for HIV in the body. HIV-1 also invades brain cells, causing dementia in over half the patients.

Immune Tolerance

Specific Immunologic Tolerance

Specific immunologic tolerance is defined as the acquired inability of a host to express specific humoral or cell-mediated immunity to an antigen to which it would normally respond. The lack of responsiveness is not caused by nonimmunogenicity of an antigen or any impairment of the immune response. To be called specific tolerance, a recipient must have two exposures to the antigen: the first tolerance-eliciting exposure followed by a second challenging exposure of the same antigen that fails to evoke an immune response. Thus, tolerance is the opposite of secondary immune response.

Some of the observations on immune tolerance are as follows: (1) High zone tolerance or immune paralysis is produced by large doses of antigen, probably by depleting the specific clones of cells. (2) Low zone tolerance is induced by repeated subimmunogenic doses of thymus-dependent antigens. (3) Aggregate-free antigens are tolerogenic, probably because they escape phagocytosis by the macrophages. (4) Tolerance is easier shortly after birth.

Tolerance to Fetus

Because of the incorporation of the paternal genes, the fetus differs in genetic makeup from its mother. It should therefore induce immune response in the mother in the same way as the fetal rhesus antigen in an Rh– mother. However, that never happens, probably for the following reasons: (1) The placenta is resistant to immune attack because after implantation, the trophoblasts lose much of their immunogenicity due to a decrease in the density of the MHC (major histocompatability) antigens or the development of an inert coating of mucoprotein on the surface of these cells. (2) The antibodies produced by the mother are absorbed by the placenta, preventing their entry into the fetal circulation. (3) Alpha fetoprotein (AFP) and progesterone produced during embryonic development are immunosuppressants.

Tolerance to Self

Tolerance to self is probably a high zone tolerance induced during fetal life when large amounts of self-antigens react with and deplete the corresponding clones.

Autoimmune diseases result when the body's immune response gets directed toward its own tissues, which are normally exempted as self-antigens. Examples of autoimmune diseases are given in **Table 30.2**. The possible mechanisms of development of autoimmunity are as follows: (1) A sequestered self-antigen that has not come in contact with, and therefore did not deplete, its corresponding clone during fetal life will elicit an immune response in the adult if it comes in contact with immunocompetent cells. This appears to be the case with lens proteins, which are enclosed in a capsule but may leak out in the adult following injury or surgery. (2) Although antibodies are highly specific, sometimes an antibody formed in response to some foreign antigen cross-reacts with some tissue of the body itself. This happens in rheumatic heart disease, where the heart is damaged by antibodies formed against streptococcal antigens. (3) With age, some tissues of the body undergo an antigenic change that is not recognized as a self-antigen. (4) The suppressor T cells may fail to check the immune process adequately.

Table 30.2 Some Autoimmune Diseases and Their Mechanism

Hashimoto disease	T cells react with the antigens on the thyroid cells
Graves disease	Autoantibodies bind to thyroid cells and stimulate them
Insulin-dependent diabetes mellitus	Autoantibodies damage the insulin-producing B cells of the pancreas
Myasthenia gravis	Autoantibodies damage the muscles
Rheumatoid arthritis	Autoantibodies damage the joints
Pernicious anemia	Autoantibodies damage the gastric mucosa
Autoimmune hemolytic anemia	Autoantibodies damage the erythrocytes
Thrombocytopenic purpura	Autoantibodies damage the platelets
Rheumatic fever	Antistreptococcal antibodies cross-react with heart valve tissues

Hypersensitivity

When an immune reaction results in considerable damage to the body, it is called hypersensitivity. There are four types of hypersensitivity reactions (**Fig. 30.2**).

Type I hypersensitivity (anaphylaxis) occurs due to mast cell degranulation and is caused by antigens that evoke a strong IgE response. Examples are allergic rhinitis (hay fever), atopic dermatitis (eczema), and acute urticaria (hives). It occurs within minutes after a repeat exposure to the offending allergen (antigen). Mast cell degranulation occurs when the IgE molecules present on them are cross-linked by the antigen. The mediators include histamine and the slow-reacting substance of anaphylaxis (SRS-A). They cause capillary dilatation and exudation and sensory nerve stimulation (itching, sneezing, and coughing).

The susceptibility to type I hypersensitivity is called *atopy*. Atopic individuals are treated by desensitization, that is, repeated administration of increasing doses of the offending allergen. The repeated exposure induces formation of IgG rather than IgE. On subsequent challenge with the allergen, the IgG reacts with the allergen before it can react with the IgE or cause mast cell degranulation.

Type II hypersensitivity (antibody-mediated cytotoxicity) is an immediate immune reaction that damages antigen-bearing cells. Examples of this are seen in incompatible blood transfusion and hemolytic disease of the newborn. When antibodies react with the antigens, they also damage the cells (erythrocytes, leukocytes, or platelets) on which the antigens are located.

Type III hypersensitivity (immune complex disorder) occurs when antigen–antibody complexes are deposited in normal tissues of the body where they fix complement. Complement activation damages the tissue cells in the vicinity (damage of "innocent bystanders"). A form of glomerulonephritis is an example of this type of hypersensitivity.

Type IV hypersensitivity (delayed-type hypersensitivity, DTH) differs from the preceding types in two ways. (1) It is not mediated by antibodies; rather, it is mediated by macrophages that have been activated by T cells. The cytokines secreted do most of the damage. (2) The hypersensitivity starts after several hours and peaks at 48 to 72 hours. DTH is characteristically associated with granuloma formation. DTH is typically seen in Koch phenomenon, the hypersensitivity to tuberculin, which is present in *M. tuberculosis*.

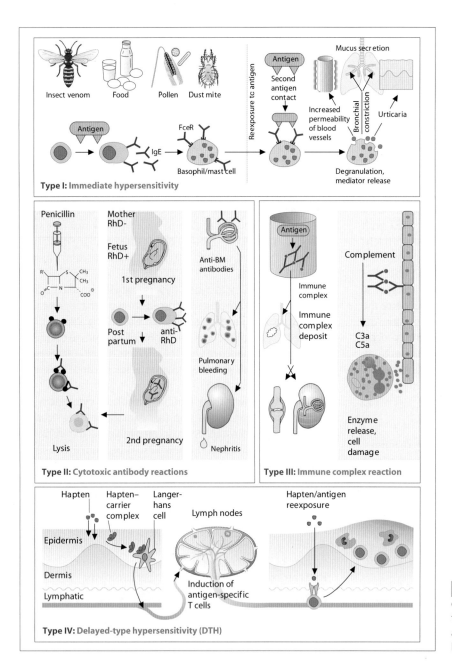

Type I: Immediate hypersensitivity

Type II: Cytotoxic antibody reactions

Type III: Immune complex reaction

Type IV: Delayed-type hypersensitivity (DTH)

Fig. 30.2 Hypersensitivity reactions: type I or anaphylaxis, type II or antibody-mediated cytotoxicity, type III or immune complex disorder, and type IV or delayed-type hypersensitivity. BM, basement membrane.

Summary

- Immunity is the body's ability to resist foreign substances that could potentially damage the body.

- Innate immunity refers to several mechanisms that defend the body against nonspecific threats.

- Acquired or adaptive immunity refers to responses targeting a specific foreign material (antigen or hapten).

Applying What You Know

30.1. Patients with autoimmune diseases, such as myasthenia gravis and pernicious anemia, are more likely than others to have other autoimmune diseases, such as type 1 diabetes and Hashimoto disease (thyroiditis). What mechanism might explain this phenomenon?

There are three phases of the immune response: the initial phase, the central phase, and the effector phase. The phases occur sequentially. The *initial phase* involves innate immunity and includes the events between the entry of antigen and its contact with specific receptors on the lymphocytic membrane. The monocyte–macrophage system is essential to this phase of immune response. The *central phase* of the immune response involves cooperation among different subsets of lymphocytes that proliferate and differentiate to form sensitized T and B lymphocytes and memory cells. The *effector phase* involves the inactivation of the antigen by the sensitized B and T cells generated during the central phase.

Initial Phase of Immune Response

T lymphocytes have specialized receptors for antigens. In B lymphocytes, the immunoglobulins (Ig) present on the cell membrane (IgM and IgD) serve as receptors for antigens. T lymphocytes fail to recognize the antigen in isolation: the antigen has to be closely associated with some major histocompatibility (MHC) molecules to be recognized by the T cells. The phenomenon is called *associated recognition*. B lymphocytes do not require MHC molecules for recognizing antigens.

MHC molecules are present on every cell in the body. Just as specific blood group polysaccharides are responsible for transfusion reaction, similarly, specific MHC molecules are responsible for graft rejection following tissue transplantation. In humans, the MHC antigens are referred to as the human leukocytic antigens (HLAs) and are located on the short arm of chromosome 6. MHC molecules are broadly of two types: class I and class II. *Class I MHC molecules* are present on all cells except macrophages and B cells. *Class II MHC molecules* are present only on macrophages and B cells.

During tissue grafting, the MHC molecules on the donor tissue cells (mostly class I molecules) themselves act as an antigen (then called MHC antigens). Antigens other than the MHC antigens have different ways of getting associated with MHC molecules (**Fig. 31.1**). (1) When a malignant tumor cell develops in the body, its mutant gene codes the synthesis of abnormal antigenic protein molecules on its surface. Thus, the tumor cell gets associated with class I MHC molecules. (2) When a virus invades a cell, it codes the synthesis of protein molecules that present themselves on the cell surface. The viral antigens thereby get associated with class I MHC molecules. (3) When a macrophage phagocytoses an antigen and fragments it, the antigenic epitopes make their way to the

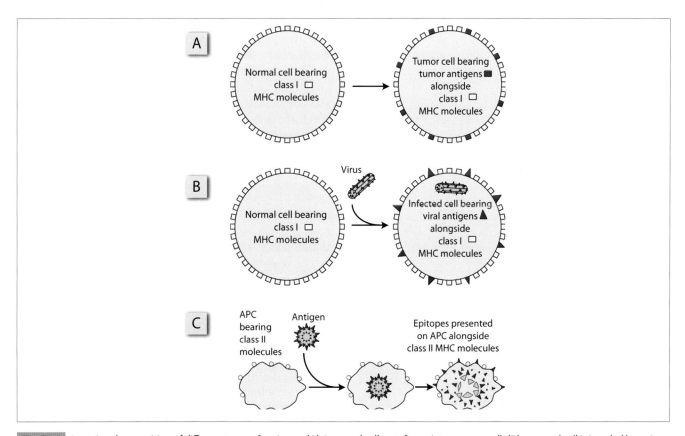

Fig. 31.1 Associated recognition of different types of antigens. **(A)** A normal cell transforms into a tumor cell; **(B)** a normal cell is invaded by a virus; **(C)** a macrophage engulfs an antigen. APC, antigen-processing cells; MHC, major histocompatibility.

surface of the macrophages. Thus, the antigenic epitopes get associated with class II MHC molecules of the macrophage.

The process of engulfing an antigen, fragmenting it, and presenting the epitopes on the cell surface is called *antigen processing*, and phagocytes that process antigens are called antigen-processing cells (APCs). Macrophages engulf tumor cells too. Thus, a tumor antigen that was originally associated with class I molecules subsequently gets associated with class II molecules. Also, tumor cells are known to shed their antigens (antigen shedding). These antigens are also phagocytosed and processed by macrophages. Therefore, nearly all antigens, including viral and tumor antigens, eventually get associated with class II MHC molecules.

Central Phase of Immune Response

A lymphocyte normally develops from a lymphoblast, which is larger in size. However, when stimulated by a suitable antigen, the lymphocyte becomes larger and looks once again like a lymphoblast. This is known as *blast transformation*. The B lymphoblast differentiates into the plasma cell, which produces immunoglobulins. The T lymphocyte differentiates into two different effector T cells, the T_H (*H* for helper) cells and T_C (*C* for cell-mediated cytotoxicity). Some of the B and T lymphocytes (T_4 subtype, see below) do not enlarge or undergo blast transformation when exposed to antigen. Instead, they only proliferate, forming a large number of small-sized *memory cells* (**Fig. 31.2**), which are responsible for the secondary immune response.

T-Cell Differentiation

Depending on the type of their surface antigens, the mature T lymphocytes are further classified into two antigenic subtypes: T_4 cells and T_8 cells (**Fig. 31.3**). Antigens associated with

class II molecules stimulate T_4 cells to differentiate into T_H cells. Antigens associated with class I molecules stimulate T_8 cells to differentiate into T_C cells. The T_C cell requires the help of the T_H cell for its activity, which is called *T-T cooperation*. Recalling that antigens associated with class I MHC molecules eventually also get associated with class II MHC molecules, it is obvious that most antigens would stimulate both T_4 and T_8 lymphocytes, resulting in the production of both T_C and T_H cells.

B-Cell Differentiation

B cells can recognize the antigen but cannot undergo proliferation and transformation into plasma cells until they receive the cooperation of the T_H cells. In other words, the B cells can decipher the "antigenic signal" but cannot proliferate until they receive the "proliferative signal" from the T_H cells. This is known as T–B cooperation. Hence, the B cells, too, are ultimately dependent on MHC molecules, without which there would be no T_H cells to enable their differentiation.

Thymus-independent (TI) antigens do not require the help of T_H for stimulating the proliferation of B cells. Examples include the ABO agglutinogens and dextran. All TI antigens have an orderly arrangement of repeating antigenic determinants. It seems that ~12 to 16 receptors on the B cell must be cross-linked by identical, properly spaced antigenic determinants to provide the proliferative signal normally provided by the T_H cell. The TI antigens induce only IgM formation; therefore, there is no "class switch" (**Fig. 30.1**) of antibody. Consequently, the secondary response, which is dependent on IgG production, is weak with TI antigens.

Theories of Immune Specificity

The antibody produced in response to an antigen is highly specific: it reacts only with the antigen that has evoked its production and not with any other antigen. Such specificity also implies that because there are innumerable antigens to which the body can be possibly exposed, there must be an equal number of antibodies in the body to match them. However, the ultimate blueprint for the production of all antibodies resides in the solitary hemopoietic stem cell, and somewhere down the line of differentiation, the cells or the antibodies acquire a bewildering range of specificity. The crucial question is, at what stage of differentiation does the specificity develop? Broadly, there are three possibilities, each of which has been shaped into a well-argued theory.

The **template (instructive) theory** (**Fig. 31.4A**) suggests that antibody specificity does not develop during the course of cell differentiation, but develops only following the contact of the antigen with antibody. The antigen acts as a template, and the antibody molds itself to fit with it. Thus, it suggests that the antigen "instructs" the production of its antibody and that immunoglobulins present in the body are nonspecific prior to antigenic exposure.

The **germline (selective) theory** (**Fig. 31.4B**) suggests that the complete range of antibodies is present on the surface of each B cell, and the antigen has only to "select" and stimulate the production of the antibody that is specific to it. In other words, the B cell itself is nonspecific, but produces the whole range of

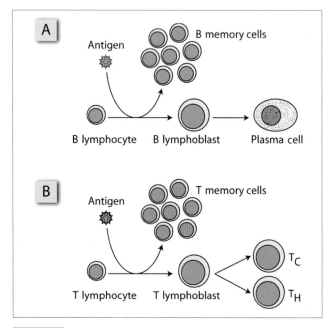

Fig. 31.2 Differentiation of B and T lymphocytes.

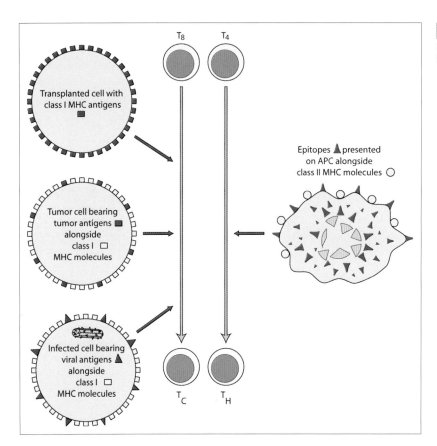

Fig. 31.3 Role of major histocompatibility (MHC) molecules in T-cell differentiation. APC, antigen-presenting cells.

specific antibodies. It, however, seems unlikely that so many genes in a single cell are devoted only to antibody production.

The **somatic mutation (clonal selection) theory** (**Fig. 31.4C**) differs from the germline theory in suggesting that the complete set of antibodies is produced, not by just one nonspecific B cell, but by a complete set of specific B cells. It proposes that during lymphocytic processing in the central lymphoid tissues, the cells proliferate massively. During proliferation, the cells mutate frequently, giving rise to genetically diverse B cells, each capable of producing a different antibody. Each specific B cell multiplies and establishes a population of genetically and immunologically identical B cells called a *clone.* An antigen has only to select and stimulate a specific clone; hence, the name "clonal selection" theory.

Effector Phase of Immune Response

The effector phase mechanisms can be classified into three stages.

The *first stage* is concerned with delivering immune cells to the site where antigens are located. This is made possible through vasodilatation and chemotaxis. (1) *Vasodilatation* causes increased movement of phagocytic cells and immunoreactive proteins from the blood vessels into the extravascular spaces. (2) *Chemotactic factors* attract the cells to the site of the antigen. Most of the factors producing vasodilatation and chemotaxis are released by mast cells.

The *second stage* of the effector phase makes the antigens and antigen-bearing cells susceptible to their final elimination. These mechanisms are as follows. (1) *Agglutination* causes clumping of antigens, increasing their vulnerability to phagocytosis. (2) *Opsonization* is the coating of antigens with antibody and complement. The coating makes the antigen vulnerable to lysis or phagocytosis (**Fig. 31.5**). (3) *Antibody-dependent cell-mediated cytotoxicity* (ADCC) is a form of cytotoxicity in which natural killer (NK) cells recognize and kill antibody-coated target cells. Opsonization is to phagocytosis as ADCC is to cytolysis.

The *final stage* is concerned with the inactivation and elimination of the antigen, all of which is ultimately dependent on the activation of B and T lymphocytes. These mechanisms are (1) *phagocytosis* of the cell on which it is present, (2) *cytolysis* of the cell on which it is present, (3) *bacteriostasis,* in the case of bacterial antigens, and (4) *neutralization,* in the case of toxic antigens.

Depending on the immune mechanisms employed for eliminating the antigen, immune mechanisms have been classified into humoral and cellular immunity. *Humoral immunity* is a major defense against bacterial infections. It includes effector mechanisms involving antibodies (γ-globulins or immunoglobulins) and complement (enzymatic plasma proteins). *Cell-mediated immunity* is mainly responsible for defense against tumor and transplant cells and infections due to viruses, fungi, and certain bacteria, such as the tubercle bacilli. It is

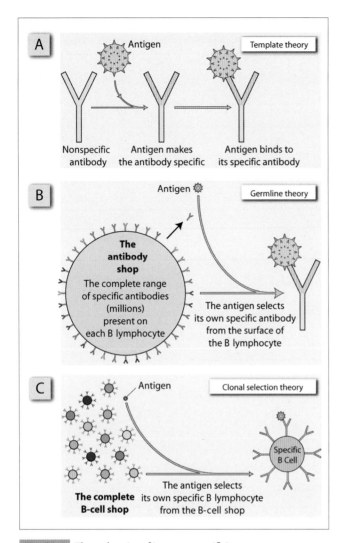

Fig. 31.4 Three theories of immune specificity.

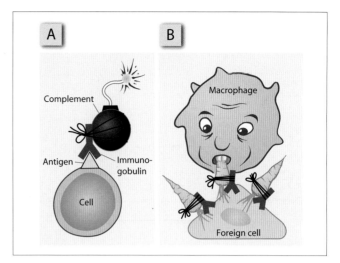

Fig. 31.5 **(A)** Cell lysis through complement. The Fc of the antibody is bound to the complement (shown here as a bomb with its fuse lighted). The Fab of the antigen binds to the antigen on the cell surface. The complement destroys the cell. **(B)** Phagocytosis induced through opsonization. The Fab of the antibody binds to a foreign cell. The Fc of the antibody is bound to some foreign materials (shown here as alluring carrots) that attract macrophages and result in the phagocytosis of the foreign cell.

mediated by T lymphocytes. The distinction between humoral and cellular immunity is blurred by the presence of extensive overlaps between the two systems.

Humoral Immunity

An **immunoglobulin** molecule is made of two heavy and two light chains (**Fig. 31.6**). Disulfide bonds anchor the light chain to the heavy chain and also hold the two heavy chains together. The heavy chains are of five subtypes: μ, γ, α, ε, and δ (constituting, respectively, IgM, IgG, IgA, IgE, and IgD). The light chains are only of two types, κ and λ.

The NH_2 terminal part of each chain (designated as V_L in the light chain and V_H in the heavy chain) has a variable sequence of amino acids and is therefore called the *variable region*. The COOH terminal part has a relatively constant sequence and is called the constant region. The variable regions bind to the antigen.

Disulfide bonds fold each chain into incomplete loops. Each light (L) chain has only two loops, V_L and C_L. The heavy (H) chain has four loops: the V_H, C_H1, C_H2, and C_H3. The V_L and V_H together form the variable (V) region, which binds to the antigen. The C_L, C_H1, C_H2, and C_H3 constitute the constant (C) region of the immunoglobulin molecule.

The immunoglobulin molecule can be split enzymatically by papain or pepsin. Papain yields the Fab (antigen-binding fraction) that bears all the variable regions and the Fc (crystallizable fraction), which determines such properties of the immunoglobulin as diffusibility, placental transfer, complement-fixation, and opsonization. Pepsin splits off a dimer of Fab from the immunoglobulin molecule.

Immunoglobulin M (IgM) comprises ~10% of the total plasma immunoglobulins. It is the first immunoglobulin produced in the primary response. Its level does not rise significantly in the secondary response. Because of its large size, it is predominantly intravascular. This, coupled with its early production, makes it important in bacteremias. IgM is the only immunoglobulin that is produced before birth. Natural antibodies such as anti-A and anti-B agglutinogens are therefore of the IgM type. IgM has a theoretical valence of 10, which is actually observed only with small haptens. With larger antigens, its effective valence drops to 5 due to steric restriction. However, it has much more affinity and avidity of binding for large antigens with multiple epitopes than for small haptens. IgM produces very effective agglutination. It fixes complement by the classical pathway, and the lysis it causes is very effective. Its opsonizing power is rather weak.

Immunoglobulin G (IgG) is the most abundant immunoglobulin, comprising ~70% of the total immunoglobulins. It is the major immunoglobulin to be synthesized during the secondary response in which the initial IgM production gives way to IgG production (**Fig. 30.1**). This change in the profile of antibody production is called a *class switch*. Unlike IgM, it is able to cross the placenta. Thus, it is able to provide passive immunity to the neonate in its first few weeks. The protection is further reinforced by the transfer of colostral IgG across the gut

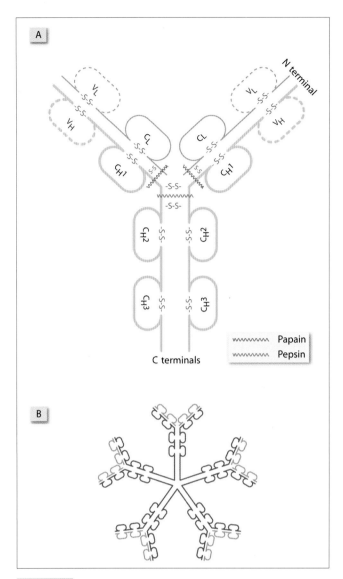

Fig. 31.6 **(A)** Structure of an immunoglobulin molecule. **(B)** The pentamer of immunoglobulin M.

Immunoglobulin E (IgE) binds to mast cells through its Fc receptor. When an antigen binds to two different IgE molecules, the cross-linking of the IgE molecules triggers the degranulation of the mast cells. Haptens with a single epitope cannot cross-link Fc receptors and therefore cannot degranulate mast cells. Rather, they inhibit IgE by blocking their Fab part. Parasites are particularly efficient in stimulating IgE production.

Immunoglobulin D molecules are present on the surface of B cells and act as the antigen receptors for the B cells.

The **complement system** is a system of nine enzymatic plasma proteins designated C1 to C9 (**Fig. 31.7**). Normally in the inactive state, their activity is triggered when C1 binds to the antigen–antibody complex. The activated C1, in turn, activates the other complement proteins in a series of cascade

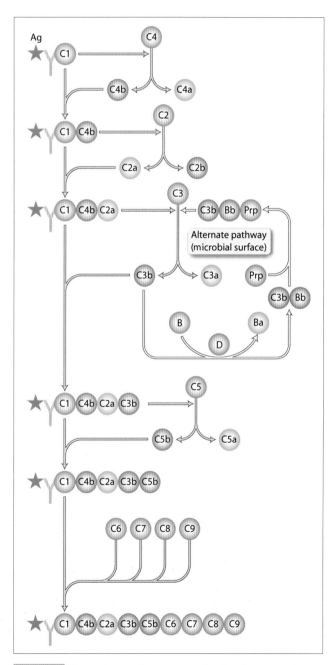

Fig. 31.7 The pathways of complement fixation. Prp, properdin.

mucosa of the neonate. After birth, the serum IgG concentration steadily falls for 2 to 3 months and then rises slowly over years. IgG readily diffuses out into the extravascular spaces, where its concentration is the same as that in the plasma. It is also found in milk, saliva, and nasal and bronchial secretions. IgG causes opsonization, ADCC, and neutralization of toxins. Although it fixes complement by the classical pathway, the lysis it produces through complement-fixation is weak. The IgG-antigen complex binds to platelets through Fc receptors, causing platelet aggregation.

Immunoglobulin A (IgA) is secreted in colostrum, saliva, nasal and lung secretions, tears, and genitourinary and gastrointestinal fluids, providing "secretory immunity." IgA brings about opsonization and neutralization. It also fixes complement by the alternative pathway. The intestinal mucosa secrete IgA bound to a secretory protein, which stabilizes it against proteolysis. It coats the microbes and inhibits their adherence to the mucosal cells, thereby preventing entry into the body tissues. *Neisseria gonorrhea,* which produces IgA protease, can penetrate the mucosal barrier even in an immune person.

reactions. Although the final product of complement activation (C5b-C6-C7-C8-C9) is cytolytic, many of the by-products cause vasodilatation, chemotaxis, opsonization, immune adherence, and mast cell degranulation (**Table 31.1**). IgM and IgG fix and activate complement by the classical pathway; IgA fixes complement by the alternative pathway.

In the *classical pathway* of complement activation, C1 cleaves C4 into C4a and C4b. C4b binds to the antigen–Ig–C1 complex. The complex cleaves C2, releasing C2b, which is a kinin (a potent vasodilator), while binding C2a to itself. The complex then cleaves C3 into C3a (an opsonin) and C3b, which causes mast cell degranulation. C3b adds on to the growing complex. The C4b-C2a-C3b fragment of the complex effects immune adherence. The complex finally cleaves C5, adding on C5b to itself and releasing C5a, which effects chemotaxis and degranulates mast cells. C6, C7, C8, and C9 then add on to the complex in successive stages. The C5b-C6-C7 fragment causes chemotaxis. The C5b-C6-C7-C8-C9 fragment is called the *membrane-attack complex*. It produces cytolysis by enzymatically digesting a part of the membrane and making a hole in it. It may be noted that the activation of C3 to C3a and C3b occupies a central position in complement activation, just as activation of factor IX occupies a central position in the blood coagulation pathway.

The *alternative pathway* of complement activation provides a feedback amplification of C3b production. It involves four plasma proteins: C3, factor B, factor D, and properdin. All reactions of the alternative pathway occur on microbial surfaces. The membranes of human cells contain sialic acid that destroys factor C3b. The cells of the host tissue are therefore spared the damage caused by complement activation.

The alternative pathway is initiated by factor D, which splits factor B into Ba and Bb. Factor Bb combines with C3b to form C3bBb, which is called the alternative pathway C3 convertase. The C3bBb complex is unstable and decays rapidly unless it is bound to a factor called properdin. The C3bBb–properdin complex splits more C3 into C3a and C3b.

Cell-mediated Immunity

In the following passages, the term *cell-mediated immunity* has been used in its restricted sense—when the immune effectors are T lymphocytes or cytokines. In its broadest sense, the term encompasses everything that is related to T lymphocytes and therefore includes the initial and central phases of immune response.

Cytotoxic T cells (Tc cells) destroy antigen-bearing cells in two ways: through the induction of apoptosis and by perfo-

rating the cell membrane. (1) The Tc cell secretes the tumor necrosis factor-β (TNF-β), which increases the calcium (Ca^{2+}) permeability of the antigen-bearing cell. The increased intracellular Ca^{2+} concentration activates intracellular enzymes that degrade the nuclear DNA with concomitant nuclear fragmentation. Apoptosis is also induced by a Ca^{2+}-independent mechanism. Activated Tc cells develop receptors for the Fas proteins that are present on the antigen-bearing cells. The binding of Fas proteins with the Fas receptors on T_c cells triggers the onset of apoptosis. (2) Activated TC cells also secrete perforin. In the presence of extracellular Ca^{2+}, perforin polymerizes on the surface of the antigen-bearing cell and dissolves parts of the membrane, forming pores in it. The pores cause cell death by disrupting cell homeostasis.

Helper cell (TH cells) | The T_H cells are of two types, T helper 1 (T_H1) and T helper 2 (T_H2).

The T_H1 cells are also called inflammatory T cells. They secrete mainly three cytokines: interleukin-2 (IL-2), γ-interferon (IFN-γ), and TNF-β. These cytokines have three functions. (1) They stimulate macrophages. The stimulated macrophages destroy antigen-bearing cells and are sometimes responsible for the delayed-type hypersensitivity. (2) They help T_8 cells to differentiate into T_c cells (T-T cooperation). (3) INF-γ has the direct ability to kill antigen-bearing cells.

The T_H2 cells are primarily concerned with T-B cooperation—enabling B cells to produce antibodies. They secrete interleukins 4, 5, and 6. The differentiation of T_H2 is dependent on interleukin-1 secreted by the macrophage and interleukin-2 secreted by T_H1.

Summary

● The initial phase of the immune response involves B and T lymphocytes recognizing the presence of an antigen.

● The central phase of the immune response involves the proliferation and differentiation of sensitized B and T cells and memory cells.

● During the effector phase of the immune response, the antigen is inactivated by the sensitized B and T cells.

Applying What You Know

31.1. There are three phases to a typical immune response: the initial phase, the central phase, and the effector phase. In what way do autoimmune diseases such as myasthenia gravis (MG) and pernicious anemia (PA) differ from a more common immune response? Explain.

Table 31.1 Effectors of the Complement System

C2b	A potent vasodilator
C3a	An opsonin
C3b	Causes mast cell degranulation
C4b-C2a-C3b	Causes immune adherence
C5b	Causes chemotaxis and mast cell degeneration
C5b-C6-C7	Causes chemotaxis
C5b-C6-C7-C8-C9	The membrane-attack complex

Answers to Applying What You Know

Chapter 20

1 Calculate Mr. Lundquist's total body water and his ICF and ECF volumes.

Mr. Lundquist is overweight but not necessarily obese. We can therefore assume that his total body water is 60% of his body weight expressed in kilograms. Because he is known to weigh 65 kg, his total body water is 39 L. ICF volume is two thirds of total body water, and ECF is one third of total body water. Thus, ICF = 26 L, and ECF = 13 L. If Mr. Lundquist were significantly obese, his total body water volume would be less that 60% of his body weight because adipose cells have a lower percentage of water in them than other cells.

2 Mr. Lundquist's hematocrit (Hct) is low. What parameters might be altered from their normal values to give rise to this state?

The hematocrit is a ratio of cells to fluid, hence, its value will change if the number of cells change or if the volume of fluid changes (or if both change). Thus, abnormal values of the Hct must be interpreted in light of what is known about the patient's state of hydration. For example, a low Hct like Mr. Lundquist's could be the result of fluid retention increasing blood volume with no change in blood cells present. Or, it is possible that some pathology is present that prevents the manufacture of a normal number of red blood cells.

Chapter 21

1 Mr. Lundquist has a hematocrit (Hct) that is significantly lower than normal. How does this relate to his chief complaint of fatigue and shortness of breath?

The Hct reflects the concentration of red blood cells in Mr. Lundquist's blood. With fewer RBCs, there will be less hemoglobin available to transport oxygen to the tissues. The lack of adequate tissue oxygen, particularly when any physical exertion is occurring, would lead to fatigue and to the sensation of shortness of breath.

Chapter 22

1 Mr. Lundquist's [Hb] = 11 g/dL, and he is clearly anemic. How does this relate his presenting symptom of fatigue?

Mr. Lundquist has an abnormally low measured value of hemoglobin concentration. Thus, his blood can carry less oxygen to the tissues, including his skeletal muscles, and the consequence is fatigue. The fact that his Hct is also known to be low leads to the same explanation for his chief complaint.

2 Calculate an approximate value for the oxygen content of Mr. Lundquist's arterial blood.

The oxygen content of blood is determined by the hemoglobin concentration, which we know from Mr. Lundquist's laboratory report, and the percent saturation of his blood, which we do not know. His breathing frequency is somewhat high, but there is no reason to believe that there is a problem with gas exchange in the lungs. Thus, we can assume that his hemoglobin is fully saturated (although in reality it is likely to be closer to 95–97% saturated).

Because 1 g of Hb can bind 1.34 mL of oxygen, and his [Hb] is 11 g/dL, the oxygen bound to his Hb amounts to ~14.74 mL O_2/100 mL blood if his saturation is 100%.

Chapter 23

1 Is Mr. Lundquist's anemia due to a decreased rate of production of red blood cells or an increased rate of destruction of red blood cells? How do you know?

Mr. Lundquist exhibits both decreased hemoglobin concentration and a decreased hematocrit. We also know that his vitamin B_{12} level is abnormally low. Vitamin B_{12} is required for DNA synthesis and hence for the production of hemoglobin. It is thus most likely that Mr. Lundquist is suffering from a reduction in the rate of red blood cell production.

Chapter 24

1 A test has revealed that Mr. Lundquist is producing antibodies against intrinsic factor. Describe the consequences that would be expected.

Intrinsic factor (IF) is required for the absorption of vitamin B_{12} in the intestine. In the absence of IF, Mr. Lundquist will have greatly reduced concentrations of vitamin B_{12}. B_{12} is required to recover folate from the "methyl trap," which is required for DNA synthesis. Because the production of RBCs requires DNA synthesis, the lack of B_{12} will cause an anemia.

Incidentally, lack of vitamin B_{12} can also give rise to neurologic deficiencies.

Chapter 25

1 If Mr. Lundquist were to need a transfusion, which blood group could he safely receive? Explain.

The laboratory report available for Mr. Lundquist does not include his ABO blood grouping. In the absence of that information, all one can say is that he could safely receive type O- blood because it contains no agglutinogens, thus minimizing the possibility of a transfusion reaction. If Mr. Lundquist's blood group were known, this would, of course, provide the needed information to select donor blood.

Chapter 26

1 Patients like Mr. Lundquist with pernicious anemia commonly also exhibit thrombocytopenia (a reduced number of platelets). How would this condition affect the clotting of Mr. Lundquist's blood? What would be the mechanism of this effect?

If the reduction in platelet numbers is large enough, Mr. Lundquist would show longer clotting times. As a consequence, he might bruise easily or have frequent nosebleeds. The mechanism of his lengthened clotting time is inhibition of the intrinsic pathway. With fewer platelets, there would be reduced activation of factor X to factor Xa, then reduced conversion of prothrombin to thrombin.

Chapter 27

1 Predict the results of subjecting Mr. Lundquist's blood to the following tests: (1) partial thromboplastin time, (2) prothrombin time, and (3) thrombin time. Explain your predictions.

The measurement of partial thromboplastin time (PTT) provides an indication of the state of the *intrinsic* and common pathway clotting mechanisms. Because Mr. Lundquist has a reduced number of platelets, his intrinsic pathway is defective, and his PTT time would be elevated. The measurement of prothrombin time (PT) provides information about the state of the *extrinsic* and common pathway mechanisms. Because Mr. Lundquist has normal extrinsic clotting mechanisms and the common pathway is normal, the PT results should be normal. The thrombin time (TT) tests the common pathway, and Mr. Lundquist's results should be normal.

Chapter 28

1 Patients with pernicious anemia often exhibit leukopenia (a reduced white cell count). What roles do leukocytes play in host defense?

There are three types of leukocytes: neutrophils, eosinophils, and basophils. Neutrophils defend against bacteria by engulfing them and essentially digesting them. Eosinophils attack invading organisms, such as parasites, that are too large to be ingested by phagocytosis by neutrophils. Eosinophils also play an important role in generating allergic responses. Basophils release mediators producing inflammation.

Chapter 29

1 Both Miss Adams, the patient with myasthenia gravis, and Mr. Lundquist, who has pernicious anemia, are likely to exhibit an increase in the number of lymphocytes. Explain why this is likely to be so.

Both myasthenia gravis (MG) and pernicious anemia (PA) are autoimmune diseases in which the body's immune system produces antibodies to parts of the body. In MG, the antibodies bind to the acetylcholine receptors in the neuromuscular junction, inactivating them. In PA, the antibodies attack the parietal cells in the stomach that produce intrinsic factor (IF), and there may be antibodies that inactivate any IF that is produced (IF is needed to absorb vitamin B_{12}). In both MG and PA, lymphocytes are the immune cells that produce these antibodies.

Chapter 30

1 Patients with autoimmune diseases, such as myasthenia gravis and pernicious anemia, are more likely than others to have other autoimmune diseases, such as type 1 diabetes and Hashimoto disease (thyroiditis). What mechanism might explain this phenomenon?

There are a number of hypotheses about the mechanisms that produce autoimmune diseases. Some invoke mechanisms that would seem to be limited to explaining single autoimmune diseases. For example, release of normally sequestered antigens from the lens of the eye may explain some eye problems, but it is not easy to see how this might be associated with other autoimmune diseases. On the other hand, the hypothesis that altered function of suppressor T cells might result in autoimmune responses could explain the occurrence of multiple autoimmune diseases in a single individual. It is relevant to note that there appears to be a reasonably strong genetic component to this phenomenon.

Chapter 31

1 There are three phases to a typical immune response: the initial phase, the central phase, and the effector phase. In what way do autoimmune diseases, such as myasthenia gravis (MG) and pernicious anemia (PA), differ from a more common immune response? Explain.

The initial phase of a typical immune response against tumor cells, viral infections, or exogenous antigens involves cell transformations so that the antigens or epitopes are presented in the cell membrane. This process does not occur in an autoimmune response because the "offending" antigens are naturally occurring molecules present in the membrane. For example, in MG, the normally expressed acetylcholine receptor molecule in the neuromuscular junction is detected by lymphocytes and attacked as though they were foreign proteins. In PA, the naturally occurring antigenic molecules are either normal constituents of the parietal cell membrane or the intrinsic factor molecule. Autoimmune diseases do exhibit a *central phase*, in which a number of processes lead to the appearance of sensitized lymphocytes, and an *effector phase*, in which the antigen is inactivated, and cell damage or death results.

Section IV Case Analysis:
Mr. Lundquist has no energy.

Clinical Overview

Review of patient condition | Erik Lundquist is suffering from pernicious anemia, a disease caused by a lack of vitamin B_{12}. Although this could be due to a dietary deficiency, it is most commonly due to a lack of intrinsic factor (IF) required for the absorption of vitamin B_{12} in the digestive tract.

Etiology | Pernicious anemia is most often an autoimmune disease in which antibodies against gastric parietal cells are present. Parietal cells secrete IF, and when the number of cells is decreased, or they are dysfunctional, absorption of vitamin B_{12} is decreased.

Prevalence | Pernicious anemia is most common among certain ethnic groups (Celts, Scandinavians) in which there may be as many as 20 cases per 100,000 people. Although once thought to be relatively rare in other ethnic groups, it is now thought that its incidence has been underestimated.

Diagnosis | The presence of a severe anemia in a patient with relatively mild symptoms and no weight loss would certainly suggest the possibility of pernicious anemia. Decreased levels of IF or the presence of antibodies against IF would confirm the diagnosis.

Treatment | Administration of vitamin B_{12} via injection will reverse the anemia that is present. Care must be taken to determine the minimum dosage to allow normal production of red blood cells. Oral vitamin B_{12} can work if a large enough dose is administered. Even in the absence of IF, absorption of 1% of a large ingested amount of B_{12} will meet the minimal daily requirements for this vitamin.

Understanding the Physiology

Hemopoietic cells divide and multiply rapidly to maintain the required number of red blood cells and white blood cells. This rapid cell division requires the synthesis of DNA. Folate is an essential factor in this process because it is used as a carrier to transform uridine to deoxythymidine, one of the four bases from which DNA is built.

In the process, folate gets "trapped" in the form of methyl tetrahydrofolate (methyl THF). Vitamin B_{12} takes the methyl group, freeing THF to function in the pathway of synthesizing DNA. By doing this, the B_{12} is methylated, but the conversion of homocysteine to methionine results in "recycled" B_{12}.

Pernicious anemia is only one example of megaloblastic anemia. It is caused by a deficiency of B_{12} due to any of several causes. In Mr. Lundquist's case, the problem is an autoimmune response, which produces IF antibodies. These antibodies bind to IF molecules, making it impossible for the IF to function properly in the absorption of B_{12}. With greatly diminished levels of IF, the intestine is unable to absorb the B_{12} in the diet, and the cascade of effects outlined above fail. The hemopoietic cell cannot multiple normally, and the result is anemia. The mechanism of pernicious anemia is illustrated in the accompanying flow chart.

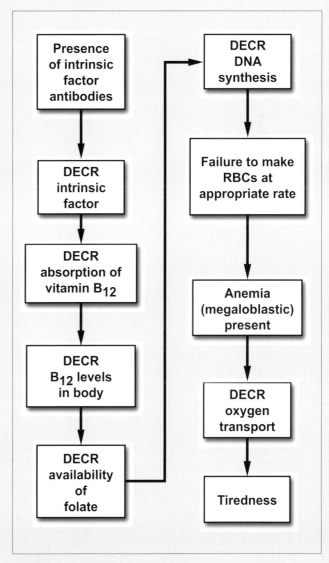

Fig. IV.1 Mr. Lundquist has an auto-immune response that produces antibodies to intrinsic factor (IF). Reduced IF causes reduced vitamin B_{12} and therefore reduced folate. The result is reduced erythropoesis (anemia). With less oxygen being carried to his tissues, Mr. Lundquist tires easily.

Section V | Cardiovascular System

Overview

Case Presentation

Chapters

Answers to Applying What You Know

Case Analysis

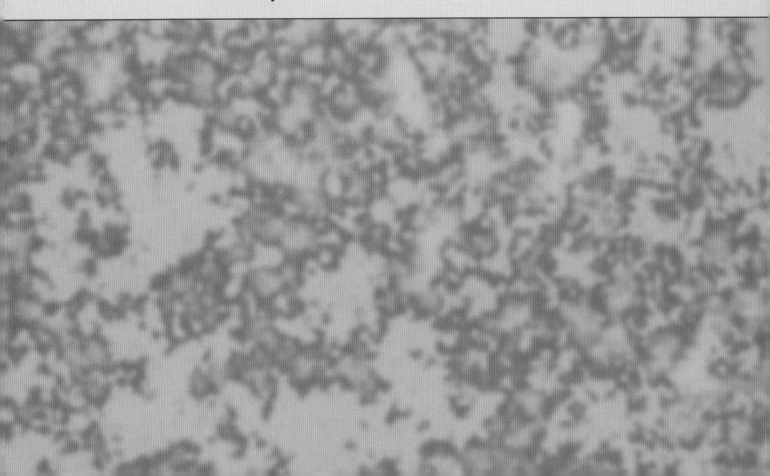

Overview

E very cell in the body must get oxygen and all the nutrients required to support its metabolism. At the same time, every cell must dispose of the waste products of its metabolism: carbon dioxide, nitrogenous wastes, and heat.

Both of these necessary functions can occur only if there is a transport system that perfuses every tissue of the body, carrying oxygen and nutrients sufficiently close to every cell so that simple diffusion can provide what each cell needs, and at the same time taking away, again by simple diffusion, the waste products generated by each cell.

The cardiovascular system carries out these functions. It consists of a muscular pump (the heart), a set of blood vessels that are distributed all over the body (the circulation), a fluid that transports the needed substances (the blood), and neural and humoral controllers to regulate and coordinate all of these functions.

To ensure that every tissue and cell receives what it needs, the cardiovascular system regulates the pressure present in the arteries and then apportions flow between various tissues by varying the flow resistance. Thus, the regulation of a constant blood pressure in the face of external perturbations and alterations of function is an essential feature of the system. Similarly, because blood pressure is, in part, a function of the volume of blood present in the system, blood volume is also a regulated parameter.

Section V Case Presentation:
Doris Daniels is short of breath.

Chief Complaint

Doris Daniels, a 45-year-old African-American secretary, has come to the clinic complaining of increasing shortness of breath.

History of Present Illness

About 3 weeks ago, she first noticed that moderate exertion, climbing two flights of stairs or running to catch a bus, made her unusually short of breath. In the past week, she has noticed mild swelling of her feet. During the past 5 days, she has noted that she becomes winded on climbing less than a half flight of stairs. For the last 3 nights, she has had difficulty breathing while lying flat on her back; she has begun to prop her head up on three pillows when sleeping at night. Today she has a cough productive of whitish sputum.

Past Medical History

In retrospect, Mrs. Daniels thinks she has been tiring easily on exertion for the last 2 years, but she has not had difficulty sleeping until now. She has always avoided seeing doctors and was hospitalized only once, at age 6. All she can recall about that hospitalization is that she had a rash and some jerky movements of her arms and legs. She is married and has no children. She does not smoke, drink alcohol, or take any drugs or medications.

Physical Examination

- *General appearance* | Well-developed, well-nourished black woman with somewhat labored breathing
- *Vital signs*
  - Temperature: 99.2°F (oral)
  - Pulse: 90/minute
  - Respirations: 26/minute
  - Blood pressure: 120/80 mm Hg
- *HEENT* (*head, eyes, ear, nose throat*) | All normal
- *Neck* | No evidence of jugular distention
- *Lungs* | Diffuse expiratory wheezing bilaterally with some bibasilar (*across the base of the lungs*) crackles (*abnormal breath sounds*)

- *Cardiac*
  Heart: Left border of cardiac dullness (*region of the chest wall where the lungs are not between the heart and the chest wall*) at left midclavicular line; no heaves or thrills noted (*palpable signs of murmurs*)
  Pulses: Auscultation (*use of stethoscope*) reveals a loud S$_1$, a prominent pulmonic component to S$_2$, a low-frequency diastolic murmur at the cardiac apex, and a harsh, blowing holosystolic (*present throughout the duration of systole*) murmur at the apex with radiation to the axilla (*armpit*)
- *Abdomen* | Normal bowel sounds, soft, nontender, non-distended; no organomegaly (*abnormally enlarged organs*) or masses
- *Extremities* | Trace pedal edema bilaterally
- *Neurologic exam* | Normal

Laboratory Studies

- CBC (complete blood count): Normal
- Blood chemistry: Normal
- Urinalysis: Normal
- Chest x-ray: Cardiac shadow is abnormal, suggesting left atrial enlargement; the pulmonary veins are enlarged and tortuous; lung markings consistent with interstitial pulmonary edema
- Electrocardiogram (ECG): Sinus rhythm; evidence of left atrial enlargement; suggestion of right ventricular hypertrophy

Mrs. Daniels is admitted to the hospital for additional testing.

Cardiac Catheterization

To evaluate Mrs. Daniels' cardiac murmur further, cardiac catheterization (both the right and left side of the heart) is ordered. (In this procedure, small tubes are inserted into the femoral vein [on the right side] and femoral artery [left side] and are pushed up into the chambers of the heart and the outflow vessels. With these catheters, pressures can be measured and small blood samples removed.)

Parameter	Results	Normal
Heart rate (beats/min)	68	
Ventilation (L/min)	7.28	6–7
O$_2$ consumption (cc/min)	262	250
Hemoglobin (g/100 mL)	14	13–14
Pulmonary a-v O$_2$ difference (cc/100 mL)	7.2	3.0–4.8
Systemic a-v O$_2$ difference (cc/100 mL)	7.2	3.0–4.8
Cardiac output (L/min)	3.6	3.0–4.8
Body surface area (m^2)	2.1	
Cardiac index (L/min/m^2)	1.7	2.6–4.0; avg. 3.2

Pressure (mm Hg)	Result	Normal
Right atrial pressure (M)	8	0–8
Right ventricle pressure (S/ED)	55/10	17–32/0–6
Pulmonary artery pressure (S/D/M)	50/20/34	15–29/5–13/ 10–18
Pulmonary wedge pressure (M)	30	2–12
Left ventricle pressure (S/ED)	130/10	90–130/5–12
Aortic pressure (S/D/M)	120/80/93	90–130/60–90/ 70–105
Central venous pressure (M)	7	0–8

Abbreviations: a-v, arterial-venous; D, diastolic; ED, end diastolic; M, mean; S, systolic.

In the course of the cardiac catheterization procedure, arterial blood gas values were obtained (breathing room air).

Parameter	Value	Normal
pH	7.36	7.35–7.45
P$_a$O$_2$	74.9 mm Hg	83–108
P$_a$CO$_2$	39.6 mm Hg	35–48 (f)
Saturation	92%	95–98

Diagnosis

Mrs. Daniels has a mitral valve that is both stenosed and incompetent (regurgitant).

Some Things to Think About

1. What is/are the mechanism(s) causing Mrs. Daniels' dyspnea and low arterial PO$_2$?

2. Why does Mrs. Daniels exhibit a tachycardia?

3. What has caused her enlarged left atrium and her hypertrophied left ventricle?

4. Mrs. Daniels' pressures from her left atrium through her right ventricle are elevated. What mechanism is producing these findings?

5. Why does Mrs. Daniels have findings suggestive of edema formation?

Cardiac Excitation

The heart as a whole obeys the all-or-none law: it contracts completely, or it does not contract at all, depending on whether the stimulus applied is of threshold or subthreshold strength. When any part of the heart depolarizes, the depolarization spreads over the entire heart ephaptically (via gap junctions), and the heart contracts as strongly as its current state allows.

General Model: Communications

The spread of electrical excitation over the heart is an example of cell-to-cell communications using bioelectric signals. In the heart, this involves both direct cell-to-cell spread of electrical activity through gap junctions (see **Fig. 7.1**) and spread of electrical activity via a specialized conduction system (see **Fig. 32.1**).

Initiation of Cardiac Excitation

Although skeletal muscle fibers are physiologically excited by an external signal, an action potential in the motor neuron innervating the muscle, some cardiac muscle cells have the property of spontaneously depolarizing and firing an action potential. This property is referred to as *automaticity*. Although many cardiac muscle cells exhibit automaticity (see below), the cells of the sinoatrial node exhibit the highest frequency of spontaneous firing and therefore normally serve as the pacemaker for the heart. The mechanism of automaticity is discussed in Chapter 19.

Conductive System of the Heart

The depolarization of the various parts of the heart proceeds in an orderly and timely way. This is made possible by the presence of the conductive system of the heart (**Fig. 32.1**), which consists of the sinoatrial node (SA node), internodal atrial pathways, atrioventricular node (AV node), bundle of His and its branches, and the Purkinje system. Most cells of the conductive system are specialized for fast conduction, although some, like the cells of the AV node, are specialized for slowing down conduction (**Table 32.1**). Cells of the conductive system also possess automaticity—the capability of spontaneous excitation. The automaticity of the SA node sets the pace of the heart, whereas the automaticity of the other parts of the conductive system normally remains suppressed. The cells of the conductive system are also contractile, though weakly.

Intrinsic automaticity is present in all of the cells making up the conductive system: the SA node, the AV node, the bundle of His and its branches, and the peripheral Purkinje system. The SA node has the highest automaticity (72/min), followed by the AV node (40/min). Other cardiac fibers have even lower intrinsic

discharge rates. The automaticity of the SA node, being the highest, paces the excitatory drive to all other cardiac fibers, suppressing their intrinsic automaticity. However, if the SA node stops discharging, the AV node, which has the next highest automaticity, takes over the role of cardiac pacemaker.

The **sinoatrial node** is a small strip of conductive tissue located in the superolateral wall of the right atrium, immediately below and lateral to the opening of the superior vena cava. The rate of SA node discharge often shows rhythmic changes with the phase of respiration, increasing with inspiration and decreasing with expiration. Such rhythmic variations in the heart rate are called *sinus arrhythmia*.

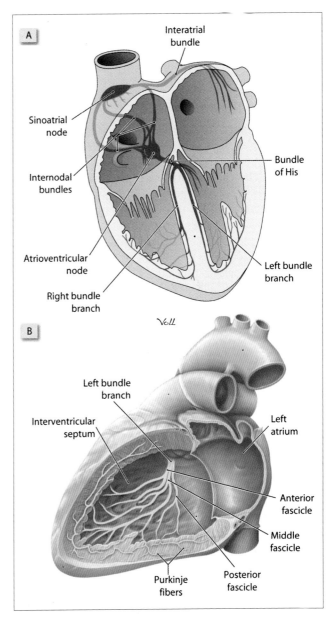

Fig. 32.1 (A) The conductive system of the heart. (B) The fascicles of the left bundle branch.

Table 32.1 Conduction Velocity of Different Conductive Tissues

Cardiac Tissue	Conduction Velocity (m/sec)
SA node	0.05
Interatrial pathways	1.00
Atrial muscle	0.30
AV node	0.05
Bundle of His	1.00
Purkinje system	4.00
Ventricular muscle	1.00

Abbreviations: AV, atrioventricular; SA, sinoatrial.

The **internodal atrial pathways** are the three strips of conductive tissues, the anterior, middle, and posterior, that connect the SA node to the AV node. Impulses from the SA node travel to the AV node along these interatrial pathways. The atrial musculature is excited by impulses spreading out from the internodal and interatrial pathways. The interatrial pathways conduct impulses at a speed of 1 m/sec, which is three times faster than the conduction speed in the contractile atrial muscle fibers. Atrial depolarization is complete in ~0.1 second.

The **atrioventricular node** is located in the posterior and inferior part of the interatrial septum. The AV node is the gateway for all action potentials traveling from the atria to the ventricles. This is because the atrium is electrically insulated from the ventricles by a fibrous partition. This partition is bridged only by the bundle of His that originates from the AV node; nowhere else can atrial depolarization enter the ventricle.

The conduction speed of AV nodal tissue is only 0.05 m/sec, so that impulses take 0.1 second to travel across the AV node. This 0.1-second delay is called the *AV nodal delay* and is critically important for allowing the atrial systole to complete itself before the onset of ventricular systole. The AV nodal delay is shortened by stimulation of the sympathetic nerves to the heart and lengthened by stimulation of the vagi. The increase in AV nodal delay caused by vagal stimulation is put to use in the differential diagnosis of certain types of arrhythmias. Commonly used bedside methods for increasing vagal activity is carotid massage, which initiates the baroreceptor reflex (Chapter 38), and pressing on the eyeball, which initiates the oculocardiac reflex.

The **bundle of His** originates from the AV node. It penetrates the fibrous barrier separating the atria and ventricle and continues downward in the interventricular septum for ~1 cm. Thereafter, it divides into the left and right bundles that run on the respective side of the septum under the endocardium. The left bundle divides further into the anterior and posterior fascicles. After reaching the apex, the bundle branches turn back toward the base of the heart, coursing through the endocardium, where it spreads the excitation to the Purkinje system.

The **Purkinje system** is a network of fast conductive fibers on the endocardial surface of the ventricles. Purkinje fibers conduct at a speed of 4 m/sec and spread the excitation quickly throughout the ventricles, which is important for enabling near-simultaneous contraction of both the ventricles. However, the Purkinje system excites only those cardiac muscle cells that are located near the endocardial surface. Thereafter, the impulses are conducted by the ventricular muscle fibers themselves, and the depolarization spreads outward radially toward the epicardium. Ventricular depolarization is completed in ~0.1 second. The spatial sequence of the spread of ventricular depolarization is described later in the context of the electrocardiogram (ECG) waves.

Electrocardiography

Cardiac Vectors

Electrically, the body fluids behave like a volume conductor. The ECG records the potential differences on the surface of the body resulting from the currents set up in body fluids by the electrical activity of the heart. The currents are set up by the array of dipoles formed at the border between the depo-

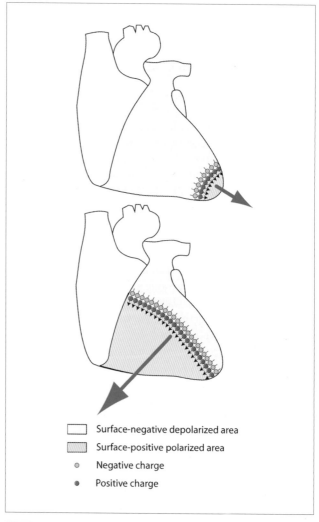

Fig. 32.2 The direction of the cardiac vector is perpendicular to the border between the depolarized and repolarized areas. The longer the border, the greater the number of dipoles; therefore, the greater is the magnitude of the cardiac vector.

larized and repolarized cardiac tissue. The direction of the current is from the depolarized (surface-negative) to the repolarized (surface-positive) areas of the heart (**Fig. 32.2**). The dipoles are formed when only a part of the heart is depolarized. They disappear when the heart is either completely depolarized or completely polarized. The physics of dipoles is discussed in Appendix A. The ECG gives an estimate of the magnitude and direction of the body currents set up by cardiac dipoles. However, what it actually measures is the potential drop along the path of the current. The potential drop recorded is taken as a measure of the current, assuming a uniform resistance of body fluids.

Instantaneous Electrical Axis of the Heart

At any moment during the cardiac cycle, the dipoles on the cardiac surface set up currents in all directions. The resultant of these currents is called the *cardiac vector* (or electrical axis). The magnitude and direction of the cardiac vector change throughout the cardiac cycle. Both depend on the contour of the border between the depolarized and polarized muscles of the heart. The direction of the resultant vector is perpendicular to the border. The magnitude of the resultant vector depends on the length of the border: the longer the border, the greater is the magnitude of the resultant vector. For example, if the left side of the heart were depolarized, and the right side were still polarized, the border between the depolarized and polarized area would be long, and a large vector would be directed toward the right. However, if all but the apex of the heart were depolarized, the border would be short, and a small vector would be directed toward the apex (**Fig. 32.2**). Thus, as the wave of depolarization sweeps across the heart, the instantaneous electrical axis keeps swinging in all directions, and its magnitude keeps changing.

The graphic recording of the swinging instantaneous electrical axis during the cardiac cycle is called *vectorcardiography*. It has never been popular with physicians who are more comfortable with the conventional ECG record. However, it retains its utility in specific situations.

Einthoven Triangle

Einthoven triangle is an imaginary triangle formed by the two shoulders and the pubis. The electrodes connected to the three corners of the Einthoven triangle are designated as LA (left arm), RA (right arm), and LL (left leg).

An electrode connected to all three corners of the Einthoven triangle will always be at zero potential, regardless of the direction of the cardiac vector. Such an electrode is called the *indifferent electrode* (or the *central terminal of Wilson*), and it serves as a convenient reference for several electrocardiographic measurements. The three limb electrodes need to be interconnected through high (5000 ohm) resistors (**Figs. 32.3** and **32.4**).

Unipolar versus bipolar recording | A pair of electrodes recording the potential difference between two different sites is called a lead. Leads are classified as unipolar and bipolar, a nomenclature that is misleading because both types of lead record the potential difference between two electrodes. In the

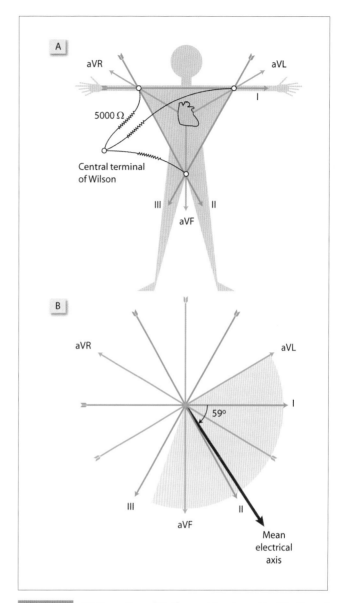

Fig. 32.3 **(A)** Formation of Einthoven triangle and justification of the orientation of the leads. **(B)** The orientation of the lead lines in the frontal plane is such that there is one lead line at an interval of every 30 degrees. The mean electrical axis is shown here as 59 degrees. aVF, augmented vector foot; aVL, augmented vector left; aVR, augmented vector right.

strictest sense, therefore, all recordings are bipolar. However, according to the conventional usage of the terms, bipolar recording involves recording the potential difference between two different sites on the body using two electrodes, one serving as the reference, and the other called the exploring or active electrode. In unipolar recording, the indifferent electrode serves as the reference.

ECG Leads in the Frontal Plane

ECG recording in the frontal plane involves the placement of six leads in such a way that there is one lead at each interval of 30 degrees (**Fig. 32.3B**). This many leads are placed so that no matter at what angle the cardiac vector is directed, it will get recorded maximally in at least one of the leads. Maximum

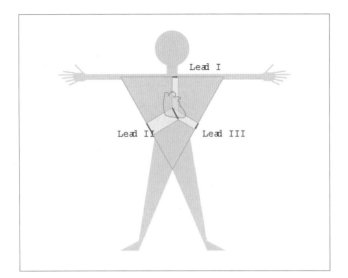

Fig. 32.4 Einthoven triangle: the potential difference recordable in the standard limb leads (I, II, and III) is proportional to the vector components of the cardiac electrical axis.

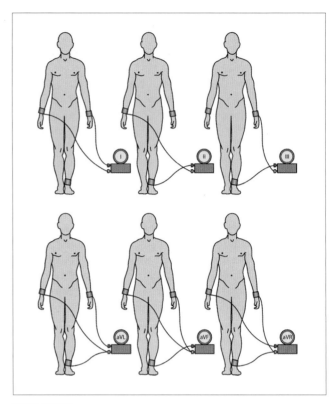

Fig. 32.5 Electrocardiogram recording with standard limb leads. Leads I, II, and III are the Einthoven leads. Leads aVL, aVF, and aVR are "augmented" leads.

amplitude is recorded in the lead that is disposed along the direction of the cardiac vector. The lead that is oriented exactly perpendicular to the cardiac vector records nothing. Conventionally, the electrocardiograph (the ECG machine) is designed to give a positive deflection when a cardiac vector is directed toward the active electrode.

Standard (bipolar) limb leads record the potential difference between any two corners of the Einthoven triangle. *Lead I* records the potential difference between the LA (active electrode) and the RA (reference electrode). Its axis is 0 degrees. *Lead II* records the potential difference between the LL (active electrode) and the RA (reference electrode). Its axis is 60 degrees. *Lead III* records the potential difference between the LL (active electrode) and the LA (reference electrode). Its axis is 120 degrees (**Fig. 32.5**).

ECG Leads in the Horizontal Plane

The **chest (precordial) leads** are placed on the chest in a transverse plane roughly at the level of the heart. They are placed at regular angular intervals, with at least one lead at every 30-degree interval (**Fig. 32.6**). Unipolar leads can also be placed at the tips of catheters and inserted into the esophagus or heart.

ECG Calibration

An ECG (**Fig. 32.7**) typically shows five waves named P, Q, R, S, and T. The amplitude and duration of these waves and the interval between them (**Table 32.2**) are of immense diagnostic significance, especially in cardiac disorders. Standardization of signal amplification (gain) is necessary for giving correct readouts of the amplitudes. The gain of the electrocardiograph (amplification of signals) is calibrated so that a 0.1 mV input signal produces a 1 mm vertical deflection. Similarly, standardization of chart speed is necessary for giving correct readouts of the durations. The chart speed of the ECG paper is mostly set at 25 mm/sec, so that 1 mm horizontal distance is equivalent to 0.04 second.

Electrocardiogram

ECG Waves

The **P wave** is produced by atrial depolarization. When its width exceeds 3 mm or its amplitude exceeds 2.5 mm, it suggests the presence of hypertrophy or dilatation of the atria or intra-atrial conduction delay.

The **Q, R, and S waves** are produced at different stages of ventricular depolarization, and they together constitute the QRS complex. If the initial deflection in the QRS complex is negative, it is called the Q wave. If the initial deflection is positive, it is called the R wave. If there is a negative deflection after the R wave, it is called the S wave. If there is a second positive deflection, it is called the R' wave. If there is another negative deflection, it is called the S' wave, and so on. If there is a single large negative deflection, and there is no R wave, the negative deflection is called the QS complex (**Fig. 32.7**).

The duration of the QRS complex is measured from the onset of the Q wave (or R wave when the Q wave is not present) to the termination of the S wave (or R' or S' when the S wave is not present). It represents the time taken for ventricular depolarization, and its upper limit is 0.1 second. The interval between the beginning of the Q wave and the peak of the R wave is called the *ventricular activation time* (VAT), which is normally less than 0.05 second. Both increase in ventricular hypertrophy and bundle branch block.

The amplitudes of the Q, R, and S waves differ considerably from lead to lead. In the chest leads, the QRS complex shows

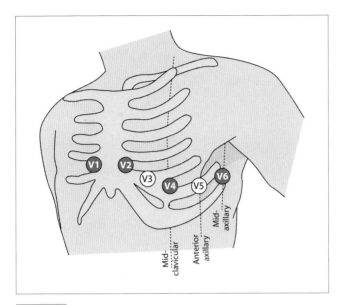

Fig. 32.6 Position of the chest leads.

a gradual increase in amplitude from V1 through V6, which is called the *R wave progression*. The amplitude of the R wave in V5 or V6 does not normally exceed 27 mm. Also, the sum of the S wave in V1 and the R wave in V6 does not normally exceed 35 mm. When they exceed these limits, they suggest ventricular hypertrophy.

The **T wave** is produced by ventricular repolarization. Because ventricular repolarization is slower and less synchronous than ventricular depolarization, the T wave is of lower voltage and longer duration than the QRS complex. The height of the T wave is usually less than 10 mm in precordial leads. Very tall T waves up to 16 or 18 mm in V2 to V4 are seen when there is vagal hyperactivity. Conversely, sympathetic hyperactivity and tachycardia tend to produce flattened T waves. Even then, when the ECG shows abnormally tall T waves, conditions like hyperkalemia (see **Fig. 59.4**) and myocardial ischemia should also be considered.

The **U wave** is only occasionally observed and is due to the repolarization of the papillary muscles. There is no ECG wave corresponding to atrial repolarization because it is obscured by the large QRS complex.

The **P-R segment** is the portion of the ECG tracing between the onset of the P wave and the onset of the QRS complex. It is normally isoelectric (i.e., it is at 0 mV) because during this interval, the ventricles are in a completely polarized state unless there is a diastolic current of injury (see below). The normal P-R interval is 0.12 to 0.2 second. It represents the total of the time taken for conduction of the impulse from SA node to AV node (10–50 msec), AV nodal conduction (90–150 msec), and conduction along the bundle of His (25–55 msec). It is prolonged in atrioventricular block and shortened in Wolff-Parkinson-White (WPW) syndrome.

The **ST segment** is the portion of the ECG tracing between the J point and the onset of the T wave. This segment is usually isoelectric, but it may vary from –0.5 to +2 mm in the precordial leads. The duration of the ST interval does not have much clinical significance. Instead, the duration of the *QT interval*, measured from the onset of the Q wave to the end of the T wave, is used as an estimate of the duration of electrical systole. Because the duration of the cardiac cycle varies with the heart rate (**Table 33.2**), the QT interval varies inversely with the heart rate. When corrected for the heart rate, it is called QT and does not normally exceed 0.43 second.

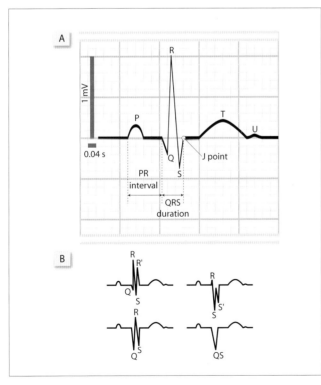

Fig. 32.7 **(A)** A typical PQRST complex of an electrocardiogram. **(B)** Abnormal QRS complexes.

Table 32.2 The Duration and Amplitude of Electrocardiogram (ECG) Waves and Intervals as Recorded on the ECG Chart*

	Duration (mm)	Range of Duration (mm)	Amplitude (mm)	Range of Amplitude (mm)
P wave	2.5	1–3	2.5	–
P-R interval	5	3–5	–	–
QRS complex	2.5	2–2.5	–	–
Q wave	–	–	1	0–4
R wave	–	–	7	2–17
S wave	–	–	1	0–5
ST interval	8	–		
T wave	5	–	4	1–6
QT interval	10	10–11	–	–

*Time in ms = time in mm × 0.04. Amplitude in millivolts = amplitude in mm × 0.1.

The **R-R interval** gives the time interval between two consecutive heart beats. If the R-R interval is 0.83 second, then the instantaneous heart rate is given by

$$60 \text{ s/min per } 0.833 \text{ s} = 72 \text{ beats/min}$$

The P-P interval, when substituted in the above formula, will give the atrial rate of contraction, which is normally equal to the heart rate. However, in arrhythmias, the two rates can differ.

ECG Changes in Myocardial Infarction

In myocardial infarction, there is irreversible ischemic damage to the myocardial cells. The damaged cells lose potassium ions to the extracellular fluid. The rise in the local interstitial potassium (K^+) concentration depolarizes the injured myocardial cells. The decrease in resting membrane potential (RMP) occurs within minutes of the infarction and results in a flow of current, called the *current of injury,* into the infarcted area from the surrounding tissues (**Fig. 32.8A**). Because this current of injury appears when the cardiac muscle is in the polarized state, it is called the *diastolic current of injury.* It results in the depression of the TP segment in the ECG recorded from the

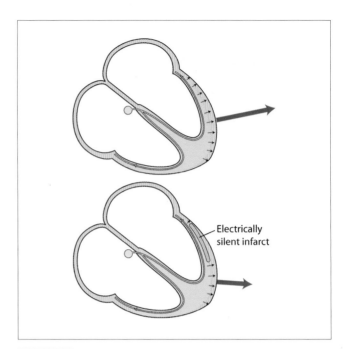

Fig. 32.9 Change in cardiac vector due to an electrically silent infarcted area. Note the change in both direction and magnitude of the vector.

chest leads overlying the infarcted area. A depression of the TP segment produces an apparent elevation of the ST segment. Most cases of ST elevation are relative elevations attributable to TP depression due to this diastolic current of injury. The diastolic current of injury disappears when the myocardium is completely depolarized.

The injured myocardial cells also show other electrophysiologic abnormalities, such as a rapid repolarization (within seconds of the infarction, **Fig. 32.8B**) and a delayed depolarization (about a half hour after infarction, **Fig. 32.8C**) . Delayed depolarization and rapid repolarization make the surface of the infarcted area positive relative to the surrounding normal area. As a result, the current of injury flows out of the infarcted area into the surrounding areas. This current of injury appears when the cardiac muscle is depolarizing or repolarizing (i.e., during electrical systole) and is therefore called the *systolic current of injury.* It produces an elevation of the ST segment in the ECG recorded from the chest leads overlying the infarcted area. The systolic current of injury disappears when the myocardium is completely repolarized.

Electrical silence | After some days or weeks, the infarcted area becomes a nonconducting zone (it is electrically silent). The current of injury stops, and the ST segment abnormalities subside. However, the presence of an area of electrical silence alters both the direction and the magnitude of the instantaneous electrical vectors during the cardiac cycle (**Fig. 32.9**) and results in changes in the Q, R, and T waves. There is an increase in the height and width of preexisting Q waves, sometimes resulting in a large QS complex. Q waves may appear in leads in which they are normally absent. R wave amplitude decreases. T waves become very tall within the first few hours, probably

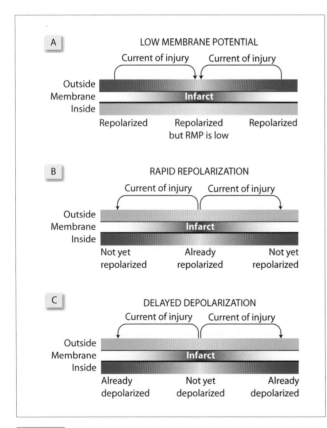

Fig. 32.8 Origin of the current of injury in myocardial infarction. Red: positive potential, blue: negative potential. Lighter shades of red and blue indicate lower positive and negative potentials, respectively. RMP, resting membrane potential.

as a result of the local rise in extracellular K⁺ concentration. Later, they gradually become inverted.

Conduction abnormalities | Atrioventricular block or bundle branch block occurs if the septum is infarcted, damaging the conduction system. Arrhythmias occur due to development of microreentrant circuits as well as increased automaticity. Increased automaticity occurs possibly because the infarct damages the autonomic fibers that course through the heart. Epicardial infarcts damage mostly the sympathetic fibers, resulting in denervation hypersensitivity to circulating catecholamines. Endocardial infarcts damage mostly the parasympathetic fibers, leaving the sympathetic activity unopposed.

ECG Isoelectric Potential

J point | Normally, both the ST segment (when the entire myocardium is depolarized) and the TP segment (when the entire myocardium is repolarized) should be isoelectric—at zero potential. However, the ST segment does not remain isoelectric when there is a systolic current of injury, and the TP segment does not remain isoelectric when there is a diastolic current of injury. Because the systolic current of injury occurs due to delayed depolarization, it manifests itself only after the J point, that is, after the rapid phase of repolarization. Hence the J point, which is the point where the S wave ends sharply, is a reference point for isoelectric potential in the ECG tracing (**Fig. 32.10**).

Abnormalities of Cardiac Excitation

Abnormalities of cardiac excitation affect the rhythm of the heart, causing arrhythmias (disruption of the normal cardiac rhythm). Arrhythmias that are associated with bradycardia

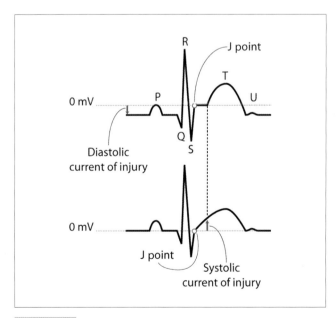

Fig. 32.10 The baseline of the electrocardiogram is indicated by the J point. A diastolic current of injury affects the potential of the TP segment; a systolic current of injury affects the potential of the ST segment.

(decrease in heart rate) are called bradyarrhythmias (*brady* = slowing). Arrhythmias that are associated with tachycardia (increase in heart rate) are called tachyarrhythmias (*tachy* = speeding). The electrocardiogram is an essential tool for the precise diagnosis of arrhythmias.

Bradyarrhythmias

Sick-sinus syndrome | The sick-sinus syndrome is a dysfunction of the SA node that results in marked bradycardia with symptoms such as dizziness and repeated episodes of syncope. It can be due to a reduction of SA node discharge frequency to 60/min or less (sinus bradycardia) that does not respond to sympathetic stimulation or vagal inhibition. It can also occur due to a blockade of impulse conduction from the SA node to the atria (sinoatrial block) or a complete stoppage of sinus discharge (sinus arrest).

Atrioventricular block | Any block or slowing down of the conduction of cardiac impulses across the atrioventricular node is called atrioventricular (AV) block or simply heart block (**Fig. 32.11**). There are three degrees of atrioventricular block.

In first-degree AV block, there is a slowing of impulse conduction from the atria to the ventricles. It results in the prolongation of the PR interval, which could be due to slow conduction of the impulse anywhere between the SA node and the AV node, in the AV node, or in the bundle of His.

In second-degree AV block, there is atrioventricular conduction failure at regular intervals: some of the impulses fail to reach the ventricle, resulting in dropped ventricular beats. Dropped beats at regular intervals result in a "regularly irregular" pulse.

In third-degree AV block, the atrioventricular conduction failure is complete; that is, none of the impulses that originate in the SA node reach the ventricle: ventricular depolarization is initiated by the AV node, and the ventricles beat at a rate determined by the intrinsic AV nodal frequency of 40 beats/min. This is called the *idioventricular rhythm*. The atria, however, continue to beat at the normal sinus rhythm of 72 beats/min.

Thus, the atrial and ventricular rhythms become entirely independent, each contracting at its own rate. This is called *atrioventricular dissociation*. The ECG shows the rate and rhythm of the P waves and the QRS complexes to be completely independent of each other.

Bundle-branch block | There may be conduction blocks in one or more branches of the bundle of His. Accordingly, there may be different types of blocks whose names are self-explanatory and include the right bundle-branch block (RBBB), left bundle-branch block (LBBB), left anterior hemiblock (LAH), left posterior hemiblock (LPH), bifascicular block (RBBB with LAH or LPH), and trifascicular block. Conduction blockade of any of the branches results in delayed depolarization of the part of the ventricle that is supplied by the branch. Irrespective of the type of block, the total QRS duration is prolonged beyond the normal limit of 0.1 second.

Tachyarrhythmias

The common types of tachyarrhythmias are premature supraventricular contractions, supraventricular tachycardia, atrial

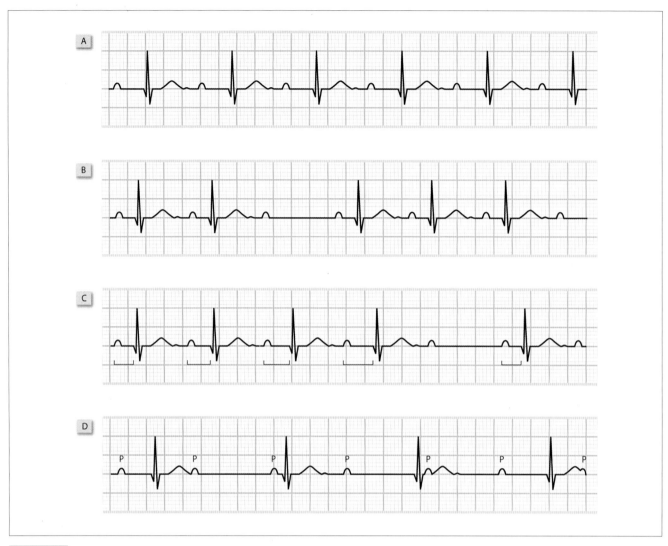

Fig. 32.11 Heart block. **(A)** First-degree heart block. **(B)** Second-degree (type I) heart block. **(C)** Second-degree (type II) heart block. **(D)** Third-degree atrioventricular block.

flutter, atrial fibrillation, premature ventricular contractions, ventricular tachycardia, ventricular flutter, and ventricular fibrillation. The term *supraventricular* is used when the site of origin of the arrhythmia could be either the atria or the atrioventricular junction. Tachyarrhythmia can originate in the SA node, in which case it is called *sinus tachycardia*. Most tachyarrhythmias, however, originate in ectopic foci, sites other than the SA node. They occur either due to increased automaticity or due to reentry of impulses in closed circuits within the heart. Increased automaticity usually produces premature atrial and ventricular contractions, but it can also lead to flutter and fibrillation when ectopics occur simultaneously at multiple sites. Similarly, reentrant circuits usually result in paroxysmal tachycardia, flutter, and fibrillation, but microreentrant circuits can also produce single, premature contractions.

Increased automaticity is present in all automatic cardiac fibers, but it usually remains suppressed due to the continuous activity of the SA node. Sometimes, the intrinsic automaticity is abnormally increased and gives rise to ectopic foci of dis-

charge. If the ectopic focus discharges at a critical moment when the cardiac tissue is not refractory, it gets conducted to large areas of the heart, resulting in depolarization and contraction of the atria or ventricles.

Reentrant circuits are closed-circuit pathways in the heart along which impulses are repeatedly conducted without cessation. Reentrant circuits are broadly of two types: the microreentrant and macroreentrant circuits. The *microreentrant circuits* are confined to a very small area in the atria or ventricles and occur due to local inhomogeneity in cardiac excitability and conductivity. The *macroreentrant circuits* pass through a large part of the heart and involve abnormal anatomical tracts.

A microreentrant circuit, for example, can occur around a postinfarction scar in the atria or the ventricles. Its mechanism is explained in **Fig. 32.12A**. The temporary block referred to in the diagram could be an ectopic focus that is still refractory after having discharged shortly before. More commonly, the microreentrant circuit resides inside the AV node. The intra-

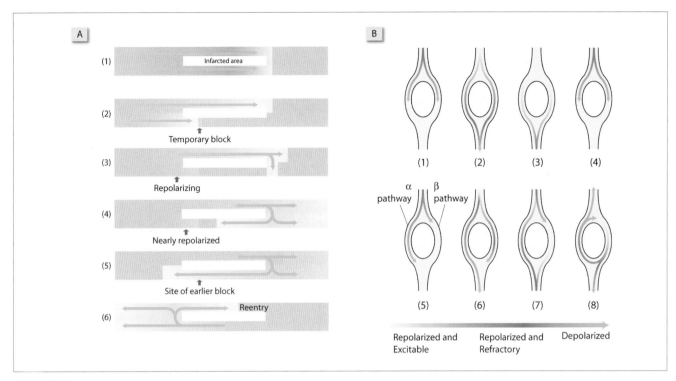

Fig. 32.12 **(A)** A microreentrant circuit around an infarct. (1) Impulse travels from left to right. The leading end is depolarized. The trailing end is repolarizing. No reentry occurs. (2) In the lower track, the impulse meets with a temporary block. (3) Impulse in the upper track spreads to the lower track, which has remained polarized due to the block. (4) Impulse in the lower track spreads both forward and backward. Also, the site of the block is now nearly repolarized. (5) The recurrent impulse travels backward in the lower tract to enter the site of the block, which by now has repolarized fully. (6) The recurrent impulse in the lower track reenters the upper track, which by now has repolarized completely. **(B)** (1–4) Normal propagation of excitation in the atrioventricular (AV) node. (5–8) A reentrant circuit in the AV node. The excitation travels along two conducting pathways inside the node, the α pathway, having faster conduction velocity but longer refractory period, and the β pathway, having slower conduction velocity but shorter refractory period. The β pathway recovers earlier from its refractory period. An ectopic impulse entering the node at this point will enter the β pathway. The α pathway recovers from its refractory period, allowing a recurrent entry to the impulse in the β pathway.

nodal reentrant circuit comprises two conducting pathways inside the node, the α pathway, having faster conduction velocity but longer refractory period, and the β pathway, having slower conduction velocity but shorter refractory period. This results in reentry, as shown in **Fig. 32.12B**.

Supraventricular Tachyarrhythmias

A **premature supraventricular contraction** is a contraction out of rhythm with the normal ongoing heartbeat. It occurs due to the discharge of an ectopic focus in the atrium (atrial premature beat) or in the AV node (junctional premature beat). The ectopic impulse not only spreads to the ventricle but also travels back to depolarize the SA node and in the process, resets the SA node. After the atrial premature beat, the SA node discharges only after the normal R-R interval has elapsed. Hence, there is no compensatory pause (**Fig. 32.13A**) as in the case of a ventricular extrasystole (see below). Because the atrial activation occurs from below upward, the P wave is inverted in those leads where it is normally upright (e.g., lead II) and upright in those where it is normally inverted (lead aVR).

Supraventricular tachycardia mostly occurs in paroxysms (*paroxysm* = a sudden outburst) and is therefore called *paroxysmal supraventricular tachycardia*. It often occurs in

healthy subjects with abrupt onset and termination, appearing as episodes lasting minutes or hours and separated by periods of days, weeks, months, or years during which no episodes occur. When the tachycardia originates in the AV node, both the atria and the ventricles beat at the same rate of ~120 to 200 beats/min (**Fig. 32.13B**). However, when the tachycardia originates in the atria, the ventricular rate is slower because many of the atrial impulses do not reach the ventricles due to AV delay.

Atrial flutter is similar to paroxysmal atrial tachycardia except that the rate of atrial contractions is much higher at 220 to 350 beats/min. It occurs mostly due to a macroreentrant circuit around the tricuspid valve or the vena caval opening. The high rate of atrial contraction is inevitably associated with AV block, and only a fraction of all atrial impulses reach the ventricles, resulting in a lower ventricular rate, which is usually regular (**Fig. 32.13C**). Atrial flutter causes a reduction in cardiac output because at such high rates, the strength of atrial contractions reduces, rendering ineffective the atrial pumping that normally contributes ~30% to the cardiac output.

Atrial fibrillation results from random excitation of various parts of the atria. In the absence of a coordinated sequence of excitation, there is no effective contraction of any of the cardiac chambers, and the atrium "quivers" instead of contracting.

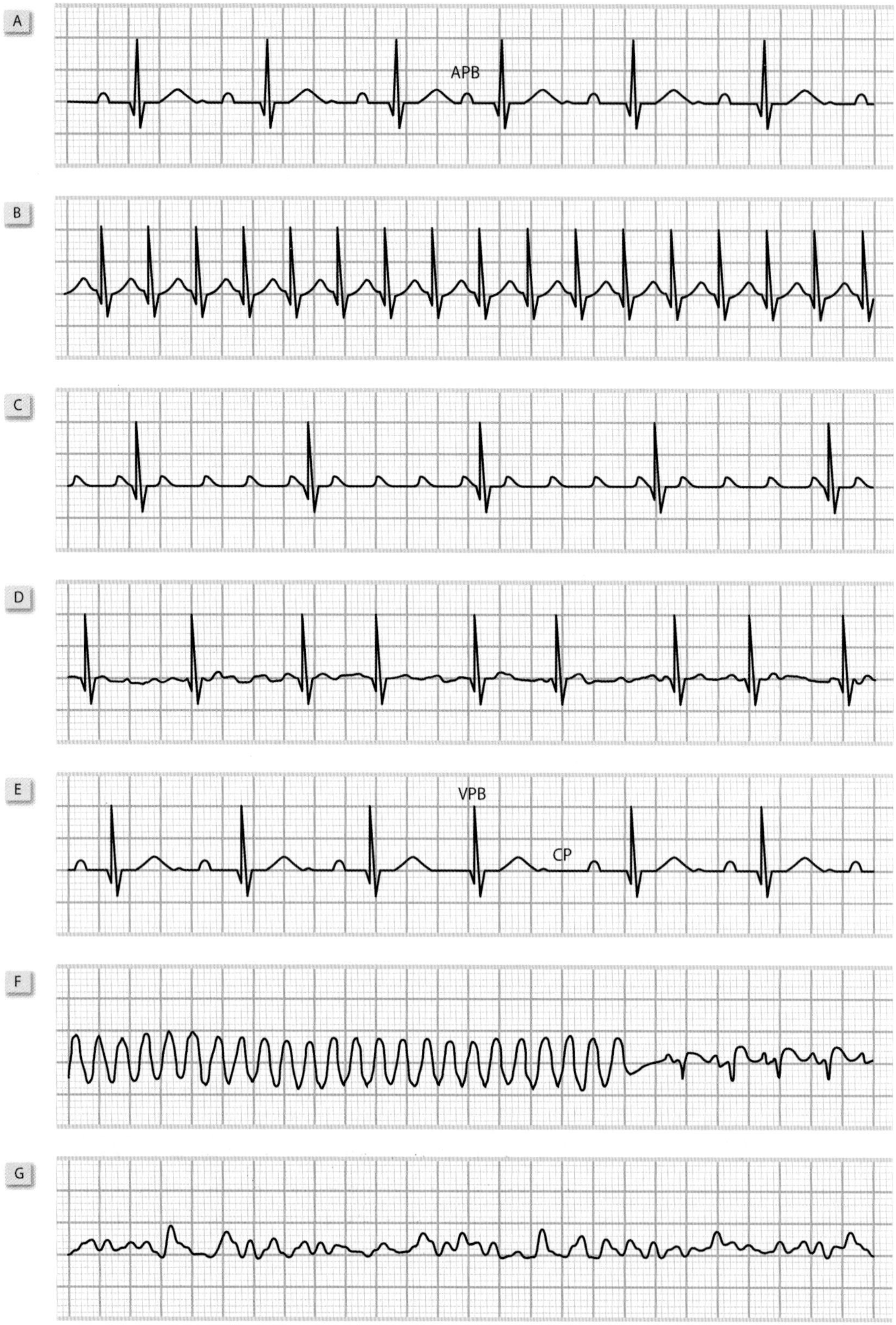

Fig. 32.13 **(A)** Atrial premature beats (APB). **(B)** Paroxysmal supraventricular tachycardia. **(C)** Atrial flutter. **(D)** Atrial fibrillation. Note the absence of definite P waves and the irregularly irregular pulse. **(E)** Ventricular premature beat (VPB) and compensatory pause (CP). **(F)** Ventricular flutter, progressing to fibrillation. **(G)** Ventricular fibrillation.

Fibrillation occurs due to numerous microreentrant circuits. There are several depolarized patches all over the heart, and the impulse wanders along the repolarized areas in between the depolarized patches. When the wandering impulse reaches the AV node, it gets conducted to the ventricle. Hence, the ventricular rate is extremely erratic and is said to be "irregularly irregular" (**Fig. 32.13D**). The ventricular rate usually does not exceed 150 beats/min.

Ventricular Tachyarrhythmias

A **premature ventricular contraction** (ventricular extrasystole) is one that is not preceded by a regular atrial contraction. The ventricular activation does not antidromically activate the atria or depolarize the SA node; therefore, the regular SA node rhythm is not disturbed. The regular sinus impulse following the premature beat does not activate the ventricle, which is still refractory from the premature contraction. Rather, the ventricle responds to the next normal sinus impulse. Hence, there is a slight pause, the *compensatory pause,* following the ventricular extrasystole. The interval between the QRS complexes immediately preceding and following the extrasystole is exactly twice the normal R-R interval (**Fig. 32.13E**).

Ventricular tachycardia occurs when premature ventricular contractions occur repetitively for more than 30 seconds. The heart rate in ventricular tachycardia ranges from 130 to 200 beats/min.

In **ventricular flutter**, the heart rate is 200 to 250 beats/min. It is characterized by wavy QRS complexes with no isoelectric line between them, and the absence of a T wave. The upstroke and downstroke of the QRS complex look the same, so that the ECG looks the same even when turned upside down (**Fig. 32.13F**). Ventricular flutter usually leads to ventricular fibrillation and is self-limiting only in exceptional cases. It is a medical emergency that has to be treated immediately. Its management involves DC cardioversion followed by appropriate antiarrhythmic drugs.

Ventricular fibrillation is similar to atrial fibrillation and results in ineffective ventricular contraction and cardiac failure. The ECG is nearly flat with small, *sawtooth waves* (**Fig. 32.13G**). Like ventricular flutter, it is a medical emergency that needs immediate cardioversion.

DC cardioversion involves passing electricity through the heart by placing electrodes on the thorax (external defibrillation) or directly on the heart (open-chest defibrillation). Defibrillation results in the simultaneous depolarization of the entire heart. Following repolarization, the normal sinus rhythm tends to resume.

Summary

- Excitation of the heart begins at the SA node, spreads to the AV node, then down the bundle of His and the Purkinje fibers to excite the ventricular muscle cells.

- The electrocardiogram (ECG) is an electrical potential recorded at the body surface originating in the changing cardiac dipole.

- The waves seen in the ECG are the P wave (atrial depolarization), the QRS complex (ventricular depolarization), and the T wave (ventricular repolarization).

- Alterations in the normal ECG result from abnormalities anywhere along the conducting system of the heart and from the death of cardiac cells.

Applying What You Know

32.1. Mrs. Daniels' ECG exhibits a normal sinus rhythm. This means that her SA node is functioning as the pacemaker. Describe the properties of the membrane of SA node cells that give rise to this pacemaker function.

32.2. Signs of atrial enlargement and ventricular hypertrophy are visible in Mrs. Daniels' ECG. Explain how these changes to her heart give rise to changes in her ECG.

32.3. Mrs. Daniels has a sinus tachycardia; her heart rate is 90 beats/min. There is no evidence that this tachycardia is due to cardiac pathology or pathophysiology. Therefore, it is most likely to be due to changes in the sympathetic and parasympathetic signals reaching her SA node. What changes in these signals do you expect to be present.

The heart has two large chambers called the ventricles and two small chambers called the atria. The ventricles pump blood into the aorta and pulmonary artery; the atria fill the ventricles. The left and right ventricles are separated by the interventricular septum. The left and right atria are separated by the interatrial septum. The pathway of blood through the heart is described in Chapter 35.

The atria and the ventricles are separated by the atrioventricular (AV) valves that prevent backflow of blood from the ventricles to the atria. The left AV valve is called the mitral or bicuspid valve, and the right AV valve is called the tricuspid valve. The free margins of the valve cusps are attached to the papillary muscles by tendinous cords called the chordae tendinae (**Fig. 33.1A**). During ventricular contraction (systole), the rise in ventricular pressure tends to push open the AV valves back into the atria. This is prevented by the contraction of the papillary muscles at the outset of systole, which restricts the movement of the cusps of the AV valves.

The passage of blood from the left ventricle into the aorta is through the aortic valve (**Fig. 33.1B**). The passage of blood from the right ventricle into the pulmonary artery is through the pulmonary valve. The aortic and pulmonary valves are called the semilunar valves. During ventricular relaxation (diastole), when blood tries to flow back into the ventricle, the cusps of the semilunar valves get distended with blood and thereby occlude the enclosed passage.

Phases of the Cardiac Cycle

A cardiac cycle refers to the interval between the onset of one heartbeat and the onset of the next heartbeat. It has two main phases: ventricular systole (contraction) and ventricular diastole (relaxation), which are often simply called systole and diastole (**Fig. 33.2A**). Although electrical systole begins with the beginning of the Q wave, the onset of mechanical systole begins with the first heart sound ("lub") and roughly coincides with the peak of the R wave. Similarly, although electrical systole ends at the end of the T wave, mechanical diastole begins a little later, with the second heart sound ("dup"). The unqualified terms *systole* and *diastole* refer to the mechanical events.

Systole and diastole are further subdivided and named after the most prominent event of that phase. The *systolic phase* is divided into (1) isovolumetric ventricular contraction, (2) rapid ventricular ejection, and (3) protodiastole. The *diastolic phase* is divided into (1) isovolumetric ventricular relaxation, (2) rapid ventricular filling, (3) diastasis, and (4) atrial systole (**Table 33.1**).

Ventricular and Atrial Events

Systole

Isovolumetric ventricular contraction | Before the onset of systole, the intraventricular pressure remains very low, a little

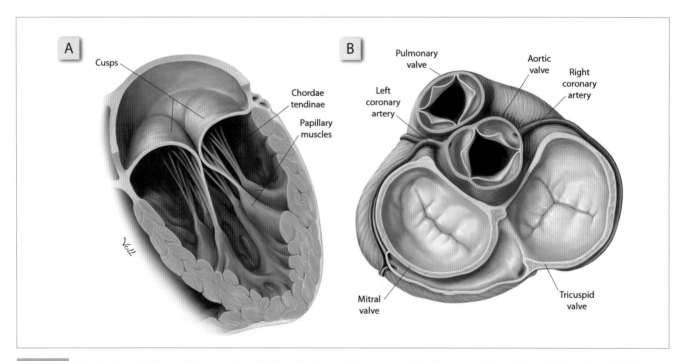

Fig. 33.1 Heart valves. **(A)** The papillary muscles with their chordae tendinae anchored to the cusps of the atrioventricular valves. **(B)** The open semilunar valves and the closed atrioventricular valves.

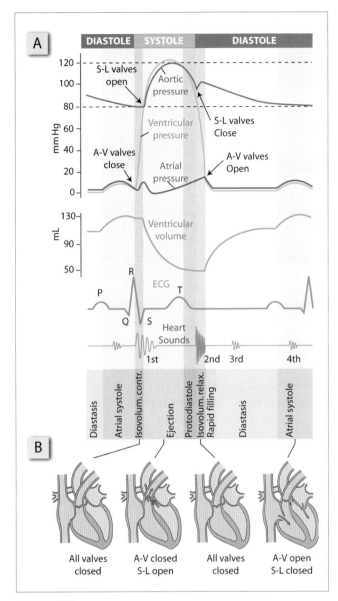

Fig. 33.2 **(A)** Events during the cardiac cycle, showing pressure changes in the left ventricle, left atrium, and the aorta, volume changes in the ventricles, the electrocardiogram (ECG), and the heart sounds. **(B)** The valvular positions in different phases. A-V, atrioventricular; S-L, semilunar.

above zero mm Hg (**Fig. 33.2A**). As the ventricle starts contracting, the intraventricular pressure rises. The rising ventricular pressure immediately closes the mitral and tricuspid valves (**Fig. 33.2B**), producing the first heart sound that marks the onset of systole. The pressure is not enough to push open the semilunar valves, but forces the closed AV valve to bulge into the atrium, causing a small but sharp rise in atrial pressure called the *c-wave*. (The *c* stands for contraction of the ventricle). With both the valves (atrioventricular and semilunar) momentarily closed, the pressure inside the ventricle rises steeply as the ventricle contracts. Because there is no change in the ventricular volume in this phase, it is called isovolumetric contraction.

Table 33.1 Duration of Cardiac Cycle Phases

Systole 0.3 second	
Isovolumetric contraction	0.05 second
Rapid ventricular ejection	0.20 second
Protodiastole	0.05 second
Diastole 0.5 second	
Isovolumetric relaxation	0.05 second
Rapid ventricular filling	0.05 second
Diastasis	0.30 second
Atrial systole	0.10 second

Ventricular ejection | When the steeply rising left ventricular pressure exceeds the aortic pressure (80 mm Hg), it is able to push open the aortic valve and eject the blood into the aorta, marking the onset of ventricular ejection. Similarly, the right ventricular pressure exceeds the pulmonary arterial pressure (8 mm Hg) and ejects blood into the pulmonary artery after pushing open the pulmonary valve. During ventricular ejection, the volume of each ventricle reduces from 130 mL (the end-diastolic volume) to 50 mL (the end-systolic volume), pumping out 80 mL of blood (the stroke volume).

Ventricular ejection is rapid at first, slowing down as systole progresses. Concomitantly, the intraventricular pressure rises to a maximum and then declines toward the end of ventricular systole. During rapid ventricular ejection, the ventricular pressure rises because the rate at which the ventricle contracts is greater than the rate at which the blood is ejected. Toward the end of ventricular ejection, however, there is no further contraction of the ventricle, but the blood continues to be ejected at a rapid rate due to its momentum set up during rapid ejection. Hence, the ventricular pressure drops. The phase toward the end of systole in which the ventricular pressure falls is called the *protodiastole*. Notwithstanding its name, it is actually the last phase of systole. Through most of the protodiastole, the atria get slowly filled with blood flowing in from the systemic and pulmonary veins, and the atrial pressure rises slowly.

When the ventricles contract, not only is the apex of the heart pulled up, but also the fibrous partition separating the ventricles from the atria (the AV ring) is pulled down. As a result, the atrial muscles get stretched, and the atria dilate. The dilatation of the atria causes a sharp fall in the atrial pressure, which is known as the *x-descent* of atrial pressure. The fall in atrial pressure probably also exerts a suction force on the venous return. As venous blood continues to flow into the atria from the great veins, the atrial pressure rises and continues to rise as long as the AV valves remain closed, that is, until the end of isovolumetric relaxation. This results in an atrial pressure wave called the *v-wave*, which peaks at the end of systole (the *v* stands for venous filling).

Another important event that occurs during this phase is the *apex beat*. Due to the spiral arrangement of the ventricular muscle fibers, the heart rotates to the right during ventricular contraction, and its apex strikes the anterior wall of the chest.

The site of the impact, which is known as the apex beat, can be detected by palpating the chest wall. The apex beat is located at or medial to the left midclavicular line in the fourth or fifth intercostal space. A shift in the location of apex beat is often of diagnostic significance.

Diastole

Isovolumetric ventricular relaxation | When the ventricles begin to relax, the intraventricular pressure falls, and the semilunar valves immediately close. With further relaxation, the AV valves open. However, there remains a small intervening period during which the semilunar valves have closed, and the atrioventricular valves have not opened. With all valves closed, no change in ventricular volume is possible during this phase, and the relaxation is isovolumetric. In the absence of any change in volume, the relaxation is associated with a steep drop in ventricular pressure.

Rapid ventricular filling | As the ventricular pressure continues to drop rapidly during isovolumetric ventricular relaxation, it reaches a point where it falls below the atrial pressure. At this point, the AV valves open, and the accumulated blood in the atria rushes into the ventricles. Filling is rapid at first; hence, the name of this phase. During rapid ventricular filling, there is a sharp fall in atrial pressure, which is known as the *y-descent*.

Diastasis | After the initial rapid ventricular filling, blood flows slowly and smoothly from the superior and inferior vena cava through the right atrium into the right ventricle without any turbulence anywhere along the path. Similarly, blood from the pulmonary veins flows into the left ventricle without any turbulence. This phase of nonturbulent ventricular filling is known as diastasis. The atrial pressure remains slightly greater than the ventricular pressure because upstream pressure must always be greater. The volume of each ventricle increases to ~105 mL. The pressure in both ventricles increases slowly, the rate of increase being determined by the ventricular compliance (the elastic properties of the ventricular walls).

During the **atrial systole,** the atria contract and pump blood into the ventricles. The onset of atrial systole coincides with the peak of the P wave of the ECG. Atrial systole, is associated with a sharp rise in atrial pressure called the *a-wave*. The ventricular volume increases sharply to the end-diastolic volume of 130 mL. The increase in volume of each ventricle during atrial systole is ~25 mL, which is ~30% of the stroke volume (80 mL). When atrial systole is ineffective, as in atrial fibrillation, the stroke volume decreases by 30% due to ineffective atrial contraction.

Arterial and Venous Events

Aortic Pressure

During the **ejection phase,** blood flows from the left ventricle into the aorta. Hence, the aortic pressure (downstream pressure) is slightly less than the left ventricular pressure (upstream pressure) during most of the rapid ejection phase. However, toward the end of the ejection phase (protodiastole), left ventricular pressure drops below the aortic pressure because blood flows out of the left ventricle at a faster rate than the rate

at which it contracts. On the other hand, blood flows into the aorta faster than it can flow out into the peripheral arteries, leading to a temporary accumulation of blood in the aorta. In other words, the aorta expands, and the elastic elements in its walls are stretched, storing energy.

General Models: Reservoir and Elasticity

The aorta is a reservoir whose volume is determined by the rate at which blood enters from the left ventricle and the rate at which blood flows out to the periphery. During cardiac systole, the flow in is greater than the flow out, and the volume of blood in the aorta increases. This increased volume stretches the elastic elements in the walls of the aorta. During diastole, the volume in the aorta falls as outflow exceeds inflow, and the recoil of the elastic elements maintains an elevated pressure.

During **isovolumetric ventricular relaxation,** there is a sharp drop in ventricular pressure. Hence, blood in the aorta tries to rush back into the ventricle, only to collide against the closed aortic valve. The collision causes a small but sharp rise in aortic pressure. This sharp pressure rise is recordable even from peripheral arteries and is called the notch or *incisura*.

During **diastasis and atrial systole** (i.e., the remainder of the diastolic phase), the aortic pressure smoothly declines, with aortic pressure being maintained by the energy being given up by the relaxing elastic elements in the aortic walls. If there had not been another systole, the pressure would have declined to ~10 mm Hg (the mean systemic filling pressure), which is the pressure present in the circulation when the heart is stopped. This is the pressure present in the system given a blood volume that is greater than the unstressed volume of the circulation. However, by the time the aortic pressure declines to ~80 mm Hg, another ventricular systole boosts the aortic pressure again.

Jugular Venous Pressure (JVP)

The variations in right atrial pressure are transmitted to the jugular veins, producing the a-, c-, and v-waves of the venous pressure pulse (**Fig. 33.3**). These waves are low-pressure waves: they are visible in an in vitro recording, but they are not palpable at the body surface. The waveform of the jugular venous pulse, when recorded, offers a diagnostic sign. In atrioventricular dissociation, the JVP is characterized by the presence of *cannon waves*—giant c-waves that are produced due to the occasional simultaneous contraction of the right atrium and right ventricle.

Heart Sounds

Heart sounds are produced by the heart valves when they close (**Fig. 33.2A**). Normally, no sounds are produced when valves open. However the opening of a stenosed AV valve is sometimes associated with an opening "snap."

The *first heart sound* (S_1) is a low, slightly prolonged lub sound and is associated with the closing of the AV valves. The

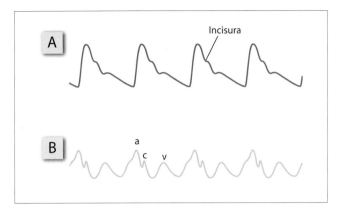

Fig. 33.3 **(A)** The brachial artery pulse. **(B)** The jugular venous pulse.

sound is caused by vibrations set up by the sudden increase in tension in the valves and the surrounding chamber walls at the onset of ventricular systole. It has a duration of ~0.15 second and a frequency of 25 to 45 Hz.

The *second heart sound* (S_2) is a shorter, louder high-pitched dup sound associated with the closing of the semilunar valves. The sound is caused by oscillations in the column of fluid in the vessels and the tensed state of their walls. It lasts ~0.12 second and has a frequency of 50 Hz.

The *third heart sound* (S_3) is a soft, low-pitched sound heard during the first third of the diastole. It is produced due to the turbulence of blood flow during rapid ventricular filling. In adults, it generally indicates a volume overload (increased preload) of the atria. However, it is often present in normal young individuals.

A *fourth heart sound* (S_4) is sometimes audible immediately before the first sound when atrial pressure is high or the ventricular compliance is low, as is the case when ventricular hypertrophy is present. It occurs late in the ventricular filling phase. Generally, S_4 indicates a pressure overload (increased afterload) of the atria.

Loud heart sound | Heart sounds become louder when the heart rate is high, the reason for which is as follows. Although the semilunar valves open fully at the onset of systole, they normally start floating back to their closed position toward the end of systole when the ejection of blood from the ventricle slows down. Hence, the sound produced by their closure at the onset of diastole is not very loud. During tachycardia, the systole is shorter (**Table 33.2**), and the ejection of blood does not slow down much toward the end of systole. The valves therefore remain wide open until the end of systole, and at the onset of diastole, they shut down from the fully open position to produce a loud S_2. For the same reason, the mitral

and tricuspid valves produce a loud S_1 during exercise. Heart sounds are also loud when the diastolic pressure in the aorta or pulmonary artery is elevated (as in systemic or pulmonary hypertension), causing the respective valves to shut forcefully.

Split heart sound | The events on the two sides of the heart are slightly asynchronous, with the left ventricle contracting slightly before the right ventricle. Hence, the mitral (M) valve closes before the tricuspid (T), resulting in the "splitting" of the first heart sound S_1 into M_1 and T_1, in that order. Although the left ventricle starts contracting earlier, the pulmonary valve opens before the aortic valve because the pulmonary arterial pressure is much lower than the aortic pressure. For the same reason, during diastole, the aortic (A) valve closes before the pulmonary (P) valve, resulting in the splitting of the second heart sound S_2 into A_2 and P_2, in that order. The splitting of S_2 widens during deep inspiration because during inspiration, right ventricular output increases slightly, keeping the pulmonary valve open longer. As a result, P_2 gets delayed further, and the split widens.

Murmurs (**Fig. 33.4**) are abnormal heart sounds caused by the presence of turbulent blood flow anywhere in the system.

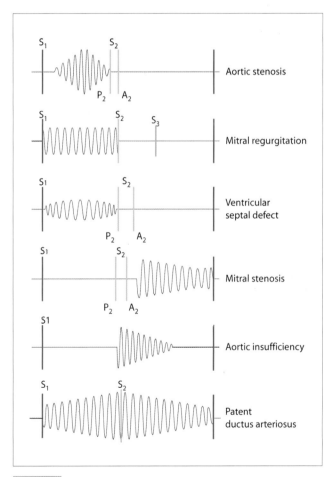

Fig. 33.4 Cardiac murmurs arising from different pathologies. S_1 and S_2 are the normal heart sounds arising from the closing of the atrioventricular (AV) and semilunar valves. In the presence of certain pathologies, the single S_2 sound may occur as a "split S_2", with the closure of the pulmonic valve (P_2) being heard before the closure of the aortic valve (A_2). Murmurs occur when flow velocity is high enough, and turbulent flow is present.

Table 33.2 Duration of Cardiac Cycle at Resting Heart Rate (HR) and in Tachycardia

Duration	HR 75/min	HR 200/min
Cardiac cycle	0.8 second	0.30 second
Systole	0.3 second	0.15 second
Diastole	0.5 second	0.15 second

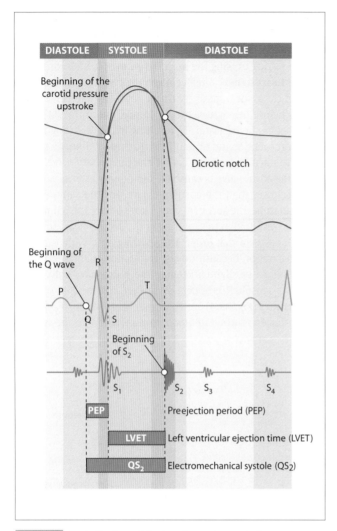

Fig. 33.5 Clinical indices of the isovolumetric ventricular contraction. Changes in the value of PEP, LVET, and QS$_2$ can occur in the presence of left ventricular dysfunction.

Flow through a defective valve can give rise to an audible murmur. Stenosed valves have a smaller than normal area when open and hence a high flow velocity. Regurgitating valves are leaky valves that do not close properly and allow backflow of blood, often with a high flow velocity. When the flow velocity is high enough, turbulent flow is present, and a murmur results.

Murmurs are produced during systole (systolic murmurs) in stenosed semilunar valves or regurgitant AV valves. Murmurs are produced during diastole (diastolic murmurs) in stenosed AV valves or regurgitant semilunar valves. Murmurs are also heard over ventricular septal defect and patent ductus arteriosus (see **Fig. 35.5**).

Duration of Cardiac Events

The durations of the various phases of the cardiac cycle depend on the heart rate. The durations at cardiac rates of 75 beats/min and 200 beats/min are given in **Table 33.2**.

Effect of heart rate | When the heart rate increases, the durations of all the phases decrease. However, the duration of diastole decreases much more than the duration of the systole. The diastole shortens due to greater automaticity of the sinus node. The systole shortens due to quicker repolarization, which reduces the duration of cardiac action potential.

The marked reduction in diastolic time during tachycardia has important clinical implications. It is during diastole that most of the ventricular filling occurs. Also, it is during diastole that most of the cardiac muscle, especially the subendocardial portions of the left ventricle, gets adequately perfused by the coronary blood flow (see Chapter 39). Hence, at heart rates greater than 150 beats/min, there is a reduction of both ventricular filling (which tends to reduce cardiac output) and cardiac perfusion (which tends to cause myocardial ischemia and infarction).

Clinical Indices
The duration of isovolumetric ventricular contraction is of considerable clinical importance. However, it is not easy to measure. Hence, certain other indices have been devised as approximations for the duration of isovolumetric contraction. These indices can be calculated by simultaneous recording of the electrocardiogram, phonocardiogram, the record of the heart sounds, and carotid pulse, which is indicative of aortic pressure changes (**Fig. 33.5**).

Electromechanical systole (QS$_2$) is the time interval between the onset of the ventricular activation (QRS complex) and the closure of the aortic valves (S$_2$). Left ventricular ejection time (LVET) is the time interval between the beginning of the carotid pressure rise and the incisura. Preejection period (PEP) is the difference between QS$_2$ and LVET and gives the duration of electromechanical events preceding systolic ejection. The normal PEP/LVET ratio is 0.35. When left ventricular function is impaired, the PEP/LVET ratio increases without a change in QS$_2$.

Ventricular Pressure–Volume Loop

The ventricular pressure–volume loop (**Fig. 33.6**) is an alternative method of representing the cardiac cycle. In this visual representation, the time dimension is eliminated; therefore, it is not possible to tell from this loop how fast the events are occurring. However, the advantage is that the work done by the heart is instantly apparent from the area enclosed by the loop. It thus enables the clinician to easily diagnose a failing heart (see **Fig. 34.10**).

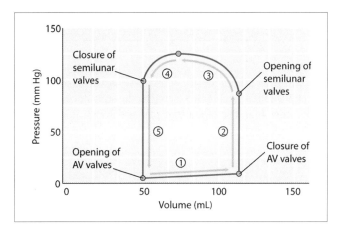

Fig. 33.6 Ventricular pressure–volume loop showing (1) ventricular filling, (2) isovolumetric contraction, (3) rapid ejection, (4) slow ejection, and (5) isovolumetric relaxation. The area inside the loop is proportional to the work done by the heart during that cardiac cycle. AV, atrioventricular.

General Model: Energy

Work can only be done through the expenditure of energy; in the case of the heart, this means the utilization of adenosine triphosphate (ATP) by the contractile machinery in ventricular muscle cells. The area of the pressure–volume loop represents the work done and hence the oxygen consumption that occurs to generate the ATP used by the contractile cardiac muscle.

Summary

- The heart is made up of two two-chambered pumps in series.

- Flow through the heart and out into the pulmonary and systemic circulation is through valves that normally ensure one-way flow. The closing of these valves produces the heart sounds.

- The cardiac cycle is all of the events that occur during a single heartbeat.

- The cardiac cycle has a systolic phase, during which the ventricles are contracting, and a diastolic phase, during which the ventricles are relaxed.

- The right heart ejects blood into the pulmonary artery, and the left heart ejects blood into the aorta.

Applying What You Know

33.1. On auscultation, Mrs. Daniels' S_2 heart sound exhibits an unusually loud pulmonic component. Explain the mechanism that is causing this component of the S_2 heart sound to be louder than normal.

33.2. Mrs. Daniels has an audible diastolic murmur. How does the stenosis alter the properties of the valve, and how does this affect flow across it? Describe the mechanism by which her stenosed mitral valve gives rise to a murmur.

Cardiac Output and Its Measurement

What Is Cardiac Output?

Cardiac output (CO) is the amount of blood pumped into the aorta by the left ventricle or into the pulmonary artery by the right ventricle per minute. The normal CO is 5 to 6 L/min. Cardiac index is the CO expressed in relation to the body surface area. The normal cardiac index is ~3.2 L/min/m².

Cardiac output is the product of stroke volume and heart rate. The *stroke volume* is the amount of blood pumped out by the left ventricle in each stroke. During a single contraction, each ventricle pumps out 80 mL of blood. Stroke volume is given by the difference between *end-diastolic ventricular volume* (130 mL) and *end-systolic ventricular volume* (50 mL).

$$\underset{(6\ \text{L/min})}{\text{Cadiac output}} = \underset{(80\ \text{mL})}{\text{Stroke volume}} \times \underset{(75/\text{min})}{\text{Heart rate}} \quad (34.1)$$

$$\underset{(80\ \text{mL})}{\text{Stroke volume}} = \underset{(130\ \text{mL})}{\text{End-diastolic ventricular volume}} - \underset{(50\ \text{mL})}{\text{End-systolic volume}}$$

$$(34.2)$$

The ejection fraction is the percentage of the end-diastolic ventricular volume that is ejected with each stroke. The ejection fraction is a valuable index of ventricular pump function. It is normally ~60% and decreases in a failing heart.

$$\text{Ejection fraction} = \frac{\text{Stroke volume}}{\text{End-diastolic ventricular volume}} \times 100$$

$$(34.3)$$

Although CO is the product of stroke volume and heart rate, it does not necessarily mean that the CO increases whenever the stroke volume or the heart rate increases. In fact, it is not uncommon for physiologic responses to generate an increased CO by increasing heart rate with a consequent small decrease in stroke volume. Nevertheless, the product of heart rate and stroke volume is increased.

Cardiac Output Measurement

The cardiac output is the blood flow that delivers to the tissues of the body the nutrients required by every cell and removes the waste products of cellular metabolism. The CO is also one of the determinants of blood pressure. It is thus important, both in the laboratory and for dealing with patients with cardiovascular disease, that CO be measured.

Fick method | The CO can be estimated by using the Fick principle, which states that blood flow (F) through an organ is given by the quotient of the rate at which a substance is added or removed from the blood ($\dot{Q}$) and the arteriovenous (A-V)

concentration difference ($C_A - C_v$) that results. This principle is not applicable if the organ exchanges the substance with anything other than the blood that passes through it. Expressed mathematically,

$$F = \frac{\dot{Q}}{C_A - C_v} \quad (34.4)$$

General Model: Reservoir

The Fick method of calculating flow is an example of the use of the *reservoir model*; the oxygen in the blood leaving the lungs came from only two possible inputs, the pulmonary artery blood and from the air. Similarly, the oxygen present in the veins draining the tissues is what is left of the oxygen in the aorta after tissue uptake of oxygen from the blood.

For calculating CO using the Fick principle, oxygen is used as the indicator substance. Thus, $\dot{Q}$ is the rate at which O_2 diffuses from the lungs into blood (mL O_2/min), C_A is the O_2 concentration in arterial blood (mL O_2/L), and C_v is the O_2 concentration (mL O_2/L) in mixed venous blood (**Fig. 34.1**). Application of the Fick principle to these parameters gives the pulmonary blood flow (F), which is essentially equal to the CO.

$\dot{Q}$ can be estimated from the volume difference between the volume of inspired air and the volume of expired air that is passed through soda lime to remove CO_2. C_A can be estimated

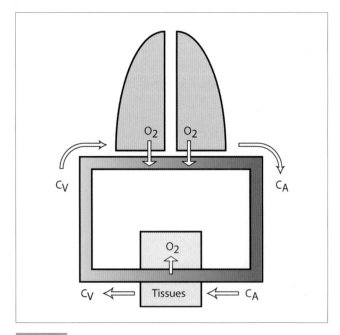

Fig. 34.1 Fick principle used to measure cardiac output.

in an arterial blood sample withdrawn from any convenient artery because all systemic arteries have roughly the same Po_2 as pulmonary venous blood. C_v is estimated in a sample of mixed venous blood obtained directly from the pulmonary artery through catheterization. This is necessary because almost every vein flowing toward the heart brings in blood with a different level of O_2 desaturation.

Example

If $\dot{Q}$ = 250 mL O_2/min, C_A= 195 mL O_2/L, and C_v = 145 mL O_2/ L, then F = 5000 mL/min = cardiac output

Dye-dilution technique | A bolus dose (Q) of indicator dye is injected into any superficial vein, and blood samples are withdrawn from an artery every few seconds (**Fig. 34.2**). The indicator must be a substance that stays in the bloodstream during the test and has no harmful or hemodynamic effects. The concentration of the dye in blood (C) is determined, and the time (T) taken by the column of dyed blood to flow across the sampling point is noted.

Suppose the total amount of dye passing under the sampling point in T seconds = q.

Then the volume of blood passing under the sampling point in T seconds = q / C.

Therefore, the volume of blood (f) passing under the sampling point in 60 seconds is given by the formula

$$f = \frac{q}{C} \times \frac{60}{T} \qquad (34.5)$$

Two corrections need to be made here. First, the flow rate (f) calculated is that of a single artery (from which blood has been sampled), which is only a fraction (say, 1/n) of the CO (F). Second, the amount of dye flowing into the artery (q) is a fraction (also 1/n) of the total amount of dye injected (Q). Applying these corrections,

$$F/n = \frac{Q/n}{C} \times \frac{60}{T} \qquad (34.6)$$

n cancels out, and the formula becomes

$$F = \frac{Q}{C} \times \frac{60}{T} \qquad (34.7)$$

However, the column of blood passing under the sampling point does not have a uniform concentration of dye in it (**Fig. 34.2C**). Moreover, there is recirculation of the dye back to the heart and into the artery from where the dye is sampled (**Fig. 34.2D**). It is therefore difficult to estimate the mean concentration of the dye passing under the sampling point and to estimate the time taken by the dye to pass under it.

The problem is tackled by obtaining multiple blood samples as the dyed blood passes under the sampling point. A graph is plotted between the dye concentration on the y-axis and time on the x-axis (**Fig. 34.3B**). The time taken (T) is read

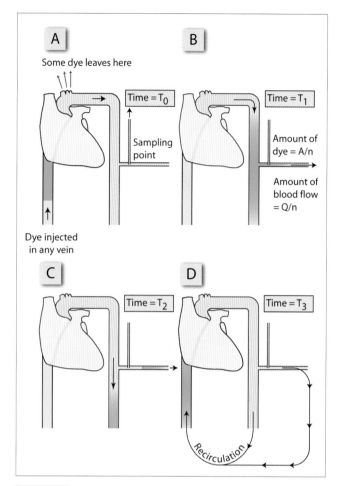

Fig. 34.2 Steps in the circulation of an indicator dye injected into a vein. **(A)** Dye injected into a vein. **(B)** Dye approaches the sampling point in an artery. **(C)** Dye passes the sampling point. **(D)** Dye recirculates and reenters the vein.

out from the graph after exponentially extrapolating the dye concentration to a very low value. The integrated value of C × T can be estimated from the area under the curve.

A modification of the dye-dilution technique is the thermodilution technique, in which cold saline is used instead of a dye, and the dilution of its temperature by blood is measured. This technique has the twin advantages that the saline is completely harmless, and the cold is dissipated in the tissues, so that recirculation is not a problem.

The **Doppler technique** measures CO by placing an electromagnetic flow meter on the ascending aorta in experimental animals. The Doppler effect is the change in sound velocity when the medium through which it is propagating is itself in motion. Thus, flowing blood changes the velocity of sound through it. The magnitude of the change indicates the velocity of blood flow. In humans, CO is measured by combining Doppler techniques with echocardiography.

The **cineradiographic technique** calculates the ejection fraction by imaging the cardiac blood pool at the end of diastole and the end of systole after injecting radiolabeled red blood cells.

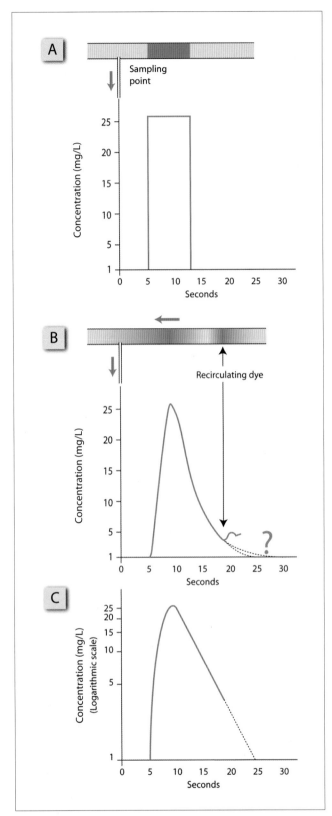

Fig. 34.3 Indicator dilution technique of cardiac output estimation. **(A)** If the dye moved like a solid block, the graph would be rectangular. **(B)** The dye concentration fades exponentially at both ends. Due to recirculation of the dye, there is as increase in dye concentration before the decline is complete. The graph has to be extrapolated exponentially to get the value of T. **(C)** Extrapolation is easier if the graph in B is plotted on a semilogarithmic scale.

Ballistocardiography measures the recoil force produced by the rapid ejection of a large amount of blood through the aorta. The magnitude of the recoil force gives a measure of the stroke volume.

Determinants of the Cardiac Output

Cardiac output is determined by cardiac factors and vascular factors. The interaction between these factors determines the *right atrial pressure* or, equivalently, the *central venous pressure* (CVP, the pressure in the superior and inferior vena cavae, also known as the great veins, just outside the heart, with a value slightly greater than the pressure in the right atrium). CVP is normally between 1 and 5 mm Hg. A vigorously pumping heart lowers the CVP by translocating a greater volume of blood from the venous to the arterial compartment. However, the heart requires an optimum CVP for its pumping action. If the CVP falls, the CO falls with it. If the CVP dropped to subatmospheric levels (below 0 mm Hg), the great veins would collapse, and no blood would enter the heart. One role of the vascular system, then, is to ensure that the CVP does not fall too low for effective cardiac pumping. The vascular factors include venous pumping, which propels blood toward the heart.

The role of the cardiac and vascular factors can therefore be summarized as follows. The cardiac factors try to prevent the CVP from rising, whereas the vascular factors try to prevent the CVP from falling. If the CVP rises above 5 mm Hg, it indicates that the heart is not pumping adequately and is probably failing. If the CVP falls below 1 mm Hg, it indicates that the vascular factors are failing in their role. The CVP can be measured directly by inserting a catheter into the right atrium. CVP is assessed clinically by examining the jugular venous pulse (see **Fig. 35.13**).

Circulatory load on the heart | When discussing the function of any pump, it is important to consider the load on it. There are two types of load on the heart: the preload and the afterload. The preload is the stretch (the length) of the cardiac fibers before they start contracting. Cardiac preload is represented by the volume of venous blood that distends the ventricle. Ventricular filling increases with the CVP. The CVP therefore determines the preload on the heart.

An afterload is the load encountered by the cardiac muscle after it starts contracting. The aortic pressure, the pressure against which the ventricle must pump blood, is an afterload. The left ventricle does not "feel" the load of the aortic pressure due to the closed aortic valve. However, as soon as the heart contracts, the aortic valve opens, and the left ventricle encounters the high aortic pressure. Hence, arterial hypertension imposes a heavy afterload on the heart.

When preload increases, the end-diastolic volume of the ventricle increases. Up to a point, an increase in preload increases cardiac contraction in accordance with the length–tension relationship of striated muscles (see Chapter 15). As a result, the CO tends to increase in proportion to the preload imposed on it. This is known as the *Frank-Starling law* of the heart, which states that the ventricular output is proportional to the ventricular end-diastolic volume.

On the other hand, when the afterload on the heart increases, the end-diastolic ventricular volume is unaffected, and the CO falls. The fall in the CO occurs despite an increase in myocardial contraction, which is known as the *Anrep effect*. The preload on the heart increases in dynamic exercise, a change in posture, and aortic regurgitation. The afterload increases in static exercise, hypertension, and aortic stenosis. However, until aortic pressure gets very high (≈160 mm Hg), the reduction in stroke volume that occurs is of little significance.

Myocardial Contraction

The contraction of cardiac muscle fibers can be increased by heterometric and homometric mechanisms. In the heterometric mechanism, the cardiac muscle fibers are stretched to increase their initial length (i.e., an increase in preload occurs). In the homometric mechanism, the active tension produced in cardiac muscle fibers is increased without increasing the initial fiber length.

Heterometric mechanism comes into play only when the preload on the heart changes. An increased preload results in a higher end-diastolic volume. In accordance with the Frank-Starling law of the heart, the increase in end-diastolic volume increases the strength of cardiac contraction, and the stroke volume increases.

Heterometric change in CO occurs, for example, immediately after a change of posture from sitting to lying, which increases the CVP. Heterometric response also occurs continuously for small, momentary adjustments necessary for keeping the outputs of the two ventricles equal. For example, if the output of the right ventricle increases momentarily, the left atrial pressure will increase, which in its turn will increase the output of the left ventricle.

Homometric mechanism increases cardiac performance without changing the initial length of the cardiac fibers. Factors that increase cardiac contractility homometrically include sympathetic stimulation of the ventricular muscle, circulating catecholamines, and tachycardia. What all three have in common is an increase in intracellular Ca^{2+} and hence greater generation of force at the cross-bridges. The relation between heart rate and cardiac contractility is known as the *staircase effect* (see **Fig. 19.4**).

In exercise, regulation of CO is largely (though not entirely) homometric and occurs through the activation of the sympathetic nervous system. Circulating catecholamines and tachycardia also contribute to the increase in contractility. Sympathetic stimulation increases the stroke volume without increasing the end-diastolic volume of the heart. In other words, it increases the ejection fraction. This is made possible by an increase in myocardial contractility and a simultaneous increase in heart rate. The increase in myocardial contractility decreases the end-systolic volume (increases the stroke volume) and reduces the duration of systole. This ensures that with each stroke, the ventricles pump out blood quickly and in larger amounts. The increase in heart rate decreases the end-diastolic volume (the heart has less time for relaxation and venous filling). By increasing both stroke volume and heart rate, sympathetic stimulation increases the CO massively without increasing the cardiac size—without increasing the end-diastolic volume.

The interaction between peripheral vasodilation and increased sympathetic stimulation of the heart that increases the CO in exercise is illustrated in **Fig. 34.4**.

Cardiac Pump Function

Myocardial contractility should not be confused with the pumping efficacy of the heart. A heart with a valvular defect, for example, will have poor pumping efficacy even if its contractility is normal or high.

Factors resulting in a *hypoeffective heart* are as follows: (1) decrease in pump power, as occurs in reduced sympathetic discharge or myocardial damage; (2) inefficient pumping, as in valvular or septal defects of the heart; (3) reduced pump filling, as in positive intrathoracic pressure (e.g., during expiration or Valsalva maneuver) and pericardial effusion or cardiac tamponade (filling of the pericardial space with blood). These conditions reduce diastolic filling of the heart. The fourth condition is increased afterload on the pump, as in hypertension.

Factors resulting in a *hypereffective heart* are as follows: (1) sympathetic stimulation of the heart; (2) inotropic drugs, such as digitalis, that increase cardiac contractility; and (3) increased intrathoracic negativity (e.g., during inspiration), which permits greater diastolic filling of the heart.

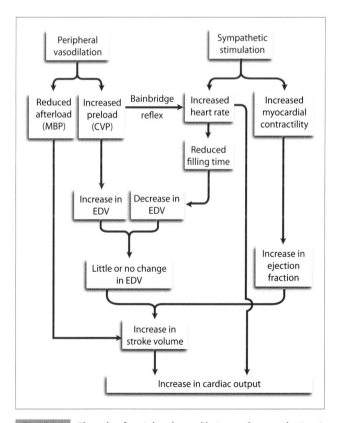

Fig. 34.4 The role of peripheral vasodilation and sympathetic stimulation of the heart in increasing cardiac output. CVP, central venous pressure; EDV, end (ventricular) diastolic volume; MBP, mean (arterial) blood pressure.

General Model: Balance of Forces

It is essential to keep in mind that the two determinants of stroke volume (and hence CO), preload or filling and contractility, do not always change in the same direction or by the same amount. Consequently, you need to be able to judge what effect the balance of the factors will have in any given situation.

Effect of cardiac pumping on CVP | The volume of blood that is pumped out by the heart each minute always equals the volume of blood that returns to the right atrium each minute. Why, then, does the CVP fall as the CO increases? Or, why does CVP rise in cardiac failure when the CO falls?

In answering the question, we shall begin from the stage where the circulation has stopped, and the blood pressure in the arteries and veins is 10 mm Hg, the mean systemic filling pressure. We shall now assume that after every second, 100 mL of blood is quickly pumped by the heart from the venous to the arterial side. (The experiment replicates a CO of 6 L/min, with a stroke volume of 100 mL and heart rate of 60/sec.)

Let us consider what happens when for the first time, the heart shifts 100 mL of blood from the venous to the arterial side. The arterial pressure will rise, and the venous pressure will fall. Because the arterial compliance is much lower than the venous compliance (see Chapter 35), the rise in arterial pressure will be higher than the fall in venous pressure. Due to the difference of blood pressure in the arteries and veins, blood starts flowing from the arteries to the veins through the capillaries. The A-V pressure difference starts narrowing. However, not all of the 100 mL of blood that was pumped into the arteries is able to flow back into the veins in 1 second, and it is time again for the heart to shift another 100 mL of blood from the venous to the arterial side. This time, the arterial pressure rises higher, and the venous pressure falls lower than before. The A-V pressure difference is greater, and blood flows back into the veins faster.

As the sequence continues, the arterial pressure keeps rising. When the blood flows back into the veins as fast as it is being pumped out of the heart (100 mL of blood each beat), and the volume of blood in the arterial and venous compartments has stabilized, the pressure in the arteries will be 120 mm Hg.

If the above steps are repeated, translocating only 50 mL of venous blood every second into the aorta, the result will be similar, but in the steady state, the arterial pressure will be lower, and the venous pressure will be higher than before (**Fig. 34.5**).

Vascular Functions

The cardiac pump is not the sole regulator of CO: even a strong cardiac pump will fail to increase the CO if the afterload on it is very high, or the preload on it is very low. The circulatory load is controlled by vascular factors. Two primary vascular factors that control the CO are the peripheral resistance and mean systemic filling pressure. Other vascular factors are venous pumping and gravity.

Peripheral resistance falls when the arterioles are dilated, allowing arterial blood to flow into the veins with greater ease. The easier A-V flow lowers the arterial pressure and raises the venous pressure. The fall in the arterial pressure reduces the afterload on the heart and therefore increases the CO. The rise in venous pressure and CVP helps the heart to sustain the high CO. Vasodilation is by far the most important mechanism that increases the venous pressure in exercise. It is through vasodilation that tissue hypoxia is able to increase the CO. The sequence of events shown in **Fig. 34.6** ensures that whenever tissues consume more O_2, the CO increases to meet their O_2 demand.

Peripheral resistance also decreases in A-V shunts and fistulas, severe anemia (and decreased viscosity of the blood), and thyrotoxicosis (due to the vasodilation caused by the increased tissue O_2 consumption). All these conditions are associated with high CO.

The **mean systemic filling pressure** is the pressure that is present in the circulation when the heart is stopped. Stated differently, it is the pressure in the circulation when it contains a volume of blood greater than its unstressed volume. Normally, the filling pressure is ~10 mm Hg. The filling pressure increases if the blood volume increases. It also increases

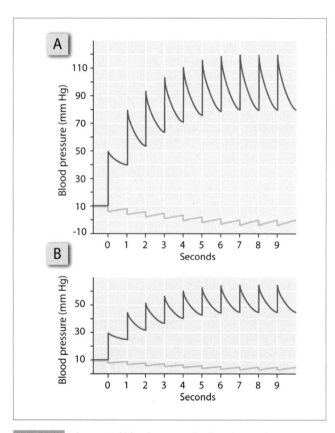

Fig. 34.5 The arterial blood pressure (red) and central venous pressure (blue) attained at two different rates of cardiac output, **(A)** 6 liters per minute and **(B)** 3 liters per minute starting from a cardiac output of 0 (the heart is stopped). With a smaller cardiac output, the arterial pressure stabilizes at a lower pressure. CVP, central venous pressure.

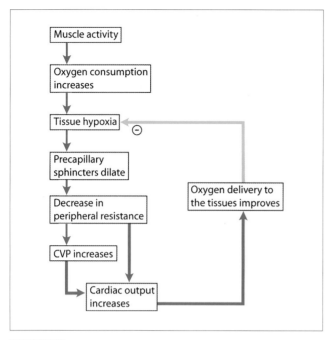

Fig. 34.6 Cardiac output changes according to the oxygen requirement of tissues, which is a major controller of cardiac output. CVP, central venous pressure.

if the venous compliance decreases, as occurs in response to sympathetic discharge. When the compliance is low, a given volume of blood would produce a greater filling pressure.

Venous return is usually defined as the amount of blood entering the right atrium per minute. Obviously, in the steady state, it is equal to the CO, ~5 L/min. The term is in wide usage and is considered to be an important factor controlling CO through changes in the diastolic filling of the heart. Thus, a fall in venous return, as occurs when the posture changes from supine to standing, reduces the CO. Similarly, in the presence of an A-V fistula, the venous return increases, and therefore the CO increases, too.

In some circumstances, the term *venous return* should be taken to mean *central venous pressure*. "Factors affecting venous return" are essentially the "vascular factors that affect the CVP." There is no inconsistency in stating that gravity reduces the CVP and therefore reduces the CO. Similarly, an A-V fistula increases the CO by reducing the peripheral resistance. It also increases the CVP, which enables the heart to sustain the high output.

Is, then, the term *venous return* a misnomer? Not quite. The CVP can rise only if there is more blood in the right atrium. More blood can be present in the right atrium only if there is less blood in the lower extremities, assuming that the amount of blood in the arterial circuit does not change much. Thus, the term *venous return* describes a *translocation of blood* from the extremities to the right atrium. To that extent, the term *return* is justifiable as long as it is not confused with a flow rate. Nonetheless, the term *venous return* has been studiously avoided in this book, if only to prevent needless confusion.

Venous "pumping" | Before discussing venous "pumping," it is important to understand the effect of steady venous compression. Application of a steady pressure on a large vein, say, the inferior vena cava, results in a biphasic response in CO. There is an *initial increase* in CO for a few seconds. The increase occurs because the blood present in the inferior vena cava gets displaced mostly toward the heart, raising the CVP. (Less blood flows back into the periphery because peripheral veins are smaller and offer more resistance to flow, whereas the central veins are larger and offer less resistance. Moreover, the limb veins have valves that prevent backflow.) The initial increase is followed by a *sustained decrease* in CO. The decrease occurs because the pressure on the inferior vena cava increases the resistance to blood flow into the atria, reducing the CVP and the filling of the heart.

We can now proceed to discuss the effect of the respiratory and muscle "pumps" that are connected in series with the heart and directly contribute to the circulatory flow rate. By propelling blood toward the heart, they increase the CVP and consequently increase the CO.

The *respiratory pump* (**Fig. 34.7**) refers to the effect of rhythmic breathing on circulatory flow rate. During inspiration, the rise in intra-abdominal pressure compresses the large abdominal veins. Because the compression is rhythmic and transient, it results in a brief increase in the CVP with each inspiration. The simultaneous inspiratory increase in intrathoracic negativity allows greater diastolic filling of the ventricles and consequently increases the CO. During expiration, the compression of the abdominal vein is relieved, and blood flows in from the periphery.

The *muscle pump* refers to the effect of intermittently contracting limb muscles on the circulatory flow rate. When limb veins are squeezed by exercising muscles, the venous blood squirts toward the heart because the venous valves prevent the blood from flowing back.

Gravity | In the upright posture, venous blood loses pressure energy and gains potential energy as it flows toward the heart (in accordance with the Bernoulli principle). The CVP is therefore low. In the recumbent position, the blood flows horizontally toward the heart; therefore, there is no conversion of pressure energy into potential energy. The CVP is thus higher.

Cardiac Output during Exercise

The cardiovascular effects of exercise depend on whether the exercise is static or dynamic (see Chapter 38).

Static exercise is associated with a massive increase in peripheral resistance because of the compression of blood vessels in the contracted muscles. This leads to a sharp reduction in CO.

Dynamic exercise is associated with a rise in CO. The hypoxia and the metabolites produced during exercise dilate the precapillary sphincter, lowering the peripheral resistance. The fall in peripheral resistance increases the CO by reducing the afterload on the heart. The higher CO would tend to lower the CVP. That, however, does not happen due to the low

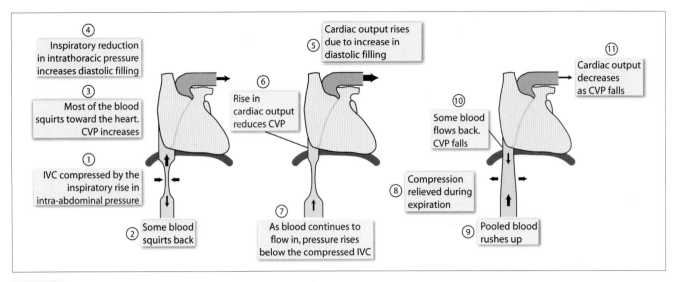

Fig. 34.7 The respiratory pump. It is observed that more blood flows from the periphery toward the inferior vena cava (IVC) (in step 9) than the amount of blood that flows back from the IVC (in step 2). Hence, although the cardiac output rises and falls during the cardiac cycle, the respiratory pump has an overall propelling effect on the circulation. The sequence of events can be followed from step 1 to 11. CVP, central venous pressure.

peripheral resistance, which also raises the venous pressure. The venous pressure is raised further by the muscle and respiratory pumping of venous blood, both of which are vigorously active in exercise. Because peripheral vasodilation increases the CO and because the vasodilation is metabolic in origin, the increase in CO, parallels the increase in tissue oxygen consumption. In athletes, the CO can rise to up to 25 L/min during exercise.

As discussed above, a rise in CO involves an increase in both stroke volume and heart rate. Tachycardia is associated with shorter diastole and reduced diastolic perfusion of coronary arteries. Hence, a healthy heart relies more on the stroke volume for increasing its output. For the same reason, a heart with low resting heart rate (bradycardia) has been called the *athlete's heart.* However, a low or moderate increase in heart rate following exercise indicates not only cardiac fitness, but also respiratory fitness. A reduction in the diffusion capacity of the lungs, for example, would cause hypoxia, resulting in a compensatory increase in CO and with it, an increase in heart rate.

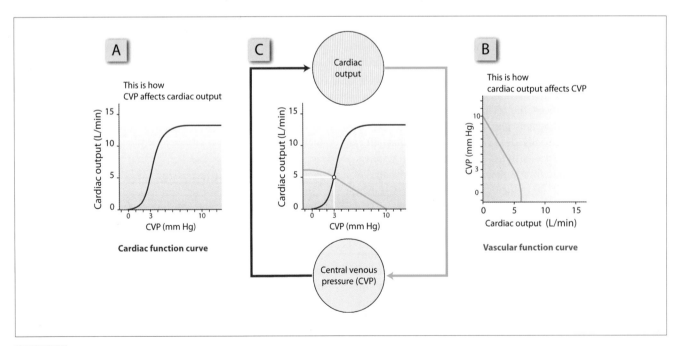

Fig. 34.8 The interdependence of cardiac output and central venous pressure (CVP). **(A)** A cardiac function curve relating CVP and the resulting cardiac output. **(B)** A vascular function curve relating cardiac output and the resulting CVP. **(C)** Both relationships plotted on a single set of axes. The point of intersection of the two curves represents the operating point for the cardiovascular system (heart and circulation).

Graphic Analysis of Cardiac Output

The graphic analysis of CO is based on the interdependence of CO and CVP. The cardiac function curve shows how the CVP affects CO. The vascular function curve shows how the CO affects the CVP. By combining the two function curves, the operant CO and CVP can be determined (**Fig. 34.8**).

Cardiac Function Curves

The cardiac function curves depict the heterometric regulation of CO: when CVP increases, there is increased ventricular filling with a consequent increase in CO. The effect plateaus off at higher levels of CVP. The cardiac function curve can be altered by several factors. There thus exists a whole family of cardiac function curves, some representing varying levels of cardiac contractility (**Fig. 34.9A**) and others representing varying levels of effective ventricular filling pressure (**Fig. 34.9B**). At any given CVP, the CO will be above normal when cardiac contractility is high and below normal when cardiac contractility is low.

Vascular Function Curves

The vascular function curve shows how changes in the CO affect the CVP. The CVP falls steeply when the CO rises. When the CO exceeds a limit (~6.0 L/min in **Fig. 34.8B**), the CVP falls steeply to zero or even below zero. At this stage, no further increase in CO is possible because the great veins get compressed by the intrathoracic pressure, which is greater than the distending pressure in the veins (CVP), effectively stopping

the flow of blood through them. Any further increase in cardiac contractility only makes the CVP more negative without increasing the CO.

The vascular factors affecting CVP have been discussed above. A rise in the *mean systemic filling pressure* shifts the vascular function curve to the right: at a given CO, the greater the filling pressure, the greater will be the CVP (**Fig. 34.9C**).

A fall in *peripheral resistance* rotates the vascular function curve clockwise about the point defined by the systemic filling pressure, as shown in **Fig. 34.9D**. Thus, at a given CO, a lower peripheral resistance is associated with a greater CVP.

Coupled Cardiac and Vascular Function Curves

The cardiac and vascular function curves can be combined into a single graph in which both cardiac and vascular function are shown as dependent on the CVP. The intersection of the two curves gives the operant values of CO and CVP. Besides its other advantages, this graphical approach corroborates that the CVP decreases whenever the CO increases due to an increase in pump efficiency, with the vascular functions remaining unchanged.

The utility of this graph is brought out best by considering the effect of sympathetic discharge on CO (**Fig. 34.10**). Sympathetic discharge causes three changes. (1) It makes the cardiac function curve hypereffective. (2) It shifts the vascular function curve to the right due to increase in filling pressure. (3) It also rotates the vascular function curve anticlockwise, due to the increased peripheral resistance caused by vasoconstriction.

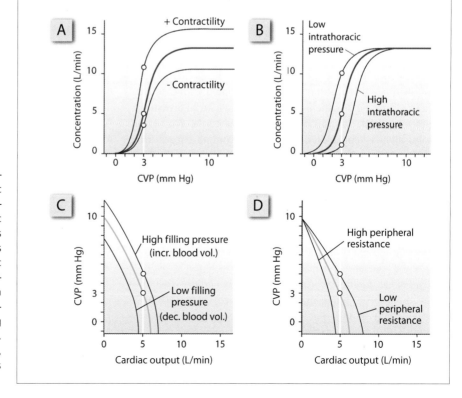

Fig. 34.9 **(A)** Cardiac function curves illustrating the effects of varying levels of cardiac contractility. **(B)** Cardiac function curves illustrating the effects of varying intrathoracic pressure. Note that at a given central venous pressure (CVP), the cardiac output increases as cardiac contractility increases or intrathoracic pressure decreases. **(C)** Vascular function curves illustrating the effects of varying the mean systemic filling pressure (altering blood volume). **(D)** Vascular function curves illustrating the effects of varying the peripheral resistance. Note that if the cardiac output is held constant, CVP increases as the filling pressure increases or the peripheral resistance decreases.

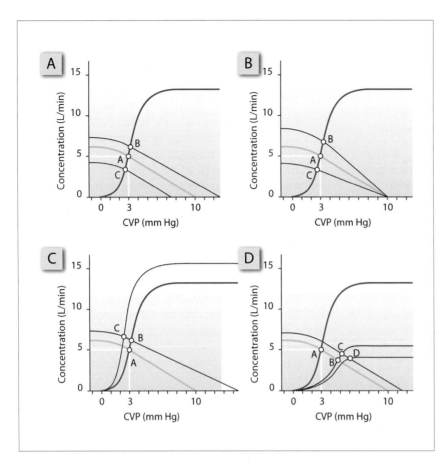

Fig. 34.10 The cardiac function curve (red) and vascular function curve (blue) intersect at A, which represents the normal cardiac output. **(A)** A rise in blood volume shifts the vascular function curve to the right and thereby increases the cardiac output from A to B. Conversely, a fall in blood volume shifts the vascular function curve to the left and reduces the cardiac output to C. **(B)** A fall in peripheral resistance rotates the vascular function curve clockwise and raises the cardiac output to B, whereas an increase in peripheral resistance lowers cardiac output to C. **(C)** During sympathetic stimulation, the vascular function curve shows the effect of simultaneous increase in blood volume and peripheral resistance: the curve shifts as well as rotates. If cardiac function is unchanged, cardiac output increases to B. If cardiac function is augmented, cardiac output rises to C. **(D)** When the cardiac function is impaired, the cardiac output falls from A to B. The compensatory increase in blood volume increases the cardiac output to C, which is still inadequate. The retention of fluid and electrolytes impairs myocardial contractility and lowers myocardial function further, and the cardiac output falls to D. The vicious cycle of decompensation continues. CVP, central venous pressure.

Cardiac Failure

Cardiac failure (or heart failure) is said to be present when the CO is not large enough to meet the demands of all of the tissues of the body.

If cardiac failure is present, then atrial pressure is high. This state is called left-sided or right-sided failure depending on whether the pressure is elevated in the left or the right atrium. In the long run, failure of one side of the heart leads to the failure of the other side. Cardiac failure is associated with cardiomegaly (cardiac enlargement) because the high atrial pressure results in greater diastolic filling of the ventricle. This can be conveniently represented by pressure–volume curves for the heart. **Figure 34.11A** represents a normal heart. **Figure 34.11B** represents a failing heart; filling is increased, as is end-diastolic volume.

Left-sided failure is associated with excess blood in pulmonary blood vessels (pulmonary congestion) and transudation of fluid into the alveolar interstitium (pulmonary edema). During physical exertion, there is a further increase in pulmonary venous pressure, resulting in dyspnea.

Right-sided failure or *congestive cardiac failure* results in accumulation of blood in the systemic veins. The CVP increases, which is apparent from the raised jugular venous pressure (JVP). Hepatomegaly (hepatic enlargement) occurs as the increased CVP is transmitted backward into the hepatic portal vein. Generalized edema occurs as the raised CVP is transmitted all the way back to the systemic capillaries. It is

prominent in the dependent portions of the body where the capillary pressure is higher due to gravity. The high CVP is also transmitted to the coronary veins, reducing the diastolic perfusion of the myocardium and predisposing to myocardial ischemia. The increase in myocardial oxygen demand due to the cardiomegaly also contributes to the risk of myocardial infarction.

Cardiac failure may be associated with a normal CO, a low CO, or a high CO. When the CO is normal, it is called a *compensated cardiac failure* to emphasize that the cardiac function is impaired and that the normal CO is being maintained through a heterometric mechanism.

When the CO is reduced, it is called a *decompensated cardiac failure*. It is associated with hypotension and poor renal perfusion, leading to renin-degranulation. The activation of the renin–angiotensin–aldosterone system leads to hypervolemia, increasing the CVP and thereby aggravating the failure. If the CO drops very low, it can lead to cardiogenic shock.

High-output cardiac failure is seen in thyrotoxicosis, large A-V fistulas, and wet beriberi. In these conditions, the peripheral resistance is markedly reduced, allowing the high arterial pressure to be transmitted to the venous side and thereby increase the CVP. The high CVP increases the CO. However, the CO does not rise high enough to reduce the CVP to a normal level.

The aim of treatment is twofold: improving cardiac contractility and reducing the load on the heart. Digitalis is used for increasing cardiac contractility. Reduction of the load on

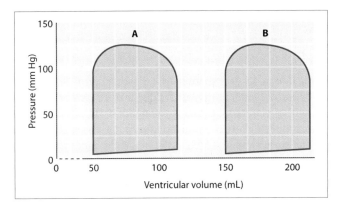

Fig. 34.11 Pressure–volume (PV) loops of cardiac function. **(A)** The PV loop for a normal heart. **(B)** The loop for a failing heart shows that the heart is doing the same amount of work (area of the loop is the same in both), but at a higher end-diastolic volume. Note also that the failing heart has greater diastolic filling.

the heart is achieved by administration of diuretics and ACE inhibitors (inhibitors of angiotensin-converting enzyme). Both reduce the blood volume.

Summary

- Cardiac output, the blood flow out of the heart each minute, is the product of stroke volume and heart rate.

- Cardiac output is determined by both cardiac and vascular functions.

- Stroke volume (and hence cardiac output) is determined by preload (the filling of the heart) and afterload (the pressure against which the ventricles must eject blood).

- Stroke volume is also determined by cardiac contractility, which is a function of the concentration of Ca^{2+} inside the myocyte.

- Cardiac output is greatly increased during exercise.

Applying What You Know

34.1. From the available data, calculate the value of Mrs. Daniels' *right* ventricular stroke output.

34.2. Mrs. Daniels stenosed mitral valve would reduce her stroke volume and hence her cardiac output if no compensation occurred. What mechanisms are helping to sustain her left ventricular stroke volume? Explain.

34.3. Although her jugular veins are *not* distended, Mrs. Daniels is showing some signs of elevated *central venous pressure* (pulmonary and pedal edema). What could be done to lower her CVP and thereby improve her condition?

35 Circulatory Pathway and Hemodynamics

Circulatory Pathway

Circulatory Pathway in the Adult

Blood is pumped by the heart through a closed circuit of blood vessels (**Fig. 35.1**). The right and left ventricles of the heart function as two pumps connected in series; the entire output of one ventricle enters the other ventricle. From the left ventricle, blood flows through the arteries, arterioles, and systemic capillaries and back through the venules and veins to the right atrium. This circuit constitutes the *systemic circulation.* From the right ventricle, blood flows through pulmonary arteries, pulmonary capillaries, and pulmonary veins to return to the left atrium. This circuit constitutes the *pulmonary circulation.*

There is a small flow of blood from the systemic circulation (in the bronchial circuit) directly into the pulmonary circulation, bypassing the right ventricle. This constitutes a *physiologic shunt.*

As the blood flows through the capillaries, a part of its plasma gets filtered into the interstitial spaces, then drains out through lymphatic channels as lymph. The lymph flows through the thoracic duct and the right lymphatic duct to drain into the subclavian veins, thereby reentering the systemic circulation. This circuit constitutes the *lymphatic circulation,* which is disposed in parallel to the systemic circulation. A similar lymphatic system exists in the lungs also, but the lymph is formed only in the pleural and bronchial capillaries and not by the alveolar capillaries. Hence, there is no separate lymphatic system that is disposed in parallel to the pulmonary circuit because bronchial and pleural capillaries belong to the systemic circulation.

Circulatory Pathway in the Fetus

In the fetus, it is the placenta and not the fetal lungs that oxygenates the blood. Deoxygenated fetal blood is carried to the placenta by the umbilical artery, a branch of the femoral artery, and oxygenated blood is brought back from the placenta by the umbilical vein (**Fig. 35.2A**). The umbilical vein passes through the liver, where it joins the portal and hepatic veins, which drain into the inferior vena cava. The umbilical vein is also connected directly with the inferior vena cava through a connecting vein called the *ductus venosus.*

Inside the right atrium, the blood from the superior and inferior vena cavae flow in two separate streams without mixing much. Blood from the superior vena cava mostly enters the right ventricle, which pumps the blood into the pulmonary arteries. Because the fetal lungs are collapsed, the pulmonary capillary resistance is very high. Hence, most of the blood pumped into the pulmonary artery flows out into the aorta through a connecting artery called the *ductus arteriosus.* A much smaller amount flows through the pulmonary capillaries into the left atrium. Blood from the inferior vena cava mostly enters the left atrium through the *foramen ovale,* a small hole

in the interatrial wall guarded by a flap that permits only one-way flow of blood. In the left atrium, it mixes with the small amount of blood brought in by the pulmonary veins and then enters the left ventricle, which pumps it into the aorta.

The aorta supplies blood to the brain and upper part of the body through the common carotids and then continues as the descending aorta to supply the lower part of the body. Significantly, the highly deoxygenated blood from the pulmonary vein flowing into the ductus arteriosus enters the aortic arch only after the origin of the common carotids, so that the brain receives relatively better oxygenated blood. It is important to note that in the fetus, both ventricles are pumping blood into the aorta. Thus, the two ventricles operate in parallel and not in series, as in the adult heart.

The mechanism of circulatory changes at birth | The umbilical cord constricts when it comes in contact with the relatively colder atmospheric air (**Fig. 35.3**). Its subsequent clamping completely stops the flow of oxygenated blood to the fetus through the umbilical vein. This asphyxiates the fetus, stimulating it to take its first breath. As air distends the lungs, the resistance of the pulmonary vessels reduces markedly, and the left atrial pressure increases. On the other hand, the elimination of the placental circulation increases the resistance of the systemic circulation. The pressure in the pulmonary artery therefore falls below the aortic pressure, causing a reversal of blood flow through the ductus arteriosus: for a few days, blood continues to flow through it from the aorta into the pulmonary artery. The rise in the partial pressure of oxygen (PO_2) caused by breathing through the lungs gradually brings about the closure of the ductus arteriosus by causing contraction of the smooth muscles in its walls. A prostaglandin, $PGE_{2\alpha}$, seems to mediate the closure. Over time, it reduces to a fibrous band called the *ligamentum arteriosum.* Similarly, the ductus venosus is reduced to a fibrous *ligamentum venosum,* and the intra-abdominal part of the umbilical vein gets converted into the *ligamentum teres* (**Fig. 35.2B**).

Another consequence of the fall in pulmonary capillary resistance is that the blood pumped by the right ventricle starts flowing easily through the pulmonary vasculature into the left atrium. This reduces the pressures in the right atrium and right ventricle due to the reduced afterload on them. The pressure in the left atrium now exceeds the right atrial pressure, and blood tries to flow from left to right through the foramen ovale. That, however, is not permitted by the flap (septum secondum) guarding the foramen ovale, which subsequently closes permanently.

Congenital defects in circulatory pathway | Any abnormal communication between the left-sided and right-sided chambers of the heart usually results in a *left-to-right shunting* of blood due to the higher pressures in the left-sided chambers (**Fig. 35.4**). This is seen in congenital heart diseases such as an *atrial septal defect* and a *ventricular septal defect.* It is also seen when the ductus arteriosus fails to get obliterated after

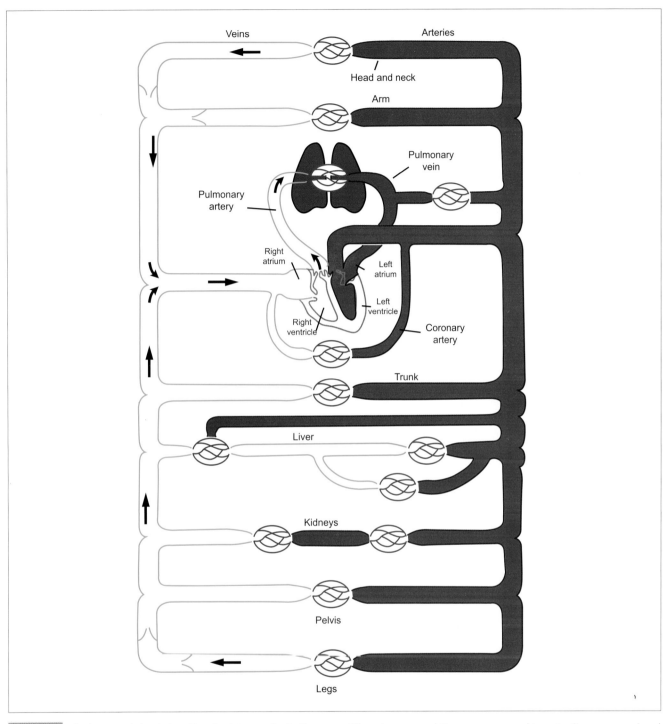

Fig. 35.1 The heart and circulation. The circulatory paths to the many different organs and tissues are arranged in series (in some cases) and parallel (most often).

birth, a condition known as the *patent ductus arteriosus.* As a result of the shunt, a part of the left ventricular output recirculates through the lungs. It thus causes volume overload of the pulmonary circulation and right ventricle but does not cause cyanosis (desaturation of blood).

Cyanosis does occur in the *tetralogy of Fallot.* Two of the four defects that characterize the tetralogy are ventricular septal defect (a hole between the ventricles) and pulmonary stenosis (a narrowing of the pulmonary artery). The pulmonary stenosis markedly increases the right ventricular pressure,

leading to the third defect, right ventricular hypertrophy. The high right ventricular pressure leads to a *right-to-left shunting* of blood through the ventricular septal defect, mixing of the deoxygenated blood in the right ventricle with the oxygenated blood in the left ventricle. The oxygenation of arterial blood therefore gets diluted, leading to central cyanosis. The fourth defect in Fallot's tetralogy is the "overriding" of the aorta on the ventricular septum. This allows right ventricular blood to move directly into the aorta, which too constitutes a right-to-left shunt.

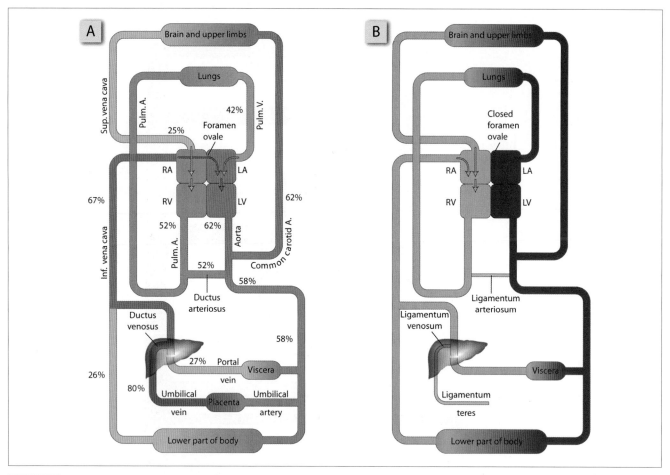

Fig. 35.2 **(A)** The fetal circulation and **(B)** circulatory changes present at birth. The fetal circulation must accommodate the placenta, which is the site at which fetal blood is oxygenated. LA, left atrium; LV, left ventricle; RA, right atrium; RV, right ventricle.

Vascular System

The vascular system begins with the aorta and the pulmonary artery, which originates from the ventricles. Each vessel ramifies separately and successively into smaller arteries, arterioles, and capillaries. The capillaries join together and drain successively into the venules and veins. The largest veins drain into the atria. The blood vessels of different types and caliber have different structural and functional characteristics (**Fig. 35.5**).

General Model: Reservoir

The vascular compartment is a reservoir in which things are transported between cells and between the external environment and the cells. The amount of any substance in the vascular compartment, whether water itself or any of the solutes dissolved in it, depends on the transport of things *into* the blood and the transport of things *out of* the blood.

Arteries and Arterioles

Arteries | All arteries and arterioles have three concentric layers in their wall (**Fig. 35.5C**): an inner layer called the tunica intima made of squamous endothelial cells, an intermediate layer called the tunica media composed of smooth muscle cells oriented circumferentially, and an outer coat called the tunica adventitia made of fibroblasts and collagen fibers. The tunica intima and tunica media are separated by the internal elastic lamina. The tunica media and tunica adventitia are separated by the external elastic lamina.

Large arteries have a lot of elastic tissues in their wall. The elastic walls prevent abrupt changes in blood pressure. The walls are stretched during systole as blood enters, stretching the elastic elements in their walls. This storage of energy slows the rise in blood pressure. During diastole, when flow into the vessels is less than flow out, the walls recoil back, maintaining the blood pressure.

General Model: Elasticity

The elastic elements of blood vessels, and the heart, behave exactly like all other elastic structures that you have encountered. When stretched, they store energy that can be used to do work.

The **medium and small arteries** contain less elastic tissue and more muscle fibers than the large elastic arteries. The

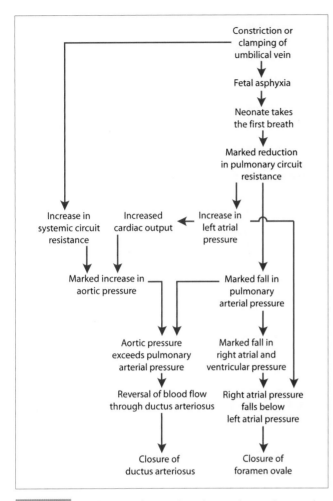

Fig. 35.3 Mechanisms that produce the circulatory changes that occur at birth.

smallest arteries terminate in the muscular arterioles, ~100 to 50 μm in diameter.

Arterioles act as resistance vessels. They are the major site of the resistance to blood flow. They are also the site at which the resistance of the circulation is controlled by chemical and neural inputs (Chapter 37). The terminal arterioles are the terminal continuation of the muscular arterioles and are ~20 μm in diameter.

Metarterioles branch off almost at right angles from terminal arterioles (**Fig. 35.6**). Their proximal portion is discontinuously coated with smooth muscle cells. Its distal segment, which is also called the *thoroughfare* or *preferential channel,* is devoid of smooth muscle coat. The thoroughfare channels open into the venules.

Capillaries and Postcapillary Venules
Capillaries branch off from metarterioles and terminal arterioles. Capillaries are of two types: the true capillaries and the thoroughfare channels (**Fig. 35.6**). The *true capillaries* form an anastomotic network before reuniting and draining into a venule. The origin of a true capillary, whether directly from the terminal arteriole or from the metarteriole, is guarded by a *precapillary sphincter,* which is made of a single layer of

single-unit smooth muscle and is well innervated by sympathetic fibers. True capillaries permit exchange of plasma and solutes through pores in their walls, which is the main function of capillaries and, indeed, of the entire circulatory system. *Thoroughfare channels* do not have any nutritive role.

Postcapillary venules are ~20 μm in diameter and are not much different from capillaries. They participate in capillary exchange and are the preferred site for leukocytic emigration. The walls of larger venules (~50 μm or more) have smooth muscles in them.

Veins
Veins, like arteries, are made of the tunica intima, tunica media, and tunica adventitia. However, the layers and the boundaries between them are less distinct. Veins show considerable venoconstriction in response to sympathetic nerves and circulating vasoconstrictors like endothelins.

Veins are easily distensible, partly because of the sparse smooth muscles in their wall and partly due to their elliptical cross-sectional contour, which becomes circular when distended. Their distensibility makes them excellent capacitance vessels or blood reservoirs (**Fig. 35.7A**). They can accommodate large amounts of blood with minimal rise of pressure and are therefore called a *low-pressure system,* unlike the arterial system, which is a *high-pressure system.* The venous system (venules and veins) accounts for more than 50% of the total blood storage capacity of the circulatory system. If 100 mL of blood is transfused into circulation, less than 1 mL of it will enter the high-pressure arterial system, and the rest will locate itself in the low-pressure systemic veins, pulmonary circulation, and heart chambers other than the left ventricle.

The intima of the limb veins are folded at intervals to form venous valves (**Fig. 35.8**) that prevent retrograde flow. Valves are absent in the great veins and the very small veins.

Arteriovenous Anastomoses
The arteriovenous anastomoses are short channels that connect arterioles to venules, bypassing the capillaries. The arterial end of the channel structurally resembles an artery, and its venous end structurally resembles a vein. They have muscular walls and are abundantly innervated by both adrenergic and cholinergic nerve fibers. They are present in the skin of fingers, palms, and earlobes, and they have an important thermoregulatory role. When they are open, they allow a large amount of blood to flow through the skin, dissipating heat to the exterior.

Hemodynamics

Determinants of Blood Flow
The flow of blood, or the amount of blood moving through a vessel each minute ($\dot{Q}$), is determined by the pressure gradient (ΔP) and by the resistance to flow (R) that is present in the system. Thus, we can write a form of Ohm's law for the circulation:

$$\dot{Q} = \frac{\Delta P}{R} \qquad (35.1)$$

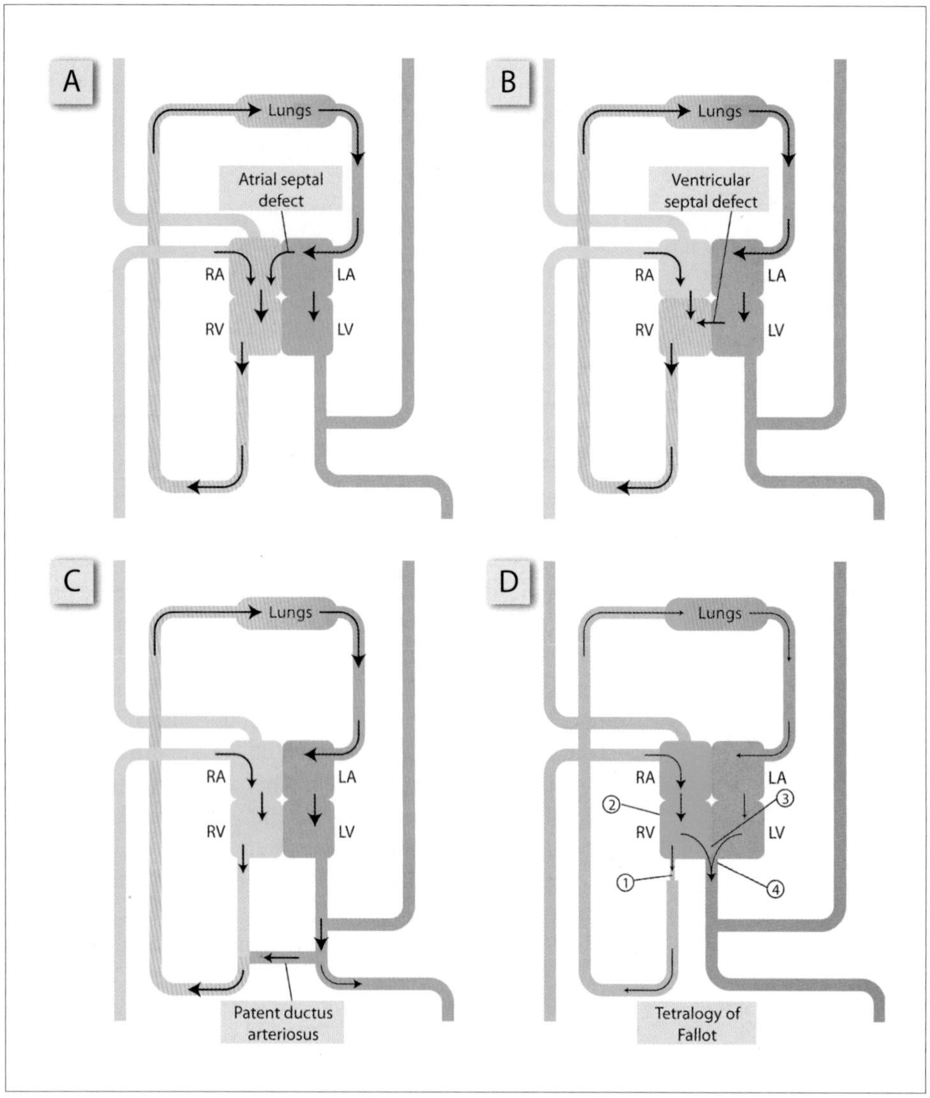

Fig. 35.4 Congenital heart diseases. **(A)** In a patient with an atrial septal defect, a patent opening is present between the left and right atria. **(B)** When a ventricular septal defect is present, there is a patent flow path between the two ventricles. **(C)** In some individuals, the ductus arteriosus remains patent after birth. **(D)** The four defects in the tetralogy of Fallot are (1) pulmonary stenosis, (2) right ventricular hypertrophy, (3) ventricular septal defect, and (4) overriding of aorta on the ventricular septum. LA, left atrium; LV, left ventricle; RA, right atrium; RV, right ventricle.

General Model: Flow

This is one of many applications of the general flow model that describes the movement of "stuff" (solutes, blood, air) in the body. We first applied this model in describing the origins of the diffusion potential across cell membranes (see Chapter 6). There the energy gradient was created by the difference in concentration inside and outside the cell (the concentration gradient), and the resistance to flow was represented by the permeability of the sodium (Na^+) and potassium (K^+) leak channels (the more permeable, the lower the resistance). Here the gradient to be considered is a hydrostatic pressure gradient, and the resistance to flow is a property of the system through which flow is occurring (as we will see, this is most powerfully determined by the diameter of the vessel we are looking at). You will encounter additional examples of this general model of flow later.

The ΔP across the ends of a vessel is generated by the contraction of the heart. R is determined by the properties of the blood and properties of the vessel in which flow is occurring.

Resistance to flow in a vessel is determined by three variables: the length of the vessel (L), the viscosity of the fluid (η) that is flowing, and the cross-sectional area of the vessel that is represented by the radius (r). Poiseuille's law describes the relationship between these variables:

$$R = \frac{8\eta L}{\Pi r^4} \tag{35.2}$$

Note that the radius is raised to the 4th power, which means that even a small change in the radius of a vessel has a large effect on its resistance to flow.

When resistances are arranged in series (see **Fig. 35.9A**), the total resistance that is present is represented by

$$R_{total} = R_1 + R_2 + \cdots + R_n \tag{35.3}$$

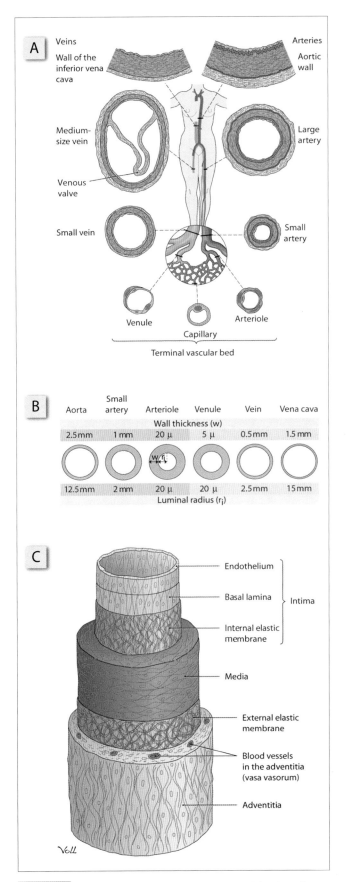

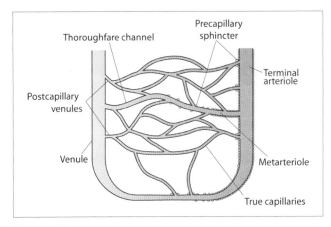

Fig. 35.6 The terminal arteriole and venule are connected through metarterioles and capillaries. The origin of true capillaries, whether directly from the arteriole or from the metarteriole, is guarded by the precapillary sphincter.

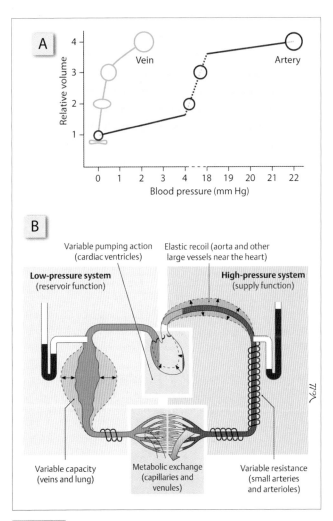

Fig. 35.5 **(A)** Different types of blood vessels and **(B)** their dimensions. **(C)** The many layers that make up the structure of an artery.

Fig. 35.7 **(A)** Contour of veins and arteries in cross section. When engorged with blood, the contour changes from elliptical to circular. **(B)** The arterial system is a high-pressure, high- (but variable) resistance, low-capacity system. The venous system is a low-pressure, low-resistance, high- (but variable) capacity system.

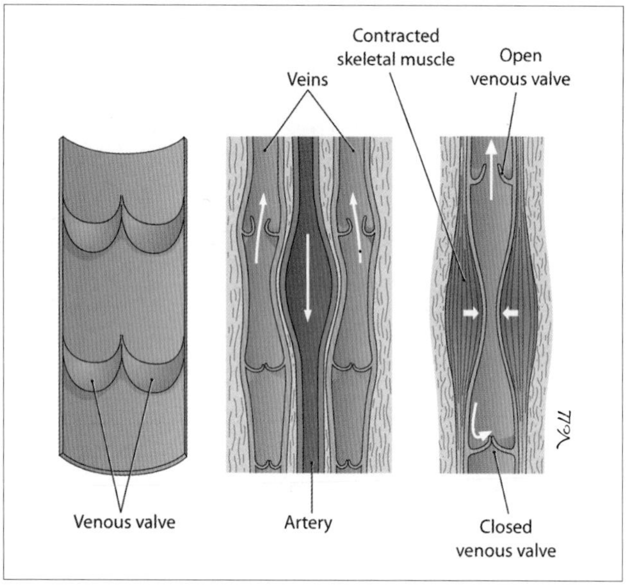

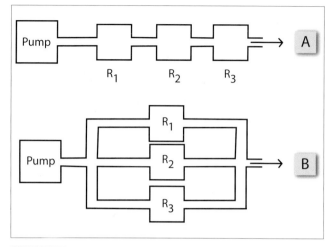

Fig. 35.8 Venous valves and muscle pumping. When the muscles surrounding a vein contract, the vein is compressed, and the pressure inside is increased. Consequently, the downstream valve closes, and blood is "pumped" toward the heart.

Thus, the total resistance is greater than any single resistance in the system.

When resistances are arranged in parallel (see **Fig. 35.9B**), the total resistance that is present is represented by

$$\frac{1}{R_{total}} = \frac{1}{R_1} + \frac{1}{R_2} + \cdots \frac{1}{R_n} \qquad (35.4)$$

Thus, the total resistance is less than the resistance of any of the resistances in the system.

In the circulation (see **Fig. 35.1**), many of the tissue beds (organs) are in parallel with one another. This means that each of them has the same ΔP across them, and the flow through each organ is determined by the resistance to flow in each pathway. Thus, as long as ΔP is held constant (see Chapter 38), each organ receives the flow required to maintain its function based on its resistance.

Determinants of Blood Flow Velocity
The velocity of flow (distance/time) is determined by the magnitude of the flow (volume/time) and the cross-sectional area of the vessel. We can express this as

$$Velocity\ (V) = \frac{flow\ (\dot{Q})}{area\ (A)} \qquad (35.5)$$

This, then, tells us that as flow in a vessel increases, the flow velocity also increases. It also says that if a vessel gets smaller (and the flow is unchanged), the flow velocity must increase.

In the circulation, the various types of blood vessels differ greatly in their size and number (**Table 35.1**). For example,

Fig. 35.9 (A) When resistances are arranged in series, all the flow goes through all the resistances. (B) When resistances are arranged in parallel, the flow is divided, with each resistance getting only a portion of the total flow.

we can see that capillaries are individually the smallest vessel type (0.008 mm in diameter), and there are an enormous number of them (1.2 × 10⁹).

From the dimensions listed in **Table 35.1**, it is possible to calculate the total cross-sectional area (TCSA in mm²), the flow rate (FR in mm³/sec), the flow velocity (F in mm/sec), and the relative resistance (assuming that the resistance of the aorta is 1) if we assume a cardiac output of 5.4 L/min (which is equivalent to 90,000 mm³/sec). The results of these calculations are tabulated in **Table 35.2**.

Two of the results in **Table 35.2** deserve special mention. The highest resistance to flow is encountered in the arterioles (7.81), not in smaller vessels, such as the capillaries (5.09). The explanation for this is that the total cross-sectional area of all of the arterioles is appreciably smaller than the total cross-sectional area of all of the capillaries. This is illustrated in another way in **Fig. 35.10**, which shows the pressure drop across the various vascular elements between the left ventricle and

Table 35.1 Comparative Dimensions of Different Types of Blood Vessels in a Dog

	Diameter (mm)	Length (mm)	Number
Aorta	10	400	1
Large arteries	3	200	40
Main arterial branches	1	100	600
Terminal branches	0.6	10	1800
Arterioles	0.02	2	40,000,000
Capillaries	0.008	1	1,200,000,000
Venules	0.03	2	80,000,000
Terminal veins	1.5	10	1800
Main venous branches	2.4	100	600
Large veins	6	200	40
Vena cava	12.5	400	1

Table 35.2 Comparison of Total Cross-sectional Area (TCSA), Flow Rate (FR), Flow Velocity (FV), and Relative Resistance (Comparison to Aortic Resistance) of Different Types of Blood Vessels

	TCSA (mm²)	FR (mm³/s)	FV (mm/s)	Relative Resistance
Aorta	79	90,000	1146	1.00
Large arteries	283	2250	318	1.54
Main arterial branches	471	150	191	4.17
Terminal branches	509	50	177	1.07
Arterioles	12,566	0.00225	7	7.81
Capillaries	60,319	0.000075	1	5.09
Venules	56,549	0.001125	2	0.77
Terminal veins	3181	50	28	0.03
Main venous branches	2714	150	33	0.13
Large veins	1131	2250	80	0.10
Vena cava	123	90,000	733	0.41

the right atrium. The largest drop in pressure occurs along the arterioles.

The other result of importance is that the velocity of flow is lowest in the capillaries (1 mm/s). The explanation is simply the enormous number of capillaries in parallel and thus the enormous total cross-sectional area that must be crossed. The significance of this lies in the function of the capillaries as the site of molecular exchange between the vascular compartment and the tissues. The very low velocity in the capillaries allows for adequate time for diffusion to transport solutes between these two compartments.

Work Done

The blood is set into motion by the pumping action of the heart. In the language of physics, work is done *by* the heart *on* the blood in the circulation. Ignoring the wastage of energy in the form of heat, the work done by the heart exactly equals the energy gained by circulating blood.

Work done by the heart | If the ventricles contract against closed valves (see the discussion of isovolumetric contraction in Chapter 33), there is no change in ventricular volume, and therefore no external work is done (the contracted myocardial cells are, however, doing internal work). External work is done by the ventricle only when its volume changes and is given by the formula

$$\text{Work done } (W) = P \times \Delta V \tag{35.6}$$

where P is the intraventricular pressure and ΔV is the change in volume. It can be estimated by measuring out the area enclosed in the pressure–volume loop of the cardiac cycle (see **Fig. 33.6**). The rise in intraventricular pressure and the de-

crease in ventricular volume are determined by the tension developed in the ventricular muscle fibers. Assuming the ventricular cavity to be spherical, the relation between fiber tension (T), ventricular radius (R), and intraventricular pressure (P) is given by Laplace's law.

$$P = \frac{2T}{R} \tag{35.7}$$

The law tells us that the rise in myocardial fiber tension results in a greater rise in ventricular pressure when the ventricular volume is low. Thus, although an increase in the end-diastolic volume increases the strength of myocardial contraction and tension (in accordance with Starling's law of the heart), the extra myocardial tension generated fails to produce greater ventricular pressure at higher end-diastolic volume (in accordance with Laplace's law). Hence, in a dilated, failing heart, the consequences of Starling's law and Laplace's law tend to cancel each other out.

The **energy gained by circulating blood** can take various forms. For example, it could lead to the compression of blood. That does not happen because blood, like any other liquid, is incompressible. The efficient circulation of blood is possible only because blood is incompressible. Had it been compressible, cardiac pumping would have compressed the blood instead of making it flow. Gases, however, are highly compressible. *Air embolism*—the entry of air into the circulation—has serious consequences. When a large amount of air enters the circulation, it fills the heart and effectively stops the circulation,

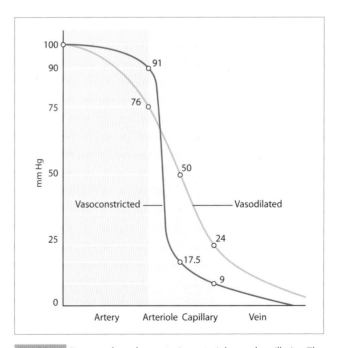

Fig. 35.10 Pressure drop along arteries, arterioles, and capillaries. The arterioles are the site of the greatest resistance and hence the greatest pressure drop. The numbers on each curve are the pressures at that point in the circulation.

causing sudden death. When a small amount of air enters the circulation, it flows in blood as bubbles that lodge in the small blood vessels, stopping the flow of blood and causing ischemia. Small air bubbles do not cause any problem in the heart or the large vessels.

Because blood is incompressible, the energy gained by the circulation is converted into other forms of energy: potential energy, kinetic energy, and pressure energy. *Potential energy* is represented by the vertical height through which a column of blood rises against gravity. *Kinetic energy* is represented by the motion of blood. *Pressure energy* is exerted laterally on the walls of the blood vessels. According to Bernoulli's principle, the total of all three forms of fluid energy will always be constant and, in this case, will equal the work done by the ventricle.

$$\begin{aligned} \text{Work done by} \atop \text{the ventricle} = {\text{Potential energy} \atop \text{of blood}} + {\text{Kinetic energy} \atop \text{of blood}} \\ + {\text{Pressure energy} \atop \text{of blood}} \end{aligned} \qquad (35.8)$$

There are several possibilities for how the total energy is apportioned among its three forms. (1) If the entire circulatory system is horizontal, as in a recumbent individual, for example, there is no possibility of the blood rising through a height. Hence, the entire work done by the ventricle will be converted partly into kinetic energy and partly into pressure energy. (2) If the blood is forced up a vertical column, its potential energy increases. The increase in potential energy must necessarily be accompanied by a decrease in pressure energy and kinetic energy. (3) Arteriolar constriction increases the blood flow velocity through the arteriole but decreases blood flow velocity in the arteries. The reduction in kinetic energy of blood in the artery is associated with a rise in arterial blood pressure. The increase in kinetic energy of blood in the arteriole is associated with a fall in arteriolar blood pressure. However, only the arterial blood pressure is important clinically. Similarly, when a vessel is narrowed by an atherosclerotic plaque, the velocity of flow in the constricted segment increases. The increase in the kinetic energy results in a reduction in the lateral pressure in the affected segment. The narrowing, therefore, tends to maintain itself.

It can thus be appreciated from Bernoulli's principle that for a given amount of energy imparted to blood circulation by the contracting heart, the rise in blood pressure depends on the *velocity and rate of blood flow* (which affect the kinetic energy of blood) and the *effect of gravity* (which affects the potential energy of blood). These two factors are discussed below.

General Model: Energy

For the heart to perform, this work requires the expenditure of energy. This energy is available to the cardiac muscle cells in the form of adenosine triphosphate (ATP) produced by the cell's metabolism (principally by the oxidation of glucose).

Effect of blood viscosity on blood flow | Although the effect of viscosity on fluid flow is given by the Poiseuille–Hagen formula, the formula is valid only for Newtonian fluids and is not precisely applicable to blood, which is not a Newtonian fluid. The viscosity of blood decreases with an increase in shear rate. This is especially marked at low shear rates. This anomalous viscosity of blood is attributable to *axial streaming* of blood cells at high shear rates. Axial streaming means that the cells occupy the central axis of the tube through which blood is flowing. This leaves a 5 μm wide cell-free zone immediately adjacent to the vessel wall. This cell-free zone produces less friction with the vessel wall; therefore, the viscosity is lower.

The involvement of axial streaming in determining the viscosity of the blood means that blood viscosity is determined by the hematocrit. Thus, the viscosity of blood when polycythemia (abnormally high number of red blood cells [RBCs]) or anemia (a lower than normal number of RBCs) is present is significantly altered.

Axial streaming also explains the *Fåhreus–Lindqvist effect:* the reduction in blood viscosity with a decrease in tube diameter. Because the cell-free zone has a constant width of ~5 μm, expressed as a percentage of the tube diameter, it is much greater for smaller tubes and therefore results in a lower viscosity.

Another consequence of axial streaming is *plasma skimming:* a vessel that branches off from the main blood vessel at a large angle carries way more plasma than cells because the cell-free zone lies at the periphery of flowing blood (**Fig. 35.11**). It explains why the hematocrit of capillary blood is ~25% lower than the whole-body hematocrit. In large vessels, a rise in hematocrit causes an appreciable rise in viscosity. However, in vessels smaller than 100 μm in diameter, like the arterioles, capillaries, and venules, the viscosity change is much less than it is in large vessels. This is why hematocrit changes have relatively little effect on the peripheral resistance except when the changes are large.

Critical closing pressure | If one goes by the Poiseuille–Hagen formula, the flow of blood through a blood vessel of finite length can never be zero unless the pressure gradient is zero. It is, however, observed that the blood flow reduces to zero well before the pressure gradient reduces to zero. The pressure gradient at which blood flow through a vessel reduces to zero

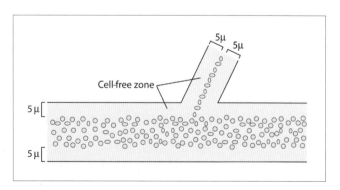

Fig. 35.11 An illustration of the phenomenon of axial streaming and plasma skimming.

is called the *critical closing pressure* or the *zero flow pressure.* When the distending pressure in a vessel is lower than the pressure outside the vessel, it must collapse, preventing flow from occurring. This is an important phenomenon to consider when thinking about blood flow in certain circulations, such as the cerebral circulation.

Turbulent flow | The flow of blood in the blood vessels, like the flow of liquids in narrow rigid tubes, is normally laminar or streamlined. The laminar flow, however, occurs only up to a certain critical velocity. At or above that velocity, flow becomes turbulent. Streamlined flow is silent, but turbulent flow creates sounds. Turbulence also depends on other factors, and these are included in the *Reynolds number*, a calculated dimensionless number. When the Reynolds number gets high, the probability of turbulent flow increases. In anemia, for example, the Reynolds number increases because the viscosity of blood is low, and the cardiac output is high. Hence, there is higher probability of turbulence, which is associated with soft systolic murmurs over the cardiac area. Constriction of an artery increases the velocity of blood flow through the constriction, producing turbulence as the Reynolds number increases. The turbulence produces sound beyond the constriction, examples of which are the bruits heard over arteries constricted by atherosclerotic plaques, the murmurs over stenosed and leaking valves, and the Korotkoff sounds that are heard during sphygmomanometry (**Table 35.3**).

Effect of Gravity on Circulation

Effect of normal gravity | Both venous and arterial pressures are affected by gravity, increasing or decreasing by an amount that is given by the formula hρg (see Pressure subsection, Appendix A). Thus, the pressure increases by 0.77 mm Hg for each centimeter below the right atrium and decreases by the same amount for each centimeter above the right atrium (**Fig. 35.12**).

Venous pressure ~5 mm above the heart is zero. Above 5 mm, all veins are in a collapsed state because the blood pressure inside them is less than zero (i.e., subatmospheric). The jugular vein rises straight up from the right atrium and acts as a manometer for the right atrial pressure, which is also called the central venous pressure (CVP). Because the CVP is greater than zero, blood is pushed up some distance into the collapsed jugular vein, which then gets distended. The upper limit of the distended jugular vein shows pulsations called the *jugular venous pulse* (JVP), which are synchronous with the atrial pres-

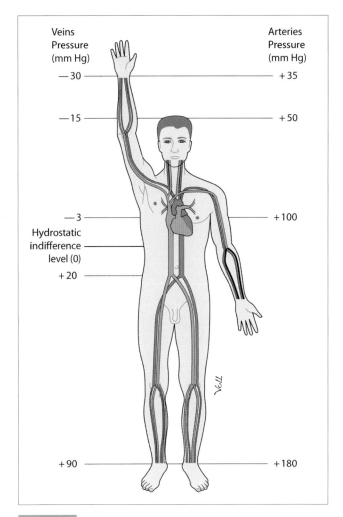

Fig. 35.12 Effect of gravity on arterial pressure. In an erect (standing) individual, pressures above the heart are decreased, and pressures below the heart are increased.

sure waves. The vertical height of the distended segment of the jugular vein gives the jugular venous pressure (**Fig. 35.13**).

In the head and neck, all the veins are in a collapsed state. The pressure is subatmospheric (about –10 mm Hg) in the dural sinuses, which do not collapse completely, as their walls are fixed to the cranium. If a dural sinus is opened up during a neurosurgical procedure with the patient seated, air is sucked into the sinus, resulting in an air embolism.

In the lower limbs, blood tends to accumulate in the more dependent parts, especially if the venous valves are incompetent. This is known as *venous pooling* (although it should be kept in mind that blood is flowing continuously, and that what has changed is the volume of blood in the veins), and its cause can be appreciated if one considers that a continuous vertical column of venous blood extending from the right atrium to the foot would exert a downward pressure of 90 mm Hg at the foot. The pressure would be transmitted back into capillaries and cause pedal edema due to transudation of fluids. If such a high pressure does not normally exist at the foot, it is because the tall column of venous blood is broken up into shorter columns by the venous valves: each venous valve bears the downward

Table 35.3 Phases of Korotkoff Sounds at Different Levels of Blood Pressure

Phase 1	Tapping sounds, as produced with the fingertips.
Phase 2	Knocking sounds, as produced by the knuckles.
Phase 3	Thumping sounds as produced with the fist.
Phase 4	Patting and wiping sounds as produced by the palm. For best simulation, pat softly and glide the palm over the surface of the table. Technically, it is described as muffled sound.

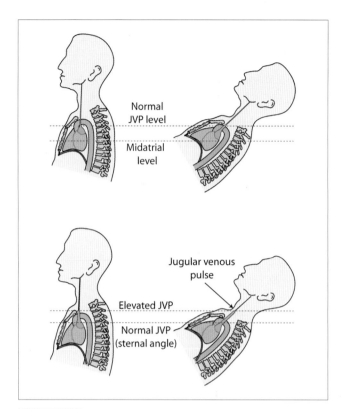

Fig. 35.13 The jugular venous pressure (JVP). Even when slightly elevated, the jugular venous pulse remains hidden behind the manubrium sterni. Tilting the patient makes the pulse visible in the neck. The jugular venous pressure is taken as the vertical height of the pulse from the right atrium.

pressure exerted by the short column of venous blood above it. When the valves are incompetent, the venous pressure at the foot rises, and venous pooling occurs.

Effect of G forces | There are situations where the body is subjected to high positive Gz, low positive Gz, zero Gz, or negative Gz. Any change in Gz changes the downward pressure exerted by a fluid column, which is given by hρg. The higher the Gz+, the heavier the fluid becomes and vice versa. Thus, at a higher Gz+, blood becomes heavier, and venous pooling increases in the dependent parts of the body. At very high Gz+ (as experienced by pilots during looping), blood becomes so heavy that arterial blood is unable to rise to the brain, causing cerebral ischemia and unconsciousness. Moments before unconsciousness, there is a *gray-out*, when everything appears gray due to ischemia of cones and loss of color vision. The gray-out is followed by a *blackout*, a total loss of vision. The gray-out serves as a warning for pilots who must slow down the aircraft and reduce the Gz+.

At zero Gz, blood becomes weightless; therefore, the venous blood reaches the brain as easily as it reaches the lower limbs. The circulatory changes associated with zero Gz are the same as the changes associated with the supine position. Gravitational force always acts vertically, and its effect on circulation is eliminated when the body is in the supine position and blood flows horizontally. For the same reason, astronauts are able to avoid the effects of high Gz or negative Gz by position-

ing themselves perpendicular to the direction of the motion of the spacecraft. The tolerance for G forces exerted across the body is much greater in the chest-to-back direction (Gx–) than in the back-to-chest direction (Gx+). Astronauts are therefore positioned to take the G forces of rocket flight in the chest-to-back direction.

In negative Gz, the weight of the blood is directed upward. This causes a rise in cerebral arterial pressure and congestion of cerebral vessels leading to *red-out* and severe throbbing headache. Despite the great rise in cerebral arterial pressure, the vessels in the brain do not rupture because there is a corresponding increase in intracranial pressure, which supports the walls of the blood vessels. In other words, the cerebrospinal fluid acts like a G-suit (see below). There is also a general increase in venous return leading to an increase in cardiac output. However, most of the cardiac output moves toward the upper parts of the body.

The *antigravity suit,* or the G-suit, in its simplest form, is a water-filled jacket that is worn by astronauts. When there is a high Gz+, there is a tendency of venous pooling. Simultaneously, the water in the G-suit rushes to the lower parts, so that there is a proportionate increase in the pressure in the G-suit. Thus, as Gz increases, the pressure in the G-suit parallels the blood pressure in the dependent parts of the body, preventing venous pooling and edema.

Hemodynamic Measurements

Measurement of Blood Flow Velocity

Doppler flow meters | Blood flow velocity can be measured with Doppler flow meters. Ultrasonic waves are sent into a vessel diagonally from one crystal, and the waves reflected from the red and white blood cells are picked up by a second, downstream crystal. The frequency of the reflected waves is higher by an amount that is proportionate to the velocity of flow toward the second crystal because of the Doppler effect.

Electromagnetic flow meters depend on the principle that a voltage is generated in a conductor moving through a magnetic field and that the magnitude of the voltage is proportionate to the speed of movement. Blood is, of course, a conductor. If a magnet is placed around the vessel, a voltage proportionate to the flow velocity can be measured with appropriately placed electrodes on the surface of the vessel.

Clinical estimation | Clinically, an approximate idea of the velocity of the circulation can be obtained by injecting a bile salt preparation into an arm vein and timing the first appearance of the bitter taste it produces. The average normal arm-to-tongue circulation time is 15 seconds. However, the normal variations are too large to allow its diagnostic use.

Measurement of Blood Flow Rate

Plethysmography (= volume recording) estimates the blood flow rate to a limb by measuring its change in volume following venous occlusion (**Fig. 35.14**). The part of the body where the blood flow is to be measured (the forearm, for example) is sealed in a watertight chamber (plethysmograph). Changes in the volume of the forearm reflect the changes in the amount of

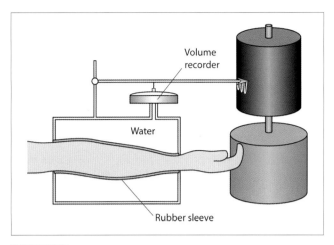

Fig. 35.14 Plethysmography of the forearm. As blood flows into the arm, the volume contained within the rubber sleeve increases, and the change in volume is displayed on the recorder.

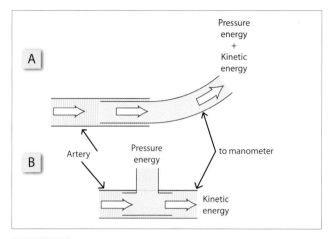

Fig. 35.15 Relevance of Bernoulli's principle in direct manometry. **(A)** Measurement of end-on pressure and **(B)** lateral pressure. The pressure recorded in **(A)** will be higher than the pressure recorded in **(B)**.

blood and interstitial fluid it contains. When the volume of the forearm increases, it displaces water. The volume of water displaced is measured with a volume recorder. When the venous drainage of the forearm is occluded, the rate of increase in the volume of the forearm is a function of the arterial blood flow (venous occlusion plethysmography).

Fick principle and indicator dilution | Indirect methods like the Fick method and dye dilution technique (Chapter 34) have already been described. Methods like the Kety nitrous oxide (N_2O) method for measuring cerebral blood flow or the estimation of renal blood flow by measuring para-aminohippuric acid (PAH) clearance are based on the Fick principle.

Measurement of Blood Pressure

In **direct manometry**, one end of a cannula is inserted into the artery, and the other end is connected to a manometer. Flow in the artery is thus blocked, and all the kinetic energy of flow is converted into pressure energy. The pressure recorded in this way is called the *end-on pressure*. If, instead, a T tube is inserted into a vessel so that the blood can flow through, and the pressure is measured in the side arm of the tube, the pressure recorded is called the *lateral pressure* (**Fig. 35.15**). It is lower than the end pressure, in accordance with Bernoulli's principle. Direct blood pressure measurement is performed clinically for CVP monitoring in patients in circulatory shock, and for pulmonary wedge pressure measurement in patients with pulmonary hypertension.

Sphygmomanometry is an indirect method of blood pressure measurement. There are three methods of performing sphygmomanometry: palpatory, auscultatory, and oscillatory. For the most part, the procedure for sphygmomanometry is the same in all three methods.

An inflatable rubber cuff (the Riva-Rocci cuff) attached to a mercury manometer (sphygmomanometer) is wrapped around the arm about an inch above the cubital fossa. The cuff is rapidly inflated until the pressure in it is well above the expected systolic pressure so that the brachial artery is occluded. The pressure in the cuff is then lowered slowly at the rate of

~1 cm H_2O/s. When the systolic pressure in the artery just exceeds the cuff pressure, blood spurts through the artery with each heartbeat. This is the point of systolic blood pressure. As the cuff pressure is lowered further, the blood flows through the brachial artery relatively smoothly, though it still passes in spurts, being unable to pass through when the blood pressure is at its lowest. Finally, when the cuff pressure falls to the level of diastolic pressure, the blood flow in the brachial artery becomes entirely free from turbulence. This marks the diastolic blood pressure. The three different methods of sphygmomanometry differ only in the criteria for identifying the systolic and diastolic blood pressures.

The sounds described above are called the *Korotkoff sounds,* and they appear at the systolic pressure and disappear at the diastolic pressure. These sounds have been attributed to the turbulence caused by the partial occlusion of the artery (**Fig. 35.16**). There are four phases of Korotkoff sounds and there are authentic descriptions of the sounds.

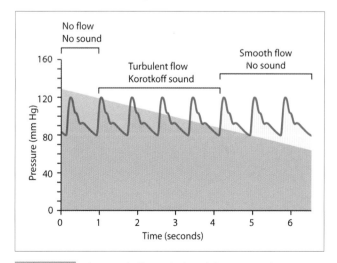

Fig. 35.16 The Korotkoff sounds, heard during auscultatory measurement of blood pressure, result from the presence of turbulent flow. The shaded area represents the gradually declining sphygmomanometer cuff pressure.

Summary

- The path of blood flow through the heart begins in the right atrium and proceeds through the right ventricle, the pulmonary circulation, the left atrium, and then out the left ventricle through the systemic circulation.

- A single vascular pathway through the circulation takes blood through the aorta, arteries, arterioles, capillaries, venules, and veins. These vessel types all have slightly different properties that relate to their function.

- The arterioles are the site of the greatest resistance (largest pressure drop) in the circulation.

- Capillaries are the site of exchange (fluid and solutes) between the vascular compartment and the tissues.

- Venules and veins have a significant capacitance function and return blood to the heart.

- Resistance to flow is determined by the viscosity of the blood (η), the length of the vessel (L), and, most powerfully, the radius raised to the 4th power.

Applying What You Know

35.1. During the cardiac catheterization procedure, Mrs. Daniels' pulmonary wedge pressure (measured when the small catheter being used is advanced through the right heart and is "wedged" tightly in the arteriolar end of the pulmonary capillary network) is measured. Under these measurement conditions, the pressure measured at the tip of the catheter reflects the pressure in the left atrium. Estimate the pressure that would be present in Mrs. Daniels' left atrium. Explain.

35.2. Mr. Lundquist (see Section IV) has pernicious anemia, which reduces his red blood cell count. As Mr. Lundquist recovers from this condition as treatment with vitamin B_{12} is begun, his red blood cell (RBC) count will increase. How will the viscosity of his blood be affected by the increasing RBC count? What will happen to his total peripheral resistance as he gets better? Explain.

Capillary Circulation

The exchange of oxygen (O_2), nutrients, and waste products between blood and the interstitial tissue takes place across the capillary walls and is known as *capillary exchange*. The diameter of true capillaries is 4 to 8 µm, which is barely enough to permit red blood cells (RBCs) to squeeze through in single file, and this facilitates gas exchange between the RBC and the interstitium. In resting tissues, most of the capillaries are collapsed (inactive capillaries), and blood bypasses them to flow through the thoroughfare vessels connecting the metarterioles to the venules. In metabolically active tissues, the precapillary sphincters dilate, and blood starts flowing through the capillaries (active capillaries). The precapillary sphincters are dilated by local metabolic vasodilators and constricted by sympathetic discharge.

Capillary Structure

All capillaries are made of a single layer of cells (the endothelial cells) placed on a basement membrane (basal lamina). Often, the entire circumference of the capillary is wrapped around by a single endothelial cell, though sometimes there are two or three cells circumferentially. The size of the solutes that diffuse out of the capillaries and the rate at which they diffuse out indicate that the capillary wall has two types of pores: a few large pores with a diameter of ~70 nm and a larger number of small pores with a diameter of 10 nm. The small pores are located at the intercellular junctions between the endothelial cells. The large pores pass through the cell itself and are

called fenestrae (windows). The fenestrations permit massive filtration of fluids and the passage of large molecules.

Capillaries that have a large number of fenestrae are called *fenestrated capillaries* (**Fig. 36.1B**). They are found in renal glomeruli and vasa recta, in exocrine and endocrine glands, choroid plexuses, intestinal villi, and in most capillaries that lie close to an epithelium, which includes the skin.

Capillaries that are not densely fenestrated are called *continuous capillaries* (**Fig. 36.1A**). They are found in muscles, brain, and connective tissues. In brain capillaries, tight junctions between endothelial cells constitute a component of the blood–brain barrier. The pores in these tight junctions are smaller, and they permit only small molecules to pass through.

A third type of capillary is found in the sinusoids of the bone marrow, liver, and spleen. In these, there are large intercellular gaps of ~600 to 3000 nm between the endothelial cells that permit the passage not only of macromolecules but also of erythrocytes. These capillaries are called *discontinuous capillaries*. The basal lamina is much reduced or absent in these capillaries.

Capillary Exchange

Capillary exchange occurs in three different ways: through filtration of fluids with their solutes (bulk flow), through diffusion of solutes, and through pinocytosis.

Capillary filtration and reabsorption | Filtration and reabsorption of fluid across the capillary membrane are determined by the balance of the hydrostatic and oncotic pressures that are called the *Starling forces*.

Figure 36.2 shows that at the arterial end of the capillary, fluid is filtered out under a filtration pressure of 16 mm Hg: at the venous end, fluid is reabsorbed under a reabsorptive pressure of 14 mm Hg. Thus, there is a mean filtration pressure of 1 mm Hg: ($+16 - 14$) ÷ 2. The above dynamics are valid for muscle capillaries. In other capillaries, the balance of Starling forces may be different. For example, fluid moves out of almost the entire length of glomerular capillaries (**Fig. 54.1B**). On the other hand, in intestinal capillaries, fluid moves into the capillaries through almost their entire length. The calculations of capillary exchange can be simplified by taking the average values of the arterial and venous sides of the capillaries. Thus, the average capillary hydrostatic pressure is taken as P_{cap}, and the average plasma osmotic pressure is represented by π_{cap}. If P_I and π_I represent the interstitial hydrostatic and oncotic pressure, respectively, the equation for the net filtration force (F) can then be written as

$$F = (P_{cap} + \pi_I) - (P_I + \pi_{cap}) \tag{36.1}$$

$$\therefore F = (25 + 3) - (2 + 25) = 1 \tag{36.2}$$

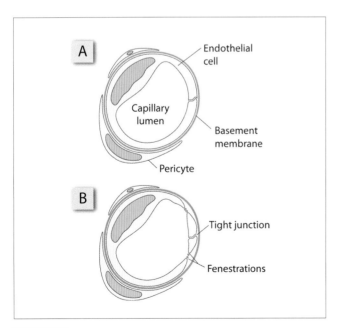

Fig. 36.1 Structure of a capillary, showing how a single endothelial cell is wrapped around its lumen. **(A)** A continuous capillary. **(B)** A fenestrated capillary.

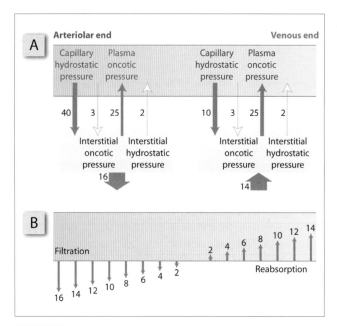

Fig. 36.2 **(A)** Starling forces of capillary exchange at the arterial and venous ends of a capillary. **(B)** Filtration at the arterial end and reabsorption at the venous end occur under the influence of the Starling forces. Compare with **Fig. 54.1**.

The volume of fluid that is filtered under a pressure of 1 mm Hg is determined by the capillary filtration coefficient (k_f), which is an index of capillary permeability. Thus, the amount of capillary filtration is given by

$$V = k_f \times F \tag{36.3}$$

or

$$V = k_f \times [(P_{cap} + \pi_I) - (P_I + \pi_{cap})] \tag{36.4}$$

Because k_f, π_I, P_I, and π_{cap} mostly remain unchanged, capillary filtration is controlled largely by P_{cap}. The capillary hydrostatic pressure increases when the precapillary sphincter dilates or the postcapillary sphincter constricts. In other words, the capillary hydrostatic pressure increases when the *pre:post capillary resistance ratio* decreases (**Fig. 36.3**). Normally, this ratio is 5:1. Sympathetic vasoconstriction increases this ratio and therefore reduces capillary hydrostatic pressure. Hence, sympathetic discharge favors movement of fluid from the interstitium into the capillary and thereby retains fluid within the circulation. Conversely, local metabolites dilate mainly the precapillary sphincter and decrease the pre:post capillary resistance ratio. Hence, the capillary hydrostatic pressure increases, favoring filtration of fluids from the capillary into the interstitium.

The fluid that is filtered out of continuous capillaries into the interstitial space does not have appreciable amounts of proteins in it. This fluid is called a *transudate*. However, if the permeability of the capillaries increases markedly, as happens during inflammation from any cause, large amounts of proteins diffuse out from the capillaries. This protein-rich fluid that comes out of the capillaries under conditions of inflammation is called *exudate*. The increase in capillary permeability in inflammation is due to the effect of inflammatory mediators like histamine. Histamine binds to receptors on endothelial cells and stimulates the cells to contract, resulting in the widening of the intercellular junctions between them. The increase in permeability can also be the direct consequence of endothelial injury.

Diffusion across the capillary wall | Diffusion is quantitatively much more important than filtration in terms of the exchange of nutrients and waste materials between blood and tissue. It may be argued that because plasma is filtered out of the capillaries and then subsequently reabsorbed, dissolved gases and nutrients would move in and out with it, making diffusion unnecessary. However, the amount of filtration is

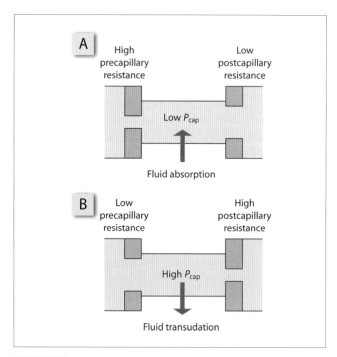

Fig. 36.3 Pre:post capillary resistance ratio and the capillary hydrostatic pressure. **(A)** High pre:post capillary resistance ratio is associated with fluid absorption in capillaries. **(B)** Low pre:post capillary resistance ratio is associated with fluid transudation in capillaries.

not enough to transport adequate gases and nutrients through bulk flow. O_2 and glucose are in higher concentration in the bloodstream than in the interstitial fluid and diffuse into the interstitial fluid, whereas CO_2 and the waste products of metabolism diffuse in the opposite direction.

The rate of diffusion of substances from the capillaries to the tissues increases with the concentration gradient of the substance, the permeability of the capillary wall, and the total number of active capillaries. The effect of blood flow rate on diffusion depends on whether the diffusion is flow-limited or diffusion-limited. The concentrations of small molecules like glucose and sodium chloride (NaCl) in plasma and the interstitial fluid usually equilibrate near the arteriolar end of the capillary. In such situations, the amount of solutes delivered or carried away by the capillary can be increased by increasing blood flow—the exchange is *flow-limited*. On the other hand, large molecules like sucrose do not reach equilibrium with the tissues during their passage through the capillaries. Their exchange is said to be *diffusion-limited*. An increase in blood flow will not increase the amount of solute exchange. The concept is explained further in **Fig. 36.4**.

General Model: Flow

Diffusion from the capillary to the interstitium is governed by the same relationship that describes all flow phenomena. Substances move down their concentration gradients into and out of the vascular compartment. The large surface area of a capillary bed maximizes the flux of any substance into or out of the vascular compartment by minimizing the resistance to flow.

Pinocytosis by the endothelial cells is responsible for the transport of large, lipid-insoluble molecules between the blood and the interstitium. A very small amount of transport across the capillary wall occurs through this mechanism.

Lymphatic Circulation

The extra fluid filtered from the capillaries enters the lymphatics as lymph. The lymph flows through a system of lymphatic vessels and finally drains into the thoracic duct, which opens into the junction of the left subclavian and internal jugular veins. Thus, all the lymph is eventually returned to the blood. The normal 24-hour lymph flow is 2 to 4 L. Agents that increase capillary permeability increase the lymph flow and are called *lymphagogues*. Agents that cause contraction of smooth muscle also increase lymph flow from the intestines.

Lymphatic vessels (**Fig. 36.5**) are of two types: the initial lymphatics and the collecting lymphatics. *Initial lymphatics* lack valves and smooth muscle in their walls. They are found in the intestine and skeletal muscle. Tissue fluid enters them through the loose junctions between their endothelial cells. The fluid is propelled by the massaging effect of muscle contractions and the pulsations of the arterioles nearby. They drain into the collecting lymphatics. Unlike capillaries, lymphatic endothelium does not have any basal lamina, and the junctions between the

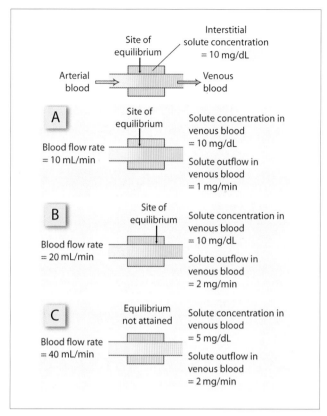

Fig. 36.4 Flow-limited transport. **(A)** Capillary blood equilibrates with the tissue at the point marked by the arrow. The solute carried away by the capillary (1 mg/min) is given by the product of the blood flow rate (10 mL/min) and the solute concentration in blood (10 mg/dL). A faster diffusion rate will shift the point of equilibrium to the left but will have no effect on the solute concentration in blood or the solute outflow. **(B)** The flow rate increases, and the point of equilibrium shifts a little to the right. Solute concentration in blood remains unchanged. The solute outflow increases proportionately with the flow rate. Hence, the solute outflow is called flow-limited. **(C)** The flow rate increases further because the capillary blood fails to equilibrate completely with the tissue. The amount of solute carried away by capillary blood remains unchanged. The solute concentration in blood falls in inverse proportion to the flow rate. The solute outflow is no longer flow-limited because it is not increased further by an increase in flow rate. Rather, it has now become diffusion-limited because a faster diffusion rate will allow the capillary blood to equilibrate with the tissue.

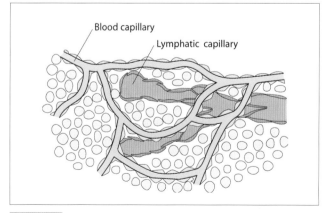

Fig. 36.5 A lymph capillary in a tissue. Note the close proximity of blood capillaries.

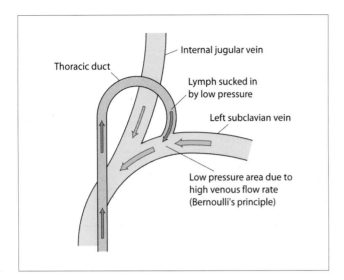

Fig. 36.6 The high rate of blood flow in a vein creates a reduced pressure area in a lymphatic vessel draining into the vein (Bernoulli's principle) and facilitates the return of lymph to the vascular compartment.

cells have no tight intercellular connections. Lymphatic endothelium does not have visible fenestrations.

Collecting lymphatics have valves and smooth muscle in their walls. They contract in a peristaltic fashion, propelling the lymph along the vessels. Flow in the collecting lymphatics is further aided by contraction of skeletal muscle, the negative intrathoracic pressure during inspiration, and the suction effect of high-velocity flow of blood in the veins in which the lymphatics terminate (**Fig. 36.6**). Of these, muscle contraction is the principal factor propelling the lymph. Collecting lymphatics traverse lymph nodes at regular intervals along their course. Lymphocytes enter the circulation principally through the lymphatics.

General Model: Flow

The flow of fluid in the lymphatic vessels, along with the return of lymph to the vascular compartment, is driven by a pressure gradient created predominantly by external forces acting on the walls of the lymph vessels. Occlusion or compression of lymph vessels must therefore reduce the removal of lymph from the tissue affected.

The **composition of lymph** is similar to plasma except that its protein content is lower due to the low permeability of the capillary walls to proteins. The walls of the lymphatics are permeable to protein macromolecules, and the composition of lymph varies with the capillary permeability in the region it drains. The lymph from liver has the highest protein content (~6.0 g/dL). The lymph from the intestine and skeletal muscle has ~4.0 and 2.0 g/dL of protein, respectively. In the intestine, fats are absorbed into the lymphatics, and the lymph in the thoracic duct after a meal is milky because of its high fat content.

Edema

Edema (**Fig. 36.7**) refers to an accumulation of excess fluids in the body. The excess fluid may be located outside the cells, or it may be confined within the cells, in which case it is called intracellular edema. The term *edema*, when unqualified as intracellular or extracellular, always implies the latter, that is, a large increase in interstitial fluid volume. The causes of edema are to be found in the factors that control the interstitial fluid volume: (1) increased capillary hydrostatic pressure, (2) reduced plasma oncotic pressure, (3) increased interstitial oncotic pressure, (4) increased capillary permeability, and (5) reduced lymphatic flow.

Increased capillary hydrostatic pressure is caused by vasodilation and increased venous pressure. The local accumulation of metabolites causes dilatation of the arteriole and the precapillary sphincter, lowering the pre:post capillary resistance ratio. Increased venous pressure is transmitted back to the capillaries, resulting in elevated capillary hydrostatic pressure. Conditions in which venous pressure is elevated include adoption of the standing posture for long periods, cardiac failure, incompetent venous valves, venous obstruction, and increased blood volume.

Reduced plasma oncotic pressure results from hypoproteinemia, the common causes of which are liver disease, nephrotic syndrome, malnutrition and starvation, and protein-losing enteropathy.

Increase in interstitial oncotic pressure promotes transudation of fluid from the capillary. Osmotically active metab-

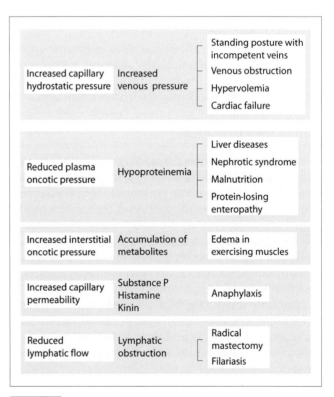

Fig. 36.7 Edema results from changes to the forces governing fluid movement across the walls of the capillary or reduced fluid drainage out of the tissue.

olites in exercising muscles accumulate faster than they can be removed by lymphatics, despite the enhanced lymph drainage during exercise. This accounts for an increase in volume of exercising muscles, which can be as much as 25%. A lowered interstitial oncotic pressure promotes the movement of fluids from the interstitial space into the capillaries. Benzopyrones increase the proteolytic activity of tissue macrophages, which leads to a lowering of interstitial oncotic pressure. They are used in the treatment of lymphedema.

Increased capillary permeability is produced by substance P, histamine, and kinins leading to exudation of large amounts of plasma and causing edema. It is typically seen in anaphylaxis.

Inadequate lymph flow is caused by lymphatic obstruction. Such edema is called lymphedema and is characterized by a high protein content of the edema fluid. Common causes of lymphedema are radical mastectomy and filariasis. *Radical mastectomy* is an operation for breast cancer in which the axillary lymph nodes are also removed. Removal of the axillary lymph nodes on one side reduces lymph drainage and results in edema of the ipsilateral arm. In *filariasis,* the filaria (a helminth) migrate into the lymphatics and obstruct them. Over a period of time, massive edema results, usually of the legs or scrotum, a condition called elephantiasis.

Summary

- Capillaries are made up of a single layer of endothelial cells (and a basement membrane) across which water and small solutes can pass.

- Movement of fluids across the walls of capillaries is determined by the Starling forces: the hydrostatic pressure gradient and the oncotic pressure gradient.

- Solutes in the blood can cross the capillary walls in three ways: (1) by the bulk flow of water, (2) diffusion, and (3) pinocytosis.

- The lymphatic system returns fluid filtered out of capillaries (and not reabsorbed) to the circulation.

Applying What You Know

36.1. Mrs. Daniels exhibits mild pedal edema (swelling of the feet and hands). Why are the hands and feet parts of the body where edema is most often visible?

36.2. Mrs. Daniels exhibits several signs suggesting that she has pulmonary edema as well as pedal edema. What is the most likely cause of her pulmonary edema? Explain.

Control of cardiovascular effectors, the heart and the blood vessels, is provided by both chemical and neural mechanisms. These mechanisms play an essential role in the homeostatic maintenance of function in the cardiovascular system.

Chemical Control of the Cardiovascular System

Chemical control of the cardiovascular system involves several different mechanisms and a variety of different chemical messengers. Some of the mechanisms act locally; others act at a distance via chemical messengers carried in the blood. Most of these chemical messengers act on the circulation.

Paracrine Control

Any vasodilator metabolite that accumulates in a tissue during activity can produce autoregulation of blood flow. When blood flow to the tissue decreases, the vasodilator metabolites accumulate, and local blood vessels dilate. The vasodilatation increases blood flow, which washes away the metabolites. The metabolic changes that produce vasodilatation include a decrease in partial pressure of oxgen (PO_2) or hydrogen ion concentration (pH) and an increase in partial pressure in carbon dioxide (PCO_2) or osmolarity. These changes cause relaxation of the precapillary sphincters. A rise in temperature exerts a direct vasodilator effect. In exercise, the heat of metabolism raises the temperature of active tissues and contributes to vasodilatation there. Potassium (K^+) and lactate ions possibly have a role in autoregulation in skeletal muscle. Similarly, adenosine may have an autoregulatory role in cardiac muscle.

Nitric oxide (NO) is produced in endothelial cells from L-arginine in the presence of the enzyme nitric oxide synthetase (NOS), which exists in three isoforms. NOS I is present in nervous tissues, NOS II is present in activated macrophages, and NOS III is present in endothelium. NO acts through group IIB hormonal mechanisms (see Chapter 75), that is, through cyclic guanosine monophosphate (cGMP) as the second messenger. NO has a very short half-life of less than 5 seconds, as it is highly reactive. NO is inactivated through oxidation into nitrite and nitrate, which are excreted in urine. The plasma and urine concentrations of nitrate and cGMP are useful indicators of NO production rates. NO has several important physiologic functions.

1. NO relaxes vascular smooth muscle cells. The constant release of NO from endothelial cells produces vasodilatation; therefore, NO deficiency causes hypertension. The drug *nitroglycerin,* which is of great value in the treatment of angina (pain caused by ischemic cardiac tissue), exerts its vasodilator action by being converted to NO.

   Many vasoconstrictors (e.g., norepinephrine, endothelin, serotonin, and thromboxane A_2), as well as vasodilator substances (e.g., acetylcholine, bradykinin, histamine, adenosine, and prostacyclin), stimulate the release of NO

from the endothelium. The release of NO potentiates the vasodilators and reduces the effect of vasoconstrictors. Moreover, NO directly interferes with the secretion and action of endothelin, a potent vasoconstrictor.

2. NO is released in response to pulsatile stretch- and flow-induced shear stress. When flow (mL/min) to a tissue is suddenly increased by arteriolar dilatation, the large arteries upstream to the tissue also dilate. This *flow-induced vasodilatation* (**Fig. 37.1A**) is due to local release of NO and occurs, for example, during physical exercise. Flow-induced vasodilatation is also responsible for *poststenotic vasodila-*

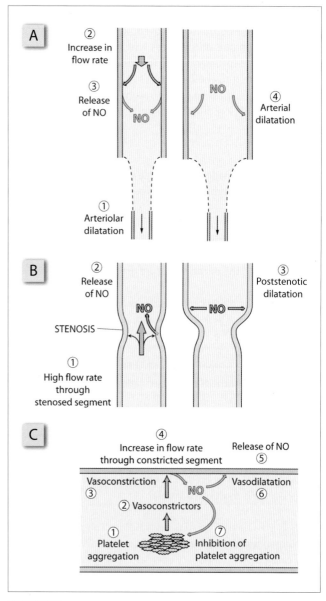

Fig. 37.1 Actions of nitric oxide (NO). **(A)** Flow-induced vasodilatation. **(B)** Poststenotic vasodilatation. **(C)** Negative feedback control of platelet aggregation by nitric oxide.

tation (**Fig. 37.1B**): any luminal narrowing of arterial vessels increases the local blood flow velocity (mm/s), which stimulates NO release and results in vasodilatation beyond the point of narrowing.

3. NO causes vasodilatation and engorgement of the corpora cavernosa, resulting in penile erection. The drug Viagra (sildenafil citrate; Pfizer Pharmaceuticals, New York, NY), a selective inhibitor of cGMP-specific phosphodiesterase, promotes penile erection by inhibiting the inactivation of NO.

4. NO inhibits platelet adhesion and aggregation. During platelet aggregation, several vasoconstrictors are released. These vasoconstrictors cause an increase in flow velocity that, in turn, stimulates the release of NO from the endothelium. The NO released inhibits platelet adhesion and aggregation, thereby exerting a negative feedback control on them (**Fig. 37.1C**). This effect, along with its vasodilatory effect, makes NO important for the maintenance of the normal flow of blood.

5. NO decreases low-density lipoprotein (LDL) oxidation and inhibits superoxide anion (O_2^-) production by inhibiting nicotinamide adenine dinucleotide phosphate (NADPH) reductase activity. These actions result in a strong *antiatherosclerotic effect.*

6. NO is necessary for the cytotoxic activity of macrophages, including their ability to kill cancer cells. NO inhibits leukocyte adhesion and migration. Production of NO, which acts as a mediator of the inflammatory response, is elevated in inflammatory diseases.

Kinins | Two forms of kinins with similar actions are found in the body, one is bradykinin, and the other is lysyl-bradykinin, also known as kallidin (**Fig. 37.2**). They are formed, respectively, from high-molecular-weight and low-molecular-weight kininogens (HMWK and LMWK) by the action of plasma and tissue kallikreins. Lysyl-bradykinin can be converted to bradykinin by aminopeptidase.

Kinins are present mostly in tissues, although small amounts are also found in the circulating blood. Their actions resemble those of histamine. Bradykinin receptors B_1 and B_2 are serpentine (membrane-spanning) receptors coupled to G proteins. They cause contraction of visceral smooth muscle, but they relax vascular smooth muscle through NO, lowering the blood pressure. They also increase capillary permeability, attract leukocytes, and mediate pain. Tissue kallikrein is formed in sweat glands, salivary glands, and exocrine pancreas during active secretion and mediates the hyperemia in these organs that is normally associated with active secretion.

Endothelins | The endothelins (ET) are a family of three highly potent vasoconstrictor peptides (ET-1, ET-2, and ET-3) synthesized and secreted by vascular endothelial cells of the brain, kidneys, and intestine. Endothelins are initially synthesized as preproendothelin, which undergoes preprocessing to proendothelin, also called big-endothelin. Big-endothelin is released and converted to active endothelin by the endothelin-converting enzyme.

Most of the endothelin-1 is secreted into the media of blood vessels, where it acts in a paracrine fashion. Endothelin secretion is increased by other vasoconstrictors, such as catecholamines and angiotensin II, and is inhibited by vasodilators like NO. Endothelin is also secreted when blood flows over the endothelium at high velocity (increased shear stress).

Endothelin is primarily a paracrine regulator of vascular tone. In the brain, endothelins play a role in regulating transport across the blood–brain barrier (which limits the diffusion of substances between the vascular compartment and the tissues of the brain). In the renal glomerulus, endothelin causes contraction of mesangial cells and thereby decreases the glomerular filtration rate. Endothelins play a role in closing the ductus arteriosus at birth. Endothelin-1 is a potent growth factor for smooth muscle and a chemoattractant for monocytes.

The vascular effects of endothelin are mediated by endothelin receptors, of which there are two subtypes (ET-A and ET-B). ET-A is found predominantly on vascular smooth muscles. It is coupled to G_s protein and when activated, stimulates slow and sustained vasoconstriction. ET-B resides on endothelial cells. It is coupled to G_i protein and when activated, stimulates release of NO and thus favors vasodilatation.

Prostaglandins are autocrine and paracrine mediators having a wide variety of actions, notably those on smooth muscles and platelets. They are synthesized in the cell from arachidonate, which is derived from membrane phospholipids through the action of phospholipase A_2 (**Fig. 37.3**). Arachidonate passes into the lipoxygenase pathway to form leukotrienes and into the cyclooxygenase pathway to form thromboxane and prostaglandins. Prostaglandins are produced from arachidonic acid by prostaglandin H synthetase (PGHS). Prostaglandins have a short half-life before being inactivated and excreted.

There are different receptors for different types of prostaglandins: IP receptors for PGI_2, TP receptors for thromboxanes, DP receptors for PGD_2, EP receptors for PGE_2, and FP receptors for PGF_2. Prostaglandins act principally through G-protein-coupled receptors.

Prostaglandins act on vascular smooth muscle cells, some causing constriction and others, dilatation. There is a high concentration of $PGE_{2\alpha}$, a vasodilator, in the fetal ductus arteriosus.

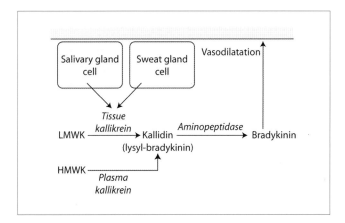

Fig. 37.2 Bradykinin is derived from low-molecular-weight and high-molecular-weight kininogens (LMWK and HMWK, respectively) catalyzed by kallikrein. Bradykinin acts on arteriolar smooth muscle to produce vasodilatation.

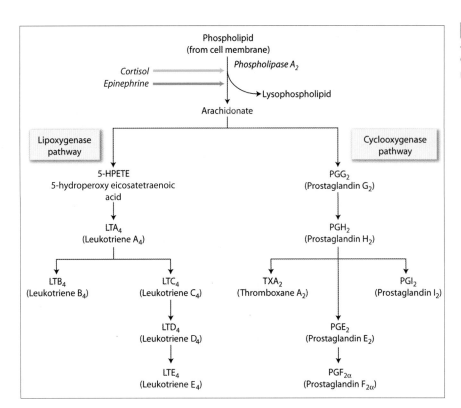

Fig. 37.3 The synthesis of prostaglandins (PDs) and leukotrienes (LTs) membrane phospholipids. Cortisol (blue) stimulates production of arachidonate, while epinephrine (red) inhibits it.

At birth, $PGE_{2\alpha}$ synthesis is inhibited due to the inhibition of cyclooxygenase, leading to the closure of the ductus arteriosus. PGF_2, a vasoconstrictor, causes the vasospasm of the uterine arteries that precedes menstrual bleeding, has a role in luteolysis, and increases the intensity of oxytocin-induced contractions of the myometrium. Prostaglandin is also an inhibitor of gastric secretion and a stimulator of renin secretion.

Prostaglandins are important inflammatory mediators; PGE_2 in granulocytes and macrophages, PGD_2 in mast cells, PGI_2 (prostacyclin) in endothelial cells, PGH_2 and thromboxane A_2 in platelets, and leukotrienes in mast cells. The thromboxane A_2 synthesized in platelets causes platelet aggregation; the PGI_2 produced by the endothelial cells inhibits platelet aggregation. Prostaglandins are therefore important for the hemostatic balance. The prostaglandins released from injured tissues act on nociceptors (pain receptors) to produce primary hyperalgesia. PGE_2 is a mediator of fever.

Synthetic prostaglandins are used to induce childbirth, to close a patent ductus arteriosus in newborns, to reduce gastric acid secretion and treat peptic ulcers, as a vasodilator in severe ischemia of a limb, and in pulmonary hypertension. Nonsteroidal antiinflammatory drugs (NSAIDs) reduce prostaglandin synthesis by inhibiting PGHS.

Endocrine Control

Paracrine control is by definition local control; it is mainly involved with matching perfusion to local tissue needs. Endocrine control of the circulation is more centralized; it is involved with the reflex (homeostatic) regulation of cardiovascular system function.

Circulating Vasodilators

Vasoactive intestinal peptide (VIP) is a circulating vasodilator, which also acts as a gastrointestinal hormone (see Chapter 72). It is a transmitter in the vagal nonadrenergic, noncholinergic fibers that mediate bronchodilatation. It is also a transmitter in the pelvic splanchnic nerve fibers to the penis and mediates penile erection.

Atrial natriuretic peptide (ANP) is a circulating vasodilator with several effects (see Chapter 61 for a discussion of its role in the kidney), but whose exact systemic physiologic role is not understood. It reduces blood pressure, and in general, its actions are opposite to those of angiotensin II.

Circulating Vasoconstrictors

Renin–angiotensin system | Renin is a protease enzyme present in the juxtaglomerular (JG) cells of the kidneys. It is released in response to circulating catecholamines and sympathetic discharge to the kidneys. Renin catalyzes the conversion of angiotensinogen to angiotensin I, which in turn is converted into angiotensin II (AII). AII causes vasoconstriction, increases thirst, and stimulates aldosterone secretion. The renin–angiotensin system has important roles in the regulation of blood pressure and extracellular fluid (ECF) volume. Its role in affecting kidney function is discussed in Chapter 61.

Vasopressin (ADH) is a potent vasoconstrictor. It also causes renal retention of water. Its actions in the kidney are discussed in detail in Chapter 61, and its role in blood pressure regulation is discussed in the next chapter.

Catecholamines include epinephrine, norepinephrine, and dopamine. Of these, epinephrine and norepinephrine act

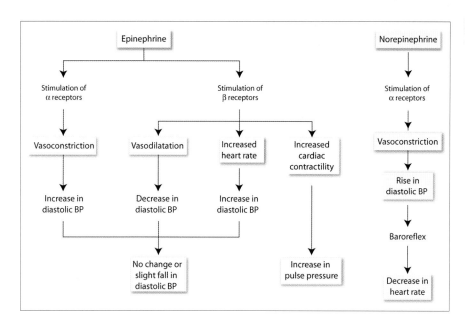

Fig. 37.4 Flow chart of the cardiovascular effects of epinephrine and norepinephrine. BP, blood pressure.

through α- and β-adrenergic receptors, whereas dopamine acts through separate dopaminergic receptors. α Receptors mediate excitation of smooth muscles, β1 receptors mediate excitation of cardiac muscle, and β2 receptors mediate inhibition of smooth muscles. The cardiovascular effects of epinephrine and norepinephrine are summarized in **Fig. 37.4** and contrasted in **Table 37.1**.

Epinephrine stimulates both α and β receptors in blood vessels. The α-induced vasoconstriction is more than nullified by the β-induced vasodilatation. Hence, the peripheral resistance and diastolic blood pressure (BP) remain unchanged or fall slightly. The β-induced increase in stroke volume and heart rate results in higher cardiac output and a rise in systolic BP. The pulse pressure increases.

Norepinephrine has much greater effect on α than on β receptors. Hence, it produces vasoconstriction with a rise in peripheral resistance and diastolic BP. Due to weak β-activation, direct cardiac stimulation is insignificant. Rather, there is a reflex decrease in heart rate due to the rise in diastolic BP. The cardiac output falls as a result of the low heart rate. The stroke volume and pulse pressure remain nearly the same.

Circulating norepinephrine is of little significance compared with the importance of the norepinephrine released from sympathetic nerves. When α adrenoceptors are blocked, sympathetic stimulation causes vasodilatation (instead of the usual vasoconstriction) because the norepinephrine released from the nerve terminals acts only on the β adrenoceptors.

The physiologic function of the dopamine in the circulation is unknown. However, its pharmacologic effects make it an important drug in the treatment of circulatory shock because (1) it produces renal vasodilatation (preventing renal shutdown), acting through dopaminergic receptors; (2) it produces vasoconstriction elsewhere (preventing hypotension), probably by stimulating the release of norepinephrine; and (3) it has a positively inotropic effect on the heart due to the action on β_1-adrenergic receptors.

Table 37.1 Differences in the Cardiovascular Effects of Epinephrine and Norepinephrine

Epinephrine	Norepinephrine
Stimulates the heart through β receptors	Due to weak β-activation, cardiac stimulation is insignificant
Due to stimulation of both α and β receptors, peripheral resistance and diastolic blood pressure remain unchanged or fall slightly	Due to predominant α-activation, peripheral resistance and diastolic blood pressure increase
Due to direct stimulation of the heart, there is increased stroke volume and heart rate	The reflex inhibition of sympathetic discharge (due to high diastolic blood pressure) results in reduced heart rate and stroke volume

General Model: Communications

The many paracrine and circulating substances that act on the circulation are each an example of cell-to-cell communication. These chemical signals act on arteriolar smooth muscle to alter the state of their contraction and hence the caliber of the blood vessel. In every case, there is a receptor (on the cell membrane or in the cell) that detects the presence of the signaling molecule.

Neural Control of the Cardiovascular System

Cardiovascular reflexes are controlled by centers located in the brainstem reticular formation. These brainstem centers are under the control of higher hypothalamic and cortical centers. The effectors of cardiovascular reflexes are the cardiac muscle (of the heart) and the smooth muscle (of the blood vessels). The receptors initiating cardiovascular reflexes are either mechanoreceptors (sensing blood pressure and volume) or chemoreceptors (sensing gas tension and blood pH). The efferent arcs are the autonomic fibers to the heart and blood vessels. The afferent arcs are in the glossopharyngeal and vagal fibers.

Efferent Control of the Cardiovascular System

Sympathetic innervation of the heart | The sympathetic nerve cells supplying the heart are located in the intermediolateral horn of spinal segments T1–T5. All parts of the heart (sinoatrial [SA] node, atria, atrioventricular [AV] node, and ventricles) receive sympathetic innervation. The sympathetic innervation on the right side is distributed primarily to the SA node; the sympathetic innervation on the left side is primarily to the AV node. Sympathetic fibers are mostly distributed to the epicardium.

Sympathetic discharge has five effects on the heart: positive inotropic (increase in the force of cardiac contraction with a constant ventricular filling), positive chronotropic (increase of the cardiac rate), positive bathmotropic (increase in automaticity), positive dromotropic (increase in conduction velocity), and inhibition of parasympathetic effect mediated by neuropeptide Y.

Sympathetic innervation of the blood vessels | Sympathetic fibers innervating blood vessels originate from the intermediolateral horns in spinal segments T1–L2. They innervate blood vessels of all calibers except the capillaries and postcapillary venules, which do not have smooth muscles in their wall. The arterioles are most densely innervated. The precapillary sphincters are also well innervated. Most sympathetic fibers produce vasoconstriction. They use norepinephrine as their neurotransmitter. Sympathetic vasoconstrictor fibers show tonic (i.e., continuous) discharge. Hence, sympathectomy produces widespread vasodilatation. Some sympathetic fibers cause vasodilatation and constitute what is called the *sympathetic vasodilator system.* They supply the arterioles to the skeletal muscles and have acetylcholine and VIP as their neurotransmitters.

Parasympathetic innervation of the heart | Parasympathetic fibers to the heart originate from the nucleus ambiguus. They reach the heart through the vagus nerve and relay in ganglia located within the cardiac muscle. The right vagus is distributed mainly to the SA node; the left vagus innervates mainly the AV node. Vagal fibers are mostly endocardial in distribution. Vagal stimulation slows the heart (has a negative chronotropic effect), but it has no inotropic effect because it does not innervate the contracting myocardial cells of the atria or the ventricles in sufficient numbers. If both noradrenergic and cholinergic systems are blocked, the heart rate is ~100 beats/min. Because the resting heart rate is ~72 beats/min, it

indicates that at rest, the vagal tone at the SA node is greater than the sympathetic tone.

Parasympathetic innervation of the blood vessels | For the most part, blood vessels do not have any parasympathetic innervation. Some parasympathetic vasodilator fibers run to restricted cranial and sacral areas, supplying vessels in the brain, tongue, salivary glands, external genitalia, bladder, and rectum. They are not tonically active and do not participate in the baroreceptor and chemoreceptor reflexes. In skin, the active vasodilatation associated with these fibers is mediated by bradykinin.

General Model: Communications

The neural inputs to the heart and the circulation are also examples of cell-to-cell communication with the particular neurotransmitter involved eliciting a response from a tissue with the corresponding receptor.

Cardiovascular Control Centers

The **spinal sympathetic center** is located in the intermediolateral horn of the spinal segments T1–L2. It has two parts: the *pressor area,* containing the intermediolateral (IML) cells from which the sympathetic fibers originate, and the *depressor area* located a little medially containing the intermediomedial (IMM) cells that inhibit the pressor area.

The **medullary sympathetic center** is also called the *vasomotor center.* It controls the output of the spinal sympathetic center. It has two parts: the *pressor area* located in the rostral ventrolateral medulla (RVLM), which increases the spinal sympathetic output, and the *depressor area,* located in the caudal ventrolateral medulla (CVLM), which reduces the spinal sympathetic output.

The **medullary parasympathetic center** gives origin to the vagal parasympathetic fibers to the heart. It is often called the *cardioinhibitory center,* and it includes the nucleus ambiguus.

The **hypothalamic autonomic center** controls the lower sympathetic and parasympathetic centers. It contains the pressor and depressor areas. The *pressor area,* also called the *defense area,* is located in the ventral hypothalamus, ventral to the genu of the corpus callosum. It is connected with the lower autonomic centers to increase the sympathetic output and reduce the parasympathetic output. The *depressor area,* which is located in the anterior hypothalamus, is connected with the lower autonomic centers to decrease the sympathetic output and increase the parasympathetic output.

The **subthalamic movement center** initiates sympathetic discharge simultaneously with the onset of motor activities. It is probably important for the augmented sympathetic discharge that occurs during exercise.

Cardiovascular Effects of Breathing

The heart rate shows small oscillations that are synchronous with the breathing cycle. During inspiration, the heart rate increases slightly. During expiration, it decreases. The oscillation in heart rate is called *sinus arrhythmia* and is partly due to the spilling over of impulses from the inspiratory center to the nucleus ambiguus. The Bainbridge reflex also contributes: during inspiration, the central venous pressure (CVP) increases due to a rise in the intra-abdominal pressure. The increased CVP initiates the Bainbridge reflex and increases the heart rate.

Breathing is also associated with rhythmic changes in the cardiac output (see **Fig. 34.6**) and therefore in blood pressure, too.

Chemical and Neural Responses to Exercise

Exercise is characterized by an increased cardiac output and a marked redistribution of blood flow throughout the body, and the magnitude of these changes is determined by the work being done during exercise (**Table 37.2**).

The initial responses to exercise are driven by neural mechanisms activated by the central nervous system (CNS) initiation of muscle contraction. A central increase in sympathetic activity (and a concomitant decrease in parasympathetic activity) increases the heart rate (which directly increases cardiac output) and cardiac contractility (that increases stroke volume and hence increases cardiac output). There is also increased vasoconstriction in nonexercising muscles and the splanchnic and renal circulations (making available the increased blood flow being shunted to the exercising muscles) and contraction of smooth muscle in veins (decreasing venous compliance and thus increasing CVP).

The increased contraction of the active muscles (and the increased ventilation that accompanies exercise) acts like a "muscle pump" that augments venous return and maintains and even increases filling of the ventricles. This contributes to the increased cardiac output that is present.

Once exercise is under way, there are later responses that help sustain the cardiovascular responses to exercise. Of particular importance is the massive vasodilatation that occurs in the exercising muscles that results from the local accumulation of vasodilating metabolites generated by the increased muscle activity (increased carbon dioxide, decreased oxygen, decreased pH, increased extracellular potassium). There is also the release of histamine and kinins that produce vasodilation.

The increased sympathetic activity that has been centrally generated also stimulates the adrenal medulla to release epinephrine that reinforces the sympathetic effects on the heart and blood vessels.

Finally, the massive dilation in the active muscles causes a fall in total peripheral resistance, a fall that is much greater than the increased resistance in those tissue beds that are being centrally vasoconstricted. This would cause blood pressure to fall were it not for activation of the baroreceptor reflex (see Chapter 38), which contributes to the increased cardiac output and vasoconstriction in the nonexercising tissue beds.

These responses are highly integrated and result in the changes seen in **Table 37.2**. Cardiac output increases as the level of exercise increases. As the level of exercise increases, the absolute flow and the percentage of the cardiac output directed to the exercising muscle increase. The increased flow to the active muscles is largely the result of the increased cardiac output, although redistribution of flow plays a significant role. Note that coronary blood flow increases as the heart works harder, producing local metabolites that maintain the flow needed to deliver oxygen and nutrients to the cardiac muscle. Cerebral blood flow is essentially unchanged and reflects the very powerful autoregulatory mechanisms at work in this tissue bed. Finally, note that skin blood flow increases

Table 37.2 The Distribution of Blood Flow at Increasing Levels of Exercise*

	Cardiac Output	Skeletal Muscle	Coronary	Cerebral	Skin	Splanchnic	Renal	Other Organs
At rest								
Flow (mL/min)	5000	1050	200	650	450	1200	950	500
% CO		21	4	13	9	24	19	10
Light exercise								
Flow (mL/min)	8200	3854	328	650	1312	984	820	328
% CO		47	4	8	16	12	10	4
Strenuous exercise								
Flow (mL/min)	15,100	10,721	604	650	1661	453	453	302
% CO		71	4	4	11	3	3	2
Maximal exercise								
Flow (mL/min)	21,550	18,964	862	650	430	215	215	108
% CO		88	4	3	2	1	1	0.5

*With maximal exercise, 88% of the cardiac output is being delivered to the muscles, with coronary flow increased in proportion to the increased work, and cerebral blood flow kept constant. (The numbers presented here are only intended to illustrate several important concepts and are not real data.)

Abbreviation: CO, cardiac output.

at lower levels of exercise as the body attempts to dispose of the heat produced by the exercising muscles (see Chapter 43). However, at maximal levels of exercise, the demand for increased blood flow to the muscles results in shunting of flow from the skin to the muscles. Consequently, there is danger of hyperthermia at high levels of exercise.

Summary

- Chemical control of the cardiovascular system is exerted primarily on the circulation.

- Locally produced (paracrine) substances act on blood vessels to alter their state of constriction (NO, kinins, endothelins, prostaglandins).

- Hormones (VIP and ANP) produced in a variety of locations circulate and produce vasodilatation, whereas others (AII, vasopressin, catecholamines) produce vasoconstriction.

- Neural control of the heart and circulation is exerted by the sympathetic and parasympathetic branches of the autonomic nervous system.

- Central neural control centers are located at the spinal, medullary, and hypothalamic levels.

- Changes in heart and circulatory function during exercise are mediated by integrated neural and chemical control.

Applying What You Know

37.1. Mrs. Daniels reports that even modest exertion (exercise) leaves her short of breath. What changes should occur in her cardiovascular system when she exercises? How can her shortness of breath be explained?

37.2. Digitoxin is a drug that inhibits the Na^+–K^+ pump in the cell membrane of cardiac cells. Thus, it results in an accumulation of Na^+ in cardiac cells. What effect will this have on the function of ventricular cells? How might this help Mrs. Daniels' condition? Explain.

Every tissue and organ must receive the oxygen and nutrients that it requires to support its basal metabolism and to carry out its particular special function(s). That is to say, it must receive the blood flow it requires at all times. Thus, the cardiac output, the volume of blood pumped each minute, must be divided between all of the tissues and organs in an appropriate way.

The cardiovascular system accomplishes this task in a way that depends on two mechanisms. First, blood pressure (the mean arterial pressure, MAP) is regulated, held more or less constant, in the face of all internal and external disturbances, by a variety of reflexes. Second, the resistance to flow to each tissue or organ is determined by the local metabolic activity. As long as a constant blood pressure can be maintained, local changes in individual tissue beds can apportion the cardiac output in a functionally appropriate manner.

General Model: Homeostasis

Blood pressure regulation is achieved by a negative feedback system that is made up of all of the components of the systems described in Chapter 4: a sensor (baroreceptor), a central site at which the desired pressure and the pressure present can be compared, and a set of controllers, which generate neural signals to determine the behavior of those components of the cardiovascular system that determine the blood pressure.

Blood Pressure

The maximum arterial pressure attained during each cardiac cycle is called the *systolic blood pressure* (SBP), and the minimum pressure recorded during diastole is called the *diastolic blood pressure* (DBP). When recorded from the brachial artery of a young adult in the sitting or supine position, the SBP is ~120 mm Hg, and the DBP is ~80 mm Hg. The difference between the systolic and diastolic pressures is called the *pulse pressure* (PP). It is normally ~40 mm Hg (120 mm Hg – 80 mm Hg).

The *mean blood pressure (or MAP)* is the average pressure during the cardiac cycle. It can be estimated by measuring out the area under a blood pressure tracing for one cardiac cycle and dividing it by its duration. Because systole is shorter than diastole, greater weight is given to the DBP in the calculation of the MAP, which is therefore slightly less than the simple average of the systolic and diastolic pressures. As an approximation, the mean pressure is weighted 2:1 in favor of the DBP. Thus, an approximate value for MAP can be obtained using the equation

$$MAP \cong DBP + 1/3\ PP \qquad (38.1)$$

For example, if the SBP is 120 mm Hg, and DBP is 90 mm Hg, the MAP is 100 mm Hg (and not 105 mm Hg, the simple arithmetic mean).

Note, however, that this calculation is only approximately correct if the duration of systole and diastole are normal; there are conditions in which the durations change, and hence this calculation yields an erroneous estimate of MAP.

Determinants of Blood Pressure

Arterial blood pressure is the product of the cardiac output and the total peripheral vascular resistance (peripheral resistance, for short).

$$\text{Mean arterial blood pressure} = \text{Cardiac output} \times \text{Peripheral resistance} \qquad (38.2)$$

If the cardiac output is expressed as a product of stroke volume and heart rate, the formula for blood pressure can be expressed as the product of three variables (the triple product).

$$\text{Mean arterial blood pressure} = \text{Stroke volume} \times \text{Heart rate} \times \text{Peripheral resistance} \qquad (38.3)$$

Blood pressure is therefore affected by conditions that affect any of these factors. However, any inference drawn from this formula must also take into account the interdependence of these three factors. For example, a rise in peripheral resistance reduces the stroke volume (by increasing the afterload on the heart) and the heart rate (through the baroreceptor reflex). Even then, a rise in peripheral resistance increases the MAP. It increases the DBP more than the SBP.

An increase in stroke volume increases the PP and the SBP. The increase in DBP is less marked. SBP is also related to the distensibility of the large arteries. For the same cardiac output, SBP is higher if the arterial distensibility is low (if the vessels are stiffer), as in elderly patients with atherosclerosed arteries.

If heart rate reaches very high levels, a reduction in stroke volume can occur due to reduced diastolic filling of the heart. After the first few seconds of such a tachycardia, the cardiac output falls, and the blood pressure falls with it.

Homeostatic Regulation of Blood Pressure

The various mechanisms that maintain a near-constant blood pressure in the body can be categorized into the short, intermediate, and long-term mechanisms (**Table 38.1**). The short-term regulatory mechanisms adjust the function of the heart

Table 38.1	Mechanisms of Blood Pressure Regulation
Short-term mechanisms	
Baroreceptor reflex	
Chemoreceptor reflex	
CNS ischemic response	
Intermediate-term mechanisms	
Renin–angiotensin mechanism	
Stress–relaxation	
Capillary fluid shift mechanism	
Long-term mechanisms	
Pressure diuresis and natriuresis	

Abbreviation: CNS, central nervous system.

and the circulation to maintain a constant blood pressure from minute to minute. The intermediate and long-term mechanisms bring about a change in blood volume, a necessarily slower process, which, in turn, corrects the blood pressure. The mechanism through which a change in blood volume changes blood pressure is shown in **Fig. 38.1**.

It is to be noted that an increase in blood volume does not by itself increase the blood pressure in a proportional way. Any additional volume of blood will locate itself mostly in the venous reservoir, and only a little will be found in the arterial system; this is a consequence of the greater compliance of the venous compartment. As shown in **Fig. 38.1**, it is the increase in cardiac output caused by increased volume that produces the rise in arterial pressure.

Short-term Mechanisms

All homeostatic, regulatory mechanisms require the presence of sensors (receptors) to measure the parameter to be regulated.

Cardiovascular receptors | The mechanoceptors of the cardiovascular system are stretch receptors that provide information about the blood pressure (the baroreceptors) or blood volume (the volume receptors). There are also chemoreceptors located in the carotid and aortic bodies (**Fig. 38.2**). These are discussed with the chemical control of pulmonary ventilation (see Peripheral Chemoreceptors subsection, Chapter 50), and their role in blood pressure regulation is discussed in the context of circulatory shock later in this chapter.

All peripheral afferents from baroreceptors and chemoreceptors end in the nucleus of the tractus solitarius (NTS). The afferents release the excitatory neurotransmitter glutamate. Cells of the NTS, in turn, relay the information to other centers that control parasympathetic and sympathetic output.

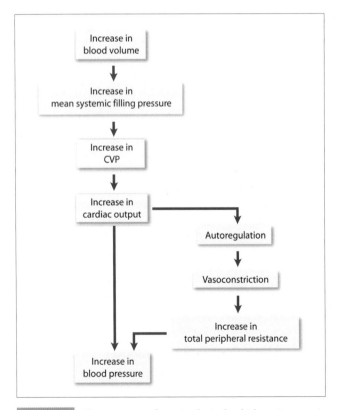

Fig. 38.1 The sequence of events through which an increase in blood volume leads to an increase in blood pressure. CVP, central venous pressure.

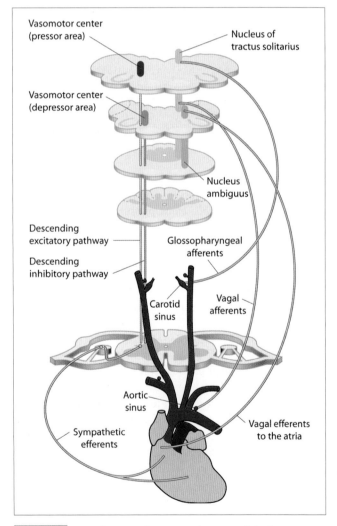

Fig. 38.2 The afferents, efferents, and centers of the baroreceptor reflex. The interconnections of the centers are shown in **Fig. 38.3**.

Baroreceptors are coiled nerve endings located in the adventitia of carotid and aortic arteries at specialized locations. The *carotid baroreceptors* are located in a small dilatation of the internal carotid artery (the carotid sinus) located just above the bifurcation of the common carotid. It is innervated by the sinus nerve, which is a branch of the glossopharyngeal nerve. The *aortic baroreceptors* are located at the transverse part of the aortic arch, adjacent to the root of the left subclavian artery. It is innervated by the left aortic (mainly) and right aortic nerves, which join the superior laryngeal branch of the vagus. The sinus nerves (from the carotid sinus) and vagal fibers (from the aortic arch) are together called the *buffer nerves* because they are the afferents of cardiovascular reflexes that buffer abrupt changes in blood pressure.

The baroreceptors are tonically active above an, MAP of ~40 to 50 mm Hg and reach their maximum firing rate at ~200 mm Hg. Their rate of firing action potentials increases as pressure rises and falls if pressure falls. They are most sensitive to changes in pressure at ~100 mm Hg (the setpoint for the cardiovascular system).

Volume receptors are located in low-pressure areas of circulation, as in the walls of the right and left atria at the entrance of the superior and inferior vena cavae and in the pulmonary veins and arteries. Collectively, they are called cardiopulmonary receptors. The immediate effect of an increase in blood volume is an increase in the central venous pressure (CVP) (**Fig. 38.1**). The rise in CVP stretches the atrial wall and stimulates the volume receptors present in it.

Baroreceptors and volume receptors are structurally and functionally similar: it is their location that determines whether they detect blood pressure or blood volume. The same stretch receptor located in the high-pressure, low-compliance, low-volume carotid sinus functions as a baroreceptor. A stretch receptor in the low-pressure, high-compliance, high-volume right side of the heart or circulation functions like a volume receptor.

Cardiovascular Reflexes

Baroreceptor reflex | At normal blood pressure, the afferent fibers in the buffer nerves discharge at a low rate. When the pressure inside the sinus or aortic arch rises, the discharge rate increases. The discharge rate reaches a plateau at 150 mm Hg. When the pressure falls, the discharge rate declines and becomes zero when the blood pressure decreases to 30 mm Hg. The carotid receptors respond both to the mean pressure and the PP. Thus, the baroreceptor discharge increases if the mean pressure rises while the PP remains unchanged, or if the PP rises while the mean pressure remains unchanged.

Whenever the blood pressure changes rapidly, the baroreceptor reflex quickly brings about a compensatory change (via a negative feedback system), correcting the original change in blood pressure. The baroreceptor reflex prevents erratic fluctuations in blood pressure. In the absence of the reflex, the blood pressure would fluctuate wildly during postural changes, emotional changes, or the Valsalva maneuver associated with defecation and coughing.

The baroreceptor reflex fails if the change in pressure is slow and sustained. This is because of baroreceptor resetting, wherein the baroreceptor readjusts itself to a different "resting" blood pressure. The reset baroreceptor reflex then tries to maintain blood pressure at the new resting blood pressure. The resetting is reversible. Because of baroreceptor resetting, the baroreceptor reflex cannot contribute to the long-term regulation of blood pressure. In chronic hypertension, for example, the baroreceptor reflex is reset at a higher blood pressure, say, 110 mm Hg. Any rapid change in blood pressure from this setpoint will be quickly restored to 110 mm Hg through the baroreceptor reflex.

The multiple cardiovascular control centers discharge in a coordinated way. The ultimate output is either sympathetic stimulation with parasympathetic inhibition or parasympathetic stimulation with sympathetic inhibition.

For example, when baroreceptor firing decreases (pressure decreases), sympathetic outflow increases. Multiple sites are involved in this response (**Fig. 38.3**): the cells of the NTS that receive the baroreceptor input (1) stimulate the intermediomedial (IMM) cells and inhibit the intermediolateral (IML) cells, (2) stimulate the vasomotor center (VMC) depressor area and inhibit the VMC pressor area, (3) stimulate the hypothalamic depressor area and inhibit the defense area, and (4) stimulate the nucleus ambiguus.

Thus, the baroreceptor reflex (**Fig. 38.4**) regulates MAP by altering the firing of the sympathetic and parasympathetic innervation of the heart and blood vessels. So, in the case of a disturbance that causes a decrease in pressure, the changes in sympathetic and parasympathetic firing bring about an increase in heart rate. This tends to increase cardiac output. However, the increase in cardiac output decreases CVP, and hence filling of the right ventricle decreases. Stroke volume falls somewhat, but not too far because the increased sympathetic stimulation of the ventricles increases cardiac contractility. The increased sympathetic activity also increases peripheral resistance. With cardiac output increased and peripheral resistance increased, mean pressure (MAP) returns toward its original level.

The baroreceptor reflex can be elicited in an experimental animal such as a dog by bilateral perfusion of the carotid sinus or by bilateral clamping of the carotid arteries distal to the carotid sinus. As already mentioned, the carotid baroreceptor reflex will cause reduction in blood pressure, heart rate, and respiratory rate. However, the fall in blood pressure will be detected by the aortic baroreceptors, which will partially restore the blood pressure and heart rate. Hence, the reflex effects of carotid baroreceptor stimulation are exaggerated by vagotomy, which abolishes the buffering effects of the aortic baroreceptors.

In humans, the baroreceptor reflex can be elicited by applying pressure on the carotid sinus and through the Valsalva and Müller maneuvers. The reflex increase in vagal discharge during baroreceptor reflex is of therapeutic value in controlling supraventricular tachycardia; therefore, the reflex is sometimes stimulated through *carotid massage*—applying

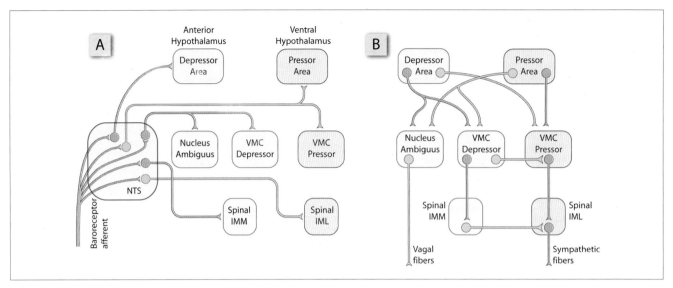

Fig. 38.3 **(A)** Central connections of the baroreceptor afferents. **(B)** Interconnections of hypothalamic, brainstem, and spinal control centers of the cardiovascular system. Red: excitation; blue: inhibition. IML, intermediolateral; IMM, intermediomedial; NTS, nucleus of the tractus solitarius; VMC, vasomotor center.

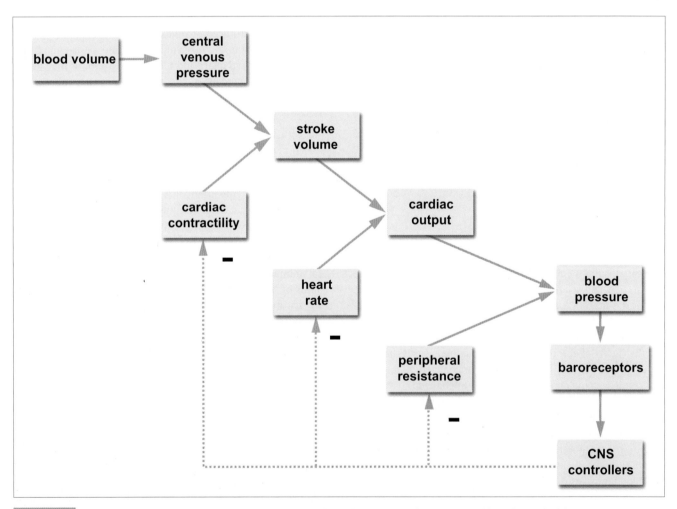

Fig. 38.4 The baroreceptor reflex. The solid lines represent physical interactions between variables. The dashed lines represent neural connections. This is a negative feedback system that regulates (holds more or less constant) mean arterial pressure. CNS, central nervous system.

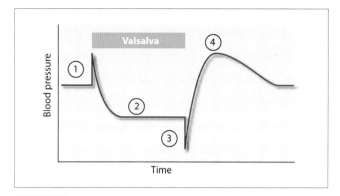

Fig. 38.5 Blood pressure changes during the Valsalva maneuver.

pressure on the area of the neck overlying the carotid sinus. The reflex is also activated on wearing a tight collar that presses upon the carotid sinus, causing reflex hypotension and fainting (carotid sinus syncope).

In the *Valsalva maneuver,* a forced expiration performed against a closed glottis results in a large rise in the intrathoracic pressure. The maneuver helps in defecation and parturition, as it is also associated with a sharp rise in intra-abdominal pressure due to the contraction of abdominal muscles. The rise in intrathoracic pressure during a Valsalva maneuver (+40 mm Hg or more) results in a series of changes in cardiac output and arterial blood pressure, which can be described in four phases (**Fig. 38.5**).

In *phase 1,* the arterial pressure increases transiently as the increase in intrathoracic pressure compresses the aorta. *Phase 2* consists of a fall in the DBP and PP because the high intrathoracic pressure prevents adequate diastolic filling of the heart. The fall in blood pressure initiates the baroreflex, which increases the heart rate slightly but fails to increase the cardiac output in the absence of adequate diastolic filling. The blood pressure therefore remains low. *Phase 3* occurs 1 to 2 seconds after release of the strain and consists of a transient fall in blood pressure. It is the reversal of phase 1, caused by the release of pressure compressing the aorta. In *phase 4,* the systolic pressure and MAP rise above the resting level within 10 seconds and return to resting value in 1 to 2 minutes. The blood pressure overshoot is caused by the continuation of the vasoconstriction initiated in phase 2.

Exactly the opposite changes occur in the Müller maneuver—forced inspiration against a closed glottis.

A common situation in which the baroreceptor reflex is activated is during venous pooling. Venous pooling occurs when the posture changes from the recumbent (supine) to the erect (standing) posture, or when the body is exposed to high Gz+ (**Fig. 38.6**). This sets off a series of responses that are summarized in **Table 38.2**.

The **Bainbridge reflex** increases the heart rate when the right atrial pressure rises above normal. The increase in CVP excites vagal afferents in the atrial wall and reflexively stimulates sympathetic discharge. The increase in heart rate reduces the diastolic filling time of the ventricles and limits the rise in stroke volume that would otherwise occur due to the increase

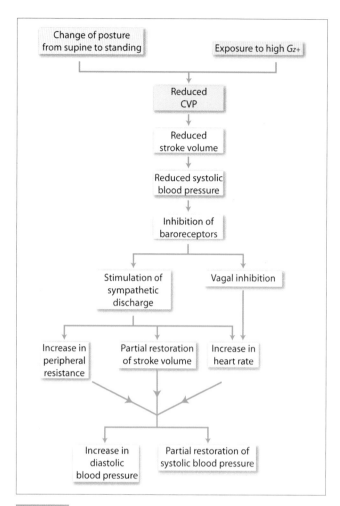

Fig. 38.6 Flow chart showing changes in blood pressure following a change of posture from supine to standing or an exposure to high Gz+. Both of these procedures cause an expansion of the venous compartment below the heart ("venous pooling"). CVP, central venous pressure.

Table 38.2 Cardiovascular Responses to Venous Pooling Brought About by the Baroreceptor Reflex

Central venous pressure	Reduced
Total peripheral resistance	Increased
Stroke volume	Reduced
Cardiac output	Reduced. Due to a rise in heart rate, the reduction in cardiac output is less marked than the reduction in stroke volume
Systolic blood pressure	Slightly reduced due to the fall in stroke volume, which remains undercorrected by the reflex sympathetic discharge
Diastolic blood pressure	Slightly elevated due to the rise in peripheral resistance
Pulse pressure	Reduced
Mean blood pressure	Nearly unchanged

in right atrial pressure. The reverse, however, is not true: the heart rate increases even when the CVP falls. At low CVP, the cardiac output and blood pressure fall, triggering the baroreceptor reflex, which now overrides a weak Bainbridge reflex (**Fig. 38.7**).

The atrial receptors that bring about the Bainbridge reflex are volume receptors. In addition to the Bainbridge reflex, stimulation of the atrial volume receptors reflexively brings about renal vasodilatation, inhibition of antidiuretic hormone (ADH) secretion from the posterior pituitary, and the release of atrial natriuretic peptide (ANP).

Chemoreceptor reflex | Hypoxic stimulation of the chemoreceptors increases blood pressure, heart rate, and respiratory rate (**Fig. 38.8**). Under experimental conditions in which the respiratory effects are prevented, there is an increase in blood pressure, but a decrease in heart rate (see below). The importance of the chemoreflex is discussed in Chapter 50.

The chemoreceptor reflex can be experimentally stimulated by perfusion of the carotid sinus with a perfusate containing 5% oxygen. As already mentioned, the reflex effects would be a rise in blood pressure, heart rate, and respiratory rate. If, however, our subject, the dog mentioned here earlier, is anesthetized to the point where the respiratory center is inhibited, keeping it alive through artificial ventilation, then the heart rate decreases instead of increasing. The reason is as follows. Chemoreceptor afferents (1) stimulate the vasomotor pressor area, resulting in a rise in blood pressure; (2) stimulate the nucleus ambiguus, resulting in a decrease in heart rate; and (3) stimulate the respiratory center, resulting in a rise in the respiratory rate. The stimulated respiratory center also inhibits the nucleus ambiguus and therefore increases the heart rate. This increase in heart rate is not seen if the respiratory center is kept inhibited by anesthesia. It is likely that the

respiratory center does not directly inhibit the nucleus ambiguus but might be blocking (gating) the excitatory impulses traveling from the NTS to the nucleus ambiguus.

The effects of stimulation of the chemoreceptor afferents (increased blood pressure, heart rate, and respiratory rate) are exactly opposite the effects of baroreceptor stimulation (decreased blood pressure, heart rate, and respiratory rate). Hence, stimulation of the sinus nerve, which contains both chemoreceptor and baroreceptor afferents, results in a mutual cancellation of their effects. On the other hand, the proximal clamping of the common carotid causes a combination of chemoreceptor stimulation (due to reduced perfusion of carotid bodies) and baroreceptor inhibition (due to reduced pressure in the carotid sinus). The result is a marked stimulation of blood pressure, heart rate, and respiratory rate.

Blood Pressure during Exercise
Whether blood pressure rises or falls during exercise depends on the type of exercise. If the exercise involves rhythmic contractions and relaxations (as occurs in rowing, for example), it is called *dynamic exercise*. If the exercise involves intense and sustained isometric contraction (as in weightlifting), it is called *static exercise*.

In **dynamic exercise,** there is a marked dilatation of the capillary bed due to metabolic autoregulation, leading to an increase in cardiac output (see **Fig. 34.4**). The DBP falls slightly because, although the cardiac output rises many fold, there is a marked fall in peripheral resistance. The PP increases due to an increase in stroke volume. The systolic pressure rises, and so does the MAP.

In **static exercise,** the muscle capillaries get squeezed by the contracting muscles; therefore, there is a marked rise in peripheral resistance. The stroke volume decreases due to the

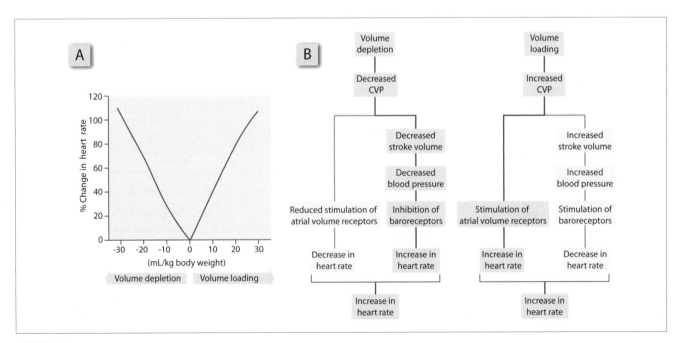

Fig. 38.7 **(A)** Changes in heart rate in response to volume depletion and volume loading of circulation. **(B)** Reflex mechanisms that mediate the biphasic response of heart rate to volume depletion and volume loading. CVP, central venous pressure.

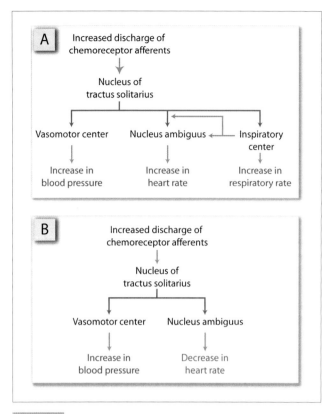

Fig. 38.8 **(A)** Chemoreceptor reflex increases the heart rate due to inhibition of the nucleus ambiguus by the stimulated respiratory center. **(B)** Chemoreceptor reflex decreases the heart rate *if its effect on the respiratory center is prevented*.

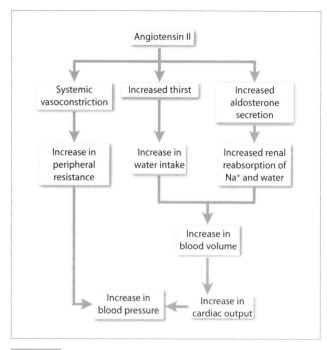

Fig. 38.9 The effects of angiotensin on blood pressure.

combination of an increase in afterload (increased peripheral resistance) and reduced preload (reduced CVP). The DBP rises due to the increased peripheral resistance, but the PP falls due to a reduction in stroke volume. The MAP rises markedly and can rise to as high as 400 mm Hg in heavy weightlifting. Static exercises cannot be sustained continuously for more than a few seconds because blood supply to the muscles ceases completely due to capillary compression.

Intermediate-term Mechanisms
Renin–angiotensin mechanisms are discussed in Chapter 61; they are briefly summarized here (**Fig. 38.9**). A fall in blood pressure results in a reflex increase in sympathetic discharge. The sympathetic discharge to the kidneys causes renin-degranulation. Renin catalyzes the formation of angiotensin I, which is then converted into angiotensin II by angiotensin-converting enzyme (ACE). Angiotensin II is a powerful vasoconstrictor that helps to restore blood pressure by increasing the peripheral resistance. Angiotensin II also brings about an increase in blood volume by increasing thirst and stimulating aldosterone secretion. It thus increases the cardiac output, which helps in restoring the blood pressure.

Capillary fluid shift mechanism | When blood pressure rises, it increases the capillary hydrostatic pressure, which causes increased capillary transudation. As a result, blood volume decreases and blood pressure falls.

Stress–relaxation mechanism | When there is a sustained increase in arterial blood pressure, the arterial and arteriolar smooth muscles yield to the sustained distending pressure (see Mechanism of Smooth Muscle Contraction subsection, Plasticity, Chapter 18), leading to a dilatation of these vessels. The vasodilatation decreases the blood pressure.

Long-term Mechanism
The long-term mechanism corrects blood pressure by causing appropriate changes in blood volume through diuresis and natriuresis (**Fig. 38.10**). In fact, it is similar to the capillary fluid shift mechanism except that only the glomerular capillaries are involved in the process.

Role of electrolytes in blood volume regulation | An increase in blood volume produced by water retention alone gets quickly corrected because it leads to changes in both volume and osmolarity of the plasma (see **Fig. 57.3**), stimulating volume receptors as well as osmoreceptors. This leads to powerful suppression of the thirst-ADH mechanism, resulting in prompt diuresis with restoration of blood volume. If the excess water intake is accompanied by excess salt intake, too, the blood volume increases but remains iso-osmolar. In such a situation, osmoreceptors are not stimulated, and the volume receptors alone bring about the suppression of the thirst-ADH mechanism. However, being stretch receptors similar to the baroreceptor, volume receptors get reset to a higher level when the rise in blood volume is slow and sustained. Hence, an increase in the sodium (Na^+) intake or a decrease in the Na^+ output can produce a sustained increase in the blood volume.

Pressure natriuresis refers to the changes in urinary output of Na^+ in response to changes in arterial blood pressure. For maintenance of a constant blood pressure, the amount of natriuresis must be balanced by an equal amount of Na^+ intake.

the impairment of pressure natriuresis in the kidneys. In disease states, increased peripheral resistance is generalized and affects the kidney, too. Increased resistance of the renal artery reduces renal blood flow, stimulates angiotensin formation, and impairs pressure natriuresis.

Some of the causes of hypertension are as follows. (1) Preeclampsia and eclampsia cause hypertension due to a pressor polypeptide secreted by the placenta. (2) Hyperaldosteronism and Cushing syndrome produce hypertension due to salt and water retention. (3) Pheochromocytomas are catecholamine-secreting tumors of the adrenal medulla. Hypertension develops when the catecholamine secreted is norepinephrine. (4) Renal hypertension is due to narrowing of the renal arteries. (5) Coarctation of the aorta, a congenital narrowing of a segment of the thoracic aorta, increases the resistance to blood flow, producing severe hypertension in the upper part of the body. The blood pressure in the lower part of the body is usually normal, but it may be elevated due to increased renin secretion. (6) Pill hypertension is produced if estrogen-containing oral contraceptives are consumed over prolonged periods. The hypertension is due to an increase in circulating levels of angiotensinogen, the production of which is stimulated by estrogens.

Hypertension of unknown origin is called *essential hypertension* and accounts for 90% of cases of hypertension. It is probably due to autonomic hyperreactivity so that there are exaggerated hypertensive responses to common stimuli, such as cold and excitement. The frequent spasms of the arterioles lead to hypertrophy of their musculature so that at later stages, the hypertension becomes sustained. In hypertension of known causes, the pathogenesis can mostly be traced to a right-shifted salt-loading curve.

Adverse Effects of Hypertension

Clinical hypertension is classified as mild, moderate, severe, and very severe, as given in **Table 38.3**. The adverse effects of hypertension are directly related to the severity of the hypertension.

Cardiac effects | Hypertension imposes a sustained high afterload on the left ventricle, leading to left ventricular hypertrophy. Ultimately, left ventricular function deteriorates, leading to left ventricular failure. There is also myocardial

Table 38.3 Clinical Classification of Blood Pressure

Category	Systolic (mm Hg)	Diastolic (mm Hg)
Normal	< 130	< 85
High normal	130–139	85–95
Mild hypertension	140–159	90–99
Moderate hypertension	160–179	100–109
Severe hypertension	180–209	110–119
Very severe hypertension	≥ 210	≥ 120

Note: When systolic and diastolic pressures are in different categories, the higher category is selected.

ischemia due to increased myocardial O_2 demand without a commensurate increase in coronary blood flow: the myocardial O_2 demand rises as the high afterload necessitates development of greater intraventricular pressure and therefore higher myocardial tension. Most deaths from hypertension are due to myocardial infarction or cardiac failure.

Vascular effects | Hypertension is associated with characteristic retinal changes, such as narrowing of arterioles, retinal hemorrhages, exudates, and papilledema. Hypertension is commonly associated with occipital headache, particularly in the morning. There may be cerebral infarction due to the increased incidence of atherosclerosis that is seen in hypertensive patients. The high blood pressure also tends to cause cerebral hemorrhage. The atherosclerosis associated with hypertension affects the renal arterioles, too, and thereby impairs glomerular filtration. About 10% of deaths from hypertension occur due to renal failure.

Treatment of Hypertension

Antihypertensive drugs include (1) α-adrenergic receptor blocking drugs, which reduce the vasoconstrictive effect of sympathetic discharge and circulating catecholamines; (2) β_1-adrenergic receptor blockers, which decrease cardiac contractility; (3) ACE inhibitors, which inhibit the activity of angiotensin-converting enzyme; and (4) calcium channel blockers, which relax vascular smooth muscle. Some patients show a marked increase in blood pressure when fed a high-sodium diet, whereas others do not. Because there is no easy test to distinguish salt-responsive from salt-resistant humans, salt restriction is advised for all patients with hypertension.

Circulatory Shock

Patients with an SBP of less than 100 mm Hg are called hypotensive. However, most of them are normal and symptom-free. Some of them may complain of lethargy, weakness, and easy fatigability. The symptoms are due to reduced perfusion of the brain, heart, skeletal muscles, and other organs. Chronic hypotension is often seen in adrenocortical insufficiency (Chapter 79).

Sometimes, however, the blood pressure drops so low that there is widespread, serious reduction of tissue perfusion, which, if prolonged, leads to general impairment of cellular function. Such a state is called *circulatory shock*. Shock is triggered by hypotension, but hypotension does not always result in shock. Conversely, shock can get triggered in the absence of hypotension. This can happen in a hypertensive patient whose blood pressure suddenly drops to normal.

Stages of Circulatory Shock

Nonprogressive (compensated) stage | The blood pressure remains more or less normal in the nonprogressive stage (**Fig. 38.12**). The cardiac output, too, is normal or is slightly reduced. Why, then, call it shock at all? It is called a shock because it requires a high rate of sympathetic discharge to maintain the blood pressure at the normal level. The high pulse rate reflects the augmented sympathetic discharge.

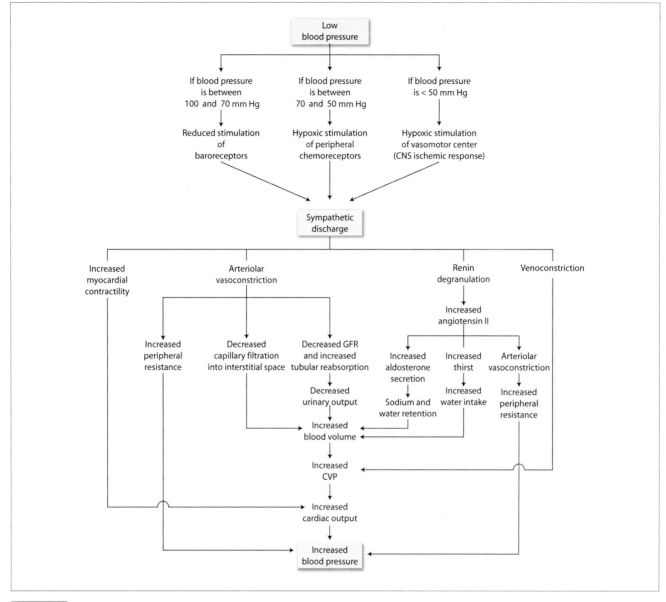

Fig. 38.12 Compensatory responses to hypotension. CNS, central nervous system; CVP, central venous pressure; GFR, glomerular filtration rate.

Sympathetic discharge increases cardiac contractility and peripheral resistance. Also, it increases the blood volume by numerous mechanisms, including fluid shift into capillaries, renal conservation of water, and increased thirst. Because of these compensatory responses, ~10% of the total blood volume can be removed with no significant effect on either arterial pressure or cardiac output, but greater blood loss usually diminishes the cardiac output first and later the blood pressure, both falling to zero when ~40% of the total blood volume has been removed. The increase in sympathetic discharge is brought about by three reflexes, which are given below.

1. The *baroreceptor reflex* is triggered by even a slight lowering of the MAP. The fall in blood pressure reduces the afferent baroreceptor discharge and disinhibits the vasomotor center. The utility of the baroreflex ends when the blood pressure falls so low that the vasomotor center is completely disinhibited. This occurs at ~70 mm Hg of blood pressure.

2. The *chemoreceptor reflex* is activated when the MAP drops below 70 mm Hg. Stimulation of chemoreceptors occurs due to severe stagnant hypoxia and anemic hypoxia (in hemorrhagic shock). When the compensatory chemoreflex becomes prominent, the blood pressure may slow fluctuations with a frequency of 1.5 to 3/min. In a continuous record of blood pressure, these fluctuations appear as the Mayer waves. The fluctuations probably occur due to a slowing of blood circulation.

3. The *CNS ischemic response* is triggered when the MAP drops to below 55 mm Hg. It is stimulated by ischemia of the brain and brings about a last bout of the most intense sympathetic discharge.

Sympathetic stimulation does not cause significant constriction of either the cerebral or the coronary vessels. In both these vascular beds, local autoregulation is excellent, which prevents even a moderate fall in arterial pressure from significantly affecting the blood flow in them. Therefore, blood flow through the heart and brain is maintained essentially at normal levels as long as the arterial pressure does not fall below ~70 mm Hg, even as blood flow in other parts of the body decreases to as low as 25% due to vasospasm.

Progressive stage | In the progressive stage, there is a measurable hypotension, indicating that even the maximum compensatory responses are inadequate (**Fig. 38.13**). As shock progresses, the cardiac output deteriorates more than the blood pressure. The reason why the blood pressure is better maintained than the cardiac output is that sympathetic discharge, which is the main compensatory mechanism, increases both cardiac output and peripheral resistance. Because blood pressure is the product of both, it improves markedly. On the other hand, the increase in cardiac output is partly thwarted by the increase in peripheral resistance.

The continuous fall in blood pressure indicates that a vicious cycle has started. Somewhere along this vicious path is a point of no return. Therapeutic interventions before this point can restore normalcy. However, beyond this point, all interventions are ineffective, and the shock is called irreversible. The vicious cycle occurs due to the following reasons.

1. *Cardiac depression* When the arterial pressure falls very low, coronary blood flow decreases, causing myocardial ischemia. This weakens the heart and decreases the cardiac output further.
2. *Vasomotor failure* In the early stages of shock, various circulatory reflexes intensify the discharge of the vasomotor center. However, in the late stages, the diminished blood flow to the vasomotor center depresses the center itself (vasomotor failure), so that the sympathetic discharge is abolished.
3. *Acidosis* The sluggish blood flow through tissues causes accumulation of vasodilatory metabolites and results in stagnant hypoxia. The hypoxia causes lactic acidosis as the cells switch to anaerobic glycolysis. Lactic acid and other vasodilatory metabolites aggravate the shock.
4. *Sludging of blood* The sluggish blood flow in the capillaries leads to thrombosis in the capillaries and a tendency for the blood cells to stick to each other, making it difficult for

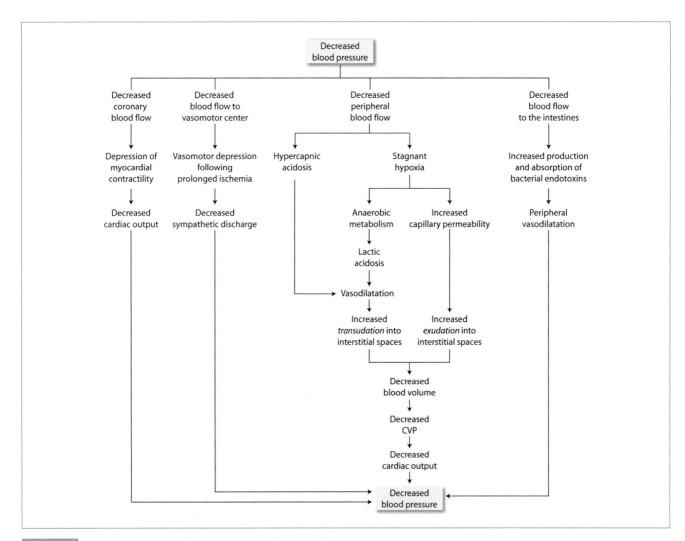

Fig. 38.13 Sequence of events leading to the progression of shock. CVP, central venous pressure.

blood to flow through and aggravating the tissue hypoxia and acidosis.

5. *Increased capillary permeability* Prolonged capillary hypoxia damages the capillary endothelium, allowing the transudation of large quantities of fluid into the tissues. This further decreases the blood volume, aggravating the shock.

6. *Release of toxins by ischemic tissues* Diminished blood flow to the intestines favors the formation of endotoxins by gram-negative bacteria and enhances their absorption. These endotoxins cause extensive vasodilatation and depress the myocardium. Endotoxins play a major role in septicemic shock.

7. *Generalized cellular deterioration* As shock becomes very severe, there is anoxic damage to the tissues, especially in the liver, lungs, and heart. The heart and liver are especially vulnerable because of their high metabolic rate. The liver is also the first organ to be exposed to toxins from the intestine through the portal vein. The lungs develop pulmonary edema and fail to oxygenate the blood adequately.

8. *Tissue necrosis* occurs in the cells worst affected by hypoxia. Hence, there is necrosis in zone 3 of hepatic acini (see **Fig. 42.4**), in the tubules of the kidney (acute tubular necrosis), in the lung (shock lung syndrome), and in the heart.

Irreversible stage | Once the shock progresses to the irreversible stage, the cardiac output and blood pressure continue to deteriorate despite transfusion and medication, culminating in death. Probably, the single most important event that marks the point of irreversibility is the depletion of cellular adenosine. The high-energy phosphate reserves, especially in the liver and in the heart, are greatly diminished in severe shock. Nearly all the adenosine triphosphate (ATP) gets degraded to adenosine diphosphate (ADP), adenosine monophosphate (AMP), and eventually to adenosine. The adenosine diffuses out of the cells into the circulating blood and is converted into uric acid. New adenosine is synthesized rather slowly so that once depleted, the high-energy phosphate stores of the cells are difficult to replenish.

Causes of Shock

Blood pressure is the product of cardiac output and peripheral resistance. Hence, causes of hypotension include conditions causing a reduction in cardiac output and conditions in which peripheral resistance is reduced. Of course, a reduction in peripheral resistance tends to increase cardiac output by reducing cardiac afterload, but so long as their product, the blood pressure, is reduced, the possibility of shock remains. If the reduction in cardiac output is due to a hypoeffective heart, it is called cardiogenic shock. If the reduction of cardiac output is due to a reduced CVP, the most common cause of which is hypovolemia, it is called hypovolemic shock. Another cause of shock is vasogenic or low-resistance shock, in which there is excessive peripheral vasodilatation. It is also called distributive shock because vasodilatation is associated with a redistribution of blood flow, with more blood accumulating in the venous compartment.

Hypovolemic shock | Common causes of hypovolemic shock are as follows: (1) loss of blood (external or internal bleeding); (2) loss of plasma (burns and exudative lesions)—in burns, large areas of the skin get denuded, and hence large volumes of plasma are exuded through these exposed areas so that hypovolemia is a common complication of burns; (3) loss of fluids (dehydration due to excessive vomiting, diarrhea, sweating)—hypovolemia due to loss of plasma or fluids creates the additional problem of raised blood viscosity, which tends to slow down circulation; (4) *traumatic shock* is a special type of hypovolemic shock in which there is associated neurogenic shock, too, caused by the severe pain that inhibits the vasomotor center.

Cardiogenic shock | Common causes of cardiogenic shock are myocardial infarction, arrhythmias, and valvular disorders.

Obstructive shock occurs due to obstruction to the diastolic filling of the heart, resulting in a decrease in cardiac output. Examples include pulmonary embolism, cardiac tamponade, and tension pneumothorax.

Distributive shock occurs due to massive exudation of plasma from the blood vessels to the interstitial spaces. It may be neurogenic, anaphylactic, septicemic, or endotoxic. (1) *Neurogenic shock* occurs due to a marked reduction in sympathetic vasomotor tone. Its causes include deep general anesthesia, spinal anesthesia affecting the thoracolumbar sympathetic outflow, spinal injury, brain concussion, and antihypertensive drugs. Some cases of neurogenic shock occur due to an increase in the vagal tone of the heart, as in vasovagal syncope. (2) *Anaphylactic shock* is associated with reduced peripheral resistance due to the release of histamine, which causes vasodilatation and increased capillary permeability. Hypovolemia occurs due to excessive exudation. (3) *Septicemic shock* is produced by bacterial toxins that produce vasodilatation, not only in the infected tissues but elsewhere, too, by stimulating cellular metabolism and producing fever. (4) *Endotoxic shock* occurs in gram-negative septicemia due to release of endotoxin. Endotoxic shock is similar in mechanism to anaphylactic shock. Additionally, endotoxin depresses myocardial contractility.

Clinical Features of Shock

The patient in shock is typically restless and tachypneic. There may be Cheyne-Stokes breathing. The pulse is rapid and thready (of low volume). The skin is pale, cold, and clammy (moist) and may show peripheral cyanosis. The SBP is less than 100 mm Hg, and the DBP is often not recordable through sphygmomanometry. There is hypothermia due to depressed metabolism. In septic shock, however, there is fever. There is severe muscular weakness.

Impaired renal function | The glomerular filtration rate decreases even in the early stages of shock. It is a part of the compensatory mechanism for restoration of blood volume. In the late stages of shock, the renal tubular epithelial cells get damaged. Certain parts of the tubule are more vulnerable, as they have a very high metabolism but receive only a moderate blood supply. The result is acute tubular necrosis with tubular cell death and sloughing, and blockage of the tubules, leading to acute renal failure.

Treatment of Shock

Patients in shock are kept in a cold room so that there is no further hypovolemia from sweating. Temperature regulation is a prepotent reflex. If exposed to warmth, there would be sweating, which would aggravate the shock further. Shock patients are usually hypothermic, and therefore naïve attendants might be inclined to cover them with blankets. This should never be done.

Replacement therapy | Depending on the cause of hypovolemia (loss of blood, plasma, or fluids), the patient is transfused, respectively, with blood, plasma (or plasma expanders like dextran solution), or isotonic saline solutions. Dextran is a large polysaccharide that does not pass through the capillary pores. It therefore promotes osmosis of water from the interstitial to the intravascular spaces, thereby restoring the plasma volume.

Sympathomimetic drugs are especially beneficial in neurogenic shock and anaphylactic shock. The sympathomimetic drug of choice is dopamine because it produces renal vasodilatation and at the same time, produces vasoconstriction elsewhere in the body. It also has a positive inotropic effect on the heart. In neurogenic shock, sympathomimetic drugs fulfill the physiologic role of the sympathetic nervous system, which is severely depressed. In anaphylactic shock, histamine plays a prominent role; therefore, sympathomimetics are useful in its treatment. Sympathomimetic drugs and histamine are said to be physiologic antagonists because the two have opposite effects. For example, sympathomimetic drugs are vasoconstrictors, whereas histamine is a vasodilator. In hemorrhagic shock, the sympathetic system is already maximally active; therefore, sympathomimetic drugs have limited value.

Glucocorticoids are frequently given to patients in severe shock for several reasons. They increase the strength of the heart in the late stages of shock. They stabilize the lysosomal membranes and prevent release of lysosomal enzymes into the cytoplasm of the cells, thus preventing tissue damage. They also aid in the metabolism of glucose by the severely damaged cells.

Trendelenburg position | Placing the patient with the head lower than the feet helps to increase the CVP, thereby increasing the cardiac output.

Oxygen therapy may be beneficial in some instances. However, the response is not marked, which is not unexpected, considering that oxygen is beneficial mostly in hypoxic hypoxia. The hypoxia of shock is of the stagnant type.

Summary

- Blood pressure is determined by cardiac output and total peripheral resistance.

- Short-term homeostatic mechanisms regulate blood pressure; these are driven by baroreceptors (measuring arterial pressure) and volume receptors (measuring pressure, or volume, in the low-pressure side of the circulation).

- Exercise (dynamic and static) results in cardiovascular changes that alter blood pressure.

- The renin–angiotensin mechanism provides intermediate-term regulation of blood pressure.

- Long-term regulation of blood pressure is dependent on the kidneys to alter blood volume by diuresis and natriuresis.

- Hypertension can be caused by a variety of different mechanisms, but whatever its origin, there are adverse effects that result.

- Shock is a low-pressure state in which tissue perfusion is inadequate to sustain tissue function. There are a variety of causes of low blood pressure that underlie this state, some reversible, others not.

Applying What You Know

38.1. Predict what will happen to central venous pressure if a reflex response generates an increase in Mrs. Daniels's cardiac output. Explain.

38.2. Mrs. Daniels asks if she can donate a pint of blood to a nephew who is to undergo surgery shortly (she has the same blood type). If she were to do this, what changes would occur in her cardiac vascular system immediately after the procedure? What changes would occur over the next day or so?

The right and left coronary arteries take their origin from the aorta at the base of the sinuses of Valsalva behind the cusps of the aortic valve (see **Figs. 33.1** and **39.1**). The right coronary artery supplies the right atrium, the free wall of the right ventricle, parts of the posterior one-third of the ventricular septum, the posterior wall of the left ventricle, the pulmonary conus, the sinoatrial (SA) node (in roughly half the cases), and the atrioventricular (AV) node. The left coronary artery further divides into the left circumflex artery and the anterior descending artery. The left circumflex artery supplies the left atrium and the interatrial septum, the lateral and posterior walls of the left ventricle, and the SA node (in roughly half the cases). The anterior descending artery supplies the free wall of the left ventricle, the ventricular septum, and the anterior wall of the right ventricle.

The left ventricular musculature is drained into the coronary sinus by coronary veins. The coronary sinus opens into the right atrium. The anterior surface of the right ventricle is drained by the anterior cardiac veins, which empty into the right atrium. The atrial muscles are drained by the thebesian veins, which empty into the lumen of the right and left atria. In addition to the veins, there are *myocardial sinusoids* that drain

the myocardial capillaries directly into the ventricles, and the *arterioluminal vessels* that drain the arterioles directly into the ventricles.

Anastomoses between the coronary vessels are usually quite small; hence, sudden occlusion of a coronary artery results in a localized area of myocardial ischemia or infarction (see below). However, if the arterial flow is gradually decreased, as in occlusive coronary artery disease, these anastomotic connections slowly dilate to develop into a collateral channel to the capillary bed of the diseased artery.

Control of the Coronary Blood Flow

The resting coronary blood flow averages ~225 mL/min (70–80 mL of blood/min/100 g of heart), which is 4 to 5% of the total cardiac output.

General Model: Energy

All of the processes involved in permitting the heart to beat continuously require the availability of energy to power the many ion pumps involved, to power the contraction of the myocardial cells, and to make it possible to continuously build the structures of the myocardial cells. Thus, it is essential that coronary blood flow be large enough to meet the metabolic demands of the heart. It also means that as the work of the heart increases (say, during exercise), coronary blood flow increases.

Myocardial oxygen demand is the main controller of coronary blood flow. The resting heart has an O_2 consumption of 8 mL/min/100 g, which is the highest of all organs. To meet this high basal demand for O_2, the myocardium extracts 70% of the O_2 carried by the resting coronary blood supply. As this is the maximum possible extraction ratio, any further increase in O_2 demand can be met only through an increase in coronary blood flow. Changes in coronary blood flow and myocardial oxygen consumption therefore parallel each other. During maximal exertion, the myocardial O_2 demand increases five times; to deliver this augmented O_2 supply, the coronary blood flow, too, must rise five times. The mechanism of this increase is as follows.

Whenever myocardial oxygen demand increases, several products of muscle metabolism, such as CO_2, H^+, potassium (K^+), and adenosine, accumulate in the myocardial tissue. These metabolites produce vasodilatation and thereby increase the coronary blood flow. Though all vasodilator metabolites play some role in adjusting the blood flow, to, the metabolic demand, adenosine seems to be the main physiologic regulator of coronary blood flow. So long as the myocardial oxygen demand remains unchanged, the coronary blood flow, too, tends to remain unchanged. This is known as the autoregulation of coronary blood flow and is seen for perfusion pressures between 60 and 180 mm Hg. As explained in the context of

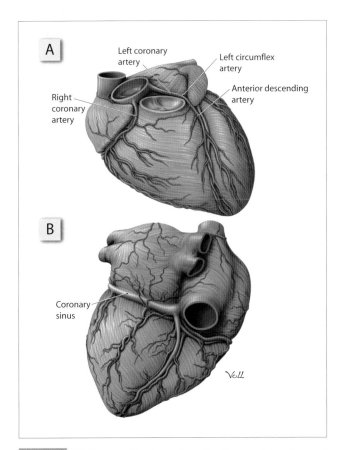

A
Left coronary artery
Left circumflex artery
Anterior descending artery
Right coronary artery

B
Coronary sinus

Voll

Fig. 39.1 **(A)** Coronary blood vessels on the sternocostal surface and **(B)** diaphragmatic surface of the heart.

muscle circulation (see Chapter 42), the mechanism of auto-regulation can be either myogenic or metabolic or both. In case of coronary blood flow, the autoregulation seems to be metabolically mediated, with adenosine as its main mediator.

Myocardial interstitial tissue pressure (intramyocardial pressure) is another major determinant of coronary blood flow. In the left ventricle, pressure in the walls of the ventricle varies widely during the cardiac cycle and causes marked changes in coronary blood flow (**Fig. 39.2**). In the right ventricle, the changes are less marked. During systole, the intramyocardial pressure of the left ventricle is very high, being highest (~120 mm Hg) in the subendocardium and less in the subepicardium (**Fig. 39.3B**). Subendocardial vessels are therefore squeezed much more than the subepicardial ones, and the blood flow to the subendocardial capillaries nearly stops during systole. The subepicardial capillaries are better perfused during systole. The subendocardial capillaries, however, are more numerous and have larger caliber. Hence, they are better perfused during diastole (**Fig. 39.3A**). Generally, the subendocardial and subepicardial capillaries are perfused equally well under normal conditions.

Neural control | Coronary blood vessels are innervated by both sympathetic and vagal fibers. Sympathetic fibers constrict and vagal fibers dilate the coronary vessels. In physiologic situations, however, sympathetic stimulation results in coronary vasodilatation because the direct vasoconstrictor effect of sympathetic discharge is overridden by the marked vasodilatation caused by the increase in myocardial oxygen demand associated with the sympathetic stimulation of the heart.

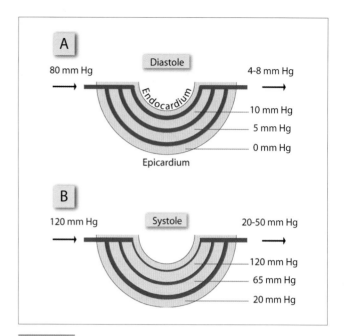

Fig. 39.3 Tissue pressures in different layers of the myocardium during **(A)** diastole and **(B)** systole.

Coronary Insufficiency

The most common cause of coronary insufficiency (reduced blood flow) is atheromatous coronary artery stenosis (commonly called coronary artery disease). It can also occur due to spasm of the coronary artery. Coronary arteries are end-arteries (they have no anastomes), which perfuse their own exclusive capillary bed. Hence, coronary insufficiency results in myocardial ischemia, especially in the subendocardial layers, which are more prone to ischemia than the subepicardial layers. Myocardial infarction (necrosis of myocardial cells) starts occurring after ~20 minutes of continuous myocardial ischemia.

The impairment of cardiac function depends on the extent of myocardial necrosis. Infarction of more than 25% of the left ventricle produces signs of cardiac failure. Infarction of more than 40% produces cardiogenic shock. The infarcted area generates ectopic impulses that can lead to ventricular fibrillation. The mechanical complications include ischemic ventricular septal defect that results from infarction and perforation of the interventricular septum, and mitral regurgitation that results from infarction and rupture of the papillary muscle.

Coronary insufficiency, however, does not always lead to ischemia or infarction. In some individuals, the myocardium adjusts to the coronary insufficiency by reducing its oxygen demand. This phenomenon is called *myocardial hibernation*. The reduced myocardial metabolism reduces the power of the cardiac pump and tends to cause cardiac failure. The exact mechanism of myocardial hibernation is not understood, though it seems to be associated with reduced entry of calcium (Ca^{2+}) into the cardiac muscle cell during contraction.

Consequences of myocardial ischemia | During ischemia, myocardial metabolism switches from aerobic to anaerobic,

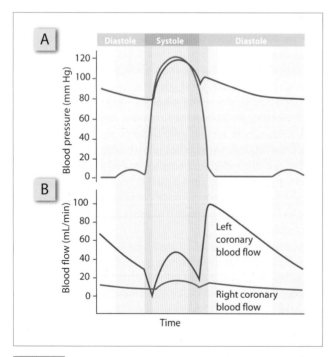

Fig. 39.2 **(A)** The aortic pressure (red) and left ventricular pressure (purple). **(B)** The left and right coronary blood flow. The left coronary blood flow is determined by aortic pressure and the resistance of the coronary vessels, which increases when the walls of the ventricles contract during systole.

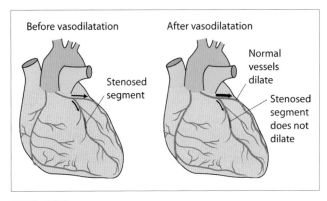

Fig. 39.4 When a stenosed coronary vessel is present, administration of a vasodilator can lead to coronary steal. The normal arteries dilate more than the stenosed artery; therefore, blood flow is shunted to the normal vessel and away from the stenosed vessel.

resulting in acidosis. The high concentration of H^+ competes with Ca^{2+} for binding sites on myosin heads, inhibiting cross-bridge cycling and reducing myocardial contractility. Because the adenosine triphosphate (ATP) yield is much lower in anaerobic metabolism, there is a progressive depletion of ATP. The ATP depletion reduces Ca^{2+} reuptake into sarcoplasmic reticulum and thereby impairs diastolic relaxation. ATP depletion also impairs ion pumps, causing loss of intracellular K^+ and accumulation of intracellular sodium (Na^+) and water. These changes depolarize the muscle, increasing its excitability and triggering arrhythmias. The characteristic anginal pain that is associated with myocardial ischemia is produced by the adenosine formed by degradation of ATP.

Treatment of myocardial ischemia | Nitrates are administered for dilating coronary arteries. However, their use is fraught with the risk of *coronary steal*, in which the flow through the stenotic coronary artery decreases instead of increasing following vasodilator administration. It occurs be-cause the vasodilator dilates other coronary arteries that are disposed in parallel to the stenosed artery but is unable to significantly dilate the stenosed artery (**Fig. 39.4**). Most of the blood therefore flows into the dilated artery (which offers less resistance) instead of flowing into the stenosed artery.

The mainstay of medical therapy is therefore to reduce the cardiac workload, thereby reducing the myocardial O_2 demand. This is achieved by controlling heart rate using β-blockers and reducing afterload and preload by using vasodilators, such as angiotensinogen-converting enzyme (ACE) inhibitors, Ca^{2+}-channel blockers, and nitrates. An interesting method of alleviating myocardial ischemia is to provide *counterpulsations* for improving diastolic perfusion. In this method, a balloon is inserted through the femoral artery and positioned below the left subclavian but above the renal arteries. The inflated balloon increases the diastolic pressure in the aorta. As coronary blood supply is mainly diastolic, this "diastolic augmentation" helps in better perfusion of the coronaries.

Surgical intervention is required only when there is more than 75% reduction in vessel diameter (**Fig. 39.5**). Stenosis of epicardial vessels can be surgically bypassed (coronary artery bypass grafting) using arterial or venous conduits taken from the internal mammary or radial artery or saphenous vein of the patient. Stenosis of the coronary artery may also be dilated by passing a balloon through the femoral or brachial artery and pushing it all the way up into the coronary artery. The balloon is inflated at the stenosis site, causing it to dilate (coronary angioplasty). To avoid recurrence of stenosis, a stent (a tiny tubular mesh of the size similar to coronary vessels) is placed at the stenosed site.

Coronary Vasodilator Reserve

Coronary stenosis may not cause myocardial ischemia at rest, as flow is maintained by compensatory poststenotic dilatation of the artery. This compensatory dilatation is possible only

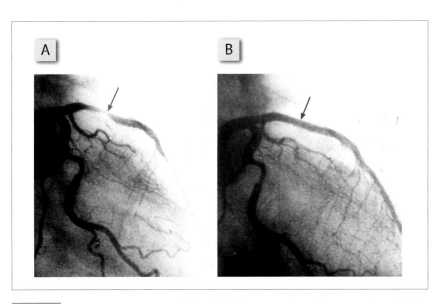

Fig. 39.5 Coronary angiogram. **(A)** Block of the left anterior descending artery (*arrow*). **(B)** Restoration of circulation after angioplasty and stenting (*arrow*).

as long as there is a coronary vasodilator reserve. When the reserve is low, myocardial ischemia appears during physical exertion. When the reserve is exhausted, myocardial ischemia occurs on the slightest exertion. It is therefore important to have an estimate of the coronary vasodilator reserve of an individual. The reserve will be low if the myocardial oxygen consumption is high or if the diastolic perfusion of coronary vessels is low.

Myocardial oxygen consumption (MVO_2) | In the heart, there is a high density of capillaries (perhaps one capillary for each myocardial fiber). With cardiac hypertrophy, the diameter of each muscle fiber increases with concomitant increase in O_2 consumption, but without a corresponding increase in vascularity. As a result, enlarged hearts have an increased vulnerability to circulatory insufficiency. MVO_2 is also high when the myocardial contractility is high.

Summary

- Blood flow to the heart (the coronary circulation) accounts for 4 to 5% of the cardiac output.

- The primary determinant of coronary blood flow is myocardial oxygen demand; the products of myocardial muscle contraction are strong vasodilators (particularly adenosine).

- The tension in the walls of the ventricles is also an important determinant of perfusion; the high pressure present during systole greatly increases resistance and therefore decreases perfusion.

Applying What You Know

39.1. Mr. Wright's (see Section III) response to anesthesia included a rapidly developing tachycardia. What effect did this have on Mr. Wright's coronary blood flow? Explain.

Cerebral Blood Flow

The blood flow to the brain is ~750 mL/min, which is 15% of the resting cardiac output. The weight of the brain is ~1500 g; therefore, the cerebral blood flow is 50 mL/min/100 g of brain tissue. Of all the organs in the body, the brain is most easily damaged by ischemia. A reduction of cerebral blood flow below 30 mL/min/100 g for ~5 seconds results in syncope (fainting). Prolonged ischemia results in neuronal dysfunction, damage, and cell death.

The brain receives blood from two pairs of large arteries: a pair of vertebral arteries and a pair of internal carotid arteries (**Fig. 40.1**). The vertebral arteries unite into a solitary basilar artery, which divides into a pair of posterior cerebral arteries (the vertebrobasal system). Together, they constitute the posterior circulation of the brain.

The carotid artery divides into the anterior and middle cerebral arteries (the carotid system) and constitutes the anterior circulation of the brain. The anterior and posterior circulations communicate through the posterior communicating artery, a branch of the middle cerebral artery. The circulations of the two hemispheres communicate through the anterior communicating artery, a branch of the anterior cerebral artery. The three cerebral arteries (anterior, middle, and posterior) and the two communicating arteries (anterior and posterior) form an arterial network called the circle of Willis below the hypothalamus.

Blood from each carotid artery is distributed largely to the ipsilateral cerebral hemisphere, and very little mixing occurs between the two circulations despite their interconnection through the circle of Willis. This separation takes place because the blood pressure is approximately equal in the two carotid arteries, so that there is no pressure gradient between them. Moreover, the communicating arteries are too small to permit significant flow when there is a sudden occlusion of one carotid artery. Hence, despite the presence of communicating arteries, occlusion of one internal carotid artery results in ipsilateral cerebral ischemia and brain damage.

The lateral surfaces of the cerebral hemisphere are supplied by the terminal branches of the anterior, middle, and posterior cerebral arteries. The border zones between the areas served by these arteries barely receive adequate blood supply and are therefore vulnerable to ischemic damage during sudden hypotension (watershed infarcts).

Measurement of Cerebral Blood Flow

Kety method | In this method, the subject breathes a gas mixture of 15% nitrous oxide (N_2O), 21% oxygen, and 64% nitrogen for 10 minutes, which is sufficient time for equilibration of N_2O between brain tissues and the cerebral venous blood. Simultaneous samples of arterial blood (from any artery) and mixed venous blood (from the internal jugular vein) are taken at the beginning and at every minute interval for 10 minutes. From these data, cerebral blood flow can be calculated by the Fick equation. Because the arterial and venous concentrations are continuously changing with time, it is necessary to get the mean arteriovenous (A-V) difference over the 10-minute period.

$$\text{Cerebral blood flow} = \frac{\substack{N_2O \text{ uptake by brain} \\ \text{in 10 min}}}{\substack{\text{Mean A-V difference of } N_2O \\ \text{over 10 min}}} \quad (40.1)$$

Autoregulation of Total Cerebral Blood Flow

The total cerebral blood flow (CBF) is held constant in the face of considerable changes in the systemic blood pressure (60–140 mm Hg). This autoregulation is important because pressures below 60 mm Hg cause syncope, whereas pressures above 140 mm Hg cause disruption of the blood–brain barrier and cerebral edema. The factors that contribute to the autoregulation of total cerebral blood flow are the rigid compartment in which the brain is located (Monro-Kellie doctrine), Cushing reflex, and myogenic autoregulation.

Monro-Kellie doctrine | There are three elements, the brain, cerebrospinal fluid (CSF), and blood, that are enclosed in the rigid cranial cavity. Fluids are, of course, incompressible. Hence, if any one of them increases, it has to be at the expense of the other two. For example, when a person stands up from a supine position, or if the body accelerates upward (high Gz+), the blood moves toward the feet, and the carotid arterial

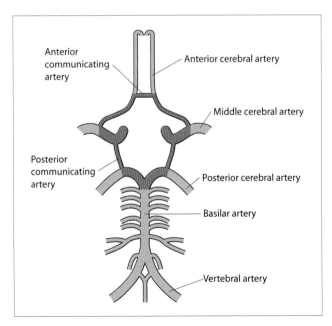

Fig. 40.1 Cerebral arteries (light red) and the circle of Willis (deep red).

Anterior communicating artery

Anterior cerebral artery

Middle cerebral artery

Posterior communicating artery

Posterior cerebral artery

Basilar artery

Vertebral artery

pressure at the level of the head decreases. However, the cerebral blood flow does not decrease much because the intracranial pressure falls simultaneously, reducing the pressure on the artery. The reverse happens with low or negative Gz when the carotid arterial pressure increases. Because the intracranial pressure also rises, the pressure differential across the vessel wall is not increased, and the vessels do not rupture.

Cushing reflex | When the intracranial pressure rises, the cerebral blood flow falls as cerebral blood vessels are compressed, leading to ischemia. The cerebral ischemia causes direct stimulation of the vasomotor area, leading to a rise in the blood pressure and restoration of adequate cerebral blood flow. The rise in blood pressure is proportionate to the rise in intracranial pressure only up to a certain limit, beyond which cerebral circulation ceases.

The rise in intracranial pressure is also associated with reflex bradycardia (produced by the rise in blood pressure through baroreflex) and abolition of the pupilloconstrictor response to light (due to the direct compressive effect on the pupilloconstrictor nerves near the aqueduct). Intracranial tension rises in the late stages of extradural hematoma, and the three signs of raised intracranial tension (blood pressure, heart rate, and pupil) are therefore of ominous significance to the surgeon.

Myogenic autoregulation | As in other circulatory beds, the cerebral precapillary sphincter is sensitive to stretch and responds to an increase in arteriolar pressure with an increase in myogenic tone, thereby limiting the rise in blood flow.

Metabolic Regulation of Regional Cerebral Blood Flow

On performing a specific mental task, the blood flow to the active cerebral area increases (**Fig. 40.2**) because the activated neurons produce metabolites that cause local vasodilatation.

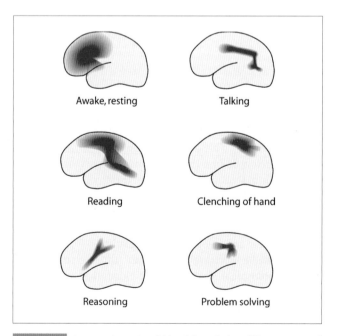

Awake, resting

Talking

Reading

Clenching of hand

Reasoning

Problem solving

Fig. 40.2 Increase in regional blood flow during different types of cerebral activities.

The total cerebral blood flow remains unaltered by localized neuronal activity.

The main metabolic factor responsible for the vasodilatation associated with cerebral activity is the CO_2 produced by the activated neurons. Cerebral vasodilatation is also produced by a rise in blood partial pressure of carbon dioxide (PCO_2) because CO_2 rapidly diffuses into the brain extracellular fluid (ECF) and CSF. Conversely, a decrease in blood PCO_2, as occurs in hyperventilation, causes a reduction in CBF.

The vasodilatory effect of CO_2 is indirect and is mediated by the formation of H^+, which has a direct vasodilatory effect on cerebral blood vessels. A fall in the pH of brain ECF or CSF is therefore equally effective in causing vasodilatation. However, a fall in arterial pH fails to cause cerebral vasodilatation if the arterial PCO_2 is held constant. Hydrogen ions cannot cross the blood–brain barrier: a rise in arterial hydrogen ion (H^+) concentration increases cerebral blood flow only when the blood PCO_2 rises simultaneously.

Other factors affecting cerebral blood flow are potassium (K^+) and adenosine. The K^+ concentration in the brain ECF and CSF increases in the initial stages of hypoxia, seizures, and electroconvulsive therapy. The initial rise in cerebral blood flow in these conditions may therefore be due to the rise in K^+. A more likely mediator of the vasodilatation is adenosine, the synthesis of which increases rapidly during tissue hypoxia and remains elevated throughout the period of hypoxia.

General Model: Energy

Neurons in the brain rely heavily on the oxidative metabolism of glucose for the ATP that provides energy for all of their activities. It is thus essential that the blood flow to the brain, carrying oxygen and glucose, matches brain activity and that the flow is uninterrupted. The cerebral circulation exhibits powerful metabolic controls and does not participate in reflex regulation of blood pressure.

Syncope

Syncope (or fainting) is a sudden and transient loss of consciousness due to inadequate CBF. It is invariably associated with falling down, which is lifesaving because the change in posture increases cerebral blood flow. Syncope can be due to cardiac or noncardiac causes. Cardiac syncope occurs due to the reduction of cardiac output. Noncardiac syncope can be due to a variety of causes, some of which are given below.

Vasovagal syncope (or the common faint) is associated with hypotension and bradycardia. It is caused by some trigger (the sight of blood, an emotional experience) that causes CNS cardiovascular controllers to increase parasympathetic activity in the vagus nerve and decrease sympathetic activity. *Postural syncope* is the fainting that occurs due to inadequate vasomotor response to the fall in blood pressure resulting from a change in posture from sitting or lying to standing. *Carotid sinus syncope* occurs due to excessive sensitivity of the carotid sinus to compression, as by a tight collar. These types of syn-

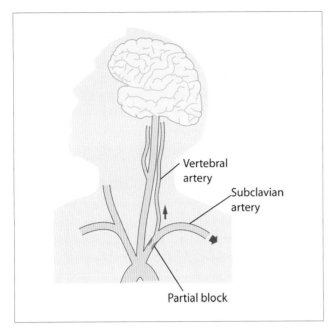

Fig. 40.3 Subclavian steal. Exercising muscles draw more blood into the left upper limb through the subclavian artery, reducing the blood flow to the brain through the vertebral artery.

copes are common in elderly patients. *Situational syncopes* may be associated with cough, micturition, or defecation. All these activities are associated with the Valsalva maneuver, which increases intrathoracic pressure. Micturition and defecation are additionally associated with a sudden reduction in intra-abdominal pressure. The two factors (high intrathoracic and low intra-abdominal pressures) together bring about a reduction in cardiac output and consequent hypotension and syncope. Other factors, for example, the orthostatic hypotension associated with getting up from bed before micturating, might contribute to situational syncopes. Hypoglycemia or hyperventilation can cause *metabolic syncope.* Hypoglycemia inhibits the vasomotor center, whereas hyperventilation causes hypocapnia, resulting in cerebral vasoconstriction and ischemia.

The *subclavian steal syndrome* is sometimes seen when the subclavian artery is blocked proximal to the origin of the vertebral artery. Exercise of the arm of the affected side may draw blood from the vertebral artery into the arm, reducing the blood flow in the basilar artery and causing cerebral ischemia (**Fig. 40.3**).

Cerebrospinal Fluid

Cerebrospinal fluid (CSF) is a clear, colorless, almost protein-free filtrate (transudate) of blood. It is present around the brain and spinal cord (in the subarachnoid space), as well as inside the brain and spinal cord (in its ventricles and the central canal, respectively).

The **subarachnoid space** lies between the arachnoid and the pia mater. It is enlarged in a few places to form subarachnoid cisterns (**Fig. 40.4**). Some of these cisterns (cisterna magna and the spinal cistern) are easily accessible to a needle inserted

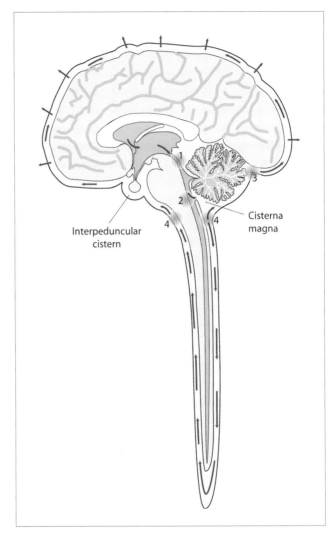

Fig. 40.4 Cerebrospinal fluid circulation within the ventricles and in the subarachnoid space. Obstruction at sites 1 (aqueduct) and 2 (foramen of Magendie and Luschka) results in internal hydrocephalus. Obstruction at sites 3 (tentorial opening) and 4 (foramen magnum) results in external hydrocephalus. Also shown are the subarachnoid cisterns.

through the skin and are therefore used for obtaining samples of CSF. The cranial nerves pierce the dura, but carry with it an investment of arachnoid and pia mater. Thus, the subarachnoid space continues along the cranial nerves. The continuation of the subarachnoid space along the optic nerve leads to the formation of papilledema in conditions of raised intracranial tension. The subarachnoid space also continues along the cerebral blood vessels as perivascular space (also known as Virchow-Robin space).

Cerebrospinal Fluid Circulation

CSF formation | CSF is secreted by the choroid plexus, which is formed by the fusion of the pia mater of the brain with the ventricular ependyma. The ventricular ependyma contains within its folds the choroid capillaries. About 500 mL of CSF is formed each day. The rapid production rate keeps up a slight pressure of ~150 mm of water within the subarachnoid space. The watery part of CSF is secreted by transudation, but each of its constituents is actively transported. Sodium (Na^+) is secreted into the CSF with the help of Na^+-K^+ ATPase. Glucose enters CSF through facilitated diffusion mediated by a membrane glucose transporter GLUT-1. Bicarbonate (HCO_3^-) is secreted into the CSF with the help of carbonic anhydrase, a mechanism also seen in renal tubules.

CSF circulation | From the lateral ventricles, CSF flows through the interventricular foramina (of Monro) into the third ventricle. From there, it flows through the aqueduct (of Sylvius) in the midbrain into the fourth ventricle. Finally, it flows out of the fourth ventricle through the median (Magendie) and two lateral (Luschka) foramina to circulate in the subarachnoid space around the brain and spinal cord.

CSF absorption | The CSF is absorbed into the venous system mostly through small villi called the arachnoid granulations projecting into the dural sinuses (**Fig. 40.5**). About 20% of the CSF is absorbed into the veins through spinal arachnoid granulations; the rest is absorbed through cerebral arachnoid granulations. The absorption is driven mainly by the difference in colloid oncotic pressure of the CSF (nearly zero) and the plasma (25 mm Hg). It is also aided by hydrostatic pressure, which is slightly greater in the CSF than in the dural sinuses.

Functions of Cerebrospinal Fluid

The brain weighs ~1500 g, but it weighs just 50 g in CSF due to buoyancy. The importance of this buoyancy is apparent from the occasional traction headache that occurs after withdrawal of CSF by lumbar puncture (see below). CSF withdrawal reduces the buoyancy and increases the weight of the brain, which pulls down on the pain-sensitive dura from which it is suspended by the cerebral veins draining into the dural sinuses. Moreover, the brain presses harder upon the floor of the cranial cavity, producing pain due to pressure on the cranial nerves at the base of the brain.

The CSF provides a cushion around the brain and protects it from injury. However, the brain still gets injured sometimes. For example, if there is a severe blow on the head, the skull

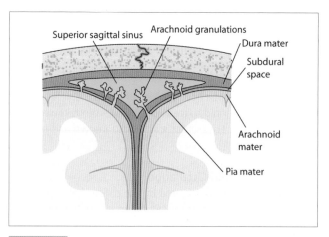

Fig. 40.5 The meninges and arachnoid granulations. (Courtesy Dr. M. Abid Geelani, Professor of Cardiothoracic Surgery, GB Pant Hospital, Maulana Azad Medical College, New Delhi, India.)

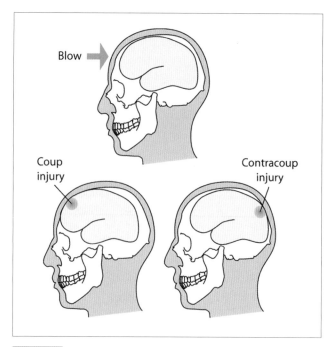

Fig. 40.6 Coup and contracoup injuries.

quickly moves in the direction of the blow, but the brain lags behind due to inertia. This results in the *coup injury*. Moments later, the movement of the skull stops, but the brain keeps moving due to inertia. As a result, the brain hits the skull at the opposite side to the blow. This is known as *contracoup injury* (**Fig. 40.6**).

The CSF provides an optimum environment (milieu intérieur) to neurons, which are highly sensitive to changes in their external environment. It acts as a medium for nutrient exchange. Proteins that leak out of capillaries into the brain interstitial fluid are drained by CSF and returned to the bloodstream. Thus, the CSF fulfills the role of the lymphatics, which are absent in the brain.

Cerebrospinal Fluid Analysis

Lumbar puncture | Although samples of CSF can be drawn by lumbar, cisternal, or ventricular puncture, the most convenient and commonly used way is the lumbar puncture (**Fig. 40.7**). It can be done safely between L3 and L4 or L4 and L5 vertebrae because the spinal cord ends at L1, whereas the dura and arachnoid continue until S2. Besides obtaining a CSF sample, lumbar puncture allows the estimation of CSF pressure by connecting the puncturing needle to a manometer.

The physical characteristics of CSF are given in **Table 40.1**, and its chemical composition is given in **Table 40.2**. Substances present in greater concentration than in plasma are chloride and CO_2. Substances present in concentrations equal to that in plasma include Na^+ and urea. Substances present in lower concentration than in plasma include K^+, calcium (Ca^{2+}), phosphates, proteins, and glucose. Most other substances do not pass from plasma to the CSF except in minute traces.

Abnormalities in the CSF include the following. (1) Turbidity indicates increased content of protein and cells, indicative of

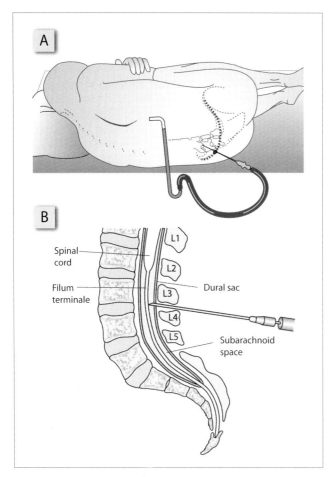

Fig. 40.7 Lumbar puncture. **(A)** Positioning of the patient for lumbar puncture. **(B)** Positioning of the needle in the spinal subarachnoid space.

meningitis. (2) CSF glucose is low in meningitis due to utilization of glucose by microbes. (3) Neutrophils in large numbers (reaching up to 1000 to 10,000 cells/mL, indicate bacterial meningitis or brain abscess. (4) Lymphocytes in large numbers (200–300/mL) suggest meningeal syphilis. (5) Red cells in large numbers indicate subarachnoid hemorrhage.

Cerebrospinal Fluid Pressure
The CSF pressure, as measured through a lumbar puncture, is ~150 mm of water when the patient is supine. The pressure recorded is higher in the sitting position. A raised intracranial

Table 40.1 Normal Physical Characteristics of Cerebrospinal Fluid (CSF)

Amount	125–150 mL
Specific gravity	1.007, a density close to that of brain tissue
pH	7.33
Pressure	70–200 mm H_2O (in the horizontal position)
Potential	+5 mV (CSF positive)
Cells	< 5 cells/mm³ (mostly lymphocytes)

Table 40.2 A Comparison of the Biochemical Compositions of Cerebrospinal Fluid (CSF) and Plasma

	Plasma Concentration (mEq/kg)	CSF Concentration (mEq/kg)
Cl⁻	100	130
PCO_2 mm Hg	40	50
K⁺	4.5	3.0
Protein	6000	20 (mainly albumin)
PO_4^{3-}	4.5	3.5
Ca^{2+}	4.5	2.5
Glucose	100	60

pressure can cause neuronal damage directly, or it can compress cerebral capillaries, leading to ischemic damage. Further damage occurs if a part of the brain herniates through openings in the cranial bones or tentorium.

A characteristic sign of raised CSF pressure is papilledema (swelling of the optic disk), which occurs when the raised intracranial pressure causes compression of the ophthalmic veins. Blood can still flow along the arteries and reach the optic disk, but its return is impeded. Fluid exudes from the capillaries, resulting in the swelling of the optic disk. Other signs associated with raised CSF pressure are those of Cushing reflex and impaired consciousness, such as disorientation, stupor, and coma.

Blood–Brain Barrier

The blood–brain barrier is a physiologic barrier to the movement of several substances in and out of the brain. It maintains a constancy of environment in and around the brain, prevents escape of neurotransmitters, and protects the neuron from harmful substances that may be present in blood. Most of the substances that gain entry into the brain ECF or the CSF are actively transported across the capillary endothelium of the cerebral capillaries. The high density of mitochondria in brain capillary endothelium reflects the higher metabolic activity of these capillaries.

The compositions of brain interstitial fluid and CSF are slightly different; hence, the blood–brain barrier (between blood and the interstitial fluid of the brain) is sometimes distinguished from the blood–CSF barrier. Substances diffusing across the *blood–CSF barrier*, that is, from the choroidal capillary to the CSF, have to cross two functionally effective barriers (**Fig. 40.8**): the tight junctions between capillary endothelial cells and the tight junctions of the choroidal epithelium. The pia mater and the capillary basement membrane do not constitute effective barriers. Substances diffusing across the *blood–brain barrier* from the cerebral capillary to the brain interstitium have to cross only the endothelial barrier, the choroidal epithelium being absent. The foot processes of astrocytes, which encircle the cerebral capillaries and form a complete sheath around them, do not constitute an effective barrier. Yet they contribute to the blood–brain barrier because they induce the formation of the tight junctions between endothelial cells.

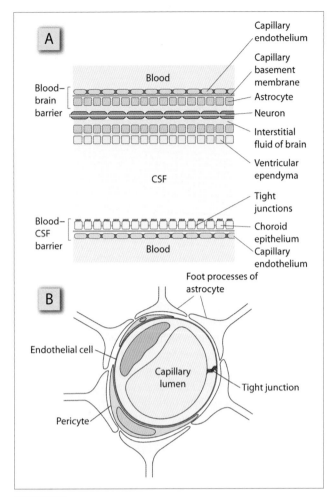

teristics are apparent from the composition of the CSF (**Table 40.2**).

Structures outside the blood–brain barrier | Certain areas of the brain have fenestrated capillaries and because of their permeability, are said lie outside the blood–brain barrier. These areas are located mostly around the third ventricle and are therefore called *circumventricular organs.* Some of them are neurosecretory organs secreting polypeptide neurotransmitters that must be able to enter the circulation freely; others are chemoreceptor areas for detecting blood-borne substances that must be able to reach the brain. The *neurosecretory areas* are the posterior pituitary and the median eminence of the hypothalamus. The *chemoreceptor areas* are the area postrema, subfornical organ, and organ vasculosum of the lamina terminalis. The pineal gland and the anterior pituitary also have fenestrated capillaries and are outside the blood–brain barrier, but both are endocrine organs and not part of the brain.

Although the blood–brain barrier is deficient in the circumventricular organs, the blood–CSF barrier in these organs is quite effective due to the presence of tight junctions between the modified ependymal cells of the third ventricle called the *tancytes.* Hence, the substances that leak out of capillaries in the circumventricular organs are unable to enter the CSF.

Summary

- Cerebral blood flow is very large, amounting to 15% of the cardiac output. The brain is highly sensitive to ischemia (reduced flow).

- Regional cerebral blood flow exhibits powerful autoregulation as the result of vasodilatation caused by local products of the metabolism.

- The blood–brain barrier prevents the diffusion of substances between the cerebral spinal fluid and the blood.

Applying What You Know

40.1. When Ms. Adams (see Section II) repetitively contracts muscles in her arms or trunk, those muscles rapidly fatigue, and their force of contraction decreases. What change in cerebral blood flow in the motor regions of the cortex would you expect to see when this phenomenon occurs? Explain.

Fig. 40.8 (A) The blood–brain and blood–cerebrospinal (CSF) fluid barriers. (B) The tight junctions and astrocyte foot processes in a cerebral capillary. Compare with **Fig. 36.1**.

Deficiency of the blood–brain barrier | The blood–brain barrier is not properly developed in infancy; therefore, a high serum bilirubin level leads to accumulation of bilirubin in the brain, causing kernicterus. The blood–brain barrier is also deficient at the site of a brain tumor because the new capillaries that proliferate in a brain tumor are not encircled by astrocytes. A radiolabeled amino acid that is injected into the circulation gets localized in the tumor and not other parts of the brain. This offers an obvious advantage in diagnostic radiography. Inflammation of the brain and meninges weakens the blood–brain barrier. Hence, antibiotics that normally do not cross the blood–brain barrier do so during inflammation. Experimental disruption of the blood–brain barrier can be produced by exposing cerebral capillaries to hyperosmolar solution. It acts by shrinking endothelial cells, thereby making the tight junctions less tight.

The blood–brain barrier is highly permeable to water, CO_2, O_2, lipid-soluble substances such as alcohol, and most anesthetics. It is slightly permeable to electrolytes, Na^+, chloride (Cl^-), and K^+ and totally impermeable to plasma proteins and large, lipid-insoluble organic molecules. These permeability charac-

Pulmonary Circulation

The pulmonary vasculature offers a relatively low resistance to the blood flowing from the right to the left ventricle. It is also a highly distensible system. The distensibility of the pulmonary circulation makes it a low-pressure (**Table 41.1**), high-capacitance system. The afterload on the right ventricle is therefore much less than the afterload on the left ventricle. Compared with the aorta, the pulmonary artery is much shorter, has a larger diameter, and has about one-third its wall thickness. This is also true for pulmonary arterioles in relation to their systemic counterparts.

The bronchi receive oxygenated blood through bronchial arteries, which are systemic arteries (**Fig. 41.1**). Some of the deoxygenated bronchial venous blood mixes with the oxygenated pulmonary venous blood (**Fig. 44.3**). This interconnection between bronchial and pulmonary circulations is called the *physiologic shunt.* This shunt reduces the oxygen (O_2) saturation of arterial blood slightly.

Lymphatics are present in the walls of the terminal bronchioles. Particulate matter entering the alveoli is partly removed via these channels. Proteins are also removed from the lung tissues, thereby helping to prevent edema.

Pulmonary blood pressure | Pressure in the pulmonary circulation is measured by inserting a catheter through the right side of the heart and into the pulmonary artery, where a pressure reading can be made. If the catheter is pushed into one of the small branches of the pulmonary artery until it wedges tightly in the artery (**Fig. 41.2**), the pressure measured there is called the *pulmonary wedge pressure,* and is ~5 mm Hg. Because the catheter stops the flow of blood into the artery and faces toward the venous side of the pulmonary circuit, what is measured is closer to the pulmonary venous pressure than the pulmonary arterial pressure. The mean pressure in pulmonary veins and the left atrium is ~2 mm Hg in the recumbent position. The wedge pressure is 2 to 3 mm Hg greater than the left atrial pressure.

The **pulmonary blood volume** is ~600 mL, which is located mostly in the pulmonary arteries and veins. When there is hemorrhage from systemic circulation, it is partly compensated for by translocation of blood from this pulmonary reservoir. The pulmonary blood volume increases when the posture changes from a standing to a lying position and decreases when the intrathoracic pressure increases, for exam-

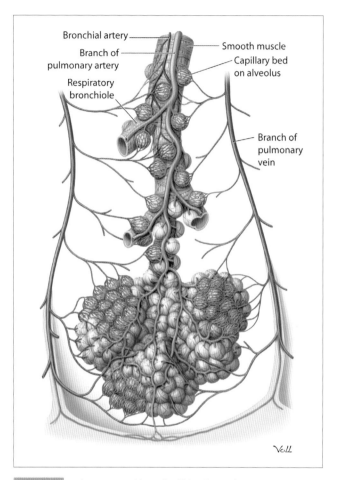

Fig. 41.1   Pulmonary and bronchial blood vessels.

ple, during a Valsalva maneuver. It also increases in pathological conditions like mitral stenosis and mitral regurgitation.

Effect of gravity | In the normal, upright individual, the pulmonary arterial pressure varies from the base to the apex of the lung (**Fig. 41.3**). Compared with the pulmonary arterial pressure at the level of the heart (which is located about at the level of the middle of the lungs), the apical pressure is 15 mm Hg less, and the basal pressure is 8 mm Hg greater. There are corresponding differences in regional blood flow that form the basis of two lung zones: a basal zone called zone 3 extending up to a distance of 10 cm above the heart level, and an apical zone called zone 2. A third zone, called zone 1, appears in disease states such as chronic obstructive pulmonary disease (COPD) (see Chapter 52).

Zone 3 has continuous blood flow because the alveolar capillary pressure remains greater than the alveolar air pressure throughout the cardiac cycle.

Zone 2 has intermittent blood flow, occurring only during the peaks of pulmonary arterial pressure. The pulmonary systolic and diastolic pressures are 25 mm Hg and 8 mm Hg when measured at the heart level. The corresponding pressures at

Table 41.1   Pressures in Pulmonary Circulation

Systolic pressure	25 mm Hg
Diastolic pressure	8 mm Hg
Mean pressure	15 mm Hg
Pulse pressure	17 mm Hg

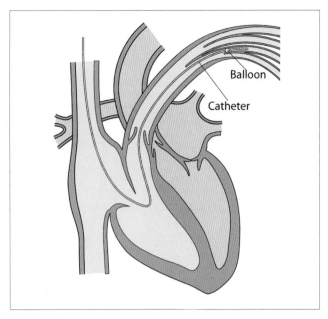

Fig. 41.2 Pulmonary artery wedge pressure measurement.

the apex, where the pressure is 15 mm Hg less, would be 10 mm Hg and –7 mm Hg, respectively. The air pressure in the alveoli is 0 mm Hg. Hence, during diastole, the alveolar capillaries collapse, and no blood flows through them. However, in the recumbent position, no part of the lung is more than a few centimeters above the level of the heart. Therefore, the entire lung, including the apex, becomes equivalent to zone 3, receiving continuous blood flow.

In *zone 1*, no blood flows at all during any phase of the cardiac cycle because the local capillary pressure in zone 1 never

rises higher than the alveolar pressure. Zone 1 is not present normally: it is present when the pulmonary systolic arterial pressure is too low (as in hypovolemic states) or the alveolar pressure is too high (as in obstructive lung disorders) to allow blood flow.

Effect of exercise | Blood flow in all parts of the lung increases during exercise, sometimes as much as sevenfold. This extra flow is made possible by the opening up (recruitment) of inactive capillaries and the expansion of the highly distensible pulmonary vessels. Together, these two factors decrease the pulmonary vascular resistance so much that the pulmonary arterial pressure rises very little, even during maximal exercise. However, the rise in pressure is enough to provide continuous blood flow to the apices so that, in effect, the entire lung becomes equivalent to zone 3 during exercise.

The ability of the lung to allow a large amount of blood to flow through it during exercise reduces the load on the right side of the heart. It also prevents a significant rise in pulmonary capillary pressure and therefore prevents development of pulmonary edema during exercise.

Effect of Left Ventricular Failure

The left atrial pressure rises concomitantly with the severity of left ventricular failure (the inability of the ventricle to produce a flow to the systemic circulation to meet the metabolic needs of the body). A rise in left atrial pressure up to 7 mm Hg does not cause a rise in the pulmonary arterial pressure due to the large compliance of pulmonary venules and the opening up of more pulmonary capillaries. The resultant increase in the pulmonary vascular capacity limits the pressure rise. However, pressures greater than 7 mm Hg are transmitted to the pulmonary arteries, imposing a high afterload on the right ventricle. As the pressure is transmitted through the capillaries, the pulmonary capillary hydrostatic pressure rises. When the left atrial pressure exceeds 25 mm Hg, the capillary pressure is sufficiently high to produce pulmonary edema.

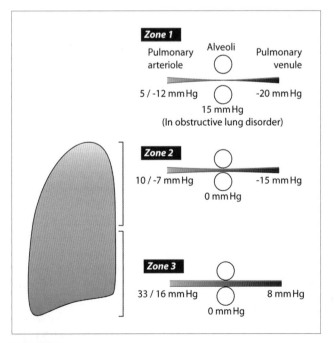

Fig. 41.3 Zones of pulmonary circulation. Zone 3 is present only in disease states such as chronic obstructive airway disorder.

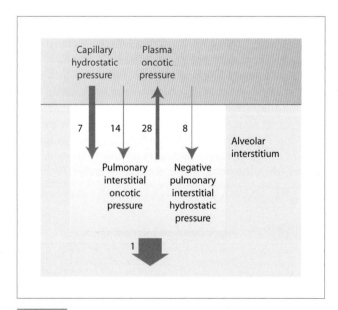

Fig. 41.4 Starling forces in pulmonary capillaries.

Neural Control of Pulmonary Circulation

Efferent control of pulmonary vessels is exerted only through sympathetic fibers, which cause a slight increase in the pulmonary vascular resistance. However, the effect is insignificant and physiologically unimportant. The main function of sympathetic discharge is to constrict the large pulmonary capacitance vessels, especially the veins, causing translocation of pulmonary blood into systemic circulation.

Afferent control | Pulmonary baroreceptors are present in the adventitia of the pulmonary trunk and the right and left pulmonary arteries. These receptors detect rises in pulmonary arterial pressure and produce reflex inhibition of sympathetic discharge to the pulmonary vasculature. The afferent arc is through the vagus.

Chemical Control of Pulmonary Circulation

Reduced PO_2 in the lung interstitium (outside the arterioles) induces pulmonary vasoconstriction. This is exactly the opposite of what happens in systemic circulation where hypoxia produces vasodilatation. The physiologic significance of this phenomenon (called *hypoxic vasoconstriction*) is to divert pulmonary blood flow from the alveoli that are poorly ventilated to alveoli that are better ventilated. The smooth muscle of pulmonary arteries contains O_2-sensitive K^+ channels that close down when the partial pressure of oxygen (PO_2) falls. K^+ channel closure is associated with depolarization and contraction of smooth muscle.

The vasoconstriction associated with chronic hypoxia causes a marked increase in pulmonary arterial pressure (pul-

monary hypertension), which imposes a heavy afterload on the right ventricle leading to its hypertrophy and eventual failure (cor pulmonale). Pulmonary hypertension is common in high-altitude dwellers and in COPD (see Chapter 52).

Pulmonary Capillary Dynamics

Pulmonary transit time | Blood passes through the pulmonary capillaries in ~0.75 second (the transit time). A rise in cardiac output during exercise shortens the transit time to ~0.3 second, which is barely adequate for complete oxygenation of blood (see **Fig. 47.7**). The transit time would be shorter if several inactive capillaries did not open up with exercise. The opening up of inactive capillaries increases the total capillary cross-sectional area, slowing down the linear velocity of blood and prolonging the transit time.

Pulmonary capillary Starling forces | The balance of Starling forces at the capillary membrane is shown in **Fig. 41.4**. Note that the pulmonary interstitial hydrostatic pressure is negative at –8 mm Hg. The net filtration pressure of 1 mm Hg (14 + 8 + 7 – 28) causes a slight filtration of fluid from the pulmonary capillaries into the interstitial spaces. Except for a small amount that keeps the alveolar lining moist, this fluid is returned to the circulation through the pulmonary lymphatic system.

Pulmonary edema | A common cause of pulmonary edema is left ventricular failure. It is associated with an increase in the pulmonary capillary hydrostatic pressure that causes transudation (increased capillary filtration) of fluids into the alveolar interstitium. Capillary permeability also increases following

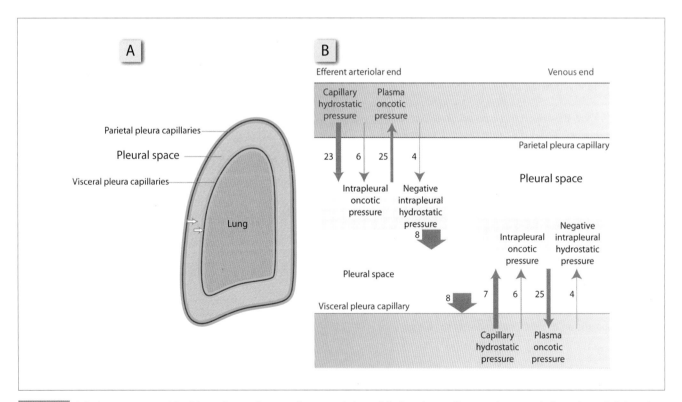

Fig. 41.5 **(A)** The movement of fluid from the capillaries in the parietal pleura (blue) to the capillaries in the visceral pleura (green). **(B)** Starling forces in pleural capillaries.

exposure to irritant gases. It results in exudation, that is, leakage of both fluid and plasma proteins out of the capillaries.

In acute cases, pulmonary edema occurs when the pulmonary capillary hydrostatic pressure exceeds 28 mm Hg. In chronic cases, there is a compensatory increase in lymphatic drainage and therefore the capillary pressure must rise higher to produce edema. The edema is initially confined to the interstitial fluid. Once the interstitial fluid pressure becomes positive, the fluid begins to enter the alveoli. Edema, wherever the fluid is located, reduces the oxygenation of blood in the lungs.

Pleural Circulation

There is a negative intrapleural pressure of ~ −4 mm Hg during normal respiration. The oncotic pressures in both parietal and visceral pleural capillaries are the same—25 mm Hg. Because there is very little protein in the normal pleural fluid, the pleural oncotic pressure is only ~6 mm Hg. The hydrostatic pressure in the parietal pleura capillaries fed by the systemic arteries is ~23 mm Hg. The hydrostatic pressure in the visceral pleura capillaries fed by the pulmonary arteries is only ~7 mm Hg (**Fig. 41.5**).

Thus, there is a net pressure gradient of 8 mm Hg pushing the pleural fluid from parietal capillaries to the pleural space. Similarly, there is a net force of 8 mm Hg driving the pleural fluid from the pleural space to visceral capillaries and lymphatics. This pressure gradient ensures that the fluid filtered into the pleural space by the parietal pleural capillaries is rapidly absorbed by the visceral pleura capillaries. The proteins and particles that enter the pleural space are slowly absorbed by lymphatics opening in the parietal pleura.

Summary

- The pulmonary circulation reaches the total cardiac output (from the right ventricle).

- It exhibits a low flow resistance and a high distensibility. One consequence is that the pressures in the pulmonary circulation are much lower than those in the systemic circulation.

- Another consequence is that pressures in the pulmonary circulation increase relatively little when cardiac output increased.

- Pulmonary arterioles vasoconstrict when hypoxia is present in the lung interstitium.

- In an erect individual, the effects of gravity result in a non-uniform perfusion of different regions of the lungs.

Applying What You Know

41.1. Mrs. Daniels has a mitral valve that is both stenosed and regurgitant. It is likely that both of these conditions developed more or less gradually and resulted in a gradual increase of left atrial volume and hence increased left atrial pressure. This, in turn, would cause pulmonary pressures to increase. Why is it likely that Mrs. Daniels's pulmonary artery pressure increased more slowly than her left atrial pressure?

41.2. If Mrs. Daniels were to visit the top of Pike's Peak (over 14,000 feet at the summit) while on vacation, how would her condition be affected? Explain.

Cutaneous Circulation

The oxygen and nutrient requirements of the skin are relatively small. Cutaneous circulation is therefore regulated less by its metabolic activity and more by thermoregulatory requirements (see Chapter 43). The metabolic control of cutaneous blood flow is revealed by the presence of *reactive hyperemia*—the increase in blood flow that occurs after a period of occlusion of blood flow. Local metabolites accumulate in the skin during the occlusion and dilate the precapillary sphincters of cutaneous capillaries, producing hyperemia when the occlusion is released. Metabolic control is overridden by thermoregulatory control; therefore, it is unable to relieve the ischemia caused by cold-induced vasoconstriction.

In shock, cutaneous vasoconstriction diverts blood to vital, more metabolically active tissues. Yet if the ambient temperature is high, the cutaneous blood flow increases at the expense of reducing the blood supply to the vital tissues. It can prevail over other reflexes that tend to reduce cutaneous blood flow. However, this is *not* always the case, and cutaneous blood flow is reduced during severe exercise even though heat production is greatly increased (see **Table 37.2**).

The resting cutaneous blood flow is the flow when a person is at thermal equilibrium with the environment, at ~25 to 27°C (the thermoneutral zone; see Chapter 43), and it is 450 mL/min or ~13 mL/min/100 g of skin tissue. At temperatures below the thermoneutral zone, the skin vessels are strongly constricted, and blood flow is directed to the deeper tissues. Depending on the amount of sweating, cutaneous blood flow varies from one-tenth to 10 times the resting blood flow. Maximal cutaneous blood flow occurring on heat exposure imposes a heavy circulatory load on the heart, which can lead to hypotension and shock.

The thermoregulatory control of cutaneous blood flow may be local or reflex. The local thermoregulatory control is brought about by the direct effect of skin temperature on vascular smooth muscles, which contract when cooled and relax when warmed. The center for reflex thermoregulation is located in the hypothalamus, which controls the sympathetic output of the brainstem vasomotor center. This explains why cardiovascular reflexes centered at the vasomotor center are overridden by the thermoregulatory reflexes controlled by the hypothalamus.

Triple response to trauma | A firm, strong stroke across the skin using a blunt point evokes three sequential responses: the red reaction, flare, and wheal. The *red reaction* is a red line that develops along the line of the stroke. It occurs due to the dilatation of precapillary sphincters. The dilatation is not neurally mediated, but caused by the histamine and bradykinin released from the injured skin. The *flare* is a warm, erythematous (red) area that develops around the red line. It occurs due to a dilatation of the arterioles, terminal arterioles, and precapillary sphincters. The dilatation is mediated by the axon

reflex in the cutaneous C fibers. The *wheal* is a swelling that develops along and around the line of the stroke. It is caused by the capillary damage, which results in increased capillary permeability and exudation of plasma.

Some of the features of cutaneous circulation are different in the apical and nonapical skin. Apical skin is found in the exposed, but poorly insulated areas of the body, like the palms of the hands, soles of the feet, face, and ears. Elsewhere, the skin is called nonapical.

Apical skin arterioles have a high degree of basal sympathetic tone, which is under corticohypothalamic control. Heat exposure reduces the sympathetic tone and dilates the arterioles. Conversely, cold exposure constricts the arterioles. However, when the skin temperature falls below 10°C, the arterioles dilate. The cold injury to the tissues causes the liberation of histamine, which excites the sensory terminals of cutaneous nerves and produces sustained vasodilatation through the axon reflex. The vasodilatation increases the cutaneous blood flow so as to warm up the skin and prevent frostbite of the highly exposed apical skin. This is known as *cold vasodilatation.*

The apical skin also contains arteriovenous (A-V) anastomoses, which are under similar neural control to the arterioles (**Fig. 42.1**). These A-V anastomoses produce quicker and larger increases in the cutaneous blood flow, which makes them especially important in cold vasodilatation. The rapid change in cutaneous blood flow caused by the A-V anastomoses also causes quick changes in skin color. Emotions are therefore promptly reflected in the color of the face: shame and anger cause sympathetic inhibition, resulting in blushing due to dilatation of these vessels, whereas fear and anxiety cause blanching due to sympathetic vasoconstriction.

Nonapical skin lacks A-V anastomoses | The neural control of arterioles in nonapical skin is similar to that in apical skin.

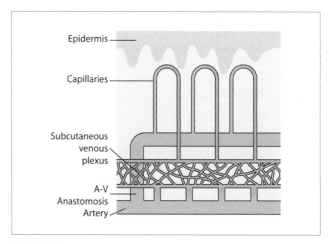

Fig. 42.1   Organization of cutaneous blood vessels. A-V, arteriovenous.

The arterioles here have a high degree of intrinsic myogenic tone and low sympathetic tone. Withdrawal of the sympathetic tone therefore does not produce much vasodilatation. Large dilatation of these arterioles is mediated by sympathetic vasodilator fibers to the sweat glands. The stimulated sweat glands release bradykinin, which causes vasodilatation (**Fig. 37.2**).

Sweat Glands

Sweat glands are of two types: eccrine and apocrine. Both are present in the dermis, and both secrete excessively in emotional states. However, they have several differences that are summarized in **Table 42.1**. There are 3 to 4 million sweat glands in the body, which would add up to the size of a kidney and can secrete up to 10 L of sweat per day in an acclimated individual. They account for the huge increase in cutaneous blood flow that occurs during heat exposure. The blood flow to the actively secreting sweat glands is increased by bradykinin. Because eccrine glands are innervated by cholinergic sympathetic fibers, sweating and the associated increase in cutaneous blood flow are inhibited by atropine and in diseases of the autonomic nervous system.

Muscle Circulation

Blood vessels of skeletal muscle constitute the largest vascular bed in the body. During exercise, the vascular resistance in muscle falls massively, allowing up to a 20 times increase in blood flow. Hence, at rest or during exercise, muscle resistance vessels have considerable effect on the arterial blood pressure.

Blood flow to tonic and phasic muscles | Unlike phasic (white) muscle fibers, tonic (red) muscle fibers employ aerobic metabolism and contract all the time. Hence, their oxygen (O_2) demand is much higher. Their resting blood flow (30 mL/min/100 g) far exceeds that of phasic muscle (3 mL/min/100 g). However, because they comprise only a fraction of the total muscle mass, their total resting blood supply is only twice that of white fibers. Red fibers have myoglobin, which allows them to overcome brief periods of ischemia that occur due to capillary compression during muscle contraction. However, during sustained contraction of 10 seconds or more, the myoglobin O_2 content is exhausted, and muscle metabolism becomes anaerobic, resulting in fatigue and ischemic pain.

Myogenic autoregulation | The precapillary resistance vessels in the muscle have a high basal myogenic tone. A rise in arterial blood pressure induces a stretch-induced contraction of the precapillary sphincter (myogenic contraction), which prevents an excessive rise in capillary pressure. The response is important in leg muscles, where it reduces the rate of capillary filtration in the erect position, preventing pedal edema.

Metabolic control | In exercising muscle, the products of metabolism accumulate faster than they can be carried away by blood flow. The accumulated metabolites, such as carbon dioxide (CO_2), potassium (K^+), and hydrogen (H^+), cause dilatation of the precapillary sphincters, resulting in marked reduction of local vascular resistance. This enormously increases the size of the capillary bed being perfused, and the blood flow increases many fold (exercise hyperemia). The blood flow increases in excess of the O_2 demand of exercising muscles. Hence, the A-V O_2 difference falls during exercise. The capillary hydrostatic pressure rises sharply, and there is increased transudation into the interstitium, reducing the plasma volume and causing hemoconcentration. After the cessation of heavy exercise, the blood flow does not subside immediately, but falls exponentially from its high level during the exercise to resting values. This is due to the oxygen debt of exercise.

Metabolic control also explains the reactive hyperemia that occurs in muscles following a period of occlusion of blood supply. The occlusion results in the accumulation of metabolites in the capillary bed, which gets maximally dilated. Release of the occlusion brings in a rush of blood through the dilated capillaries, washing out the metabolites.

Neural control | The resistance vessels of muscle possess a high basal tone, which is largely attributable to the intrinsic myogenic tone of vascular smooth muscle. The neurogenic tone due to sympathetic discharge is much less. Hence, sympathetic discharge is very effective in causing vasoconstriction (there is a wide margin for increase), but is rather poor in causing vasodilatation (there is little margin for decrease). It is obvious, therefore, that a reduction in sympathetic discharge cannot be responsible for the massive exercise hyperemia, which is entirely due to metabolic factors. Rather, sympathetic discharge limits the exercise hyperemia in muscle.

The role of sympathetic discharge to muscle capillaries lies elsewhere. (1) Sympathetic discharge increases the precapillary:postcapillary resistance ratio and thereby promotes the absorption of interstitial fluid into the capillaries. In exercise, there is transudation of fluids from the capillaries to the interstitial fluid. Sympathetic discharge reduces the transudation, though it is not able to stop it completely. (2) During circulatory shock, sympathetic vasoconstriction reduces muscle blood flow profoundly. Because the muscle capillary bed is very large, these help in diverting substantial amounts of blood toward the heart, which helps to raise the blood pressure in circulatory shock.

Table 42.1 Differences between Eccrine and Apocrine Sweat Glands

Eccrine	Apocrine
Present all over the body, but dense on the head and densest on the palms and soles	Present in the axilla, perianal region, around the nipples, in mons pubis, and labia majora
Open on the skin surface	Open into the canal of a hair follicle
Secrete profuse watery, hypotonic sweat	Secrete a milky fluid that is acted upon by bacteria to release a characteristic odor
Innervated and stimulated by cholinergic sympathetic fibers; important in thermoregulation	Not innervated but stimulated by circulating epinephrine; no role in thermoregulation

Intermingled with the sympathetic fibers to the muscle are certain special types of sympathetic fibers that have acetylcholine and not norepinephrine as their neurotransmitter. These *sympathetic vasodilator fibers* are activated by cortico-hypothalamic–reticulospinal pathways that are quite different from the vasomotor center–thoracolumbar spinal pathway. They are not influenced by the baroreceptor and chemoreceptor afferents and do not participate in the usual cardiovascular reflexes. Rather, they produce muscle vasodilatation in emotional states.

Sympathetic vasodilator fibers do not increase nutritive blood flow to the muscles, either during or before exercise (**Fig. 42.2**). Their importance lies in preventing an excessive rise in blood pressure before the onset of exercise. Confrontation with a fight-or-flight situation triggers the "defense reaction" that is associated with considerable sympathetic discharge, causing widespread vasoconstriction in the muscle beds. As a result, the total peripheral resistance and blood pressure tend to rise to dangerous levels. At this time, the discharge of the sympathetic vasodilator nerves lowers the blood pressure to safe levels. It does so by dilating the arterioles in the muscle. Opening of these arterioles does not improve nutritive flow to the muscles because most of the precapillary sphincters are still closed, and the extra blood that flows into the muscles through dilated arterioles flows out into the veins through the thoroughfare channels. Once exercise commences, the precapillary sphincters are dilated by local metabolites, and most of the blood flows from the arterioles into the muscle capillaries, which now offer less resistance than the thoroughfare channels. The importance of sympathetic vasodilatation has

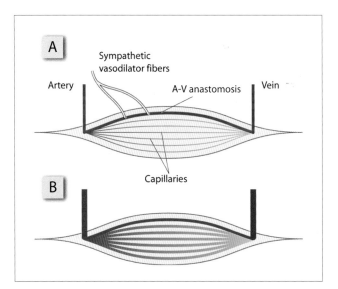

Fig. 42.2 Role of sympathetic vasodilator fibers in muscle. **(A)** Before exercise, the arterioles are dilated by the discharge of sympathetic vasodilator fibers. Blood flow through capillaries is minimal, as most of it flows through the thoroughfare channels. **(B)** Following exercise, capillary blood flow increases markedly due to autoregulation and far exceeds the blood flow through the thoroughfare channels. Note that oxygen denaturation of blood occurs only in the capillaries and not in the thoroughfare channels. A-V, arteriovenous.

not been established in humans, though it probably underlies vasovagal syncope.

Muscle pump | The rhythmic muscle contraction of dynamic exercise has a propulsive effect on circulation (see Venous "Pumping" subsection, Chapter 34). On the other hand, the strong sustained muscle contraction of static exercise compresses the vascular bed and stops the flow of blood through muscles.

Splanchnic Circulation

The vascular beds of the gut, liver, and spleen are together called the *splanchnic circulation*. The total splanchnic blood flow is ~1.5 L/min. In the gut, the mucosa receives approximately four times the amount of blood as the smooth muscle in its walls. If the entire gastrointestinal tract became simultaneously active, the splanchnic blood flow would have increased to ~4.0 L/min. However, because during digestion and absorption different parts of the gastrointestinal tract are sequentially activated, the maximum splanchnic circulation is only ~3.0 L/min.

Mesenteric Circulation

Hormonal control | Food ingestion increases intestinal blood flow. The mediators of this hyperemia include gastrin, cholecystokinin, and products of digestion, such as glucose and fatty acids. Intestinal blood flow is also increased by the process of absorption of food. Undigested food has no vasoactive influence.

Neural control of the mesenteric circulation is almost exclusively sympathetic. Increased sympathetic activity constricts both the mesenteric arterioles and veins. Both α-adrenergic and β-adrenergic receptors are stimulated, but the α-adrenergic (vasoconstrictive) effect predominates.

The sympathetic fibers to the gut are tonically active. When stimulated, these fibers bring about a rise in systemic blood pressure. The main reason for this rise is not an increase in peripheral resistance but venoconstriction, which squeezes out blood from mesenteric circulation and increases the CVP and cardiac output. This translocation of blood is beneficial in a fight-or-flight situation, where more blood must be available to the heart, muscles, and brain than to the intestines.

Autoregulation of blood flow in the intestinal circulation is not as well developed. The principal mechanism responsible for autoregulation is metabolic, although a myogenic mechanism probably also contributes. Adenosine is a potent vasodilator of the mesenteric vascular bed and may be the principal metabolic mediator of autoregulation. However, potassium concentration and altered osmolarity of the plasma may also contribute to autoregulation.

Villous countercurrent system | The direction of blood flow in the capillaries and venules in a villus is opposite to that in the main arteriole. This arrangement constitutes a countercurrent exchanger that has both advantages and disadvantages (**Fig. 42.3**).

1. Absorbed lipid-soluble substances that are carried in the venous limbs of the vascular hairpin loop diffuse into the

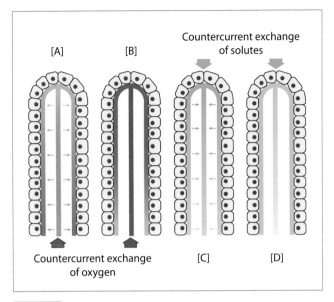

Fig. 42.3 Countercurrent exchanges in the villi. **(C,D)** Due to countercurrent exchange, the arterial blood reaching the tip of the villus is richer in solutes (shown in *green*) and therefore is able to absorb less solute from the lumen. **(A,B)** Due to countercurrent exchange, arterial blood entering the villus is less oxygenated, and venous blood is less deoxygenated than it would be without the exchange.

arterial limb because of a concentration gradient. High concentrations of absorbed substances are thus attained in the outer parts of the villi, and these substances leave relatively slowly through the venous drainage. Such a system automatically slows down the entrance of rapidly absorbed solutes into the blood so that the liver can handle them effectively.

2. The countercurrent exchange also permits diffusion of O_2 from arterioles to venules. At low flow rates, a substantial portion of blood O_2 is shunted from arterioles to venules near the base of the villus. Thus, the supply of O_2 to the mucosal cells at the tip of the villus is reduced. When intestinal blood flow is very low, the shunting of O_2 is exaggerated and may cause extensive necrosis of the intestinal villi.

Hepatic Circulation

The definition of the **functional unit of the liver** has changed over the years (**Fig. 42.4**). The earliest concept was a functional unit called the *hepatic lobule,* which was polygonal with a vein (called the central vein) at its center. During the first half of the 20th century, the concept of a triangular *portal lobule* was preferred. It was centered on the portal triad. Presently, the functional unit of the liver is called the *hepatic acinus,* which is somewhat ellipsoidal in shape. It is symmetrically disposed on either side of the line connecting two central veins. Because the central vein does not occupy a central position in

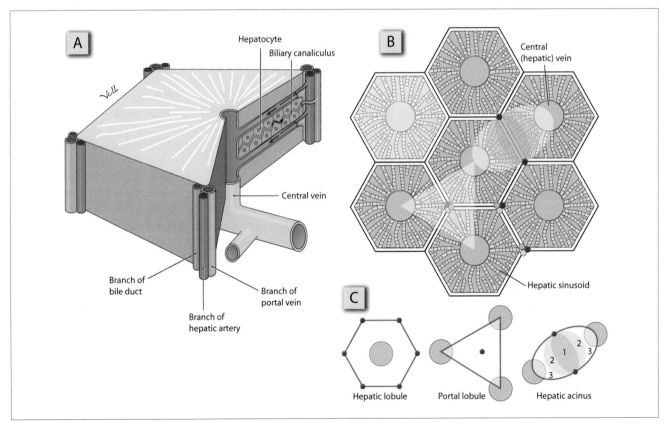

Fig. 42.4 **(A)** A classical (structural) representation of an hepatic lobule showing the arrangement of the vessels carrying blood to the liver, the branches of the hepatic artery and the portal vein, and the vessel carrying blood away from the liver, the central hepatic vein. **(B)** A section through the liver showing three models of the functional unit of the liver. **(C)** Three models of the functional unit of the liver: an hepatic lobule, a portal lobule, and an hepatic acinus.

the hepatic acinus, it has been renamed the terminal hepatic vein.

The concept of hepatic acini as the functional unit helps explain the pattern of cell degeneration seen in hypoxic and toxic damage to the liver. The hepatic acinus has three concentric zones. *Zone 1* is an ellipsoid area immediately surrounding the arteriole and terminal portal venule. The cells here are well oxygenated. The area contains mainly those enzymes that are involved in oxidative metabolism and gluconeogenesis. *Zone 2* is intermediate in all respects. It contains a mixed complement of enzymes. *Zone 3* is the peripheral zone of the acinus. It is the least oxygenated zone; therefore, it is most susceptible to anoxic injury. It is rich in enzymes involved in glycolysis and lipid and drug metabolism.

The small branches of the portal vein and hepatic artery give rise to terminal portal venules and hepatic arterioles, respectively. These terminal vessels enter the hepatic acinus at its center. Blood flows from these terminal vessels into the sinusoids, which constitute the capillary network of the liver. The sinusoids radiate toward the periphery of the acinus, where they connect with the terminal hepatic venules. Blood from these terminal venules drains into progressively larger branches of the hepatic veins, which are tributaries of the inferior vena cava.

Dual blood flow to the liver | Despite having a low O_2 demand, the liver has a relatively high blood supply. This is because only 25% of its blood supply is brought in by the hepatic artery and caters to its metabolic requirements. The remaining 75% is brought in by the portal vein. Both the streams meet in the sinusoids. Blood flows in the portal venous and hepatic arterial systems vary reciprocally; when one reduces, the other compensates partially. The hepatic blood flow is autoregulated. The portal blood flow is not autoregulated; it increases after a meal.

The mean hepatic arterial pressure is ~90 mm Hg; the pressure in the hepatic vein is only 5 mm Hg. Both the hepatic arterial and portal systems converge on the sinusoids (**Fig. 42.5**). One would therefore expect the sinusoidal pressure to be very high. However, this is not the case due to the high presinusoidal resistance in the hepatic arterioles. The sinusoidal pressure

is only 10 mm Hg. On the other hand, the postsinusoidal resistance is low, and any change in the hepatic venous pressure is promptly transmitted to the sinusoids, profoundly affecting the transsinusoidal exchange of fluids. This phenomenon is of clinical importance in the understanding of ascites and portocaval anastomosis, as explained below.

Ascites, the presence of fluid in the abdominal cavity, occurs in congestive heart failure because the elevated central venous pressure (CVP) is transmitted backward to the hepatic veins, portal veins, and mesenteric capillaries. A rise in hydrostatic pressure in mesenteric circulation results in extensive fluid transudation into the abdominal cavity.

Ascites also occurs in hepatic cirrhosis in which there is extensive fibrosis of the liver. The fibrosis leads to a marked rise in hepatic sinusoidal resistance. The consequent increase in the portal venous pressure is transmitted backward to the mesenteric circulation.

The reverse occurs when a collateral circulation is established between the portal and systemic veins (portocaval anastomosis). In such cases, the pressure rises substantially in systemic veins that anastomose with the portal vein. Such anastomosis can develop, for example, at the lower end of the esophagus and may enlarge considerably to form esophageal varices. These varices may rupture and lead to severe, frequently fatal internal bleeding.

Oxygen supply to the liver | Nearly 70% of the O_2 used by the liver is derived from the portal blood. This is possible because the portal blood entering the liver is three times the volume of hepatic arterial blood entering the liver. Moreover, portal blood is not markedly desaturated because of the low O_2 demands of gastrointestinal tissues. Thus, it contains ~17 mL O_2/dL of blood compared with the 19 mL O_2/dL of hepatic arterial blood.

One point of view is that the portal venous blood is more desaturated during digestion and therefore represents an undependable source of oxygen, supplying least during digestion when hepatic activity is greatest. The counter viewpoint is that there is a marked increase of portal blood flow during digestion so that, although the partial pressure of oxygen (PO_2) of portal blood is reduced, the total oxygen supply is increased due to hyperemia. Although the oxygen delivery to the liver keeps varying, the liver maintains a constant O_2 consumption, and the O_2 extraction varies with it.

Blood storage in the liver | The liver serves as a blood reservoir, with ~400 mL of blood present in its sinusoids. The sympathetic nerves cause constriction of portal veins, causing, in turn, a marked reduction in the capacitance of the portal system that helps to divert blood toward the heart.

Summary

- The skin exhibits low metabolic activity, and the cutaneous blood flow is determined by the need to regulate body temperature.

- Muscle blood vessels exhibit a high basal myogenic tone but are controlled both by metabolic and neural controls.

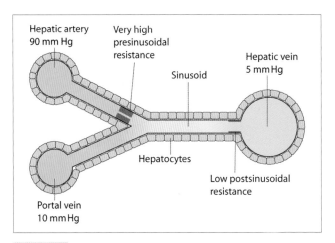

Fig. 42.5 Hydrostatic pressures in the hepatic artery, portal vein, and hepatic vein.

- The splanchnic circulation (gut, liver, spleen) is controlled by gastrointestinal hormones and the sympathetic nervous system; there is little autoregulation.

- The hepatic circulation is unusual in that it perfuses the liver from both the high-pressure hepatic artery and the low-pressure portal vein.

Applying What You Know

42.1. Mr. Wright (see Section III) responds to the anesthetic being administered during surgery by dumping the calcium (Ca^{2+}) stored in the sarcoplasmic reticulum of his muscles. The increase in intracellular Ca^{2+} concentration causes sustained contraction of the muscles affected. What effect does this have on blood flow to these muscles? Explain.

42.2. Mr. Lundquist (see Section IV) plays tennis regularly. What might be a consequence of eating a large meal before a tennis match?

Humans, as indeed all mammals and birds, are temperature regulators: they have the capability to maintain a constant body temperature in the face of changes in environmental temperature and changes in internal heat generation. They are therefore called *homeothermic*. All lower animals are temperature conformers: their body temperature conforms to (equals) the environmental temperature and are called *poikilothermic*. Because enzymes regulating metabolism have a narrow range of optimum temperature that coincides with the normal body temperature, any change in body temperature adversely affects metabolism.

There are many processes involved in maintaining body temperature, but the exchange of heat at the body surface, a process mediated by the cutaneous circulation, is one of the central ones.

The Body Must Lose Heat All the Time

Maintenance of a constant body temperature is possible only if the net heat lost by the body exactly matches the amount of heat generated in the body and any heat gained from the environment. The body surely loses heat to the exterior in winter, but is there a net heat loss to the exterior in summer, too? Yes. Because the body constantly produces metabolic heat, the body must also constantly lose heat to the environment if it is to maintain a constant body temperature. If the body temperature is 37°C, and it makes a net gain of heat from the environment, the body temperature will rise and culminate in death. Even when we gain heat standing out in the sun or in front of a fire, heat is also lost to the environment simultaneously. The result must necessarily be a net loss of heat. If there is a net heat gain, it is uncomfortable, and we instinctively move away from the heat source. A continuous net heat gain from the environment spells certain death.

General Model: Reservoir

The body is a reservoir for heat, and the more heat in it, the higher its temperature. Thus, to maintain a constant body temperature, the amount of heat in it must be constant. This means that the heat lost and the heat gained must be equal.

How can a net heat loss be possible if the ambient temperature is 45°C? The answer lies in the evaporative cooling of the body through sweating. Evaporative cooling is practically the sole method that prevents the body temperature from rising when the ambient temperature is high. That is why one feels hotter on a humid day when there is decreased evaporation of sweat. That is also why the simple fan is so effective in cooling the body. Obviously, the maintenance of body temperature in a cold environment is far easier than in a hot environment, and the adaptive mechanisms responding to cold far out-

number adaptive mechanisms responding to warm temperature. It is common experience that ambient temperatures several degrees lower than the body temperature—even subzero temperatures—can be comfortably borne using simple behavioral methods, whereas temperatures a few degrees higher than the body temperature kill.

Normal Body Temperature

The temperature of the body surface (shell temperature) is not the same as the temperature inside the body (core temperature) or inside the cranium (the intracranial temperature).

The *shell temperature* is represented by the skin temperature. The practical way of measuring the skin temperature is to measure the armpit temperature. The skin temperature is less in the extremities.

The *core temperature* is best represented by the aortic blood temperature. The practical way of measuring the core temperature is to note the rectal temperature. The oral temperature (37°C) is lower than the rectal temperature (37.5°C), and it is affected by many factors, including ingestion of hot or cold fluids, gum chewing, smoking, and mouth breathing.

The *intracranial temperature* is best represented by the tympanic membrane temperature. The central thermoreceptors located in the hypothalamus sense the intracranial temperature rather than the general core temperature.

Physiologic variations in body temperature (1) The normal human core temperature undergoes a diurnal fluctuation of 0.5 to 0.7°C, being lowest at ~6 AM and highest in the evening. A change in the sleep–wake cycle (i.e., working on night shifts) reverses the temperature curve. Physical activity may be contributory to the temperature curve; it cannot be the sole factor because it is present even during continuous bed rest. (2) In women, there is a monthly cycle of temperature variation, with a rise in basal temperature at the time of ovulation (see **Fig. 84.2**). (3) Temperature regulation is less precise in young children. Their body temperature is 0.5°C higher than that of adults. The elderly have a lower normal temperature and are intolerant to extremes of ambient temperature. (4) Body temperature rises with physical activity, sometimes as high as 40°C. This rise is partly due to the resetting of the hypothalamic thermostat to a higher temperature during exercise. Body temperature also rises slightly during emotional excitement, probably due to unconscious tensing of the muscles. (5) When the body temperature is chronically elevated in normal adults, it is called *constitutional hyperthermia*.

Body Heat Exchange with Exterior

The heat exchange between the body and its environment can be viewed as a two-step process. The first step is the transfer of heat between the core of the body and its shell (the skin). The second step is the heat transfer between the body shell and the exterior (**Fig. 43.1**).

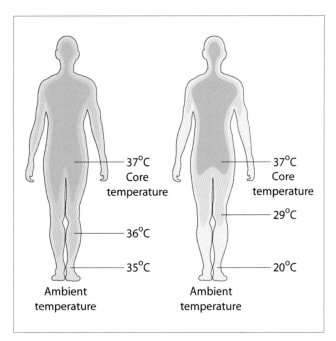

Fig. 43.1 Core and shell temperatures. Regardless of the ambient temperature, the core temperature is maintained at 37°C.

The transfer of heat from the core to the shell occurs almost entirely through convection and is regulated by the cutaneous blood flow. When the cutaneous vessels are dilated, blood flows into the skin, carrying the heat from the core to the shell. When the cutaneous vessels are constricted, blood does not flow into the skin, and the heat remains trapped in the core of the body. The arteries supplying the limbs have accompanying veins (venae comites) that serve as countercurrent heat exchangers. These exchangers minimize the convective heat transfer from the core to the shell.

The transfer of heat from the shell to the exterior occurs through conduction, convection, radiation, and evaporation. The conductive heat loss is partly regulated by the layer of hair on the skin. Heat is conducted from the skin to the air trapped between hairs and from the trapped air to the exterior. Convective heat loss is determined by the movement of air over the skin (whether from the wind or a fan). Evaporative heat loss is regulated by the amount of sweating. Radiative (nonevaporative) heat loss is proportional to the temperature difference between the skin and the external environment.

A large amount of heat is lost from the scalp due to its high vascularity. At subzero temperatures, up to 50% of the body heat is lost from the scalp of bald persons. It explains why the elderly, who have a relatively less efficient thermoregulation, should wear a cap in winter, especially if bald.

Thermoregulatory Mechanisms

The temperature of the body is determined by a "thermostat" located in the hypothalamus. The set-point of the hypothalamic thermostat is 37°C, but it can be reset. When the body temperature rises above or falls below the set-point, the thermostat activates appropriate effector mechanisms for restoration of the body temperature.

The various effector mechanisms activated by the hypothalamus (**Table 43.1**) broadly fall into three categories: the sympathetically mediated mechanisms (vasoconstriction or vasodilatation, sweating, chemical thermogenesis), somatic mechanism (shivering), and behavioral mechanisms (hyperactivity or lethargy, hyperphagia or hypophagia).

Following transverse damage to the spinal cord above the thoracolumbar sympathetic outflow, the sympathetic and somatic thermoregulatory mechanisms do not remain under hypothalamic control. Some local vasodilatation and sweating are still possible through spinal reflexes, but these are too weak for effective control of body temperature. Such patients have to depend largely on conscious behavioral thermoregulatory mechanisms.

Body Heating Mechanisms

Cutaneous vasoconstriction is sympathetically mediated and occurs reflexively in response to cold. It reduces the cutaneous blood flow. Thus, the heat loss from the body core to the body shell is minimized. Cutaneous vasoconstriction occurs through a direct effect on smooth muscles and local reflexes, as well as in response to descending hypothalamic command. When cutaneous blood vessels are cooled, they become more sensitive to catecholamines and the arterioles and venules constrict. This local effect of cold directs blood away from the skin.

Chemical (nonshivering) thermogenesis | Sympathetic discharge and adrenaline cause an immediate increase in the rate

Table 43.1 Thermoregulatory Effector Mechanisms

Mechanisms activated by cold
Increase heat production
Shivering
Hyperphagia
Hyperactivity
Increased secretion of norepinephrine and epinephrine
Decrease heat loss
Cutaneous vasoconstriction
Curling up
Horripilation
Mechanisms activated by heat
Increase heat loss
Cutaneous vasodilatation
Sweating
Increased respiration
Decrease heat production
Anorexia
Lethargy

of metabolism due to uncoupling of oxidative phosphorylation, that is, the oxidation of foodstuffs is associated with release of heat rather than generation of adenosine triphosphate (ATP). Heat produced in this way is called chemical thermogenesis.

The amount of chemical thermogenesis is proportional to the amount of brown fat in the tissues. Brown fat contains large numbers of special mitochondria where the uncoupled oxidation occurs. These cells have sympathetic innervation. Adults do not have brown fat; therefore, chemical thermogenesis contributes less than 15% to the total heat production in them. Infants have some brown fat in the interscapular region and are therefore able to double their heat production through chemical thermogenesis. Chemical thermogenesis is promoted by thyroxine (see Chapter 77). Cold temperature stimulates hypothalamic release of thyrotropin-releasing hormone (TRH), which, in turn, stimulates the secretion of thyroid-stimulating hormone (TSH), which stimulates the secretion of thyroxine. However, several weeks of cold exposure are required before the thyroid gland secretes more thyroxine.

Shivering is a cortical reflex in which stimulation of cold receptors in the skin reflexively increases the muscle tone of the body. When the muscle tone increases above a certain threshold, it results in muscle clonus, which is commonly known as shivering. Shivering, or even the increase of muscle tone, is associated with greater metabolic activity and greater heat generation. A primary motor center for shivering is located in the posterior hypothalamus.

Horripilation is the fluffing of the feathers or erection of the hairs seen in animals in response to cold: it traps air in its layers, reducing heat loss from the skin. Horripilation is not seen in humans; what is seen instead is piloerection—the cold-induced contraction of the piloerector muscles attached to the hairs on the skin, resulting in "goose bumps."

Behavioral mechanisms | Cold environmental temperature also stimulates several behavioral mechanisms like hyperactivity and hyperphagia. Hyperphagia helps because the thermic effect of food increases the body metabolism. Hyperactivity generates excess body heat. A particular type of hyperactivity is the rubbing of palms: it generates frictional heat in the palms and keeps them warm. A behavioral mechanism for minimizing heat loss is curling up while sleeping. Curling up reduces the body surface area in contact with the environment. Behavioral responses in winter also include seeking out heat sources and putting on warm clothes. Heat-seeking behavior includes standing out in the sun or by a fire and consumption of hot food and drinks.

Body Cooling Mechanisms
Nonevaporative heat loss is radiative heat loss. It is proportional to the difference between body temperature and the ambient temperature. As the ambient temperature decreases, there is a linear rise in heat loss.

Insensible perspiration | About 50 mL of water evaporates every hour from the skin at all times. This is called insensible perspiration and results in an obligatory evaporative heat loss.

Vasodilatation and sweating | A rise in the ambient temperature produces cutaneous vasodilatation and sweating. The sweating causes evaporative cooling of the skin. Vasodilatation increases the cutaneous blood flow and promotes heat transfer from the core to the cooler surface. Like vasoconstriction, vasodilatation and sweating are produced by a local response, a spinal reflex, and a hypothalamic reflex. Persons acclimatized to hot climates can sweat much more than others. Their sweat has a low sodium (Na^+) concentration due to increased aldosterone secretion; therefore, they can sweat while slowly depleting the body of sodium.

Behavioral mechanisms | A rise in ambient temperature also activates behavioral responses like lethargy and hypophagia. There is also a search for shade and a preference for cold food and drinks. Some mammals lose heat by panting. This rapid, shallow breathing greatly increases the amount of water that evaporates in the mouth and respiratory passages; therefore, the amount of heat lost also increases. Because the breathing is shallow, there is not much change in the alveolar air composition.

Thermoneutrality and Thermal Comfort

The thermoneutral zone (TNZ), also called the zone of least thermoregulatory effort, is defined as the range of ambient temperature (normally 25°–27°C) within which the heat produced in the body is balanced by the nonevaporative and obligatory evaporative heat losses, without stimulating any reflex heating or cooling mechanisms of the body. The lower limit of the TNZ is called the *critical temperature*, below which the metabolic heat production increases to maintain thermal balance.

The zone of thermoneutrality is not the same as the *preferred ambient temperature*, which is the range of ambient temperature associated with thermal comfort. When the humidity is high, the preferred temperature is lower than the TNZ, whereas if there is brisk air movement, the preferred ambient temperature is higher than the TNZ. Thermal comfort also depends on the level of activity and the amount of clothing. Thermal comfort is maximum when the skin temperature is ~33°C.

Figure 43.2 shows the thermal balance at increasing environmental temperature. Several points are to be appreciated in the graph. (1) The deep body temperature is maintained remarkably constant through a large range of environmental temperatures. It changes only at extremes of environmental temperature, resulting in hypothermia or hyperthermia. (2) Any fall in the environmental temperature below the critical temperature is associated with progressive increase in metabolic heat production. Above the critical temperature, the metabolic heat production remains constant at a minimum level necessitated by the basal metabolic rate. The heat production increases again at high environmental temperature if there is hyperthermia, leading to an unregulated increase in the metabolic rate of the body. (3) The nonevaporative heat loss is zero at 37°C. It rises linearly as the environmental temperature decreases. The rise is less in the thermoneutral zone due to cutaneous vasoconstriction, which minimizes the heat flow from the body core to body surface. (4) At environmental

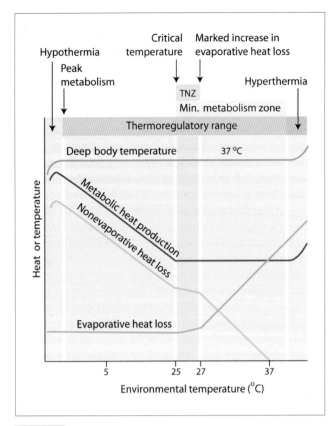

Fig. 43.2 Changes in the intensity of thermoregulatory mechanisms with increase in environmental temperature.

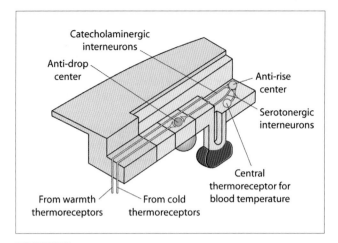

Fig. 43.3 Hypothalamic thermoregulatory centers. TNZ, thermoneutral zone.

calculates an integrated temperature from the information obtained from both the central and peripheral thermoreceptors.

Hypothalamic Thermoregulatory Mechanisms

The hypothalamus has two thermoregulatory mechanisms built into it, one for raising and the other for lowering the body temperature (**Fig. 43.3**). Both systems have their own cut-off temperature at which the heating or cooling mechanisms are activated or deactivated (**Fig. 43.4**).

Antirise center | The anterior or rostral hypothalamus acts as a heat-loss (heat-dissipating or antirise) center and opposes any rise of body temperature. Stimulation of this region, especially the preoptic area, produces heat loss by cutaneous vasodilatation, sweating, and panting, and probably by reducing heat production. The antirise center receives catecholaminergic afferents from peripheral and central thermoreceptors. Destruction of the rostral hypothalamus results in hyperthermia (neurogenic fever).

Antidrop center | The posterior or caudal hypothalamus, near the mamillary body, is concerned with heat production (antidrop center). Stimulation of this region activates heat production through shivering and increased TSH secretion. It also reduces heat loss by causing cutaneous vasoconstriction.

temperatures below the thermoneutral zone, the evaporative heat loss is minimal and attributable to the evaporation of insensible perspiration. Above the thermoneutral zone, the evaporative heat loss rises linearly due to sweating and its evaporation.

To summarize, there is a steep rise in metabolic heat production when the ambient temperature falls below the thermoneutral zone, and there is a steep rise in evaporative heat loss when the temperature rises above the thermoneutral zone. Both the processes are at their minimum within the thermoneutral zone. The thermoneutral zone can therefore be defined as the ambient temperature range in which a person neither shivers nor sweats.

Temperature Receptors

Temperature regulation is dependent on information originating in both central and peripheral receptors. *Central thermoreceptors* are present in the hypothalamus and spinal cord. They sense the temperature of blood flowing through them. Peripheral *thermoreceptors* are of two types: the cutaneous thermoreceptors that sense the ambient temperature and the visceral thermoreceptors present in the abdominal viscera and in or around the great veins. Both cutaneous and visceral thermoreceptors detect cold rather than warmth.

The central and peripheral thermoreceptors rarely provide identical information about body temperature. In dealing with body temperature, therefore, the posterior hypothalamus

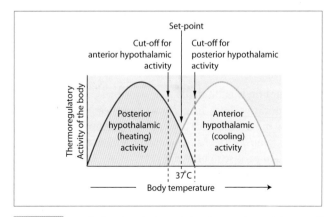

Fig. 43.4 Graph showing the hypothalamic set-point and the cut-off temperatures for posterior and anterior hypothalamic activity.

The antidrop center receives serotonergic afferents from the peripheral cold thermoreceptors. It does not have any direct input from the central thermoreceptors, but it is inhibited by impulses from the anterior center that arise when the blood temperature rises. It is also stimulated by blood-borne pyrogenic substances like viruses and toxins.

Disorders of Thermoregulation

Hyperthermia

Hyperthermia is an elevation of the body temperature above the normal range. It can occur for several different reasons.

Fever is a sudden increase in body temperature that occurs when the hypothalamic set-point is reset to a higher temperature, resulting in the activation of heat-producing and heat-conserving mechanisms of the body until the body temperature equals the hypothalamic set-point. The hypothalamic set-point is elevated by fever-producing substances called pyrogens. These substances are produced as part of the body's response to infection.

Lipopolysaccharide endotoxins derived from bacterial cell membranes are called *exogenous pyrogens*. The cytokines, interleukin- (IL-) IB, IL-6, β-interferon (IFN), γ-IFN, and tumor necrosis factor (TNF-) α, released from actively phagocytosing monocytes and macrophages are called *endogenous (leukocytic) pyrogens*. The cytokines act by inducing the synthesis and release of prostaglandin E_2. Antipyretics like aspirin prevent the formation of prostaglandin E_2 from arachidonic acid. The cytokines act on the OVLT (organ vasculosum of the lamina terminalis), which is outside the blood–brain barrier. The activated OVLT, in its turn, raises the hypothalamic set-point.

The onset of fever is signaled by the "chills" and its termination, by the "crisis." *Chills* are felt in fever when the heat-generating and heat-conserving mechanisms of the body are active. These mechanisms continue to be active until the body temperature rises to the elevated hypothalamic set-point of fever. *Crisis* is characterized by sudden sweating. It occurs when the hypothalamic set-point suddenly drops to normal, and the heat-dissipating mechanisms are activated.

The septal nuclei located anterior to the preoptic area serve as the antipyretic area. The area contains vasopressin-secreting neurons that reset the thermostat. Injection of vasopressin into this area reduces fever directly.

Fever is presumably beneficial because many microbes grow best at a specific temperature, and a rise in temperature inhibits their growth. Moreover, antibody production increases when body temperature is elevated. Before the advent of antibiotics, fever was artificially induced for the treatment of neurosyphilis and proved to be beneficial. Hyperthermia also slows the growth of some tumors.

Body temperatures above 41°C (hyperpyrexia) are harmful. Hyperpyrexia is accompanied by tachycardia, tachypnea, weakness, headache, mental confusion, and finally brain damage with loss of consciousness. A persistent temperature of over 43°C is not compatible with life.

Malignant hyperthermia is a condition that is triggered by administration of gaseous anesthesia during surgery in individuals with a defective ryanodine receptor. The response consists of spontaneous calcium release and hence sustained muscle contraction. The resulting muscle contracture greatly increases heat production, leading to hyperthermia, which is fatal if not treated.

Exercise-induced hyperthermia can occur during severe exercise, particularly if environmental temperature and humidity are high. The body is producing and gaining heat at a rate greater than can be balanced by heat loss.

Heat exhaustion and heatstroke | *Heat exhaustion* occurs due to excessive sweating leading to circulatory failure. *Heatstroke* occurs at very high ambient temperatures that upset the normal thermal balance of the body, leading to a rise in body temperature. The hyperthermia impairs the thermoregulatory capability of the hypothalamus, leading to a further rise in body temperature. A vicious cycle is thus set off, culminating in loss of consciousness.

Hypothermia

Thermoregulatory mechanisms fail when the body temperature falls below 32°C. Death usually occurs when the core temperature falls below 25°C. The temperature-regulating mechanism of old people is often defective, which is why in cold countries many elderly people die each winter of hypothermia.

Hypothermia of ~27°C is sometimes induced artificially so that the oxygen (O_2) demand of tissues is greatly reduced, and circulation can be stopped for 15 to 20 minutes, permitting surgical operations on the heart and large blood vessels. The induction of hypothermia during surgery is made easier with the use of anesthesia and muscle relaxants, both of which abolish shivering. The patient is warmed up slowly during recovery. Ventricular fibrillation is a common complication of hypothermia.

Poikilothermia

Thermoregulation can be impaired in hypothalamic lesions and in brainstem lesions that interrupt descending hypothalamic fibers to the spinal cord. The body temperature becomes labile, rising and falling frequently. The patient becomes poikilothermic: if he or she is covered with blankets, the body temperature quickly rises and may reach a dangerous level. An experimental lesion of the caudal hypothalamus produces poikilothermia because efferents from both antirise and antidrop centers descend through the caudal hypothalamus.

Summary

● Body temperature is held more or less constant by a homeostatic mechanism.

● Under most circumstances, the body must lose heat to maintain a constant temperature.

● Body temperature can be decreased (heat can be lost) by cutaneous vasodilatation (allowing greater heat loss between the body and the environment) and by sweating and evaporative heat loss.

- Body temperature can be increased (heat gained) by cutaneous vasoconstriction reducing the heat loss to the environment) and shivering (uncoordinated contraction of skeletal muscle fibers).

- Temperature receptors are located centrally (in the hypothalamus and spinal cord) and peripherally (in the skin).

- The hypothalamus is the site of the body temperature controller.

Applying What You Know

43.1. When Mr. Wright's (see Section III) core temperature became dangerously high, ice packs were used to lower his temperature. By what mechanisms did this alter his temperature?

43.2. Mr. Lundquist (see Section IV) plays tennis on a hot and sunny but also humid day. What happens to his body temperature? Explain the mechanisms that are at work.

Answers to Applying What You Know

Chapter 32

1 Mrs. Daniels' electrocardiogram (ECG) exhibits a normal sinus rhythm. This means that her sinoatrial (SA) node is functioning as the pacemaker. Describe the properties of the membrane of SA node cells that give rise to this pacemaker function.

The membrane of SA node cells (and atrioventricular [AV] node cells) is clearly different than the membrane of ventricular muscle cells. Ventricular cells have a very rapidly depolarizing phase 1, a long phase 2 plateau, and a stable phase 4 resting potential. SA node cells show a phase 4 in which the membrane potential is not constant; after the completion of the action potential, the SA node membrane slowly depolarizes until threshold is reached. At this point, an action potential is triggered. This phase 4 "pacemaker" potential is the consequence of the properties of membrane channels carrying potassium (K^+), sodium (Na^+), and calcium (Ca^{2+}) currents. See Chapter 19 for a more complete description of this phenomenon.

2 Signs of atrial enlargement and ventricular hypertrophy are visible in Mrs. Daniels' ECG. Explain how these changes to her heart give rise to changes in her ECG.

The size and orientation in the space of the cardiac dipole are determined by the size of the boundary between the depolarized portion of the heart and the resting or repolarizing portions of the heart. The increased size of the atrium and the ventricle (whether from an increase in the size of the chamber—distention—or an increase in the number and size of cells—hypertrophy—or both) will change the orientation of the cardiac dipole. The greater number of ventricular cells will change the amplitude of the dipole. The result is a recognizable change in the waveform of the ECG.

3 Mrs. Daniels has a sinus tachycardia; her heart rate is 90 beats/min. There is no evidence that this tachycardia is due to cardiac pathology or pathophysiology. Therefore, it is most likely due to changes in the sympathetic and parasympathetic signals reaching her SA node. What changes in these signals do you expect to be present?

A tachycardia with a normal sinus rhythm (the SA node is functioning as the pacemaker) is most likely the result of reflex changes to the autonomic innervation of the SA node. A reflex increase in heart rate is the result of *increased* sympathetic activity and simultaneously *decreased* parasympathetic activity. These changes in the neural inputs to the SA node cells alter the rate at which the membrane depolarizes during the phase 4 pacemaker potential (see Chapter 19).

Chapter 33

1 On auscultation Mrs. Daniels' S2 heart sound exhibits an unusually loud pulmonic component. Explain the mechanism that is causing this component of the S2 heart sound to be louder than normal.

The pressures in Mrs. Daniels' pulmonary circulation are elevated because of the stenosed and regurgitant mitral valve. Consequently, the afterload on the right ventricle is elevated (it has to pump against a higher pressure), and it has hypertrophied. This enables it to generate the higher pressure needed to open the pulmonic valve during systole. Because pulmonary artery pressure is high, when the right ventricle relaxes (diastole) and the pressure there drops sharply, the higher than normal pressure in the pulmonary artery closes the pulmonic valve more "forcefully," and a louder sound is generated.

2 Mrs. Daniels has an audible diastolic murmur. How does the stenosis alter the properties of the valve, and how does this affect flow across it? Describe the mechanism by which her stenosed mitral valve gives rise to a murmur.

The stenosed valve has a smaller cross-sectional area than a normal valve. This has two hemodynamic consequences. (1) The resistance to flow, R, presented by the valve is greatly increased because R is proportional to $1/r^4$. This leads to a larger pressure drop ($P_{LA} - P_{LV}$) across the mitral valve. (2) The velocity of flow through the valve increases because the area is reduced much more than any reduction in flow that might be present. If flow velocity through the opened mitral valve increases sufficiently, turbulent flow will be present, and a murmur will be generated during diastole when the left ventricle is filling. Note that, although the reduced size of the valve changes both resistance and velocity of flow, the change in resistance is *not* directly responsible for changing the velocity of flow.

Chapter 34

1 From the available data, calculate the value of Mrs. Daniels' right ventricular stroke output.

The simplest way to do this is to recognize that the output of Mrs. Daniels's right and left ventricles are identical (in the absence of any abnormal flow path). You know that the cardiac catheterization data yielded a cardiac output (CO) of 3.6 L/min. Therefore, her cardiac output, 3.6 L/min, divided by her heart rate (HR) 68 beats/min during the procedure, will yield her stroke volume, ~53 mL/beat.

If you do not know whether there is an abnormal flow path present, you can use the Fick method to calculate right ventricular output using the pulmonary arteriovenous (A-V) O_2 difference. In this case, the calculation yields the same cardiac output and therefore the same stroke volume.

$$CO = \frac{O_2 \text{ consumption}}{A-V\ O_2 \text{ content difference}}$$

$$CO = \frac{262\ mL\ O_2/min}{7.2\ mL\ O_2/100\ mL\ blood}$$

$$CO = 3600\ mL/min = 3.6\ L/min$$

$$SV = \frac{CO}{HR}$$

$$SV = \frac{3600\ mL/min}{68\ beats/min}$$

$$SV = 53\ mL/beat$$

2 Mrs. Daniels' stenosed mitral valve would reduce her stroke volume and hence her cardiac output if no compensation occurred. What mechanisms are helping to sustain her left ventricular stroke volume? Explain.

It is most likely that Mrs. Daniels has both elevated contractility and elevated filling. An uncompensated fall in cardiac output would reduce blood pressure and elicit a baroreceptor reflex response with increased sympathetic firing to the heart. This would increase heart rate and also increase cardiac contractility. We do know that heart rate is elevated, so it seems likely that contractility is also up. There is also evidence that filling is increased; the left ventricle end-diastolic pressure is certainly on the high end of normal. So both contractility and filling are increased, and thus a near normal cardiac output is maintained.

However, this response can become counterproductive if filling increases too far. The dilated ventricle does not pump as effectively as a normal ventricle, and thus at some point cardiac output begins to fall again.

3 Although her jugular veins are not distended, Mrs. Daniels is showing some signs of elevated central venous pressure (CVP, pulmonary and pedal edema). What could be done to lower her CVP and thereby improve her condition?

An increase in cardiac output produces a decrease in CVP as a greater volume of blood is transferred from the venous compartment into the arterial compartment. Thus, any procedure that increases her cardiac output will decrease her CVP. There are at least two categories of drugs that will act on the heart to increase cardiac output: (1) drugs acting to increase contractility by stimulating catecholamine receptors on ventricular myocytes, and (2) cardiac glycosides that increase contractility by increasing intracellular Ca^{2+} concentration.

Chapter 35

1 During the cardiac catheterization procedure, Mrs. Daniels' pulmonary wedge pressure (measured when the small catheter being used is advanced through the right heart and is "wedged" tightly in the arteriolar end of the pulmonary capillary network) is measured. Under these measurement conditions, the pressure measured at the tip of the catheter reflects the pressure in the left atrium. Estimate the pressure that would be present in Mrs. Daniels' left atrium. Explain.

The measured pulmonary wedge pressure was 30 mm Hg. Because flow into the atrium is occurring, the downstream pressure in the left atrium must be less than 30 mm Hg.

2 Mr. Lundquist (see Section IV) has pernicious anemia, which reduces his red blood cell count. As Mr. Lundquist recovers from this condition as treatment with vitamin B_{12} is begun, his red blood cell (RBC) count will increase. How will the viscosity of his blood be affected by the increasing RBC count? What will happen to his total peripheral resistance as he gets better? Explain.

According to Poiseuille's law, the viscosity of blood (η) is one of the determinants of resistance to flow in the circulation. Viscosity is a function of the number of red blood cells in the blood. As Mr. Lundquist produces more RBCs, the viscosity of his blood will increase, and hence his total peripheral resistance will increase. The baroreceptor reflex will, of course, compensate by reducing cardiac ouput and by vasodilating arterioles.

Chapter 36

1 Mrs. Daniels exhibits mild pedal edema (swelling of the feet and hands). Why are the hands and feet parts of the body where edema is most often visible?

When Mrs. Daniels is erect, there is a vertical column of fluid (blood) in the circulation of her hands and feet. The effect of gravity is to increase the pressures in both the arterial and venous compartments. Although this leaves the artery-to-vein pressure gradient unchanged, the increased venous hydrostatic pressure increases capillary hydrostatic pressure and promotes edema formation.

Edema is particularly visible in the hands and feet because these are relatively bony structures with a small amount of soft tissue arranged around a set of bones. The accumulation of even a small amount of fluid in the tissues of the extremities will thus be visible.

2 Mrs. Daniels exhibits several signs suggesting that she has pulmonary edema as well as pedal edema. What is the most likely cause of her pulmonary edema? Explain.

Mrs. Daniels's pulmonary edema is the result of pulmonary hypertension. The hydrostatic pressure in all of her pulmonary vessels is higher than normal as a result of the mitral stenosis (see the cardiac catheterization data in the Case Presentation). There is no reason to believe that any of the other Starling forces acting at the capillaries are abnormal.

Mrs. Daniels is now sleeping on three pillows because this keeps her lungs more vertical, and the effect of gravity on lung perfusion minimizes pulmonary edema formation and reduces shortness of breath.

Chapter 37

1 Mrs. Daniels reports that even modest exertion (exercise) leaves her short of breath. What changes should occur in her cardiovascular system when she exercises? How can her shortness of breath be explained?

During exercise, heart rate increases, as does cardiac contractility. Both of these changes contribute to increasing CO. With CO increased, perfusion of the exercising muscles can be increased, thus delivering the oxygen and nutrients needed to sustain the exercise.

Mrs. Daniels' mitral valve damage (stenosis and regurgitance) prevents her heart from increasing her CO to the level required to sustain even modest levels of exertion.

In addition, Mrs. Daniels' arterial PO_2 is low (74.9 mm Hg), and her hemoglobin saturation is somewhat low (92%). Thus, the oxygen content of her blood is somewhat low, probably aggravating her sensation of shortness of breath.

2 Digitoxin is a drug that inhibits the Na+–K+ pump in the cell membrane of cardiac cells. Thus, it results in an accumulation of Na+ in cardiac cells. What effect will this have on the function of ventricular cells? How might this help Mrs. Daniels' condition? Explain.

Digitoxin brings about an increased concentration of Ca^{2+} in ventricular cells. Slowing of the Na^+–K^+ pump raises intracellular Na^+ concentration. This, in turn, slows the Na^+–Ca^{2+} antiporter, which moves Ca^{2+} out of the cell. The result is a higher concentration of Ca^{2+} in the myocytes. This is, of course, a positive inotropic effect: cardiac contractility increases, and stroke volume goes up.

Mrs. Daniels would be able to increase her level of exertion (exercise) because she would now be able to increase her cardiac output more than she could previously.

Chapter 38

1 Predict what will happen to central venous pressure if a reflex response generates an increase in Mrs. Daniels' cardiac output. Explain.

When CO increases, the flow of blood out of the venous compartment increases. The increased flow in the arterial compartment takes some time (up to a minute) to reach the venous compartment. During this lag time, the volume of the venous compartment decreases (more blood is leaving than is being returned), and the pressure in the compartment must decrease. Hence, the increase in cardiac output will result in a decrease in central venous pressure.

2 Mrs. Daniels asks if she can donate a pint of blood to a nephew who is to undergo surgery shortly (she has the same blood type). If she were to do this, what changes would occur in her cardiac vascular system immediately after the procedure? What changes would occur over the next day or so?

Loss of one pint of blood (~0.5 L) will lower central venous pressure and hence reduce ventricular filling. Stroke volume will decrease, as will CO. The result will be a fall in blood pressure.

The reduced rate of firing of the baroreceptors will elicit a baroreceptor reflex. This will consist of increased firing in sympathetic nerves innervating the heart, thus increasing heart rate and contractility. There will also be increased firing in the sympathetic nerves innervating arteriolar smooth muscle in blood vessels. Total peripheral resistance increases. Sympathetic nerves innervating venous vessels will also increase, decreasing the capacitance of the venous compartment and mobilizing some volume of blood to restore a more normal blood pressure.

The result is a reflex return of blood pressure toward its normal level. This response takes only a few minutes to occur.

The increase in sympathetic firing will cause increased release of renin from the kidney and thus an increase in circulating angiotensin II (AII). This is a very potent vasoconstrictor and will help to restore blood pressure. In addition, AII will stimulate the adrenal cortex to release aldosterone (see Chapter 79), which will cause the kidneys to reabsorb more Na^+, hence reabsorbing more water. This will partially restore the lost blood volume. This response takes much longer to have its effect than does the baroreceptor reflex.

Chapter 39

1 Mr. Wright's (see Section III) response to anesthesia included a rapidly developing tachycardia. What effect did this have on Mr. Wright's coronary blood flow? Explain.

Mr. Wright's tachycardia results in the heart having to do more work. Thus, the metabolic needs of the myocardium increase. To meet these needs, the coronary blood flow will increase as locally produced vasodilators reduce coronary artery resistance.

There is, however, another effect to consider. Coronary blood flow is greatest during cardiac diastole when the compression of coronary vessels by contracting cardiac muscle is minimal. Increased heart rate occurs with a reduction in the diastolic period. The reduction in the duration of diastole will tend to decrease coronary blood flow if the heart rate were to get high enough.

In a normal heart, the increase in coronary blood flow due to metabolic vasodilatation will be larger than any decrease in blood flow due to the increased physical compression of the blood vessels in the walls of the heart.

Chapter 40

1 When Ms. Adams (see Section II) repetitively contracts muscles in her arms or trunk, those muscles rapidly fatigue, and their force of contraction decreases. What change in cerebral blood flow in the motor regions of the cortex would you expect to see when this phenomenon occurs? Explain.

Voluntary motor acts involve firing of cortical motor neurons. The increased metabolic activity of these neurons will cause local vasodilatation and increased local (cerebral) blood flow.

The decrease in muscle contraction that Ms. Adams experiences is, of course, not a cortical phenomenon, but rather a peripheral phenomenon occurring at the neuromuscular junction. So, if Ms. Adams attempts to continue to contract a set of muscles, blood flow in her motor cortex will remain elevated even though the contractions soon cease to occur.

Chapter 41

1 Mrs. Daniels has a mitral valve that is both stenosed and regurgitant. It is likely that both of these conditions developed more or less gradually and resulted in a gradual increase of left atrial volume and hence increased left atrial pressure. This, in turn, would cause pulmonary pressures to increase. Why is it likely that Mrs. Daniels' pulmonary artery pressure increased more slowly than her left atrial pressure?

The pulmonary vasculature is highly compliant (distensible) and thus can accommodate large changes in fluid volume with small changes in pressure. Two features of the pulmonary circulation make this possible. First, there are a large number of parallel flow paths that are normally not open, but which can open when volume or flow increases. Second, individual pulmonary vessels are highly distensible (more so than comparable systemic blood vessels).

Thus, mitral stenosis and regurgitation cause increased left atrial volume and increased left atrial pressure. However, the pressure in the pulmonary circulation will increase much less for each additional volume of blood that is displaced to it than occurs in the left atrium.

2 If Mrs. Daniels were to visit the top of Pike's Peak (over 14,000 feet at the summit) while on vacation, how would her condition be affected? Explain.

At high altitudes, the partial pressure of oxygen in the air is reduced. Consequently, hypoxic vasoconstriction will occur, increasing pulmonary blood pressure. This will be added to the increased pulmonary blood pressure due to the increased volume in the pulmonary vessels. Thus, going to the top of Pike's Peak will aggravate Mrs. Daniels' pulmonary hypertension and her pulmonary edema. Her shortness of breath would be aggravated by decreased partial pressure of oxygen in the inspired air and the increased pulmonary edema.

Chapter 42

1 Mr. Wright (see Section III) responds to the anesthetic being administered during surgery by dumping the Ca^{2+} stored in the sarcoplasmic reticulum of his muscles. The increase in intracellular Ca^{2+} concentration causes sustained contraction of the muscles affected. What effect does this have on blood flow to these muscles? Explain.

When Mr. Wright's muscles begin to contract, their metabolic activity increases. That is, they use oxygen at a faster rate and produce carbon dioxide at a faster rate. These and other products of exercise cause local vasodilatation and increased muscle blood flow.

However, at the same time the sustained contraction of his muscles must compress the blood vessels there, thus limiting the increase in blood flow that can occur.

As in the heart, the metabolic controls on muscle blood flow are normally stronger than the effects of physically compressing the blood vessels.

2 Mr. Lundquist (see Section IV) plays tennis regularly. What might be a consequence of eating a large meal before a tennis match?

Mesenteric blood flow increases after eating. This increased flow facilitates the absorption of the products of digestion. To the extent that mesenteric blood flow is increased when exercise begins (and blood flow is shunted to the exercising muscles), there is going to be "competition" for blood flow. The massive metabolic dilatation in the exercising muscles is likely to shunt flow away from the gastrointestinal tract, resulting in disruption of all of the digestive processes that are occurring there.

Chapter 43

1 When Mr. Wright's (see Section III) core temperature became dangerously high, ice packs were used to lower his temperature. By what mechanisms did this alter his temperature?

Ice packs cool Mr. Wright by conduction. They create a skin temperature that is lower than his core temperature and thus create a temperature gradient, causing increased heat flow through his tissues. However, by cooling the skin in this way, the vascular smooth muscle in the cutaneous vessels will contract, causing cutaneous vasoconstriction and limiting blood flow from the hot core to the cold skin. Nevertheless, there is rapid loss of heat, and his temperature decreases.

2 Mr. Lundquist (see Section IV) plays tennis on a hot and sunny, but also humid, day. What happens to his body temperature? Explain the mechanisms that are at work.

An individual exercising on a hot, sunny, and humid day will experience a rise in body temperature. The exercising muscles will generate heat at a faster than normal rate, thus raising body temperature. Heat will also be gained by radiation from the sun and from all heated objects in the environment (the tennis court, etc.). Conduction of heat from the air will occur if the air temperature is greater than skin temperature. The only mechanism by which he can lose heat is sweating and evaporative cooling. However, if the humidity is high, only limited evaporation is possible. There is thus a real danger of hyperthermia and heat exhaustion or heat stroke.

Clinical Overview

Review of patient condition | Mrs. Daniels has a problem with her mitral valve; it is both stenosed (smaller in cross-sectional area of the valve) and regurgitant (leaky). Consequently, she has pulmonary hypertension and pulmonary edema.

Etiology | Rheumatic fever ("strep throat"), a streptococcal infection, is still among the most common causes of mitral valve problems, although it has become quite rare since the availability of diagnostic tests for the presence of the bacteria and antibiotics with which to treat it.

Prevalence | The occurrence of mitral valve problems from rheumatic fever is much less frequent than it was 50 years ago. Nevertheless, the number of surgical procedures to correct severe valve problems is between 1000 and 2000 each year.

Diagnosis | The signs and symptoms presented by the patient (tiring on exertion, dyspnea, both systolic murmur and a diastolic rumble, signs of left ventricular and left atrial enlargement) point to the diagnosis. Confirmation of this diagnosis and determining the severity of the condition can be accomplished by cardiac catheterization.

Treatment | The treatment for valvular disease of this kind (stenosis and regurgitation) requires surgical replacement of the damaged valve.

Understanding the Physiology

Mitral stenosis (reduction in the cross-sectional area of the valve) has several important consequences. The outflow resistance across the valve is increased. This results in an increase in the pressure gradient (P_{LA} to P_{LV}) across the valve. With the area of the valve reduced, the velocity of flow through the valve must increase. This increases the likelihood of turbulence and the presence of a diastolic murmur.

Because the resistance to flow through the mitral valve is increased, filling of the left ventricle is reduced. This has two consequences. The left atrium is not emptying as much as it normally does, and hence its volume increases. This means that left atrial (LA) pressure increases, as do the pressures in the pulmonary circulation. At the same time, the reduced filling of the left ventricle (LV) means that stroke volume decreases, as does cardiac output. Mean arterial pressure (MAP) will decrease, and tissue perfusion will be reduced. Of course, the fall in MAP elicits a baroreceptor reflex, which increases the contractility of the heart (SV increases) and increases peripheral resistance. Thus, there is at least partial compensation for the fall in MAP.

Mitral regurgitation has the following consequences. During systole, there will be flow back through the partially open mitral valve. If flow velocity is high, turbulence will be present, and a systolic murmur will be present. The flow back into the left atrium further enlarges this chamber and raises left atrial pressure. At the same time, the left ventricle stroke is reduced (some of the volume present at the end of diastole returns to the right atrium; hence, it is available to be pumped into the systemic circulation).

Mrs. Daniels' mitral valve is both stenosed and regurgitant. Both problems result in increased left atrial pressure and elevated pulmonary pressures. The elevated pulmonary capillary pressure results in pulmonary edema and reduced gas exchange in the lungs. Thus, there is a reduced uptake of oxygen. The consequence is shortness of breath that is aggravated by exertion (when oxygen utilization is increased). When the edema is severe enough, the hydrodynamic changes in pulmonary perfusion that occur when lying down increases edema formation still further, and the individual can only sleep with his or her head and chest elevated (near vertical). This is called three-pillow orthopnea.

If the stenosis and regurgitation are severe enough, the elevated pressures extend to the right side of the heart. Increased right atrial pressures will increase central venous pressure, and the result will be pedal edema.

The accompanying flow chart illustrates the physiologic relationships that give rise to Mrs. Daniels' signs and symptoms (**Fig. V.1**).

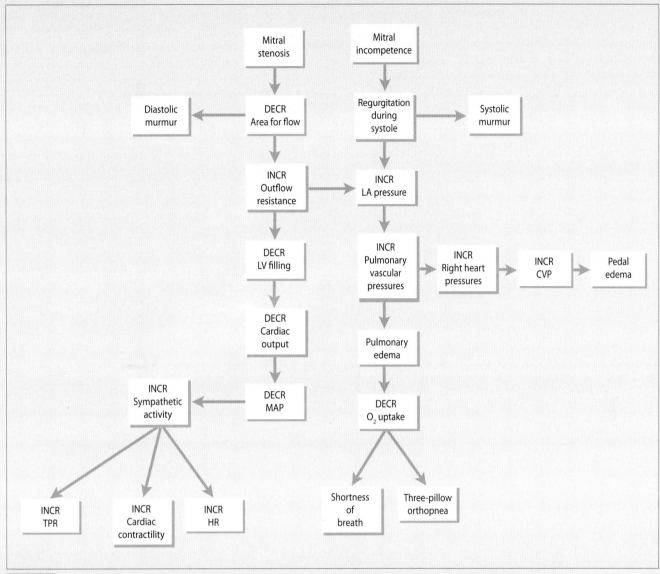

Fig. V.1 Mrs. Daniels has a mitral value with two defects. Her mitral stenosis causes a decreased MAP and a baroreceptor reflex that partially compensates. Her mitral incompetence causes elevated pulmonary vascular pressures, pulmonary edema, and shortness of breath.

Section VI | Respiratory System

Overview

E very cell in the body requires oxygen with which to generate the energy needed to power all of its processes (pumping ions, synthesizing compounds, contracting, etc.). The carbon dioxide that results from those metabolic processes is a waste product that must be eliminated from the body.

The job of the respiratory system is to obtain the needed oxygen and to dispose of the unwanted carbon dioxide.

This is accomplished by an interacting set of mechanisms. The lungs and chest wall function like a pump, creating a pressure gradient that causes airflow into and out of the lungs (ventilation). The air entering the lungs is brought into contact with a very thin diffusional barrier with a very large surface area. This structure maximizes the transfer of gases between the blood and the air in the lungs.

Oxygen is transported around the body, almost all of it bound to hemoglobin. The carbon dioxide to be eliminated is carried in the blood in a variety of forms.

The respiratory system homeostatically regulates the partial pressure of oxygen and carbon dioxide in arterial blood. The values of these two parameters are measured by sensors and used to control the rate of ventilation by varying the contraction of the respiratory muscle. The respiratory system also makes an important contribution to the homeostatic regulation of the pH (acidity) of the body.

The availability and utilization of oxygen by the cells of the body thus involve the integrated function of systems ranging over all levels of organization from the molecular to the whole organism.

Section VI Case Presentation:
Evelyn Eng is short of breath.

Chief Complaint

Evelyn Eng, a 24-year-old Asian-American newspaper writer, has been brought to the emergency room with severe shortness of breath. She is wheezing, coughing, and can barely get out two or three words without gasping for breath.

History of Present Illness

She manages to give you the following history. She was visiting a friend's house, and while chatting in the living room, two Siamese cats jumped into her lap. She immediately began to wheeze, and despite using her albuterol (a β_2-adrenergic receptor agonist) inhaler, she has gotten progressively worse.

Past Medical History

She has suffered from "hay fever" since childhood and has a tendency to have prolonged upper respiratory infections.

After several years of episodic shortness of breath, she was diagnosed as having asthma 6 months ago. She was told to use an albuterol inhaler whenever she experienced any chest tightness. She was also told to use it prior to exposure to anything that she thought might trigger an attack, such as cold air, cigarette smoke, cats, or stressful situations. She had been doing well until early autumn, about 1 month ago. At this time she began requiring her inhaler three or four times a day.

Family History

Her older sister has reported having a similar problem with cats and other pets.

Physical Examination

- *General appearance* | Ms. Eng is a thin, young woman in obvious respiratory distress.
- *Vital signs*
  - Blood pressure: 160/100 mm Hg
  - Pulse: 130/min
  - Respirations: 35/min
  - Temperature: 99.0°F (oral)
- *HEENT (head, eyes, ears, nose, throat)* | Examination is unremarkable. Specifically, there is no sinus tenderness, no nasal polyps, and a normal nasopharynx. There are no neck masses.
- *Lungs* | Examination reveals the use of accessory muscles of respiration, intercostal retractions, and tachypnea. There is inspiratory and expiratory wheezing throughout both lung fields, with a prolonged expiration.
- *Cardiovascular* | The heart examination is normal except for the tachycardia.
- The remainder of the physical examination is normal.

Stat Laboratory Studies

Complete Blood Count	Value	Normal
WBC	15.2×10^3/mL	$4–10 \times 10^3$
RBC	5.26×10^6/mL	$4.0–5.2 \times 10^6$ (f)
[Hb]	15.5 g/dL	12–16 (f)
Hct	45.1%	36–46 (f)
MCV	86 fL	80–100
MCH	29.5 pg/cell	26–34
MCHC	34.3 g/dL	31–37
Blood Gas Analysis (Room Air)	**Value**	**Normal**
pH	7.39	7.35–7.45
PCO$_2$	37 mm Hg	32–45 (f)
PO$_2$	66 mm Hg	83–108
[HCO$_3$]	22.5 mM/L	24
Sat	91%	95–98

Abbreviations: WBC, white blood cell; RBC, red blood cell; Hb, hemoglobin; Hct, hematocrit; MCV, mean corpuscular volume; MCH, mean corpuscular hemoglobin; MCHC, mean corpuscular hemoglobin concentration.

Radiology Study

Chest x-ray shows mild hyperinflation of the lungs. There are no signs of parenchymal infiltrates.

Treatment in the Emergency Room

The patient was placed on supplemental oxygen, and an intravenous line was established. She was given 300 mg of aminophylline (an adrenergic agonist) over 30 minutes and then a continuous infusion at a rate of 0.5 mg/kg/hr. Terbutaline (an adrenergic agonist) 0.25 mg was administered intramuscularly. The terbutaline was repeated 45 minutes later because the patient was still in marked distress. Atropine (a muscarinic antagonist) 3 mg in 3 cc of saline was administered by a medical nebulizer (a device that turns a liquid into very small airborne particles) when she still had not improved after 90 minutes.

After several hours, she started to feel better and said her breathing had improved. An hour later she was feeling perfectly normal, and an exam was free of wheezes.

She was sent home with instructions to continue to use her inhaler and to avoid exposure to Siamese cats. She was asked to make an appointment for a follow-up visit in your office in 1 week.

Office Visit

When you see Ms. Eng in the office 1 week later, she is in no obvious respiratory distress, although you note a slight bilateral expiratory wheeze.

To obtain baseline data on this patient, you refer her to the pulmonary function laboratory. The results of this testing are seen below.

	Actual	Predicted	% Predicted
Vital capacity (L)	3.80	4.30	88
FEV_1 (L)	2.47	3.46	71
FEV_1/FVC (× 100%)	65	80	
FEF_{25-75} (L/sec)	1.90	3.88	49
Peak flow (L/min)	280	409	57
FRC (L)	3.35	3.12	107
RV (L)	2.23	1.73	129
TLC	6.00	6.03	100

Abbreviations: FEV_1, forced expiratory volume in 1 second; FVC, forced vital capacity; FEF, forced midexpiratory flow rate; FRC (L), functional residual lung capacity; RV (L), residual lung volume; TLC, total lung capacity.

Administration of a bronchodilator and a repeat of the above tests resulted in a significant improvement of FEV_1 and FEV_1/FVC.

You again advise her to avoid exposure to things or situations likely to trigger an episode of breathing difficulty. You assure her that there are additional drugs that can be used to control her problem. Before leaving, Ms. Eng asks if she will be able to continue her participation in water sports. You assure her that asthma should not prevent her from swimming.

Some Things to Think About

1. It is noted that Ms. Eng is using her accessory respiratory muscles. How does activity in the respiratory muscles produce the normal pattern of inspiration and expiration?

2. Ms. Eng exhibits a prolonged expiration. What factors determine the time it takes for an expiration to be completed?

3. Ms. Eng has a low arterial partial pressure of oxygen (PO_2). What are the determinants of arterial PO_2?

4. The patient was brought to the emergency room suffering from shortness of breath. What does this mean, and what mechanisms can produce this sensation?

5. What is the role of the respiratory system? Which, if any, respiratory parameters are homeostatically regulated?

The process of respiration comprises external respiration—the intake of oxygen (O_2) and removal of carbon dioxide (CO_2) from the body—and internal respiration—the consumption of O_2 for energy release, production of CO_2 by cells, and the gaseous exchanges between the cells and their extracellular fluid environment.

Respiratory Passages

The respiratory passages are functionally divided into the upper and lower respiratory tracts. The upper respiratory tract is composed of the nasal and oral cavities, the pharynx and the larynx. The lower respiratory tract is composed of the tracheobronchial tree and the lung parenchyma.

Upper Respiratory Tract

The nasal cavity warms up the air to the body temperature, humidifies the air to 100% saturation, and cleans and filters the air of its particulate contents by channeling the air through a tortuous path between the turbinates. The particles are deposited at the bends, where they adhere to the mucus lining the cavity.

The intrinsic muscles of the larynx are broadly divided into the abductors (which open the glottis) and the adductors (which close the glottis). They are innervated by the recurrent laryngeal branch of the vagus nerve. The abductor muscles (posterior cricoarytenoid) contract early in the inspiratory phase, pulling the vocal cords apart and opening the glottis. When the abductors are paralyzed, there is inspiratory stridor. (Stridor is a harsh, high-pitched whistling sound produced during breathing if there is airway obstruction.) In unconscious or anesthetized patients, or when abductors are paralyzed, glottis closure may be incomplete, and vomitus may enter the trachea, causing an inflammatory reaction in the lung (aspiration pneumonia). The adductor muscles begin to contract early in expiration, but their contraction is not complete. Their main function is protective. During swallowing, there is reflex contraction of the adductor muscles that closes the glottis and prevents aspiration of food, fluid, or vomitus into the lungs. Another protective function of the glottis is its role in the cough reflex (see below). By contracting during the early compressive stage of cough, adductors allow a high intratracheal pressure to be developed.

Maintenance of upper airway patency | Keeping the upper airway patent (open, unobstructed) is an important step in any form of resuscitation. The victim is placed in the supine position, and the airway is opened by placing a hand under the neck and lifting while keeping pressure with the other hand on the victim's forehead. This extends the neck and lifts the tongue away from the back of the throat (**Fig. 44.1**).

Lower Respiratory Tract

Tracheobronchial tree | After passing through the nasal passages and pharynx, where it becomes warm and moist, the inspired air passes down the trachea and through the bronchioles, respiratory bronchioles, and alveolar ducts into the alveoli. Between the trachea and the alveolar sacs, the airways divide 23 times (**Fig. 44.2**). The first 16 generations of passages form the *conducting zone* of the airways. They are made up of bronchi, bronchioles, and terminal bronchioles. The remaining seven generations form the *respiratory zone*. They are made up of respiratory bronchioles, alveolar ducts, and alveoli. The exchange of gases with blood occurs only in the respiratory zone.

By definition, *bronchioles* are airways with diameter less than 1 mm, and the term *small airways* is used for airways less than 2 mm in diameter (i.e., small bronchi and bronchioles). Airways in the conducting zone have smooth muscle in their walls. Bronchioles and smaller airways have cuboidal epithelium; larger airways have columnar epithelium. Alveolar epithelium is made of flat, squamous cells. The trachea and bronchi have cartilage in their walls but relatively little smooth muscle. The walls of bronchioles and terminal bronchioles do not contain cartilage; instead, they contain more smooth muscle.

Alveoli | The alveoli are surrounded by pulmonary capillaries. The structures between alveolar air and capillary blood, across which O_2 and CO_2 diffuse, are exceedingly thin and constitute the *respiratory membrane* (see **Fig. 47.6**). There are 300

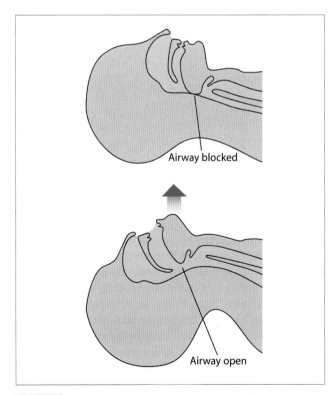

Airway blocked

Airway open

Fig. 44.1 Upper airway obstruction caused by the soft tissue (tongue) falling back. Neck extension and chin elevation clears the upper airway obstruction caused by soft tissue.

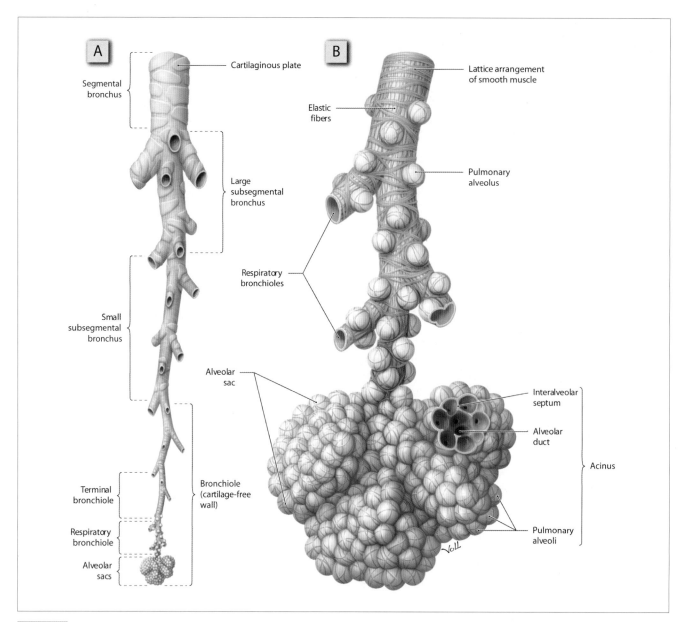

Fig. 44.2 **(A)** The tracheobronchial tree from segmental bronchus to alveoli. **(B)** The structure of the exchange portion of the respiratory tree.

million alveoli in a human, and the total area of the alveolar walls in contact with capillaries in both lungs is ~50 to 100 m². The alveoli are lined by two types of epithelial cells or pneumocytes. *Type I pneumocytes* (squamous alveolar cells) are the primary lining cells. *Type II pneumocytes* (granular alveolar cells) are thicker and contain numerous lamellar inclusion bodies. They are located commonly near the angles between neighboring alveolar septa. These cells secrete surfactant (see next chapter). The lungs also contain pulmonary alveolar macrophages (PAM) or the dust cells, lymphocytes, plasma cells, Clara cells (see below), APUD (amine precursor uptake and decarboxylation) cells, and mast cells.

Blood supply | The entire right ventricular output passes through the pulmonary artery to the pulmonary capillary bed, where it is oxygenated and returned to the left atrium via the pulmonary veins. The smaller bronchial arteries are systemic

arteries arising from the aorta: they supply bronchial smooth muscles and pleura and drain into the bronchial veins (one-third) and the bronchopulmonary veins (two-thirds) (**Fig. 41.1**, see **Fig. 44.3**). The bronchial veins drain into the right atrium. The deoxygenated bronchial capillary blood in the bronchopulmonary veins mixes with the oxygenated blood in the pulmonary vein, resulting in a *physiologic shunt*. Lymphatic channels are more abundant in the lungs than in any other organ.

Nerve supply | Bronchi and bronchioles are kept in a state of slight constriction (the bronchomotor tone) due to the tonic discharge of parasympathetic (cholinergic) fibers in the vagus. The sympathetic (adrenergic) control, which causes bronchodilatation, is feeble. Bronchodilatation is mainly under the control of a *nonadrenergic, noncholinergic* (NANC) system that has VIP (vasoactive intestinal peptide) as its neurotrans-

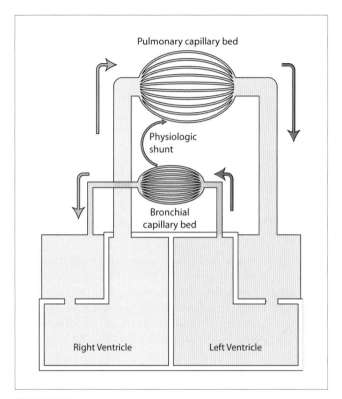

Fig. 44.3 The physiologic shunt, produced by the mixing of deoxygenated bronchial capillary blood with the oxygenated pulmonary capillary blood.

mitter. Nerve fibers belonging to the NANC system reach the lungs through the vagus.

The vagus also contains afferent fibers originating in the bronchial epithelium. These afferents are stimulated by a variety of physical and chemical factors. Chemical factors include common air pollutants like sulfur dioxide (SO_2) and nitrogen dioxide (NO_2) that produce bronchoconstriction. Physical factors include foreign bodies in the trachea that trigger cough. Another potent physical stimulus is cold air, which causes bronchoconstriction. The bronchoconstriction caused by cold air is not due to a neural reflex as with other physical or chemical factors: low temperature acts directly on smooth muscle to cause contraction. Exercise, too, causes bronchoconstriction, possibly due to the excessive ventilation of airways with cool air.

Although the sympathetic innervation of the bronchi and bronchioles is sparse, adrenergic receptors are as abundant in these airways as are the cholinergic receptors. Hence, drugs that stimulate adrenergic receptors (sympathomimetic drugs) are as effective in relieving bronchospasm as are drugs that block cholinergic receptors (anticholinergic drugs). The adrenergic receptors are predominantly of the β_2 subtype (see Chapter 12). Also present on the bronchial smooth muscles are histamine receptors. Numerous drugs and allergens cause mast cell degranulation with release of large amounts of histamine. The histamine released binds to the histamine receptors present on bronchial smooth muscles, producing bronchoconstriction.

Nonrespiratory Functions

Physical Protection

The respiratory passages humidify and warm or cool the inspired air so that by the time it reaches the alveoli, it is at (or near) body temperature. The respiratory passages also have various mechanisms to prevent particulate matter from reaching the alveoli (**Fig. 44.4**). Particles larger than 10 μm in diameter are strained out by the hairs in the nostrils. Most of the remaining particles of this size settle on mucous membranes in the nose and pharynx. Because of their inertia, they do not follow the airstream as it curves downward into the lungs but instead fall on the tonsils and adenoids, which dispose of these particles. Particles 2 to 10 μm in diameter generally fall on the walls of the bronchi as the airflow slows in the smaller passages. There they are expelled by mucokinesis and coughing. Particles less than 2 μm in diameter generally reach the alveoli, where they are ingested by the PAM cells.

Mucokinesis | Inhaled particulate matter gets trapped in the mucus layer that covers the respiratory passage, starting from the nose and covering the tracheobronchial tree epithelium up to the terminal bronchioles. The surfactant layering the alveolar epithelium drains into the bronchiolar mucus layer.

The mucus layer consists of a superficial gel layer that is secreted by the bronchial mucus glands and goblet cells and a deeper sol layer ~5 μm in thickness (**Fig. 44.5**) that mainly comes from the Clara cells. The cilia, which are covered with mucus, beat in a coordinated fashion (**Fig. 44.6**), moving the gel layer at a rate of 1 to 2 cm/min toward the larynx and into the pharynx, where it is swallowed. The moving of the mucus layer is called mucokinesis.

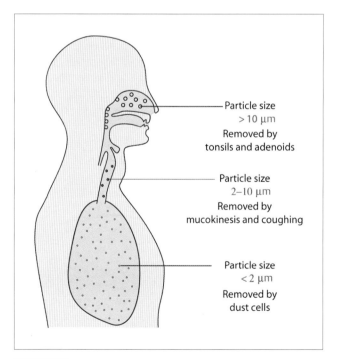

Fig. 44.4 The structures and mechanisms that remove particulate matter from the respiratory tract and lungs.

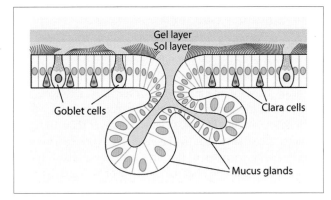

Fig. 44.5 Bronchial epithelium showing the gel and sol layers, goblet cells, and submucosal mucus glands.

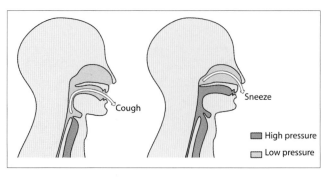

Fig. 44.7 When a cough occurs, the air pressure builds up below the closed glottis. When a sneeze occurs, the air pressure builds up below the nasopharynx.

When ciliary motility is defective, mucokinesis is almost absent, leading to retained secretions that provide an excellent medium for bacterial growth (stasis pneumonia). The retained secretions also cause plugging of bronchioles, leading to collapse (atelectasis) of the connected alveoli.

Coughing and sneezing are concerned with the cleansing of the air passages by removing secretions or inhaled material. Both are reflexes that have their centers in the medulla. Efferent (motor) impulses of both the reflexes travel down the vagus to the larynx (or soft palate) and by spinal nerves to diaphragm, abdominal, and pelvic muscles that contract during cough (or sneeze). Both involve the following sequence of events: (1) a deep inspiration; (2) trapping of air by shutting off its exit; (3) initiation of expiratory effort, raising the intrathoracic pressure; (4) augmentation of the pressure of the trapped air (the compressive stage); and (5) sudden release of the trapped air at high pressure by opening up the exit passages.

The differences between the two reflexes are as follows. (1) Sneezing is stimulated by irritation of the nasal mucosa. The impulses travel up via the trigeminal nerve. Cough occurs due to irritation of sensory receptors in the tracheobronchial tree. Impulses travel up via the vagus and glossopharyngeal nerves. (2) In sneezing, the air is trapped by shutting off its exit passages through the nasopharynx (by raising the soft palate to the posterior pharyngeal wall) and the oral cavity (by raising the tongue to the hard palate). In coughing, the air is trapped behind the closed glottis by contraction of the laryngeal ad-

ductor muscles (**Fig. 44.7**). (3) In sneezing, the air is released by opening the nasopharynx. The jet of air passing through the nasopharynx can be decreased if necessary by releasing some air through the mouth by lowering the tongue. In coughing, the air is released by opening the glottis. (4) Sneezing always occurs reflexively, but coughing can be performed voluntarily also.

There are two types of cough, depending on the type of receptor stimulated. (1) In the mucosa of large airways (larynx, trachea, and bronchi), there are rapidly adapting stretch receptors or irritant receptors sensitive to mechanical stimuli. They initiate a forceful expiration without a preceding inspiration. Absence of the preceding inspiration helps prevent aspiration of noxious material. (2) Distal to the large airways up to the acinus, there are chemical receptors. When stimulated, these receptors first initiate a deep inspiration, which is followed by a forceful expiration. This type of cough helps in expectoration of mucus containing chemical irritants.

Immunologic Protection

Bronchial secretions contain immunoglobulin A (IgA) that helps resist infections. In addition, the epithelium of the paranasal sinuses produces nitric oxide that is bacteriostatic.

Pulmonary alveolar macrophages (PAM) or the dust cells are a component of the monocyte–macrophage system. They are actively phagocytic and ingest inhaled bacteria and small particles. They process antigens and secrete cytokines that attract granulocytes and stimulate granulocyte and monocyte formation in the bone marrow. PAM produces α_1-antitrypsin, which offers protection against emphysema (by inhibiting the enzyme that breaks down elastic tissue). When the macrophages ingest large amounts of pollutants, such as cigarette smoke, silica, and asbestos particles, they release lysosomal enzymes into the extracellular space, causing inflammation.

Metabolic and Endocrine Functions

The lungs have several metabolic functions. (1) Type II pneumocytes synthesize surfactant. (2) The lungs contain a fibrinolytic system that lyses clots in the pulmonary vessels. (3) The angiotensin-converting enzyme (ACE) responsible for the activation of angiotensin I into angiotensin II is located on the surface of the endothelial cells of the pulmonary capillar-

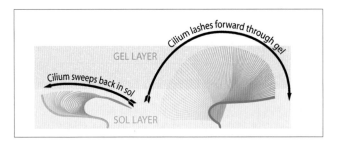

Fig. 44.6 The function of the cilia in clearing inhaled particulate matter from the respiratory tract. The cilia slowly arch backward, moving through the sol layer. Thereafter, they lash forward, sweeping through the gel layer and propelling it forward.

ies. ACE also inactivates bradykinin. (4) The lungs release several substances (e.g., histamine and kallikrein) into systemic circulation and remove several others (e.g., serotonin and norepinephrine) from circulation. Prostaglandins are both secreted into and removed from the circulation by the lungs.

Summary

- External respiration is the uptake of oxygen into the body and the disposal of carbon dioxide in the atmosphere; internal respiration is the use of oxygen in energy-producing reactions and the production of carbon dioxide.

- Airflow proceeds from the upper respiratory tract (nose and pharynx) to the lower respiratory tract (trachea and bronchioles), then to the alveoli (where gas exchange occurs).

- The respiratory tract has several nonrespiratory functions, including warming and humidifying the air and trapping, expelling, or neutralizing noxious materials.

Applying What You Know

44.1. When Ms. Eng's symptoms first appear, she uses her albuterol inhaler. Where along the respiratory tree will albuterol have its effect?

44.2. Which, if any, of Ms. Eng's vital signs are abnormal?

The lungs are elastic, nonmuscular organs that get inflated (when air enters through the trachea) or deflated (by expelling air through the trachea) when the thorax expands or contracts. The lungs are separated from the chest wall by a thin layer of pleural fluid that allows the lung and the thoracic wall to glide easily on each other. Nevertheless, the lung resists being pulled off the chest wall in the same way as two wet glass slides are not separated easily. Hence, when the thorax expands or contracts, so do the lungs.

Mechanism of Thoracic Expansion

Changes in Chest Wall Dimensions

During inspiration, all three dimensions of the thoracic cavity expand: the vertical (superoinferior) diameter, the anteroposterior diameter, and the transverse diameter. There is a different mechanism for expansion in each direction.

The **vertical diameter of the thoracic cavity** increases when the diaphragm descends into the abdominal cavity. The diaphragmatic descent ranges from 1.5 cm (in eupnea—normal breathing) to 7.0 cm (deep breathing) and accounts for nearly 75% of the thoracic expansion during quiet breathing. The extent of diaphragmatic descent, illustrated in **Fig. 45.1,** can be assessed in a plain radiograph and is of diagnostic importance.

The **anteroposterior diameter** of the thorax increases during inspiration when the upper ribs (2nd to 6th ribs), which normally slope obliquely downward and forward, swing upward to assume a more horizontal position from their joints with the spine. This is called the *pump-handle movement* because of its obvious resemblance to the movements of the handle of a hand pump (**Fig. 45.2**).

The **transverse diameter** also increases during inspiration, but to a lesser degree. This occurs due to the movements of the lower ribs (7th to 10th ribs) that swing outward and upward in inspiration. This is called the *bucket-handle movement* due to its obvious resemblance to the movements of a bucket handle (**Fig. 45.2**).

Muscles of Inspiration

The diaphragm or the external intercostal muscles alone can maintain adequate ventilation at rest. However, some other muscles called *accessory muscles of inspiration* must contract when greater inspiratory force is required during exercise.

The **diaphragm** consists of a central tendinous dome with muscle fibers attached to its periphery. The muscle fibers are attached to the xiphisternum and the inner surfaces of the lower six ribs (costal attachment), and to the lumbar vertebrae (crural attachment). The descent of the diaphragm is brought about by the contraction of its peripheral muscular part pulling down its central tendinous part. The costal and crural parts of the diaphragmatic muscles are innervated by different parts of the phrenic nerve (spinal roots C3–C5) and can contract separately.

The **quadratus lumborum** is a posterior abdominal muscle that serves a synergistic role with the diaphragm, acting as a stabilizer (**Fig. 45.3**). When the diaphragmatic muscles contract, the dome of the diaphragm tends to flatten out (action). Simultaneously, the lower ribs to which the diaphragm is attached get pulled up (reaction), which would elevate the diaphragm instead of lowering it. This is prevented by the quadratus lumborum muscle, which anchors the 12th rib to the iliac crest and prevents it from moving up during inspiration.

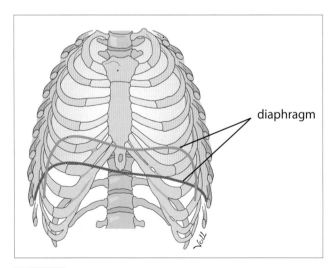

Fig. 45.1 An illustration of the change in position of the diaphragm in inspiration (red) and expiration (blue).

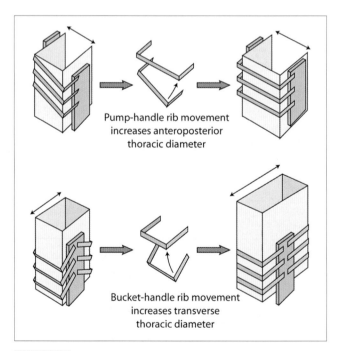

Pump-handle rib movement increases anteroposterior thoracic diameter

Bucket-handle rib movement increases transverse thoracic diameter

Fig. 45.2 Pump-handle and bucket-handle movements of the rib cage.

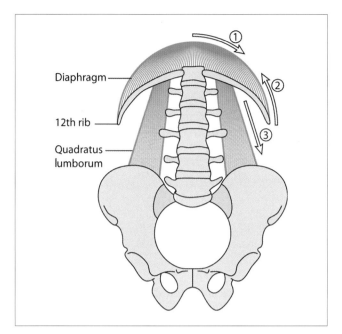

Fig. 45.3 The action of the quadratus lumborum muscle as an inspiratory muscle. Contraction of the diaphragm flattens the dome of the diaphragm, thereby lowering it (1), but simultaneously pulls up the 12th rib (2), thereby minimizing the effect on the vertical thoracic diameter. The elevation of the 12th rib is prevented by the quadratus lumborum (3).

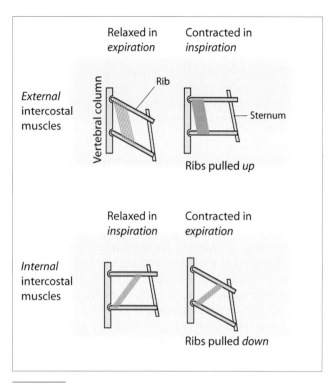

Fig. 45.4 Direction of rib movement caused by contraction of the external and internal intercostal muscles.

The **external intercostal muscles** pass obliquely forward and downward from the upper rib to the lower rib. When the external intercostals contract, the lower ribs move up (**Fig. 45.4**). Although the upper ribs would be expected to move down simultaneously, that does not happen for two reasons. The first reason is the mechanical advantage available to the upper ribs due to the direction of the muscle fibers that move away from the fulcrum as they reach the lower ribs. The second reason is the simultaneous contraction of the scalenus muscles (see below).

Two prominent **accessory muscles of inspiration** are the scalenus and sternocleidomastoid muscles. The scalenus muscles originate in the cervical transverse process and are inserted into the first rib. They are supplied by spinal nerves C3–C8. The sternocleidomastoid extends from the mastoid process above to the manubrium sterni and medial part of the clavicle below. It is supplied by the 11th cranial nerve and spinal nerve C2. When the scalenus and sternocleidomastoid contract during inspiration, they tend to elevate the first rib, thereby counteracting the downward pull exerted on the ribs by the external intercostal muscle.

General Models: Energy and Communications

The respiratory muscles are made up of cells that are specialized for the transformation of biochemical energy into the mechanical energy of contraction. Contraction of these muscles is triggered by neural activity, one form of cell-to-cell communication.

Muscles of Expiration

Normal expiration occurs due to the passive recoil of the lungs and thoracic wall and does not require any muscle action. Muscle action is required only during forced expiration. The muscles for forced expiration are the anterolateral abdominal muscles and the internal intercostal muscles.

The **anterolateral abdominal muscles** (obliquus externus abdominis, obliquus internus abdominis, transversus abdominis, and rectus abdominis) are the most important muscles involved in forced expiration. They have two actions that aid expiration: they pull the ribs downward, reducing the transverse and anteroposterior diameter of the thorax. They also increase the intra-abdominal pressure, thereby pushing the diaphragm upward.

Contraction of the **internal intercostal muscles** pulls the upper ribs down. Although the lower ribs would be expected to move up simultaneously, that does not happen for two reasons. The first reason is the mechanical advantage available to the lower rib due to the direction of the muscle fibers (**Fig. 45.4**). The second reason is the simultaneous contraction of the abdominal muscles and the quadratus lumborum.

Respiratory Resistance

To inflate or deflate the lung requires that work be done to overcome the "respiratory resistance" presented by the resistance to airflow in the airways, pulmonary tissue "resistance," and thoracic "resistance." We can then say that

Total "respiratory resistance" =

$$\underset{\text{resistance}}{\text{Airway}} + \underset{\text{"resistance"}}{\text{Pulmonary tissue}} + \underset{\text{"resistance"}}{\text{Thoracic}} \quad (45.1)$$

The airway resistance and pulmonary tissue resistance are together called pulmonary resistance. Therefore,

$$\underset{\text{resistance"}}{\text{Total "respiratory}} = \underset{\text{resistance}}{\text{Pulmonary}} + \underset{\text{"resistance"}}{\text{Thoracic}} \quad (45.2)$$

Factors affecting "respiratory resistance" The *pulmonary tissue resistance* is higher in the recumbent position due to the engorgement of the pulmonary vascular bed with blood, which increases the stiffness of the lung tissue. It also increases when lung surfactant is deficient or in diseases affecting lung tissue, such as interstitial fibrosis.

The *thoracic resistance* comes from the rib cage, diaphragm, and abdominal contents. It is increased in the recumbent position as the abdominal contents press on the diaphragm.

Of the total *airway resistance* during quiet mouth breathing, 10% is contributed by the peripheral airways (smaller than 2 mm in diameter), 50% by the larger airways, and 40% by the nasal cavity. The resistance of a fluid (liquid or gas) flowing through a tube varies inversely with the fourth power of the tube radius. Yet the resistance of the peripheral airways is low because several of them are disposed in parallel. Moreover, the length of the peripheral airways is much smaller than that of the central airways.

General Model: Flow

Flow of a fluid, whether a liquid (e.g., blood) or a gas (air), is determined by the pressure gradient and the resistance to flow that are present. For a more detailed discussion of fluid resistance, see Chapter 35 (which describes blood flow in the circulation).

The resistance offered by the nasal cavity is higher due to the turbulence of air in it. The resistance increases markedly during exercise, making it necessary to breathe through the mouth.

Airway resistance changes with lung volume: it does not decrease much when the lung volume increases, but it increases markedly when the lung volume decreases below its functional residual capacity (i.e., ~2 L) due to compression of the small airways. It is also affected by the bronchomotor tone. Fine particles of carbon, chalk, and cigarette smoke, when inhaled, cause bronchoconstriction and increase airway resistance. Finally, the small airways, which do not have rigid walls, are kept open by the traction exerted by the elastic tissue in the lung. When these elastic tissues are destroyed, as in chronic obstructive pulmonary disease (COPD), the smaller airways tend to collapse, and the peripheral airway resistance

increases. Loss of elastic tissues affects the resistance of the larger airways also, though to a lesser degree.

Compliance

We can quantitate the "resistance" to being distended posed by the lungs or thorax by measuring what is called the compliance of each of these structures.

General Model: Elasticity

The compliance of a system (whether we consider the lungs, the chest wall, or the combination of the two) is one way of quantitating the elastic properties of the system. The lungs and chest wall behave like elastic structures, such as balloons.

Lung compliance is defined as the change in lung volume (ΔV) in response to a unit change in the transpulmonary pressure (ΔP), that is the pressure difference inside and outside the lungs (**Fig. 45.5**). The term *compliance* can be extended to the whole respiratory system (lung + thorax combined).

Compliance is the reciprocal of resistance. Hence, the relationship among lung compliance, thoracic compliance, and total (lung + thorax) compliance can be derived as follows:

$$\underset{\text{resistance"}}{\text{Total "respiratory}} = \underset{\text{resistance}}{\text{Pulmonary}} + \underset{\text{"resistance"}}{\text{Thoracic}} \quad (45.3)$$

or

$$\frac{1}{\textit{Total compliance}} = \frac{1}{\textit{Lung compliance}} + \frac{1}{\textit{Thoracic compliance}} \quad (45.4)$$

The compliance rates of lung and thorax are each ~200 mL/cm H_2O. Their combined compliance is therefore 100 mL/cm H_2O (or 147 mL/mm Hg).

The compliance that is measured is called the static or the dynamic compliance, depending on how the test is performed. If the lung is inflated or deflated in very small steps, and the measurements are made only after allowing the lung volume to stabilize completely at each step, then the recorded graph gives the *static compliance*. The graph is curvilinear. On the other hand, if the measurements are made during rhythmic breathing, it gives the *dynamic compliance*. It is calculated from only two sets of pressure–volume measurements, one each at the end of inspiration and expiration. Dynamic compliance varies significantly with the breathing rate in patients with obstructive lung disease.

Static Lung Compliance

Static lung compliance can be calculated by asking the subject to breathe in a measured volume of air (ΔV) and recording the associated fall in intrapleural pressure (ΔP) while the breath is held in inspiration. Lung compliance is not uniform over a range of pressures. This becomes apparent when the lung is dis-

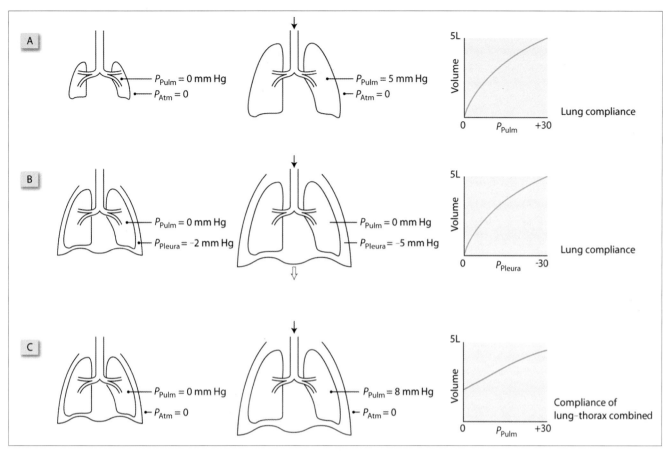

Fig. 45.5 Measurement of compliance. **(A)** The lungs are excised from the thorax and inflated by increasing the intrapulmonary pressure (P_{Pulm}). The distending pressure is given by the difference between P_{Pulm} and atmospheric pressure (P_{Atm}). Because the P_{Atm} is taken as zero, the distending pressure equals P_{Pulm}. **(B)** The lungs inflate in response to the negative intrapleural pressure (P_{Pleura}). The pressure producing airflow is given by the difference between P_{Pulm} and P_{Pleura}. Because P_{Pulm} = 0, this pressure equals P_{Pleura}. Note that the compliance curve remains identical regardless of whether the volume changes are plotted against P_{Pulm} or P_{Pleura}. **(C)** The lungs and thorax are distended together by increasing P_{Pulm}, and the distending pressure is given by P_{Pulm} minus P_{Atm}. Because P_{Atm} = 0, the distending pressure equals P_{Pulm}. On plotting the volume changes against P_{Pulm}, what is obtained is the compliance of the lung–thorax combined.

tended in small steps, and at each step, the pressure and volume of the lung is noted and plotted on a graph. The line obtained is not straight, but flattens out at higher pressures. The flattening of the compliance curve occurs due to the marked increase in pulmonary tissue resistance at high lung volumes.

The compliance at any point on the pressure–volume curve is given by the slope ($\Delta V/\Delta P$) at that point; the steeper the slope, the higher the compliance (**Fig. 45.6**). The pressure–volume curve can be extended below by forced expiration and noting the volume of expired air and the increase in intrapleural pressure.

Specific compliance | A lung compliance of 200 mL/cm H_2O means that when the intrapleural pressure changes by 1 cm H_2O, the volume of both the lungs taken together changes by 200 mL. For the same pressure change, each lung expands by 100 mL; therefore, the compliance of each lung would be 100 mL/cm H_2O. The compliance of a single lobe of lung would be even less. This difference in compliance does not represent any difference in the lung tissue stiffness, the assessment of

which is the primary objective of compliance measurements. Hence, the term *specific compliance* has been introduced.

$$\text{Specific compliance of the lungs} = \frac{\text{Compliance of the lungs}}{\text{Functional residual capacity (FRC)}} \quad (45.5)$$

The specific compliance of the lungs is 200 ÷ 2000 = 0.1 mL/cm H_2O. The specific compliance of the lungs in neonates is ~0.065 mL/cm H_2O, indicating that their lungs are stiffer.

Static Compliance of Lung–Thorax Combined
Clinically, the lung–thorax static compliance can be measured by asking the subject to breathe in measured volumes of air and then release it, keeping the nose closed, into a manometer that records the pressure. The subject is instructed not to exert force while breathing out. The pressure recorded in the manometer is the *intrapulmonary pressure*, and when it is recorded under relaxed conditions (without exerting extra pressure), it is called the *relaxation pressure*. Measuring the

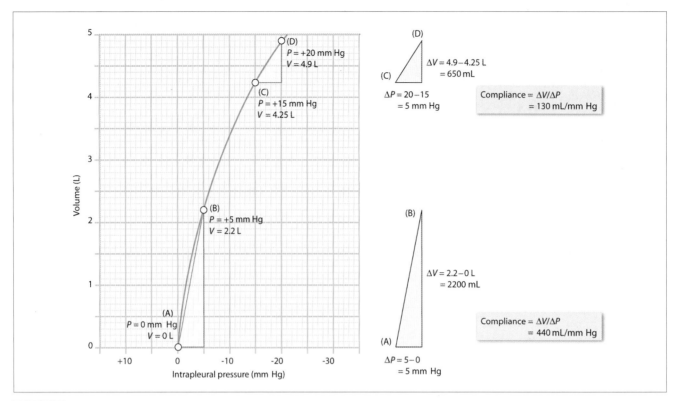

Fig. 45.6 Lung compliance is nonuniform over a range of pressures. Between points A to B, compliance is 440 mL/mm Hg; between points C and D, compliance is 130 mL/mm Hg. The average compliance between points A and D can be calculated to be 245 mL/mm Hg, or 180 mL/cm H_2O (245 ÷ 1.36 = 180).

relaxation pressure at a given volume is an indirect method of estimating the intrapulmonary pressure required to distend the lung–thorax combined to the same volume.

The compliance curve of the lung–thorax combined (**Figs. 45.5C** and **45.7A**) can be understood by noting that the distending pressure required to maintain the lung–thorax combined at any volume is the algebraic sum of the distending pressures required to maintain the lung and thorax separately at the same volume. Thus, to maintain the lung–thorax combined at 2 L, the pressure required is the sum of –4 mm Hg (the pressure required to contract the thorax to 2 L) and +4 mm Hg (the distending pressure required to expand the lung to 2 L). Because the sum is zero, it means that in the absence of any distending pressure, the lung–thorax combined has a volume of 2 L. This volume is known as the functional residual capacity (FRC). In the same way, the pressures required to maintain the volume of lung–thorax combined at 1.5 L and 5 L are shown both graphically and diagrammatically in **Fig. 45.7B**.

Figure 45.7A shows that in the absence of any distending pressure (when intrapulmonary pressure = 0 mm Hg), the resting volume of the lung–thorax combined is 2 L (point C_0 in the graph, which is equal to the functional residual capacity). The resting volume of the thorax, if unattached to the lungs, is ~4 L (point T_0 in the graph). The resting volume of the lung is zero: the lungs, unless kept distended, would collapse completely (point L_0 in the graph). This means that the lungs are continuously trying to collapse completely, while the thorax is continuously trying to spring back to its actual size of 4 L. When

the volume of lung–thorax combined is 2 L, the recoil pressure of the lung that is trying to collapse it (4 mm Hg) is precisely counterbalanced by the recoil pressure of the thorax that is trying to distend it (also 4 mm Hg). If the lung elasticity decreases, as in emphysema, the thoracic cage increases in size, resulting in the characteristic barrel-shaped chest.

The compliance curve can be extended below by removing air from the lungs and the thorax. When the negative pressure is sufficiently high, the lung or the thorax reaches its minimum volume, below which it cannot be collapsed. The thoracic volume can be reduced to its minimum of 1 L by applying a pressure of –20 mm Hg, below which the thorax caves in. The lung, as already mentioned collapses completely if there is no distending pressure. At high pressures, the curves terminate abruptly because the lung or the thorax ruptures, and no further measurements are possible.

Dynamic Lung Compliance
During quiet breathing, the intrapleural pressure decreases from –2 to –6 mm Hg (becomes more negative). The 4 mm Hg fall in intrapleural pressure should be associated with an increase of 588 mL in lung volume because the static lung compliance is ~147 mL/mm Hg (147 × 4 = 588). The actual increase in lung volume is only 500 mL. The lung compliance would therefore be 125 mL/mm Hg (500 ÷ 4 = 125), only 85% of the static compliance. This reduced lung compliance observed during actual breathing is called dynamic lung compliance. The decrease in compliance is attributable to the limitation of time

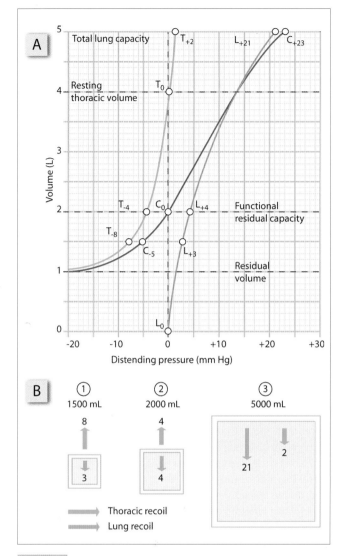

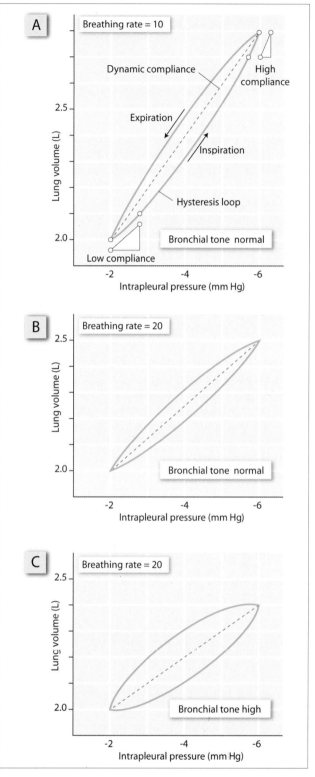

Fig. 45.7 **(A)** Static compliances of the thoracic cage, the lungs, and the lung–thorax combined. **(B)** The recoil pressures (in mm Hg) of the thorax and the lungs at different volumes when the two are attached together by the pleura. (Adapted from Rahn H. Otis AB, Chadwick LE, Fenn WO. The pressure-volume diagram of the thorax and lung. Am J Physiol, 1946, 146:170.)

available for inspiration: at a respiratory rate of 15 per minute, each breath lasts for 4 seconds or less. Thus, inspiration lasts for only 2 seconds or less, which permits only 500 mL of air to enter the lungs. If the respiratory rate is higher, even less time is available to the lungs for expansion. Moreover, because the air tries to rush in and out in a shorter time, the airway resistance increases, adding further to the reduction in dynamic lung compliance.

The effect of emphysema on compliance is unique in that it results in an increase in static compliance, but a decrease in dynamic compliance. Static compliance increases due to destruction of elastic tissues in the alveolar wall. The reduction in elastic tissue makes it easier for the lung to expand in response to a distending pressure. However, the loss of elastic tissue in the walls of the smaller airways makes them vulnerable

Fig. 45.8 Dynamic compliance and hysteresis. **(A)** A slow breathing rate of 10 breaths per minute allows adequate time for the lung to inflate and deflate completely. The dashed line connecting the end-inspiratory and end-expiratory points represents the dynamic compliance. **(B)** When the breathing rate increases to 20 breaths per minute, less time is available for lung inflation and deflation, which remain somewhat incomplete; therefore, the dynamic compliance decreases. **(C)** Bronchoconstriction slows down inspiration and expiration; therefore, the dynamic compliance falls further. Also, the hysteresis loop enlarges due to higher airway resistance.

to dynamic airway compression (see below). This increases the airway resistance with consequent decrease in dynamic compliance.

Hysteresis of Lung Compliance

Measurement of compliance requires that the change of volume be recorded for a unit change in pressure. The experimenter has the freedom to make the measurements by either increasing or decreasing the pressure. Experimenters, however, soon realized that in the case of the lungs, the compliance measured depended on whether measurements were made during inflation or deflation. Thus, instead of getting a single compliance curve, experimenters obtained two curves, one for inspiration and the other for expiration (**Fig. 45.8**). Together, the curves formed a loop called the hysteresis loop. This phenomenon is called hysteresis (from the Greek *hysterein* = to fall short, to lag behind) because the volume change lags behind the pressure change. Hysteresis occurs due to the presence of viscous resistance to changes in lung volume. Viscosity is the frictional resistance of fluids (liquids or gases). Frictional resistance occurs only during motion: the faster the motion, the greater is the friction. There are two main sources of viscous resistance: the movement of air in and out of the lungs, and the presence of surfactant.

Hysteresis of dynamic compliance | When airflow rate through respiratory passages increases, the airway resistance increases markedly, and with it, the hysteresis increases. Inspiratory and expiratory forces are highest at the beginning of the respective phases (**Fig. 45.9**). Hence, airflow rate and airway resistance are highest at the beginning of inspiration and expiration. Because resistance reduces compliance, the compliance curve is flatter (low compliance) in early inspiration and steeper (high compliance) near its termination. Similarly, the curve is flatter (low compliance) in early expiration and steeper (high compliance) in late expiration. The hysteresis loop occurs due to these variations in compliance with the phase of breathing. In obstructive lung disorders, the dynamic compression of the airways further accentuates the hysteresis loop.

Hysteresis of static compliance | During measurement of static lung compliance, the lung is inflated in very small steps, and the measurements are made only after the airflow has stopped. Therefore, airway resistance has no effect on static compliance. Yet there remains a slight amount of hysteresis in the static lung compliance, which is attributable to the presence of surfactant in the lung. Finally, even when the surfactant is washed out with saline solution, some hysteresis still remains. This residual hysteresis is due to the viscous resistance of the lung parenchyma itself, attributable to the intracellular fluid and the fluidity of membranes. The single static compliance curve shown in **Fig. 45.7** is the compliance recorded during expiration, which experimenters find to be more consistent than the inspiration curve.

Dynamic Airway Compression

Rapid, forceful expiration results in compression, and often closure, of the small airways, especially of the respiratory bronchioles. The closure results in trapping of air in the alveolus (air trapping) during expiration. In emphysema, the elastic tissues in the walls of the small airways are destroyed. These airways collapse due to dynamic compression in early expiration, resulting in considerable air trapping. The consequent increase in the FRC and reduction in vital capacity are often observed in obstructive airway diseases (see Table 52.1).

Equal Pressure Point Theory

Why do the respiratory bronchioles tend to collapse before the alveoli have emptied completely? An explanation to this is offered by the *equal pressure point theory* (**Fig. 45.10**). Suppose the intrapleural pressure at the end of a deep inspiration is –15 mm Hg. Although the intraalveolar pressure is negative initially, it soon becomes equal to atmospheric pressure as air rushes into the alveoli. Hence, if the breath is held in inspiration, the airway pressure becomes uniformly atmospheric (**Fig. 45.10A**).

At the end of quiet expiration, the intrapleural pressure increases by 10 mm Hg to become –5 mm Hg. The intraalveolar pressure too rises by 10 mm Hg, only to be restored to atmospheric pressure as the alveolar air rushes out. The flowing alveolar air sets up a pressure gradient along its path, with the elevated alveolar pressure (10 mm Hg) at one end and the atmospheric pressure (0 mm Hg) at the other (**Fig. 45.10B**).

At the end of a forced expiration, the intrapleural pressure becomes positive, increasing by 35 mm Hg (from –15 mm Hg) to become +20 mm Hg. Intra-alveolar pressure also increases to 35 mm Hg, and air rushes out of the alveoli, setting up a pressure gradient as before (**Fig. 45.10C**). Although the intraalveolar pressure is higher than the intrapleural pressure, somewhere near its exit, the intra-airway pressure drops below the intrapleural pressure. The airway collapses distal to this site, which is called the equal pressure point (**Fig. 45.10D**). Airway collapse does not occur so long as the intrapleural pressure remains negative, as during quiet expiration.

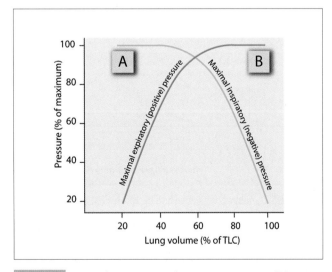

Fig. 45.9 Maximal inspiratory and expiratory pressures. **(A)** Inspiratory pressure is maximum at low lung volume and declines at higher volumes. **(B)** The reverse is true for expiratory pressure. TLC, total lung capacity.

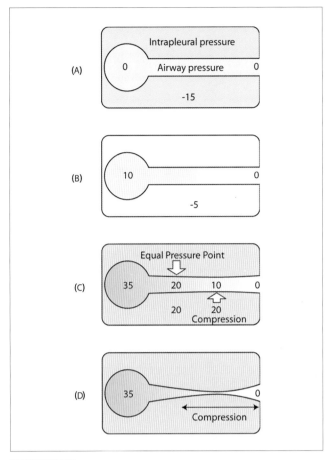

Fig. 45.10 Mechanism of airway closure. **(A)** At end-inspiration, intrapleural pressure is negative, while airway pressure is atmospheric. **(B)** After quiet expiration, intrapleural pressure is still negative, and airway pressure is mostly above atmospheric. **(C)** After forced expiration, intrapleural pressure becomes positive and exceeds the pressure in the distal segment of the airway. **(D)** The positive intrapleural pressure compresses the distal airway. (Negative pressures are shown in blue, and positive pressures are shown in red.)

General Model: Balance of Forces

This phenomenon is an example of the balance of forces determining the state of a system (whether the airway is open or closed during expiration). Changes in any property of the system will, of course, alter the point at which collapse occurs.

Intrapleural Pressure

At the end of a normal expiration, there is no distending pressure inside the lungs. The volume of the lung–thorax combined is therefore 2 L, and it is said to be in its resting state. However, as explained above, at zero distending pressure, the lungs are trying to collapse, and the thorax is trying to expand. These opposite pulls result in a negative (i.e., subatmospheric) pleural pressure of about –2.5 mm Hg. If the elastic recoil of the lung is reduced, as in older people or in patients with chronic lung disease, the intrapleural pressure may not be negative.

Intrapleural versus intrathoracic pressure | When the thorax and the lungs try to move in opposite directions, the

entire space separating the two (see **Fig. 45.11**) is subjected to a negative pressure. Not only the pleural space, but also everything else that lies in that space (the heart and the mediastinum), is subjected to the negative pressure, which is called the *intrathoracic pressure*. The intrathoracic pressure is equal to the intrapleural pressure, and the two terms are used synonymously. The heart has a thick muscular wall; therefore, the pressure in the heart chambers is relatively unaffected by the negative intrathoracic pressure. However, the pressure in great veins decreases as they enter the thorax. Even the pressure inside the thoracic aorta is affected by large intrathoracic pressure changes during the Valsalva maneuver (see below). The intraluminal pressure of the esophagus, which has a soft wall, faithfully reflects the intrathoracic pressure and offers a convenient method for the measurement of the intrathoracic pressure.

Intrapleural pressure can thus be measured with an intraesophageal balloon. However, because the esophagus opens to the exterior through the mouth, the pressure in its lumen equilibrates quickly with atmospheric pressure. Hence, for measuring intraesophageal pressure, it is important to keep the mouth closed, sealing off the esophageal cavity from the exterior. The intrapleural pressure can also be recorded by inserting a needle directly into the intrapleural space. A small air bubble is injected into the pleural space, and the tip of the needle is kept in the bubble. This ensures that the tip of the needle does not get blocked by the pleural membranes.

Intrapulmonary Pressure
It has been discussed that the intrapulmonary pressure recorded during a relaxed expiration is called the relaxation pressure. The relaxation pressures at different lung volumes give the compliance of the lung-thorax combined.

Forced Intrapulmonary Pressures
The intrapulmonary pressure can be maximized by exerting extra inspiratory or expiratory efforts against an obstruction. A strong expiratory effort against a closed glottis is called the *Valsalva maneuver*. It can raise the intrathoracic and intrapulmonary pressures to +100 mm Hg. A strong inspiratory effort against a closed glottis is called the *Müller maneuver*. It can reduce these pressures to –80 mm Hg. The maximal pressures that can be achieved by forceful inspiration and expiration indicate the strength of the inspiratory and expiratory muscles, respectively, and are called the *maximal (forced) inspiratory and expiratory pressures*. Thus, relaxation pressures indicate lung–thorax compliance, whereas forced pressures indicate the strength of respiratory muscles.

Maximal expiratory pressures can be developed only when the thoracic volume is large. Conversely, maximal inspiratory pressures can be developed only when the thoracic volume is minimal. One reason is that an inflated chest exerts a high relaxation pressure. More important, the muscles of expiration are at their "resting length" (see Muscle length–tension relationship subsection, Chapter 15) when the thorax is inflated. Conversely, the inspiratory muscles are at their resting length when the thoracic volume is low (**Fig. 45.11**). When

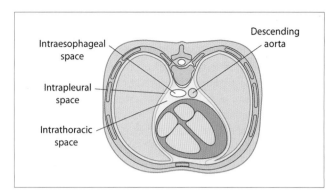

Fig. 45.11 Intrathoracic, intrapleural, and intraesophageal spaces. Because these spaces are separated by thin walls, the pressures in them are nearly equal.

respiratory muscles are severely stretched, they contract with less strength. They can also become fatigued and fail (pump failure), leading to inadequate ventilation.

Breathing Cycle

Pressure–Volume Changes during Breathing

Intrapleural pressure | At the end of quiet expiration, the intrapleural pressure is –2.5 mm Hg (**Fig. 45.12**). When the thorax expands, the intrapleural pressure tends to decrease. The lungs comply: they respond to the fall in intrapleural pressure by expanding. Had the lungs not expanded, there would have been a drastic fall in intrapleural pressure. The intrapleural pressure therefore depends on lung compliance and is affected by the hysteresis of the compliance curve. During forceful breathing, lung compliance decreases due to a sharp rise in viscous resistance; therefore, the pleural pressure changes are accentuated. It can fall as low as –30 mm Hg during mid-inspiration. During normal breathing in a healthy subject, the fall in intrapleural pressure at the end of a maximal inspiration is only 4 mm Hg (from –2 to –6 mm Hg).

It is observed in **Fig. 45.12** that the intrapleural pressure falls to its peak negativity a little before end-inspiration. The reason for this can be easily demonstrated in a lung–thorax–diaphragm analog model (**Fig. 45.13**); it takes some time for the air to move into the lungs expanding them. Conversely, the intrapleural pressure becomes positive a little before end-expiration.

Intrapulmonary pressure | The intrapulmonary pressure drops to about –3 mm Hg during mid-inspiration but returns to 0 mm Hg by end-inspiration due to rapid flow of air into the lungs. During quiet expiration, the elastic recoil of the lung raises the intrapulmonary pressure to about +3 mm Hg by mid-expiration. As air flows out of the lungs, the intrapulmonary pressure returns to atmospheric levels by the end of quiet expiration. The changes in intrapulmonary pressure are much greater when airway resistance is high.

Work of Breathing

Work is performed by the respiratory muscles in overcoming the elastic and viscous resistances offered by the chest wall,

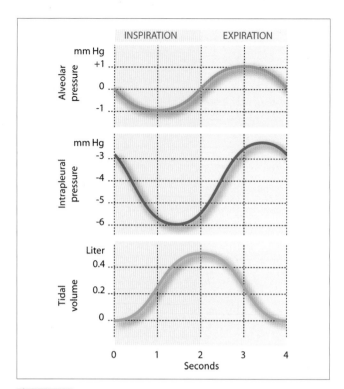

Fig. 45.12 Cyclic changes in alveolar pressure, intrapleural pressure, and tidal volume during normal breathing.

lungs, and airways. During heavy breathing, the work of breathing can increase considerably. The work of breathing done in overcoming the viscous resistance can be estimated graphically by measuring the area enclosed by the hysteresis loop (**Fig. 45.14**). The elastic work of breathing, the viscous work during inspiration, and the viscous work of expiration can be separately estimated, as shown in **Fig. 45.14**.

One way to think about the work of breathing is to consider the rate at which oxygen is used by the respiratory muscles. With quiet breathing at rest, the oxygen used to produce ventilation is less than 2% of the total oxygen being consumed by the body. Because the work of breathing is determined by

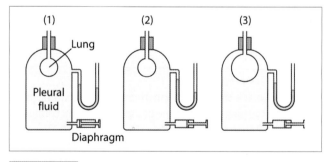

Fig. 45.13 A lung–thorax–diaphragm analog model (after TF Sherman) explaining the changes in pleural pressure during inspiration (1). If the plunger is pulled suddenly (diaphragm contracts), the intrapleural pressure falls sharply before the lung is able to expand (2). As air moves into the lungs, the lung expands, and the pleural pressure rises slightly (3). (Adapted from Sherman TF. A simple analog of lung mechanics. Am J Physiol. 1993;265:S33.)

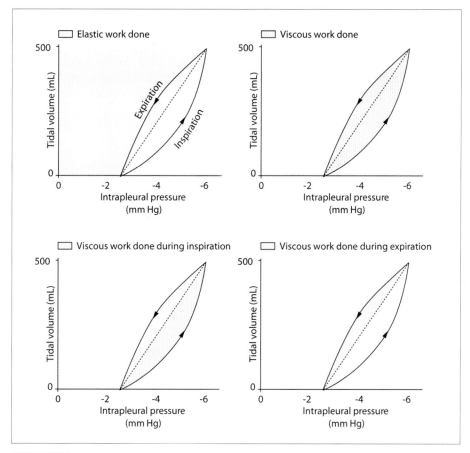

Fig. 45.14 Graphic measurement of work of breathing. The areas ($\Delta P \times \Delta V$) represent the work done.

both breathing frequency and tidal volume, changes in these variables will change the respiratory muscle oxygen consumption. For example, during voluntary hyperventilation, oxygen consumption increases to 30% of the total oxygen consumption. Oxygen consumption by the respiratory muscle thus increases substantially during exercise. The work of breathing, the percentage of the total oxygen consumption being used by the respiratory muscles, is greatly increased in diseases such as emphysema, asthma, and congestive heart failure with dyspnea and orthopnea.

> **General Model: Energy**
>
> Because the work of breathing arises from the activity of the respiratory muscles transforming biochemical energy into mechanical energy, it is essential that these specialized cells receive oxygen and glucose from the blood perfusing them.

Dyspnea, or breathlessness, is the unpleasant awareness of breathing effort and usually occurs whenever the work of breathing increases. The theory of length–tension inappropriateness holds that there is a constant subconscious comparison between ventilation required and ventilation achieved, and between muscle tension exerted and change in muscle length achieved. Dyspnea occurs when this inappropriateness reaches a certain threshold. Dyspnea may be evoked by stimu-

lation of receptors in the upper airways, lungs (see J receptors), respiratory muscles, or chest wall. In a supine position, the abdominal contents tend to press on the diaphragm and cause dyspnea. This is one mechanism leading to dyspnea, which occurs upon assuming a supine position. Dsypnea on lying down, whatever the cause, is called orthopnea. In this case, sitting up takes this load off the diaphragm. A severely dyspneic patient therefore tends to sit up and bend forward.

Pulmonary Surfactant

Surfactant is a soaplike substance secreted by the type II pneumocytes of the alveolar epithelium. It is a mixture of dipalmitoyl phosphatidylcholine (a phospholipid), other lipids, and proteins. The surfactant molecules form a thin layer on the internal surface of the alveoli (**Fig. 45.15**), with the hydrophilic heads layering the alveolar membrane and the hydrophobic fatty acid tails facing the alveolar lumen.

Functions of Surfactant
Surfactant reduces the alveolar surface tension. This has three important physiologic consequences. (1) It reduces the tendency of the lungs to collapse. (2) It reduces the natural tendency of the smaller alveoli to collapse and empty into the larger ones (**Fig. 45.16**). (3) It reduces the tendency of the alveolar interstitial fluid to enter the alveolar space. Each of these is explained below.

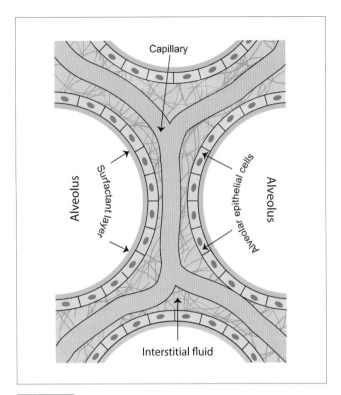

Fig. 45.15 Alveoli, internally lined by surfactant and externally separated by interstitial fluid. If alveoli shrink in size, the interstitial fluid pressure becomes more negative.

The collapsing tendency of an alveolus (P) is given by the Laplace law, $P = 2T/R$, where R is the radius of the alveolus, and T is the alveolar surface tension. By reducing T, surfactant reduces the collapsing tendency of the alveoli. A reduced collapsing tendency also means that a given distending pressure would cause greater lung expansion. In other words, surfactant increases lung compliance.

The surfactant molecules are farther apart in large alveoli and closely spaced in smaller alveoli (**Fig. 45.16**). Because the surface tension of the surfactant fluid is inversely proportional to the concentration of surfactant (phospholipid) molecules per unit area, the surfactant is more effective in reducing the collapsing tendency of the smaller alveoli than of the larger alveoli. This compensates for the naturally greater tendency of the smaller alveoli to collapse and is called *alveolar stabilization*. Another cause of alveolar stabilization (unrelated to surfactant) is *interdependence*—several alveoli share a common wall so that when one tends to collapse, it is prevented from doing so by the adjacent alveoli.

When adjacent alveoli try to collapse simultaneously, the hydrostatic pressure of the interstitial fluid between them decreases. Reduction in interstitial fluid hydrostatic pressure pulls out fluid from the alveolar capillaries in accordance with the dynamics of capillary fluid exchange. Presence of surfactant reduces alveolar collapsing tendency. Hence, less fluid is sucked out of the alveolar capillaries, and the alveoli are kept dry.

Deficiency of surfactant occurs in cigarette smokers and in patients on long-term 100% O_2 inhalation. It is seen in pre-

mature infants not secreting adequate amounts of pulmonary surfactant (*infant respiratory distress syndrome* or the *hyaline membrane disease*). Deficiency of surfactant leads to collapse (atelectasis) of parts of the lung. It is possible that other cases of atelectasis, such as those occurring following bronchial or pulmonary artery obstruction, are also due to surfactant deficiency.

Assisted Ventilation

Assisted ventilation can be life-saving when breathing stops, as in acute asphyxia due to drowning, carbon monoxide poisoning, electrocution, or anesthetic accidents. It should always be attempted because respiration stops before the heart stops. Of the several methods of artificial ventilation, mouth-to-mouth breathing is the simplest and can be delivered at short notice. When there is more time at hand, or when long-term ventilatory support is required, mechanical ventilators are preferred (**Fig. 45.17**). However, patients on long-term ventilatory support have disuse atrophy of the respiratory muscles, and it takes time for their respiratory muscles to regain their strength once assisted ventilation is withdrawn.

Negative-pressure breathing | The first event in a normal inspiration is thoracic expansion that makes the intrathoracic pressure negative. This is followed by lung inflation and suction of air into the lungs. Ventilators that simulate this mechanism are called negative-pressure ventilators. The patient's

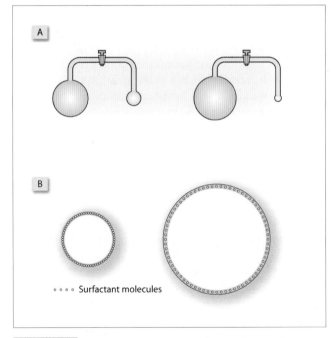

Fig. 45.16 **(A)** When two inflated balloons of unequal sizes are interconnected, the smaller balloon will collapse and empty completely into the larger one so that at the end, there will be a single large balloon left. It occurs in accordance with the Laplace law, which states that the smaller the radius, the greater is the collapsing tendency. **(B)** Alveolar stabilization. (*Left*) Surfactant molecules lightly packed in a small alveolus. (*Right*) The same number of surfactant molecules are spaced apart in a large alveolus, and the surfactant concentration falls.

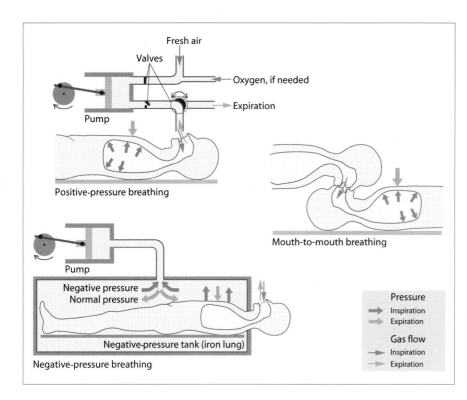

Fig. 45.17 Three different mechanisms of producing artificial breathing: pumps (on the left) can be used to produce either positive- or negative-pressure breathing; mouth-to-mouth breathing is a form of positive-pressure breathing.

body is placed inside a chamber (the "iron lung") that can produce a subatmospheric pressure. The head remains outside the chamber; therefore, when a subatmospheric pressure is produced around the chest wall, a pressure gradient between ambient atmosphere and the alveoli is produced. Negative-pressure ventilators are rarely used today.

Positive-pressure breathing In positive-pressure breathing, the physiologic mechanics of breathing are reversed. Air is forced into the patient's lung through the mouth. The lung expands first, followed by thoracic expansion. The intrathoracic pressure never becomes negative; rather, it becomes positive. The positive intrathoracic pressure impedes venous return and tends to reduce the cardiac output. For providing long-term positive-pressure ventilation, an artificial airway (endotracheal tube or tracheostomy tube) is provided. It is used for acutely ill patients and is of value especially when the lungs are diseased because it opens up previously unventilated alveoli.

Mouth-to-mouth breathing takes advantage of the fact that the expired air of a normal subject has enough oxygen left in it for reviving a critical patient. It is a form of positive-pressure breathing in which the rescuer seals his mouth to the victim's mouth and forcefully expires into the victim's airways about twice the normal tidal volume of air at the rate of 12 per minute. In doing so, attention must be paid to the maintenance of patency of the airways (see **Fig. 44.1**) and occlusion of the nostrils of the victim.

Summary

- Inspiration requires the expansion of the thorax and lungs resulting from the contraction of the primary inspiratory muscles.

- Expiration (at rest) occurs when the passive recoil of the lungs reduces the volume of the thorax.

- To produce inspiration, work must be done to overcome the "resistance" of the respiratory system.

- The compliance of the respiratory system (the ΔV that results from a ΔP) is the sum of the compliance of the lungs and the thorax.

- The pressure in the pleural space is negative (subatmospheric) because of the inward elastic recoil of the lungs and the outward elastic recoil of the thorax.

- Pressure in the alveoli decreases during inspiration and increases during expiration (which constitutes one respiratory cycle).

- The amount of work done during one respiratory cycle depends on the tidal volume and the breathing frequency.

- Pulmonary surfactant reduces the surface tension in the air–fluid interface in the alveoli and thereby reduces the work of breathing and the tendency for alveoli to collapse.

Applying What You Know

45.1. Ms. Eng is coughing when she comes to the emergency room. Which of the respiratory muscles contract to produce the explosive expiration that is seen when someone coughs?

45.2. When Ms. Eng comes into the emergency room, she is suffering from bronchoconstriction, which causes an increase in airway resistance. What effect would you expect this condition to have on her functional residual capacity (FRC)? Explain your prediction.

45.3. What is shortness of breath, and what are possible mechanisms that could cause it? Which mechanism is most likely causing this in Ms. Eng?

Measurements of pulmonary ventilation are broadly of two types. One set of measurements tells us about the size of the lungs and the extent to which they can inflate or deflate. These may be called the static lung functions. Another set of measurements tells us the rate at which the lungs are ventilated in health and disease. These measurements have to be timed and are called dynamic lung functions.

A simple device called the *spirometer* makes possible quite a few ventilatory measurements, static as well as dynamic. Spirometry has both diagnostic and therapeutic uses. It affords a simple and reliable method for diagnosis of restrictive and obstructive lung disorders (see Chapter 52). It is also used for providing patients with feedback on the state of their respiratory problem, thereby motivating them to continue with their prescribed management activities. This is known as *incentive spirometry.*

In its simplest form, the spirometer is an inverted light metal cylinder floating on water, trapping some air under it. As the subject breathes the trapped air in and out, the cylinder sinks and rises. (Breathing should be through the mouth, with the nose kept pinched with a clip.) The movements of the cylinder are recorded on a moving drum through a pulley system with a writing lever (**Fig. 46.1A**). The system involves rebreathing the same air over and over again; therefore, it cannot be used for long periods. To permit rebreathing, the breathing tube is passed through a soda lime tower to remove carbon dioxide. Spirometers used in clinical practice today employ airflow transducers and a computer to produce spirograms.

Static Lung Volumes

Spirometric Measurements

The terms *lung volumes* and *lung capacities* (**Fig. 46.1B, C**) have different connotations. Capacities are composite volumes representing the sum of two or more lung volumes.

Tidal volume (V_T) is the volume of air that moves into the lungs with a relaxed inspiration after a passive expiration. In other words, it is the volume of air that moves in or out of the lung with each normal breath. It has a value of ~500 mL. *Inspiratory reserve volume* (IRV) is the volume of air in excess of the

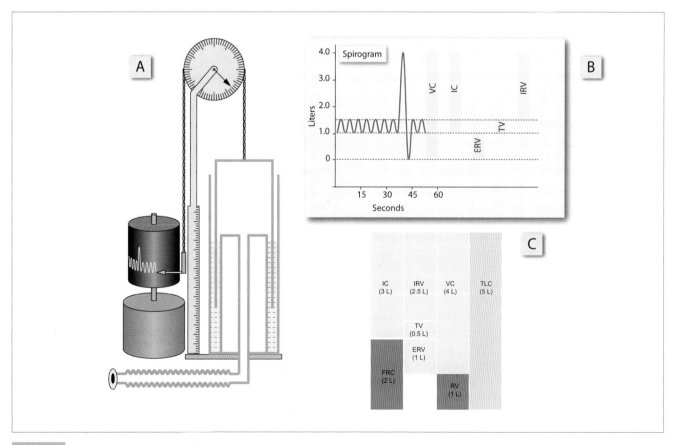

Fig. 46.1 **(A)** A simple spirometer. **(B)** A normal spirogram. The normal lung volumes and capacities are given in brackets in milliliters. **(C)** The relationship between lung volumes and lung capacities. ERV, expiratory reserve volume; FRC, functional residual capacity; IC, inspiratory capacity; IRV, inspiratory reserve volume; RV, residual volume; TLC, total lung capacity; TV, tidal volume; VC, vital capacity.

tidal volume that can be inspired with a maximal inspiratory effort. It is ~2500 mL. *Expiratory reserve volume* (ERV) is the volume of air that can be expelled with a maximal expiratory effort, commencing after a passive expiration. It is ~1000 mL. *Inspiratory capacity* (IC) is the maximum volume of air that can be inspired after a passive expiration. It is ~3000 mL. *Expiratory capacity* (EC) is the maximum volume of air that can be expired after a relaxed inspiration. It is ~1500 mL. *Vital capacity* (VC) is the maximum volume of air that can be inspired after a maximal expiration. It is ~4000 mL. These static lung volumes are interrelated as follows:

$$IC = V_T + IRV \tag{46.1}$$

$$EC = V_T + ERV \tag{46.2}$$

$$VC = V_T + IRV + ERV \tag{46.3}$$

Expiratory versus inspiratory vital capacity | There are two accepted methods of determining vital capacity. In one, the subject takes a maximally deep breath and expires slowly and completely. The volume of expired air is called the *expiratory vital capacity*. In the other method, the subject does the reverse, expires completely and then takes a maximally deep inspiration. The volume of inspired air represents the *inspiratory vital capacity*. In normal individuals, both methods give the same result. However, in the presence of any airway obstruction, expiration is more difficult than inspiration, and the expiratory vital capacity becomes less than the inspiratory vital capacity.

Slow versus forced vital capacity | *Forced vital capacity* (FVC) is the vital capacity recorded when expiration is made forcefully and quickly. When the subject expires slowly but completely, the vital capacity recorded is called *relaxed* or *slow vital capacity* (SVC), or simply, the vital capacity. In obstructive airway disorders, FVC is less than SVC due to dynamic compression of airways and associated air trapping.

Nonspirometric Measurements

Even after maximal expiration, a certain volume of air, called the residual volume, always remains in the lungs and cannot be expelled. This volume cannot be estimated through spirometry, and it requires special techniques to estimate it. The same is true for lung capacities that have residual volume as one of its components, such as the functional residual capacity and the total lung capacity. *Residual volume* (RV) is the volume of air (~1000 mL) that remains in the lungs after maximal expiration. *Functional residual capacity* (FRC) is the volume of air (~2000 mL) that remains in the lungs after passive expiration. *Total lung capacity* (TLC) is the volume of air (5000 mL) present in the lungs at the end of a maximal inspiration.

$$FRC = ERV + RV \tag{46.4}$$

$$TLC = IRV + V_T + ERV + RV \tag{46.5}$$

The presence of residual air in the lungs has an important consequence: the alveolar partial pressure of oxygen (PO_2) and carbon dioxide (PCO_2) does not fluctuate excessively. Without the residual air, alveolar PO_2 would have increased to atmospheric levels (150 mm Hg) during inspiration and reduced to nearly zero during expiration. However, the PO_2 of the alveolar air actually remains fairly stable at ~100 mm Hg. In the same way, the alveolar PCO_2 would have dropped to atmospheric levels (0.3 mm Hg) during inspiration. This would have reduced the respiratory drive that is provided mainly by CO_2. The residual air also helps to dilute the effect of any toxic gases that might be inhaled in small amounts.

The residual air also prevents the lungs from collapsing at the end of each expiration. Reexpansion of the lung from a totally collapsed state would have required tremendous breathing effort in accordance with the law of Laplace. Moreover, the collapsed lung would have increased the pulmonary vascular resistance and imposed a heavy afterload on the right ventricle.

The commonly employed methods for FRC estimation are the gas-dilution methods (helium dilution and nitrogen-washout techniques) and plethysmography. Plethysmography has a distinct advantage over the gas-dilution methods, which fail to record the volume of any gas that may be trapped in an isolated compartment inside the lung and therefore give a false-low value of the FRC. The value obtained through plethysmography is unaffected by such trapped gases. In fact, a large, nonventilating bleb can be detected by noting the discrepancy between the values obtained by gas dilution and plethysmography.

Helium-dilution (closed circuit) technique | Using this method, beginning after a normal expiration, the subject is given a known volume of gas mixture containing 80% oxygen and 20% helium to rebreathe. As rebreathing progresses, the gas mixture gets diluted by the air inside the lungs, and the helium concentration falls. The helium concentration stabilizes in ~5 minutes. The fall in helium concentration indicates the extent of dilution, which increases with the FRC.

Example

A subject rebreathes into a 2 L reservoir containing 20% helium and 80% oxygen (**Fig. 46.2A**). The total amount of helium in the reservoir is 2 L × 20/100 = 400 mL. After equilibrium, the helium concentration in the reservoir drops to 10% (**Fig. 46.2B**). Knowing that the total amount of helium was 400 mL, it must have been distributed in 400 mL ÷ 10/100 = 4000 mL of gaseous space (the volume of distribution). Because the volume of the reservoir is 2 L, the remaining 2 L of space must be the FRC.

Nitrogen-washout (open circuit) technique | In this method, the subject breathes in 100% oxygen from a cylinder and breathes it out into a large bag. The process is repeated several times. Initially, the expired air contains a high concentration of nitrogen (80%). As the breathing continues, the concentration of nitrogen in the expired air decreases. The breathing is continued until the nitrogen concentration in the expired air is negligible. At this stage, it can be said that

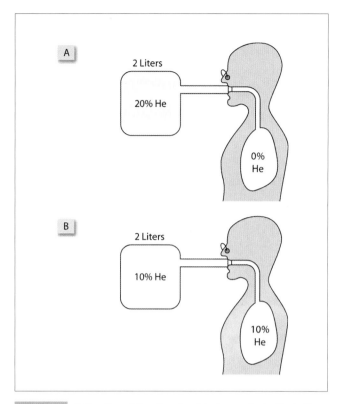

Fig. 46.2 Estimation of functional residual capacity by the helium-dilution method. **(A)** Before taking a breath, the helium (He) is all in the bag. **(B)** When the subject breathes, the He quickly distributes itself uniformly throughout the system (bag + lungs).

the nitrogen that was present in the lungs has been completely washed out.

The product of the total volume of air collected (V) and the concentration of nitrogen (C) in it gives the total amount of nitrogen (Q) washed out of the lungs.

$$Q = C \times V \quad (46.6)$$

Knowing that the concentration of nitrogen in the alveolar air was 80%, the FRC can be calculated using a similar formula:

$$Q = 80\% \times FRC \quad (46.7)$$

Example
A subject breathes in 40 L of oxygen, and the expired gas mixture has a nitrogen concentration of 5%. The total volume of nitrogen in the 40 L of expired gas mixture (V) would be 40 L × 5% = 2 L. Because the entire 2 L of nitrogen must have been present in the lungs at a concentration of 80%, the resting volume of the lungs (FRC) must have been 2 ÷ 80/100 = 2.5 L.

Plethysmography | In this method, the subject sits in an airtight chamber made of transparent plastic (the whole-body plethysmograph) and tries to breathe against a tube connected to a pressure gauge. As the subject makes the breathing movements, the changes in alveolar pressure (ΔP) are recorded by the pressure gauge connected to the mouthpiece, and the lung volume changes (ΔV) are recorded by the volume gauge connected to the chamber (**Fig. 46.3A**).

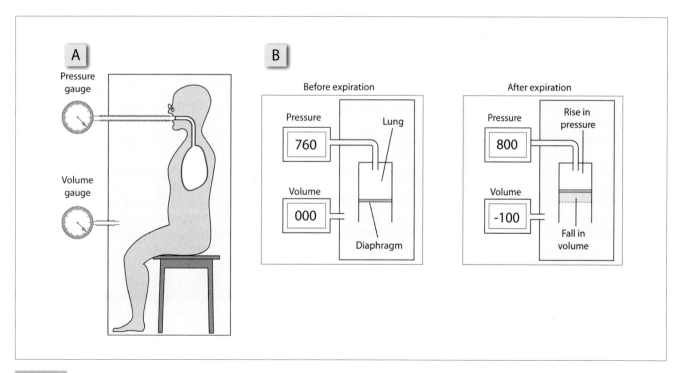

Fig. 46.3 Whole-body plethysmography. **(A)** A subject sitting inside a whole-body plethysmograph. **(B)** The initial and final measurements after the subject breathes against the pressure gauge.

Let V be the FRC (which is to be measured). Using Boyle's law, we have

$$PV = (P + \Delta P) \times (V - \Delta V) \qquad (46.8)$$

or

$$PV = -\Delta P \Delta V - P\Delta V + V\Delta P + PV \qquad (46.9)$$

or

$$V\Delta P = P\Delta V + \Delta P \Delta V \qquad (46.10)$$

Dividing throughout by ΔP, we have

$$V = P\Delta V/\Delta P + \Delta V \qquad (46.11)$$

Example

While blowing into the pressure gauge, a subject records a rise in pressure from 760 to 800 mm Hg, a rise of 40 mm Hg. Simultaneously, the plethysmograph records a decrease in volume by 100 mL (**Fig. 46.3B**). The FRC of the subject can be calculated as:

$$760 \times (1004 \div 40) + 100 = 2000 \text{ mL}$$

Factors Affecting Static Lung Volumes

FRC denotes the resting volume of the lung. It is the volume at which the inward recoil force of the lung balances the outward recoil force of the thorax. The end-expiratory diaphragmatic tone also affects the FRC. If the diaphragm does not relax fully at the end of expiration, the FRC will remain somewhat high. Hence, during anesthesia, the FRC decreases by ~400 mL due to the complete relaxation of the diaphragm.

Change in posture also affects FRC (**Fig. 46.4**). In the supine position, FRC decreases by ~25% due to the pressure of the abdominal contents on the diaphragm and the restriction of thoracic cage movements by the bed or floor below. Had it not been for the end-expiratory diaphragmatic tone, the reduction in FRC in the supine position would have been greater. In the supine position, the VC decreases mainly due to the congestion of the pulmonary vessels with blood, which displaces an equal volume of air from the lung. However, the inspiratory capacity increases because, while the FRC decreases by nearly 25% in the supine position, the VC decreases by only 5%. The RV is not reduced.

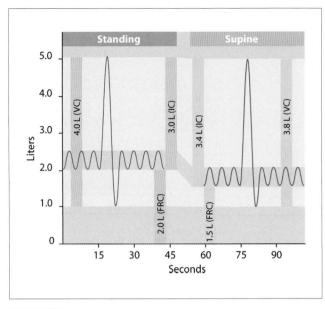

Fig. 46.4 Effect of posture on vital capacity (VC), functional residual capacity (FRC), and inspiratory capacity (IC).

FRC increases with body height and shows a slight increase with age. Obesity is associated with a reduction in FRC and ERV and a compensatory increase in IC. The RV is not reduced. The reduction in FRC is due to reduced thoracic compliance caused by the weight added to the chest wall. The TLC and VC do not change much. Thus, on the whole, the changes associated with obesity are similar to the changes associated with the supine position.

The tidal volume is equal in both sexes. However, all other lung volumes, the TLC and IC in particular, are greater in men. The difference in lung volumes is not entirely due to difference in height: the FRC is slightly more in men than in women of the same height. Measurements of lung volumes and capacities are always compared with normal, expected values and expressed as a percentage of normal. These normal values are calculated from the sex, age, and height of the subject.

In pregnancy, the RV is reduced due to the gravid uterus pushing the diaphragm up (**Fig. 46.5**). Although the gravid uterus impedes the inspiratory lowering of the diaphragm, there is a compensatory increase in the rib excursions, resulting in a normal or slightly increased VC. Accordingly, the TLC may be slightly reduced or remain unchanged. Pregnancy is also associated with an increase in the respiratory rate and a greater increase in the tidal volume so that there is an increase in respiratory minute volume (see below). A similar increase in minute ventilation occurs during the luteal phase of the menstrual cycle.

The inspiratory capacity, and therefore the vital capacity, is increased by activities that strengthen the accessory muscles of inspiration, such as swimming and rowing.

Dynamic Lung Functions

Dynamic lung functions are measured with reference to time. Measurements that are made on a single breath are timed in

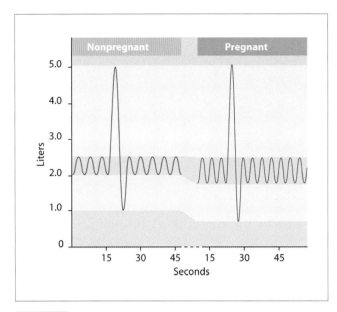

Fig. 46.5 In pregnancy, the vital capacity is increased at the cost of functional residual capacity. Tidal volume increases.

seconds and signify the airflow rate. Measurements that are made over multiple breaths are timed in minutes and signify ventilatory capacity.

Expiratory Flow Rates

Airflow rates can be estimated using a spirometer. The subject is initially asked to breathe normally into a spirometer, while the spirogram is recorded on a moving drum. Thereafter, the subject breathes in maximally, holds his or her breath as the drum speed is set to ~20 mm/sec, then expires maximally as fast as possible.

The graph thus obtained (**Fig. 46.6**) is almost identical to a typical spirogram (**Fig. 46.1B**) except for a small part of it that has been stretched out in time. The graph permits the measurement of all the spirometric volumes and capacities. As explained above, the vital capacity recorded is the FVC.

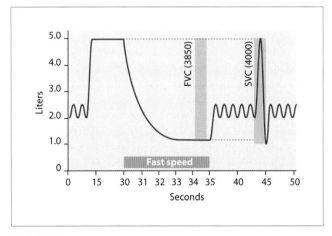

Fig. 46.6 Spirogram showing forced vital capacity (FVC) recorded at high speed. SVC, slow vital capacity.

For measurement of airflow rates, the expiratory phase is broken up into smaller segments. The segmentation can be done in two ways (**Fig. 46.7A**): either the entire duration of expiration is segmented into 1-second intervals, or the entire volume of expired air is segmented into four quarters. In the first case, the indices obtained are called *forced expiratory volumes.* In the second case, the indices obtained are called *forced expiratory airflow rates.* Notwithstanding their different names, both signify flow rates.

Forced expiratory volumes | The most commonly measured forced expiratory volume (also called timed vital capacity) is the FEV_1, which is the maximum volume of air that the subject can breathe out in the first second of a forced expiration. **Figure 46.7B** shows how FEV_1 is measured out from the spirogram. The other forced expiratory volumes are FEV_2 and FEV_3. FEV_1 becomes more meaningful when it is expressed as a percentage of the FVC: it is the FEV_1/FVC ratio and not FVC that is the cornerstone of diagnosis of obstructive airway disease. Normally, FEV_1/FVC is 83%, FEV_2/FVC is 94%, and FEV_3/FVC is 97%.

The time taken for completing the expiration forcefully (~4 seconds) is called *forced expiratory time* (FET). Although not a very precise index, it provides a useful bedside test to the clinician: the forced expiration is heard by auscultating (hearing through the stethoscope) the lungs and is timed using the wristwatch. When FET exceeds 4 seconds, airway obstruction is suspected, and when it exceeds 6 seconds, the clinician is almost sure.

Expiratory flow rates ($\Delta V/\Delta t$) can be measured out from a spirogram, as shown in **Fig. 46.7C**. During the first 25% of the expiration, the airflow rate is determined almost entirely by the strength of the expiratory muscles. Hence, it is called *effort-dependent flow rate.* During the last 25% of the expiration, the airflow rate is determined almost entirely by the caliber of the smaller airways and cannot be increased no matter how hard the subject expires. Hence, it is called *effort-independent flow rate.* Accordingly, two different indices of airflow rates are designed to measure different points of the expiratory flow curve: the peak expiratory flow rate (PEFR) and maximal mid-expiratory flow rate (MMEFR).

The PEFR measures the initial part of expiratory flow when the lungs are full to more than 75% of the FVC (somewhere between point A and point B in **Fig. 46.7C**). The MMEFR measures the middle part of the expiratory flow when the lungs are full to exactly 50% of the FVC (point C in **Fig. 46.7C**). It can be estimated graphically by considering the average flow between 75% and 25% of the FVC. Hence, it is also called $FEFR_{25-75\%}$ (FEFR = forced expiratory flow rate).

The PEFR is effort-dependent: the greater the expiratory effort, the greater is the PEFR attained. Because the force of expiration is greater at large lung volumes (see **Fig. 45.9**), the PEFR should be attained right at the onset of expiration. That, however, does not happen, and the flow rate takes a little while to rise to its peak (**Fig. 46.8**).

The PEFR also depends on airway resistance. Because the bronchi and larger bronchioles account for 50% of the airway resistance, the caliber of these airways is another major

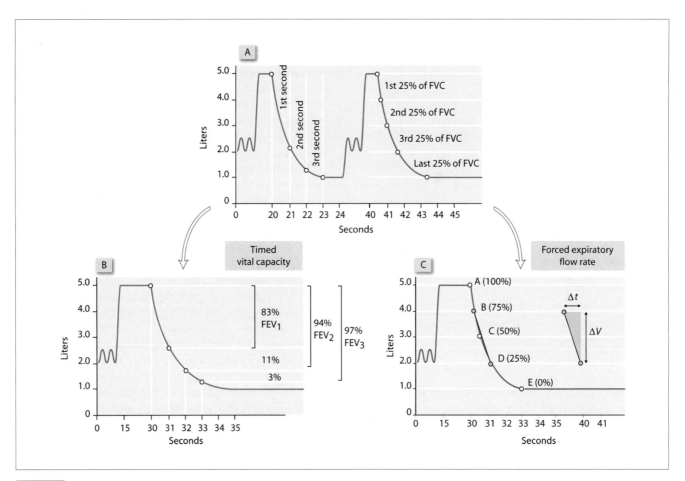

Fig. 46.7 Dynamic lung function tests. **(A)** The forced vital capacity (FVC) can be segmented in two different ways: at fixed time intervals or at fixed fractions of the FVC. **(B)** Measurement of timed vital capacity (FEV$_1$, FEV$_2$, and FEV$_3$). **(C)** Measurement of maximal midexpiratory flow rate (FEF$_{25-75\%}$) from the volume-time curve. Point A denotes that the lungs are full to their capacity, point B denotes that the lungs are full to 75% of the FVC, and so on. The flow rate ($\Delta V/\Delta t$) between any two points can be calculated, as shown here. FEV$_1$, forced expiratory volume in 1 second; FEF$_{25-75\%}$, forced midexpiratory flow rate between 25 and 75% of expiration.

determinant of PEFR. Hence, the test is widely used to monitor patients with asthma who have variable degrees of bronchoconstriction. However, being effort-dependent, it may be reduced if the respiratory muscles are weak. For the same reason, it is also low if the TLC is reduced (i.e., in restrictive lung disorder) because at low lung volumes, expiratory force produced is less. Measuring PEFR alone is therefore a poor substitute for complete spirometry. Its only advantage is that it can be measured using a small, handy instrument (**Fig. 46.8A**) and is therefore used for monitoring airway obstruction for mass health surveys or when a spirometer is not available. PEFR ranges from 5 to 15 L/sec in men and 2.5 to 10 L/sec in women. Much higher flow rates are recordable during cough. Hence, the subject must not "cough" into the mouthpiece.

The graphic method for measurement of airflow rate, as shown in **Fig. 46.7**, fails when the time interval is very small. In other words, the graphic method allows the calculation of flow rate between two points, but not at a single point. The latter, denoted by $\Delta V/\Delta t$, is recorded directly with *respiratory anemometers* (devices for measuring airflow). The expiratory

flow rate thus measured is plotted against the lung volume, resulting in the flow volume graphs (**Figs. 46.8** and **46.9**).

Clinicians prefer the flow volume curves because they assume characteristic shapes in certain abnormal conditions, allowing almost instant diagnosis. The flow volume loops give direct readouts of both flow rates and lung volumes. The only information that cannot be obtained from the loops is the duration of inspiration or expiration. However, the information is redundant to clinicians when the flow rates are known. Mostly, it is only the expiratory half of the flow volume loop that interests the clinician.

The flow volume graph can be generated directly with an instrument called the pneumotachograph. **Figure 46.9** shows a series of loops obtained at different levels of respiratory efforts, keeping the depth of breathing unchanged. It is observed that the greater the effort, the larger are the expiratory and inspiratory loops. However, there is an important difference between the inspiratory and expiratory curves. Although all the inspiratory curves are distinct, all the expiratory curves merge together toward the end, indicating that their terminal slopes are equal. In other words, no matter how high the

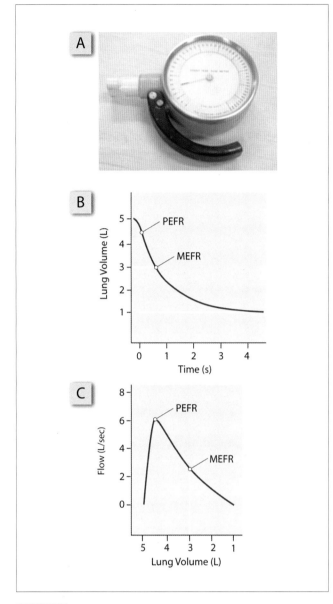

Fig. 46.8 **(A)** A peak flow meter. **(B)** A spirogram showing the points of peak expiratory flow rate (PEFR) and mid-expiratory flow rate (MEFR). **(C)** A flow volume curve showing the corresponding PEFR and MEFR.

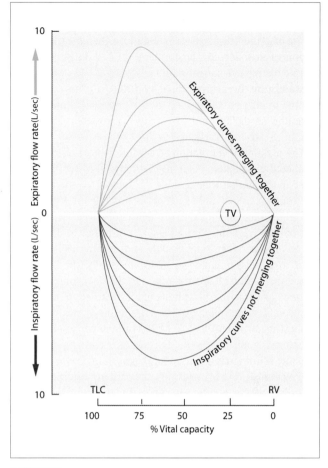

Fig. 46.9 Six superimposed flow volume loops recorded at different levels of inspiratory and expiratory efforts while the depths remain equal. For comparison, the flow volume loop recorded during tidal breathing (TV) is also shown.

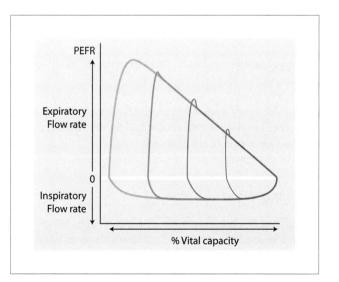

Fig. 46.10 Four superimposed flow volume loops at different depths of slow inspiration followed by maximal expiration. PEFR, peak expiratory flow rate; IC, inspiratory capacity; V_T, tidal volume; IRV, inspiratory reserve volume.

expiratory effort is, the terminal part (last 35%) of expiration has the same flow rate. The terminal flow rate is therefore effort-independent and depends on the resistance in the small airways—the small bronchi and bronchioles. Normal flow volume loops at different depths of breathing are shown in **Fig. 46.10.**

Ventilatory Capacity

Minute ventilation ($\dot{V}_E$) is the volume of air expired over a period of 1 minute when the subject is breathing normally.

Minute ventilation = Tidal volume × Respiratory rate

(46.12)

V_E can be measured simply by asking the subject to breathe in through the nose and expire the air through the mouth into a large bag (the Douglas bag) for 1 minute, then measuring the volume of air collected. The normal $\dot{V}_E$ is 6 L. V_E must be known for calculating alveolar ventilation.

Maximum breathing capacity (MBC) is the maximum volume of air that the subject can expire in 1 minute when breathing as deeply and as rapidly as possible. Maximum breathing capacity is attained during exercise.

The maximum ventilation achievable when not exercising is called the *maximum voluntary ventilation* (MVV). It is measured in the laboratory by asking the subject to rebreathe into a spirometer as fast and as deeply as possible for 15 seconds. The rebreathing ensures that the ventilatory drive is not inhibited by CO_2 washout. The subject is permitted to determine the balance between tidal volume and respiratory frequency so as to achieve maximal ventilation. Usually, the breathing frequency is 40 to 70 breaths/min, and the tidal volume is 50% of the vital capacity. The volume of air breathed in (or out) in 15 seconds is multiplied by 4, and the results are expressed in L/min. The normal MVV is 125 ± 25 L/min in young men.

Before the introduction of FEV_1, MVV used to be the major dynamic spirometric test used for diagnosis of airway obstruction. Not only is the MVV less in such patients, but the pattern of the spirogram is different. An asthmatic who voluntarily ventilates maximally does so by increasing the frequency at relatively low tidal volume, and the end-expiratory volume is higher than normal (see **Fig. 52.1**). However, the test is exhausting and causes faintness. It is affected by the motivation and endurance of the subject. Other factors affecting it are the compliance of the lung and thorax and the strength of respiratory muscles. After the advent of FEV_1, MVV is left with very little utility.

Summary

- Spirometry is a technique for measuring static and dynamic lung volumes.

- Lung capacities can be calculated from the measured lung volumes.

- Spirometry is a major component of pulmonary function testing, an important diagnostic tool for determining the presence of pulmonary disorders.

Applying What You Know

46.1. Ms. Eng presents in the emergency room with wheezing, the production of an abnormal breath sound. What conditions are present in the respiratory system when wheezing is occurring?

Dead Spaces

Anatomic Dead Space

During quiet breathing, ~500 mL of air is inspired and expired (the tidal volume). Not all the air that is breathed in enters the alveoli. About 150 mL of inspired air remains in the upper airways, trachea, and bronchi, and therefore does not participate in exchange with pulmonary blood. This is called the anatomic dead space (V_D) and can be measured by the *single-breath nitrogen (N_2) method,* which is depicted in **Fig. 47.1**.

At the end of a quiet expiration, the subject takes in a deep breath of pure oxygen (O_2) and breathes it out slowly and steadily. The exhaled air is instantaneously monitored for its N_2 concentration. The initial volume of air that is entirely N_2 free gives the anatomic dead space. The air exhaled thereafter, which comes from the alveoli, has a higher concentration of N_2.

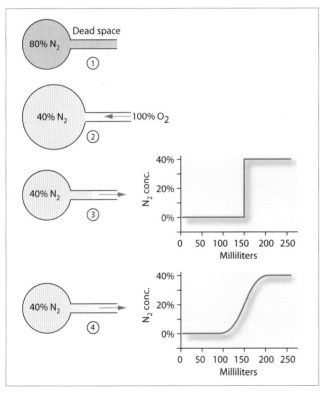

Fig. 47.1 Measurement of anatomic dead space. (1) Normally, the dead spaces and alveoli remain filled with air containing 80% nitrogen (N_2). (2) Breathing in pure oxygen (O_2) fills the dead spaces with 100% O_2 and dilutes the alveolar N_2 to 40%. (3) During exhalation, 150 mL of pure O_2 in the dead spaces comes out first, followed by 40% N_2. (4) Due to mixing of N_2 with O_2 inside the dead spaces, the transition is not abrupt, as shown in (3). The O_2 concentration starts rising from 100 mL and peaks at 200 mL. The mean value of 150 mL is taken as the dead space volume.

Physiologic Dead Space

Normally, ~350 mL of air enters the alveoli with each breath. Not all the air that enters the alveoli necessarily participates in alveolar gas exchange. This is because the alveoli might not be getting adequate blood supply, or their walls might not permit adequate diffusion. Such spaces in the alveoli constitute the *alveolar dead space.* The sum of anatomic dead space and alveolar dead space is called the physiologic dead space. Hence, the physiologic dead space is the volume of inspired air, either in the airways or in the alveoli, that does not participate in gaseous exchange. The physiologic dead space (PDS) is normally slightly larger than the anatomic dead space. It can be calculated using the Bohr equation:

$$PCO_{2[EXP]} \times V_T = PCO_{2[Art]} \times (-V_T - PDS) + PCO_{2[Ins]} \times PDS \quad (47.1)$$

where $PCO_{2[Exp]}$ is the partial pressure of carbon dioxide (PCO_2) in expired air; $PCO_{2[Art]}$ is PCO_2 in arterial blood; $PCO_{2[Ins]}$ is PCO_2 in inspired air; and V_T is tidal volume. Ignoring $PCO_{2[Ins]}$ because it is very small, the formula reduces to

$$PCO_{2[Exp]} \times V_T = PCO_{2[Art]} \times (V_T - PDS) \quad (47.2)$$

Example:

$$PCO_{2[Exp]} = 28 \text{ mm Hg}$$
$$PCO_{2[Art]} = 40 \text{ mm Hg}$$
$$V_T = 500 \text{ mL}$$
$$28 \times 500 = 40 \times (500 - PDS)$$
$$\therefore PDS = 150 \text{ mL}$$

The derivation of the Bohr equation is based on the knowledge that all the CO_2 in expired tidal air ($PCO_{2[Exp]} \times V_T$) comes from the alveoli. It is also known that the amount of air (nearly CO_2-free) in each breath that equilibrates with blood is V_T minus PDS. The PCO_2 of this alveolar air equals the PCO_2 of pulmonary arterial blood, that is, $PCO_{2[Art]}$. Hence, $(V_T - PDS) \times PCO_{2[Art]}$ is equal to the amount of CO_2 entering the alveoli from pulmonary capillaries and leaving with each breath. This must be equal to the total amount of CO_2 exhaled with each breath, which is given by $PCO_{2[Exp]} \times V_T$.

Alveolar Ventilation

Alveolar ventilation ($\dot{V}_A$) is defined as the amount of inspired air entering the alveoli per minute during normal breathing. It is given by

Alveolar ventilation =
(Tidal volume – Anatomic dead space) × Respiratory rate
$$= (500 \text{ mL} - 150 \text{ mL}) \times 14/\text{min}$$
$$= 4900 \text{ mL/min} \quad (47.3)$$

Alveolar air composition can be estimated by alveolar air sampling, that is, analyzing the last few milliliters of air that issue from the lungs during expiration. The alveolar air composition represents a dynamic equilibrium between the rate at which atmospheric air ventilates the alveoli and the rate at which pulmonary arterial blood perfuses the alveoli and exchanges its gases with them. Thus, the alveolar air composition depends on the *ventilation–perfusion ratio* (**Fig. 47.2**).

If alveolar perfusion decreases or alveolar ventilation increases, the alveolar composition will become closer to that of the inspired air. On the other hand, if alveolar perfusion increases or alveolar ventilation decreases, the alveolar partial pressure of gases will become closer to the corresponding partial pressures in arterial blood.

General Model: Reservoir

The alveoli (collectively, the alveolar space) is a reservoir into which oxygen enters from the atmosphere and diffuses into the blood, and carbon dioxide enters from the blood and is exhaled to the air. The partial pressures of these gases in the alveolar space (which is related to their concentrations) are determined by the rate of entry in and the rate of removal of these gases from this space.

Because alveolar PO_2 and alveolar PCO_2 are both related to alveolar ventilation, it stands to reason that the two will be interrelated. The relationship between alveolar PO and PCO_2 is given by the alveolar gas equation below.

$$PO_{2[Alv]} = PO_{2[Ins]} - PCO_{2[Alv]} \times \left[FO_2 + \frac{1 - FO_2}{RQ} \right] \quad (47.4)$$

where $PO_{2[Alv]}$ is the alveolar PO_2 (normally 100 mm Hg); $PO_{2[Ins]}$ is the PO_2 in inspired air (normally 150 mm Hg); $PCO_{2[Alv]}$ is the alveolar PCO_2 (normally 40 mm Hg); FO_2 is the fraction of O_2 in dry air (normally 0.2); and RQ is the respiratory quotient (normally 0.8).

It is the ratio of CO_2 output and O_2 intake by tissues per minute. By substituting the normal values of $PO_{2[Ins]}$, FO_2, and RQ, the formula simplifies to

$$PO_{2[Alv]} = 150 - PCO_{2[Alv]} \times \left[0.2 + \frac{1 - 0.2}{0.8} \right] \quad (47.5)$$

or

$$PO_{2[Alv]} = 150 - (PCO_{2[Alv]} \times 1.2) \quad (47.6)$$

The formula can be verified by substituting normal values of $PO_{2[Alv]}$ and $PCO_{2[Alv]}$.

$$102 = 150 - (40 \times 1.2)$$

Effect of Gravity on Alveolar Ventilation

Gravity reduces the ventilation of the apical alveoli, the alveoli that are nearer to the apex of the lungs. The reason is twofold: (1) gravity causes the apical alveoli to operate over a volume range where their compliance is reduced, and (2) gravity increases the intrapleural pressure near the base of the lungs.

Effect of gravity on alveolar compliance | In the erect posture, the apical alveoli are larger but poorly ventilated, whereas the basal alveoli are smaller but better ventilated (**Fig. 47.3**). This is because the weight of the lungs stretches the apical

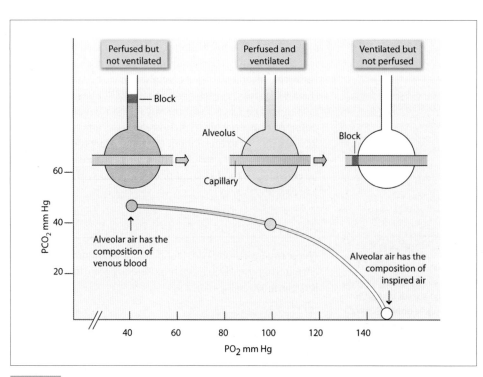

Fig. 47.2 Ventilation–perfusion ratio affects alveolar air composition.

alveoli to nearly their maximum size, leaving little room for further expansion during inspiration. In other words, apical alveoli have lower compliance. Although apical alveoli are poorly ventilated, the PO_2 of apical alveoli is higher. This is because of the effect of gravity on alveolar perfusion (see below).

A clinical correlate of the effect of gravity on ventilation is that arterial oxygenation improves in unilateral lung diseases when the patient lies on his or her side so that the good lung is in the dependent position. For reasons not understood, the situation is opposite in infants, who seem to do better with the diseased lung in the dependent position.

Effect of gravity on intrapleural pressure | Gravity also affects the intrapleural pressure. Near the apex, the entire weight of the lungs acts to pull the lungs away from the thorax. Near the base, the lungs tend to "sit" on the thoracic floor, and the weight of the lungs tends to make the intrapleural pressure positive.

At the end of a forced expiration, intrapleural pressure at the base of the lungs can exceed the atmospheric pressure in the airways. This high pressure causes the respiratory bronchioles near the base of the lungs to collapse (airway closure). The respiratory bronchioles near the apex, however, remain open because the intrapleural pressure is more negative near the apex and also because the weight of the lungs keeps the bronchiolar lumen stretched open. In disorders like emphysema that are associated with reduction in lung elasticity, airway closure at the base may occur even at the end of a quiet expiration.

The lung volume at which the basal airways start closing down is called the *closing volume* and can be estimated by the single-breath O_2 method. The subject takes a deep breath of 100% O_2 and exhales it slowly, while the N_2 concentration of

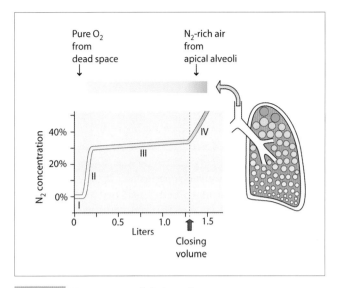

Fig. 47.4 Measurement of closing volume.

the exhaled air is monitored continuously. As explained above, most of the O_2 inspired enters the basal alveoli, greatly diluting the alveolar N_2. Much less O_2 enters the apical alveoli, where the air remains rich in N_2. A graph of the N_2 concentration plotted against the volume of expired air therefore shows four distinct phases (**Fig. 47.4**).

In phase I, the pure O_2 present in the dead spaces is exhaled, and there is no N_2 in the expired air. In phase II, there is a sharp rise in N_2 as the alveolar air is exhaled. The N_2 concentration reaches a plateau in phase III. However, there is a slight rise in N_2 concentration during phase III due to the progressive closure of the basal alveoli, which have less N_2, so that relatively more air comes from the N_2-rich apical alveoli. In phase IV, the N_2 concentration rises abruptly again, as most of the exhaled air now comes from the N_2-rich apical alveoli. By now, the basal alveoli have closed down completely, and the lung volume at the beginning of the fourth phase denotes the closing volume of the lung.

The normal closing volume is ~10% of the vital capacity plus residual volume. It increases when there is a narrowing of the small airways, or there is a reduction in lung elasticity that normally keeps the small airways patent. The elasticity decreases with age, and the closing volume can be as high as 25% by the age of 50 years. Closing volume is also high in chronic smokers.

Alveolar Perfusion

The normal pulmonary blood flow is the same as the right ventricular output—~5.0 L/min. However, not all of the blood that flows into the lungs perfuses the alveoli. Some of the blood supplies the bronchi and gets further deoxygenated instead of getting oxygenated. This blood, which bypasses the alveoli (gets shunted) to supply the bronchi and returns to the left atrium, constitutes a physiologic shunt (see **Fig. 44.3**). The deoxygenated blood from bronchial circulation drains into the pulmonary veins and mixes with oxygen-rich blood (with a

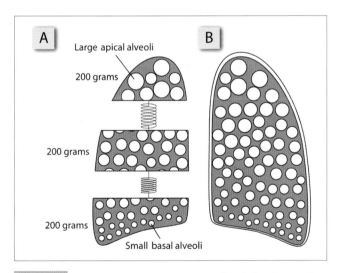

Fig. 47.3 **(A)** Apical alveoli are larger than basal alveoli. Assuming the weight of the lungs to be 600 g, the alveoli in the upper third of the lungs are pulled down by 400 g of lung tissue, whereas alveoli in the middle third are pulled down by only 200 g of lung tissue. **(B)** The lungs "sit" on the diaphragmatic pleura. Hence, the intrapleural pressure at the apex is more negative than the intrapleural pressure at the base.

PO_2 of 97 mm Hg) from the alveoli. Hence, the PO_2 of mixed pulmonary venous blood is slightly lower, at 95 mm Hg.

> **General Model: Flow**
>
> Blood flow to the alveoli is driven by the pressure gradient across the pulmonary circulation (see **Table 41.1**).

Effect of gravity on alveolar perfusion | In the erect posture, the basal alveoli are much better perfused than the apical alveoli. The PO_2 and PCO_2 of the well-perfused basal alveoli become equal to that of pulmonary arterial blood: it has low PO_2 and high PCO_2. Conversely, the alveolar air composition of the poorly perfused apical alveoli approximates more that of inspired air: it has high PO_2 and low PCO_2. The high PO_2 in apical alveoli is the reason for the vulnerability of apical areas of the lungs to infection by *Mycobacterium tuberculosis,* which is an aerobic bacterium.

Ventilation–Perfusion Ratio

Considering that the cardiac output is 5.0 L/min, and alveolar ventilation, too, is ~5.0 L/min, the overall ventilation:perfusion ($\dot{V}/\dot{Q}$) ratio is 1:1. Ideally, therefore, each alveolus should have a $\dot{V}/\dot{Q}$ ratio of 1:1. However, that is not so even in normal lungs.

Due to gravity, the apical alveoli are both underventilated and underperfused, whereas the basal alveoli are both overventilated and overperfused (**Fig. 47.5**). However, gravity affects perfusion much more than it affects ventilation. Hence, apical alveoli are more underperfused than underventilated ($\dot{V}/\dot{Q}$ = 3), whereas the basal alveoli are more overperfused than overventilated ($\dot{V}/\dot{Q}$ = 0.6). These regional disparities in ventilation and perfusion get exaggerated in diseases, resulting in gross impairment of alveolar gas exchange with consequent hypoxic hypoxia.

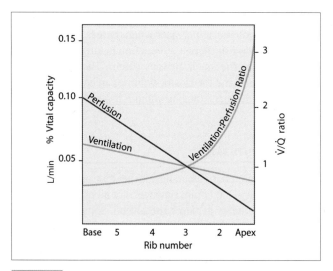

Fig. 47.5 Both ventilation and perfusion decrease in the upper part of the lungs, but perfusion decreases more than ventilation. Hence, the ventilation:perfusion ratio increases toward the apex.

> **General Model: Flow**
>
> The diffusion of gases (flow) between the alveolar space and the blood is determined by the partial pressure gradient for each gas and the properties of the barrier that determine the rate of diffusion (the permeability to the gases).

Alveolar Gas Exchange

The **respiratory membrane** (or the alveolocapillary membrane) is made up of six layers (**Fig. 47.6**). From the alveolar to the capillary side, they are (1) surfactant layer, (2) alveolar epithelium, (3) alveolar basement membrane, (4) alveolar interstitial space, (5) capillary basement membrane, and (6) capillary endothelium. It is ~0.5 µm thick, and its total surface area in the two lungs equals ~50 to 100 m². The gases have to pass through these layers while diffusing from the alveoli to pulmonary blood.

Flow-limited versus diffusion-limited transport | Blood spends ~0.75 second (the transit time) in the pulmonary capillaries (**Fig. 47.7**). This time is more than double the time taken by O_2 (~0.3 second to completely equilibrate with the pulmonary blood). CO_2 takes even less time to equilibrate. Transport of these gases across the respiratory membrane is therefore flow-limited (see **Fig. 36.4**). In other words, if the pulmonary blood flow increases, the amount of O_2 and CO_2 diffusing across the respiratory membrane will increase with it. Of course, the diffusion of oxygen is flow-limited as long as the transit time is greater than 0.3 second. At higher flow rates (lower transit times), it becomes diffusion-limited. This can limit oxygen

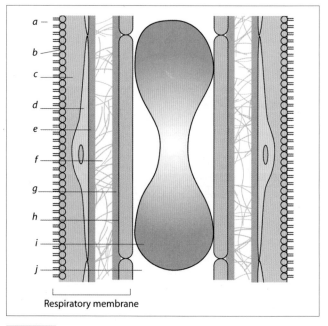

Fig. 47.6 The respiratory membrane. a. Alveolar space, b. surfactant molecules, c. water layer, d. alveolar epithelial cells, e. alveolar basement membrane, f. alveolar interstitium, g. capillary basement membrane, h. capillary endothelium, i. red blood cell, and j. capillary lumen filled with fluid.

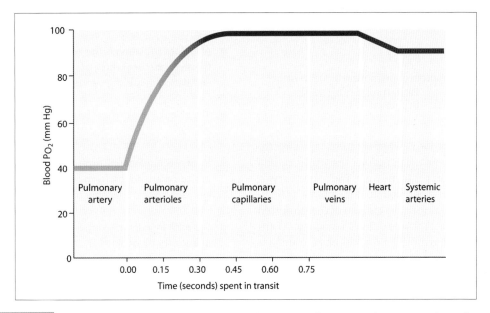

Fig. 47.7 Time course of gaseous equilibration in pulmonary capillaries. Note that oxygen takes only ~0.3 second to equilibrate completely with the pulmonary blood, though it remains in the pulmonary capillaries for 0.75 second.

uptake during severe exercise when cardiac output is very high, and the velocity of blood flow is high. It is also a problem if diffusion is limited by pathology (as occurs in pneumonia).

Conversely, carbon monoxide, which does not reach equilibrium in 0.75 second, will have a diffusion-limited transport: its transport across the respiratory membrane will increase only if the rate of diffusion increases.

Diffusion Capacity of the Lung

The volume (V) of a gas that diffuses across the respiratory membrane is (1) directly proportional to the partial pressure gradient, ΔP, across the respiratory membrane, (2) directly proportional to the duration (t) of the diffusion, (3) directly proportional to the surface area (A) of the respiratory membrane, (4) directly proportional to the solubility (S_{gas}) of the gas in the respiratory membrane, (5) inversely proportional to the thickness (d) of the respiratory membrane, and (6) inversely proportional to the square root of the molecular weight (W_{gas}) of the gas.

$$V \propto \frac{\Delta P \times t \times A \times S_{gas}}{d \times \sqrt{W_{gas}}} \qquad (47.7)$$

$$V = K \times \frac{\Delta P \times t \times A \times S_{gas}}{d \times \sqrt{W_{gas}}} \qquad (47.8)$$

where K is the proportionality constant. The formula can be reduced to

$$V = \Delta P \times t \times D_L \qquad (47.9)$$

where D_L is the *diffusion capacity* of the respiratory membrane, and is given by

$$D_L = K \times \frac{A \times S_{gas}}{d \times \sqrt{W_{gas}}} \qquad (47.10)$$

Equation 47.9 gives the definition of diffusion capacity because D_L equals V when $t = 1$ and $\Delta P = 1$. Hence, the diffusion capacity of the lung for a given gas is defined as the volume of gas diffusing across the respiratory membrane in 1 minute when the pressure gradient is 1 mm Hg. The formula for D_L can be reduced to

$$D_L = K \times \frac{A}{d} \times \text{Diffusion coefficient} \qquad (47.11)$$

where

$$\text{Diffusion coefficient} = \frac{S_{gas}}{\sqrt{W_{gas}}} \qquad (47.12)$$

It may be noted that the diffusion coefficient is dependent entirely on the characteristics of the gas. The diffusion coefficients of O_2 and CO_2 are in a ratio of 1:20. On the other hand, diffusion capacity is dependent not only on gaseous characteristics but also on the area and thickness of the respiratory membrane. The diffusion capacity for O_2 = 20 mL/min/mm Hg; the diffusion capacity for CO_2 = 400 mL/min/mm Hg. The diffusion capacity for O_2 increases in exercise and is markedly reduced in emphysema and interstitial lung disorder.

Measurement of diffusion capacity for O_2 | From equation 47.3, we have

$$V = \Delta P \times t \times D_L \qquad (47.13)$$

or

$$D_L = \frac{V/t}{\Delta P} \qquad (47.14)$$

For a gas that diffuses from the alveoli into blood, the formula can be written as

$$D_L = \frac{\text{Increase in the gas content of pulmonary blood in 1 min}}{\substack{\text{Partial pressure of} \quad \text{Partial pressure of the gas} \\ \text{the gas in alveolar air} \; - \; \text{in pulmonary capillary blood}}}$$

(47.15)

The diffusion capacity for O_2 is rarely measured directly. Instead, it is calculated from the diffusion capacity for carbon monoxide (CO), which is easier to measure. The reason is twofold: (1) O_2 diffusion across the respiratory membrane is flow-limited, and therefore measuring the amount of O_2 transferred to blood will underestimate the true diffusion capacity. CO diffusion, on the other hand, is diffusion-limited, and the amount of CO transferred to the blood is a correct estimate of the diffusion capacity. (2) CO has an added advantage that once in blood, it reacts with hemoglobin to form carboxyhemoglobin. Hence, it has a negligible partial pressure in pulmonary capillary blood, and equation 47.15 reduces to

$$D_L = \frac{\text{Increase in the gas content of pulmonary blood in 1 min}}{\text{Partial pressure of carbon monoxide in alveolar air}}$$

(47.16)

The diffusion capacity measured for CO at rest is ~17 mL/min/mm Hg. Because the diffusion coefficient of O_2 is 1.23 times greater than that of CO,

$$D_L \text{ for } O_2 = 17 \times 1.2 = 20 \text{ mL/min/mm Hg}$$

Diffusion capacity in exercise | The diffusion capacity (D_L) increases about threefold in exercise due to the opening up of inactive capillaries, resulting in an increase in the total area of the respiratory membrane.

Diffusion rate in exercise | Diffusion rate (V/t) is the product of diffusion capacity (D_L) and the pressure gradient (ΔP) of gases between the alveoli and pulmonary venous blood. This is obvious from equation 47.14, which can be rewritten as

$$\frac{V}{t} = D_L \times \Delta P$$

(47.17)

In exercise, there is an increase in the pressure gradient (ΔP) of gases between the alveoli and pulmonary venous blood. Hence, in exercise, the rise in diffusion rate (V/t) of gases is more marked than the rise in diffusion capacity (D_L).

Volume of gaseous diffusion in exercise | Referring to equation 47.3, it is obvious that the total volume of gaseous diffusion (V) depends on the time (t) spent in the pulmonary capillaries. During exercise, blood spends only 0.3 second in the pulmonary capillaries. During rest, although the blood remains longer (0.75 second in pulmonary capillaries), the gaseous diffusion is completed in only 0.3 second. Hence, the time factor does not reduce gaseous diffusion in exercise.

Summary

- Alveolar ventilation is the volume of air per minute entering the alveolar space where gas exchange can occur. It is minute ventilation minus the ventilation of the dead space.

- The alveolar space is perfused by blood in the pulmonary artery.

- In an erect individual, both alveolar ventilation and alveolar perfusion are nonuniform from the top to the bottom of the lungs because of the effects of gravity on the lungs.

- Gas exchange (O_2 moving from the air in alveoli to the pulmonary blood and CO_2 moving from the blood into alveolar air) occurs solely by passive diffusion down a partial pressure gradient.

- The diffusing capacity of the lungs is a measure of the effect of surface area, the thickness of the diffusional barrier, and the properties of the tissues on gas transport.

Applying What You Know

47.1. Ms. Eng has an increased breathing frequency (tachypnea). What effect will this have on her tidal volume? Explain your prediction.

47.2. Ms. Eng has a markedly decreased P_aO_2 but an essentially normal P_aCO_2. Such a state can only result from what kind of disturbance in the respiratory system? Explain your answer.

Transport of Oxygen in Blood

Oxygen (O_2) is transported in blood in two forms: bound to hemoglobin as oxyhemoglobin and in solution in plasma. The volume of O_2 that is dissolved in plasma is directly proportional to the partial pressure of oxygen (PO_2) (**Fig. 48.1A**). It is given by the formula

$$\text{Volume of dissolved } O_2 = 0.003 \times PO_2 \text{ (mL/dL of blood)}$$
$$(48.1)$$

The amount of O_2 transported in plasma is only ~1.5% of the total amount transported. However, there is no limit to the amount of O_2 that can be carried in plasma provided the PO_2 is sufficiently high. This is a distinct advantage over O_2 transport as oxyhemoglobin, which is limited by the availability of hemoglobin. Dissolved O_2 at high PO_2 (hyperbaric oxygen) is used by therapists for the oxygenation of the tissues when hemoglobin gets denatured in carbon monoxide (CO) poisoning.

The bulk of oxygen in blood is normally transported as oxyhemoglobin. (The mechanism of hemoglobin oxygenation is discussed Chapter 22.) Its only disadvantage is that there is a ceiling on the amount of oxygen that can be transported. When 100% saturated, 1 g of hemoglobin can carry a maximum of 1.34 mL of oxygen. The amount is actually higher (1.39 mL) for pure hemoglobin-A. However, under normal conditions, some of the O_2 binding sites are unavailable, and thus the clinically measured value is lower than this theoretical limit.

General Model: Flow

Oxygen diffuses (flows) from the alveoli into the pulmonary capillary blood down a partial pressure gradient. The rate of flow depends on the magnitude of the gradient and the properties of the diffusional barrier. Changes in either of these will affect the transport of oxygen in the blood.

Oxygen Dissociation Curve

The amount of oxyhemoglobin formed is proportional to the PO_2. Plotting the amount of oxyhemoglobin against the PO_2 of blood gives the oxygen dissociation curve (**Fig. 48.1B**). The curve is not straight (as is the case for dissolved O_2), but sigmoidal in shape.

If the arterial and venous PO_2 are known, the amount of O_2 carried by hemoglobin in arterial or venous blood can be read out from the O_2 dissociation curve. The amount of oxyhemoglobin is often expressed as the percentage saturation: the percentage of total available oxygen-binding sites on hemoglobin that are, in fact, binding oxygen.

The amounts of O_2 bound to hemoglobin and dissolved in plasma in arterial and venous blood are given in **Table 48.1**.

Coefficient of O_2 utilization As shown in **Table 48.2**, each minute, 5 L of blood carrying 990 mL of O_2 delivers 230 mL of oxygen to the tissues. Thus, only ~25% [(230 ÷ 990) × 100] of the O_2 carried by the arterial blood is released to the tissues. This fraction is called the *coefficient of utilization*.

The coefficient increases in exercise. In severe exercise, it increases to 65% or higher. The reasons for this increase are threefold: (1) Exercise causes metabolic dilatation of the muscle capillary beds, which increases the surface area of exchange and also slows the flow velocity of blood, allowing equilibration of PO_2 between the blood and the tissues to occur completely. (2) The PO_2 gradient between arterial blood and the tissues becomes very high, the tissue PO_2 being reduced nearly to zero. (3) The O_2 dissociation curve shifts to the right in tissues (see below).

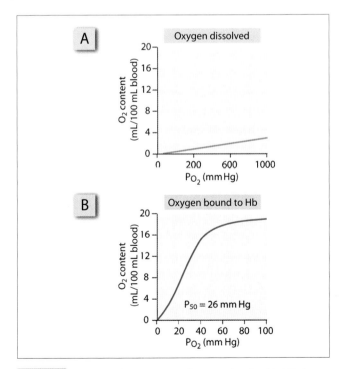

Fig. 48.1 Transport characteristics of oxygen dissolved in **(A)** plasma and **(B)** bound to hemoglobin (Hb). Note the difference in the scale of the x-axes; oxygen content bound to hemoglobin is very much greater at any partial pressure of oxygen than that which can be carried in solution.

Table 48.1 Oxygen (O_2) Content of 100 mL of Blood with 15 g/dL Hemoglobin

	Arterial Blood (PO_2 = 95 mm Hg)	Venous Blood (PO_2 = 40 mm Hg)
Hemoglobin-bound	19.5 mL	15.08 mL
Dissolved	0.29 mL (= 95 × 0.003)	0.12 mL (= 40 × 0.003)
Total	19.8 mL	15.2 mL

Table 48.2 Oxygen (O_2) Delivery to Tissues

	Arterial Content	Venous Content	Delivery
O_2 transported in 100 mL of blood	19.8	15.2	4.6 mL
O_2 transported in 5 L of blood	990 mL (19.8 × 50)	760 mL (15.2 × 50)	230 mL (990 − 760)

Shifts in O_2 dissociation curve | Several factors alter the affinity of hemoglobin for O_2 and thereby shift the O_2 dissociation curve to the left or right (**Fig. 48.2**). Such shifts affect the amount of O_2 taken up at the lungs and delivered to the tissues. A convenient way of expressing the extent of right or left shift is the P_{50}, which is the PO_2 at which hemoglobin is 50% saturated. It is higher in right-shifted and lower in left-shifted hemoglobin. Thus, the P_{50} of normal adult hemoglobin is 26 mm Hg, whereas that of the left-shifted fetal hemoglobin is 20 mm Hg.

A *shift to the right* is caused by factors that decrease the affinity of hemoglobin for O_2. At a given PO_2, the oxygen saturation of right-shifted hemoglobin is somewhat lower than in the normal curve. A right shift would be disadvantageous in the lungs because blood would take up less oxygen. However, it is advantageous in the tissues because the blood can offload more oxygen. Normally, the advantage outweighs the disadvantage, and the amount of O_2 delivered to the tissues improves with a right shift.

The body exploits this advantage in mild-to-moderate hypoxia: in hypoxia, the O_2 dissociation curve automatically shifts to the right for reasons explained below. However, this right shift proves to be disadvantageous in severe hypoxia when the PO_2 falls to 40 mm Hg or less. Hence, as one ascends to higher altitudes where the PO_2 progressively decreases, the right shift is beneficial only up to a point. Thereafter, the right shift turns disadvantageous.

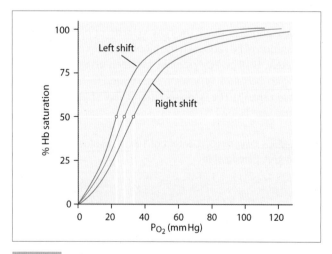

Fig. 48.2 Shifts in the oxygen dissociation curve. Also shown are the P_{50} (the partial pressure of oxygen at which hemoglobin is 50% saturated) values of the three curves.

Factors causing right shift are high PCO_2 (the Bohr effect), (2,3-diphosphoglycerate) acidic pH, rise in temperature, and a rise in red blood cell DPG concentration. The cause of the shift is discussed Chapter 22. Hypoxia increases DPG concentration by inhibiting the Krebs cycle. Thyroid hormones, growth hormones, and androgens increase DPG concentration in red blood cells (RBCs).

A *shift to the left* is caused by factors that increase the affinity of hemoglobin for O_2. At a given PO_2, the oxygen saturation of left-shifted hemoglobin is somewhat greater than in the normal curve. A left shift is advantageous in the lungs because blood can take up more oxygen. However, it is disadvantageous in the tissues because the blood would offload less oxygen. Normally, the disadvantage outweighs the advantage, and the amount of O_2 delivered to the tissues reduces with left shift. Left shift, however, becomes advantageous in severe hypoxia, when the arterial PO_2 is 40 mm Hg or less. Such low arterial PO_2 is normal in the fetus in utero. The tissue O_2 delivery remains adequate in the fetus because fetal hemoglobin has a markedly left-shifted O_2 dissociation curve.

Factors causing left shift are low PCO_2 and high pH, fall in temperature, and a fall in RBC DPG concentration. Fetal hemoglobin is left-shifted because it has a low affinity for DPG.

Effect of acute versus chronic acidosis | Although acidosis shifts the O_2 dissociation curve to the right, chronic acidosis decreases the DPG concentration in the RBCs by inhibiting glycolysis and thereby tends to shift the dissociation curve to the left. Hence, chronic changes in pH usually do not shift the dissociation curve either way. This knowledge is of importance in diabetes ketoacidosis. An overenthusiastic correction of the acidosis in acidotic patients may leave unopposed the effect of lowered DPG content of the RBCs on the O_2 dissociation curve of hemoglobin, which would shift to the left and cause hypoxia. The acidosis therefore has to be corrected slowly to allow the recovery of the DPG levels in the RBCs.

Effect of exercise | During exercise, there is a left shift of the O_2 dissociation curve in the lungs, but a right shift occurs in the tissues. Thus, O_2 uptake is facilitated in the lungs, whereas O_2 delivery is facilitated in the tissues. The right shift in the tissues occurs because the local PCO_2, temperature, and H^+ concentration increase in exercising muscles. Conversely, the left shift in the lungs occurs due to a relatively lower PCO_2, temperature, and H^+ concentration in the alveolar interstitium.

Transport of Oxygen in Tissue

Myoglobin is found in red muscle fibers engaged in slow and sustained contractions, as in postural skeletal muscle. These muscles have low PO_2 in them because sustained contraction of muscles compresses the capillaries, compromising their own blood supply. The role of myoglobin is thus to bind to O_2 at very low PO_2 and release them at even lower PO_2. Myoglobin is an iron-containing pigment that is similar to hemoglobin except that it contains only one polypeptide chain instead of four. Consequently, it does not exhibit the sigmoidal O_2 dissociation curve that is seen with hemoglobin. Its O_2 dissociation curve is a rectangular hyperbola and is markedly left-shifted as compared with hemoglobin (**Fig. 48.3**). This makes it especially suitable

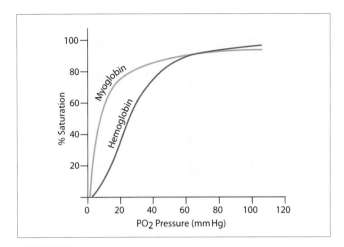

Fig. 48.3 The oxygen dissociation curve of myoglobin is left-shifted compared with that of hemoglobin.

for taking up O_2 at low PO_2. Myoglobin does not show the Bohr effect, which, if present, would defeat its very purpose.

Transport of Carbon Dioxide in Blood

CO_2 is transported in the blood in three forms: as bicarbonate, as carbamino compounds of hemoglobin and plasma proteins, and as dissolved CO_2. One hundred mL of venous blood carries 53 mL of CO_2; the same volume of arterial blood carries 49 mL of CO_2. Thus, 100 mL of blood takes away 4 mL of CO_2 (53 – 49 mL) from the tissues. Therefore, 5 L blood transports 200 mL of CO_2 from the tissues each minute.

> **General Model: Flow**
>
> Carbon dioxide diffuses (flows) from the blood into the alveoli down a partial pressure gradient. The mechanism is identical to that moving oxygen into the blood, although the direction of flow is obviously different.

As plasma bicarbonate, RBCs contain the enzyme carbonic anhydrase that catalyzes the reaction $CO_2 + H_2O \rightleftarrows HCO_3^- + H^+$ (**Fig. 48.4**). Hence, when CO_2 diffuses into the RBC, it reacts chemically with water to generate the bicarbonate ion (HCO_3^-) and hydrogen ions. The H^+ ions are taken up by hemoglobin, which is an excellent buffer. This enables the reaction to proceed in the forward direction (to the right). The bicarbonate ions generated diffuse out into the plasma in exchange for chloride (Cl^-) ions that diffuse into RBCs simultaneously. The movement of chloride ions into the RBC is called the chloride shift. The above events result in a small increase in the total number of ions inside the RBC, and water enters the RBC to maintain osmotic balance. The RBCs carrying CO_2 in bicarbonate form are therefore somewhat larger than normal. This is manifest in the slightly higher (~3%) volume of packed red cells (VPRC) of venous blood.

Carbaminohemoglobin CO_2 binds to hemoglobin to form carbaminohemoglobin. Carbamino compounds are formed with plasma proteins, too.

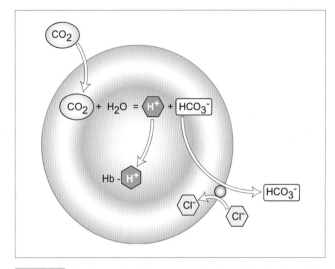

Fig. 48.4 The formation of bicarbonate in the red blood cell and the chloride shift.

Blood is saturated with carbaminohemoglobin at a PCO_2 of 10 mm Hg. At higher PCO_2, most of the CO_2 is transported as bicarbonates, and the H^+ generated in the process blocks the NH_2 groups of hemoglobin that are essential to the formation of carbaminohemoglobin.

$$R-N-H+CO_2 \rightleftarrows R-N-COO^- + H^+$$
$$\quad\ \ | \qquad\qquad\qquad |$$
$$\quad\ \ H \qquad\qquad\qquad H$$

As dissolved CO_2, the volume of dissolved CO_2 is proportional to the PCO_2. It accounts for ~6% of the total volume of CO_2 carried in blood (**Table 48.3**).

Carbon Dioxide Dissociation Curve

As with O_2, the dissociation curve of CO_2 can be obtained by plotting the CO_2 content of hemoglobin against the PCO_2 (**Fig. 48.5**).

Shifts in the CO_2 dissociation curve (1) Oxygen shifts the curve to the right, which means that oxyhemoglobin has less CO_2-binding capacity. The effect is called the CDH effect (after Christiansen, Douglas, and Haldane) or simply the Haldane effect (**Fig. 48.5**). The Haldane effect occurs because, as compared with

Table 48.3 The Carbon Dioxide (CO_2) Content of 100 mL of Blood

	Arterial Blood (mL)	% of Total Arterial CO_2	Venous Blood (mL)	% of Total Venous CO_2
CO_2 present in the form of:				
Dissolved CO_2	2.6	5	3.0	6
Bicarbonate	43.8	90	46.3	88
Carbamino Hb	2.6	5	3.4	6
Total CO_2 (all forms)	49.0	100	52.7	100

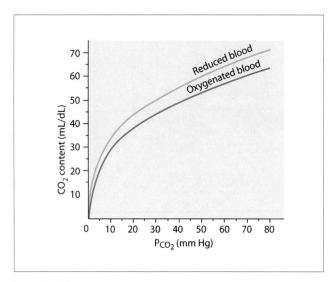

Fig. 48.5 The carbon dioxide dissociation curve and the Haldane effect.

hemoglobin, oxyhemoglobin has less affinity for CO_2 and H^+. (2) DPG shifts the curve to the right, especially that of reduced blood. The shift occurs because both DPG and CO_2 bind to the terminal α-NH_2 groups (valine) of the p chains of hemoglobin.

Gas Transfer

Figure 48.6 provides a convenient summary of the partial pressures and content of the blood gases in the lungs, arterial compartment, tissues, and venous compartment.

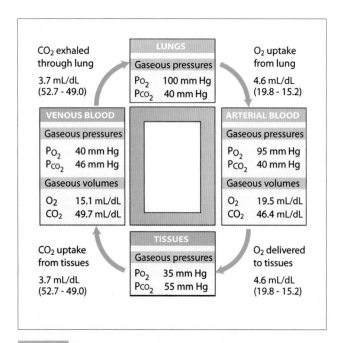

Fig. 48.6 Summary of partial pressures and volumes of oxygen and carbon dioxide in lungs, arterial blood, tissues, and venous blood.

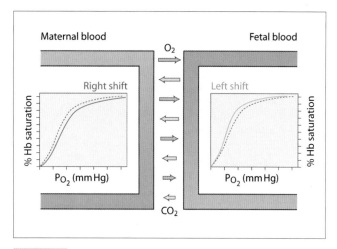

Fig. 48.7 The double Bohr effect in placental gas transfer.

Placental Gas Transfer

Double Bohr effect | In the placenta, gaseous exchange takes place directly between two different blood streams: the maternal and fetal. This provides a situation wherein the Bohr effect has double benefit (**Fig. 48.7**): (1) The CO_2 liberated by fetal blood shifts the O_2 dissociation curve of maternal blood to the right. (2) The lowering of PCO_2 of fetal blood shifts its own O_2 dissociation curve to the left. Thus, there is a simultaneous increase in O_2 delivery by maternal blood and O_2 uptake by fetal blood. This is known as the double Bohr effect.

Summary

- Oxygen is transported in the blood as dissolved gas (small amount) and bound to hemoglobin (chief form of transport).

- The binding of oxygen to hemoglobin is a sigmoidal function of the oxygen partial pressure.

- The oxyhemoglobin dissociation curve is shifted right or left by several physiologic factors.

- Carbon dioxide is transported in blood in solution, as carbamino compounds, predominantly as bicarbonate ions.

- The CO_2 dissociation curve is shifted by the Haldane effect.

Applying What You Know

48.1. Calculate the value of Ms. Eng's total oxygen content when she is in the emergency room.

48.2. Ms. Eng has a partial pressure of oxygen in arterial blood (P_aO_2) value that is significantly reduced (down from a normal value of 100 mm Hg to 66 mm Hg), although her hemoglobin saturation is only slightly reduced (down from a normal value of 98–99% to 91.5%). Explain the mechanism that accounts for this discrepancy.

Central Respiratory Rhythm

Respiratory Centers

The two main brainstem areas involved in the control of respiration are the dorsal respiratory group of neurons (DRG), located in the dorsal part of the medulla, and the ventral respiratory group of neurons (VRG), located midway between the dorsal and ventral surfaces of the medulla (**Fig. 49.1**).

General Model: Communication

Breathing is controlled by neural information from the central nervous system to the respiratory muscles. This is another example of the importance of cell-to-cell communication mechanisms.

The **dorsal respiratory group of neurons** comprises mainly the ventrolateral nucleus of the tractus solitarius (VLN-TS) and has both sensory and motor functions. The DRG contains upper motor neurons that descend to terminate on the spinal motor neurons innervating the primary muscles of inspiration: the diaphragm and the intercostals. Sensory fibers from the pe-

ripheral chemoreceptors (Chapter 50) and pulmonary mechanoreceptors (see below) that reach the brainstem through the glossopharyngeal and vagus nerves also terminate in the DRG, where they modulate respiration. Also present in the DRG are short interneurons that connect it to the VRG.

The **ventral respiratory group of neurons** extends through the entire length of the medulla. It is subdivided into three parts, caudal, intermediate, and rostral, and contains both inspiratory and expiratory neurons. The *caudal VRG* contains upper motor neurons that descend to terminate on the spinal motor neurons innervating the accessory muscles of expiration: the internal intercostals and abdominal muscles. The *intermediate VRG* contains (1) the pre-Botzinger complex, which is probably the center for the generation of respiratory rhythm; (2) upper motor neurons that descend on spinal motor neurons supplying the accessory muscles of inspiration; and (3) lower motor neurons that leave the brainstem through the vagus to directly innervate the muscles of the pharynx, larynx, and upper airways and help in dilating the upper respiratory passages during inspiration. The *rostral VRG* comprises the Botzinger complex or the nucleus retrofacialis. It is concerned mainly with driving the expiratory activity of the caudal VRG.

Generation of Respiratory Rhythm

One of the basic questions that remains unanswered is the site of the respiratory pattern generator. Some believe the site to be restricted to a single center in the brainstem (restricted site model) and consider the pre-Botzinger complex to be that site. Others believe that there are multiple centers, each of which is capable of producing the characteristic respiratory rhythm (distributed oscillator model) and serves as a backup should the others fail. Proponents of this model draw an analogy with the multiple pacemakers in the heart, each capable of taking over the function of pacing the heart. Still others believe that respiratory pattern generation occurs through the interaction of multiple centers, and that none of them can individually produce the characteristic respiratory rhythm (emergent property model). Discussed below is a simple emergent property model of respiratory rhythm.

The **emergent property model** assumes that the respiratory rhythm is generated by the coordinated activity of three types of medullary neurons: neurons with central inspiratory activity (CIA), neurons with inspiratory off-switch (IOS) activity, and neurons that act as the integrator (**Fig. 49.2**). The CIA neurons fire at a steadily increasing rate, a discharge pattern that has been called the inspiratory ramp. The CIA discharge has two effects: (1) It drives the motor neuron pool that is responsible for the inspiratory movements. Thus, as the firing rate increases, the tidal volume also increases. (2) The CIA depolarizes the integrator neurons.

The IOS neurons are responsible for terminating the inspiratory ramp. They discharge when the integrator neurons depolarize to a threshold level. It follows, therefore, that the

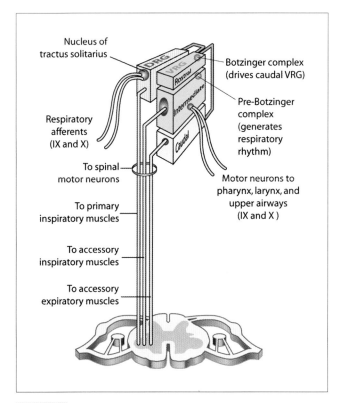

Fig. 49.1 Organization of central respiratory neurons and their motor output to the spinal cord, shown schematically. VRG, ventral respiratory group of neurons.

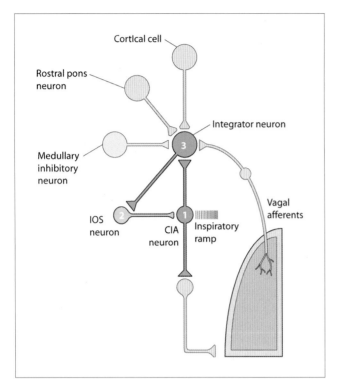

Fig. 49.2 A simple emergent property model of respiratory rhythm. The basic circuit consists of three neurons: (1) the central inspiratory activity (CIA) neuron, (2) the inspiratory off-switch (IOS) neuron, and (3) the integrator neuron. The discharge rate of the CIA neuron increases with time and is called the inspiratory ramp. Multiple inputs to the integrator neuron modulate the respiratory rhythm. If all excitatory inputs (apart from the CIA) are removed, apneustic breathing results. If any two excitatory inputs are removed, breathing becomes deep and slow.

CIA triggers the IOS indirectly through the integrator, thereby terminating its own discharge. This forms the basic circuitry for the generation of the respiratory rhythm.

The integrator receives additional excitatory and inhibitory inputs. Three main sources of excitatory inputs to the integrator are the cerebral cortex, the nucleus parabrachialis medialis (NPBM) in the rostral pons (earlier called the pneumotaxic center), and the vagal afferents from the pulmonary stretch receptors. The sources of inhibitory input include a group of cells in the medulla previously called the apneustic center.

In the presence of excitatory inputs, the integrator depolarizes quickly to the threshold and triggers the IOS, resulting in an early termination of the inspiratory ramp. Hence, inspiration is shortened, and the tidal volume decreases. Conversely, in the absence of these excitatory inputs and/or in the presence of inhibitory inputs, the integrator takes longer to depolarize to its threshold, and the inspiratory ramp continues that much longer. Hence, inspiration is prolonged, and the tidal volume increases.

Apneustic breathing | The term *apneusis* means sustained inspiration, whereas *apneustic breathing* refers to periods of apneusis interrupted by brief expiration. As mentioned above, the apneustic center inhibits the integrator neuron and

thereby delays the onset of expiration. Hence, stimulation of the apneustic center produces apneustic breathing. Apneustic breathing can occur even without the stimulation of the apneustic center. Normally, the vagal afferents from pulmonary stretch receptors do not discharge during slow breathing: they start firing only when the tidal volume exceeds 800 mL. Thus, in the simplified model presented above, there are only two excitatory inputs to the integrator in addition to the CIA neurons. However, if one of the two excitatory inputs is absent, the tidal volume increases, and the vagal afferents start discharging, providing an additional excitatory input. The total number of excitatory inputs still remains two, and breathing is not significantly affected. This is seen in normal subjects during anesthesia when the cortical excitatory input is abolished. If, however, two excitatory inputs are abolished, the breathing becomes deep and slow. This happens when the vagus is cut in an anesthetized dog: the anesthesia minimizes the cortical excitatory input, while vagotomy removes the excitatory inputs from the pulmonary stretch receptors. Another example is when an experimental midpontine section is made in the dog. The section removes excitatory inputs descending from the NPBM as well as the cortex. At this stage, the tidal volume exceeds 800 mL, and the vagal afferents start firing, providing additional excitatory inputs to the integrator. If the vagus, too, is sectioned, removing all excitatory inputs from the integrator, the breathing becomes apneustic.

The classical explanation of apneustic breathing (**Fig. 49.3**) was different. It assumed the presence of four centers, an inspiratory center, which produces inspiration; an expiratory center,

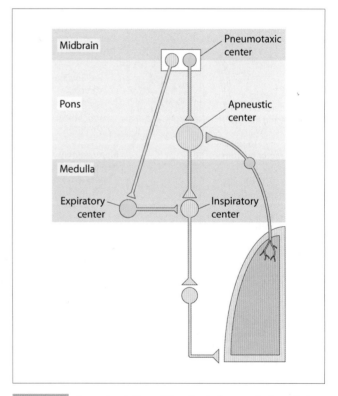

Fig. 49.3 A representation of the classical concept of respiratory centers.

which terminates inspiratory activity; the apneustic center, which stimulates the inspiratory center; and the pneumotaxic center, which stimulates the expiratory center and inhibits the apneustic center. The theory also assumed that vagal afferents from the stretch receptors in the lungs inhibited the apneustic center once the lung expansion exceeded a certain volume.

According to the classical theory, (1) vagotomy produces deep and slow breathing in anesthetized dogs because vagal afferents normally inhibit the apneustic center; (2) the midpontine section produces deep, slow breathing because it cuts off the descending inhibitory influence of the pneumotaxic center on the apneustic expiratory center; and (3) the midpontine section together with vagotomy produces apneustic breathing in an anesthetized animal because the apneustic center is totally disinhibited.

The Final Common Respiratory Motor Signal

The respiratory muscles, inspiratory and expiratory, are striated skeletal muscles that are innervated by motoneurons that leave the spinal cord at the cervical and thoracic levels. The diaphragm, the main inspiratory muscle, is innervated by the phrenic nerve (which leaves the spinal cord at the C3–C5 level). The external intercostals are innervated by nerves that leave the spinal cord at the thoracic level.

The contraction of skeletal muscle is, of course, solely determined by the neural activity stimulating it. Breathing frequency is determined by the rate at which bursts of action potentials travel down the motor nerves to the muscles; the greater the number of bursts/minute, the higher the breathing frequency. The depth of breathing, the tidal volume, is determined by the temporal pattern of action potentials making up each burst. The higher the firing rate within the burst, the greater the force of contraction of the innervated muscle fibers (see Chapter 15). Additionally, recruitment of motor units, activation of additional motor neurons, increases the tidal volume.

Afferent Neural Control

Numerous inputs from the periphery are known to affect breathing. A large number of them reach the brainstem through the vagus. They are summarized below.

Pulmonary Stretch Receptors

Pulmonary stretch receptors are located in the smooth muscle of the bronchial wall, especially at points of bronchial branching. The receptors are slow-adapting. They are responsible for the *Hering-Breuer inflation reflex*, in which inflation of the lung to a volume greater than 800 mL initiates reflex expiration. The reflex tends to limit the tidal volume while increasing the respiratory frequency. The reflex also results in bronchodilatation. It seems that the physiologic role of the Hering-Breuer reflex is to adjust the tidal volume and respiratory rate under different conditions of lung compliance and airway resistance.

Lung Irritant Receptors

Lung irritant receptors are located in the intrapulmonary bronchi and bronchioles, underneath the mucosal epithelium.

They cause reflex hyperpnea. These receptors are activated by several stimuli: (1) inhalation of irritant gases, such as ammonia (chemical irritant) or smoke (mechanical irritant), (2) large inflations of the lung that distort the bronchial epithelium, and (3) large deflations of the lung that distort the bronchial epithelium. The reflex hyperpnea in response to deflation is called the *Hering-Breuer deflation reflex* and is seen in pneumothorax and lung collapse (atelectasis). The reflex may be responsible for initiating the sighs (deep breath) or yawning in response to the decrease in compliance that occurs periodically due to the collapse of the smaller alveoli. The reflex helps in reopening collapsed alveoli. The cough receptors in the trachea and larynx are structurally and functionally similar to the lung irritant receptors.

J-Receptors

Juxtapulmonary (J) receptors (also called C-fiber receptors) are present in the alveolar interstitium adjacent to pulmonary capillaries or in the walls of the capillaries and are innervated by vagal fibers. They are stimulated by an increase in the alveolar interstitial fluid volume. Irritant gases stimulate J-receptors either directly or by causing exudation of alveolar interstitial fluid. J-receptors are also stimulated by multiple microemboli in small pulmonary vessels, but they are not stimulated by the embolization of the larger pulmonary vessels.

Stimulation of the J-receptors reflexively brings about severe tachypnea, bronchoconstriction, hypotension, and bradycardia. Stimulation of J-receptors also causes reflex muscle weakness. The reflex is known as the *J-reflex*, and it prevents inadvertent overexercise, as follows. When severe exercise causes pulmonary interstitial edema, the J-receptors are stimulated. Stimulation of the J-receptors causes reflex reduction of muscle tone and thereby terminates the exercise (**Fig. 49.4**).

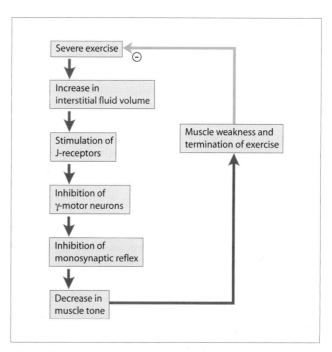

Fig. 49.4 The J-reflex.

Other Respiratory Reflexes

The swallowing reflex briefly suspends breathing in whichever phase (inspiration or expiration) the swallowing occurs. The afferent fibers of the reflex run in the superior laryngeal and trigeminal nerves. Afferents from baroreceptors and chemoreceptors also affect breathing. Nociceptive afferents stimulate breathing. The reflex is employed by the pediatrician for initiating the first breath in the newborn by slapping it. Joint afferents are thought to have an important role in the hyperventilation that occurs during exercise. Afferents in the trigeminal nerve and olfactory nerve modulate the breathing pattern during the sneezing reflex.

The First Breath

Fetal respiratory movements begin as early as the 11th week of gestation. Initially irregular, they become regular toward full term. At birth, the constriction (or clamping) of the umbilical cord asphyxiates the neonate, evoking strong gasps. The temperature of cold air, the touch of hands, and the pressure of the bed below are some of the afferent sensory stimuli that contribute to respiratory stimulation. Respiratory stimulation is also facilitated by the reduction of endorphin levels in blood: endorphins are produced by the placenta and exert an inhibitory effect on the respiratory center. Also, the norepinephrine secreted by the neonate during birth sensitizes the peripheral chemoreceptors to hypoxia: neonatal breathing is driven more by hypoxic drive than by hypercapnic drive.

The fetal lungs are filled with fluid. Some of this fluid is squeezed out as the neonate passes through the birth canal. As air enters the lungs, some of the fluid evaporates, and the rest gets absorbed into the pulmonary capillaries as the dynamics of capillary fluid exchange changes with lung expansion.

Summary

- The rhythmic neural activity that produces the pattern of inspiration and expiration is generated in the medulla.

- The descending motor pathways innervate the muscles involved in all aspects of ventilation.

- There are several sensory receptors located in the upper and lower respiratory pathways that give rise to reflex modulation of the resting breathing pattern.

Applying What You Know

49.1. When examined in the emergency room, Ms. Eng had a respiratory rate of 35/min, considerably higher than normal. What change in the motor output from the medulla occurs when breathing frequency increases? If Ms. Eng increases her tidal volume, what change in neural output occurs?

The chemical control of breathing is aimed at maintaining the partial pressure of oxygen (PO_2) and carbon dioxide (PCO_2) in arterial blood at ~95 mm Hg and 40 mm Hg, respectively. This is achieved by readjusting the rate and depth of breathing (thus changing alveolar ventilation—$\dot{V}_A$) whenever there is a change in the arterial PO_2 or PCO_2.

General Models: Homeostasis and Communications

This is another example of homeostasis, the maintenance of a constant internal environment. Respiratory homeostasis functions much like the maintenance of a constant mean arterial pressure by the cardiovascular system. Information flow (cell-to-cell communications) from chemoreceptors to the central nervous system (CNS) and from the CNS to the respiratory muscle is essential for the homeostatic mechanism to function.

Respiratory Chemoreceptors

Respiratory chemoreceptors are sensory receptors for the detection of PO_2, PCO_2, and pH of blood. Their location may be central (within the CNS) or peripheral (in the peripheral nervous system). They bring about reflex changes in the rate and depth of breathing in response to hypoxia, hypercapnia, and acidemia. The response to hypoxia is mediated entirely by peripheral chemoreceptors; the response to hypercapnia and acidemia is mediated mainly (75%) by central chemoreceptors and partly (25%) by peripheral chemoreceptors.

Peripheral Chemoreceptors

Peripheral chemoreceptors are the carotid and aortic bodies (**Fig. 50.1**). These are located in the connective tissue associated with the vessel wall, at the bifurcation of the common carotid and on the arch of the aorta, respectively. Both are stimulated by a low PO_2 and high PCO_2 in the arterial blood perfusing them, but the response of the aortic bodies is weaker.

The carotid and aortic bodies are made of two types of cells, type I and type II cells. The type I, or glomus, cells resemble the chromaffin cells of the adrenal glands (see Chapter 80) and release dopamine in response to hypoxia. The cells synapse with the afferent nerve endings bearing dopamine (D_2) receptors on them. The type II cells are glia-like supporting cells.

Type I glomus cell membranes have a population of potassium (K^+) channels that close down at low arterial PO_2, high PCO_2, or low pH. This results in the depolarization of the glomus cell. The exact mechanism of how these three different stimuli act on the K^+ channels remains uncertain. Depolarization of the glomus cell opens up the L-type Ca^{2+} channels in the glomus cell membrane, leading to a rise in Ca^{2+} influx. The Ca^{2+} influx triggers the release of dopamine as a neurotransmitter, which excites the afferent nerve endings. Like most other cells,

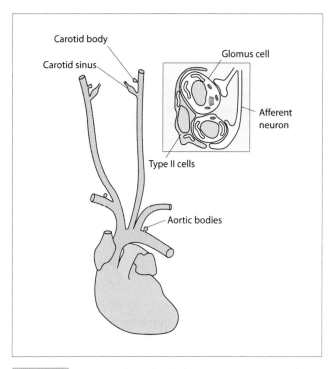

Fig. 50.1   Location of peripheral chemoreceptors. (*Inset*) Glomus cells present inside the chemoreceptors.

glomus cells also depolarize when the plasma K^+ increases. The depolarization initiates increased afferent nerve discharge even in the absence of hypoxia. Because the plasma K^+ level rises during exercise, this may be a contributory mechanism in exercise-induced hyperpnea (see below).

Afferent neurons from the carotid bodies pass through the carotid sinus nerve and glossopharyngeal nerve to reach the medullary respiratory center. Afferent fibers from the aortic bodies reach the medulla through the vagus nerve. The frequency of discharge in the afferent nerve fibers arising from the glomus cells is proportional to the fall in PO_2 or the rise in PCO_2 of arterial blood.

Central Chemoreceptors

Central chemoreceptors are located on the ventral surface of the medulla oblongata and are therefore also called medullary chemoreceptors (**Fig. 50.2**). The central chemoreceptors are distinct from the respiratory neurons that are located deeper inside the medulla and generate the respiratory rhythm.

Central chemoreceptors are not stimulated by hypoxia; rather, like any other cell, they are depressed by hypoxia. Central chemoreceptors are stimulated by a fall in pH of the cerebrospinal fluid (CSF) and the brain interstitial fluid. The magnitude of the stimulation is proportionate to the rise in hydrogen (H^+) concentration. A rise in arterial PCO_2 stimulates the chemoreceptors because the CO_2 readily diffuses from arterial blood into the CSF and reacts with water to generate H^+.

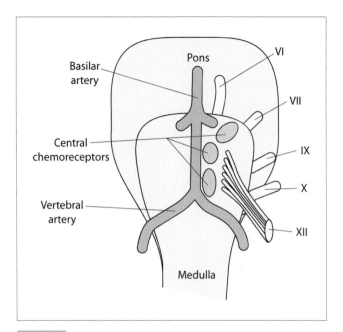

Fig. 50.2 Central chemoreceptors are located in the medulla but are distinct from the neurons that generate the respiratory rhythm.

A fall in arterial pH also stimulates the chemoreceptors. However, if the arterial PCO_2 is held constant experimentally, a decrease in arterial pH fails to stimulate the chemoreceptors because neither H^+ ions nor bicarbonate (HCO_3^-) ions cross the blood–brain barrier readily or in sufficient amounts to affect the CSF pH. Thus, a fall in arterial pH stimulates the central chemoreceptors in three stages. First, the low arterial pH results in a high arterial PCO_2. Next, the CO_2 diffuses into the CSF to lower its pH. Finally, the low CSF pH stimulates the chemoreceptors.

The central chemoreceptors exhibit the phenomenon of adaptation; a maintained increase of arterial PCO_2 does not continue to stimulate the central receptors. This occurs because of mechanisms in the blood–brain barrier that begin to "pump" bicarbonate ions into the CSF, which reduces the concentration of hydrogen ions that are present. This phenomenon takes many hours or days to occur.

Chemical Regulation of Breathing

Maintenance of Respiratory Equilibrium

The respiratory control system attempts to regulate arterial PO_2 and PCO_2 within a normal range. This is achieved by controlling the breathing frequency and tidal volume to change alveolar ventilation. Hyperpnea (increased ventilation) and hypopnea (decreased ventilation) are responses intended to restore arterial PO_2 and PCO_2 to normal values. If increased ventilation is present, and if it causes arterial PCO_2 to decrease below its normal level, this represents a state of hyperventilation.

Respiratory disorders are commonly associated with a fall in arterial PO_2, a rise in arterial PCO_2, and a fall in arterial pH. The low arterial PO_2 stimulates only the peripheral chemoreceptors, whereas the high arterial PCO_2 and low pH stimulate both peripheral and central chemoreceptors. Of the three, hy-

percapnia provides the strongest respiratory drive. The stimulated chemoreceptors reflexively increase breathing, as explained above. The hyperventilation produced raises the PO_2, lowers the PCO_2, and raises the arterial pH. The homeostatic mechanism regulating partial pressure of oxygen (P_aO_2) and carbon dioxide in arterial blood (P_aCO_2) can be seen in **Fig. 50.3**.

There are situations where the reflex increase in ventilation may not have a corrective effect. Take the example of interstitial lung disease (Chapter 52) in which the diffusion capacity of the respiratory membrane is reduced. The low diffusion capacity does not significantly affect the diffusion of CO_2, which is highly diffusible because of its lipid solubility. However, the diffusion of O_2 is impaired, resulting in hypoxia. The hypoxia reflexively stimulates hyperventilation, which restores the PO_2 to normal but lowers the PCO_2 below normal level.

Combined effect of O_2, CO_2, and pH on ventilation | Pulmonary ventilation varies linearly with the increase in PCO_2 (**Fig. 50.4**). In hypoxic states, a small rise in arterial PCO_2 produces a greater increase in ventilation. In other words, the linear relationship between PCO_2 and ventilation becomes steeper at low arterial PO_2. Thus, for each value of PCO_2, there is a family of lines, with each line representing the PCO_2–ventilation relationship at a different PO_2. A fall in pH shifts the entire family of CO_2-response lines to the left. In other words, if the pH is low, the same amount of respiratory stimulation is produced at a lower arterial PCO_2 level.

The combined effect of PO_2, PCO_2, and arterial pH explains why ventilation is stimulated only when the arterial PO_2 falls below 60 mm Hg (**Fig. 50.5**). Between a PO_2 of 100 and 60 mm Hg, there is considerable stimulation of the carotid and aortic chemoreceptors. Yet there is little increase in ventilation because any increase in ventilation reduces the hypercapnic ventilatory drive due to CO_2 washout. Respiratory drive is also reduced due to a slight rise in arterial pH that is associated with the increased deoxygenation of hemoglobin in hypoxia. The arterial pH rises because deoxyhemoglobin is a weaker acid than oxyhemoglobin. For hypoxic drive to be effective, it must be strong enough to overcome the respiratory inhibition caused by hypocapnia and a rise in blood pH.

Respiratory Correction of Acidosis and Alkalosis

The lungs can compensate for both acidosis and alkalosis that are of nonrespiratory (renal and/or metabolic) origin. The related aspects of renal correction of acid–base balance are discussed in Chapter 58.

Respiratory response to acidosis | In metabolic acidosis, the PCO_2 is high. The high PCO_2 stimulates hyperventilation, causing blood CO_2 washout. As a result, the PCO_2 decreases, and the pH is restored to normal. For example, in diabetic ketoacidosis, there is pronounced respiratory stimulation (Kussmaul breathing). The hyperventilation causes CO_2 washout, producing a compensatory rise in pH.

Respiratory response to alkalosis | In metabolic alkalosis, the PCO_2 is low. The low blood PCO_2 depresses ventilation, resulting in CO_2 retention. As a result, the PCO_2 and the pH are restored to normal. For example, excessive vomiting with loss of hydrochloric acid (HCl) from the stomach results in meta-

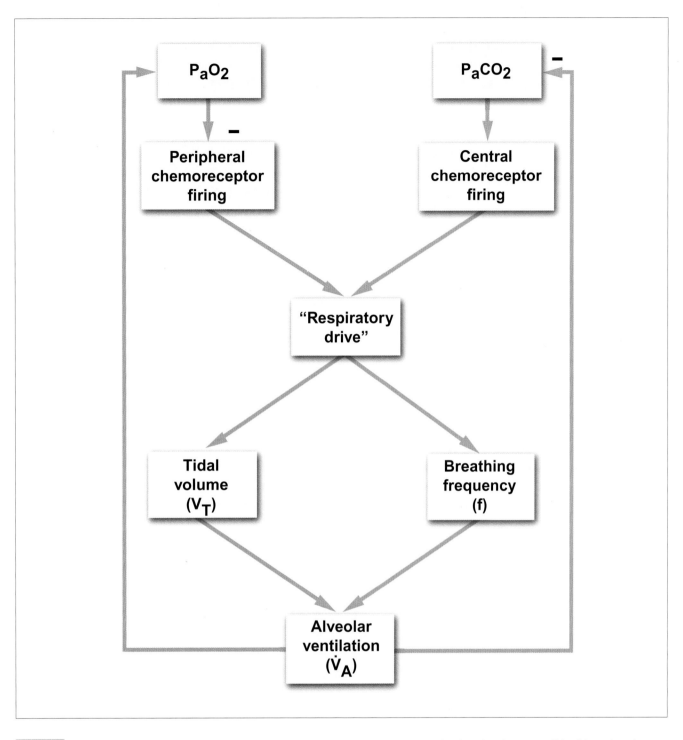

Fig. 50.3 Both the partial pressure of oxygen in arterial blood (P_aO_2) and the partial pressure of carbon dioxide in arterial blood (P_aCO_2) are homeostatically regulated by a reflex mechanism that changes breathing frequency and tidal volume in a direction that will restore the regulated variables to their desired levels.

bolic alkalosis. The alkalosis depresses ventilation, and the arterial PCO_2 rises, lowering the pH toward normal.

Exercise-induced Hyperpnea

Why is exercise associated with hyperpnea? The increased ventilation is unlikely to be due to stimulation of the central or peripheral chemoreceptors because the PO_2, PCO_2, and pH of arterial blood remain almost unchanged in exercise. In the venous blood, however, the PO_2 is low, PCO_2 is high, and pH is low, and it is possible that these are sensed by chemoreceptors in the large systemic veins or pulmonary artery. It is also possible that a metabolite produced by exercising muscles,

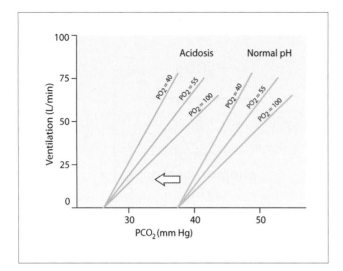

Fig. 50.4 Combined effects of carbon dioxide (CO_2), oxygen (O_2), and acidity (pH) on pulmonary ventilation. At any arterial partial pressure of carbon dioxide (PCO_2), decreasing arterial partial pressure of oxygen (PO_2) increases ventilation.

for example, K^+, enters the blood and stimulates the central or peripheral chemoreceptors. The rise in blood temperature during exercise could also stimulate the respiratory center. Yet another possibility is that when the motor cortex sends voluntary commands to the exercising muscles, it simultaneously sends direct stimulatory impulses to the respiratory centers. The respiratory center could also be stimulated by afferents from moving joints and the stretch receptors of exercising muscles. Finally, the epinephrine released during exercise could be increasing the sensitivity of the respiratory center so that even small changes in arterial PO_2, PCO_2, and pH cause hyperventilation.

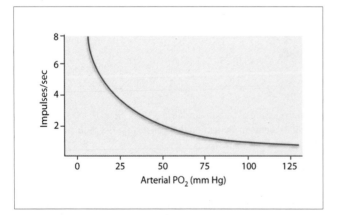

Fig. 50.5 Effect of oxygen on peripheral chemoreceptor afferents. As arterial partial pressure of oxygen (PO_2) falls, the firing rate increases. Note that the right-hand side of this curve is not really flat, and increases of arterial PO_2 above the normal value of 100 mm Hg causes decreased firing.

Respiratory Disequilibria

The PO_2 and PCO_2 of blood are normally maintained within a narrow physiologic range that is determined by the equilibrium between the rate of O_2 consumption and CO_2 production, on the one hand, and the rate and depth of breathing, on the other. When this equilibrium is disrupted, it results in respiratory disequilibria, the examples of which are hypocapnia, hypoxia, hypercapnia, and oxygen toxicity.

Hypoxia

Hypoxia is O_2 deficiency at the tissue level. There are four types of hypoxia. In hypoxic hypoxia, the PO_2 of the arterial blood is low. In anemic hypoxia, the O_2 content of blood is low despite a normal arterial PO_2. In stagnant hypoxia, the O_2 delivery to the tissues is low despite a normal O_2 content of blood. In histotoxic hypoxia, the tissues suffer from hypoxia despite an adequate delivery of O_2. The principal signs and symptoms of hypoxia are hyperventilation, cyanosis, and cerebral symptoms.

Hyperpnea occurs when peripheral chemoreceptors are stimulated by low arterial PO_2. Hence, increased ventilation occurs in hypoxic hypoxia and also in histotoxic hypoxia if the glomus cells are poisoned. Hyperpnea is not seen in anemic hypoxia so long as the arterial PO_2 remains normal. Hyperpnea is not seen in stagnant hypoxia either, because the blood supply to the carotid bodies is extremely high (2000 mL/100 g of tissue, the highest for any tissue), and the glomus cells rarely if ever suffer from O_2 deficiency so long as the blood PO_2 is normal.

Cyanosis is a bluish discoloration of the skin and mucous membranes. It is seen when the deoxyhemoglobin concentration in blood exceeds 5 g/dL. There are two types of cyanosis: peripheral and central. *Peripheral cyanosis* is seen in the nail beds and is suggestive of stagnant hypoxia. The distal parts of the body are very poorly perfused in hypotensive states and extract large amounts of O_2 from hemoglobin, raising the concentration of deoxyhemoglobin. *Central cyanosis* is seen in the mucous membranes of the tongue tip and lips and in the earlobes where the skin is thin. These areas normally receive high blood supply and become cyanotic only if the O_2 saturation of blood is low, as in hypoxic hypoxia. Cyanosis does not occur in anemic hypoxia. In fact, it cannot occur in severe anemia if the hemoglobin concentration is 5 g/dL or less. Cyanosis does not occur in histotoxic hypoxia either because the O_2 saturation of hemoglobin is normal.

Cerebral symptoms of hypoxia resemble those of alcohol toxicity with impaired judgment, drowsiness or excitement, dulled pain sensibility, disorientation, and headache. Other symptoms include nausea, vomiting, tachycardia, and hypertension.

Hypoxic hypoxia is the most common form of hypoxia seen. The causes of hypoxic hypoxia are (1) reduced PO_2 in atmospheric air at high altitudes (high-altitude hypoxia), (2) reduced ventilation due to restrictive or obstructive lung disorders, and (3) reduced diffusion capacity of O_2 across the respiratory membrane. This occurs when the respiratory membrane becomes thicker, as in interstitial lung disorders, or when there is a marked reduction in the area of the respiratory membrane, as in emphysema. In addition, there is yet another mechanism, (4) shunting of blood, bypassing the well-ventilated alveoli. This occurs due to alveolar ventilation–perfusion mismatch. It also occurs when there is a right-to-left shunt in the heart: deoxygenated blood from the right side of the heart bypasses the lung to enter the left ventricle. This is seen in congenital heart diseases like the tetralogy of Fallot.

Anemic hypoxia occurs in severe anemia. Mild to moderate anemia usually does not produce hypoxia due to compensatory increase in red cell 2,3-diphosphoglycerate (DPG). However, such patients usually become hypoxic during exercise. Anemic hypoxia also occurs in carbon monoxide poisoning and methemoglobinemia.

Carbon monoxide (CO) poisoning results in the formation of carboxyhemoglobin (COHb), which reduces the amount of Hb available for O_2 transport. CO has a very high affinity for hemoglobin and once bound, is difficult to dislodge from hemoglobin. Moreover, the COHb shifts the O_2 dissociation curve of the remaining Hb to the left, decreasing the amount of O_2 that can be released. Hence, inactivation of Hb by CO poisoning is worse than having a reduced Hb concentration. Both hyperventilation and cyanosis are absent in CO poisoning. The cherry-red color of COHb that is visible through skin and mucous membranes can, however, be confused with cyanosis. Death results due to hypoxic brain damage. Management of CO poisoning includes termination of exposure to CO and initiation of O_2 therapy, with hyperbaric O_2 if necessary.

Stagnant hypoxia occurs during circulatory shock (decreased blood pressure with decreased tissue perfusion; see Chapter 38). The most severely affected organs are the kidneys and heart, which have high O_2 demand. Stagnant hypoxia also occurs in congestive heart failure, especially in the liver and brain, which are seriously affected by venous congestion.

Histotoxic hypoxia occurs when the tissue cells cannot make use of the O_2 supplied to them. It is caused, among other things, by cyanide poisoning, which inhibits cytochrome oxidase. The general treatment for histotoxic hypoxia is hyperbaric oxygen therapy. Specific treatment for cyanide poisoning includes nitrites and methylene blue, which act by forming methemoglobin from hemoglobin. Methemoglobin detoxifies cyanide by converting it to cyanmethemoglobin. However, overenthusiastic treatment with nitrites can cause anemic hypoxia by forming too much methemoglobin and reducing the hemoglobin concentration.

Oxygen Treatment

Oxygen-rich gas mixture is useful when the blood PO_2 is low, either due to reduced alveolar PO_2 or due to inadequate diffusion of O_2 across the respiratory membrane. Hence, it is administered in most types of hypoxic hypoxia and is commonly used in chronic obstructive pulmonary diseases. For the same reason, it is of little use in those types of hypoxia (stagnant, anemic, and histotoxic) in which there is no reduction in blood PO_2. Breathing O_2 is also useless in hypoxic hypoxia if it is due to ventilation–perfusion mismatch (i.e., the deoxygenated blood bypasses the well-ventilated alveoli).

Caution is required while giving O_2 therapy to patients with severe pulmonary failure and high PCO_2. The central chemoreceptors in these patients have adapted to the high PCO_2 that is present; hence, breathing is driven by hypoxic stimulation of peripheral chemoreceptors. Oxygen therapy in such a situation may produce apnea by taking away this hypoxic drive.

Hyperbaric 100% O_2 raises the amount of O_2 dissolved in plasma; therefore, it is unaffected by hemoglobin concentration. It is useful in the treatment of carbon monoxide poisoning, decompression sickness and air embolism, severe anemia, and wounds with poor blood supply. For therapeutic use, hyperbaric 100% O_2 should not be administered at pressures higher than 3 atmospheres or for more than 5 hours.

Oxygen Toxicity

One hundred percent oxygen has toxic effects due to the production of the superoxide anion (a free radical) and H_2O_2. When administered for 8 hours or more, it causes irritation of the airways.

If it is administered chronically to infants, they may develop bronchopulmonary dysplasia (characterized by lung cysts and opacities) and retrolental fibroplasia (formation of opaque vascular tissue in the eyes, which can lead to serious visual defects). Normal retinal vascularization is stimulated by mild hypoxia. Oxygen therapy always tends to reduce the hypoxic drive, and the normal vascular pattern fails to develop. Vitamin E, an antioxidant, has been used for the treatment of retrolental fibroplasia.

Hyperbaric 100% O_2 produces, in addition to airway irritation, nervous symptoms such as muscle twitching, tinnitus, convulsions, and coma. The greater the pressure, the faster is the onset of symptoms.

Hypercapnia and Respiratory Acidosis

Hypercapnia is retention of CO_2 in the body. It can occur as a compensatory response to metabolic alkalosis; but when hypercapnia is the primary problem, it is associated with respiratory acidosis because any increase in CO_2 promptly generates excess H^+.

An increase in CO_2 production rarely produces hypercapnia because it is promptly washed out by the resulting increased ventilation. The PCO_2 does not rise even when there is considerable reduction in the diffusion capacity of the lung because CO_2 is lipid soluble and promptly diffuses out across the respiratory membrane. Hence, hypercapnia occurs essentially in two types of conditions: (1) hypoventilation, as occurs in restrictive lung disorders and in respiratory depression due to drugs and cerebral diseases; and (2) ventilation–perfusion mismatch, which is commonly present in chronic obstructive pulmonary disease (COPD).

The principal signs of hypercapnia are hyperpnea and CO_2 narcosis. *Hyperpnea* occurs reflexively due to the stimulation of respiration by hypercapnia. Reflex hyperpnea may not be possible in a restrictive lung disorder. In such case, when the arterial PCO_2 reaches high enough levels, *CO2 narcosis* can occur. This condition is characterized by symptoms of central nervous system (CNS) depression, such as confusion, diminished sensory acuity, respiratory depression, and coma.

Hypocapnia and Respiratory Alkalosis

Hypocapnia is a reduction of CO_2 in the body. It can occur as a corrective response to metabolic acidosis; but when hypocapnia is the primary problem, it is associated with respiratory alkalosis because any decrease in CO_2 results in a decrease in H^+ concentration.

Hypocapnia occurs due to hyperventilation. It is seen in hypoxic conditions that are not associated with restrictive lung disorders, for example, high-altitude hypoxia or the early stages of interstitial lung disease—the latter does not affect diffusion of CO_2, which is highly lipid soluble, but impairs O_2 diffusion, producing hypoxia. The hypoxia stimulates hyperventilation with consequent CO_2 washout and hypocapnia. In restrictive lung disorders, however, the hyperventilation is not possible; therefore, hypocapnia is uncommon. It is seen in compulsive hyperventilation due to hysteria; excessive stimulation of the respiratory center due to fever, anxiety, cerebral tumors, or in pregnancy; overenthusiastic artificial ventilation; and excessive exercise.

The respiratory alkalosis associated with hypocapnia causes cerebral vasoconstriction, resulting in faintness. Alkalosis also lowers the ionized Ca^{2+} in plasma, resulting in tetany and/or paresthesias.

Asphyxia

Asphyxia is the simultaneous development of acute hypercapnia and hypoxia. It occurs due to airway obstruction as in choking or drowning. It is associated with violent respiratory efforts, acidosis, and increased catecholamine secretion, causing high blood pressure and heart rate, and predisposing the hypoxic myocardium to ventricular fibrillation. Eventually the respiratory efforts cease, the blood pressure falls, and cardiac arrest occurs within 5 minutes.

Drowning | Only 10% of deaths in drowning occur due to asphyxia. The asphyxia occurs initially due to breath holding and after breathing resumes due to the laryngospasm triggered by the cold water. The lungs remain dry in these deaths. In others, the lungs are flooded with water. Freshwater drowning causes plasma dilution and intravascular hemolysis. Drowning in hypertonic seawater results in hypovolemia. If rescued and resuscitated, these circulatory effects have to be reversed.

Respiratory Dysrhythmias

Blood gases have an important role in determining the breathing pattern. Given the conditions that predispose to oscillations in a control system, they can cause respiratory dysrhythmias, some of which are discussed below.

Cheyne-Stokes Breathing

Cheyne-Stokes breathing is periodic breathing characterized by a regular waxing and waning of ventilation at a constant frequency, punctuated by periods of apnea (**Fig. 50.6A**). The arterial PO_2 and PCO_2 fluctuate during each cycle of Cheyne-

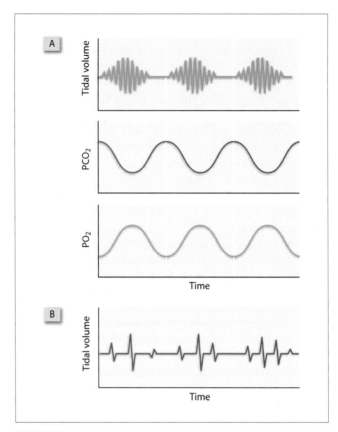

Fig. 50.6 **(A)** Cheyne-Stokes breathing. **(B)** Biot breathing.

Stokes breathing. The PO_2 is lowest and the PCO_2 highest at the end of the apnea. The factors producing Cheyne-Stokes breathing are discussed below.

Hypoxia from any cause predisposes to Cheyne-Stokes breathing if the hypoxic drive is greater than the hypercapneic drive. When driven by hypercapnia, ventilation is too tightly controlled to allow any oscillation. A reduction in the functional residual capacity (FRC) or total lung capacity (TLC) results in larger changes in alveolar PO_2 and PCO_2, with any change in breathing predisposing to oscillations. Cheyne-Stokes breathing occurs when the circulation time is prolonged, as in circulatory shock. It may also appear if there is cerebrovascular disease, and the sensitivity of central chemoreceptors to hypercapnic drive is impaired. If there is a prolonged circulation time, it, too, will contribute to the frequent appearance of Cheyne-Stokes breathing in otherwise normal older subjects. Cheyne-Stokes breathing is common in sleep and in subjects over the age of ~45.

Sedative drugs and any disorder that reduces the level of consciousness may also precipitate Cheyne-Stokes breathing. Premature infants whose cerebral functions are still immature may develop Cheyne-Stokes breathing.

Biot Breathing

Also called ataxic breathing, this is a pattern of slow and irregular breathing with impaired ventilatory response to both CO_2 and O_2 (**Fig. 50.6B**). It occurs due to the disruption of the

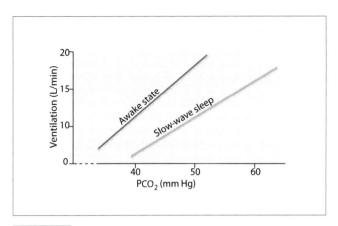

Fig. 50.7 Effect of arousal state (awake/asleep) on hypercapnic respiratory drive.

- Peripheral chemoreceptors sense arterial PO_2, but also arterial PCO_2 and pH.

- Central chemoreceptors sense arterial PCO_2, although the actual stimulus to the sensors is the H^+ ions in the cerebrospinal fluid. The central receptors exhibit adaptation.

Applying What You Know

50.1. Predict (increase/decrease/no change) the changes in the following respiratory parameters that will occur 60 minutes after Ms. Eng is started on supplemental oxygen: P_aO_2, P_aCO_2, tidal volume, and breathing frequency.

normal medullary rhythmicity of breathing and is seen in a wide variety of medullary pathology.

Breathing during Sleep

The control of the cerebral cortex over respiration is reduced in sleep, and the ventilatory response to hypercapnia changes (**Fig. 50.7**). During stages 1 and 2 of nonrapid eye movement (NREM) sleep, there may be periodic breathing, but in stages 3 and 4, the rate and rhythm become normal. In REM sleep, both rate and rhythm become erratic, especially when there are rapid eye movements. There may be phases of hyperventilation and apnea. These respiratory disturbances are attributable to reduced central inspiratory drive, reduced sensitivity of peripheral chemoreceptors, and reduced tone of respiratory muscles.

Posthyperventilation Periodic Breathing

When a subject hyperventilates until there is a feeling of faintness, it is followed by a period of apnea. There is a slow recovery from apnea. However, after a few breaths, apnea follows again. This continues for a few cycles until breathing stabilizes at the normal level. A possible mechanism of the period breathing is explained as follows.

Hyperventilation causes apnea due to CO_2 washout. During the apneic phase, the PCO_2 rises slowly, while PO_2 falls faster because the respiratory quotient (the ratio of CO_2 produced to O_2 consumed) is usually less than 1. Feeble breathing resumes due to the hypoxic drive even before the PCO_2 has been completely restored. However, a few breaths again take away the hypoxic drive with resultant apnea. The cycle continues until the arterial PCO_2 rises to the normal level and provides sustained respiratory drive.

Summary

- Regulation of arterial PO_2 and PCO_2 is achieved by a control system that incorporates peripheral and central chemoreceptors.

Breathing in unusual environments such as underwater or at high altitude poses special problems for the respiratory system. A consideration of these challenges and how they are solved can illuminate many important aspects of respiratory physiology.

Breathing under Water

Obviously, one cannot breathe normally while under water. There are, however, several ways to sustain underwater activities; these are discussed below.

Breath-holding is the oldest method of surviving under water. Following a deep inspiration, the breath can be held for 4 to 5 minutes (with training). The duration is shorter if the breath is held at end-expiration. The breath-holding time can be prolonged by hyperventilation (although there are dangers to this) or breathing pure O_2 prior to breath-holding. Hypoxia and hypercapnia cannot be the sole factors limiting the breath-holding time because rhythmic respiratory movements against a closed glottis prolongs the breath-holding time by a few seconds beyond the normal breakpoint before breath-holding gives way. For the same reason, breathing a high CO_2–low O_2 gas mixture allows breathing for longer durations than the usual breath-holding time. Encouragement prolongs breath-holding time, implying a role for psychologic factors.

Breathing through a snorkel | A snorkel is a breathing tube extending above the surface of the water, used in swimming just below the surface. The tube represents an extension of the anatomic dead space; the tidal volume must be increased to ensure that adequate alveolar ventilation is generated. Moreover, the work of breathing increases due to the additional effort required to expand the chest against the pressure of the surrounding water.

Breathing air from a tank | It is, of course, possible to carry underwater a tank containing air or oxygen. However, it will not be possible to breathe from the container if the air in it is at 1 atmosphere (atm) of pressure. The water pressure is very high at greater depths (the pressure increases by 1 atm for every 10 m of depth in seawater, so that at a depth of 30 m, the pressure will be 4 atm). At such high pressure, the thorax gets compressed. The intrathoracic pressure rises and becomes nearly equal to the surrounding water pressure. Hence, a few millimeters of pressure reduction caused by inspiratory expansion of the thorax cannot suck in air from a container that contains air at 1 atm pressure. For breathing from a container, it is necessary to carry pressurized air or gas mixtures.

For breathing underwater, therefore, divers use the SCUBA equipment (self-contained underwater breathing apparatus) consisting of one or two compressed-air tanks strapped to the back and connected by a hose to a mouthpiece. The SCUBA gear allows the diver to stay underwater for long periods.

Problems of High-Pressure Breathing

In compressed air, say, at 4 atm (~3000 mm Hg), all the gases have partial pressures that are four times their normal value.

Thus, the partial pressure of oxygen (PO_2) in the compressed air will be ~600 mm Hg; the partial pressure of nitrogen (PN_2) will be ~2400 mm Hg. The corresponding figures in the alveoli and arteries will be somewhat less, but still very high. The gases distribute themselves throughout the body in all body fluids, remaining dissolved at high pressure. Their presence in the body at high pressure causes undesirable symptoms. An additional problem is that compressed gases have higher density and require much larger respiratory effort to be moved in and out of the lungs (i.e., the work of breathing increases).

If a diver breathes compressed air, the increased PO_2 can cause oxygen toxicity, the increased PN_2 can cause nitrogen narcosis, and the increased partial pressure of the inert atmospheric gases (which includes helium) can cause high-pressure nervous syndrome, or HPNS. Breathing a high-pressure O_2–helium mixture is more likely to cause HPNS.

Nitrogen narcosis | At pressures of 4 to 5 atm (i.e., at depths of 30–40 m in the ocean), 80% N_2 produces euphoria; therefore, nitrogen narcosis is also known as "rapture of the deep." At greater pressures, the symptoms resemble alcohol intoxication. Manual dexterity may be maintained, but intellectual functions are impaired.

High-pressure nervous syndrome | At high pressure, inert gases have a nonspecific anesthetic effect on nerve membranes. HPNS is characterized by tremors and drowsiness. Unlike nitrogen narcosis, intellectual functions are not severely affected, but manual dexterity is impaired.

Problems of Rapid Drop in Pressure

Decompression sickness occurs when a diver, for whatever reason, ascends to the surface too rapidly. It occurs only if the diver is breathing pressurized air. If the diving is done using breath-holding, decompression sickness will not occur no matter how rapid the ascent is.

Decompression sickness is characterized by bends, chokes, and strokes. *Bends* are intense joint pains that occur when gas bubbles form in tissues. There is associated paresthesia and itching. *Chokes* are the choking sensation and dyspnea that occur due to gas bubbles in pulmonary capillaries. *Strokes* affect the cerebral or coronary vasculature; they occur due to gas bubbles in cerebral or coronary microcirculation, resulting in ischemia. In explosive decompression, as occurs when an aircraft flying at a great height gets suddenly depressurized, a fatal air embolism can form. The reason why gas bubbles form in blood and tissues is as follows.

As a diver breathing 80% N_2 ascends from a dive, the elevated alveolar PN_2 falls, and with it, the PN_2 of the arterial blood and body fluids also falls. It is important to recall here that the partial pressure of a dissolved gas is the ambient pressure that keeps the gas in solution. Thus, when the partial pressure of N_2 decreases, it is unable to keep in solution the large volume of N_2 that was dissolved at a much higher pressure. The N_2 therefore bubbles out rapidly from blood, in much the same way that CO_2 bubbles out of a fizzy soft drink when the bottle is opened, releasing the pressure.

If the PN_2 falls slowly, the N_2 comes out of blood slowly and is exhaled without bubble formation. This is called *slow decompression.* However, during rapid ascent through water, the decompression is fast, and bubbles form in the tissues and blood, causing decompression sickness.

Treatment of decompression sickness is prompt recompression in a pressure chamber, followed by slow decompression. Recompression is frequently lifesaving. Recovery is often complete, but there may be residual neurologic signs as a result of irreversible damage to the nervous system.

For prolonged dives at great depths, SCUBA divers use oxygen–helium mixtures instead of air. Helium has one-fifth the solubility of nitrogen and therefore dissolves less in body fluids. Being much less dense than nitrogen, compressed helium offers much less resistance to breathing than nitrogen. Finally, pressurized helium produces much less intellectual impairment than pressurized nitrogen.

Breathing at High Altitude

Breathing at high altitudes, where the atmospheric pressure is low, poses a different set of problems than breathing underwater. The problems of ascending to high altitude with or without carrying oxygen are summarized in **Table 51.1**.

If a person ascends to high altitudes without oxygen, he develops hypoxic symptoms at 4000 m and loses consciousness at 6000 m. He can climb higher only if he carries 100% O_2. However, if the O_2 cylinder is not pressurized so as to provide O_2 at 760 mm Hg, the PO_2 will still fall as the ambient pressure decreases. For example, at an altitude of 10,000 m (which is a little higher than Mount Everest), the ambient atmospheric pressure, and therefore the alveolar pressure, too, is 187 mm Hg. The aqueous tension in alveolar air is 47 mm Hg, and the alveolar PCO_2 is 40 mm Hg. Therefore, even on breathing 100% O_2, the alveolar PO_2 will be 187 – 47 – 40 = 100 mm Hg. Thus,

Table 51.1 Signs and Symptoms at High Altitudes

Altitude	P_{atm}	Effects on Body
Ascent without oxygen		
3000 m	530	Hyperventilation starts
4000 m	460	Hypoxic symptoms appear
5000 m	400	Hypoxic symptoms become severe
6000 m	350	Consciousness is lost
Ascent with oxygen at ambient pressure		
10,000 m	187	Body at the brink of hypoxia
14,000 m	100	Consciousness is lost
20,000 m	< 47	Blood begins to boil*

*This is entirely a theoretical proposition because a person trying to climb to this height without pressured air will die long before the blood begins to boil, not to mention that the highest mountain is only 9000 m. *Abbreviations*: m, meter; P_{atm}, atmospheric pressure (mm Hg).

Table 51.2 Compensatory Responses to High-Altitude Hypoxia

Increased oxygenation of blood through
- Persistent hyperventilation
- Increased diffusion capacity of lungs

Increased O_2 delivery to the tissues through
- Increased cardiac output
- Polycythemia produced by increased erythropoietin secretion
- Right shift of O_2 dissociation curve (due to high DPG content)
- Increased tissue capillary density
- Increase in myoglobin

Enhancement of the tissue oxidative machinery through
- Larger number of mitochondria
- Increase in the tissue content of cytochrome oxidase

Abbreviations: DPG, diphosphoglycerate; O_2, oxygen.

the atmospheric pressure of 187 mm Hg (at 10,000 m altitude) is the lowest barometric pressure at which the normal alveolar PO_2 of 100 mm Hg is possible even when breathing 100% oxygen. If the person continues to climb higher than 10,000 m, breathing unpressurized 100% oxygen, he will become hypoxic and will finally lose consciousness at 14,000 m.

Acute exposure to high altitude results in some immediate physiologic responses, such as hyperventilation and an increase in cardiac output. These responses often produce unpleasant symptoms, such as breathlessness and palpitation, and have been called *transient mountain sickness,* which must be distinguished from the more ominous sickness that can develop after a lag of 6 hours to 4 days and is called *acute mountain sickness.*

Acute Mountain Sickness
Acute mountain sickness usually develops within a day of arrival at high altitude and lasts about a week. It is characterized by oliguria, cerebral edema, and pulmonary edema, which are explained below. Treatment includes rest, O_2 therapy, and calcium (Ca^{2+}) channel-blocking drugs (e.g., nifedipine) that lower pulmonary arterial pressure.

Oliguria | The susceptibility to mountain sickness is highly variable and seems to be related to the ability to produce diuresis: individuals who develop diuresis at high altitude do not develop mountain sickness. Conversely, urine volume is decreased in individuals who develop the condition. However, treatment with diuretics does not prevent mountain sickness. The cause of the oliguria could be the diversion of blood flow to hypoxic muscles, resulting in reduced splanchnic and renal blood flow. It could also be due to a stress-related increase in antidiuretic hormone (ADH) secretion.

Cerebral edema | The low PO_2 at high altitude causes arteriolar dilation, and if cerebral autoregulation does not compensate, there is an increase in cerebral capillary pressure that favors increased transudation of fluid into brain tissue.

Pulmonary edema | Hypoxia, low PO_2 in the alveoli, causes localized vasoconstriction of pulmonary vessels (precapillary). However, because the entire right ventricular output must pass through the pulmonary capillaries, the pulmonary capillary hydrostatic pressure rises. This causes disruption of the walls of the weaker capillaries, resulting in exudation of protein-rich fluid into the lung tissues. High-altitude pulmonary edema remains a major problem that still eludes a satisfactory prevention or cure.

Acclimatization

Over time, acclimatization to high altitude occurs due to compensatory responses to hypoxia (**Table 51.2**). Thus, there is human habitation at altitudes as high as 5500 m. The inhabitants are barrel-chested and markedly polycythemic. They have low alveolar PO_2, but have no hypoxic signs or symptoms. Two of the compensatory responses are discussed below.

Persistent hyperventilation | Unacclimatized individuals are unable to keep up the hyperventilation due to the effects of CO_2 washout. The CO_2 washout not only takes away the respiratory drive, but also causes faintness. Persons acclimatized to high altitudes are, however, able to hyperventilate unabated even when their alveolar and arterial PCO_2 is low due to CO_2 washout. This is because acclimatized people have a normal arterial pH due to renal compensatory mechanisms. This ensures that their peripheral chemoreceptors are adequately driven by hydrogen (H^+) ions. More important, acclimatized persons are able to maintain a slightly acidic cerebrospinal fluid (CSF) pH. This is made possible by a bicarbonate (HCO_3^-) pump located at the blood–brain barrier, which pumps out HCO_3^-. The acidic CSF helps maintain adequate respiratory drive of the central chemoreceptors. It also prevents cerebral vasoconstriction and faintness.

Shift of O_2 dissociation curve to the right | The right shift in the O_2 dissociation curve is due to an increase in the 2,3-DPG content of red cells. However, the concomitant alkalosis produced by hyperventilation tends to produce a left shift. The net result is a small right shift that helps in unloading O_2 to the tissues. The alkalosis due to hyperventilation is corrected by the renal excretion of excess HCO_3^- so that in acclimatized individuals, the alkalosis is minimal.

Chronic Mountain Sickness

Chronic mountain sickness develops in some high-altitude settlers. It probably develops when the peripheral chemoreceptors become insensitive to hypoxia, resulting in severe hypoxic symptoms. There is intense pulmonary vasoconstriction, leading to cor pulmonale. In the absence of hyperventilation, the other adaptive changes become exaggerated, accounting for some of the problems associated with chronic mountain sickness. For example, a severe polycythemia can cause circulatory failure.

Summary

- Breathing at high pressure is most commonly encountered underwater, and several possible problems can arise, including increased work of breathing, nitrogen narcosis, and the bends.

- Breathing at high altitude results in reduced partial pressure of oxygen in arterial blood (P_aO_2), which produces hyper-

ventilation. When P_aO_2 falls far enough, the function of the central nervous system is degraded, and death eventually follows.

Applying What You Know

51.1. Ms. Eng vacations in Hawaii. The weather is perfect, and the water looks quite inviting, so she decides to try snorkeling. Predict the consequences of breathing through a snorkel for 30 minutes on the following parameters: dead space volume, tidal volume, breathing frequency, P_aO_2, P_aCO_2, and the work of breathing.

Pulmonary Function Tests

Pulmonary function tests (PFTs) permit an accurate and reproducible assessment of the functional state of the respiratory system and allow quantification of the severity of disease. They include measurement of lung volumes, airflow rates, lung compliance, and diffusion capacity.

PFTs are used to confirm clinical diagnosis. For instance, the presence of a low 1-second forced expiratory volume (FEV_1) value that is reversed with bronchodilators along with normal diffusion capacity suggests the diagnosis of bronchial asthma when a consistent clinical history is present. However, a similar decrease in FEV_1 in the presence of poor reversal with bronchodilators, decreased elastic recoil, and decreased diffusion capacity with a relevant clinical history would instead suggest a diagnosis of emphysema. PFTs allow early diagnosis, sometimes even before clinical symptoms appear. Decreased diffusion capacity is the earliest change seen in interstitial lung disease.

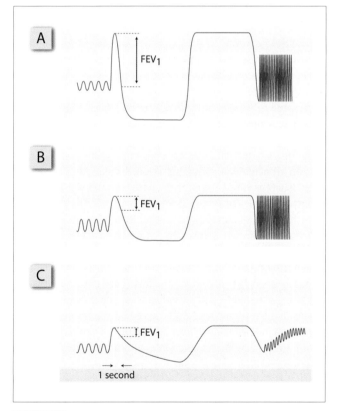

Fig. 52.1 Spirograms recording forced vital capacity, forced expiratory volume in 1 second (FEV_1), and maximum voluntary ventilation in **(A)** a normal subject, **(B)** a restrictive disorder, and **(C)** an obstructive disorder. Note that in an obstructive disorder, hyperventilation is done with reduced tidal volume and at a higher functional residual capacity. (Adapted from Ganong WF. Review of Medical Physiology. Boston: McGraw-Hill; 2005.)

Table 52.1 Comparison of Obstructive and Restrictive Lung Disorders

Obstructive	Restrictive
TLC normal; VC normal, but may be reduced at the expense of increased FRC due to air trapping	TLC and VC are always reduced
FEV_1/FVC is reduced	FEV_1/FVC is normal
The flow–volume curve reduces in height	The flow–volume curve reduces in width

Abbreviations: FEV_1, forced expiratory volume in 1 second; FRC, functional residual capacity; FVC, forced vital capacity; TLC, total lung capacity; VC, vital capacity.

PFTs help in assessing the severity of a respiratory disease; they also help in monitoring the response to treatment. For instance, the severity of asthma is best assessed by measuring FEV_1, and the level of hypoxemia is best assessed by blood gas analysis. Assessment of the severity of airway obstruction helps in fine-tuning drug therapy from time to time. PFTs are also used for the evaluation of fitness and predicting the safety of taking part in strenuous physical exercise. They can indicate which patients with preexisting lung disease can safely undertake long-distance flights because passengers flying at high altitude are exposed to lower partial pressure of oxygen (PO_2) even in pressurized cabins. PFTs are also performed as part of a preanesthetic check-up.

Based on the results of PFTs, respiratory disorders can be categorized into three types: obstructive disorders of ventilation, restrictive disorders of ventilation, and disorders of abnormal gas transfer. The three types of defects often coexist. The differences between obstructive and restrictive lung disorders show up in a spirogram (**Fig. 52.1**) and are summarized in **Table 52.1**.

Obstructive Airway Disorders

Obstructive airway disorders occur due to blockage of airflow anywhere from the large upper airways to the small peripheral airways. Large and small airway obstructions produce different PFT patterns (**Figs. 52.1** and **52.2**). However, obstructive lung disorders primarily are associated with both large and small airway obstructions (**Table 52.2**).

At large lung volumes, the bulk of the resistance to airflow is offered by the large airways. It is therefore the large airway resistance that limits the peak flow rate that can be attained. Hence, in large airway obstruction, the peak expiratory flow rate (PEFR) and FEV_1 decrease. Accordingly, the height of the flow–volume loop decreases, but the slope of the expiratory curve at low lung volumes remains unchanged.

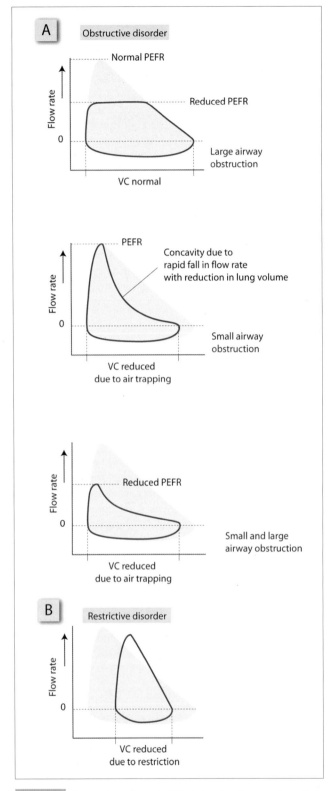

Fig. 52.2 Flow–volume loops in **(A)** obstructive (large and small airways) and **(B)** restrictive disorders. The normal loop is indicated by the yellow shadow. PEFR, peak expiratory flow rate; VC, vital capacity.

The contribution of small airways to airway resistance increases at low lung volumes. Hence, in small airway obstruction, the FEV_1 remains normal, but the FEV_3 and forced expiratory flow rate from 25 to 75% ($FEFR_{25-75\%}$) are abnormally low. Ac-

| Table 52.2 | Common Causes of Obstructive Lung Disorders |

Disease Process	Anatomic Location of Lesion	Cause of Reduced Airflow
Asthma	Large and small airways	Narrowing of airways by smooth muscle contraction, edema, retained secretion
Chronic bronchitis	Large and small airways	Narrowing of airways by fibrosis, secretions, and edema
Emphysema	Large and small airways	Loss of lung elastic recoil
Upper airway obstruction	Large airways (trachea and main bronchi)	Narrowing of large airways – the larynx, trachea, and the lobar bronchi

cordingly, the flow–volume loop does not show any reduction in height, but the expiratory curve becomes concave due to a rapid fall in flow rate with reduction in lung volume. Small airway obstruction is also associated with high closing volume and air trapping; therefore, the vital capacity is reduced.

Bronchial Asthma

Bronchial asthma is clinically defined as an airway disorder that makes the airways prone to bronchoconstriction in response to a wide variety of provoking stimuli. The airway narrowing occurs due to smooth muscle contraction, mucosal edema, and mucus plugging. Characteristic features of this airway narrowing are its spontaneous variability, aggravation on exposure to triggering factors (allergens, cold air, exercise, etc.), and alleviation on bronchodilator administration. Exposure to a provoking agent such as an allergen or exercise initiates an immediate bronchoconstriction followed several hours later by progressive bronchial wall inflammation (predominantly eosinophilic) and mucosal swelling. It is this latter state that is seen in chronic asthma. In the presence of chronic inflammation, the airways respond by bronchoconstriction even to nonspecific irritants, such as a strong smell, cold air, and dust, even if the individual is not allergic to them. Exercise-induced asthma occurs due to the drying of the respiratory passage caused by mouth breathing.

The main reason for airflow limitation is an enhanced bronchomotor tone, which is reversible with bronchodilator drugs. Another reason is dynamic airway obstruction: the collapse of small airways early in expiration. Unlike enhanced bronchomotor tone, the dynamic airway compression does not respond to bronchodilators.

Chronic Bronchitis

Chronic bronchitis is defined clinically. It is diagnosed when there is persistence of cough and excessive mucus secretion on most days over a 3-month period for at least 2 successive years. There is scarring (replacement of elastic tissues with collagen) and distortion of the terminal bronchioles. About 10 to 15% of these patients have a variable degree of airway obstruction and are diagnosed as having *chronic obstructive bronchitis*. It is this chronic obstructive variety of bronchitis that forms a component of chronic obstructive pulmonary disease (COPD) (see below). Some patients of chronic obstructive bronchitis show significant improvement (more than a 20% increase in FEV_1) with bronchodilators. Because reversibility with bronchodilator is characteristic of asthma, these cases of chronic obstructive bronchitis have been called *asthmatic bronchitis*.

Emphysema

Emphysema (**Fig. 52.3**) is defined on the basis of pathologic criteria. It is diagnosed when there is airspace enlargement distal to the terminal bronchiole and destruction of the alveolar wall, provided that the airspace enlargement is irreversible and not associated with fibrosis. The destruction of the alveolar wall reduces lung elasticity; therefore, it reduces the lung's elastic recoil. The reduction in elastic recoil of the lung allows the thorax to enlarge, resulting in the characteristic barrel-chested appearance of a patient with emphysema.

About 5% of cases of emphysema occur due to a genetic deficiency of the enzyme α_1-antitrypsin, which is synthesized by hepatocytes and macrophages. α_1-Antitrypsin inhibits trypsin and elastase; thus, it limits the damage caused by elastases released by neutrophils in inflammatory conditions of the lungs. Hence, patients who are deficient in α_1-antitrypsin are vulnerable to extensive lung damage by neutrophils. Smoking inactivates α_1-antitrypsin and thereby predisposes to emphysema and accelerates its progress in genetically vulnerable patients.

Chronic Obstructive Pulmonary Disease

Chronic obstructive bronchitis and emphysema tend to coexist, probably because both are of inflammatory origin and share some common etiology. Both are characterized by increased airway resistance, and it is difficult to assess the relative contributions of chronic obstructive bronchitis and emphysema to the overall obstructive features. Therefore, the two conditions are together termed chronic obstructive pulmonary disease (COPD).

A part of the increased airway resistance in COPD is reversible with bronchodilators and is attributable to asthmatic bronchitis. Occasionally, chronic obstructive bronchitis and emphysema occur in relatively pure form and show certain distinctive features (**Table 52.3**).

Increasing Airway Resistance

The most characteristic feature of COPD is increased airway resistance in both large and small airways. Normally, the small peripheral airways contribute only 10% of the total airway resistance. In COPD, the contribution of small airways is much higher. There are three reasons for the increased airway resistance.

1. The main reason is dynamic airway obstruction: the collapse of small airways early in expiration. The small airways are more prone to collapse in COPD than in asthma because of a loss of elasticity of the small bronchioles (which are scarred in chronic bronchitis) and loss of support from surrounding alveolar walls (which are destroyed in emphysema).
2. Airflow limitation is also partly due to enhanced bronchomotor tone, which is reversible with bronchodilator drugs. In contrast, the dynamic airway compression does not respond to medications.
3. There is some increase in resistance in the large (intrathoracic) airways, too. This is because the loss of alveolar septa in emphysema results in reduction in elastic recoil of the lung. The loss of elastic recoil reduces the distending force on intrathoracic airways and therefore increases the airway resistance.

Dynamic airway obstruction makes expiration more difficult than inspiration, leading to air trapping with consequent increase in the residual volume at the expense of the forced vital capacity (FVC) (**Fig. 52.1**). This leads to breathing at higher lung volumes. The advantage of breathing at higher lung volumes is that it keeps the intrathoracic pressure more

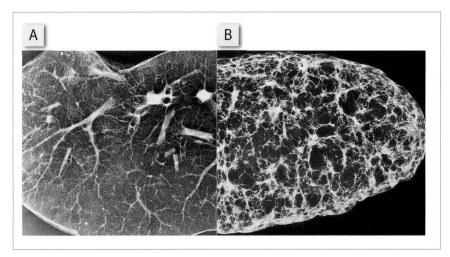

Fig. 52.3 **(A)** Structure of a normal lung and **(B)** an emphysematous lung.

Table 52.3 Comparison of Predominantly Bronchitis and Predominantly Emphysema

	Predominantly Bronchitis	Predominantly Emphysema
Appearance	Blue bloaters	Pink puffers
Onset	Cough with sputum	Dyspnea
FEV_1/FVC	Reduced	Reduced
FRC	Mildly increased	Markedly increased
TLC	Normal	Increased
Static lung compliance	Normal	Increased
Diffusion capacity	Normal	Low
Hypoxia and hypercapnia	Usually present	May not be present

Abbreviations: FEV_1, forced expiratory volume in 1 second; FRC, functional residual capacity; FVC, forced vital capacity; TLC, total lung capacity.

negative, which helps in keeping the airways patent. However, it handicaps the patient in three ways. (1) The inspiratory capacity decreases. (2) The work of breathing increases due to higher elastic recoil of the lungs at higher lung volumes. (3) The inspiratory muscles become increasingly ineffective due to the adverse length–tension relationship, leading to progressive fatigue and eventually respiratory arrest.

Reduced Diffusion Capacity

The destruction of alveolar walls reduces the diffusion capacity, resulting in hypoxemia and hypercapnia, and patients develop cyanosis. Due to their poor exercise tolerance, they exercise less and therefore gain weight. Hence, they are called "blue bloaters" (blue due to cyanosis and bloated due to obesity) or type B COPD patients. However, some patients are able to prevent hypoxemia and hypercapnia by hyperventilating. They are not cyanotic, but they lose weight due to their excessive work of breathing. They are called "pink puffers" (pink due to adequate oxygenation and puffers because they hyperventilate) or type A COPD patients. For reasons not understood, patients with predominantly chronic bronchitis tend to be blue bloaters, whereas those with predominantly emphysema tend to be pink puffers.

Ventilation–Perfusion Mismatch

Pulmonary ventilation is not uniform in COPD. The destruction of the alveolar septa with their capillaries results in diversion of blood to the intact alveoli, which consequently get excessively perfused. On the other hand, the large alveoli formed by the breaking down of alveolar septa are overventilated as they have higher compliance (Laplace's law), and the smaller, intact alveoli remain underventilated. Thus, in emphysema, the normal alveoli are overperfused and underventilated. This ventilation–perfusion mismatch results in greater reduction in the diffusion capacity than would have resulted from a reduction of alveolar surface area alone.

Pulmonary Hypertension

COPD is also associated with pulmonary hypertension for the following reasons. Hypoxia leads to compensatory increase in cardiac output. This augmented output must pass through a reduced pulmonary bed because large areas of the vascular bed are destroyed along with the alveolar septa. Hence, the resistance to blood flow is higher. The resistance is further increased by vasoconstriction of pulmonary capillaries in hypoxic areas of the lungs. The combination of increased cardiac output and increased pulmonary capillary resistance results in pulmonary hypertension. An important contribution to pulmonary hypertension comes from abnormality in vascular endothelium. The nitric oxide released by the endothelium prevents the rise in pulmonary vascular tone that is normally associated with hypoxia. In COPD, there is decreased synthesis and release of nitric oxide by endothelial cells in response to hypoxia, which results in an increase in the pulmonary vascular tone, thereby contributing to pulmonary hypertension. The pulmonary hypertension imposes greater afterload on the right ventricle and results in right ventricular hypertrophy (cor pulmonale).

Restrictive Lung Disorders

Restrictive airway disorders occur due to a reduction in the total lung capacity. Restrictive abnormality is also indicated by a reduced vital capacity, provided that air trapping has been ruled out. The PEFR may be reduced in restrictive disorder because PEFR is effort-dependent and because high expiratory efforts cannot be developed at low lung volumes (see **Fig. 45.11**). The typical flow volume loop in a restrictive disorder is shown in **Fig. 52.2**. The common causes of restrictive disorders are listed in **Table 52.4**, some of which are explained below.

Atelectasis

Atelectasis is a condition in which there is partial or total loss of alveolar air (alveolar collapse) in a part or the whole of a lung. It is a restrictive lung disorder and is associated with a reduction in gas transfer.

Atelectasis occurs when the airway supplying a part or the whole of a lung is obstructed. The obstruction can be due to

Table 52.4 Common Causes of Restrictive Lung Disorders

Disease Process	Example
Primary disease of lung parenchyma	Pneumonia, atelectasis, fibrosis, tumor
Surgical removal of lung tissue	Lobectomy
Disease of pleura and chest wall	Pleural effusion, pleural fibrosis, kyphoscoliosis, obesity
Reduced generation of expiratory force	Disorders of the neuromuscular system or the central nervous system

compression of the airway from outside, for example, by an enlarged lymph node. More often, the obstruction is inside the airway lumen, caused by foreign body aspiration, mucus plugs, or a malignant growth such as a bronchogenic carcinoma. Obstruction by a mucus plug is often seen in patients on mechanical ventilators who are unable to cough out their airway mucus. Atelectasis also occurs due to improper tracheal intubation during anesthesia. The tip of the endotracheal tube should be located in the trachea to allow positive pressure ventilation of both lungs. An inexperienced anesthetist might inadvertently push the endotracheal tube farther into the right bronchus, which is in more direct continuation of the trachea than the left bronchus, which branches off at a sharper angle. The left lung therefore remains unventilated during anesthesia, leading to atelectasis.

Consolidation

Consolidation of parts of the lung parenchyma refers to the filling up of alveolar spaces with inflammatory exudates. This is usually an infective process (bacterial or viral), as in pneumonia (**Fig. 52.4**), but it can also result from chemical or radiation injury to the lungs. The consequences are twofold. (1) A restrictive abnormality results as the alveolar gases are replaced by inflammatory exudates. (2) Hypoxemia and hypercapnia occur due to decreased diffusion of gases.

Interstitial Lung Disease

Interstitial lung disease, also called fibrosing alveolitis (**Fig. 52.5**), is characterized by two major abnormalities: thickening of the respiratory membrane due to cellular thickening and fibrosis, and the presence of large mononuclear cells within the alveolar spaces. These represent unregulated inflammatory response mostly of unknown origin (idiopathic). The thickening and fibrosis of the respiratory membrane reduce the diffusion

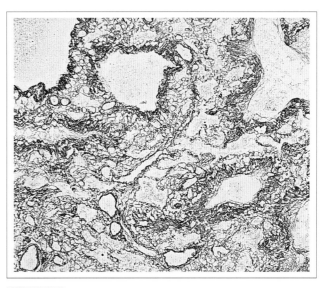

Fig. 52.5 Microscopic appearance of a section of the lung in an advanced stage of fibrosis.

capacity with consequent hypoxic hypoxia, make the lung stiff, reduce its compliance, and increase the work of breathing. All the lung volumes are reduced, resulting in a restrictive abnormality.

Pleural Effusion

In pleural effusion, pleural fluid accumulates in the pleural space. The accumulation of fluid can be due to increased transudation into the pleural space, which is due to changes in vascular pressure (increased hydrostatic pressure as in cardiac failure or decreased oncotic pressure as in hypoproteinemia). It can also occur when there is increased exudation as in any inflammatory condition, for example, infection. Finally, it can occur due to impaired lymphatic drainage of parietal pleura in neoplastic or inflammatory conditions.

Pleural effusion produces a restrictive abnormality with reduction in all the lung volumes. If the effusion develops quickly or is large, it is associated with hypoxemia with consequent hyperventilation and hypocapnia. It can also reduce the cardiac output and cause hypotension. A moderate to massive effusion causes shift of the mediastinal structures to the opposite side.

Pneumothorax

In a pneumothorax (**Fig. 52.6**), air enters the pleural space at atmospheric pressure. A primary spontaneous pneumothorax can occur in an otherwise healthy person without underlying lung disease. A secondary spontaneous pneumothorax is a complication of an underlying lung disease. Pneumothorax that occurs following injury to the chest is called traumatic pneumothorax.

Normally, the lung and pleura are held together by the pleural fluid. When air enters the pleural space, the lung and the thorax are able to move apart because air is expansible. The chest therefore recoils to a larger size, and the lung recoils to a smaller size. The pleural pressure becomes less negative. The

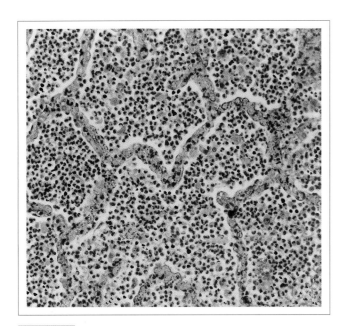

Fig. 52.4 Microscopic appearance of a section of the lung in an advanced stage of pneumonia.

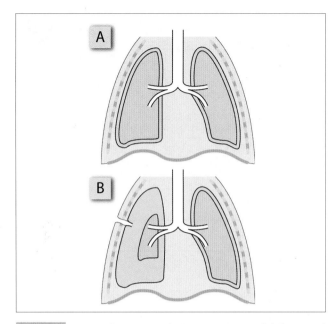

Fig. 52.6 Pneumothorax. Note that in comparison to **(A)** the normal lungs and pleural space, the lung is collapsed, and **(B)** the pleural space is enlarged in pneumothorax.

total lung capacity and the vital capacity decrease, resulting in a restrictive disorder.

Normally, any pneumothorax gets slowly absorbed spontaneously because the partial pressure of gases in the pleural capillaries is ~60 mm Hg less than atmospheric pressure (**Table 52.5**). The pressure difference that favors reabsorption of the gas from pneumothorax into the pleural capillary is maximum for O_2 (100 – 40 = 60), marginal for N_2 (573 – 569 = 4), and adverse for CO_2 (40 – 46 = –6). However, as O_2 is absorbed from the pneumothorax, the PN_2 and PCO_2 in the pneumothorax increase, resulting in a favorable gradient for the absorption of these gases into pleural capillaries. It has been estimated that roughly 5% of the pneumothorax gets absorbed every 24 hours.

In the case of *tension pneumothorax,* a valvelike tear in the visceral pleura allows air to enter the pleural cavity with each inspiration but prevents its exit during expiration. As the intrapleural pressure keeps rising, the mediastinum is pushed to the opposite side, and the lungs of both sides get squeezed, leading to restricted ventilation. The increase in intrapleural (intrathoracic) pressure results in a fall in cardiac output.

Table 52.5 Partial Pressures of Gases (in mm Hg) in Pneumothorax (Same as in Alveolar Air) and in Pleural Capillaries

	Pneumothorax	Pleural Capillaries	Difference in Partial Pressures
PN_2	573	569	4
PO_2	100	40	60
PCO_2	40	46	–6
Total	713	655	58

Clinical Diagnosis

Clinical diagnosis of respiratory disorders is based mainly on the following observations (**Table 52.6**). (1) Breathing characteristics, (2) shape of thorax, (3) shift of mediastinum (trachea and heart), (4) percussion note, (5) vocal resonance and fremitus, (6) breath sound intensity, (7) breath sound quality, and (8) adventitious sounds.

Breathing characteristics | The normal respiratory rate is ~14 to 18 per minute. Higher breathing rate is called *tachypnea* if there is no change in the depth of breathing. An increase in the depth of breathing without a change in the breathing rate is called *hyperpnea.* Neither tachypnea nor hyperpnea is necessarily associated with *hyperventilation,* which refers to any pattern of ventilation that causes P_aCO_2 to decrease below its normal level. Breathing movements are normally symmetrical: they are equal on both sides. Any asymmetry of breathing movements, especially when the subject is asked to breathe deeply, suggests the presence of lung or pleural disease on the side moving less.

An excessive inspiratory effort, which occurs in obstructive airway diseases, is often apparent from the prominence of the contracting sternocleidomastoid muscles. Excessive inspiratory effort also increases the negativity of intrapleural pressure, resulting in the retraction of suprasternal and supraclavicular fossae during inspiration. Retraction of intercostal spaces may also be observed.

Shape of the thorax | The normal chest has a transverse anteroposterior diameter of 2:1. When this ratio decreases, the thorax looks barrel-shaped and indicates hyperinflation of the lung. Hyperinflation is typically seen in patients with COPD.

Mediastinal shift | In fibrosis or collapse of the lung, the mediastinum is pulled toward the affected side. In pleural effusion and pneumothorax, the mediastinum is pushed away from the affected side. The most obvious manifestation of mediastinal shift is the shift of the trachea from its midline location in the neck, along with a shift in the apex beat. Both can be detected through palpation.

Percussion note is the sound produced by tapping the chest with the fingertips. When the finger strikes the chest wall, the chest wall tends to vibrate as a resonant cavity that is partially damped by the thoracic contents. If the underlying lung alveolar air is replaced by fluid in the pleural cavity or by exudative fluid in the alveolar space, as in pneumonia, the percussion sound becomes dull: it has a low amplitude and short duration. Conversely, if the underlying lung is replaced by air, as in pneumothorax, the percussion sound is tympanic – of high amplitude and longer duration.

Vocal resonance is assessed by placing the stethoscope on the chest wall and asking the patient to vocalize. The voice sounds are conducted from the airways to the chest wall. Because solids conduct sound better, vocal resonance is heard better in lung consolidation and is reduced in pneumothorax, pleural effusion, and hyperinflated lungs. If the airway ventilating the auscultated lung region is obstructed, for example, by a cancerous growth, the vocal resonance is reduced. The sound associated with vocalization may also be felt as the

Table 52.6 Clinical Signs in Common Respiratory Disorders

	Emphysema	Pneumothorax	Atelectasis	Consolidation	Fibrosis	Pleural Effusion
Breathing characteristics	Rapid and shallow	Rapid and shallow	Rapid and shallow	Rapid	Rapid and shallow	Rapid and shallow
Shape of thorax	Barrel-chested	Size increased ipsilaterally	Size decreased ipsilaterally	Normal	Normal	Size may be increased ipsilaterally
Tracheal shift	Pushed deeper	Pushed contralaterally	Pulled ipsilaterally	None	Pulled ipsilaterally	Pushed contralaterally
Percussion note	Hyperresonant	Tympanitic	Dull	Dull	Dull*	Stony dull
Vocal resonance/ fremitus	Decreased	Decreased	Decreased	Increased	Normal or increased	Decreased
Breath sound intensity	Decreased	Decreased	Decreased	Normal	Normal	Decreased
Breath sound quality	Vesicular	Vesicular	Vesicular	Bronchial	Vesicular	Vesicular
Adventitious sounds	Wheeze*	None	Crackles (when partial)	Crackles	Velcro crackles	Pleural rub

*May or may not be present.

vocal fremitus by placing the ulnar border of the hand on the intercostal spaces while the patient is asked to vocalize.

Breath sounds | Auscultation over the trachea and major bronchi reveals a hollow sound with a "tubular" quality. It is called *bronchial sound* and is generated in the upper airways between the nasal cavity and principal bronchi. Auscultation over normal lungs over the chest wall reveals a soft sound called the *vesicular sound*. It originates in the smaller airways. The inspiratory phase of this sound is longer than the expiratory phase (normal inspiration to expiration ratio is 2:1), the latter being nearly silent. If bronchial sound is heard over the lung fields, it indicates consolidation of lungs (**Table 52.7**).

Table 52.7 Difference between Vesicular and Bronchial Breath Sounds

Vesicular	Bronchial
Has a soft, low-pitched, "rustling" quality	Harsh and high-pitched; has a hollow, "tubular" quality
The expiratory sound is softer than the inspiratory sound	The expiratory sound is harsher than the inspiratory sound
Duration of expiratory sound is twice that of inspiration	Duration of inspiratory sound is equal to that of expiratory sound
There is no gap between the inspiratory and expiratory sounds	There is a definite gap between the inspiratory and expiratory sounds
The inspiratory sound originates within the lungs, whereas the expiration-phase sound comes partly from the larger airways	It is generated in the larger airways
Normally heard on the chest wall over the lungs	Normally not transmitted to the chest wall. When present, signifies consolidation of lungs. Normally heard over trachea

Summary

● Pulmonary function testing provides a means of differentiating (diagnosing) different types of respiratory disorders.

● Obstructive airway disease is present whenever airway resistance is increased, a condition that is present in asthma, bronchitis, emphysema, and chronic obstructive lung disease (bronchitis plus emphysema).

● Restrictive lung disease is present when total lung capacity is reduced and is due to changes in the mechanical properties of lung tissue.

Applying What You Know

52.1. Ms. Eng has no nasal polyps (abnormal growths of mucosal tissue) when first seen in the emergency room. However, people with asthma are more likely to develop them. What would be the consequence for respiratory function of the presence of a large nasal polyp?

52.2. Under what conditions would the duration of expiration be increased above the normal value? What is the most likely cause of Ms. Eng's increased expiratory duration?

52.3. Emphysema is a disorder characterized by destruction of the elastic tissue in the lungs. Predict the changes that will occur to the following pulmonary function test values in a patient with emphysema: forced expiratory volume in 1 second (FEV_1), FEV_1/forced vital capacity (FVC), peak flow, functional residual capacity (FRC), residual volume (RV), and total lung capacity (TLC).

52.4. A chest x-ray taken in the emergency room showed that Ms. Eng had "mild hyperinflation." The results of her pulmonary function test show an increased RV. Explain the mechanism giving rise to both of these findings.

Answers to Applying What You Know

Chapter 44

1 When Ms. Eng's symptoms first appear, she uses her albuterol inhaler. Where along the respiratory tree will albuterol have its effect?

Albuterol binds to β_2-adrenergic receptors found on bronchiolar smooth muscle. Thus, albuterol acts on the *conducting airways*. When β_2 receptors bind epinephrine, the bronchiolar smooth muscle relaxes, and the bronchioles get larger, thus relieving Ms. Eng's symptoms.

2 Which, if any, of Ms. Eng's vital signs are abnormal?

Ms. Eng's blood pressure is markedly high, at least in part, because her heart rate (pulse) is very high. Her tachycardia is a consequence of hypoxia (her P_aO_2 is only 66 mm Hg). Her breathing frequency is also very high, 2 to 3 times a normal value. This, too, is a consequence of her hypoxia.

Chapter 45

1 Ms. Eng is coughing when she comes to the emergency room. Which of the respiratory muscles contract to produce the explosive expiration that is seen when someone coughs?

At rest, expiration results from the passive recoil of the expanded lungs and chest wall. However, when greater expiratory effort is required to produce a cough (or during the increased ventilation that occurs during exercise), contraction of the abdominal muscles compresses the contents of the abdominal cavity, displacing the diaphragm upward and producing a forced expiration.

2 When Ms. Eng comes into the emergency room, she is suffering from bronchoconstriction, which causes an increase in airway resistance. What effect would you expect this condition to have on her functional residual capacity (FRC)? Explain your prediction.

FRC is the volume in the lungs when the elastic recoil of the lungs inward is exactly balanced by the elastic recoil of the chest wall outward. If the compliance of the lungs or the chest wall changes, the value of FRC will change.

Asthma and its increased airway resistance will have little or no direct effect on FRC because the compliance of the lungs or chest wall is unaffected. However, the increased airway resistance does make it difficult for Ms. Eng to exhale. To overcome this increased resistance to flow may call for a forced expiration. If this occurs, there is a likelihood of dynamic airway compression and the trapping of air in the lungs. With the residual volume (RV) increased, FRC will get larger.

3 What is shortness of breath (SOB), and what are possible mechanisms that could cause it? Which mechanism is most likely causing this in Ms. Eng?

Shortness of breath is a sensation that one is "not getting enough air." It can arise when hypoxia is present (P_aO_2 is too low), and tissues cannot obtain the oxygen they need, and/or when the respiratory effort to get adequate oxygen uptake is greater than normal. Both of these mechanisms probably contribute to Ms. Eng's SOB; her P_aO_2 is low, and the respiratory effort required to generate an appropriate alveolar ventilation is higher than normal (to overcome the increased resistance of her airways).

Chapter 46

1 Ms. Eng presents in the emergency room with wheezing, the production of an abnormal breath sound. What conditions are present in the respiratory system when wheezing is occurring?

The presence of abnormal sounds during breathing means that turbulent flow is occurring somewhere in the respiratory tree. Turbulence results when airflow velocity increases to a sufficiently high value. The Reynolds number increases to a greater than threshold value. The normally present laminar flow (silent) is converted into turbulent flow (noisy). Thus, when Ms. Eng is experiencing bronchoconstriction due to an allergic reaction, airflow velocity in the narrowed airways increases, turbulent flow is present, and a wheeze is produced.

Chapter 47

1 Ms. Eng has an increased breathing frequency (tachypnea). What effect will this have on her tidal volume? Explain.

Breathing frequency and tidal volume are two independently determined respiratory variables. Both are determined by the neural output of the respiratory controllers in the brainstem.

Reflex responses that increase breathing frequency also increase the tidal volume at the same time. Increased breathing frequency does decrease the time available for each breathing cycle. However, because the muscular effort to produce inspiration also increases, a more negative intrapleural pressure is created; hence, there is a larger pressure gradient driving air into the lungs.

Thus, tachypnea will have no effect on tidal volume unless breathing frequency gets very high.

2 Ms. Eng has a markedly decreased P_aO_2 but an essentially normal P_aCO_2. Such a state can only result from what kind of disturbance in the respiratory system? Explain.

Many different disturbances in the respiratory system can give rise to decreased P_aO_2 and increased P_aCO_2: decreased alveolar ventilation, decreasing diffusing capacity, a severe ventilation/perfusion imbalance, and increased left-to-right shunt will each produce this state.

Although Ms. Eng does have a low P_aO_2, her P_aCO_2 is near normal. The explanation for her state is as follows. The hypoxia present is clearly causing a reflex increase in breathing frequency (35/min) and probably tidal volume (unmeasured, but likely to be the case). The increased alveolar ventilation that is present partially compensates for the hypoxia (she is not as hypoxic as she would be without the reflex response). Her elevated alveolar ventilation is also adequate to allow her to blow off enough CO_2 to keep her P_aCO_2 near normal; CO_2 crosses the diffusional barrier in the lungs more readily than O_2.

Chapter 48

1 Calculate the value of Ms. Eng's total oxygen content when she is in the emergency room.

Total oxygen content is the sum of the *dissolved oxygen content* and the *oxygen bound to hemoglobin (Hb)*.

> *Dissolved O_2 content* (mL O_2/100 mL blood) =
> the solubility of O_2 in blood × partial pressure of O_2 =
> 0.003 mL O_2/100 mL blood/mm Hg × P_aO_2 =
> 0.003 mL O_2/100 mL blood/ mm Hg × 66 mm Hg =
> 0.198 mL O_2/100 mL blood
> The *Hb-bound O_2* =
> Binding capacity of Hb × Hb concentration × % saturation =
> 13.4 mL O_2/g Hb ×15.5 g Hb/100 mL blood × 0.915 =
> 19.0 mL O_2/100 mL blood
> Ms. Eng's total O_2 content is thus 0.198 + 19.00 =
> 19.20 mL O_2/100 mL blood.

Note that despite Ms. Eng's P_aO_2 being quite low, she is still able to transport an essentially normal amount of oxygen in her blood.

2 Ms. Eng has a partial pressure of oxygen in arterial blood (PaO_2) value that is significantly reduced (down from a normal value of 100 mm Hg to 66 mm Hg), although her hemoglobin saturation is only slightly reduced (down from a normal value of 98–99% to 91.5%). Explain the mechanism that accounts for this discrepancy.

Because of the sigmoid shape of the oxyhemoglobin dissociation curve, percent saturation does not fall a great deal as P_aO_2 decreases until the partial pressure falls to ~60 mm Hg (see **Fig. 48.1**).

Chapter 49

1 When examined in the emergency room, Ms, Eng had a respiratory rate of 35/min, considerably higher than normal. What change in the motor output from the medulla occurs when breathing frequency increases? If Ms. Eng increases her tidal volume, what change in neural output occurs?

When breathing frequency is increased, the number of bursts of action potentials per minute in the phrenic nerve innervat-

ing the diaphragm increases. This increases the diaphragm's number of contractions per minute, thus increasing breathing frequency. To increase tidal volume, the frequency of firing action potentials in each burst in the phrenic nerve is increased. Tetanic summation then results in a stronger contraction of the muscles making up the diaphragm. The diaphragm is lowered further, increasing the volume of the thorax and resulting in a larger tidal volume.

Chapter 50

1 Predict (increase/decrease/no change) the changes in the following respiratory parameters that will occur 60 minutes after Ms. Eng is started on supplemental oxygen: P_aO_2, P_aCO_2, tidal volume, and breathing frequency.

P_aO_2 will obviously increase because the PO_2 of the inspired air has increased. The increase in P_aO_2 will cause the peripheral chemoreceptors to fire more slowly; hence, the breathing frequency and tidal volume will both decrease. This, of course, means that alveolar ventilation will fall. Breathing a gas mixture high in O_2 does not, in any direct way, produce a change in P_aCO_2, but the fall in alveolar ventilation will result in some increase in P_aCO_2.

Chapter 51

1 Ms. Eng vacations in Hawaii. The weather is perfect, and the water looks quite inviting, so she decides to try snorkeling. Predict the consequences of breathing through a snorkel for 30 minutes on the following parameters: dead space volume, tidal volume, breathing frequency, P_aO_2, P_aCO_2, and the work of breathing.

Breathing through a snorkel results in a direct increase in dead space volume because air moving through the tube cannot undergo gas exchange; therefore, a larger volume of air must be moved through the tube to reach the alveolar space. This would decrease alveolar ventilation [$\dot{V}_A = f (\dot{V}_T - \dot{V}_D)$], leading to hypoxia and hypercapnia. Both of these changes are sensed by the chemoreceptors, and alveolar ventilation will be increased. That is, there will be a reflex increase in breathing frequency and tidal volume. If the respiratory controller can fully compensate for the disturbance (the increase in dead space), there will be no change in P_aO_2 or P_aCO_2. However, if the volume of the snorkel is large enough, the controller will not be able to fully compensate, and alveolar ventilation will be decreased. This would cause P_aO_2 to decrease and P_aCO_2 to increase. The work of breathing will be increased because both the elastic work of breathing will be greater (a big tidal volume is being produced) and the viscous work will be greater (the air must move faster).

Chapter 52

1 Ms. Eng has no nasal polyps (abnormal growths of mucosal tissue) when first seen in the emergency room. However, people with asthma are more likely to develop them. What would be the consequence for respiratory function of the presence of a large nasal polyp?

A large nasal polyp represents an obstruction to airflow, and like any obstruction, it will increase the resistance to flow, at least while breathing through the nose.

2 Under what conditions would the duration of expiration be increased above the normal value? What is the most likely cause of Ms. Eng's increased expiratory duration?

The duration of airflow during expiration will be increased if (1) the resistance of the airways is sufficiently increased above normal, or (2) the elastic recoil of the lungs is reduced (their compliance increases). Increased airway resistance will result in less air being moved per unit time; hence, more time is required to expire a tidal volume. Decreased elastic recoil would result in less compression of the alveoli and therefore a lower alveolar pressure; the smaller pressure gradient would slow the exit of air from the lungs.

Because Ms. Eng has asthma, we know that her prolonged expiration is the result of increased airway resistance.

3 Emphysema is a disorder characterized by destruction of the elastic tissue in the lungs. Predict the changes that will occur to the following pulmonary function test values in a patient with emphysema: forced expiratory volume in 1 second (FEV_1), $FEV_1/$forced vital capacity (FVC), peak flow, functional residual capacity (FRC), residual volume (RV), and total lung capacity (TLC).

The destruction of elastic tissue in the lungs increases the compliance of the lungs (they become more easily distended, but their elastic recoil is reduced). The loss of elastic tissue also reduces the traction exerted on the airways, which tends to keep them open.

Thus, with the airways relatively narrowed, airway resistance is increased, and FEV_1 will decrease. FEV_1/FVC will also be reduced, a sure sign that airway resistance is elevated.

Peak flow will be decreased because of the increase in airway resistance.

FRC represents the volume in the lungs when the elastic recoil of the lungs inward is exactly balanced by the elastic recoil of the chest wall outward. With lung elastic recoil reduced, FRC will be larger than normal.

RV is increased because without the elastic tissue to hold open the airways, the tendency for dynamic airway collapse during forced expiration is increased, and air trapping occurs.

TLC is increased because of the increased compliance of the lungs.

4 A chest x-ray taken in the emergency room showed that Ms. Eng had "mild hyperinflation." The results of her pulmonary function test show an increased RV. Explain the mechanism giving rise to both of these findings.

Ms. Eng's narrowed airways have a higher resistance to flow. One consequence of this is a greater tendency for dynamic air-way collapse to occur during a forceful expiration. This is, of course, exactly what Ms. Eng must produce to expire at the end of a breathing cycle. To do this, the accessory expiratory muscles are contracted, increasing the intrapleural pressure and making it positive. As a result, the pressure drop down the length of the airway is steeper, and the equal pressure point (where the pressure in the pleural space and the pressure in the airway are equal) occurs in a region of the respiratory tree where airways can collapse. The result is the inability to expire all of the air. Hyperinflation (or a larger RV) is present.

Section VI Case Analysis:
Evelyn Eng is short of breath.

Clinical Overview

Review of patient condition | Evelyn Eng suffers from asthma, a condition in which airway obstruction is episodically triggered by several possible stimuli. Her presenting problem is clearly of allergic origin, a response to her exposure to cats.

Etiology | The airway obstruction present in asthma results from bronchoconstriction (contraction of bronchiolar smooth muscle) and bronchiolar inflammation with edema formation and increased mucus secretion. Acute asthma attacks are reversible with elimination of the triggering stimulus and treatment. Chronic inflammation can lead to permanent structural changes known as airway remodeling (hypertrophy of bronchiole smooth muscle and hyperplasia of mucous glands).

Prevalence | Asthma is an increasingly prevalent disease, particularly among minority and low-income inner-city dwellers. The number of deaths per year in the United States is 5000 or more. The morbidity is high, with increasing numbers of visits to emergency rooms and hospitalizations.

Diagnosis | The diagnosis of asthma is based on the patient's history, particularly reports of triggers for the patient's symptoms. A history of airborne allergies is significant. Pulmonary function testing is of great importance in establishing the diagnosis; decreases in FEV_1/FVC certainly support a diagnosis of asthma. Acute reversibility of pulmonary function tests results supports the diagnosis.

Treatment | There are basically two avenues for treatment. The acute changes in respiratory function due to airway obstruction can be alleviated with administration of bronchodilating agents (β_2 agonists). It is also important that the allergic responses from the triggering agent (in Ms. Eng's case, cat dander) be minimized with topical steroids. It is, of course, critical that, to the extent possible, the patient avoid exposure to the allergens that trigger the asthma.

Understanding the Physiology

Narrowing of the airways, as occurs when bronchiolar constriction is present, has several important physiologic consequences.

First, airway resistance is increased, and even small decreases in airway diameter will cause large increases in resistance because resistance is proportional to $1/r^4$. The increase in airway resistance results in decreased airflow during inspiration and hence a decrease in alveolar ventilation. This, in turn, can result in decreased P_aO_2 and increased P_aCO_2. Another consequence of the increase in airway resistance is an increase in the work of breathing.

The narrowing of the airways also results in an increased velocity of airflow and an increased tendency for airflow to become turbulent, and hence the development of wheezing.

However, asthmatics may have a greater problem during expiration. The narrowed airways slow expiration (prolonged expiration is an easily measured parameter in the doctor's office). The increased resistance also increases the work that must be done and may result in the use of accessory expiratory muscles. There is also a greater tendency for dynamic airway collapse to occur (the resistance to outflow is higher than normal, and the equal pressure point is likely to be reached in the collapsible airways). The result is air trapping (an increase in RV that was seen in Ms. Eng's pulmonary function tests).

The accompanying flow chart illustrates the interactions between mechanisms resulting in Ms. Eng's symptoms (**Fig. VI.1**).

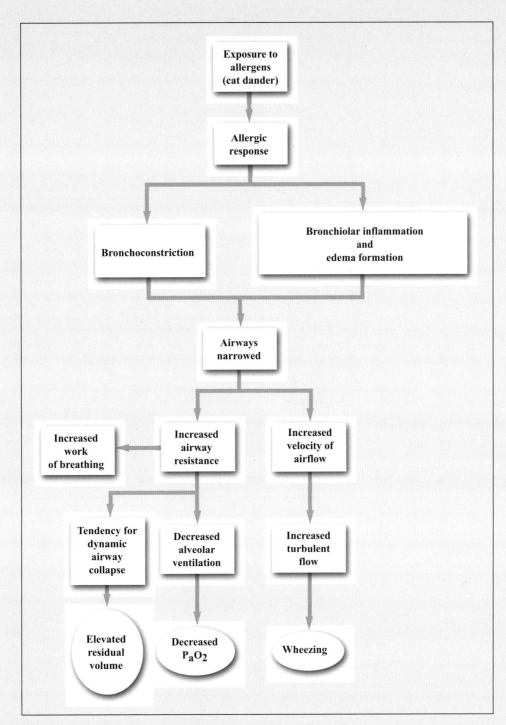

Fig. VI.1 Ms. Eng's allergy to cat dander triggers any asthma attack whose signs and symptoms all arise from her narrowed airways (bronchoconstriction).

Section VII | Renal System

Overview

The body attempts to maintain a constant internal environment, with the extracellular concentrations of many solutes held more or less constant.

The kidneys play an important role in maintaining homeostasis by (1) regulating the concentration of many solutes, (2) regulating body fluid osmolarity, (3) contributing to the regulation of pH, (4) contributing to the regulation of plasma volume and blood pressure, and (5) excreting many of the waste productions of metabolism.

The kidneys are made up of approximately two million functional units called nephrons. They are perfused by 25% of the cardiac output. Each nephron forms an ultrafiltrate of plasma at the glomerulus, the first component of the nephron. As this fluid flows through the tubule, a variety of transport processes reabsorb several solutes, with water following, while at the same time secreting other solutes.

Several mechanisms ensure that the process of glomerular filtration remains constant in the face of changes to blood flow. Neural and hormonal inputs control the transport processes involved in moving solutes into or out of the nephron.

The end result of these processes is urine, which is collected in the urinary bladder. Voiding of urine is a process that involves a local reflex that is inhibited by decreasing signals from the central nervous system.

Section VII Case Presentation:
Frank Fisher is not making any urine.

Chief Complaint

Reverend Frank Fisher is an 80-year-old retired clergyman. He has been hospitalized in the intensive care unit for the past 5 days, and it has been noted that his urine output has been falling for the past 2 days.

History of Present Illness

Reverend Fisher was originally admitted with pneumonia, for which he was treated with cephalothin and gentamicin intravenously (IV). On the second hospital day, he suffered an acute anterior myocardial infarction with cardiopulmonary arrest. He was without a pulse for several minutes and required cardiopulmonary resuscitation. Since then he has been hemodynamically stable, and his pneumonia has apparently improved.

Past Medical History

His previous medical history is remarkable only for the surgical removal of a kidney 10 years ago because of a primary renal malignancy. He had no problems subsequent to surgery.

Physical Examination

- *General appearance* | On examination at the bedside, Reverend Fisher appears well nourished, but he is lethargic and slightly confused.
- *Vital signs*
  - Temperature: 98.2°F (oral)
  - Blood pressure: 130/80 mm Hg (supine)
  - Pulse: 80/min
  - Respirations: 25/minute
- *Cardiac exam* | A regular rhythm and no murmurs. Pulses are strong and symmetric.
- *Lungs* | Lung fields reveal crackles in the right base (the site of his healing pneumonia), which seems unchanged since yesterday.
- *Abdomen* | Suprapubic palpitations reveal no bladder distention.

There is mild presacral edema, which is new since yesterday.

Laboratory Results: Plasma

Value	Today	On Admission (5 Days Ago)
Sodium	122 mM/L	123
Potassium	4.8 mM/L	3.6
Chloride	96 mM/L	97
Bicarbonate	22 mM/L	25
Urea nitrogen (BUN)	73 mg/dL	28
Creatinine	5.9 mg/dL	1.9
Protein, total	5.3 g/dL	
Albumin	2.7 g/dL	
Calcium	8.1 mg/dL	
Phosphorus	6.2 mg/dL	
Cholesterol	164 mg/dL	
Glucose, fasting	111 mg/dL	
Uric acid	13.4 mg/dL	
Bilirubin, total	1.0 mg/dL	
Alkaline phosphatase	75 IU/L	
LDH	124 IU/L	
SGPT	33 IU/L	
SGOT	36 IU/L	
Serum osmolarity	280 mOsm/L	

Abbreviations: LDH, lactate dehydrogenase; SGOT, serum glutamic oxaloacetic transaminase; SGPT, serum glutamic pyruvic transaminase.

Urinalysis

	Today	On Admission	Normal
Color	Yellow	Yellow	Yellow
Clarity	Hazy	Hazy	Clear
Specific gravity	1.011	1.023	1.002–1.030
pH	5.0		5.0–8.0
Protein	1+	Trace	Negative
Glucose	Negative	Negative	Negative
Ketones	Negative	Negative	Negative
Occult blood			Negative
Bilirubin			Negative
Nitrite			Negative
Urobilinogen			Negative
Microscopic exam			
WBC	1–2	1–2	0–5/HPF
RBC	1–2	1–2	0–5/HPF
Bacteria	Few	1+	None
Squamous epithelial cells	Many	Few	0–5/HPF
Casts	2–5 pigmented cell casts	1+	None
Mucus		1+	

Abbreviations: HPF, high-power field; RBC, red blood cell; WBC, white blood cell.

Urinalysis: Input/Output Study

	Oral and IV In	Urine Out	Weight
Yesterday	3050 cc	1050 cc	66 kg
Today	1540 cc	420 cc	68 kg

Abbreviation: IV, intravenous.

Urine Chemistries

Sodium	60 mEq/L
Urea	150 mg/dL
Creatinine	115 mg/dL
Osmolality	308 mOsm/kg
Total volume	420 cc

Ultrasound Report

Spleen is well identified. No evidence of left kidney is seen in the upper left quadrant of the abdomen (consistent with surgical history). Right kidney is normal in size and configuration. No abnormal masses are seen in the right kidney. No evidence of hydronephrosis.

Serum Gentamicin Levels

Peak (30 min after dose) 9.1 μg/mL (therapeutic 5–10)
Trough (30 min before dose) 5.8 μg/mL (0–2.0)

Urine Culture

No growth after 48 hours

Treatment

The gentamicin is stopped, and the cephalothin dose is adjusted for his renal function. After 10 days, Reverend Fisher is discharged.

Laboratory Results (at Discharge)

Serum

Sodium	130 mM/L
Potassium	4.0 mM/L
Chloride	97 mM/L
Bicarbonate	26 mM/L
BUN	30 mg/dL
Creatinine	1.9 mg/dL

Urinalysis
Within normal limits

Some Things to Think About

1. Reverend Fisher is retaining water. What effect does this have on the function of his kidney?

2. The results of his laboratory tests show Reverend Fisher to have an abnormally low osmolarity. What is the role of the kidneys in regulating osmolarity?

3. During his hospitalization, Reverend Fisher's electrolyte concentrations are abnormal. What renal mechanisms control electrolyte balance?

4. It appears that Reverend Fisher's renal problems were exacerbated by his myocardial infarct. How would changes in renal blood flow affect renal function?

5. On admission to the hospital, Reverend Fisher has high concentrations of nitrogenous waste products. What mechanisms are involved in the kidneys eliminating these substances from the body?

6. Despite his many problems, there is no indication that Reverend Fisher has an acid–base imbalance. What is the role of the kidneys in whole-body regulation of pH?

The main function of the kidney is homeostasis, the maintenance of the constancy of the *milieu interior* (the extracellular environment). In doing so, the kidney has to deal appropriately with the products of protein metabolism, as well as with water and electrolytes. It also plays a role in the homeostasis of certain other substances, such as calcium and phosphate.

Products of protein metabolism are urea, uric acid, sulfate (SO_4^{2-}), phosphate (PO_4^{3-}), creatinine, and several other substances that must be effectively eliminated from the body. Accumulation of these metabolites, mostly nitrogenous compounds, in blood is called *azotemia*. It occurs in kidney dysfunction and is diagnosed when the serum BUN (blood urea nitrogen) level is elevated. Metabolism of carbohydrates and fats produces only water and carbon dioxide (CO_2); therefore, the kidney is not loaded with metabolites. Hence, in kidney dysfunction, only protein restriction is advised.

Water, sodium (Na^+), and potassium (K^+) are dealt with according to whether there is a surplus or deficit in the body. The kidney regulates water and electrolyte balance, and also the blood and extracellular fluid (ECF) volume. The kidney also contributes to the regulation of blood pH by controlling the excretion of bicarbonate (HCO_3^-) ions, which are an important blood buffer.

Other functions of the kidney are (1) long-term and intermediate-term (through renin secretion) regulation of blood pressure; (2) regulation of erythropoiesis; (3) regulation of Ca^{2+} homeostasis and bone metabolism through the activation of 25-hydroxycholecalciferol to 1,25-dihydroxycholecalciferol and the controlled reabsorption of calcium and phosphate; (4) synthesis of metabolic substrate, such as L-arginine, which is the precursor for nitric oxide (NO); and (5) under exceptional conditions, a significant contribution to the body's gluconeogenetic capability.

The Kidneys

A longitudinal section of the kidney (**Fig. 53.1**) shows two distinct zones: the outer cortex and the inner medulla. The cortex contains most of the glomeruli (see below). The medulla comprises the renal pyramids, 4 to 14 in number, separated by the cortical columns of Bertin. One renal pyramid and its bounding renal columns constitute a renal lobule. The pyramid shows radial striations, which are due to the straight portions of the nephrons. These striations extend some distance upward into the cortex, where they are called the medullary rays. The apex of the pyramid is called the papilla. The tip of the papilla has visible pores, which are the openings of the collecting ducts into the minor calyx.

The medulla can be subdivided into an outer medulla, which is further subdivided into the outer and inner strips, and an inner medulla, also called the papillary zone (**Fig. 53.2**). The papillae end in the minor calyces. The minor calyces join together to form major calyces, which, in turn, drain into

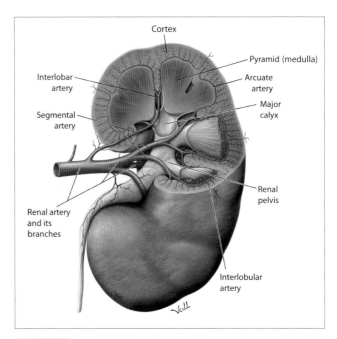

Fig. 53.1 A partial longitudinal section of the kidney, showing the renal pyramids and the arterial supply.

the pelvis. The pelvis narrows down to continue as the ureter, which drains into the bladder.

Each kidney is made up of about a million nephrons. Each nephron consists of the Bowman's capsule and the renal tubule, a part of which forms a loop called the loop of Henle. Eighty-five percent of the nephrons are located superficially in the cortex and are called *cortical nephrons*. Nephrons filter plasma into the tubule and then reabsorb the plasma solutes in required amounts so that any excess solute present in the blood is eliminated in the urine. The copious reabsorption from these tubules is made possible by a dense peritubular capillary plexus. The cortical tubules do not loop down into the inner medulla.

The remaining 15% of the nephrons are called *juxtamedullary nephrons*. Their glomerulus is located deep inside the cortex near the corticomedullary junction. They have long tubules that loop through the inner medulla, reaching up to the papilla. These nephrons help in producing a concentrated urine by building up an extremely high osmolarity in the renal medulla. The morphologic differences between the two types of nephrons are shown in **Fig. 53.3**.

Renal blood vessels | The renal artery enters the hilus and divides into anterior and posterior divisions, which give rise to segmental arteries (**Fig. 53.2**). The segmental arteries divide into the lobar arteries, one for each renal pyramid. The lobar arteries divide into two interlobar arteries and run in the cortical columns. At the corticomedullary junction, each interlobar artery divides into two arcuate arteries that run parallel to the surface of the kidney. The arcuate arteries give off the cortical radial arteries (earlier called interlobular arteries),

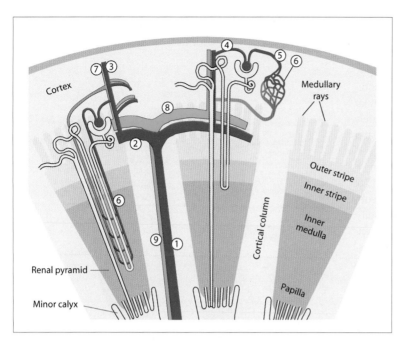

Fig. 53.2 Renal blood vessels: (1) interlobar artery, (2) arcuate artery, (3) cortical radial (interlobular) artery, (4) afferent arteriole, (5) efferent arteriole, (6) peritubular capillary network, (7) deep cortical vein, (8) arcuate vein, and (9) interlobar vein. The subdivisions of the medulla can be seen on the right.

which ascend radially toward the cortex. The cortical radial arteries give off the afferent arterioles. The afferent arterioles ramify into a tuft of capillaries called the glomerulus inside the Bowman's capsule. Glomerular capillaries reunite to form the efferent arteriole, which takes different courses in the superficial and deep cortical nephrons.

In the cortical nephrons, the efferent arterioles ramify into a dense peritubular capillary network. The capillaries of the outermost zones of the cortex are drained toward the surface by the radially arranged superficial cortical veins that join the stellate veins on the surface of the kidney. The stellate veins are drained by interlobular veins that are confluent at their inner end with arcuate veins. Capillaries in the deeper portion of the cortex drain into radially oriented deep cortical veins running parallel to the interlobular arteries. The deep cortical veins drain directly into the arcuate veins. The arcuate veins drain into interlobar veins that join to form the renal vein.

In the juxtamedullary nephrons, efferent arterioles are larger and branch into long and straight capillaries called the *vasa recta*. The vasa recta follow the course of the loop of Henle. The descending and ascending limbs of the vasa recta run close together, facilitating a countercurrent exchange (see Chapter 56). Between the descending and ascending limbs lies the peritubular capillary network of the medulla, which is less dense than the cortical network.

Renal Blood Flow and Oxygen Consumption

The *O₂ consumption* per 100 g of renal tissue is 5 mL/min, which is next highest only to that of the heart (8 mL/min). Renal O_2 consumption is determined by the rate of Na^+ reabsorption and therefore by the tubular load of Na^+.

The total *renal blood flow* (RBF) is ~1200 mL/min. The range of RBF is rather narrow as compared with other organs; only a 25% increase (300 mL/min) over the basal RBF of 1200 mL/min occurs.

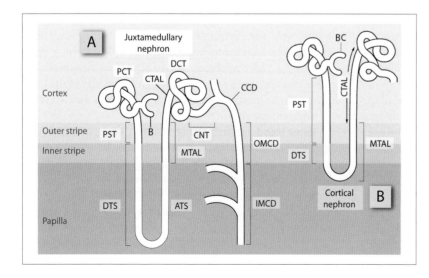

Fig. 53.3 Anatomic differences between **(A)** juxtamedullary and **(B)** cortical nephrons. ATS, ascending thin segment; BC, Bowman's capsule; CCD, cortical CD; CD, collecting duct; CNT, connecting tubule; CTAL, cortical TAL; DCT, distal convoluted tubule; DST, distal straight tubule; DTS, descending thin segment; IMCD, inner medullary CD; MTAL, medullary TAL; OMCD, outer medullary CD; PCT, proximal convoluted tubule; PST, proximal straight tubule; TAL, thick ascending limb.

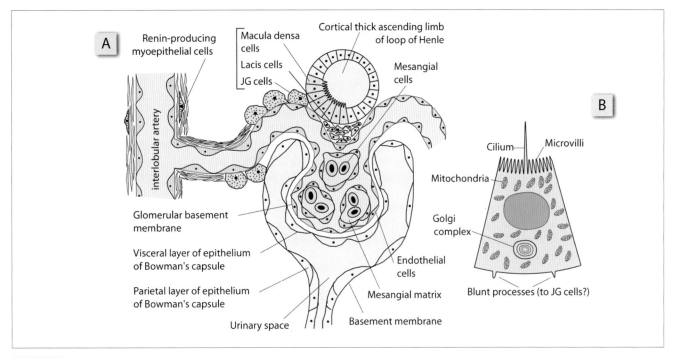

Fig. 53.4 **(A)** The Bowman's capsule, glomerulus, and distal segment of the loop of Henle. Also shown are the interlobar artery, the afferent and efferent arterioles, and the juxtaglomerular apparatus. **(B)** A macula densa cell. JG, juxtaglomerular.

The RBF per 100 g tissue is ~400 mL/min, which is disproportionately high as compared with that of the heart, which is only 80 mL/min. This indicates that more blood flows into the kidney than is required for meeting its oxygen demand. Because renal blood flow is far in excess of the renal O_2 demand, the *arteriovenous (A-V) O_2 difference* in the kidneys is only 1.5 mL O_2/100 mL of blood flow, which is much lower than in the heart, which is ~10 mL O_2/100 mL, or than the systemic average of 4 to 5 mL O_2/100 mL.

Intrarenal distribution of blood flow | Ninety percent of the RBF goes to the renal cortex, 9% goes to the outer medulla, and 1% goes to the inner medulla. The factors responsible for the low inner medullary blood flow are to be found in the Poiseuille–Hagen formula. These factors are (1) the length of the vasa recta (vascular resistance is proportional to the length of the vessel), (2) the sharp rise in the viscosity of blood in the inner medulla due to the loss of large amounts of water into the hyperosmolar interstitium, and (3) the low capillary hydrostatic pressure in the vasa recta because the efferent arterioles of the juxtamedullary nephrons are small in diameter.

The Nephron

Bowman's Capsule
The Bowman's capsule has a parietal layer and a visceral layer of epithelium. The space enclosed between the two layers is continuous with the lumen of the uriniferous tubule (**Fig. 53.4**). The cells of the visceral layer have fingerlike processes that encircle the glomerular capillaries, leaving between them slitlike gaps called *slit pores*. These Bowman's epithelial cells are called podocytes (**Fig. 53.5**).

The **glomerular membrane** (or the filtration barrier) comprises the capillary endothelium, basement membrane, and Bowman's visceral epithelium. (1) The *capillary endothelium* is fenestrated. The fenestrae are 50 to 100 nm wide. (2) The *basement membrane* is acellular. It contains hydrated channels ~6 nm wide. These channels account for the selectivity of the glomerular membrane. The basement membrane contains negatively charged proteoglycans, such as chondroitin sulfate proteoglycans and heparin sulfate proteoglycans (HSPG). HSPG is particularly important in imparting selectivity to the glomerular basement membrane. Normally, polyanions like

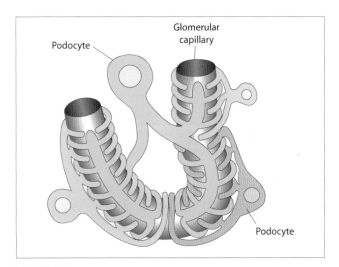

Fig. 53.5 The large and small processes of four podocytes interdigitate around a glomerular capillary, leaving between them the slit pores through which plasma gets filtered.

HSPG act as "anticlogging" agents that prevent the absorption of plasma proteins so that the pores are not choked. (3) The *Bowman's visceral epithelium* is made of podocytes that are separated by slits ~25 nm wide (**Fig. 53.5**). Cells called the *mesangial cells* are present between the capillary endothelial cells and the basement membrane, especially where the basement membrane encloses more than one capillary.

The Renal Tubule

The renal tubule is subdivided into the proximal tubule or loop of Henle, the intermediate tubule, the distal tubule, and the collecting system (**Fig. 53.3**).

The **proximal tubule** is the longest part of the nephron. It is further subdivided into (1) the proximal convoluted tubule (PCT) located in the cortex and (2) the proximal straight tubule (PST) located in the medullary rays and the outer stripe of the medulla.

The **loop of Henle** (intermediate tubule) is divided into three segments. (1) The descending thin segment (DTS), which traverses the inner stripe and extends deep into the inner medulla, and (2) The DTS loops around and becomes the ascending thin segment (ATS). In juxtamedullary nephrons, the DTS loops around as the ATS to reach the junction of the outer and inner medulla. In cortical nephrons, the DTS is continuous at the bend of the loop with the distal tubule; therefore, there is no ATS. (3) The thick ascending limb (TAL) extends across the outer medulla. It is subdivided into the medullary thick ascending limb (MTAL) and the cortical thick ascending limb (CTAL).

The **distal tubule** has two segments. (1) The distal convoluted tubule (DCT) lies in the cortex and it is connected by (2) a short connecting tubule (CNT) to the collecting duct (CD).

The **collecting duct** is not, embryologically, a part of the nephron, as it is derived from the ureteric bud. It consists of the connecting tubule and collecting duct. (1) The connecting tubule (CNT) lies entirely in the cortex. In this segment, several tubules coalesce to form the collecting duct. (2) The collecting duct (CD) runs through the cortex, medulla, and papilla, finally opening at the tip of the papilla. Accordingly, it is subdivided into the cortical collecting duct (CCD), the outer medullary collecting duct (OMCD), and the inner medullary collecting duct (IMCD) or the papillary collecting duct. In the IMCD region, several collecting ducts coalesce before finally opening at the tip of the renal papilla.

Table 53.1 contains a list of the various segments of the nephron and their abbreviations.

Juxtaglomerular Apparatus

The juxtaglomerular apparatus is located at the angle of the afferent and efferent arterioles, where it comes in contact with the cortical part of the thick ascending limb (**Fig. 53.6**). It comprises the macula densa, the juxtaglomerular (JG) cells, and the lacis cells (**Fig. 53.4**).

The part of the distal tubule that comes in contact with the afferent arteriole is made of a specialized epithelium called the *macula densa*. The cells of the macula densa have blunt processes at its base, extending toward the juxtaglomerular cells in the afferent arteriole. The Golgi complex is usually located between the nucleus and the cell base. In other tubular cells, the Golgi complex is located near the apical membrane. These structural characteristics suggest the presence of some secretory activity at the base of the cell.

The *juxtaglomerular (granular) cells* are modified smooth muscle cells in the scala media of the terminal part of the afferent arterioles. They contain large granules that secrete renin. In conditions requiring increased renin secretion, additional smooth muscle cells located in the wall of afferent arteriole and even cortical radial artery are transformed into granular cells. Granular cells are densely innervated by sympathetic

Table 53.1 The Components of the Nephron in Anatomic Order and Their Abbreviations

The Proximal Tubule	
PCT	Proximal convoluted tubule
PST	Proximal straight tubule
Thin Segment (aka the loop of Henle)	
DTS	Descending thin segment
ATS	Ascending thin segment
TAL	Thick ascending limb
MTAL	Medullary TAL
CTAL	Cortical TAL
The Distal Tubule	
DCT	Distal convoluted tubule
CNT	Connecting tubule
The Collecting Duct	
CCD	Cortical collecting duct
OMCD	Outer medullary collecting duct
IMCD	Inner medullary collecting duct

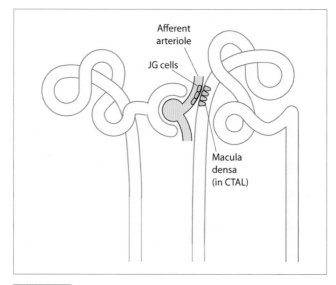

Fig. 53.6 Location of the juxtaglomerular (JG) apparatus. CTAL, cortical thick ascending limb.

nerve terminals, and they release their renin content in response to sympathetic discharge.

The *lacis cells* (extraglomerular mesangial cells) are derived from smooth muscle cells. They are present in the angular space between the glomerulus and the diverging afferent and efferent arterioles. Structurally, lacis cells may be important as a "plugging" device at the glomerular entrance, which protects the glomerulus against distending forces exerted by the high intra-arteriolar pressure. Functionally, lacis cells possibly relay the signals from the macula densa to granular cells after modulating the signals.

Tubular Cells

The cells of the nephron are mostly cuboidal except in the thin segment, where they are flat and squamous. The cells rest on a basement membrane. The apical surfaces (which face the tubular lumen) of all the cells bear a few microvilli, but in the proximal tubule these microvilli are numerous and dense, giving the apex the appearance of a brush border. The basal cell membrane (which faces the renal interstitial space) of all the cells shows fairly extensive invaginations or infoldings except in the thin segment. These infoldings create narrow "gutters" of extracellular spaces called the *basal space.* The lateral surfaces of the cells bear the lateral cell processes that interdigitate with the corresponding processes of adjacent cells. In between the interdigitations there are small spaces called the *lateral intercellular spaces.* Lateral spaces communicate with each other, but they do not freely communicate with the basal extracellular space (**Fig. 53.7**).

The apical surfaces of all cells interdigitate with neighboring cells, forming "tight junctions," or zona occludens.

Functionally, however, they are not necessarily tight. Hence, they are of two types. The *"leaky" tight junctions* permit water and solutes to diffuse across them. These are present in the proximal tubule. The *"tight" tight junctions* do not permit water and solutes to diffuse across them easily. These are present in the distal tubule.

The different types of tubular cells present in a nephron segment are (1) the proximal tubular cell, (2) the intermediate tubular cell, (3) the distal tubular cell, and (4) the collecting duct cells that are of two types, the principal cells and the intercalated cells (**Fig. 53.8**).

Tubular Potentials

An electrical potential difference is recordable across the tubular wall, between the lumen of the tubule and its exterior. This potential difference, which is called the *transepithelial potential difference* (TEPD), varies in different segments of the tubule (**Fig. 53.9**). The potential in the proximal tubule is very slight (–2 mV in the convoluted part, +2 mV in the straight part). In the thick ascending limb, it is lumen positive (+6 to +10 mV). In the distal tubule, it is highly lumen negative (–70 mV). Tubular potentials, like most other membrane potentials, are produced due to unequal diffusion of anions and cations across the tubular wall. Some of these potentials are important in the tubular transport of certain ions.

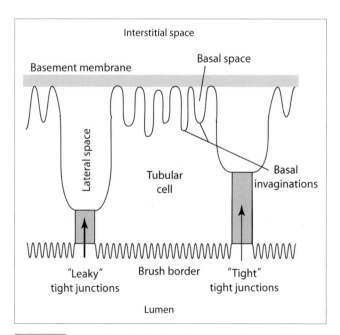

Fig. 53.7 A typical renal tubular cell. Note that the apical (luminal) and basolateral membranes have different properties.

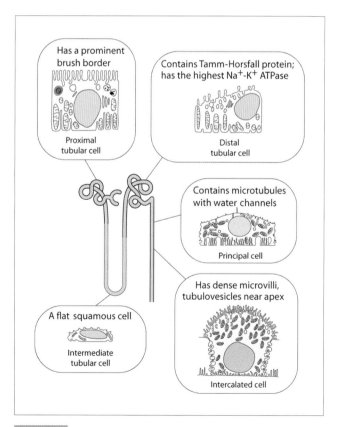

Fig. 53.8 The different types of tubular cells present in a nephron segment.

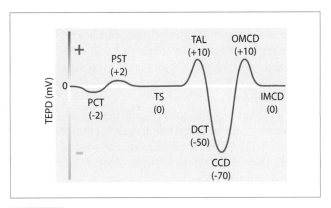

Fig. 53.9 Graphic representation (not to scale) of the transepithelial potential difference (TEPD) in different segments of the nephron. The highly negative TEPD in the cortical connecting duct (CCD) has several important physiologic consequences. PCT, proximal convoluted tubule; PST, proximal straight tubule; TS, thin segment; TAL, thick ascending limb; DCT, distal convoluted tubule; OMCD, outer medullary connecting duct; IMCD, inner medullary connecting duct.

Summary

- The kidneys receive a large fraction of the cardiac output via the renal arteries and consume a large fraction of the O_2 used by the body.

- The function units of the kidneys are the nephrons, which are made up of the glomerulus, the proximal tubule, the loop of Henle, the distal tubule, and the collecting duct.

- The epithelial cells of the nephron are polarized, with the apical (luminal) membrane having different properties than the basolateral membrane.

Applying What You Know

53.1. Reverend Fisher had a myocardial infarct and an episode of cardiac arrest. What effects would this have on his kidney functions?

In the glomerular capillaries, fluid is filtered out from blood into the uriniferous tubule. The filtered fluid, called the glomerular filtrate, is mostly protein-free. Only low-molecular-weight proteins whose size is smaller than that of albumin are present in the filtrate. The electrolyte composition of the filtrate is identical to that of the plasma. Most of the glomerular filtrate gets reabsorbed by the nephron and enters the peritubular capillaries. Both glomerular filtration and tubular reabsorption of fluids are governed by Starling forces of capillary exchange. Although the solutes in the plasma are freely filtered into the tubules, their reabsorption is active and selective.

Glomerular Filtration

The Starling forces that operate at the glomerular capillary level (**Fig. 54.1A**) are the same as in systemic capillaries but are different in magnitude. The salient differences are as follows. (1) There is no significant drop in hydrostatic pressure along the glomerular capillaries despite the filtering out of fluids. (2) There is considerable rise in plasma oncotic pressure along the glomerular capillaries. (3) The oncotic pressure of the glomerular filtrate is nearly zero. (4) The capsular hydrostatic pressure is higher than that in the tissue interstitial fluid pressure. (5) The Starling forces equilibrate toward the efferent arteriolar end of the glomerular capillaries. As a consequence of the Starling forces, fluid is filtered out from the arteriolar side of the glomerular capillaries under a net outward pressure of 10 mm Hg; there is no reabsorptive or filtrative force at the efferent arteriolar end.

Glomerular Filtration of Solutes

The concentration ratio of a substance in the Bowman's space and plasma is called its glomerular sieving coefficient. Molecules less than 4 nm in diameter are freely filtered, whereas molecules larger than 8 nm (molecular weight greater than 70,000 D) are excluded from the glomerular filtrate. The glomerular filtration barrier for solutes resides at the glomerular basement membrane, which contains negatively charged proteoglycans. Hence, negatively charged molecules have greater difficulty passing through it. This explains why albumin, which is ~7 nm (69,000 D), is largely excluded from the filtrate. Loss of the negative charge on the basement membrane even without any structural damage to the membrane is enough to produce albuminuria. It explains why albuminuria is such a sensitive indicator of glomerular damage.

Glomerular Filtration of Fluids

The glomerular filtration rate (GFR) is proportional to the effective filtration pressure that results from the Starling forces.

$$GFR \propto [(P_{glomerulus} + \pi_{Bowman}) - (P_{Bowman} + \pi_{glomerulus})] \quad (54.1)$$

$$GFR = K_f \times [(P_{glomerulus} + \pi_{Bowman}) - (P_{Bowman} + \pi_{glomerulus})]$$
$$(54.2)$$

where K_f is the *filtration coefficient*.

General Model: Balance of Forces

The movement of fluid in and out of capillaries, wherever they are located, is always the result of a balance of forces, the hydrostatic pressure gradient causing filtration out and the oncotic pressure gradient causing reabsorption.

K_f depends on the permeability of the glomerular membrane as well as its surface area. The effective surface area of the glomerular membrane is regulated physiologically by the mesangial cells, which are contractile and can constrict adjacent capillaries.

Any factor that affects the Startling forces changes the GFR. (1) A rise in systemic blood pressure increases the capillary hydrostatic pressure and therefore increases the GFR. (2) An increase in renal blood flow reduces the rise in colloid osmotic pressure along the glomerular capillary (**Fig. 54.1B**) and therefore increases the GFR. (3) The hydrostatic pressure in the Bowman's capsule increases in ureteric obstruction or renal edema, resulting in a fall in the GFR. (4) The plasma oncotic pressure increases in dehydration and decreases in hypoproteinemia. Hence, GFR decreases in dehydration and increases in hypoproteinemia. (5) GFR is also reduced by renal diseases that reduce the permeability and effective surface area of the glomerular basement membrane. Sympathetic discharge reduces glomerular filtration, the reasons for which are discussed below.

Autoregulation of Glomerular Filtration

The GFR is normally well autoregulated in the range of 70 to 180 mm Hg of systemic pressure (**Fig. 54.2**). However, this autoregulation can be overridden by renal nerves. There are two plausible hypotheses for explaining the autoregulation of GFR.

The **myogenic hypothesis** of autoregulation suggests that the afferent arterioles constrict in response to increased blood pressure. Arteriolar constriction restores GFR to normal levels. Possibly, the stretching of arterioles leads to the opening of stretch-sensitive calcium (Ca^{2+}) channels on the arteriolar smooth muscle cells, resulting in a Ca^{2+} influx that causes the cells to contract.

Tubuloglomerular feedback hypothesis | When the GFR increases, it results in increased delivery of NaCl to the distal

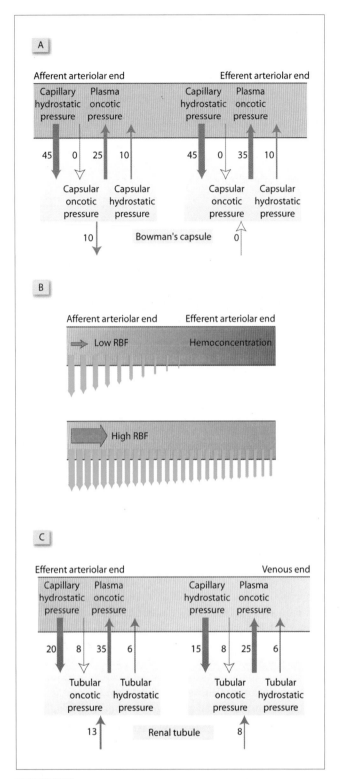

A

Afferent arteriolar end   Efferent arteriolar end

Capillary hydrostatic pressure	Plasma oncotic pressure		Capillary hydrostatic pressure	Plasma oncotic pressure
45	0	25	10	45	0	35	10

Capsular oncotic pressure | Capsular hydrostatic pressure | Capsular oncotic pressure | Capsular hydrostatic pressure

10 | Bowman's capsule | 0

B

Afferent arteriolar end   Efferent arteriolar end

Low RBF   Hemoconcentration

High RBF

C

Efferent arteriolar end   Venous end

Capillary hydrostatic pressure	Plasma oncotic pressure		Capillary hydrostatic pressure	Plasma oncotic pressure
20	8	35	6	15	8	25	6

Tubular oncotic pressure | Tubular hydrostatic pressure | Tubular oncotic pressure | Tubular hydrostatic pressure

13 | Renal tubule | 8

Fig. 54.1 **(A)** Starling forces (in mm Hg) in the glomerular capillary. **(B)** Effect of renal blood flow on glomerular filtration. **(C)** Starling forces (in mm Hg) in the peritubular capillary. RBF, renal blood flow.

tubule. The concentration of Cl^- in the distal tubule is sensed by the macula densa and signaled to the afferent arteriole (see **Fig. 53.6**). Infusion of Na^+ salts other than NaCl does not produce tubuloglomerular feedback. The signal is transmitted

from the macula densa to the afferent arteriole probably by some adenosine or eicosanoid compound that causes vasoconstriction of the afferent arteriole by opening up Ca^{2+} channels of the smooth muscles.

General Model: Communications

This is an example of a cell-to-cell signaling mechanism that enables cells and organs to coordinate their activities in a way needed to maintain function.

The ultimate purpose of renal autoregulation is to hold the GFR constant. This usually necessitates that the RBF, too, is held constant. That, however, is not always true. Often, the renal blood flow (RBF) increases or decreases to maintain a constant GFR. For example, in hypoproteinemia, the GFR increases, but RBF remains unchanged. The autoregulatory mechanisms cause arteriolar vasoconstriction, which restores GFR but decreases the RBF. Similarly, in ureteric obstruction, the GFR decreases, but the RBF remains unchanged. Due to autoregulatory mechanisms, there is arteriolar dilatation, which restores the GFR but increases the RBF.

When renal perfusion pressure increases, the GFR does not change much due to autoregulation. Yet the urinary output increases dramatically. Because the kidney is enclosed in a tough capsule that is not easily stretched, any increase in the renal perfusion pressure also increases the renal interstitial hydrostatic pressure. An increase in interstitial hydrostatic pressure decreases the reabsorption of tubular fluids and increases the urinary output.

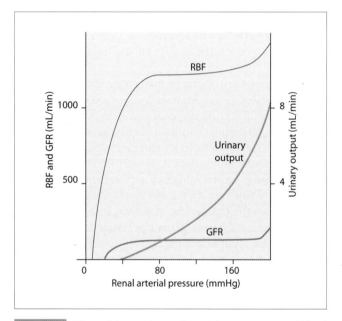

Fig. 54.2 Effect of changes in renal arterial pressure on renal blood flow (RBF), glomerular filtration rate (GFR), and urinary output. The autoregulation of renal blood flow (RBF) and GFR is evident.

Tubular Transport

Tubular Reabsorption of Water

Of the 180 L of fluid filtered into the glomerulus each day, all but 1.5 L are reabsorbed from the tubules. The Starling reabsorptive forces at the peritubular capillaries account for only a small part of this reabsorption, providing 8 to 13 mm Hg of net reabsorptive force (**Fig. 54.1C**). The bulk of the water reabsorption occurs secondary to the active sodium (Na^+) reabsorption in the tubules.

Obligatory water reabsorption | Eighty-five percent of the water reabsorption occurs irrespective of the body water balance and is called *obligatory* (must occur). About 65% of the obligatory reabsorption occurs in the proximal tubules, and 20% of the obligatory reabsorption occurs in the distal tubules.

Facultative water reabsorption | The remaining 15% of the water may or may not be reabsorbed, depending on the body water balance. It is called *facultative reabsorption* (optional). The facultative reabsorption occurs from the collecting tubule as it courses through the renal medulla. It is under the control of the antidiuretic hormone (ADH), which controls the permeability of the collecting tubule to water.

The interstitium of the renal medulla has a very high osmolarity and would normally extract water from the collecting tubules. In the presence of ADH, the collecting tubule epithelium is permeable to water, which is reabsorbed in large amounts. However, in the absence of ADH, the collecting tubule is impermeable to water; therefore, no water is reabsorbed.

Tubular Handling of Solutes

Proximal tubular handling of solutes | In the proximal tubule, different solutes are handled differently. Most solutes are reabsorbed, but some are secreted. About 60% of the tubular load of Na^+, Ca^{2+}, potassium (K^+), phosphate (PO_4^{3-}), chloride (Cl^-), and urea are reabsorbed. Bicarbonate (HCO_3^-) reabsorption is more than 60%; glucose and amino acids are reabsorbed nearly completely. Sulfate (SO_4^{2-}) is poorly reabsorbed. Reabsorption of almost all solutes is linked directly or indirectly to the active reabsorption of Na^+. Small proteins and peptides are also reabsorbed in the proximal tubules through endocytosis. Substances such as creatinine and inulin (an exogenous substance used in measuring kidney function) are not reabsorbed at all.

General Model: Energy

Active transport of Na^+, moving Na^+ against its concentration gradient, requires the expenditure of energy in the form of adenosine triphosphate (ATP). Renal cells must make a lot of ATP; hence, the kidneys have a very high blood flow relative to their mass.

The amount of water reabsorption can be estimated from the extent to which inulin or creatinine is concentrated in the tubule (**Fig. 54.3**). These solutes, which are not reabsorbed at all, are concentrated 2.5-fold in the proximal tubule, indicating

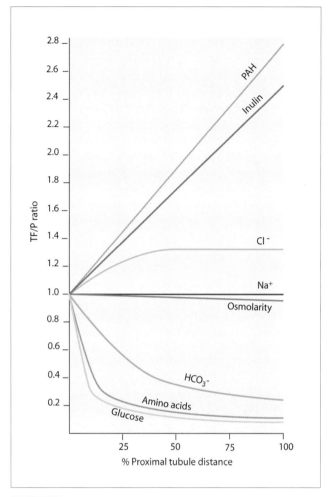

Fig. 54.3 The tubular fluid/plasma (TF/P) ratio for various solutes as a function of the distance it travels in the proximal tubule.

that ~60% of the water load is reabsorbed in the proximal tubules. Sodium ions, too, are 60% reabsorbed in the proximal tubule, indicating that the reabsorption of Na^+ is iso-osmotic—following the reabsorption of Na^+, its tubular concentration does not fall. Hence, the ratio of Na^+ concentration in the tubular fluid (TF) and plasma (P) remains 1.0 throughout the proximal tubule. Not all solutes are reabsorbed isoosmotically. Glucose, amino acids, and bicarbonates are reabsorbed relatively more than water. The TF/P ratio for these substances drops sharply along the proximal tubule. Chloride ions are reabsorbed relatively less than water, and the TF/P ratio shows a rise. Hydrogen ions are secreted into the proximal tubule. The H^+ secretion is associated with bicarbonate reabsorption. Organic acids such as para-aminohippuric acid (PAH) are secreted into the tubules. The TF/P ratio of these acids is greater than 2.5.

Distal tubular handling of solutes | The distal tubule has to handle mainly Na^+, Cl^-, K^+, H^+, HCO_3^-, and urea. Reabsorption of Na^+ in the thick ascending limb (TAL) of the loop of Henle is the prime driving force for the countercurrent multiplier system (see Chapter 56), which makes the medullary interstitium hyperosmolar. Medullary hyperosmolarity is important for urine concentration. Na^+ reabsorption in the distal tubule is stimulated by aldosterone and is also associated with reciprocal secretion of K^+ and H^+. Chloride reabsorption accompanies Na^+ reabsorption. Potassium ions are both reabsorbed and secreted in the distal tubule. The amount of K^+ secretion in the distal tubule is reciprocally related to the amount of H^+ secretion. Bicarbonate reabsorption is completed in the distal nephron, and therefore the urinary HCO_3^- concentration is zero. Hydrogen ions are secreted in the distal tubule. The H^+ secretion in the distal tubule is not necessarily linked to bicarbonate ions. Urea reabsorption occurs in large amounts in the collecting duct and contributes considerably to the inner medullary hyperosmolarity. Urea reabsorption, like that of water, is affected by ADH. In the absence of ADH, urea reabsorption decreases, and with it, the medullary hyperosmolarity also decreases.

Renal Sympathetic Discharge

Renal sympathetic discharge results in salt and water retention in the body. The mechanism is the same as the one that operates at other systemic capillaries, where sympathetic discharge also causes movement of fluid into capillaries. Afferent arteriolar vasoconstriction decreases RBF and GFR. The result is a decrease in urinary output with consequent water retention. Efferent arteriolar vasoconstriction results in a decrease in peritubular capillary pressure, which increases tubular water reabsorption and decreases urinary output, producing water retention.

Renal sympathetic discharge also stimulates the juxtaglomerular (JG) cells to release renin. Renin degranulation and the consequent formation of angiotensin II have three effects. (1) It constricts the efferent arterioles and, to a lesser degree, the afferent arterioles. Hence, it decreases RBF and, to a lesser degree, the GFR. Consequently, urinary output decreases, leading to water retention. (2) It stimulates aldosterone secretion from the adrenals, resulting in increased retention of Na^+ and water in the body. (3) It stimulates the thirst center in the brain to promote water intake.

General Model: Communications

The activity in renal sympathetic nerves is transmitted to vascular smooth muscle and to JB cells by a neurotransmitter. The renin released from the JG cells by sympathetic stimulation is a humoral agent that has widespread effects in the kidney. Both mechanisms are examples of cell-to-cell communications.

At moderate stimulation rates, sympathetic nerve stimulation causes more vasoconstriction in the efferent arteriole than in the afferent arteriole, resulting in a moderate decrease in renal blood flow with little change in the glomerular filtration rate. At higher stimulation rates, sympathetic nerve stimulation causes vasoconstriction predominantly at the afferent arterioles, resulting in a marked decrease in both renal blood flow and GFR. The effects are summarized in **Table 54.1**.

Table 54.1 Effect of Sympathetic Discharge on the Renal Regulation of Body Fluid and Electrolytes

Sympathetic discharge on the kidney results in
Decreased glomerular filtration rate
Increased reabsorption of Na^+ and water from the PCT
Increased reabsorption of Na^+ and water from the DCT
Thirst (due to angiotensin II production).

The overall effect is fluid and electrolyte retention due to
Decreased urinary output
Decreased urinary Na^+ excretion
Increased water intake

Abbreviations: DCT, distal convoluted tubule; PCT, proximal convoluted tubule.

Summary

- Filtration occurs at the glomerular capillaries, where the hydrostatic pressure gradient exceeds the oncotic pressure gradient along the entire length of the capillary.

- Both renal blood flow and glomerular filtration rate are autoregulated.

- The renal tubules are responsible for the reabsorption of filtered water and solutes.

Applying What You Know

54.1. Reverend Fisher has protein in his urine, and his total plasma protein and plasma albumin are both reduced. What can you conclude from these data?

54.2. During the time that Reverend Fisher was hypotensive, what changes occurred to his renal blood flow and his glomerular filtration rate (GFR)? Explain.

54.3. Gentamicin, one of the antibiotics used to treat Reverend Fisher, is known to be nephrotoxic, and it is particularly damaging to the proximal tubule. Predict the changes in the kidney functions listed that you would expect to see in a patient treated with gentamicin: Na^+ excretion, K^+ excretion, urine flow rate, and osmolarity.

54.4. Predict the changes that were present in GFR following Reverend Fisher's myocardial infarct, knowing that he had a markedly elevated plasma creatinine and blood area nitrogen (BUN) concentration. Explain your prediction.

About 50% of the filtered load of sodium (Na^+) is actively reabsorbed in the proximal convoluted tubule (PCT), and another 10% of the filtered Na^+ load is passively reabsorbed in the proximal straight tubule (PST). In the thick ascending limb (TAL), another 30% of Na^+ is actively reabsorbed. About 7% of the tubular Na^+ load is reabsorbed in the distal convoluted tubule (DCT) and connecting tubule (CNT): the reabsorption here is increased by aldosterone. In the collecting duct, ~3% of the Na^+ load is actively reabsorbed.

The Na^+, which is actively pumped out from the thick TAL into the outer medullary interstitium, mostly enters the descending thin segment (DTS), resulting in a *recycling of Na^+* in the loop of Henle and the accumulation of Na^+ in the interstitium of the renal medulla (**Fig. 55.1**).

Mechanisms of Na^+ Reabsorption

Almost all renal tubular cells, except the intercalated cells in the collecting ducts, reabsorb Na^+ actively. The reabsorption is driven by the Na^+–K^+ pump located on the basolateral membrane, which pumps Na^+ into the paracellular spaces and lowers the intracellular Na^+ concentration. However, the mechanisms of Na^+ transport across the apical membrane differ in the different segments of the tubule. Accordingly, there are various mechanisms of Na^+ reabsorption (**Fig. 55.2**).

> **General Model: Energy**
>
> Active transport moves a solute *against* its electrochemical gradient; therefore, it requires the expenditure of energy. Pumps producing active transport are adenosine triphosphatases (ATPases) that generate the needed energy from the high-energy phosphate bond in ATP.

Unitransport of Na^+ ions occurs in the proximal tubule (PCT and PST), as well as in the collecting duct (CNT, cortical collecting duct [CCD], outer medullary CD [OMCD], inner medullary CD [IMCD]). It involves the following steps (**Fig. 55.2A**). (1) Na^+ is actively transported by Na^+–K^+ ATPase across the basolateral surface. (2) Na^+ passively diffuses across the brush border to restore intracellular electroneutrality and Na^+ concentration. (3) chloride (Cl^-) passively diffuses across the "leaky" tight junctions to restore the transepithelial electrochemical balance. (4) The Na^+ in the basolateral spaces largely enters the peritubular capillaries and partly leaks back into the tubule (through the leaky junctions).

Unitransport of positively charged Na^+ ions from the tubular lumen tends to create a lumen-negative TEPD (transepithelial potential difference). Hence, Na^+ unitransport is also called *electrogenic Na^+ transport*. Due to the leaky tight junctions in the proximal tubules, Cl^- is reabsorbed through paracellular pathways and nearly nullifies the TEPD. Hence, no signifi-

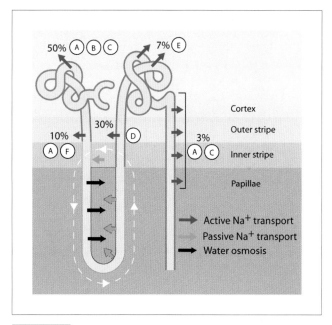

Fig. 55.1 Sodium reabsorption from different tubular segments. Letters *A* to *F* relate to the absorptive mechanisms of Na^+, which are explained in **Fig. 55.2**. See also **Fig. 53.3**.

cant TEPD develops (± 2 mV). In the distal tubules, however, the "tight" tight junctions do not permit easy passage of Cl^- through them. As a result, Cl^- reabsorption is much slower, and the TEPD, which is about –70 mV, is not nullified. The Na^+ uniport channels in the distal nephron (not in the proximal nephron) are blocked by *amiloride* and stimulated by *aldosterone*. Hence, amiloride and *spironolactone* (an aldosterone antagonist) are used as diuretics. They not only decrease the distal tubular Na^+ reabsorption, but also markedly decrease the TEPD.

Sodium cotransport with organic substrates occurs only in the PCT because glucose, amino acids, and organic anions are reabsorbed completely in the PCT. Both glucose and amino acids are cotransported with Na^+ in the proximal tubule (**Fig. 55.2B**).

The organic anion that is cotransported with Na^+ is a dicarboxylate or a tricarboxylate organic anion. Other organic ions are coupled to the transport of di/tricarboxylates and thereby are indirectly coupled to Na^+ transport. For example, para-aminohippuric acid (PAH) is transported by a PAH-anion antiport working together with a Na^+-di/tricarboxylate symporter.

Na^+-H^+ antiport with bicarbonate-chloride antiport occurs in PCT as well as in the CNT and CD. It involves the following steps (**Fig. 55.2C**). (1) Na^+ is actively extruded across the basolateral surface, producing intracellular negativity. (2) Na^+ diffuses inside across the brush border along the

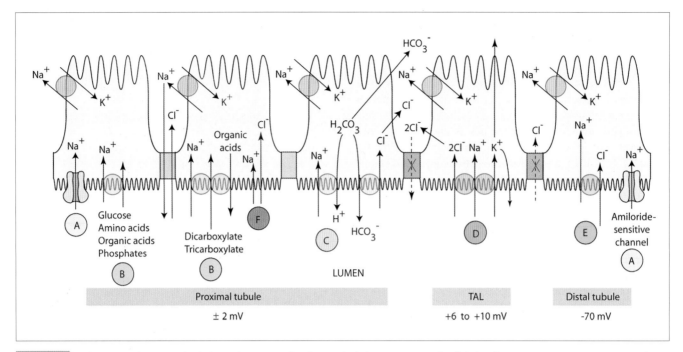

Fig. 55.2 Different mechanisms of tubular reabsorption of sodium ions. **(A)** Unitransport of Na^+; **(B)** Na^+ cotransport with non-Cl^-, non-H^+ substrates; **(C)** Na^+–H^+ exchange, usually with a parallel Cl^-–HCO_3^- uniport; **(D)** Na^+/K^+–$2Cl^-$ cotransport, **(E)** Na^+–Cl^- cotransport; and **(F)** chloride-driven Na^+ transport. TAL, thick ascending limb of the loop of Henle.

electrochemical gradient with coupled extrusion of H^+ (Na^+–H^+ antiport). The H^+ is produced, along with HCO_3^-, by the intracellular reaction of CO_2 with water. The electrical gradient persists. (3) The HCO_3^- either diffuses out across the basolateral surface to restore electroneutrality, or diffuses out across the brush border with coupled entry of Cl^- (*parallel HCO_3^-–Cl^- antiport*). Cl^- diffuses out across the basolateral surface to restore electroneutrality.

Coupled extrusion of H^+ is limited by the intracellular availability of H^+. Thus, it is increased by a high PCO_2 and decreased by diamox (carbonic anhydrase inhibitor), both of which affect H^+ production. In alkalosis, H^+ secretion decreases, and the Na^+–H^+ antiport is reduced. Hence, Na^+ reabsorption decreases in alkalosis.

Conversely, because HCO_3^- reabsorption in the proximal tubule is linked to Na^+ reabsorption, bicarbonate appears in the urine whenever Na^+ reabsorption decreases in the proximal tubule, resulting in slight acidosis. Hence, diuretics (including water diuresis) result in not only increased Na^+ excretion, but also a slight loss of bicarbonate in the urine and acidosis.

Chloride-driven sodium transport occurs in the PST alone, and its mechanism is as follows (**Fig. 55.3**). In the glomerular filtrate, the Na^+ concentration is ~110 mEq/L, and the HCO_3^- concentration is ~24 mEq/L. The Cl^-:HCO_3^- concentration in the glomerular filtrate is therefore ~4.5:1. In the PCT, Cl^-, and HCO_3^- are reabsorbed in a ratio of 3:1 because for every four Na^+ ions, three Cl^- and one HCO_3^- are reabsorbed. The Cl^-:HCO_3^- concentration in the peritubular fluid is also similar. Therefore, by the time the filtrate reaches the PST, the chloride concentration in the tubule is higher than in the peritubular capillary.

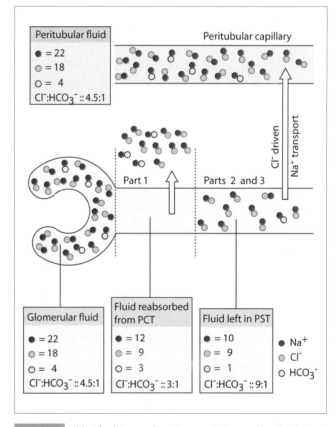

Fig. 55.3 Chloride-driven sodium transport. See explanation in text. PCT, proximal convoluted tubule; PST, proximal straight tubule.

Cl⁻ therefore diffuses passively into the peritubular capillaries. The passive diffusion of Cl⁻ across the brush border sets up an electrical gradient along which Na⁺ diffuses in. Cl⁻ ions, which lead the diffusion, tend to produce a lumen-positive TEPD. Na⁺ ions, which follow Cl⁻, nearly nullify the TEPD so that the TEPD in the PST is only +2 mV.

Sodium cotransport with chloride and potassium ions is confined to the TAL only (**Fig. 55.2D**). (1) Na⁺ is actively extruded across the basolateral surface. (2) Na⁺ passively diffuses inside with coupled cotransport of two Cl⁻ ions and one K⁺. This is termed the Na⁺/K⁺–2Cl⁻ cotransport system. (3) Two Cl⁻ and one K⁺ ion diffuse out across the basolateral surface to restore electroneutrality. (4) Due to the presence of "tight" tight junctions, Na⁺ is unable to leak back from the lateral spaces into the tubule to produce a luminal potential. (5) Some of the K⁺ that enters the cell leaks back across the apical membrane into the tubular lumen, generating a lumen-positive TEPD of +6 to +10 mV.

A group of diuretics called the *loop diuretics* inhibit the Na⁺/K⁺–2Cl⁻ system. Loop diuretics include *furosemide* and *ethacrynic acid*. The Na⁺ reabsorbed from this segment is the main driving force behind the countercurrent multiplier system, which concentrates Na⁺ and urea in the medullary interstitium. Hence, loop diuretics diminish the medullary hyperosmolarity that is essential for urine concentration. Thus, they act as very effective diuretics and are also called high-ceiling diuretics. ADH stimulates Na⁺/K⁺–2Cl⁻ and thereby enhances the urine-concentrating ability of the kidneys.

Sodium–chloride cotransport occurs in the DCT alone. It involves the following steps (**Fig. 55.2F**). (1) Na⁺ is actively extruded across the basolateral surface of the tubular cell. (2) Na⁺ diffuses across the brush border through Na⁺–Cl⁻ cotransport. (3) The chloride diffuses out into the basolateral spaces.

Na⁺–Cl⁻ cotransport is inhibited by a group of compounds called the benzothiazides. Thiazides therefore produce natriuresis with diuresis.

Factors Affecting Na⁺ Reabsorption

There are three primary factors controlling sodium reabsorption: the apical sodium transport, the activity of the basolateral Na⁺–K⁺ ATPase, and the Starling forces. It might appear unusual that although Na⁺ reabsorption is an active process, it is affected by the passive Starling reabsorptive forces. The reason for it is that the movement of Na⁺ from the basolateral spaces into the peritubular capillary is essentially passive. The movement of water from the basolateral spaces into the peritubular capillaries "drags" with it Na⁺ (due to bulk flow) and lowers the Na⁺ concentration in the lateral space. Hence, factors that increase water reabsorption into the peritubular capillaries (e.g., decreased hydrostatic pressure and increased oncotic pressure) also enhance Na⁺ reabsorption. Conversely, the extracellular fluid (ECF) volume expansion that occurs following ingestion of large amounts of water reduces water reabsorption from the proximal tubules due to alteration in the Starling forces. Concomitantly, there is also a reduction in Na⁺ reabsorption from the proximal tubules.

> **General Model: Flow**
>
> The bulk flow of water out of the basolateral space is an example of passive flow down a pressure gradient; the hydrostatic pressure in the lateral space is higher than the hydrostatic pressure in the capillaries.

Glomerulotubular balance | Na⁺ reabsorption in *proximal tubule* is load-dependent; that is, it is proportional to the Na⁺ concentration in the tubule. This is known as glomerulotubular balance, and it occurs because the tubular Na⁺ reabsorption is flow-limited. Because of glomerulotubular balance, the urinary Na⁺ output does not increase massively when the GFR increases. The following example will illustrate the point.

Example
When the glomerular filtration rate (GFR) is 125 mL/min, the amount of Na⁺ entering the tubule each minute is ~20 mOsm, of which 19.25 mOsm gets reabsorbed, and 0.75 mOsm gets excreted in urine. The Na⁺ reabsorption is associated with 124 mL of water reabsorption, and the urinary output is 1 mL/min – 1.44 L/day. Now, suppose the GFR increases by 20%, to 150 mL/min. If the Na⁺ and water reabsorption remains unchanged, the urinary output increases to 26 mL/min – 37 L/day. However, due to glomerulotubular balance, the Na⁺ reabsorption increases proportionately to 23.1 mOsm, and the water reabsorption increases to 148.8 mL. Thus, both urinary Na⁺ excretion and urinary output increase only by 20%, to 0.9 mOsm and 1.2 mL/min, respectively.

Na⁺ reabsorption in the *distal nephron*, too, is load-dependent. Thus, when proximal tubular Na⁺ reabsorption decreases, the distal tubular Na⁺ load increases, and the Na⁺ reabsorption increases proportionately. Hence, Na⁺ delivery to the distal tubules is an important controller of distal tubular Na⁺ reabsorption.

Transepithelial Potential Difference

Transepithelial potential difference (TEPD) is the electrical potential recorded between the tubular lumen and its exterior. It is recordable in all segments of the nephron that are involved in active Na⁺ transport. *Lumen-negative TEPD* is produced by active Na⁺ reabsorption that is unaccompanied by transport of equivalent amounts of anions. The high TEPD in the CCD is due to Na⁺ unitransport that is not associated with any paracellular Cl⁻ reabsorption. *Lumen-positive TEPD* is produced in the PST (by the Cl⁻ reabsorption, which exceeds Na⁺ reabsorption), in the TAL (by the back diffusion of K⁺ into the tubule), and in the OMCD (by active, electrogenic secretion of H⁺ into the tubule).

The high-negative TEPD in the CCD is of considerable physiologic importance. As already mentioned, an increased Na⁺ delivery to the distal nephron increases Na⁺ unitransport and thereby increases the TEPD. (1) Factors that increase distal Na⁺ delivery and thereby increase the TEPD include ECF volume expansion and diuretics acting on the proximal tubule. (2) *Aldosterone* increases the activity of the Na⁺–K⁺ pump in the distal nephron, thereby promoting Na⁺ unitransport and with it, the TEPD. (3) *Impermeable anions* such as sulfate (SO_4^{2-}) and nitrate (NO_3^-), which are not reabsorbed with Na^+, increase the TEPD when present in large amounts in the tubular fluid. (4) The secretion of K^+ into the lumen decreases the lumen-negative TEPD. Hence, *K$^+$ depletion,* which is associated with reduced tubular secretion of K^+, increases TEPD. (5) The secretion of the positively charged H^+ into the lumen decreases the lumen-negative TEPD. *Alkalosis* makes the TEPD more negative because H^+ secretion decreases in alkalosis. H^+ and K^+ secretion rates are reciprocally related because both are facilitated by the TEPD, and on secretion, both tend to neutralize the potential difference. For example, when H^+ secretion increases, the H^+ ions tend to neutralize the luminal negativity. The reduction in TEPD reduces K^+ secretion. In the same way, when K^+ secretion is high, the H^+ secretion decreases.

Diuretics

Diuretics are drugs that increase the rate of urine flow. They are used to adjust the volume and composition of body fluids in conditions such as hypertension and edema. The diuresis produced is almost always secondary to natriuresis (increased Na^+ losses in urine). Most diuretics have undesirable side effects, including hypokalemia and pH disturbances (**Table 55.1**).

Diuretics act on specific nephron segments (**Fig. 55.4**) and inhibit specific Na^+ transport mechanisms (**Table 55.1**). Diuretics acting on the proximal tubule have limited efficacy because the TAL, which has a great reabsorptive capacity, compensates for any decrease in Na^+ and H_2O reabsorption that might occur in the proximal tubule. Diuretics acting on sites distal to the TAL also have limited efficacy because only a small part of the filtered solute load and fluid reaches the distal tubule. Diuretics acting on the TAL are called loop diuretics or high-ceiling

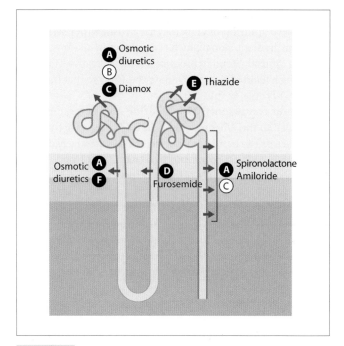

Fig. 55.4 Sodium reabsorption mechanisms (**Fig. 55.2A–F**) and the effects of various diuretics on Na^+ reabsorption (and hence water reabsorption).

diuretics. They are the most efficacious of all diuretics. They abolish the urine-concentrating ability of the nephron.

Most of the diuretics (amiloride, spironolactone, thiazide, and furosemide) have been discussed above with Na^+ reabsorption. Only osmotic diuretics are discussed here.

Osmotic diuretics | Commonly used osmotic diuretics (**Fig. 55.5**) are glycerin, mannitol, and urea. Being nonreabsorbable, they hold water in the tubule. They are most effective in the proximal tubule, where the maximum amount of water is reabsorbed. The water retained in the tubule dilutes the tubular concentration of Na^+ and other electrolytes, thereby reducing their reabsorption, too. Hence, osmotic diuretics increase the urinary excretion of nearly all electrolytes, including Na^+, K^+ (kaliuresis), Cl^-, HCO_3^- (resulting in acidosis), calcium (Ca^{2+}), magnesium (Mg^{2+}), and phosphate (PO_4^3).

As already explained above, the movement of Na^+ from the tubules into the tubular cells and from the lateral spaces to the peritubular capillaries occurs through passive diffusion. Dilution of the tubular fluid not only slows down the movement of Na^+, but also tends to reverse their direction: Na from the lateral spaces diffuses back into the tubules, and Na^+ from the peritubular capillaries diffuses back into the lateral spaces.

Summary

- Active reabsorption occurs in all segments of the tubule driven by the Na^+–K^+ pump in the basolateral membrane.

- Na^+ crosses the apical membrane from the lumen into the cell via several different transport processes, most of them associated with the cotransport of other solutes.

Table 55.1 The Mechanism of Action of Diuretics and Their Side Effects*

Diuretic	Segment and Mechanism	K$^+$ Depletion	Acidosis/ Alkalosis
Osmotic diuretics	1-(A), 2-(A), 2-(F)	Yes	Acidosis
CA inhibitors	1-(C)	Yes	Acidosis
Loop diuretics	3-(D)	Yes	Alkalosis
Thiazides	4-(E)	Yes	Alkalosis
Aldosterone antagonists	5-(A)	No†	Acidosis
Na$^+$ channel inhibitors	5-(A)	No†	Acidosis

*The numbers 1 to 5 indicate the site of diuretic action.
†These are called potassium-sparing diuretics.
Note: 1 = proximal convoluted tubule (PCT); 2 = proximal straight tubule (PST); 3 = thick ascending limb (TAL); 4 = distal convoluted tubule (DCT); 5 = collecting duct (CD). The letters refer to the Na+ transport mechanisms described in **Fig. 55.2**.
Abbreviation: CA, carbonic anhydrase.

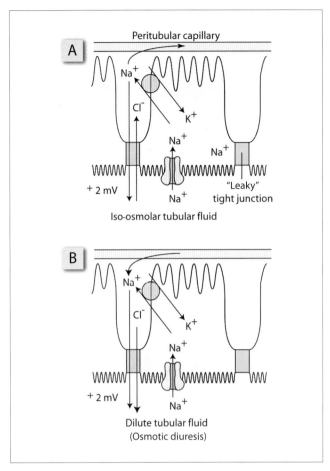

Fig. 55.5 Mechanism of action of osmotic diuretics. **(A)** Under normal conditions (iso-osmolar tubular fluid), Na^+ is reabsorbed. **(B)** When an osmotically active agent is filtered, it prevents water reabsorption, thus diluting the Na^+ that is present in the tubule. Under these conditions, Na^+ will move from the peritubular capillary to the tubular lumen.

- Na^+ absorption in the proximal and distal tubule depends on the Na^+ load presented to it; this is called glomerulotubular balance.

- Diuretics, drugs that increase the urine flow rate, almost always produce their effect by decreasing Na^+ reabsorption; with less Na^+ reabsorbed, less water is reabsorbed.

Applying What You Know

55.1. Reverend Fisher's laboratory report shows that he is hyponatremic. This may mean that his kidney is not doing a good job of reabsorbing filtered sodium. There are several different mechanisms by which Na^+ is reabsorbed. What do they all have in common?

55.2. What other possible explanation can you provide for Reverend Fisher's hyponatremia?

Osmolarity Changes in the Tubule

In the proximal tubules, solutes and water are reabsorbed in iso-osmolar proportions. Hence, the tubular fluid remains iso-osmotic to body fluids (290 mOsm/L, often rounded off to 300 mOsm/L for convenience) up to the end of the proximal tubule (in the cortex). However, as the tubule descends into the medulla, its osmolarity changes (**Fig. 56.1**).

As the thin segment descends into the deeper parts of the renal medulla, the tubular fluid increases in osmolarity until, at the papilla, it becomes hyperosmolar (as high as 1200 mOsm/L). This happens because the interstitium of the renal medulla is extremely hyperosmolar. As a result, water moves out of the tubular fluid into the hyperosmolar medulla. As the thin segment ascends back from the hyperosmotic medulla, the tubular fluid again becomes nearly iso-osmolar. The thin ascending limb is impermeable to water. Hence, the osmolarity changes occur due to the diffusion of sodium (Na^+) from the tubular fluid into the interstitium of the outer medulla and not by the diffusion of water in the reverse direction. The entire sequence of osmolar changes in the thin segment (first becoming hyperosmolar and then iso-osmolar again) might appear purposeless. On the contrary, the sequence of osmolar changes is a part of a larger mechanism called the countercurrent multiplier, and it is the countercurrent multiplier that makes the medulla hyperosmotic.

In the thick ascending limb (TAL), the urine becomes hypo-osmolar because TAL cells actively pump out Na^+ from the tubular fluid into the interstitium. Water cannot follow because the TAL is impermeable to water.

The permeability of the collecting duct to water is variable. In the presence of ADH (antidiuretic hormone or vasopressin; see Chapter 61), it is highly permeable to water. In the absence of ADH, it is impermeable to water. Accordingly, as the collecting tubule descends through the hyperosmolar medulla, the osmolarity of the tubular fluid can change in one of the two following ways. *In the absence of ADH,* the osmolarity of the tubular fluid remains unchanged. The urine formed is hypo-osmolar. *In the presence of ADH,* the osmolarity of the tubular fluid tends to equal that of the inner medulla. The urine formed is therefore hyperosmolar. It is in the collecting tubule that the urine becomes hyperosmolar a second time. (It becomes hyperosmolar for the first time in the thin segment.) The maximum possible osmolarity of the tubular fluid is 1200 mOsm/L, equal to the osmolarity in the innermost medulla. Thus, although urine invariably gets diluted in the distal tubule, it may or may not get reconcentrated in the collecting tubule.

Renal Medullary Hyperosmolarity

The interstitial fluid in the renal cortex has the same osmolarity as that of the plasma: 300 mOsm/L. In the renal medulla, however, it is much higher, and more so in the inner medulla, where it is 1200 mOsm/L. This hyperosmolarity is generated by a mechanism called the countercurrent multiplier system that operates in the loop of Henle.

The solutes concentrated in the medulla diffuse into the blood that flows through the medulla in the vasa recta. The flowing blood therefore carries away extra solutes with it and reduces the medullary osmolarity. This dissipation of medullary hyperosmolarity is minimized by the countercurrent exchanger system that operates between the ascending and descending limbs of the vasa recta.

The main driving force behind the countercurrent multiplier system is called the *single effect*; it is the osmotic gradient of ~200 mOsm/L, which exists between the tubular fluid in the ascending limb of the loop of Henle and the adjacent interstitium. The mechanisms of the single effect in the outer medulla and the inner medulla are different. *In the outer medulla,* the single effect is produced by the active reabsorption of Na^+ from the TAL. *In the inner medulla,* the thin segment cannot reabsorb Na^+ actively. Hence, the mechanism of the single effect remains unknown.

Countercurrent Multiplier in the Tubule

The operation of the countercurrent multiplier system can be better understood by considering a step-by-step approach to the processes involved (**Fig. 56.2**); this is, of course, fictitious in that flow through the nephron is continuous. (1) Initially,

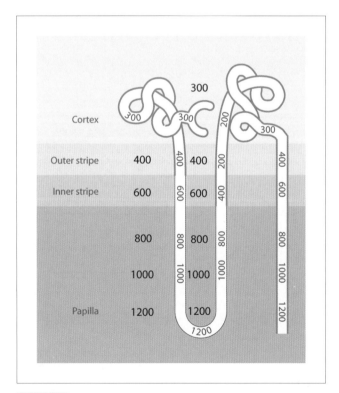

Fig. 56.1 Osmolarity of the filtrate at different sites in the tubule.

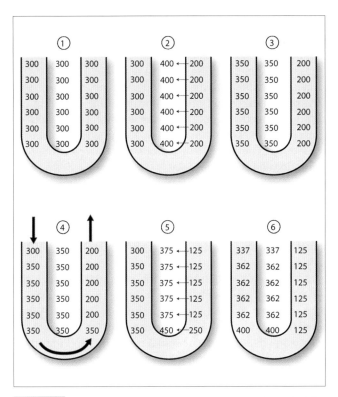

Fig. 56.2 Step-by-step changes in the osmolarity of tubular fluid due to the countercurrent multiplier effect. See text for a fuller explanation.

the tubular fluid and the renal interstitium have uniform osmolarity of 300 mOsm/L. (2) The TAL pumps out Na^+ ions (along with chlorine [Cl^-] and bicarbonate [HCO_3^-]) into the adjacent areas of the medullary interstitium. Because the TAL is impermeable to water, the osmolarity of the medullary interstitium rises and that of the tubular fluid in the TAL decreases. The maximum difference in osmolarity between the interstitium and the tubular fluid that can be established is around 200 mOsm/L, which is limited by the power of the Na^+–K^+ pump. Establishment of this osmotic gradient is the single effect. (3) The descending thin segment (DTS) is permeable to water, which flows into the osmotic gradient that exists until the osmolarity of the fluid in the DTS is in equilibrium with the osmolarity of the interstitium. (4) Fresh iso-osmolar filtrate (300 mOsm/L) flows down into the descending loop and pushes some of the hyperosmolar fluid into the ascending limb round the bend. (5) As the cycle of the above steps are repeated several times over, the tubular fluid and the medullary interstitium in the deeper regions of the medulla become more and more hyperosmolar. (6) Water moves out of the DTS to equilibrate its osmolarity with that of the interstitium. The consequence of the operation of this system is that there is a gradient of interstitial osmolarity from the top to the bottom of the renal medulla.

There is a simpler way of understanding it. Consider that Na^+ is continuously flowing in from the glomerulus into the tubule. However, most of the Na^+, instead of flowing out, gets trapped in a circular path and recycles between the ascending and descending limbs of the loop of Henle. Consequently, the Na^+ concentration becomes very high at the tip of the loop.

The above approach to understanding the countercurrent system cannot explain why a longer loop of Henle produces a higher medullary osmolarity, as observed in desert rats. An alternative approach explains the importance of the length of the loop of Henle. If all the NaCl pumped out at the TAL accumulated locally, the Na^+–K^+ pump would stop after creating a concentration gradient of 200 mOsm. However, because the countercurrent system removes the sodium chloride (NaCl) to a distant site, the Na^+–K^+ pump can continue to pump, while the NaCl concentration at the tip of the loop of Henle continues to rise.

Single effect in the inner medulla | Unlike the TAL, the inner medullary ascending thin segment (ATS) does not have the ability to actively reabsorb NaCl. The single effect in the inner medulla is therefore produced passively (**Fig. 56.3**). In the inner medulla, the osmolarity rates of the tubular fluid and the interstitium are initially the same. Although their osmolarities are the same, the composition of the tubular fluid is different from the composition of the interstitium. The tubular fluid in the thin ascending limb is rich in NaCl but has less urea in it. The adjacent interstitium is rich in urea but has less NaCl in it. Consequently, urea moves into the tubular fluid. Simultaneously, NaCl moves out of the thin ascending limb into the inner medullary interstitium. However, the rate at which NaCl diffuses out far exceeds the rate at which urea diffuses into the tubule. Hence, there is a *net solute reabsorption* from the thin ascending limb into the interstitium, which provides the single effect that is required for driving the countercurrent multiplier in the inner medulla. This hypothesis of the single effect in the inner medulla is called the *passive equilibration model*.

The countercurrent multiplier discussed above increases the Na^+ concentration in the renal medulla and occurs due to the *recycling of Na^+* between the ascending and descending

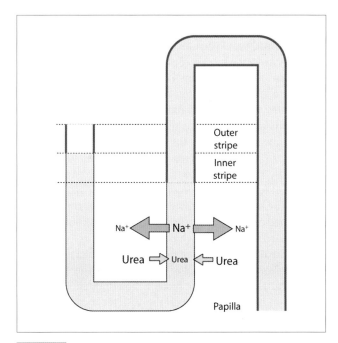

Fig. 56.3 Passive countercurrent multiplier in the inner medulla due to urea recycling.

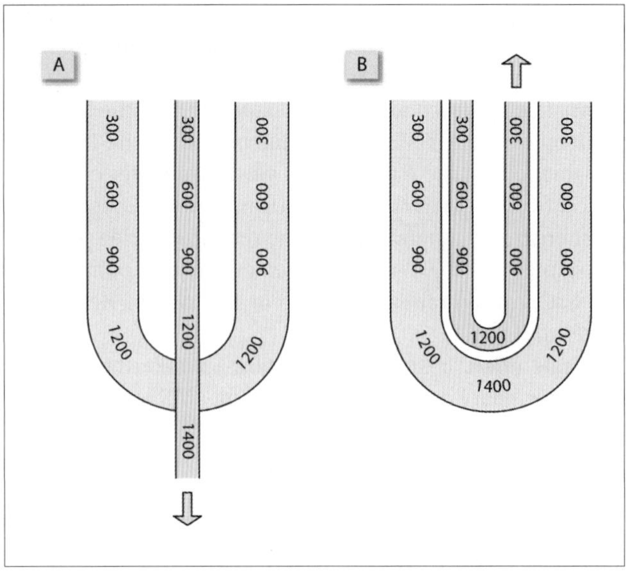

Fig. 56.4 Countercurrent exchange system in the vasa recta. **(A)** A blood vessel flowing past the loop of Henle. **(B)** A blood vessel looping with the loop of Henle.

loops of Henle. There is another countercurrent multiplier that concentrates urea in the renal medulla, and it occurs due to the *recycling of urea* between the collecting duct and the loop of Henle (see **Fig. 60.2**). Urea accounts for nearly half the osmolarity in the inner medulla.

Countercurrent Exchange in the Vasa Recta

Countercurrent exchange is essentially a physical principle that has several laboratory and industrial applications. In the human body, too, exchangers are found in the scrotum, skin, and intestinal villi. The basic principle of countercurrent exchange in the renal medulla is as follows.

If blood flowed through the hyperosmolar medulla as shown in **Fig. 56.4A**, it would equilibrate with medullary interstitium and carry away the solutes concentrated in the medulla. However, what actually happens is shown in **Fig. 56.4B**. As the vasa recta dips into the hyperosmolar medulla, the blood equilibrates with the surrounding interstitium and becomes hyperosmolar. Thereafter, as the vasa recta loops around and ascends toward the cortex, the osmolarity of the blood keeps decreasing as it equilibrates with the surrounding interstitium. By the time the vasa recta leaves the medulla, the blood in it is only slightly more hyperosmolar than when it entered the medulla. In other words, the solutes concentrated in the medulla are not washed away in significant amounts by the blood flowing through the medulla.

Because the blood flowing through the medulla equilibrates completely with the medullary interstitium, the amount of solutes carried away by the blood is flow-limited. Hence, the low rate of blood flow through the vasa recta contributes to the conservation of medullary hyperosmolarity. Conversely, a high blood flow rate through the medulla reduces medullary hyperosmolarity.

Factors Affecting Medullary Hyperosmolarity

Urea concentration in urine | Urea reabsorption from the inner medullary collecting duct (IMCD) is dependent on a urea-transport protein. Because the urea reabsorbed from IMCD is a major contributor to medullary hyperosmolarity, a genetic lack of urea-transport protein impairs urine-concentrating ability. Factors that reduce plasma urea concentration, such as a low protein diet, also affect the urine-concentrating ability of the kidneys. Conversely, a high protein diet increases the concentrating ability of the kidney.

Extracellular fluid (ECF) volume expansion increases the renal blood flow (RBF) and glomerular filtration rate (GFR) and suppresses ADH secretion. Each of these factors contributes to the reduction of medullary hyperosmolarity with consequent impairment of the urine-concentrating ability of the kidney.

An *increase in RBF* increases the blood flow through the vasa recta and washes out solutes from the renal medulla.

An *increase in GFR* increases the tubular flow rate. When tubular flow is high, the active transport of Na^+ is not able to sufficiently dilute the tubular fluid in the TAL, and the single effect is reduced in magnitude. Similarly, the reabsorption of water from the collecting tubule is not able to sufficiently concentrate urea in the IMCD if the tubular flow is high. Thus, the medullary hyperosmolarity decreases.

In the *absence of ADH,* the cortical collecting duct (CCD), the outer medullary collecting duct (OMCD), and the initial part of the IMCD become impermeable to water. Hence, urea does not get concentrated in the collecting duct. As a result, urea reabsorption from the terminal part of the collecting duct is markedly reduced (to ~20%), and urea concentration in the papillary interstitium is lowered.

Summary

● The osmolarity of the tubular fluid varies from the proximal tubule to the collecting duct.

● The interstitium of the renal medulla exhibits an osmolarity that increases from the near cortical region (~300 mOsm/L) to the tip of the papilla (as high as 1200 mOsm/L).

● The countercurrent multiplier (arising from the transport properties—pumps and permeabilities—is responsible for the gradient of interstitial osmolarity.

● The countercurrent exchanger (the vasa recta) is necessary to maintain this gradient.

Applying What You Know

56.1. Reverend Fisher's plasma osmolarity is 280 mOsm/L, slightly lower than normal. What changes to the normal mechanisms determining osmolarity might cause such a change? Explain.

Body water balance | The body gains ~2.5 L of water daily from food, drinks, and metabolism and loses the same amount in urine, insensible perspiration, sweat, and feces (**Fig. 57.1**). Nearly 7 L of water would be lost daily in gastrointestinal (GI) secretions (see **Fig. 70.4**) had the same amount not been completely reabsorbed in the intestine. When there is a GI obstruction, large volumes of secretions accumulate in the GI tract. These accumulated secretions represent losses of fluid and electrolytes from the body.

General Models: Reservoir and Balance of Forces

The body is a reservoir, with its water content determined by the balance between the input of water and various losses of water.

Body sodium balance | The daily dietary intake of sodium ions is ~100 to 400 mM. Most of this amount is lost daily in urine. A small amount is lost in sweat. Negligible amounts are also lost in feces.

Fluid and Electrolyte Homeostasis

Derangements of fluid and electrolyte balance result in changes in *blood volume* and *plasma osmotic pressure*. These changes set off a series of *readjustments* and *reflexes,* leading to the restoration of normal fluid and electrolyte composition of the body.

Readjustments in capillary exchange | Any change in the volume and oncotic pressure of the body fluids leads to changes in

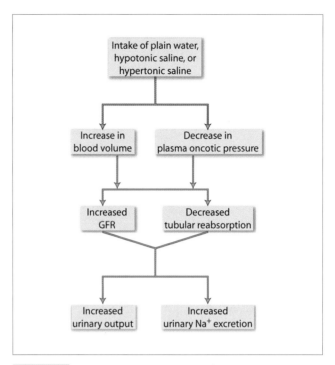

Fig. 57.2 Readjustments in renal filtration and reabsorption that correct changes in blood volume and plasma oncotic pressure. GFR, glomerular filtration rate.

the Starling forces operating at the renal glomeruli and renal tubules. The end result is a readjustment of glomerular filtration and tubular reabsorption so that the normal volume and oncotic pressure are restored (**Fig. 57.2**). Starling mechanisms affect tubular reabsorption mainly in the proximal tubule, where large amounts of water and Na$^+$ are reabsorbed. Hence, these mechanisms are more suited for large-scale adjustments in fluid and electrolyte balance. These readjustments are not initiated by changes in Na$^+$ concentration, nor do they maintain the constancy of body Na$^+$ concentration.

General Models: Flow and Balance of Forces

Fluid flow across the walls of the capillary is determined by a balance of forces between the hydrostatic pressure gradient and the oncotic pressure gradient.

The reason why an increase in blood volume results in an increased glomerular filtration rate (GFR) is explained in Chapter 54. The reason why an increase in blood volume reduces tubular reabsorption of fluids is that the peritubular capillary hydrostatic pressure increases when the blood volume is more. Finally, urinary excretion of Na$^+$ rises whenever GFR increases. This happens despite glomerulotubular balance, as explained and exemplified in Chapter 55.

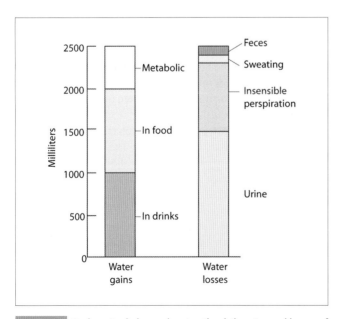

Fig. 57.1 Body water balance showing the daily gains and losses of water in the body.

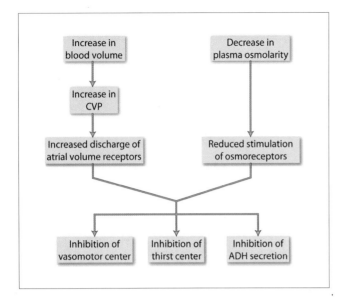

Fig. 57.3 Neurohormonal reflexes initiated by osmoreceptors and volume receptors. ADH, antidiuretic hormone; CVP, central venous pressure.

Neurohormonal reflexes | Any change in the volume and osmolarity of blood is sensed by volume receptors and osmoreceptors, respectively. These receptors in turn activate neural, hormonal, and behavioral mechanisms that correct the original disturbances (**Fig. 57.3**). The effector mechanisms include changes in renal function mediated by neural (sympathetic discharge) and hormonal (antidiuretic hormone [ADH] and aldosterone secretion) signals, and behavioral mechanisms (thirst and salt craving).

> **General Model: Homeostasis**
>
> Extracellular fluid (ECF) volume and various electrolyte concentrations are homeostatically regulated by negative feedback mechanisms, with the kidneys acting as the effector (varying its reabsorption or secretion of the substance).

Receptors for Fluid Osmolarity and Volume

Osmoreceptors are located in the anterior hypothalamus near, but distinct from, the supraoptic nuclei. They increase their discharge rate in response to as little as 1% rise in the osmolarity. Impulses from osmoreceptors reach the thirst center and the center where ADH is produced. The osmoreceptors do not respond to hypertonic solutions of urea or glucose, as these easily enter the osmoreceptor cell. That is significant because if it did, a rise in plasma urea concentration would stimulate the osmoreceptors, leading to a fall in the urinary output (see below) that would hamper the excretion of urea.

Volume receptors are located in the right atrium. When the blood volume increases, the venous pressure and with it, the right atrial pressure increase. The rise in the right atrial pressure increases the firing rate of the right atrial volume receptors. Impulses from the volume receptors travel through the vagus nerve and reach the medulla, where they inhibit the

pressor area of the vasomotor center and thereby suppress the sympathetic discharge. Conversely, a decrease in the blood volume would increase the sympathetic discharge. The afferents from the atrial volume receptors also reach the hypothalamus to inhibit thirst and ADH secretion.

The blood volume must decrease by as much as 10% to produce an increase in the sympathetic discharge, or thirst. Volume receptors are thus less sensitive than osmoreceptors. However, volume receptors bring about much stronger effects than osmoreceptors. This is apparent when a decreased plasma volume coexists with a decreased osmolarity. In such a situation, water is retained (by stimulation of thirst and ADH) to restore the blood volume at the expense of decreasing the osmolarity further; hence, the axiom volume overrides tonicity.

> **General Model: Homeostasis**
>
> The body's attempt to maintain homeostasis can result in situations in which the competing needs of the organisms must be dealt with simultaneously. In this case, the need to maintain plasma volume has precedence over the need to maintain osmolarity.

Effectors of Fluid and Electrolyte Homeostasis

Antidiuretic hormone is secreted largely by the neurons of the suprachiasmatic nuclei and also by the supraoptic nuclei in the hypothalamus, but it is released from axon terminals in the posterior pituitary gland (see **Fig. 76.3**). ADH secretion is stimulated by inputs from osmoreceptors as well as volume receptors. ADH promotes water reabsorption from the collecting duct and makes it isotonic or hypertonic, as required.

Aldosterone secretion is stimulated by (1) circulating angiotensin II formed as a result of sympathetic activation (the main stimulus), (2) rise in plasma K^+ concentration (a moderately strong stimulus), and (3) fall in plasma Na^+ concentration (a weak stimulus). Aldosterone promotes reabsorption of Na^+ from the distal convoluted tubule (DCT). Both ADH and aldosterone act on the distal tubule, where the amount of H_2O and Na^+ reabsorbed is much less than in the proximal tubule. Hence, these mechanisms are more suited for fine adjustments in fluid and electrolyte balance.

Thirst is the most prompt and effective mechanism for correcting a rise in plasma osmolarity. The center for thirst is located in the vicinity of the subfornical organ (SFO) and the organ vasculosum of the lamina terminalis (OVLT) in the hypothalamus. It results in an urge to drink water. It is stimulated by impulses from the osmoreceptors, inhibited by impulses from atrial volume receptors, and stimulated by angiotensin II. Astronauts at zero G do not get thirsty because their atrial volume receptors are continually stimulated. The importance of thirst can be appreciated from **Fig. 57.4,** which shows that at the normal plasma osmolarity of 290 mOsm/L, ADH secretion is nearly at its peak with little scope for further rise. Thus, it is thirst that is most important when osmolarity rises above 290 mOsm/L. It should also be clear that even complete reab-

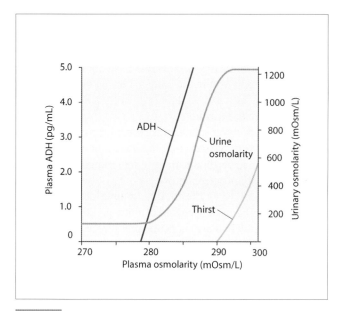

Fig. 57.4 Effect of plasma osmolarity on plasma antidiuretic hormone (ADH) and urinary osmolarity.

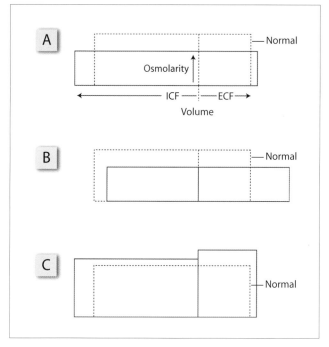

Fig. 57.5 Darrow-Yannet diagram for the graphic representation of the volume of the body fluid compartments and body fluid osmolarity. The intracellular fluid (ICF) and extracellular fluid (ECF) volumes are represented on the x-axis; the body fluid osmolarity is represented on the y-axis. **(A)** The normal status is shown in dotted lines; a fluid or electrolyte imbalance is shown in solid lines. Note that osmolarity is *always* the same in the two compartments. **(B)** An example of an unphysiologic situation, one in which the ECF volume equals the ICF volume. **(C)** Another example of an "impossible" situation, where the ECF osmolarity does not equal the ICF osmolarity.

sorption of filtered water cannot produce a gain of water content of the body; only increasing the water content by drinking can do this.

Salt craving is an intense desire for excessive consumption of NaCl evoked by a decrease in plasma Na^+ concentration. The change in plasma Na^+ concentration is sensed by receptors that are probably located in the amygdala of the brain.

Sympathetic discharge to the kidneys is stimulated by hypovolemia due to reduced stimulation of atrial volume receptors. It brings about retention of Na^+ and water (see **Table 54.1**).

Fluid and Electrolyte Imbalances

There are broadly four types of fluid and electrolyte disturbances. These are discussed below. It may be noted that in all disturbances, the volume and osmolarity of blood are affected first. The disturbance then spreads to the ECF and finally affects the intracellular fluid (ICF). Regardless of the type of imbalance, the ECF osmolarity and ICF osmolarity *always* remain equal in the steady state because water is free to move between compartments whenever an osmotic gradient is present. The changes in body fluid volume and osmolarity can be usefully depicted by Darrow-Yannet diagrams, which graphically display both fluid volume of the ICF and ECF and body fluid osmolarity (**Fig. 57.5**).

Water and Hypotonic or Isotonic Fluid Intake

Ingestion of water and hypotonic or isotonic fluids normally replenishes the obligatory amounts of salt and water that are lost in urine, expired air, and insensible perspiration (1200 mL per day). However, in certain situations, fluid intake can exceed fluid loss. For example, excess cold water or isotonic soda drinks may be ingested in summer to maintain body temperature.

Consequences | (1) The plasma volume increases. If hypotonic fluids are consumed, the plasma osmolarity decreases slightly. If isotonic electrolyte solutions are consumed, the plasma osmolarity is unaffected. (2) The plasma colloid osmotic pressure decreases irrespective of the changes in plasma osmolarity. (3) Due to the fall in colloid osmotic pressure, water and electrolytes move out of capillaries and are distributed in the interstitial compartment. (4) If the plasma osmolarity is also decreased, water moves into the intracellular compartment. Finally, all the body water compartments have a slightly higher volume and a slightly lower osmolarity. **Figure 57.6A** illustrates the consequences of drinking 3 L of distilled water (no electrolytes).

Corrective response | The changes in plasma volume and osmolarity are sensed by the atrial volume receptors and osmoreceptors, respectively. When activated, both of them bring about water diuresis: the excretion of large volumes of hypotonic urine that gradually restores the plasma volume and osmolarity to normal.

It is noteworthy that when plain water is consumed, a perfect correction of the resultant hypo-osmolarity would entail renal excretion of electrolyte-free water, but this never happens. The urine excreted is hypotonic but never salt-free; therefore, the renal response fails to correct the osmolarity. Hence,

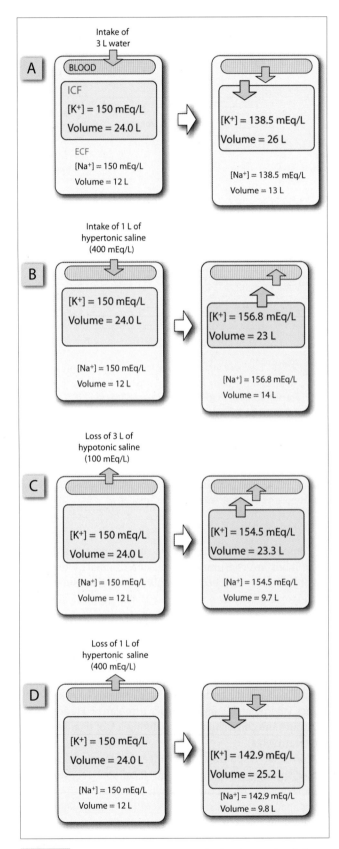

Fig. 57.6 Disruption and restoration of fluid and electrolyte balance. **(A)** Effect of excessive water intake. Note that of the 3 L of water ingested, 2 L enters the intracellular fluid (ICF), and 1 L enters the extracellular fluid (ECF). The ECF:ICF ratio remains 1:2. **(B)** Effect of intake of hypertonic saline; 1 L of water leaves the ICF and further expands the ECF. **(C)** Effect of loss of hypotonic saline; water is lost from the ICF. **(D)** Effect of loss of hypertonic saline; water enters the ICF from the diluted ECF.

plain water consumption over a period of time leads to salt depletion in the body, which must be replenished by salt intake. For the same reason, consumption of large amounts of water when hypernatremia is present would flush out the extra salts from the body and restore the body to normal osmolarity.

Hypertonic Saline Intake

Instances of hypertonic saline intake occur when salt is mistakenly added instead of sugar into the bottles of infants. Excessive amounts of hypertonic saline are sometimes administered to comatose patients erroneously.

Consequences | (1) The plasma volume and plasma osmolarity rise. The plasma colloid osmotic pressure decreases. (2) Due to the fall in plasma oncotic pressure, water and electrolytes move out of the capillaries into the interstitial spaces, uniformly increasing the ECF volume and osmolarity. (3) The electrolytes are not freely diffusible across the cell membrane. Hence, the raised osmotic pressure of the ECF extracts water from the cells into the ECF. (4) The final result is an increase in the osmolarity in all body fluids, a decrease in the volume of the ICF (with shrinking of cells), and an increase in the volume of the ECF (**Fig. 57.6B**).

Corrective response | An increase in plasma osmolarity promotes water retention, whereas an increase in plasma volume inhibits the same. In such conflicting situations, *volume overrides tonicity*; that is, the effects of volume prevail over those of tonicity. Hence, the increased plasma volume would suppress thirst and ADH, leading to the excretion of large volumes of hypotonic urine, which brings down the plasma volume. However, excretion of hypotonic urine would increase the plasma osmolarity further. The only way the osmolarity can be restored is by the natriuretic hormone, which is secreted in response to osmolarity and not volume changes. It promotes Na^+ excretion. However, the sequence of events is different if the consumption of hypertonic saline is immediately followed by drinking of plain water. The result, then, would be the same as that of consumption of isotonic or hypotonic fluids.

Water and Hypotonic or Isotonic Fluid Loss

Loss of hypotonic fluids occurs during profuse sweating because sweat is hypotonic. Loss of isotonic fluids occurs in diarrhea, intestinal obstruction (due to the accumulation of intestinal secretions above the site of obstruction), ascites and burns (plasma is sequestered in the peritoneal cavity and blisters, respectively), and hemorrhage. In effect, loss of hypotonic fluids is also caused by *water deprivation* because the daily obligatory water losses in urine, expired air, and insensible perspiration (totaling ~1200 mL of hypotonic fluid) are not replenished by water intake.

Consequences | (1) ECF volume is reduced. (2) Plasma volume is less affected than interstitial fluid volume due to the presence of plasma proteins, which "hold" fluids inside blood vessels. (3) ECF osmolarity rises if the fluid lost is hypotonic. ECF osmolarity is unchanged if the fluid lost is isotonic. (4) The rise of ECF osmolarity draws out water from the cells. After equilibrium, both ECF and ICF have reduced volume and increased osmolarity (**Fig. 57.6C**). (5) Shrunken cells suffer intracellular protein breakdown and loss of potassium (K⁺), often resulting in painful cramps of the muscles.

Corrective response | An increase in plasma osmolarity stimulates the osmoreceptors; the reduction in plasma volume inhibits the volume receptors. Both of them in turn restore the plasma volume and plasma osmolarity to normal levels. It is, however, important that the thirst (produced by osmoreceptors and volume receptors) is quenched with hypotonic or isotonic salt solutions instead of plain water. If plain water is ingested to correct the plasma volume, it will overcorrect (i.e., dilute) the plasma osmolarity. Over time, however, rehydration with plain water will lead to serious sodium chloride (NaCl) depletion in the body.

Hypertonic Fluid Loss or Salt Depletion

Hypertonic fluid loss is caused by vomiting or aspiration of gastric secretions. Simple NaCl depletion (without fluid depletion) occurs if any loss of salt and water (whether in hypotonic, isotonic, or hypertonic solutions) is followed by rehydration with only plain water. It can also be produced by completely excluding salt from the diet.

Consequences | (1) There is a uniform decrease in the ECF osmolarity. The decrease in ECF volume depends on the amount of water lost. In simple sodium chloride depletion, the ECF volume does not decrease initially. (2) Due to the fall in ECF osmolarity, water moves from the interstitial fluid into the cells. Consequently, ECF volume falls, and ICF volume rises (**Fig. 57.6D**). The cells swell up. (3) The cells of the thirst center also swell up. The thirst center interprets this as the presence of excess water in the body. Consequently, thirst is inhibited. (4) The volume and osmolarity changes of plasma tend to parallel those of the ECF. However, a decrease in plasma volume raises the plasma protein osmotic pressure. Hence, plasma volume is relatively better preserved than interstitial fluid volume. In severe cases, plasma volume reduces sufficiently to produce the grave salt deficiency syndrome, a shocklike state with signs of renal failure. However, unlike in shock, there is no sensation of thirst.

Corrective response | Although the ECF volume is reduced, thirst is absent. This is fortunate because any water ingested would promptly leave the ECF and expand the ICF further. The only appropriate response is the intense salt appetite or salt craving, which leads to consumption of large amounts of NaCl and restores the sodium osmolarity to normal. Restoration of the ECF osmolarity draws out water from the ICF and partly restores the ECF volume. As the cells lose water, thirst is restored, and any residual reduction in ECF volume is corrected through fluid intake.

Summary

- Water and electrolyte balance can only be maintained if the input (water and solutes drunk) and output (urine) are equal.

- Body fluid osmolarity and vascular volume are regulated by reflex mechanisms driven by hypothalamic osmoreceptors and atrial volume receptors.

- These reflexes employ hormones (ADH and aldosterone), thirst, and neural signals to alter kidney function so as to maintain homeostasis.

- The osmolarity of all the body compartments are the same because water moves down any osmotic gradient that might be created.

- When imbalances in water and solutes are present, water will move, creating several problems and giving rise to several compensatory responses.

Applying What You Know

57.1. Reverend Fisher is observed to have mild presacral edema, an accumulation of interstitial fluid in the soft tissue over his sacrum. What are the factors that have led to the development of edema here?

57.2. Reverend Fisher has been retaining fluids. His urine output has been significantly less than his fluid intake from drinking and from the intravenous (IV) line that is in place. Where will this retained fluid be found? Explain your reasoning.

Hydrogen (H^+) ions are being produced continuously by the metabolism of the body. By far the largest single source is carbon dioxide (CO_2) produced by aerobic metabolism of carbohydrates and most amino acids; the reaction of CO_2 and water (H_2O) then yields H^+ ions and bicarbonate (HCO_3^-) ions. However, the respiratory system normally removes CO_2 as fast as it is produced; hence, there is no net addition of H^+ ions to the body. Thus, CO_2 is often referred to as a volatile acid because it is "blown off" by the lungs.

The metabolism of proteins and fatty acids also produces sulfuric and phosphoric acids, as well as various organic acids, which are referred to collectively as nonvolatile acids (to contrast them with CO_2). The formation of nonvolatile acids, of course, creates H^+ ions. Finally, some bicarbonate formed in the pancreas is lost in feces, leaving an "excess" of H^+ ions.

If these excess H^+ ions are not removed from the body, the concentration of H^+ will rise. This means that the pH, the $-\log[H^+]$, will decrease (the lower the pH, the greater the $[H^+]$). The kidneys are responsible for eliminating these nonvolatile H^+ ions and preventing a change in the body's pH.

There is yet another problem. Bicarbonate ions are freely filtered at the glomerulus; hence, the daily filtered load of HCO_3^- is very large. If any appreciable fraction of this filtered bicarbonate were excreted, the pH of the body would become very low. Thus, the kidneys must reclaim or reabsorb most of the filtered bicarbonate.

Finally, there are a variety of disturbances, some the consequence of normal physiologic (homeostatic) responses, and some the consequence of pathology, that create changes in pH. As will be described in Chapter 68, the kidneys respond to these disturbances in a way that restores pH toward its normal value.

It is important to keep in mind the fact that the *absolute concentration* of H^+ present in the body at a normal pH of 7.4 is very small, only 40 nmol/L (40×10^{-9} mol/L). In comparison, the normal concentration of HCO_3^- ions is 24 mmol/L (24×10^{-3} mol/L), a factor of 10^6 greater.

General Models: Reservoir and Balance of Forces

The body is a reservoir in which there are various mechanisms generating H^+ ions, as well as various mechanisms by which H^+ ions are eliminated. The pH of body fluid is thus determined by the balance between these mechanisms.

Renal Secretion of H^+

The kidneys accomplish both tasks, eliminating the nonvolatile acids produced by the body and reclaiming the bicarbonate that is filtered, by mechanisms that begin with the secretion of H^+ ions into the tubular lumen. Three different transport mechanisms (see **Fig. 58.1**) are available to secrete H^+ ions

into the tubular lumen across the apical membrane of tubular cells: (1) a Na^+–H^+ exchanger or antiporter, (2) a H^+ pump, and (3) a H^+–K^+ exchange pump. In operation, the two exchangers are electroneutral, whereas the H^+ pump is electrogenic.

The Na^+–H^+ antiporter and the H^+ pump (**Fig. 58.1A**) are found predominantly in the cells of the proximal tubule (PT) and thick ascending limb (TAL). Secretion of H^+ in the PT accounts for reabsorption of 80% of the filtered bicarbonate. The TAL reabsorbs 10% of the filtered bicarbonate. In the distal tubule (DT) and collecting duct (CD), H^+ secretion is accomplished by the H^+–K^+ exchange pump (**Fig. 58.1B**); an H^+ pump is also found there. The CD reabsorbs 6% of the filtered bicarbonate, and the CD reabsorbs the remaining 4%.

Factors affecting proton secretion | H^+ secretion is affected primarily by three factors: blood pH, luminal pH, and transepithelial potential difference (TEPD). A low *blood pH,* as occurs in acidosis, is associated with higher rates of H^+ secretion. This is important in the regulation of *body pH.*

A fall in *luminal pH* reduces H^+ secretion. A steep fall in luminal pH is prevented by a high tubular flow rate (which washes out the secreted H^+) and a high concentration of urinary buffers, both of which increase the tubular secretion of H^+.

Luminal negativity increases the tubular secretion of H^+. Situations in which the TEPD, especially in the cortical CD (CCD), is altered include the following. (1) A decrease in Na^+ reabsorption in the proximal tubule results in the delivery of a greater Na^+ load to the distal tubule. The increase in Na^+ unitransport in the distal tubule increases the luminal negativity. (2) An increase in K^+ secretion in the distal tubule (as occurs in hyperkalemia) reduces luminal negativity because K^+ is positively charged. (3) The luminal negativity increases if greater amounts of impermeant anions are present in the distal tubular fluid. (4) Aldosterone stimulates Na^+ unitransport and thereby increases luminal negativity.

Bicarbonate Reabsorption

In the proximal tubule and TAL, the H^+ secreted into the lumen is buffered entirely by HCO_3^-, forming H_2CO_3. The brush border of the proximal tubule and TAL contains carbonic anhydrase (CA); therefore, the carbonic acid (H_2CO_3) dissociates into CO_2 and H_2O. The CO_2 rapidly diffuses into the tubular cell, where it reacts with water to produce HCO_3^- and H^+. The H^+ formed is recycled as it is secreted again into the tubule. The HCO_3^- formed in the tubular cell diffuses out through the basolateral membrane into the peritubular capillary via two different transport systems: a Na^+–$3HCO_3^-$ symporter and a Cl^-–HCO_3^- antiporter (**Fig. 58.1A**). Thus, when a secreted H^+ ion is buffered by bicarbonate, one HCO_3^- appears in the peritubular fluid for each HCO_3^- that disappears from the tubular fluid. This is called HCO_3^- reclamation or, less appropriately, HCO_3^- reabsorption. The proximal convoluted tubule (PCT) reclaims 80%

Fig. 58.1 Mechanisms of hydrogen (H$^+$) secretion. **(A)** In the proximal tubule and thick ascending limb, H$^+$ is secreted by a sodium–(Na$^+$) H$^+$ exchanger and an H$^+$ pump; as a consequence, a bicarbonate ion is effectively reabsorbed (reclaimed). **(B)** In the distal tubule and collecting duct, H$^+$ is secreted by a H$^+$–potassium (K$^+$) exchanger and an H$^+$ pump; a new bicarbonate ion is created using phosphate and ammonia acting as buffers. CA, carbonic anhydrase.

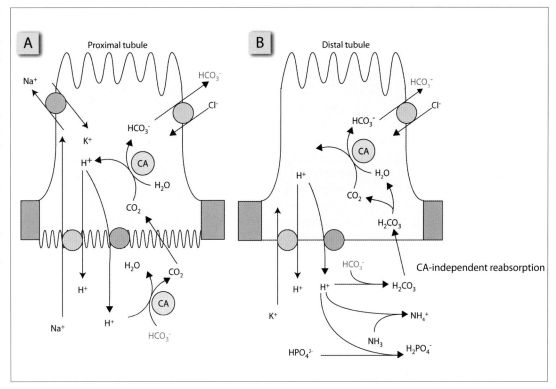

of the filtered load of bicarbonate. Another 15% of the filtered bicarbonate load is reclaimed in the TAL.

Generation of New Bicarbonate

Secretion of H$^+$ ions to reclaim filtered bicarbonate does not reduce the body's load of H$^+$ ions because the process described above regenerates H$^+$ for each one that is secreted. To deal with the excess H$^+$ from nonvolatile acids, some tubular buffer other than bicarbonate has to be used (see **Fig. 58.1B**).

Phosphate buffers comprise a mixture of monobasic and dibasic phosphates. The monobasic phosphates bind H$^+$, forming dibasic phosphates (H$^+$ + HPO$_4^{2-}$ = H$_2$PO$_4^-$). Phosphates are quite effective as urinary buffers, especially in the distal tubule, because they are not reabsorbed proximally in significant amounts and therefore become concentrated in tubular fluid. They are also effective because their pK (the negative log of the dissociation constant) is quite near the urinary pH.

Ammonia buffers bind H$^+$, producing ammonium ion (H$^+$ + NH$_3$ = NH$_4^+$). The ammonia is produced in the proximal tubular cells from glutamine.

$$\text{Glutamine} \xrightarrow{\text{Glutaminase}} \text{Glutamate} + \text{NH}_3$$

$$\text{Glutamate} \xrightarrow{\text{Glutamate } \alpha\text{-dehydrogenase}} \alpha\text{-ketoglutarate}$$

Ammonia normally buffers more of the H$^+$ from nonvolatile acids than does phosphate. The tubular secretion of NH$_3$ is stimulated in chronic acidosis, resulting in the increased production of new bicarbonate. The amount of new bicarbonate that can be generated is limited by the existing pH (which in part determines the availability of H$^+$ ions) and P$_a$CO$_2$ (the hydration of carbon dioxide is a source of bicarbonate ions). This mechanism has an important role in the regulation of body pH (see Chapter 63).

Summary

- Hydrogen ions are produced by a variety of metabolic processes, but their concentration in the body must be kept constant.

- The kidneys secrete H$^+$ using three different transport mechanisms.

- The secreted H$^+$ is buffered by filtered HCO$_3^-$ in the process of bicarbonate reclamation (reabsorption).

- Secreted H$^+$ ions are also buffered by filtered phosphate and ammonia produced by renal tubule cells.

Applying What You Know

58.1. Reverend Fisher's bicarbonate concentration is somewhat low (22 mL/L). What does this suggest about how his kidneys are handling bicarbonate ions?

Renal Handling of K⁺

The renal handling of potassium (K⁺) is summarized in **Fig. 59.1A**. The proximal convoluted tubule (PCT) has the largest reabsorptive capacity for K⁺; the connecting tubule (CNT) and the initial part of the cortical collecting duct (CCD) have the greatest capacity for K⁺ secretion. The overall result may be net K⁺ reabsorption or net K⁺ secretion. The distal convoluted tubule (DCT) cells can tilt the balance between net reabsorption and net secretion because these cells can reabsorb as well as secrete K⁺ depending on the body's potassium balance.

General Model: Balance of Forces

To understand the kidney's handling of K⁺ requires a clear understanding of the balance between K⁺ reabsorption and secretion by all available mechanisms in all segments of the nephron.

The **cellular mechanisms** of K⁺ transport are summarized in **Fig. 59.1B**. Unlike the transport mechanisms of sodium (Na⁺), which have important implications in diuretic mechanisms, the different K⁺ transport mechanisms have no such clinical importance and therefore are not discussed further.

All renal tubular cells have, on their basolateral membrane, a Na⁺–K⁺ adenosine triphosphatase (ATPase) that accumulates K⁺ inside the cell. A cell secretes K⁺ if the K⁺ leaves the cell through the apical membrane. Conversely, a cell reabsorbs K⁺ if the K⁺ enters through the apical membrane using K⁺–H⁺ ATPase and exits through the basolateral membrane. If all the K⁺ that enters the cell through the basolateral membrane exits through basolateral K⁺ channels, neither reabsorption nor secretion is occurring; the K⁺ merely recycles across the basolateral membrane.

Factors affecting potassium secretion | In the distal nephron, there may be net reabsorption or secretion of K⁺, depending on the K⁺ balance in the body. K⁺ secretion increases when (1) the activity of the apical K⁺–H⁺ ATPase is low, (2) the intracellular K⁺ concentration is high (due to increased activity of the basolateral Na⁺–K⁺ ATPase), (3) the tubular K⁺ concentration is low (due to increase in the tubular flow of filtrate), and (4) the transepithelial potential difference (TEPD) is highly negative (due to high Na⁺ unitransport).

A *fall in plasma* [K⁺] stimulates K⁺ reabsorption by stimulating the apical K⁺– H⁺ ATPase in the intercalated cells of the collecting duct. This change in K⁺ secretion in response to plasma [K⁺] is an important chronic response to external K⁺ imbalance.

Aldosterone increases K⁺ secretion because it stimulates Na⁺–K⁺ ATPase, increases lumen negativity by stimulating Na⁺ unitransport, and increases the permeability of the apical membrane to K⁺. Aldosterone-mediated change in K⁺ secretion is an important acute response to external K⁺ imbalances.

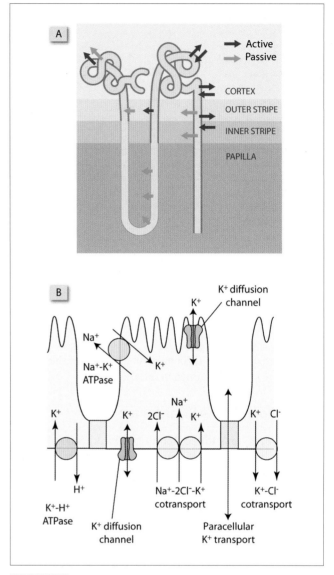

Fig. 59.1 **(A)** Sites of potassium ion (K⁺) reabsorption and secretion in the nephron. **(B)** Cellular mechanism of K⁺ reabsorption and secretion.

Acidosis decreases the basolateral Na⁺–K⁺ ATPase activity. Acidosis is also associated with increased H⁺ secretion, which reduces the luminal negativity. Both factors contribute to the reduction in K⁺ secretion in acidosis.

Body Potassium Balance

The total body K⁺ content is ~4500 mM. More than 95% of K⁺ is located within cells, mostly muscle cells, with smaller quantities in liver cells and blood cells based on number of cells (**Fig. 59.2**). The normal serum [K⁺] ranges from 3.5 to 5.3 mM/L, and large deviations from this normal range have serious consequences.

External Potassium Balance

External K⁺ balance refers to the constancy of total body K⁺ and is achieved when the daily intestinal absorption of K⁺ equals its daily urinary excretion (**Fig. 59.2**). A normal external balance ensures long-term constancy of body K⁺ content. However, rapid losses of large amounts of K⁺ can cause serious hypokalemia.

General Model: Reservoir

Here is another example of the body considered as a reservoir; the K⁺ content depends on balancing the K⁺ ingested and the K⁺ lost in urine and feces (and under some conditions, in sweat).

The average diet contains ~100 mM/day of potassium (5 g/day). Ninety percent of ingested potassium is absorbed, and the remaining 10% appears in the stool. Most of the gastrointestinal tract absorbs as well as secretes K⁺. In the colon, secretion is highly developed. Diarrheal states in which colonic K⁺ secretion is stimulated are associated with severe hypokalemia. Gastrointestinal absorption of K⁺ is not physiologically regulated; hence, the external K⁺ balance is maintained entirely through renal regulation of K⁺ excretion.

K⁺ reabsorption in the proximal tubule is load-dependent, always absorbing nearly 90% of the filtered K⁺ load. Hence, the proximal tubules play no role in the regulation of extracellular K⁺ balance. The appropriate renal response to K⁺ imbalance occurs in the DCT and the collecting duct. The renal response has both short-term and long-term mechanisms.

In the *short-term mechanism*, an increase in plasma K⁺ stimulates aldosterone secretion. Aldosterone acts on the distal nephron and increases K⁺ excretion within 2 hours.

The *long-term mechanism* takes several hours and is aldosterone-independent. An increase in plasma K⁺ inhibits the apical K⁺–H⁺ ATPase in the intercalated cells of the collecting duct and thereby increases K⁺ secretion, restoring normal plasma K⁺ levels. Conversely, K⁺ deprivation stimulates K⁺–H⁺ ATPase.

General Model: Homeostasis

Here, as in many other instances, the kidneys are the effector for homeostatically regulating the state of the internal environment (the extracellular [K⁺]).

Internal Potassium Balance

Internal K⁺ balance refers to the constancy of the distribution of K⁺ in the intracellular and extracellular compartments. What makes internal balance important is that even a small leak of intracellular K⁺ drastically raises the plasma K⁺ levels, with potentially lethal consequences. This does not happen because any acute change in plasma K⁺ results in a rapid (occurring within minutes) redistribution of K⁺ between the extracellular (ECF) and intracellular fluid (ICF), a process that acts as a buffer against extreme changes in plasma K⁺ concentration. As in the case of external balance, the internal K⁺ balance also has short-term and long-term mechanisms.

The *short-term mechanism* of restoration of the internal K⁺ balance is initiated by the membrane depolarization that occurs when the plasma K⁺ increases (see **Fig. 6.5A**). The sequence of events is depicted in **Fig. 59.3**.

In the *long-term mechanism*, chronic hypokalemia decreases the number of Na⁺–K⁺ ATPase molecules in the membrane.

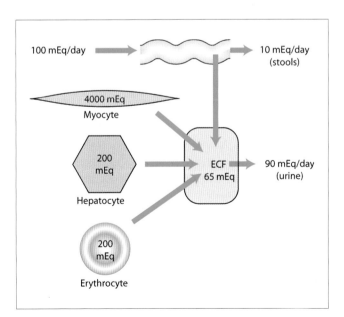

Fig. 59.2 External potassium balance. One milliequivalent (mEq) is the same as one millimole (mmol) because potassium has a single charge. ECF, extracellular fluid.

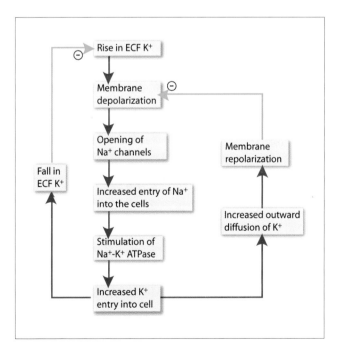

Fig. 59.3 Short-term mechanism of internal potassium balance. ECF, extracellular fluid. The pumping of K⁺ into the cell occurs at a much faster rate than the increased leak of K⁺ out of the cell.

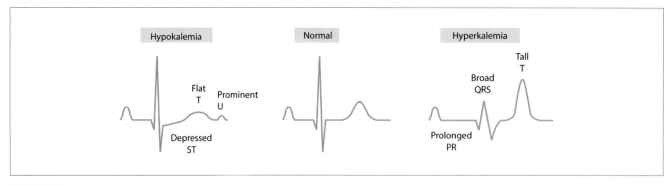

Fig. 59.4 Electrocardiographic changes associated with changes in serum potassium ion concentration. See also **Fig. 32.7**.

This reduces the intracellular K^+ concentration and increases the extracellular K^+ to a normal level.

Disorders of Potassium Homeostasis

Body K^+ balance is disturbed in several clinical situations (**Table 59.1**). The pathophysiology of some of them is discussed below.

Pathophysiology | *Diabetic ketoacidosis* results in hyperkalemia with reduced intracellular stores of K^+. The reason is twofold. (1) Insulin promotes the entry of K^+ into cells. Hence, in diabetes mellitus, K^+ moves out of the cells into the ECF. (2) The loss of insulin's growth factor activity diminishes intracellular ribonucleic acid (RNA). Normally, intracellular anions, such as organic phosphates, deoxyribonucleic acid (DNA), and RNA, counterbalance the positive charge of intracellular K^+; therefore, the loss of these anions is associated with the loss of K^+ from the cells.

Metabolic acidosis results in entry of H^+ into the ICF. The rise in intracellular H^+ concentration may or may not be associated with a fall in intracellular K^+. In the case of mineral acids, the conjugate bases, such as chloride (Cl^-), sulfate (SO_4^{2-}) and nitrate (NO_3^-), are unable to enter the cell simultaneously with H^+. The rise of intracellular H^+ therefore depolarizes the membrane, allowing intracellular K^+ to diffuse outward along a more favorable electrochemical gradient. However, organic acids (e.g., lactate and acetoacetate) enter cells readily along with H^+, so that the membrane potential remains unchanged, and there is no redistribution of K^+. *Respiratory acidosis* has very little effect on serum K^+ levels because the membrane potential does not change when CO_2 (which is electroneutral) enters the cells or when it reacts with water to form H^+ and HCO_3^- (cation–anion pair) inside the cell.

The internal K^+ balance is also disturbed during *exercise*. During the depolarization that accompanies muscle contraction, K^+ exits from cells. Most of the K^+ released enters the T tubules, from which K^+ is rapidly taken back into the cell on repolarization. Very little K^+ enters the interstitial fluid and plasma. With vigorous exercise, however, there is a rise in plasma K^+ levels. The local hyperkalemia in muscle causes vasodilatation and activation of glycogenolysis, both of which are useful in exercise. Patients with disturbed T tubule architecture may develop hyperkalemia with the slightest exercise, like fist clenching.

Clinical features | *Neuromuscular symptoms* are prominent in hypokalemia. It ranges from muscle weakness to total paralysis. *Cardiac symptoms* such as arrhythmias are more prominent in hyperkalemia. Electrocardiographic changes are present in both hypokalemia and hyperkalemia (**Fig. 59.4**). *Gastrointestinal tract symptoms* of hypokalemia include abdominal distension due to paralytic ileus.

Summary

- K^+ is both reabsorbed and secreted by the tubule; the balance between the two is determined by the state of K^+ that is present in the body.

- External (whole body) K^+ balance requires that K^+ ingested is balanced by K^+ lost in the urine.

- Internal (cellular) K^+ balance is maintained by appropriate transport of K^+ into or out of the cell.

- Changes in extracellular K^+ concentration can have profound, even life-threatening effects on the function of all excitable cells (nerve and muscle).

Table 59.1 Causes of Hypokalemia and Hyperkalemia

Causes of Hypokalemia	Causes of Hyperkalemia
Decreased dietary intake	Excessive dietary intake
	Vigorous exercise
	Tissue damage (muscle crush, hemolysis, internal bleeding)
Metabolic alkalosis	Metabolic acidosis
Renal tubular acidosis	
Hyperaldosteronism	Hypoaldosteronism
Cushing disease	Addison disease
Diuretics	Potassium-sparing diuretics
Renal failure (ARF, CRF)	

Abbreviations: ARF, acute renal failure; CRF, chronic renal failure.

Applying What You Know

59.1. Reverend Fisher's laboratory report reveals that his plasma K^+ is on the high side of normal. He is also retaining water. How can you explain his slightly elevated $[K^+]$ in the face of his being in positive water balance?

59.2. The initial laboratory report for Reverend Fisher shows him to have a low $[Na^+]$ and a $[K^+]$ that is at the high end of the normal range. How might the state of these electrolytes contribute to his appearing lethargic and confused on physical examination?

60 Renal Handling of Miscellaneous Substances

Glucose

Glucose is freely filtered into the glomerular filtrate and is completely reabsorbed in the proximal tubule. At the apical membrane of the proximal tubular cell, there is a carrier-mediated Na^+–glucose cotransporter. The carrier is called the sodium-dependent glucose transporter (SGLT). The cotransport derives its energy from the Na^+ concentration gradient that exists between the high tubular Na^+ concentration and the low intracellular Na^+ concentration produced by the pumping out of Na^+ through the basolateral surface.

General Model: Energy

Glucose is the common energy source for all cells of the body. It therefore makes sense that all filtered glucose normally will be reabsorbed rather than allowing some to be lost from the body.

The glucose that enters the cell through the apical membrane diffuses out of the basolateral membrane by facilitated diffusion. The carrier for facilitated diffusion across the basolateral membrane is called the glucose transporter (GLUT), which belongs to a different family of glucose transporters than the SGLT.

In the proximal convoluted tubule (PCT), where the tubular concentration of glucose is high, the apical glucose carrier is SGLT-2, which is a high-capacity, low-affinity SGLT. The basolateral glucose carrier is GLUT-2, which is a high-capacity, low-affinity GLUT.

In the proximal straight tubule (PST), the tubular glucose concentration is low. Appropriately, the glucose carrier is SGLT-1, which is a high-affinity, low-capacity $2Na^+$–glucose–galactose cotransporter (**Fig. 60.1**). The glucose reabsorbed

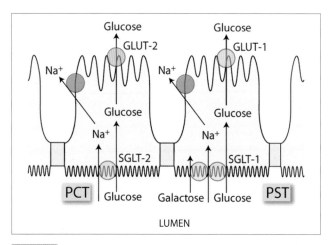

Fig. 60.1 Tubular reabsorptive mechanisms for glucose. SGLT, sodium-dependent glucose transporter; GLUT, glucose transporter; PCT, proximal convoluted tubule; PST, proximal straight tubule.

here is mostly used for cellular nutrition. Some of it exits the basolateral membrane using GLUT-1.

Although glucose reabsorption is an active process involving high-capacity transporters, it is possible to saturate them when the filtered load of glucose (that is to say, the plasma concentration of glucose because it is freely filterable) gets too high (see Chapter 62 for a discussion of this phenomenon). This situation can easily arise in a diabetic patient whose blood glucose control is not good.

Proteins

Amino acids are normally completely reabsorbed in the proximal tubule. They are transported across the apical border of proximal cells through secondary active transport. There are different carrier proteins for neutral, basic, and acidic amino acids and imino acids. Cystine and methionine have specific carriers.

Peptides and small proteins that are filtered into the tubules are endocytosed by the proximal tubular cells. Inside the cell, they are cleaved into the constituent amino acids, which diffuse out into peritubular capillaries.

Urea

Urea is filtered freely into the glomerular filtrate. About half of the filtered urea is reabsorbed passively in the proximal tubule. In the proximal straight tubule (PST) and the thin segment, urea diffuses into the tubular lumen from the medullary interstitium, where it is present in high concentration. The remaining part of the tubule, except its terminal part, has a low permeability to urea and therefore loses water to the hyperosmolar medullary interstitium. As water is reabsorbed from the cortical collecting duct (CCD), the outer medullary collecting duct (OMCD), and the initial part of the inner medullary collecting duct (IMCD), the urea in the collecting duct becomes more and more concentrated. When the urea-rich tubular fluid reaches the urea-permeable terminal IMCD, a large amount of urea is reabsorbed into the interstitium using a special *urea transport protein*. The synthesis of this protein is stimulated by antidiuretic hormone (ADH).

From the medullary interstitium, most of the urea enters the vasa recta and is carried up toward the renal cortex by the ascending vasa recta. From there, urea diffuses out to enter the PSTs of cortical nephrons. The urea is carried back to the OMCD, where it diffuses out again, resulting in a constant recycling (**Fig. 60.2**). This *recycling of urea* concentrates it in the inner medulla and explains why nearly 50% of the medullary hyperosmolarity is attributable to urea.

Uric Acid

Urate is freely filtered into the glomerular filtrate. The tubular transport of uric acid is confined almost exclusively to the

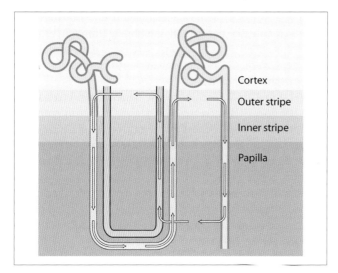

Fig. 60.2 Urea recycling.

proximal tubule and involves both reabsorption and secretion. In the initial and middle part of the PCT, the reabsorption far exceeds secretion, and the urates are reabsorbed almost completely. In the distal portion of the PCT and the beginning of the PST, moderate amounts of urates are secreted. In the remaining part of the PST, moderate amounts of urates are reabsorbed again: this is known as postsecretory reabsorption (**Fig. 60.3A**).

Tubular reabsorption of uric acid occurs both transcellularly and paracellularly. The transcellular reabsorption occurs through secondary active transport, whereas the paracellular reabsorption is passive. The apical membrane of the cells of the proximal tubule contain a *urate transport protein* involved in the countertransport of urate with intracellular anions such as Cl^- and HCO_3^-, and also organic anions such as lactate. The urates move out through the basolateral membrane using another anion exchanger. The same anion exchangers are employed for urate secretion as well (**Fig. 60.3B**).

Because urate reabsorption in the proximal tubules is linked to Na^+ reabsorption, *diuretics* that decrease the reabsorption of Na^+ and water in the proximal tubule decrease urate reabsorption, too. On the other hand, diuretics acting on the distal tubules decrease the extracellular fluid (ECF) volume, which, in turn, increases the Na^+ reabsorption in the proximal tubule. Hence, these diuretics increase urate reabsorption and tend to cause hyperuricemia.

Analgesics such as salicylates and phenylbutazone, when administered in low doses, reduce urate excretion by inhibiting urate secretion. When administered in higher doses, these analgesics also inhibit urate reabsorption and therefore increase urate excretion.

Organic Acids and Bases

In the ionized form, organic acids and bases are secreted through secondary active transport. For example, para-aminohippuric acid (PAH) is secreted across the apical membrane by PAH–anion antiport coupled with Na^+–anion symporter. The anion is a dicarboxylate or a tricarboxylate. The entire transport mechanism is nonelectrogenic (see **Fig. 55.2B**). These transport systems are nonspecific: one anion transporter can transport several endogenous (bile salts, hippurate, urate) and exogenous (PAH, penicillin, probenecid, aspirin) substances. There is competition among substances sharing the same transport system for elimination. For example, probenecid inhibits the tubular secretion of penicillin.

In the *nonionized form,* organic acids and bases are sufficiently lipid-soluble to diffuse passively across the tubular epithelium. Passive diffusion is faster than transport of the ionized forms. Many drugs and their metabolites are weak acids or bases that are predominantly nonionized and therefore diffuse out into the tubules quickly. Alkalinization of urine ionizes the weakly acidic drug in the tubular fluid, resulting in a reduction of its nonionized form in tubular fluid. This increases the concentration gradient of the nonionized drug between blood and tubular fluid; therefore, this favors its passive diffusion from blood into the tubule. This process is known as *nonionic diffusion* with *diffusion trapping* (**Fig. 60.4**).

Calcium and Phosphates

About 45% of the plasma calcium is bound to plasma proteins and therefore does not get filtered into the tubules. The free

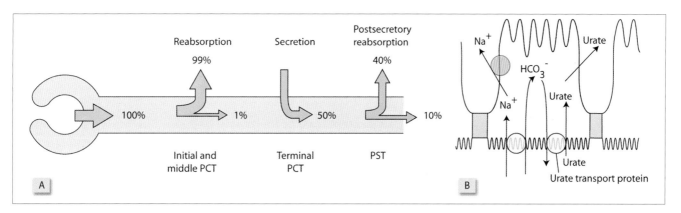

Fig. 60.3 **(A)** Postsecretory reabsorption of urates in the proximal tubule. **(B)** Tubular reabsorptive mechanism for urates. PCT, proximal convoluted tubule; PST, proximal straight tubule.

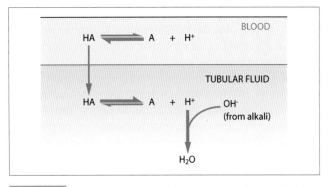

Fig. 60.4 Nonionic diffusion and diffusion trapping produced by urine alkalinization.

calcium (Ca^{2+}) that is filtered into the tubules is almost completely reabsorbed.

The cellular mechanisms of calcium and phosphate handling are summarized in **Fig. 60.5**. The reabsorption of Ca^{2+} is both paracellular and transcellular. In transcellular transport, the apical transport is mostly through facilitated diffusion and partly through Ca^{2+} channels that are responsive to parathyroid hormone (PTH) and calcitonin. The facilitated diffusion

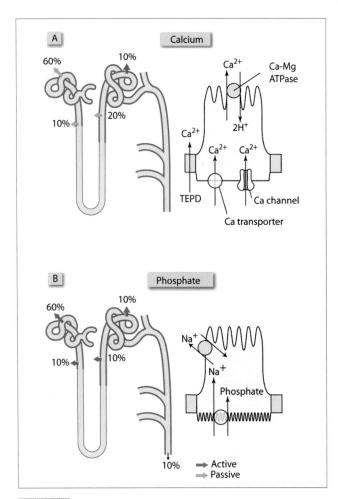

Fig. 60.5 Tubular reabsorption of calcium and phosphates. ATPase, adenosinetriphosphatase; TEPD, transepithelial potential difference.

employs a carrier protein called calbindin. Ca^{2+} is actively extruded across the basolateral membrane through primary active transport using Ca^{2+}–Mg^{2+} ATPase, a Ca^{2+}-stimulated, Mg^{2+}-dependent ATPase. Phosphate is reabsorbed through a Na^+-phosphate symport.

PTH stimulates Ca^{2+} reabsorption in the distal tubules. However, because PTH increases the plasma Ca^{2+} concentration through its actions on bones and the gastrointestinal tract, large amounts of Ca^{2+} are filtered into the tubules, and the net excretion in the urine might actually increase. PTH also increases the excretion of phosphates.

Vitamin D promotes the reabsorption of both Ca^{2+} and phosphates. Vitamin D increases the synthesis of calbindin and thereby increases Ca^{2+} reabsorption. It also stimulates the activity of Ca^{2+}-Mg^{2+} ATPase.

Loop diuretics produce a large increase in Ca^{2+} excretion by reducing the transepithelial potential difference in the thick ascending limb. Thiazide diuretics markedly reduce Ca^{2+} excretion by increasing Ca^{2+} reabsorption in the distal convoluted tubule and have been used in the treatment of hypercalcuria.

Summary

● The kidneys are responsible for controlling the concentration of a great many solutes found in body fluids, including glucose, proteins, nitrogenous waste products such as urea and uric acid, organic acids and bases, and calcium and phosphate.

Applying What You Know

60.1. Proteins are found in Reverend Fisher's urine. This is undoubtedly the result of ischemic damage to his kidneys. Where might the damage have occurred that results in protein in his urine?

60.2. Reverend Fisher has elevated BUN (blood urea nitrogen) and creatinine. What mechanism is causing an accumulation of nitrogenous waste products in his blood?

Antidiuretic Hormone

Antidiuretic hormone (ADH), also called *arginine vasopressin* (AVP), is a neurohormone, a hormone secreted into the circulation by nerve cells. The principal action of ADH (see below) is to help regulate body fluid osmolarity. The precursor of ADH is *prepropressophysin,* which is synthesized in the cell bodies of the neurons in the *supraoptic* and *paraventricular nuclei* (see **Fig. 76.3**). Prepropressophysin is cleaved in the endoplasmic reticulum to form ADH and packaged into secretory granules (called *Herring bodies*) in the Golgi apparatus. The Herring bodies are transported down the axons by axoplasmic flow to their endings in the posterior pituitary. ADH is released from the neurons when they are stimulated by neural signals arising from the osmoreceptors and volume receptors.

There are two types of ADH (vasopressin) receptors. V_1 receptors act through the group II-C hormonal mechanism; V_2 receptors act through the group II-A mechanism (see Chapter 75).

V_1 *receptors* mediate smooth muscle contraction.

Activated V_2 *receptors* promote antidiuresis in three ways. (1) They stimulate Na^+/K^+-2Cl cotransport in the thick ascending limb (TAL), augmenting the renal medullary hyperosmolarity through the countercurrent multiplier system. (2) They increase the permeability of the collecting duct to urea by activating urea transport proteins, further increasing the medullary hyperosmolarity through urea recycling. (3) They increase the permeability of the collecting duct to water by causing the insertion of water channels (aquaporins) into the luminal membrane of collecting duct cells. This increases the water reabsorption from the hyperosmolar renal medulla.

In the **syndrome of inappropriate ADH secretion (SIADH)**, secretion of excess ADH results in the retention of large amounts of water in the body with consequent dilutional hyponatremia. The extracellular fluid (ECF) expansion increases Na^+ excretion through the Starling mechanism (see **Fig. 57.2**) and aggravates the hyponatremia. The normal plasma level of ADH is 0 to 10 pg/mL. In SIADH, the plasma osmo-larity is low, and the plasma level of ADH is at its maximum: 10 pg/mL. Although in the normal range, it actually signifies a high rate of ADH secretion because it occurs despite a low plasma osmolarity, which normally should inhibit the ADH secretion completely. SIADH occurs in cerebral diseases and ADH-secreting lung tumors. SIADH can be treated with demeclocycline, which reduces the renal response to ADH.

Diabetes insipidus is associated with the formation of large volumes of urine with a low specific gravity. Diabetes insipidus may be neurogenic, nephrogenic, or gestational.

There are several causes of *neurogenic diabetes insipidus.* Cranial surgery can create conditions that reversibly or irreversibly cause failure to release ADH. Pituitary tumors are another cause of this condition. Finally, head trauma can result in severe damage to the pituitary stalk, leading to retrograde degeneration of the ADH-secreting neurons. Neurogenic diabetes insipidus can also occur as an autosomal dominant disease. Whatever its origin, it is treated by administering ADH.

Nephrogenic diabetes insipidus is usually genetic and may be an X-linked recessive disorder, in which V_2 receptors in the kidneys are not responsive to ADH, or an autosomal recessive disorder, in which aquaporin-2 formation in tubule cells is impaired.

Gestational diabetes insipidus occurs in pregnancy due to an abnormal increase in plasma vasopressinase levels. It is treated by giving desmopressin, an analogue of vasopressin, which is resistant to inactivation by vasopressinase.

Renin–Angiotensin System

The chemical messengers that make up this system play a role in the homeostatic maintenance of a constant blood volume and a constant K^+ concentration.

Renin is a protease enzyme. Its primary source is the juxtaglomerular (JG) cells of the kidneys. Renin production also occurs in unspecialized smooth muscle cells in the afferent arteriole up to the interlobular arteries in fetal kidneys and in adults when there is increased demand for renin secretion.

The principal regulators of renin release (degranulation) are as follows. (1) The JG cells themselves are probably the sensors of the afferent arteriolar pressure. They release renin when the pressure rises. (2) Increase in sodium chloride (Cl^- in particular) in the distal convoluted tubule (DCT) decreases renin secretion. The amount of NaCl in the tubular fluid is sensed by the macula densa. The information is signaled to the JG cells. Adenosine is a probable mediator of the signal. (3) The JG cells are innervated by sympathetic fibers. They release renin in response to sympathetic discharge and circulating catecholamines. (4) Prostacyclin (PGI_2) stimulates renin secretion through a direct action on the JG cells.

The renin released from the JG cells enters circulation and acts on an α_2-globulin plasma protein called *angiotensinogen* and splits off from its N terminal a decapeptide called *angiotensin I.* An enzyme called *angiotensin converting enzyme* (ACE) then acts on angiotensin I to split off from it an octapeptide called *angiotensin II.* The enzyme is found on the surface of capillary endothelium in the lungs and kidneys.

$$\text{Angiotensinogen} \xrightarrow{\text{Renin from JG cells}} \text{Angiotensin I}$$
$$(\alpha_2\text{-globulin}) \qquad\qquad (\text{decapeptide})$$

$$\text{Angiotensin I} \xrightarrow[\text{lungs and kidneys}]{\substack{\text{ACE on the capillary} \\ \text{endothelium of the}}} \text{Angiotensin II}$$
$$(\text{decapeptide}) \qquad\qquad (\text{octapeptide})$$

Central effects | Angiotensin II acts through angiotensin receptors present in the subfornical organ (SFO) and the organ vasculosum of the lamina terminalis (OVLT) to increase thirst and stimulate ADH release. Angiotensin II also acts through angiotensin receptors located in the area postrema of the brain to bring about an increased sympathetic discharge.

Renal effects | Angiotensin receptors are present on many cells making up the kidneys and their circulation. Through these receptors, angiotensin II exerts the following effects.

Effect on renal arterioles Angiotensin II constricts both afferent and efferent arterioles, thereby reducing both the glomerular filtration rate (GFR) and renal blood flow (RBF). The efferent arterioles, however, are somewhat more sensitive to angiotensin II than are the afferent arterioles. Hence, angiotensin II causes greater constriction of the efferent arterioles, thereby increasing the filtration fraction.

Effect on glomerular basement membrane Angiotensin II alters the pore size of the glomerular basement membrane and thereby alters the filtration barrier that limits filtration of proteins.

Effect on glomerular mesangial cells Angiotensin receptors are present on the mesangial cells. Angiotensin II results in mesangial cell hypertrophy and an increase in the extracellular matrix production by the mesangial cells. Because both mesangial cell hypertrophy and extracellular matrix expansion are observed in diabetes mellitus, angiotensin II has been implicated in the pathophysiology of diabetes mellitus. ACE inhibitors tend to retard these changes in diabetic nephropathy.

Effect on adrenals | Angiotensin receptors are present on the zona glomerulosa of the adrenal glands. Through these receptors, angiotensin II causes stimulation of aldosterone secretion.

Vascular effect | Angiotensin II is a powerful vasoconstrictor. Its vasoconstrictor effect, along with its other effects such as thirst and stimulation of aldosterone secretion, leads to a rise in blood pressure (**Fig. 61.1**). The role of angiotensin in the regulation of blood pressure is discussed in Chapter 38.

Aldosterone

The secretion of aldosterone and the factors affecting it are discussed in Chapter 71. The renal effects of aldosterone on Na^+ and K^+ homeostasis are discussed here.

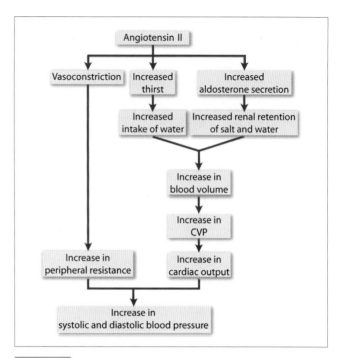

Fig. 61.1 Effect of angiotensin II on blood pressure. CVP, central venous pressure.

The actions of aldosterone are localized to the distal tubular and collecting duct cells. (1) It stimulates the basolateral Na^+–K^+ ATPase, (2) increases the permeability of the apical membrane to Na^+ unitransport channels, and (3) increases the permeability of the apical membrane to K^+. As a result of these actions, aldosterone increases the reabsorption of Na^+ and with it, of water, too. The increased Na^+ reabsorption makes the transepithelial potential difference (TEPD) highly negative. The increase in K^+ secretion produced by aldosterone is due to the combined effects of the highly negative TEPD and the increased apical permeability to K^+.

Despite its effect on Na^+ and water reabsorption, aldosterone is a relatively *weak regulator* of body Na^+ and water balance, the important regulator being the thirst-ADH mechanism (**Fig. 61.2**). In the absence of the aldosterone-feedback mechanism, the thirst-ADH mechanism maintains a near-perfect Na^+ balance in the body. In the absence of the thirst-ADH mechanism, however, aldosterone is unable to maintain proper Na^+ balance because of the *mineralocorticoid escape,* which is as follows.

A decrease in plasma Na^+ weakly stimulates aldosterone secretion (provided that the ECF volume is normal). Aldosterone increases the tubular reabsorption of Na^+, with water following. Water retention expands the ECF volume. Expansion of ECF volume produces natriuresis (see **Fig. 57.2**). Hence, aldosterone by itself is unable to produce significant amounts of Na^+ and water retention. A compensatory increase in atrial natriuretic peptide (ANP) secretion probably contributes to the escape.

Aldosterone is the sole regulator of the external potassium balance. An increase in plasma K^+ stimulates aldosterone secretion, which, in turn, restores plasma K^+ levels by promoting

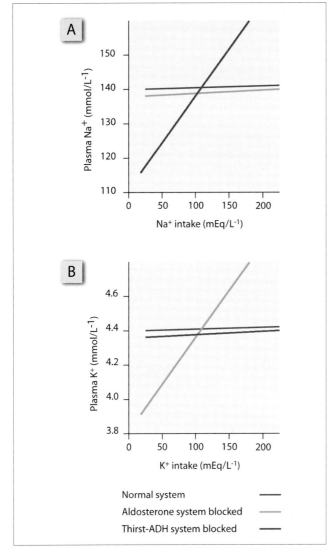

Fig. 61.2 Relative importance of the aldosterone system and the thirst–antidiuretic hormone (ADH) system on the homeostasis of sodium (Na^+) and potassium (K^+) ions. **(A)** Na^+ homeostasis is markedly impaired by blocking the thirst-ADH mechanism but is relatively unaffected by blockage of the aldosterone mechanism. **(B)** K^+ homeostasis is markedly impaired by blockage of the aldosterone mechanism but is relatively unaffected by the blockage of the thirst-ADH mechanism.

kaliuresis. An absence of this aldosterone-feedback mechanism would result in fatal hyperkalemia.

Natriuretic Hormone

The ANPs play an important role in blood volume and Na^+ concentration regulation; they are present as granules in the atrial muscle cells. There are two other related peptides, the brain natriuretic peptide (BNP) and the C-type natriuretic peptide (CNP). ANP is released in response to the stretch of the walls of the atria when atrial volume increases. In general, the effects of ANP are physiologically antagonistic to those of angiotensin II.

ANP causes natriuresis due to an increase in glomerular filtration. ANP causes relaxation of the mesangial cells of the

glomerulus, thus increasing the surface area of the glomerular membrane. It also acts on the medullary collecting duct to decrease the reabsorption of Na^+. ANP also decreases the secretion of renin, aldosterone, and ADH. It decreases the responsiveness of vascular smooth muscle to vasoconstrictors and therefore lowers blood pressure.

There are neurons in the brain that have ANP as their neurotransmitter. An ANP-containing neural pathway projects from the hypothalamus to the lower brainstem areas concerned with cardiovascular regulation. The pathway appears to be involved in lowering blood pressure and promoting natriuresis.

Calcium-Regulating Hormones

The calcium-regulating hormones and their effects on the renal handling of Ca^{2+} and phosphates are discussed in Chapter 78.

Summary

- Antidiuretic hormone (ADH) determines the permeability of the collecting duct to water and urea and is involved in regulating blood fluid osmolarity.

- The renin–angiotensin system is involved with controlling the glomerular filtration rate and the filtration fraction.

- Angiotensin has a role in blood pressure regulation.

- Aldosterone acts on the distal tubules and collecting ducts and alters the reabsorption of Na^+ and the secretion of K^+.

- Atrial natriuretic hormone peptides promote the excretion of Na^+ by the kidneys and contribute to maintenance of blood volume.

Applying What You Know

61.1. Reverend Fisher's serum osmolarity is 280 mOsm/L, a value that is slightly low. Predict whether his antidiuretic hormone (ADH) concentration will be increased, decreased, or normal.

61.2. Reverend Fisher is both hyponatremic and slightly hyperkalemic. Predict whether his aldosterone concentration will be increased, decreased, or normal. Explain your prediction.

Understanding renal contributions to homeostasis, whether in a healthy individual or a patient, is aided by measurements of renal functions, and many of the tests use simple applications of an understanding of the properties of the kidneys.

Renal Clearance and Its Applications

The clearance of a substance X is defined as the volume of plasma that is completely cleared of X in 1 minute. Obviously, what is cleared from the plasma appears in the urine. Clearance is a "virtual" volume because blood is never cleared completely of any of its constituents. The unit of clearance is mL/min and is calculated by the formula

$$\frac{U_X V}{P_X} \tag{62.1}$$

where U_X is the urinary concentration of the substance, V is the rate of flow of urine, and P_X is the plasma concentration of the substance.

Determining the clearance of certain substances can provide measurements of important aspects of kidney function (see below).

Osmolar clearance is the volume of plasma that is cleared of all its electrolytes in 1 minute. If the urine excreted is isoosmolar to the plasma, then the osmolar clearance is equal to the urinary output in 1 minute.

Osmolar clearance is given by the formula

$$C_{Osm} = \frac{U_{Osm} V}{P_{Osm}} \tag{62.2}$$

where U_{Osm} is the osmolarity of urine, P_{Osm} is the osmolarity of plasma, and if $U_{Osm} = P_{Osm}$, then $C_{Osm} = V$.

Thus, defined in another way, osmolar clearance is the volume of isoosmolar urine that must be excreted per minute to eliminate the excretory solute load.

Free-water clearance (CH_2O) is defined as the amount of pure water that must be removed from or added to the urine volume excreted to render it isotonic with plasma. It is given by the formula

$$C_{Osm} = V - CH_2O \tag{62.3}$$

or

$$V = C_{Osm} + CH_2O \tag{62.4}$$

In other words, the urine volume can be viewed as the sum of the volume of electrolyte-free urine (CH_2O) and the volume of isoosmolar urine (C_{Osm}). A positive free-water clearance occurs when urine is hypoosmolar and a negative free-water clearance when urine is hyperosmolar. When the urine is isoosmolar, $C_{Osm} = V$; therefore, $CH_2O = 0$.

The use of the term *clearance* in this case is a little misleading because what is being measured here are the properties of the urine, not the removal of substances from the plasma.

Example
The volume of urine excreted in 24 hours is 2 L. Plasma osmolarity is 300 mOsm/L. Calculate the free-water clearance when the urine osmolarity is (i) 1200 mOsm/L, (ii) 150 mOsm/L, and (iii) 300 mOsm/L.

Solution

$$CH_2O = V - C_{Osm} \tag{62.5}$$

or

$$CH_2O = V - \frac{U_{Osm} V}{P_{Osm}} \tag{62.6}$$

(i)
$$CH_2O = 2.0 - \frac{1200 \times 2.0}{300}$$
$$= -6.0 \text{ L/day}$$

(ii)
$$CH_2O = 2.0 - \frac{150 \times 2.0}{300}$$
$$= 1.0 \text{ L/day}$$

(iii)
$$CH_2O = 2.0 - \frac{300 \times 2.0}{300}$$
$$= 0 \text{ L/day}$$

Plasma Concentration and Clearance
The general formula for urinary excretion of solutes is

$$UV = (GFR \times P) - Tr + Ts \tag{62.7}$$

where Tr is the rate of reabsorption from the tubule, Ts is the rate of *secretion* into the tubule, GFR (glomerular filtration rate) × P is the rate of filtration into the tubule per minute, and U × V is the rate of solute excretion in urine per minute.

Dividing throughout by P:

$$UV/P = GFR - Tr/P + Ts/P \qquad (62.8)$$

If a substance is neither secreted into the tubule nor reabsorbed from the tubule, the formula reduces to

$$UV/P = GFR \qquad (62.9)$$

Inulin and, to a lesser extent, creatinine meet the above criteria. Hence, the GFR can be estimated by measuring inulin clearance or creatinine clearance. Because the values of Tr or Ts cannot increase indefinitely (they are limited by the transport maximum [Tm]), Tr/P and Ts/P approach zero at very high values of P. Hence, the clearance of all substances approaches the value of GFR (inulin clearance) at higher values of P (**Fig. 62.1**).

The clearance of glucose is normally zero because the normal urinary concentration of glucose (U) is zero. However, as the plasma level of glucose exceeds the threshold, its clearance exceeds zero. At higher plasma levels the clearance of glucose, too, like that of other substances, approaches the value of inulin clearance. For the same reason, the clearance of para-aminohippuric acid (PAH) only at low plasma levels gives the renal plasma flow (see below); at higher values, it will approach the value of GFR.

PAH Clearance and Renal Plasma Flow

If a dye is infused into the blood, and its arterial and venous concentrations are estimated, it is possible to calculate the renal plasma flow (RPF) using the Fick principle:

$$RPF = \frac{Q}{(P_a - P_v)} \qquad (62.10)$$

where Q is the amount of dye removed from the kidney, P_a is the dye concentration in the renal artery, and P_v is the dye concentration in the renal vein.

The amount of dye (Q) removed from the kidney is equal to the amount of dye excreted in the urine.

$$\therefore Q = UV \qquad (62.11)$$

where U is the urinary concentration of the dye, and V is the rate of urine formation.

$$RPF = \frac{UV}{(P_a - P_v)} \qquad (62.12)$$

The concentration of the dye in the renal artery is the same as in the other systemic arteries. Hence, P_a can be estimated by sampling blood from any systemic artery that can be conveniently accessed. However, it is difficult to obtain blood from the renal vein. Hence, it is expedient to use a dye that is completely excreted into the urine in a single passage through the kidney so that the concentration of the dye in renal venous blood is zero. If $P_v = 0$, then Eq. 62.15 reduces to

$$RPF = \frac{UV}{P_a} \qquad (62.13)$$

The dye that comes nearest to satisfying the condition of complete extraction in a single passage through the kidney is PAH. Hence, RPF equals the renal clearance of PAH. However, PAH is only 90% excreted in the urine in a single passage. In other words, its extraction ratio is 90%. Hence, its concentration in renal venous blood is ~10% of its concentration in the renal arterial blood:

$$P_v = P_a \times (1 - \text{extraction ratio})$$

$$= P_a - (P_a \times \text{extraction ratio}) \qquad (62.14)$$

Substituting Eq. 62.17 in Eq. 62.16, we have

$$RPF = \frac{UV}{(P_a \times \text{extraction ratio})} \qquad (62.15)$$

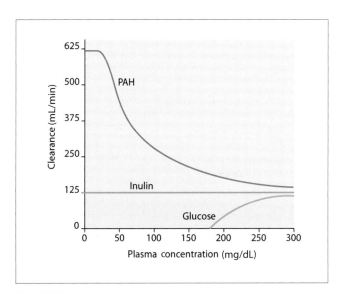

Fig. 62.1 Changes in renal clearance of para-aminohippuric acid (PAH; secreted into tubule), glucose (reabsorbed from tubule), and inulin (neither secreted nor reabsorbed) as a function of plasma concentration.

The RBF (renal blood flow) can be calculated from RPF using the formula

$$RBF = \frac{RPF}{(1 - hematocrit)} \qquad (62.16)$$

Inulin Clearance and the GFR

Inulin is a polysaccharide whose clearance gives an estimate of the GFR because it is freely filtered into the glomerular filtrate and is neither secreted nor reabsorbed in the kidneys. It also satisfies the basic requirements of a good indicator dye; that is, it is neither metabolized nor stored in the kidneys, is nontoxic, has no effect on the filtration rate itself, and can be easily estimated in the laboratory.

Inulin clearance (GFR) is given by the formula

$$\text{Inulin clearance (GFR)} = \frac{UV}{P_a} \qquad (62.17)$$

where U is the urinary concentration of inulin, V is the rate of urine flow, and P_a is the arterial concentration of inulin.

In making this measurement, it is important to maintain a constant plasma concentration of inulin. This is achieved by giving a single bolus dose of inulin solution followed by a continuous intravenous (IV) inulin infusion.

GFR is more easily estimated by using creatinine as an indicator. Creatinine is an endogenous substance having a fairly constant plasma value (P) of ~0.6 to 1.5 mg/dL, and therefore does not need continuous IV infusion. Creatinine, however, is slightly secreted into the tubules, increasing its urinary concentration (U). The value of GFR obtained, although not accurate, is still acceptable to clinicians. All clearance techniques depend on accurately timed collections of urine, which is the major source of error.

The **filtration fraction** (FF) is given by the ratio of GFR and RBF. It serves as an approximate index of glomerular filtration coefficient (Kf).

$$FF = \frac{GFR}{RPF} \qquad (62.18)$$

Urea Clearance

The concept of clearance originally developed around efforts to use urea excretion as an index for renal function. Part of the problem in such efforts was that urea excretion even by a normal kidney varies greatly depending on the rate of urinary outflow. Two empirical indices were therefore developed, one for urinary flow less than 2 mL/min (called the standard clearance), and the other for urinary flow more than 2 mL/min (called the maximal clearance). These indices are fairly constant as long as there is no impairment of renal function.

$$\text{Standard urea clearance} = \frac{U\sqrt{V}}{B} \qquad (62.19)$$

$$\text{Maximum urea clearance} = \frac{UV}{B} \qquad (62.20)$$

It was realized later that UV/B actually signified the "volume of blood" that was cleared of urea per minute. The blood concentration (B) was later replaced by plasma concentration (P), and the term *clearance* was extended to other solutes, some of which more accurately indicated the GFR or RBF. Maximal urea clearance underestimates GFR because urea is reabsorbed from the collecting duct. Standard urea clearance does not denote a volume of blood and therefore cannot be called clearance according to its present definition.

Renal Threshold for Glucose

Like any other active process, the rate of active tubular transport cannot exceed a certain maximum called the transport maximum (Tm). It is expressed in g/min or mM/min. The concept of transport maximum is explained below with reference to glucose.

At the normal plasma glucose level of 60 to 100 mg/dL, the glucose filtered into the urine is totally reabsorbed. As the plasma concentration of glucose increases, more glucose is filtered into the tubule, and the tubular concentration of glucose rises. The tubular reabsorption of glucose increases concomitantly; therefore, no glucose appears in urine initially (**Fig. 62.2**). However, after the plasma level exceeds a certain limit (usually the limit is 180 mg/dL) called the renal threshold for glucose, the amount of glucose filtered into the tubule exceeds the maximal rate at which glucose can be reabsorbed from the tubules (normally ~375 mg/min, called the *transport*

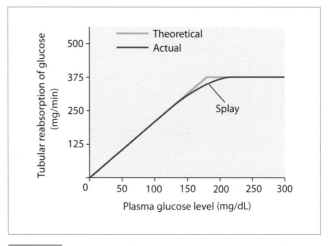

Fig. 62.2 Increase in tubular reabsorption as a function of plasma glucose level, showing transport maximum for glucose (TmG) and splay.

maximum for glucose, or TmG). Hence, glucose starts appearing in the urine. The TmG can be calculated from the formula

$$U_GV = (GFR \times P_G) - Tr \qquad (62.21)$$

where U_G is the urinary concentration (g/dL) of the glucose, V is the urinary output (mL/min), GFR is the glomerular filtration rate (mL/min), P_G is the plasma glucose concentration (g/dL), and Tr is the rate of tubular reabsorption of glucose (g/min).

When P_G is sufficiently high (i.e., greater than the renal threshold for glucose), the rate of tubular reabsorption (Tr) will be maximal and will equal the TmG.

$$U_GV = (GFR \times P_G) - TmG \qquad (62.22)$$

or

$$TmG = (GFR \times P_G) - U_GV \text{ (when } P_G \text{ exceeds renal threshold)} \qquad (62.23)$$

Estimation of renal threshold for glucose | Before starting the test, the patient voids, and the baseline plasma glucose is determined. An IV infusion of 50% dextrose is given at the rate of 1 to 2 mL/min so that plasma glucose concentration remains above 550 mL/dL for 2 hours. Sequential half-hourly blood and urine samples are collected, and the glucose concentration

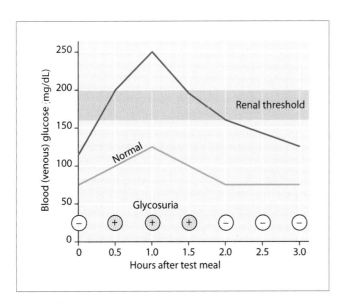

Fig. 62.3 Estimation of renal threshold. It can be inferred from the graph that the renal threshold is somewhere between 160 and 200 mg/dL (indicated by the shaded strip). The range of the estimate can be narrowed down by more frequent estimation of blood and urinary glucose concentrations.

is estimated. The renal threshold for glucose is estimated by plotting the blood and urine glucose concentrations simultaneously (**Fig. 62.3**).

Splay | The term *splay* refers to the divergence of the measured value (as described above) and the calculated value of renal threshold (as explained below). The renal threshold for glucose can be calculated from the formula

$$Tr = (GFR \times P_G) - U_GV \qquad (62.24)$$

When the plasma concentration (P_G) equals the renal threshold, the tubular reabsorption (Tr) reaches its maximum (i.e., the TmG) and exactly balances the filtered load of glucose. At that stage, P_G is renal threshold for glucose, Tr is the TmG, and U_GV is 0.

$$\therefore TmG = GFR \times \text{renal threshold} \qquad (62.25)$$

or

$$\text{Renal threshold} = TmG/GFR \qquad (62.26)$$

There is, however, a discrepancy between the calculated and the measured values of the renal threshold. The renal threshold calculated from TmG would be

$$\frac{375 \text{ mg/min}}{125 \text{ mL/min}}$$

$$= 3 \text{ mg/mL}$$

$$= 300 \text{ mg/dL}$$

Thus, glucose would be expected to appear in urine when the arterial concentration of glucose exceeds 300 mg/dL, which corresponds to a venous glucose concentration of ~200 mg/dL. However, the measured value is lower, at ~180 mg/dL. This is because the calculated value represents the average value of 2 million nephrons. A nephron can have a TmG that is either higher or lower than the average of 375 mg/min. Nephrons with a lower TmG leak glucose into urine at plasma glucose levels below the calculated threshold. This discrepancy shows up graphically as the splay (see **Fig. 62.4**).

Renal Function Tests and Their Clinical Uses

Glomerular Function Tests
Electrophoresis of urinary proteins helps to distinguish the high-molecular-weight proteins (HMWPs) from the low-

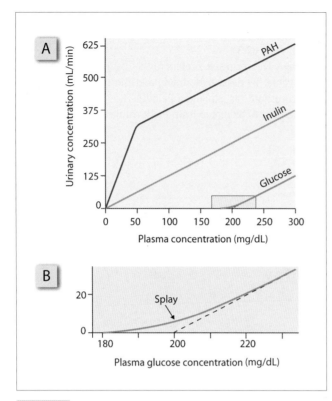

Fig. 62.4 **(A)** Changes in the urinary concentration of para-amino-hippuric acid (PAH; secreted into tubule), glucose (reabsorbed from tubule), and inulin (neither secreted nor reabsorbed) as a function of plasma concentration. **(B)** The splay, showing the divergence between the calculated renal threshold for glucose (200 mg/dL) and the measured renal threshold for glucose (180 mg/dL).

molecular-weight proteins (LMWPs) that are normally present in the urine in fairly large amounts. When present in excess of 2 g/24 hours, high-molecular-weight proteinuria indicates the presence of glomerular disease. If the urine deposit contains red cell casts, then glomerular inflammation is virtually certain.

GFR measurement | Clearance of inulin or creatinine can be measured for estimating the GFR. However, they are not routinely estimated in the clinics. The plasma levels of urea and creatinine are used instead.

Plasma urea and creatinine | Neither blood urea nor plasma creatinine increases much until the GFR falls below 30 mL/min. Thereafter, the plasma creatinine is an accurate and sensitive guide to further changes in renal function.

Plasma urea may give a false high in conditions of low urine flow rates like dehydration, heart failure, and nephrotic syndrome. In these conditions, the urea diffuses out of the tubular lumen to reenter the blood. Plasma urea is also abnormally high following consumption of a high protein diet, gastrointestinal bleeding (blood proteins are digested), and catabolic states such as infection and steroid therapy.

Plasma creatinine levels are less affected by extrarenal causes, though the urinary excretion of creatinine is proportional to the whole body muscle mass.

Proximal Tubular Function Tests
Electrophoresis of urinary proteins helps to detect LMWPs in the urine. Damage to the proximal tubule is associated with low-molecular-weight proteinuria. Large amounts of light chains of immunoglobulin can also appear in the urine in multiple myeloma and lymphoma. One differentiating feature is that in tubular dysfunction, all classes of light chains appear in the urine, but in immunologic disorders, they are monoclonal: they all belong to the same class (κ or λ). This can be easily be ascertained through immunoelectrophoresis.

Urine chromatography for amino acids helps in detecting the presence of abnormal amounts of amino acids. The presence of *N*-acetyl β-glucosaminidase (NAG) and γ-glutamyl transferase (γGT) in the urine indicates damage to the proximal tubular epithelial cells.

The **renal threshold for glucose** is a fairly good index of proximal tubular function. The renal threshold is an easily measurable index of glucose reabsorption in tubules. TmG is a more stable index than the renal threshold: the threshold is affected by the splay, but the TmG is not (**Fig. 62.2**).

Distal Tubular Function Test
Tests for renal water handling | The *specific gravity* and *free-water clearance* give preliminary information about the osmolarity of the urine. More diagnostic clues are obtained on studying the urine-diluting and urine-concentrating ability of the kidney.

The *oral water-loading* test gives accurate information regarding the urine-diluting ability of the kidneys. After voiding, the subject drinks 20 mL/kg of body weight of water over 15 minutes. Half-hourly samples are collected over the next 5 hours. Normally, more than 75% of the administered water load is excreted by 4 hours. Urine osmolarity falls to < 100 mOsm/kg. The ability to produce a dilute urine is lost in chronic renal failure, which is associated with isosthenuria. Urine-diluting ability is also lost in cardiac failure because the impaired renal perfusion causes excessive proximal reabsorption of Na⁺. In chronic liver diseases, there is secondary hyperaldosteronism, leading to an inability to concentrate urine.

The *water-deprivation test* gives accurate information regarding the urine-concentrating ability of the kidneys. Oral fluids are withheld for a period of 12 hours, after which a urine sample is collected and analyzed for its volume and osmolarity. To prevent serious and life-threatening dehydration, the test should be abandoned if body weight falls by 3% at any time during the test. Normally, urine osmolarity is > 900 mOsm/L. In diabetes insipidus, urine osmolarity is < 300 mOsm/L. If the diabetes insipidus is nephrogenic, subsequent ADH administration will not improve it. If the polyuria is due to compulsive water drinking, the osmolarity would be normal following a water-deprivation test.

Renal acidification tests indicate the H⁺ concentrating ability of the kidney. They are unnecessary if the early morning sample has a pH of < 5.3, which is sufficient proof of the renal concentrating ability.

In the *oral ammonium chloride test,* ammonium chloride is administered in gelatin capsules to maximally acidify the plasma. Hourly urine samples are collected and tested for pH. Normal subjects can reduce the urine pH to < 5.0 in 2 hours. The nausea and vomiting due to ammonium chloride can be troublesome. Liver patients should not be given ammonium salts. Alternative acidifying agents include arginine hydrochloride and calcium chloride.

The *sodium sulfate infusion test* helps to differentiate whether the impaired renal acidification is due to reduced H^+ secretion as in renal tubular acidosis or due to increased back leakage from the tubules. Sodium sulfate solution is infused slowly. Hourly urine volumes are collected and tested for pH. Normal subjects can reduce urine pH to < 5.0. If the distal tubular defect is due to the back diffusion of hydrogen ions, then urine can be normally acidified. This is because sulfates, being nonreabsorbable ions, trap hydrogen ions in the tubular lumen. If the problem is failure to secrete hydrogen ions, then the urine is not acidified even in the presence of sulfate ions.

Urine Analysis

Examination of a urine specimen is always performed during routine health check-ups and is the first test performed on patients with suspected renal disorders. However, many of the tests performed in a urine examination may not be indicative of renal functions.

Physical Examination

The normal volume of urine passed per day ranges from 500 to 2500 mL. It increases after meals, after drinks, and on exposure to cold, and decreases if water intake is low and after excessive sweating. Polyuria occurs in diabetes insipidus, diabetes mellitus, and the diuretic phase of acute renal failure. Oliguria occurs in acute glomerulonephritis, hypotension, and dehydration. Anuria occurs in lower urinary tract obstruction.

Color and turbidity | Urates precipitate in acidic urine on standing, making the urine cloudy. Urinary urate excretion increases when purine metabolism in the body increases, as in gout. Strongly alkaline urine appears cloudy due to the precipitation of tricalcium phosphate $[Ca_3(PO_4)_2]$. The cloudy appearance increases on warming the urine, which makes it more alkaline as the CO_2 bubbles off from it. Urinary tract infection increases the pus cells and bacteria in urine, giving it a cloudy appearance (**Table 62.1**).

Hematuria means the presence of red blood cells in the urine. Hematuria does not necessarily indicate a renal abnormality: the blood can come from the urinary tract. Red cells that enter urine through the damaged glomerulus are usually distorted, which helps in differentiating glomerular from nonglomerular bleeding. *Hemoglobinuria* refers to the presence of free hemoglobin in the urine.

The normal specific gravity of urine is 1.003 to 1.030, and the normal urine osmolarity is 100 to 1000 mOsm/kg. If the early morning urine sample after an overnight fast has an osmolarity of > 600 mOsm/kg (specific gravity > 1.018), it indicates that the patient has a normal urine concentrating ability. If the osmolarity remains constant at 300 mOsm/kg (specific gravity 1.009), it is called *isosthenuria*. It occurs in chronic

Table 62.1 Causes of Urine Color and Turbidity

Normal tint	Urochrome, uroerythrin urobilin (formed on standing)
Cloudy	Strongly alkaline urine, excessive urates, infection
Smoky	Hematuria
Frothy	Proteinuria
Milky	Chyluria
Orange	Excess urobilin
Brown	Bilirubinuria
Red–dark brown	Porphyrins (on standing), frank hematuria
Red–dark brown–black	Hemoglobinuria, melanin (on standing)

renal failure. Urine is normally slightly acidic except shortly after a meal due to the postprandial alkaline tide. Abnormal causes of alkaline urine include alkali consumption, impairment of tubular acidification, and urinary tract infection (UTI) with urea-splitting organisms.

Chemical Analysis

Proteins | Up to 150 mg of protein is excreted daily in urine. Of this, 15 mg is albumin. The rest comprises LMWPs. About 25 mg of the LMWPs are Tamm-Horsfall protein derived from the cells of the thick ascending limb (TAL). The remainder of the LMWPs is derived from plasma proteins, such as β_2 microproteins, retinal binding protein, and light chains of immunoglobulin. Excretion of > 150 mg per day of proteins is called proteinuria. *Transient proteinuria* can occur in fever and after exercise. *Orthostatic proteinuria* occurs only on standing and is not associated with any renal damage. The clinically important proteinurias are glomerular proteinuria, tubular proteinuria, overflow proteinuria, and nephrogenic proteinuria.

In *glomerular proteinuria*, large amounts of albumin and other HMWPs are filtered into the tubule. Hence, glomerular proteinuria is also called high-molecular-weight proteinuria. Massive glomerular proteinuria is called *nephrotic syndrome*.

In *tubular proteinuria*, the LMWPs that are normally filtered into the tubule in fairly large amounts are not reabsorbed. Hence, this type of proteinuria is also called low-molecular-weight proteinuria.

Overflow proteinuria is the name given to the low-molecular-weight proteinuria that occurs when the plasma concentration of LMWPs rises markedly, as in multiple myeloma, rhabdomyolysis, and intravascular hemolysis. The proteins appear in urine when the protein reabsorptive capacity of the tubules is exceeded.

Nephrogenic proteinuria is the name given to the appearance of tubular enzymes such as *N*-acetyl β-glucosaminidase (NAG) and gamma-glutamyl transferase (γGT) in the urine. These enzymatic proteins are released when the proximal tubular cells are damaged.

Sugars are normally absent in the urine. *Glycosuria* may be due to diabetes mellitus, renal glycosuria, or alimentary glycosuria. *Galactosuria* and *fructosuria* occur due to inborn errors of metabolism. Lactosuria occurs in late pregnancy and lactation. Pentosuria is caused by consuming large quantities of plums, cherries, or grapes.

Ketones are normally absent in urine. *Ketonuria* occurs in diabetic ketoacidosis, starvation, and prolonged diarrhea and vomiting.

Bilirubin is normally absent in urine but appears in conjugated hyperbilirubinemia. The daily urobilinogen excretion is normally 1.0 to 3.5 mg.

Heme pigments are normally absent in urine They appear following intravascular hemolysis and hemolysis in renal tubules. They also appear following crush injury to muscles and in myopathies that release heme from myoglobin.

Nitrites | Urine normally contains nitrates (NO_3^-) but not nitrites (NO_2^-). Urinary nitrites suggest the presence of UTI tract infection because organisms infecting the urinary tract produce nitrites from urinary nitrates.

Microscopic Examination

The common types of *cells* found in the urine are leukocytes, tubular epithelial cells, and squamous epithelial cells. *Crystals* are usually of no pathologic significance. However, uric acid crystals and cystine crystals, when present in large amounts, have diagnostic importance. Casts are formed within the nephron and are washed out by the flow of tubular fluid. Casts may be cellular or noncellular (**Fig. 62.5**).

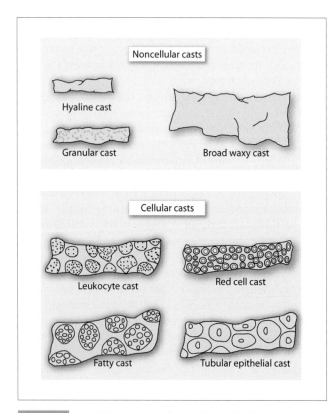

Fig. 62.5 The different types of noncellular and cellular casts found in the urine.

Cellular casts | *Leukocyte casts* are typically found in acute bacterial pyelonephritis. Fatty casts are found in nephrotic syndrome. They contain epithelial cells laden with fat droplets. *Red cell casts* are pathognomonic of glomerular bleeding and are almost diagnostic of acute glomerulonephritis. *Tubular epithelial cell casts* are most commonly present in acute tubular necrosis.

Noncellular casts | *Hyaline casts* are structureless, transparent proteinaceous plugs, made largely of Tamm-Horsfall protein. Up to 1 hyaline cast per low power field (×10) is normal. They increase in proteinuria. *Granular casts* are similar to hyaline casts except that granular aggregates of proteins are embedded in them. Fewer than 1 granular cast per low power field of the microscope is considered normal. *Broad waxy casts* (*renal failure casts*) are formed in chronic renal failure in the dilated nephrons.

Summary

● Renal clearance is the rate at which plasma would have to be completely cleared of a substance to produce the excretion rate for that substance.

● The clearance of certain substances can be used to measure the glomerular filtration rate and renal blood flow.

● Glucose is actively reabsorbed from the filtrate, and at normal plasma glucose concentrations, no glucose is seen in the urine. However, glucose reabsorption exhibits a transport maximum that can be measured.

● Clinically, there are several tests that are performed to assess kidney function; these include a test for water handling and the capacity to acidify the urine.

● Examination of urine specimens (urinalysis) is a commonly performed test to diagnose the presence of renal disease.

Applying What You Know

62.1. Analysis of a urine sample from Reverend Fisher reveals many squamous epithelial cells and several pigmented casts. Where did these come from?

The Importance of pH Regulation

It is extremely important that the pH of body fluids remain more or less constant within some range of values. The viability and function of every cell in the body depends on the functioning of the myriad of enzymes found within the cells. The activity of enzymes, the rate at which they function, is strongly determined by pH. Deviations of pH from an acceptable level will result in dysfunction along many different metabolic pathways.

The Challenges to pH Homeostasis

Metabolic Production of Carbon Dioxide
The production of energy in every cell results in the production of carbon dioxide (CO_2). When CO_2 dissolves in water, the following chemical reaction occurs:

$$CO_2 + H_2O \leftrightarrows H_2CO_3 \rightleftarrows H^+ + HCO_3^-$$

Thus, H^+ is continuously being produced.

However, in its normal operation, the respiratory system removes ("blows off") the CO_2 as fast as it is being produced (see Chapter 50). Thus, there is no retention of CO_2 and no buildup of H^+. However, changes in respiratory function, whether the result of physiologic responses or of pathology in the respiratory system, can result in either increases or decreases in CO_2 and hence changes in pH.

Metabolic Production of Acids
There are several sources of H^+ ion that arise in the operation of certain metabolic pathways. Sulfuric and phosphoric acids are generated when certain proteins and lipids are metabolized. When cells are forced to produce energy anaerobically, lactic acid is a by-product. Under certain conditions, the liver is stimulated to oxidize fatty acids released from adipose cells. The result is the production of keto acids.

As we will see below, the body has several defense mechanisms that minimize the change to body H^+ concentration, pH, thus maintaining homeostasis.

Loss of Gastrointestinal Secretions
The loss of gastrointestinal (GI) secretions can also pose a challenge to the maintenance of a constant pH. The contents of the stomach, gastric juice, is extremely acidic, and the loss of this gastric secretion in vomiting creates a significant alkalosis (pH increases). The secretions of the pancreas, on the other hand, contain a high concentration of bicarbonate, and loss of these secretions when diarrhea occurs makes the body quite acidotic (pH decreases).

Mechanisms to Regulate Whole Body pH

Buffering
The first line of defense against changes in pH is chemical buffering. Buffers are substances that readily bind or release H^+ ions depending on the pH of the environment.

Buffering is the fastest mechanism to respond to changes in H^+ concentration and thus is literally the first to do so.

The carbonic acid (CA) buffer system | The chemical system represented by

$$CO_2 + H_2O \leftrightarrows H_2CO_3 \rightleftarrows H^+ + HCO_3^-$$

is a buffering system. If H^+ ions are added to the solution from outside the system, or if H^+ ions are removed from the system, shifts in the reaction to the right or the left will remove or add H^+ ions, respectively. That is to say, the system has buffered (minimized) the change in $[H^+]$ or pH.

The CA buffer system represents an important defense against changes in pH because there is so much of it (its concentration in plasma is 24 mmol/L). Two of its components are also physiologically controlled (HCO_3^- by the kidneys and CO_2 by the respiratory system).

But it is important to recognize that the CA buffer system cannot buffer changes in its own behavior. For example, changes in partial pressure of carbon dioxide (P_aCO_2) cannot be buffered by the system, nor can the consequences of loss of HCO_3^- in the kidneys be buffered by the system.

The hemoglobin buffer | Hemoglobin (Hb) is another important buffer. It will bind or release H^+ ions depending on the pH around it. The NH_2 (amine) groups on intermediate histidine residues of the Hb molecule provide most of the buffering capacity. Changes in P_aCO_2 and the consequent changes in pH are buffered by Hb.

Respiratory Compensation for pH Changes
A change in pH will directly alter the firing of the peripheral chemoreceptor and indirectly alter the firing of the central chemoreceptor (see Chapter 50). Thus, if the body becomes acidotic (pH falls), the increased rate of firing of the chemoreceptors will cause increased alveolar ventilation, and P_aCO_2 will decrease. This will, of course, result in the reduced production of carbonic acid and hence the reduced production of H^+. If the pH becomes too alkalotic, the firing of the chemoreceptors will slow, and ventilation will decrease. The consequence is increased retention of CO_2 and hence greater production of H^+ ions.

There are two important limitations of the respiratory compensatory response. First, it cannot correct pH changes that are the result of a primary disturbance in the respiratory system. For example, a patient with emphysema (see Chapter 52) becomes hypercapnic for several different reasons. That elevated P_aCO_2 results in a significant decrease of pH, but no respiratory compensation is possible because the problem originates within the respiratory system. Second, respiratory compensation can never restore pH fully back to its normal level (see below).

General Model: Homeostasis

Homeostasis always attempts to restore a regulated parameter to its desired level. However, it usually cannot produce full compensation. Respiratory compensation for an acid–base disturbance can never, by itself, completely restore pH to its normal value.

Acid–base disturbances that are *not* the results of a respiratory disturbance are referred to as being metabolic. This label actually encompasses two quite different kinds of disturbances: (1) problems causes by renal (i.e., nonrespiratory) dysfunction and (2) problems that arise from metabolic production or losses of acids.

Renal Control of Bicarbonate

Just as the respiratory system can alter pH by changing P_aCO_2, the kidneys can change pH by altering their reabsorption of filtered HCO_3^- ions and the production of new bicarbonate. When a nonrenal disturbance alters pH, the kidneys can compensate to restore pH to normal. For example, if an individual develops a respiratory alkalosis (P_aCO_2 falls, hence H^+ decreases), the kidneys will reduce their reabsorption of HCO_3^-, causing the pH to decrease as less H^+ is secreted.

Time Course of Responses to Disturbances of pH

The CA buffer system reacts completely within minutes in plasma and within no more than 30 minutes in the extracellular fluid compartment. The Hb buffer completes its reaction within a matter of minutes. Respiratory compensation takes up to 12 hours to achieve its full effect. Renal excretion of H^+ (to reabsorb bicarbonate and make new bicarbonate) takes much longer to reach its full effect, as long as 3 days. Decreasing H^+ secretion, thus reducing bicarbonate reabsorption ("dumping" bicarbonate), is somewhat quicker.

The Davenport Nomogram

Whole body acid–base status, and the various responses to acid–base imbalances, can be visually represented by the Davenport nomogram. The nomogram is derived from the Henderson-Hasselbalch equation, which quantitatively describes the chemical reaction of CO_2 and H_2O. The equation describes the possible relationships between the concentrations of CO_2, H^+, and HCO_3^- that can occur.

$$pH = 6.1 + \log\left(\frac{[HCO_3^-]}{0.03\ PaCO_2}\right) \quad (63.1)$$

We can then create a graph of HCO_3^- as a function of pH (**Fig. 63.1A**). On this graph we can plot the normal values for these two physiologic parameters, pH = 7.4 and $[HCO_3^-]$ = 24 mmol/L. If we now solve the Henderson-Hasselbalch equation for the value of $[HCO_3^-]$ when P_aCO_2 = 40 mm Hg and pH = 7.4, we find that it is equal to 24 mmol/L (**Fig. 63.1B**). If we maintain P_aCO_2 constant at 40 mm Hg and systematically change pH in 0.1 unit steps and solve for $[HCO_3^-]$, we get a series of points that can be connected in a curved line (**Fig. 63.1C**) that is called the P_aCO_2 = 40 isobar (equal pressure). This line represents all the combinations of pH and $[HCO_3^-]$ that can be present when P_aCO_2 = 40 mm Hg. If these calculations are repeated with different values for P_aCO_2, a family of isobars can be plotted (**Fig. 63.1D**).

We can also represent the buffering ability of Hb on this graph. If we take a sample of blood with a Hb concentration of 15 g/L, we can systematically add H^+ ions and determine the value of $[HCO_3^-]$ that results. When these points are plotted, they yield the Hb buffer line (**Fig. 63.1E**).

Responses to a respiratory acidosis | If we increase P_aCO_2 in an individual and measure pH and $[HCO_3^-]$, we observe that the pH decreases (they become acidotic), and the $[HCO_3^-]$ increases. These changes occur along the Hb buffer line because they are the consequence of Hb buffering the change in H^+ production when P_aCO_2 increases.

If we cause P_aCO_2 to increase to a value of 80 mm Hg, the subject's pH, $[HCO_3^-]$, and P_aCO_2 will move from the normal value represented by point A in **Fig. 63.2** to point B. As long as P_aCO_2 is maintained at a value of 80, nothing will change.

However, we know that the kidneys will respond to restore pH to its normal level because the original disturbance is *not* the result of a kidney problem. The kidneys will increase their reabsorption of HCO_3^-, with the result that $[HCO_3^-]_a$ increases, and H^+ ions are effectively lost in the urine, thus increasing pH_a. The subject's P_aCO_2 remains fixed at 80 mm Hg because the primary

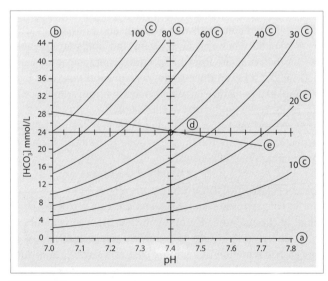

Fig. 63.1 The basic Davenport nomogram displaying the relation between pH (axis **A**), $[HCO_3^-]$ (axis **B**), and a family of P_aCO_2 isobars (lines labeled **C**). **(D)** represents normal values for all three parameters. The hemoglobin buffer line **(E)** has been included.

respiratory disturbance has not been corrected (point B, **Fig. 63.2**), but their [HCO$_3^-$] increases along the 80 mm Hg isobar. This causes a small, but significant, increase in pH. In addition, if the acidosis lasts long enough, the kidneys will begin to produce new, additional HCO$_3^-$ ions using ammonia as a buffer to take up the H$^+$ ions secreted into the tubular lumen. This will push the [HCO$_3^-$] still higher up the 80 mm Hg isobar (B to C in **Fig. 63.2**).

However, there is a limit to how much new bicarbonate the kidneys can make. This limit can be represented on the Davenport nomogram by the MKC (maximum kidney compensation) line (see **Fig. 63.2**). As long as the disturbance is maintained and P$_a$CO$_2$ continues to be 80 mm Hg, the subject will continue to be acidotic, although less so than without renal compensation, and bicarbonate will remain elevated (which does not matter because it is essentially inert in the body).

Responses to a metabolic alkalosis | Let us consider another acid–base disturbance, this time one that is the result of vomiting and the loss of H$^+$ in the vomitus. Initially, the respiratory system is holding the P$_a$CO$_2$ at the normal level of 40 mm Hg. But the subject will clearly become alkalotic (the "alkaline tide," see Chapter 68, is unopposed by the absorption of H$^+$ ions, which are now missing), and pH and [HCO$_3^-$] will increase as the subject moves up the 40 mm Hg isobar (A to B in **Fig. 63.3**). Of course, the change in pH will decrease the firing of the peripheral chemoreceptors (which respond to changes in both arterial PO$_2$ and pH), and ventilation will decrease, thus increasing arterial PCO$_2$ (B to C in **Fig. 63.3**). As CO$_2$ accumulates, pH will fall (more H$^+$ is being produced) along a trajectory that is parallel to the Hb buffer line (because Hb is releasing H$^+$; i.e., it is buffering the change that occurred). This means that pH is decreasing.

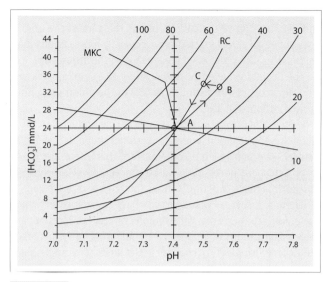

Fig. 63.3 The response to a metabolic (but nonrenal) alkalosis. [HCO$_3^-$] increases up the 40 mm Hg isobar (from **A** to **B**). When respiratory compensation occurs, it slows ventilation, increasing PCO$_2$ until the respiratory compensation (RC) line is reached (**B** to **C**). The kidneys then decrease the reabsorption of bicarbonate (**C** to **A**), and pH returns to normal.

This respiratory compensation (remember, the disturbance here is *not* a respiratory one) cannot restore pH to normal. How far can it increase pH? The compensatory response here is a decrease in ventilation and the retention of CO$_2$ (P$_a$CO$_2$ increases). However, this process cannot fully compensate because, as ventilation slows, arterial PCO$_2$ increases and stimulates the central chemoreceptors and increases their firing rate. Thus, there are two opposing mechanisms acting to change ventilation in opposite directions. The maximum compensatory response that is possible is represented by the respiratory compensation (RC) line see in **Fig. 63.3**. So, the subject's pH is lower than it was, but not normal. The kidneys will now slow their reabsorption of HCO$_3^-$, thus slowing the secretion of H$^+$ ions. As [HCO$_3^-$] falls along the RC line, pH returns to its normal value (C to A in **Fig. 63.3**).

> **General Model: Balance of Forces**
>
> The phenomenon of respiratory compensation is clearly an example where a balance between two competing influences (the respiratory drive generated by the central and peripheral chemoreceptors) determines the quantitative change that is possible.

The Davenport nomogram is a tool with which to think about all simple (one disturbance) acid–base disturbances.

Anion Gap

In any sample of plasma, a state of electroneutrality exists; there are exactly as many cations as anions. However, a typical laboratory report (see the case of Reverend Fisher) provides the

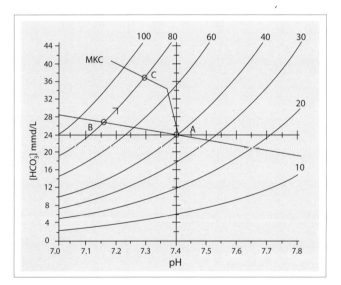

Fig. 63.2 The response to respiratory acidosis. PCO$_2$ increases to a value of 80 mm Hg along the Hb buffer line from **A** to **B** (primary disturbance). The kidneys increase their reabsorption of bicarbonate and generate new bicarbonate. [HCO$_3^-$] increases (along the 80 isobar —from **B** to **C**) until the maximum kidney compensation (MKC) line is reached, at which point the kidneys can make no more new bicarbonate. The individual can only return to normal pH (point **A**) if the respiratory problem is corrected and PCO$_2$ decreases back to normal.

concentrations of the cations Na^+ and K^+ and the anions HCO_3^- and Cl^-. The sum of the cations minus the sum of the anions does not equal zero. In fact, there are usually more cations than anions. This difference is what is meant by the **anion gap**.

The normal value of the anion gap is 12 ± 2 mEq/L. Plasma albumin accounts for as much as 80% of the anion gap under normal circumstances.

However, it is important to recognize that no such gap actually exists in the blood, which is, as stated previously, electroneutral. The gap results from the fact that there are many anions that are not usually measured and therefore not reported. It is these "missing" anions that give rise to the gap.

There are several states of acid–base imbalance in which the anion gap increases. For example, in keto- or lactacidosis, the concentrations of ketones or lactate are greatly increased but not measured. Thus, changes in the anion gap can be helpful in arriving at the correct identification of an acid–base disturbance.

The **urine anion gap** provides an indirect way of estimating the urinary ammonium (NH_4^+). It is given by the formula

$$\text{Urine anion gap} = \text{urinary } Na^+ + \text{urinary } K^+ - \text{urinary } Cl^-$$
$$(63.2)$$

It assumes that the major cations in urine are sodium (Na^+), potassium (K^+), and NH_4^+, whereas the major anion is only chloride (Cl^-) because urinary HCO_3^- is zero at pH more than 6.5. Normally, the urinary anion gap is negative and gives the urinary NH_4^+ concentration. It becomes zero if renal ammonium production is defective and becomes positive in bicarbonaturia.

Summary

- The pH of the body must be regulated to preserve the function of enzymes.

- There are several different challenges to pH that must be countered.

- The first line of defense against changes in pH is chemical buffering, with the carbonic acid buffering system and hemoglobin being the two most important extracellular buffers.

- The respiratory system can compensate, at least partially, for changes in pH produced by any nonrespiratory disturbance.

- The kidneys can compensate, in some circumstances completely and in others only partially, for pH changes that are not produced by the kidneys.

- The Davenport nomogram is a useful visual tool for analyzing the responses to acid–base disturbances.

Applying What You Know

63.1. If Reverend Fisher's renal failure had continued longer, he would have developed a frank metabolic (renal) acidosis. What compensatory responses would be generated to restore pH to normal?

Types of Renal Syndromes

Nephritic Syndrome

Nephritic syndrome is characterized by hematuria, red cell casts in urine, moderate proteinuria, edema, hypertension, and occasionally oliguria. Nephritic syndrome occurs due to immunologic damage to the glomerular basement membrane. The initiating cause of this damage is mostly unknown except for *acute poststreptococcal glomerulonephritis* that follows an infection with group-A β-hemolytic streptococci. It occurs due to a cross-reaction of antistreptococcal antibodies with the glomerular basement membrane.

Nephritic syndrome occurs in three forms that differ in their mode of onset and clinical course. *Acute glomerulonephritis* (AGN) is diagnosed when the onset is abrupt and is not due to an acute exacerbation of a previously existing disease. AGN is mostly reversible and self-limiting. Less commonly, it progresses to rapidly progressive glomerulonephritis, chronic glomerulonephritis, or nephrotic syndrome. *Rapidly progressive glomerulonephritis* (RPGN) is diagnosed when the symptoms deteriorate rapidly, leading to chronic renal failure in a matter of weeks or months. *Chronic glomerulonephritis* (CGN) is diagnosed when the symptoms persist and progress over years or decades to chronic renal failure.

The above terms are clinical syndromes and are not to be confused with the actual disease processes (glomerulopathies), the names of which are based on the pathologic changes in the glomeruli. For example, the most common form of glomerulopathy associated with AGN, especially acute poststreptococcal glomerulonephritis, is *diffuse endocapillary glomerulonephritis*. The most common form of glomerulopathy associated with RPGN is *crescentic glomerulonephritis*. The glomerulopathies associated with CGN are not identifiable except in the early stages. In late stages of CGN, all glomerulopathies look alike as the glomeruli become hyalinized.

Nephrotic Syndrome

Nephrotic syndrome is diagnosed when proteinuria exceeds 4 g/day. The differences between nephritic syndrome and nephrotic syndrome are summarized in **Table 64.1**. Most cases of nephrotic syndrome are of immunologic origin due to unknown causes. The most common glomerulopathy associated with nephrotic syndrome is *minimal change* GN or *lipoid nephrosis*. Some cases of nephrotic syndrome are secondary to known causes, such as diabetes mellitus, amyloidosis, exposure to allergens (e.g., bee stings) and toxins (e.g., mercury), infections, and drugs.

Nephrotic syndrome is characterized by *hypoalbuminemia* (due to heavy proteinuria), *edema* (because plasma oncotic pressure decreases due to hypoalbuminemia), *hyperlipidemia* (probably because the reduction in plasma oncotic pressure stimulates hepatic lipoprotein synthesis), *microcytic hypochromic anemia* (due to urinary loss of transferrin), *increased ten-*

Table 64.1 Differences between Nephrotic and Nephritic Syndromes

	Nephrotic Syndrome	Nephritic Syndrome
Proteinuria	Gross	Moderate
Plasma albumin	Markedly reduced	Slightly reduced
Hematuria	Absent or traces	Marked
Blood pressure	Normal or low	Raised
Edema	Marked	Moderate
Urine volume	Normal/reduced	Reduced
Plasma lipid	Grossly elevated	Minimal increase

dency to thrombosis, especially of renal veins (due to urinary loss of antithrombin III), *vitamin D deficiency* (due to urinary loss of cholecalciferol-binding protein), *thyroid abnormalities* (due to urinary loss of thyroid-binding globulin), and *susceptibility to infections* (due to urinary loss of immunoglobulin G [IgG]).

Defects in Tubular Transport

Renal glycosuria is an autosomal recessive disorder in which there is impaired reabsorption of glucose from the tubules. As a result, glycosuria occurs in the presence of normal blood glucose, and the measured renal threshold for glucose is low. Renal glycosuria is of two types: *type A* is characterized by a low transport maximum for glucose (TmG), and *type B* is characterized by an increased splay (**Fig. 64.1**).

Renal tubular acidosis is a condition in which systemic acidosis occurs either due to inadequate hydrogen (H^+) secretion by the tubules or due to excessive back-diffusion of the secreted H^+ from lumen to blood (see sodium sulfate infusion test, Chapter 63). Impaired H^+ secretion reduces bicarbonate reclamation. There is therefore a compensatory increase in chloride (Cl^-) reabsorption that accompanies sodium (Na^+) reabsorption. Hence, the acidosis is hyperchloremic, and the anion gap is normal.

In **nephrogenic diabetes insipidus,** the tubules respond poorly to circulating ADH, resulting in polyuria.

Fanconi syndrome results from a defect in proximal tubular transport of several ions (Na^+, K^+, bicarbonate [HCO_3^-], calcium [Ca^{2+}], and phosphate [PO_4^{3-}]) and organic substances (glucose, uric acid, proteins, and amino acids). It usually occurs as an autosomal recessive disorder.

Acute Renal Failure

Acute renal failure (ARF) is defined as an abrupt but reversible impairment of renal function, which is always associated with an increase in blood urea nitrogen (BUN) and serum creatinine and is usually associated with oliguria.

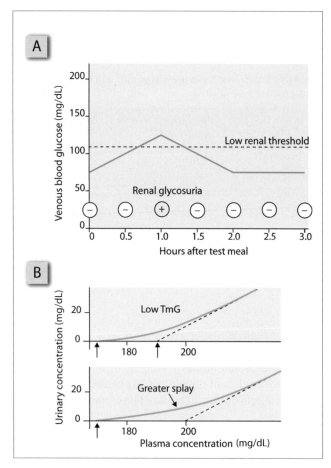

Fig. 64.1 **(A)** Glucose tolerance test graph in a case of renal glycosuria, the cause of which could be **(B)** a low transport maximum for glucose (TmG) or a greater splay.

In a broad sense, acute renal failure includes prerenal azotemia, intrinsic renal failure, and postrenal azotemia. In *prerenal azotemia,* there is inadequate renal perfusion, resulting in a rise in nitrogenous waste products in the blood, but without causing ischemic necrosis of renal tubules. Intrinsic renal failure is due to some renal disease, the most common being acute tubular necrosis (see below). Other causes include rapidly progressive glomerulonephritis. *Postrenal azotemia,* obstruction to the flow of urine, causes renal dysfunction and azotemia.

In a more restricted sense, ARF is used synonymously with acute tubular necrosis, which is by far the most common cause of ARF.

Clinically, **acute tubular necrosis** goes through the following phases. The *initiating phase* (*stage of onset*) lasts for ~36 hours. The signs of the underlying cause, for example, shock or a toxin, are prominent in this phase. The *maintenance phase* (*oliguric stage*) lasts from a few days to up to 3 weeks. It is characterized by oliguria less than 400 mL/day (anuria is rare), salt and water overload with dilutional hyponatremia, hyperkalemia, uremia, and acidosis. The *recovery phase* (*diuretic stage)* is characterized by polyuria and natriuresis, hypokalemia, and decrease in BUN.

The mainstay of the management, besides treating the underlying cause, is to overcome the oliguric phase so as to allow spontaneous recovery. Hemodialysis may be required during the crisis period. However, for the most part, the management comprises (1) restricting water intake to match urinary output and eliminating electrolytes from administered fluids and (2) restricting dietary proteins to reduce the load on the kidneys, while allowing plenty of carbohydrates and fats to provide energy.

Chronic Renal Failure

Chronic renal failure (CRF) is defined as a slowly progressive impairment of renal function associated with a reduction in the functioning renal mass. The decreased functioning renal mass has two broad effects: decreased excretion and decreased biosynthesis. The *decreased excretory capacity* results in clinical features such as azotemia, fluid imbalance and/or hypertension, hyperkalemia, and metabolic acidosis. The *decreased biosynthetic capacity* results in normocytic normochromic anemia (due to reduced erythropoietin secretion) and renal osteodystrophy (due to decreased activation of vitamin D). Management of CRF includes hemodialysis and kidney transplantation.

The ions and metabolites that are affected by the decreased excretory capacity of the kidney can be classified into three groups. (1) Substances such as *creatinine* and *urea* depend largely on glomerular filtration for their excretion into urine. Therefore, as the glomerular filtration rate (GFR) falls, the plasma levels of urea and creatinine rise progressively and serve as useful indicators of GFR impairment. Even so, the plasma levels of creatinine and urea do not start rising until the GFR falls to ~30% of the normal. (2) Substances such as PO_4^{3-}, K^+, H^+, and urate are excreted into urine at least partly through tubular secretion. Hence, the plasma levels of these substances rise only when the GFR falls to very low levels. (3) Substances such as Na^+ and Cl^- do not show any change in their plasma level even when the GFR drops to very low levels. The net urinary excretion of these ions does not change due to compensation by surviving nephrons.

The **fluid and electrolyte imbalances** associated with CRF are due largely to the reduction in the total nephron mass in the kidneys. With a decrease in nephron mass, the GFR decreases, and with it, the filtration fraction decreases because the RBF does not decrease as much as the GFR. The GFR in the individual surviving nephrons (the *single nephron GFR*) increases; therefore, there is a rapid flow of tubular fluid in these nephrons, which reduces the tubular reabsorption of water. Hence, despite the reduced GFR, the volume of urine excreted might actually increase, resulting in polyuria. Another consequence of the rapid tubular flow is that the composition of the tubular fluid is less affected by tubular reabsorption of fluids and electrolytes. Hence, urine osmolarity is limited to a narrow range of 250 to 350 mOsm/L (specific gravity of ~1.008). The excretion of urine within a narrow range of osmolarity is called *isosthenuria.*

The surviving nephrons also show a compensatory *natriuresis* for two reasons: (1) The peritubular capillary hydrostatic pressure rises due to the arterial hypertension that is usually present in CRF. (2) The peritubular capillary oncotic pressure decreases due to a decrease in the filtration fraction and due to the hypoalbuminemia that is commonly present in CRF. Due to compensatory natriuresis, the total Na^+ concentration is unaffected in CRF.

The natriuresis is somewhat exaggerated in certain forms of CRF associated with *salt-wasting nephropathies.* In these nephropathies, the renal medulla (which contains most of the tubules) is affected more than the cortex (which contains most of the glomeruli). Hence, the GFR is relatively unaffected, but the Na^+ reabsorption is greatly impaired, resulting in natriuresis.

Acidosis | The reduction of renal mass results in reduced production of ammonia, which is a major source of urinary buffer. Reduction in urinary ammonia buffers in the tubules decreases new HCO_3^- generation and results in acidosis. Because the Na^+ concentration is unaffected in CRF, so also must be the total concentration of anions. However, because the plasma HCO_3^- level is decreased, other anions must increase in plasma. In advanced CRF, the drop in plasma HCO_3^- level is compensated by an increase in sulfates and phosphates that are retained in large amounts. Hence, a large anion gap develops. In less severe CRF, the drop in plasma HCO_3^- levels is compensated by an increase in Cl^- reabsorption, and the anion gap remains normal.

Potassium balance | The plasma K^+ level is fairly well maintained in CRF. A decrease in renal mass would be expected to decrease the tubular secretion of K^+. However, there is a compensatory increase in the distal tubular secretion of K^+ for three reasons: (1) The rapid flow of tubular fluid keeps the tubular concentration of K^+ low. This facilitates tubular secretion of K^+. (2) The presence of high amounts of sulfates and phosphates in the tubular fluid increases the luminal negativity of the tubule, which promotes potassium secretion. (3) Any increase in plasma K^+ level increases aldosterone secretion. Aldosterone increases the tubular secretion of K^+.

Toxic metabolites | Although a high concentration of blood urea is characteristic of CRF, the urea is relatively nontoxic. However, urea does cause anorexia, nausea, vomiting, and hiccups, which, in turn, contribute to protein-calorie malnutrition in CRF. The actual toxic substances are the products of protein, amino acid, and nucleic acid catabolism. The bleeding tendency in CRF is caused mainly by guanidinosuccinic acid, which interferes with the activation of platelet factor III.

Calcium and phosphate imbalances | The Ca^{2+} level decreases for two reasons. (1) The kidney is normally a major site for the activation of vitamin D (Chapter 78). The decrease in renal mass is associated with a decrease in the circulating levels of calcitriol and a consequent decrease in the Ca^{2+} absorption from the gastrointestinal tract. (2) Decreased GFR also results in decreased PO_4^{3-} excretion and thereby causes a slight hyperphosphatemia. The increase in plasma PO_4^{3-} causes a reciprocal decrease in the ionized Ca^{2+} levels in the plasma due to deposition of tricalcium phosphate $[Ca_3(PO_4)_2]$ in the bone and other tissues. The hypocalcemia stimulates high levels of parathyroid hormone secretion, resulting in the bone changes described below.

Bone changes | CRF results in hypocalcemia and hyperphosphatemia, which lead to two types of pathologic changes: *renal osteodystrophy* and metastatic calcification (see Bone Chemistry subsection, Chapter 78). Renal osteodystrophy is the collective name given to several bone changes characteristically associated with CRF. It is caused by parathyroid hormone, the secretion of which is persistently elevated in CRF due to the decrease in plasma Ca^{2+}. Renal osteodystrophy can take the form of osteomalacia or rickets, osteitis fibrosa cystica, or osteosclerosis (see Bone Disorders subsection, Chapter 78).

Dialysis

Dialysis is a term of physical chemistry. It is the process of separation of colloids from crystalloids in a complex solution. In clinical medicine, it refers to the process by which some of the excess crystalloids and other toxic waste products that accumulate in blood in renal failure are eliminated from the plasma, while colloids like plasma proteins and the cellular elements are retained in the plasma.

Hemodialysis is done by interposing a semipermeable membrane between the patient's blood and the dialysate, an electrolyte solution with a composition similar to that of normal plasma. As the blood equilibrates with the dialysate, its crystalloid composition becomes similar to that of the dialysate. By varying the dialysate composition, the plasma composition can be modified as desired by the clinician.

In *peritoneal dialysis,* the dialysate is infused into the peritoneal cavity and allowed to equilibrate with blood across the peritoneal membrane, which thereby acts as the dialyzing membrane.

Dialysis involves transport of both solute and water. Hence, by appropriately altering the colloid composition of the dialysate, it is also possible to use dialysis for removal of extra water from the body. Concepts of osmolar clearance, free-water clearance, and clearance of specific substances are applicable to dialysis, too, for quantifying its effectiveness.

Summary

- Renal syndromes can be categorized as arising either from damage to the glomerulus (nephrotic and nephritic syndromes) or from damage to the tubules (proximal or distal).

- Acute and chronic renal failure differ in their speed of onset and the extent of the dysfunction that is present. In both cases, there is decreased excretory capacity and increased plasma concentrations of a variety of solutes.

Applying What You Know

64.1. What is Reverend Fisher's anion gap? Is it normal? How would you explain the value you calculate?

Urinary Bladder

The urinary bladder stores urine at a low pressure. The wall of the bladder has a serous, a muscular, and a mucous coat. The muscular coat is made of the detrusor muscle and consists of the outer, middle, and inner layers of smooth muscle fibers. Bladder smooth muscle cells are of the single unit type, with adjacent cells being electrically coupled. As a result, stimulation of the bladder during micturition results in a nearly synchronous contraction of the bladder.

General Model: Elasticity

The bladder is a structure whose elastic properties make it possible to store large volumes of urine with only a small tension in its walls.

The *mucous membrane* epithelium is of the transitional variety. There are no muscularis mucosae in the bladder wall. The transitional cell epithelium stretches as the bladder distends, prevents the loss of fluids and electrolytes, and secretes a glycosaminoglycan barrier that prevents bacterial adherence.

Urinary Sphincters

There are two urinary sphincters preventing emptying of the bladder as it fills: the *internal sphincter*, which is made up of the smooth muscle, and the *external sphincter, which is made up of skeletal muscle* (**Fig. 65.1** and **Table 65.1**).

The **internal sphincter** is simply the wall of the bladder as it narrows toward the urethra. Contraction of the smooth

Table 65.1 Comparison of the Urinary Sphincters	
Urinary Sphincter	**Function**
Sphincter vesicae	Prevents retrograde ejaculation
Intrinsic rhabdomyosphincter	Main provider of tonic continence

muscle in this part of the wall of the bladder closes the opening and prevents urine from entering the urethra.

The **external sphincter** is a skeletal muscle that wraps around the exterior of the urethra, where it joins the bladder.

Sensory Innervation of the Urinary Tract

Sensory afferents from the bladder wall reach the spinal cord (T10–L2) through the pelvic splanchnic nerve (nervi erigentes) and the hypogastric plexus (**Fig. 65.2A**). Sensory afferents

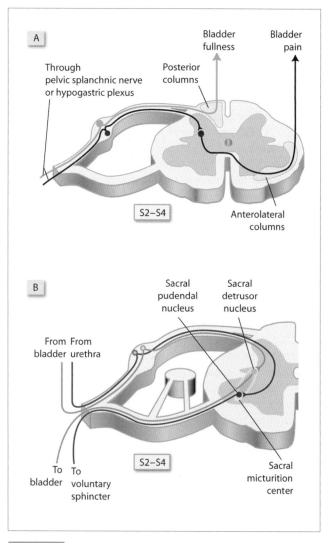

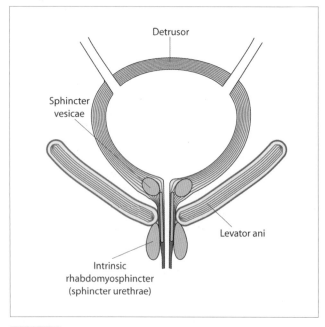

Fig. 65.1 Urinary sphincters.

Fig. 65.2 **(A)** Afferent pathway for conscious bladder sensations. **(B)** The reflex arc for the micturition reflex.

from the urethra reach the spinal cord through the pudendal nerve.

The sensation of bladder distention arises from the stretch receptors found in the walls of the bladder. The sensation of imminent voiding associated with maximal bladder filling originates in the periurethral striated muscle. These sensations ascend in the dorsal columns of the spinal cord to reach the pontine and suprapontine micturition centers.

The pain fibers from the bladder ascend in the anterolateral columns of the spinal cord. Bladder pain is therefore relieved by cutting the anterolateral columns of the spinal cord. After the anterolateral cordotomy, the patient is still aware of bladder filling and of the desire to micturate.

Motor Innervation of the Urinary Tract

The **sympathetic innervation** of the bladder originates from the intermediolateral gray horn of the spinal cord at the level of T10–L2 segments of the cord. They travel via the hypogastric nerves to the bladder and urethra. Sympathetic fibers are inhibitory to the detrusor and the internal sphincter but excitatory to the external sphincter.

The **parasympathetic innervation** originates from the sacral detrusor nucleus located in the intermediolateral gray horn of the sacral spinal cord (S2–S4). The nucleus is formed by the soma of preganglionic parasympathetic neurons. Parasympathetic efferents from the sacral detrusor nucleus leave the cord through its ventral root, pass through the pelvic splanchnic nerve, and relay in the ganglia near or within the bladder and urethra. The postganglionic fibers innervate the muscles of the bladder and urethra. The parasympathetic fibers are excitatory to the detrusor muscle and the internal sphincter and inhibitory to the external sphincter.

Somatic motor innervation | The somatic motor nerves originate from the *sacral pudendal nucleus,* also known as the nucleus of Onuf, located in the ventral horn of the S2 segment of the spinal cord. They reach the external sphincter through the perineal branch of the pudendal nerve (S2–S4), and the inferior hypogastric plexus and the pelvic splanchnic nerve.

The efferent bladder control is summarized in **Table 65.2**.

General Model: Communications

Control of bladder emptying is exerted by neural (cell–cell communications) signals in both the autonomic nervous system ("involuntary") and the somatic motor system ("voluntary").

Micturition Centers

The **sacral micturition center** (S2–S4) is the spinal center for the micturition reflex (**Fig. 65.2B**). It consists of the sacral detrusor nucleus and the sacral pudendal nucleus. Afferent impulses from the detrusor and urethra reach the *sacral micturition center* (SMC) through the dorsal root of the sacral cord. In the SMC, the afferents excite the *sacral detrusor nucleus,* causing detrusor contraction. They also inhibit the *sacral pudendal nucleus,* thereby relaxing the intrinsic and extrinsic rhabdomyosphincters.

The **pontine micturition center** (also called Barrington's center) corresponds to the locus ceruleus of the rostral pons (**Fig. 65.3**). Neurons from the pontine micturition center (PMC) descend in the reticulospinal tracts and exert control over the sacral micturition center and thoracolumbar sympathetic outflow. The PMC coordinates the activity of the bladder and urinary sphincter and relays inputs from suprapontine centers. Any lesion involving the PMC or its descending pathways to the SMC causes detrusor-sphincter dyssynergia—loss of coordination between the bladder and distal sphincteric mechanism. The associated disruption of suprapontine influences results in decreased storage and incomplete voiding.

The **cerebral cortex** has a detrusor motor area that is located in the medial frontal lobe (superior-frontal gyrus). The limbic area of the cerebral cortex (anterior cingulate gyrus and anterior genu of the corpus callosum) excites the SMC. It provides the anatomical basis for the effect of emotions on voiding.

The **basal ganglia** inhibit the SMC and hence the detrusor activity as well.

The Micturition Reflex

As the bladder slowly fills, the bladder wall stretches, and the tension in the walls is increased. Stimulation of the stretch receptors results in increased firing of sensory nerves that travel to the spinal cord, where parasympathetic fibers are stimulated. This increases parasympathetic stimulation of the bladder and increases pressure still further.

However, once past infancy, voiding of urine, emptying the bladder, is under conscious control. Descending inhibitory signals from the brain inhibit the external sphincter, preventing emptying of the bladder. The bladder then relaxes, and the tension in its walls decreases, while it continues to fill with urine being delivered by the ureters. With each "cycle" of filling and relaxing, the tension in the wall of the bladder increases still further; at some point the reflex can no longer be voluntarily inhibited, and voiding of the bladder will occur.

Table 65.2 Efferent Nervous Controls of the Bladder

Nerve Supply	Origin	Passes Through	Contracts	Relaxes
Sympathetic fibers	Intermediolateral spinal gray horn (T10–L2)	Hypogastric plexus	Sphincter vesicae	Detrusor
Parasympathetic fibers	Sacral detrusor nucleus (S–S4)	Pelvic splanchnic nerve	Detrusor	Sphincter vesicae
Somatic fibers	Sacral pudendal nucleus (S2–S4)	Hypogastric plexus and pelvic splanchnic nerve	Rhabdomyosphincters	

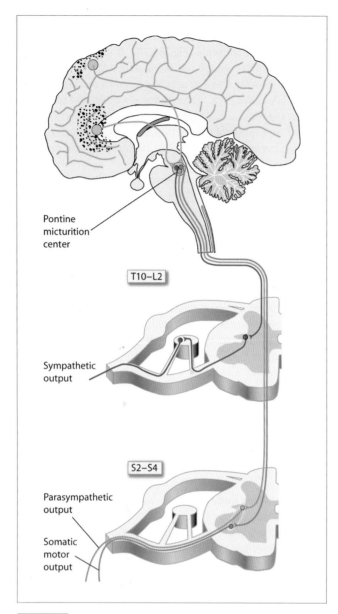

Fig. 65.3 Supraspinal control centers for micturition.

Initiation of Micturition

Common experience tells us micturition is a voluntary action. Yet in certain situations, the voluntary initiation of micturition may be difficult, for example, if the bladder is not full, or for some people, if there is an awareness of being watched in the act. Thus, micturition is not entirely voluntary, but is dependent on certain involuntary reflexes.

Micturition is voluntarily initiated by relaxing the pelvic diaphragm and the external urethral sphincter. Relaxation of the pelvic diaphragm reduces the support under the bladder, which therefore sags under its own weight. The sagging pulls open the bladder neck. As the bladder neck opens, urine trickles into the urethra through the relaxed external sphincters. The presence of urine in the urethra triggers reflex contraction of the detrusor, which forces more urine down the urethra. This sets up a positive feedback cycle that ends with the complete emptying of the bladder.

Neuropathic Bladders

A **flaccid neuropathic bladder** results from deafferentation of the bladder. In the absence of the micturition reflex, the bladder is flaccid and becomes overfilled until urine starts leaking out (overflow incontinence). The bladder always remains full, and the residual urine is high, but the intravesical pressure remains low. Due to overfilling, the bladder wall is thin and distended.

A **hypertrophic flexic bladder** results when there is damage to both the afferents and efferents of the bladder. In other words, it occurs in a decentralized (autonomous) bladder. Due to the abolition of the micturition reflex, decentralization initially results in a flaccid neuropathic bladder with overflow incontinence, as occurs in a deafferentated bladder. Subsequently, the detrusor develops denervation hypersensitivity and results in a small, hypertrophic areflexic bladder. Due to decreased bladder distensibility, bladder filling is associated with a steep rise in bladder pressure with consequent overflow incontinence. The bladder never voids reflexly and always remains full. Residual urine is low.

A **spastic neuropathic bladder** occurs when the SMC is isolated from the brain due to a suprasacral spinal cord injury. *Immediately following the injury,* there is abolition of the micturition reflex, resulting in a flaccid neuropathic bladder with all its attendant features, for example, overflow incontinence. *In the initial stages of recovery,* the reflex excitability of the striated muscle of the sphincters is restored. The incontinence disappears, and there is urinary retention. *In the later stages of recovery,* the reflex excitability of the smooth muscle returns, and the bladder capacity is reduced. In the absence of supraspinal inhibition, the micturition reflex is exaggerated, resulting in spasticity. The micturition reflex is triggered whenever the bladder is distended, resulting in incontinence. Sphincter spasticity and detrusor-sphincter dyssynergia lead to detrusor hypertrophy and high voiding pressures (i.e., intravesical pressure at which voiding is initiated). A few patients develop the ability to empty the bladder reflexly by using trigger techniques, such as by tapping or scratching the pubic area or external genitalia (**Table 65.3**).

Autonomic dysreflexia occurs in patients with spinal cord lesions above the level of sympathetic outflow—above T1. In these patients, afferent impulses to the sacral spinal cord can trigger a series of sympathetically mediated responses, including hypertension, headache, piloerection, and sweating. This phenomenon is known as *autonomic dysreflexia.* The triggering stimuli could be visceral (overdistention of bowel or bladder, penile erection) or somatic (spasm of lower extremities,

Table 65.3 Comparison of Neuropathic Bladders

Bladder Disorder	Reflexes	Overflow	Bladder Size
Flaccid neuropathic	Absent	Present	Large
Hypertrophic areflexic	Absent	Present	Small
Spastic neuropathic	Exaggerated	Absent	Small

insertion of a catheter, dilatation of the external urethral sphincter, ejaculation) in origin. Treatment includes bladder catheterization (for immediate relief), sphincterotomy, and bladder deafferentation.

Cystometry

Cystometry is one of a battery of tests called the *urodynamic studies* that record the urinary bladder activity, urethral sphincter activity, and urinary flow rate. The urodynamic studies relating to the bladder function are cystometry and radiographic (cinefluoroscopy) studies. The latter is now done only infrequently. There are two methods of doing cystometrography: voiding cystometry and static cystometry.

Voiding cystometry allows physiologic filling of the bladder with urine. Intravesical pressure is recorded through a urethral catheter, starting when the patient's bladder is empty and continuing until the bladder is full. The patient is then asked to urinate. The disadvantage with this method is that the bladder volume is inferred from the amount of urine voided, assuming that there is no residual urine.

In **static cystometry,** the bladder is progressively filled with water through a urethral catheter, and the intravesical pressure is recorded either through the catheter itself or through a suprapubic cannula. This method permits accurate determination of the bladder volume and pressure at each level of filling. The disadvantage with this method is that the fluid is introduced at a more rapid rate than occurs naturally through urine, which could affect bladder function.

In both methods, the pressure recorded from the bladder is actually the sum of both intra-abdominal and intravesical pressure. Hence, true detrusor pressure is the intravesical pressure minus the intra-abdominal pressure. Intra-abdominal pressure is recorded simultaneously by a small balloon catheter inserted high in the rectum and connected to a separate transducer. In clinical practice, however, it is usually sufficient to make a note of when the patient is straining (by observing the abdominal

contractions) and take them into consideration while interpreting the cystometrogram.

A normal cystometrogram shows three phases of filling (**Fig. 65.4**). *Phase Ia* is the initial phase of filling up to 50 mL. It is associated with a slight increase in pressure to ~10 cm of water. *Phase Ib* is the next phase of filling that lasts until the bladder volume is ~400 mL. As the bladder fills up, the bladder smooth muscles relax (due to smooth muscle plasticity), permitting an increase in the bladder volume. Thus, the pressure remains unchanged in accordance with Laplace's law. *Phase II* is denoted by a sharp rise in pressure as voiding is initiated. Normally, the voiding contractions raise the intravesical pressure by ~30 cm of water, which is called the voiding pressure. In the figure, the dotted lines beyond phase II denote the intravesical pressure changes with further filling if voiding is not initiated.

Cystometry is done to ascertain the following bladder functions. (1) The *bladder capacity* is the bladder volume at which voiding is irresistible. It is normally 400 to 500 mL. It is higher in women who have trained themselves to retain large volumes of urine. (2) *Accommodation* is the ability of the bladder to accommodate large volumes of urine without a significant rise in the intravesical pressure. Normally, the bladder pressure remains almost constant during filling up to the point of voiding. (3) *Bladder sensations* enable the perception of bladder fullness. The sensation of fullness is first perceived when the volume reaches 150 to 250 mL. There is a definite sense of fullness at 350 to 450 mL. The desire to void occurs when the bladder feels full. (4) *Bladder contractions* are assessed from the ability of the bladder to contract when full, to sustain a contraction until it is empty, and to contract in response to parasympathomimetic drugs. Normally, there is no residual urine in the bladder after voiding. Bladder contractions are not present during the filling phase, and the presence of premature bladder contractions during filling is called unstable bladder activity. (5) *Voluntary bladder control* is the ability to initiate voiding even before filling is complete, to inhibit voiding until the bladder capacity is maximal, and to stop voiding in midstream.

Summary

- The bladder is a vessel made of smooth muscle, which holds the urine produced by the kidneys.

- It is innervated by components of the autonomic nervous system and by the somatic motor system.

- It is supplied with sensory receptors sending information to the spinal cord and to the brain.

- Emptying of the bladder is controlled by two sphincters, an internal sphincter composed of smooth muscle and an external sphincter that is made of skeletal muscle.

- As the bladder fills, stretch in the walls sends afferent information.

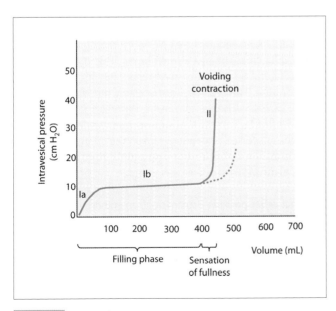

Fig. 65.4 A normal cystometrogram.

Answers to Applying What You Know

Chapter 53

1 Reverend Fisher had a myocardial infarct and an episode of cardiac arrest. What effects would this have on his kidney functions?

The kidneys receive a very large fraction of the cardiac output and a very high blood flow per gram of tissue. This reflects the kidneys' high metabolic rate, which is largely due to the activity of the tubular pumps involved in reabsorption of sodium and other solutes. The ischemia present during cardiac arrest will therefore reduce pump function and lead to alterations in electrolyte concentrations. If the ischemia lasts long enough, then damage to the tubular cells can be expected to occur, perhaps even the death of some cells. The debris (pieces of dead cells) that accumulates can affect fluid flow in the tubular lumen.

Chapter 54

1 Reverend Fisher has protein in his urine, and his total plasma protein and plasma albumin are both reduced. What can you conclude from these data?

The fact that plasma protein is reduced and there is protein in the urine suggests that the glomerular filtration barrier is damaged, and larger molecules are now being filtered out of the glomerular capillaries and into Bowman's capsule. It is also possible that the tubular mechanisms responsible for reabsorption of small proteins, which are normally filtered, have also been are damaged.

2 During the time that Reverend Fisher was hypotensive, what changes occurred to his renal blood flow and his glomerular filtration rate (GFR)? Explain.

Renal blood flow and glomerular filtration rate (GFR) both exhibit autoregulation. That is, as long as renal artery pressure is greater than ~60 mm Hg, renal blood flow (RBF) and GFR are both more or less constant. Two possible mechanisms of this autoregulation are (1) myogenic changes in resistance to flow countering any change in driving pressure, and (2) feedback from the macula densa signaling changes in tubular delivery of sodium chloride (NaCl).

If Reverend Fisher's blood pressure fell below 60 mm Hg, almost inevitable given the long period of cardiac arrest that occurred, his RBF and GFR would both fall. One consequence of the blood in RBF would be ischemia and tissue damage.

3 Gentamicin, one of the antibiotics used to treat Reverend Fisher, is known to be nephrotoxic, and it is particularly damaging to the proximal tubule. Predict the changes in the kidney functions listed that you would expect to see in a patient treated with gentamicin: Na$^+$ excretion, K$^+$ excretion, urine flow rate, and osmolarity.

If the function of the proximal tubule is compromised by gentamicin, the obligatory reabsorption of Na$^+$, K$^+$, and water will not occur. This must mean that excretion of Na$^+$ and K$^+$ is increased, and urine flow rate is increased. Osmolarity may not change because the reabsorption in the proximal tubule is normally iso-osmotic.

However, the cell damage caused by the gentamicin may lead to obstruction of the tubular lumen. If this occurs in any appreciable number of nephrons, the flow of tubular fluid would be reduced, and hence urine flow would be reduced.

4 Predict the changes that were present in GFR following Reverend Fisher's myocardial infarct, knowing that he had a markedly elevated plasma creatinine and BUN (blood urea nitrogen) concentration. Explain your prediction.

The kidneys' handling of creatinine involves filtration at the glomerulus and very little reabsorption. Hence, whatever is filtered is excreted (appears in the urine). An elevated plasma creatinine is most likely due to a decrease in GFR. Plasma creatinine values provide a generally useful measure of GFR.

The kidneys' handling of BUN is more complex, and we cannot easily use knowledge of plasma BUN to estimate changes in GFR.

Chapter 55

1 Reverend Fisher's laboratory report shows that he is hyponatremic. This may mean that his kidneys are not doing a good job of reabsorbing filtered sodium. There are several different mechanisms by which Na+ is reabsorbed. What do they all have in common?

Na$^+$ reabsorption requires that Na$^+$ from the lumen enter the tubule cell across the apical membrane. This occurs because the basolateral Na$^+$–K$^+$ pump maintains a low intracellular Na$^+$ concentration. The pathway for Na$^+$ entry into the tubule cell is quite varied, with several transport proteins facilitating the movement of Na$^+$ across the luminal membrane (along with other cotransported or countertransported solutes). Thus, the common feature is the Na$^+$–K$^+$ pump and the need for adenosine triphosphate (ATP) to power this pump.

2 What other possible explanation can you provide for Reverend Fisher's hyponatremia?

Reverend Fisher has a very low urine output and is clearly retaining water. This retained water is, at least in part, in his extracellular fluid compartment, where it will dilute *all* solutes, lowering their concentrations. This could be causing, or at least contributing to, Reverend Fisher's hyponatremia.

Answers to Applying What You Know | 411

Chapter 56

1 Reverend Fisher's plasma osmolarity is 280 mOsm/L, slightly lower than normal. What changes to the normal mechanisms determining osmolarity might cause such a change? Explain.

If antidiuretic hormone (ADH) were reduced in concentration, the permeability of the collecting duct to water would decrease, and less water would be reabsorbed. The result would be water retention and reduced plasma osmolarity.

If the osmoreceptors fire faster, the release of ADH will increase. This would lead to increased reabsorption of water; hence, body fluid osmolarity would increase.

Increased blood flow to the renal medulla would remove more solute from the interstitium, washing out (reducing) the gradient of hyperosmolarity created by the countercurrent multiplier. The result would be less water reabsorption and hyperosmolarity of blood fluids.

With shorter juxtamedullary nephrons, the countercurrent multiplier would be able to create only a small gradient of osmolarity. Thus, less water would be reabsorbed, and the body's osmolarity would increase.

In Reverend Fisher's case, the problem is reduced filtration and reduced urine flow; both are the result of mechanical obstruction of the tubular lumen by debris from the damaged or dead tubular cells. The water retention that is occurring is diluting *all* solutes and lowering Reverend Fisher's osmolarity.

Chapter 57

1 Reverend Fisher is observed to have mild presacral edema, an accumulation of interstitial fluid in the soft tissue over his sacrum. What are the factors that have led to the development of edema here?

The formation of edema fluid is driven, in part, by the increase in capillary hydrostatic pressure that occurs from the effect of gravity on fluid columns. Reverend Fisher has been in bed for many days, and gravity will affect the capillary pressure at the "lowest point" of his body, the small of his back. It would be unlikely that pedal edema (hands or feet) would be present because of his supine position.

2 Reverend Fisher has been retaining fluids. His urine output has been significantly less than his fluid intake from drinking and from the intravenous (IV) line that is in place. Where will this retained fluid be found? Explain your reasoning.

The fluids that Reverend Fisher is drinking are undoubtedly hypo-osmotic; that is, they contain much less solutes than body fluid. The IV he has been receiving is probably iso-osmotic, with the NaCl and other solutes, glucose perhaps, adjusted so that the osmolarity of the IV fluid is 300 mOsm/L. This combined fluid

intake is thus hypo-osmotic. Because water *always* moves down any osmotic gradient that is created, water will move from the vascular compartment into the interstitial compartment and then into the intracellular compartment. Thus, the fluid he is retaining will be divided (see **Fig. 20.1**) between the extracellular fluid (ECF; 40%) and the intracellular fluid (ICF; 60%).

Chapter 58

1 Reverend Fisher's bicarbonate concentration is somewhat low (22 mL/L). What does this suggest about how his kidneys are handling bicarbonate ions?

The fact that Reverend Fisher's bicarbonate concentration is low may mean that his kidneys are not fully reabsorbing the filtered bicarbonate. This might be the consequence of the damage to his kidneys sustained during his treatment with nephrotoxic antibiotics and/or from his cardiac arrest. Damage to the proximal tubule where most of the bicarbonate is reabsorbed (coupled with the reabsorption of Na^+) would certainly lower his plasma bicarbonate.

There will also be some dilution of bicarbonate from the retained water.

Finally, it is also possible that Reverend Fisher's low bicarbonate is a normal response to the presence of a metabolic acidosis (see Chapter 63).

Chapter 59

1 Reverend Fisher's laboratory report reveals that his plasma K^+ is on the high side of normal. He is also retaining water. How can you explain his slightly elevated $[K^+]$ in the face of his being in positive water balance?

Concentration = amount/volume and we know that Reverend Fisher's K^+ concentration is "high" and that his water volume is increased. This must mean that Reverend Fisher is retaining a lot of K^+ presumably because his kidney failure has reduced their ability to secrete and hence excrete K^+.

2 The initial laboratory report for Reverend Fisher shows him to have a low $[Na^+]$ and a $[K^+]$ that is at the high end of the normal range. How might the state of these electrolytes contribute to his appearing lethargic and confused on physical examination?

The resting membrane potential of neurons and the amplitude of the action potential are determined by the concentration gradients for Na^+ and K^+ across the membrane. Changes in resting potential can make neurons hypo- or hyperexcitable, altering their likelihood of firing. Changes to the amplitude of the action potential will change the conduction velocity along all axons. This will alter the timing of electrical activity in the nervous system. Any or all of these changes can lead to dysfunction in the central nervous system that could manifest itself as confusion.

Chapter 60

1 Proteins are found in Reverend Fisher's urine. This is undoubtedly the result of ischemic damage to his kidneys. Where might the damage have occurred that results in protein in his urine?

Protein in the urine could result from damage to the glomerulus and the normal diffusion barrier there, or it could result from failure to reabsorb small proteins in the proximal tubules. It is known that gentamicin, the antibiotic used to treat Reverend Fisher's pneumonia, is nephrotoxic, with the proximal tubules being particularly likely to be damaged.

2 Reverend Fisher has elevated BUN and creatinine. What mechanism is causing an accumulation of nitrogenous waste products in his blood?

BUN and creatinine are freely filtered at the glomerulus. However, during Reverend Fisher's period of cardiac arrest (and perhaps for some time afterwards), glomerular filtration was stopped or was very small. Hence, with little BUN being filtered, the blood is not cleared of these nitrogenous waste products. Plasma creatinine is used by clinicians as a useful measure of changes in GFR.

Chapter 61

1 Reverend Fisher's serum osmolarity is 280 mOsm/L, a value that is slightly low. Predict whether his antidiuretic hormone (ADH) concentration will be increased, decreased, or normal.

Reverend Fisher's osmolarity is slightly low because he is retaining fluid (his fluids in are greater than his fluids out), and his ECF (and hence vascular compartment) is expanded. His low osmolarity and expanded blood volume will result in a decrease in the firing of the osmoreceptors and volume receptors and cause a decreased release of ADH. This, of course, will result in greater water excretion and a return of the osmolarity to its normal value.

2 Reverend Fisher is both hyponatremic and slightly hyperkalemic. Predict whether his aldosterone concentration will be increased, decreased, or normal. Explain your prediction.

Reverend Fisher's significant hyponatremia (acting via increased release of renin and thus increased angiotensin II) and mild hyperkalemia (acting directly on the adrenal cortex) is most likely to cause an increase in the secretion of aldosterone. This will act on the distal nephron to promote the reabsorption

of Na^+ (restoring its concentration to normal) and the excretion of K^+ (restoring its concentration to normal).

Chapter 62

1 Analysis of a urine sample from Reverend Fisher reveals many squamous epithelial cells and several pigmented casts. Where did these come from?

The squamous cells and casts seen in Reverend Fisher's urine came from damaged cells affected by both the gentamicin and the episode of cardiac arrest. Both of these "disturbances" damage or destroy tubule cells, and the cellular debris created appears in the urine.

Chapter 63

1 If Reverend Fisher's renal failure had continued longer, he would have developed a frank metabolic (renal) acidosis. What compensatory responses would be generated to restore pH to normal?

The damage to Reverend Fisher's kidneys would prevent the tubules from secreting (excreting) H^+, and thus the body's store of H^+ would increase. He would become acidotic. The trajectory of the development of this problem would be down the $PCO_2 = 40$ mm Hg isobar. The change in pH would stimulate peripheral chemoreceptors and cause ventilation to be increased. This would result in decreased PCO_2. His acid–base status would move to a lower isobar on a trajectory parallel to the hemoglobin (Hb) buffer line because Hb would be taking up some of the excess H^+. Respiratory compensation can only correct the problem to the extent defined by the respiratory compensation (RC) line. Until the kidney problem is resolved, there can be no further correction.

Chapter 64

1 What is Reverend Fisher's anion gap? Is it normal? How would you explain the value you calculate?

Reverend Fisher's electrolytes are
$[Na^+] = 122$ mM/L
$[K^+] = 4.8.$ mM/L
$[HCO_3^-] = 22$ mM/L
$[Cl^-] = 96.0$ mM/L

Thus, his anion gap is 8.8, somewhat lower than one might expect. A possible explanation for this is his low albumin concentration of 2.7. Albumin accounts for a very large fraction of the unmeasured anions; thus, the hypoalbuminemia would cause a smaller anion gap.

Section VII Case Analysis:
Frank Fisher isn't making any urine.

Clinical Overview

Review of patient condition | Reverend Fisher has had a rather difficult time recently. He was hospitalized for pneumonia and treated with antibiotics. During his hospital stay, he suffered a myocardial infarct and a cardiac arrest. Resuscitation was successful. He is now found to be suffering from acute renal failure.

Etiology | His renal failure is probably the result of the antibiotic administered for his pneumonia. Gentamicin, an aminoglycoside antibiotic, is known to be nephrotoxic. It can produce acute renal necrosis. The resulting renal dysfunction (see below) compounds the problem because gentamicin is cleared from the body by the kidneys. The result can be a positive feedback cycle, with gentamicin levels increasing and causing further damage to the kidneys. The myocardial infarct and subsequent cardiac arrest could have resulted in significant renal ischemia leading to further renal damage.

Prevalence | From 2 to 5% of hospitalized patients develop acute renal failure.

Diagnosis | The diagnosis of acute renal failure is made when the onset of the condition is sudden, elevated plasma BUN and creatinine are present, and urine flow rate is decreased (oliguria).

Treatment | If there is a known primary cause of the renal failure, it must be eliminated or corrected. In Reverend Fisher's case, this clearly meant stopping the administration of the gentamicin. It is also important that use of agents known to negatively impact renal function be avoided (nonsteroidal antiinflammatory drugs, radiologic contrast media). It is important that urine flow be increased, although this alone will not suffice to stabilize the patient's condition. Careful control of fluid intake/output must be established. Electrolyte balance, particularly for potassium, must be maintained, or corrected if necessary. Dialysis may be necessary while the damaged kidneys repair themselves.

Understanding the Physiology

Gentamicin is an antibiotic known to be capable of damaging the kidneys. In particular, it damages the proximal tubules. The acute tubular necrosis has several effects. The tubules become filled with cell debris, posing a high resistance to fluid flow. Consequently, the pressure in Bowman's capsule increases, and GFR therefore decreases. Any damage done to the glomerulus by the antibiotic merely compounds this problem.

With the tubules filled with debris and GFR reduced, there is less urine flow. The damage done to the tubule cells makes the walls of the tubule "leaky," and tubular fluid can flow into the interstitial space and then into the peritubular capillaries. This also reduces urine flow.

Reverend Fisher is receiving IV fluids (at least some) and is drinking liquids. With his urine output very much reduced, and his fluid intake continuing, he begins to retain water. This causes two problems: (1) his $[Na^+]$ falls as his body store of sodium is diluted, and (2) the balance of the Starling forces at the capillaries favors filtration, and edema formation occurs. In a patient generally confined to bed, the location where such edema is most visible will be in the presacral region.

The decreased GFR means that the excretion of nitrogenous waste products such as blood urea nitrogen (BUN) and creatinine is reduced, and their blood levels must increase. Similarly, the excretion of K^+ is reduced, and K^+ is retained, increasing its concentration.

The role of Reverend Fisher's myocardial infarct and the episode of cardiac arrest is difficult to assess precisely. However, the kidneys use a large fraction of the total O_2 consumed by the body to power the solute pumps that reabsorb Na^+, bicarbonate, calcium, and so on. With no or reduced blood flow to the kidneys, the resulting ischemia can certainly contribute to damage to renal tubules.

With cessation of gentamicin administration, the damaged kidneys will repair themselves, and the acute renal failure will reverse. By the date of Reverend Fisher's discharge, the laboratory report shows that kidney function is nearly back to normal.

A flow chart (**Fig. VII.1**) illustrating the interactions between mechanisms that produced Reverend Fisher's condition is given on the next page.

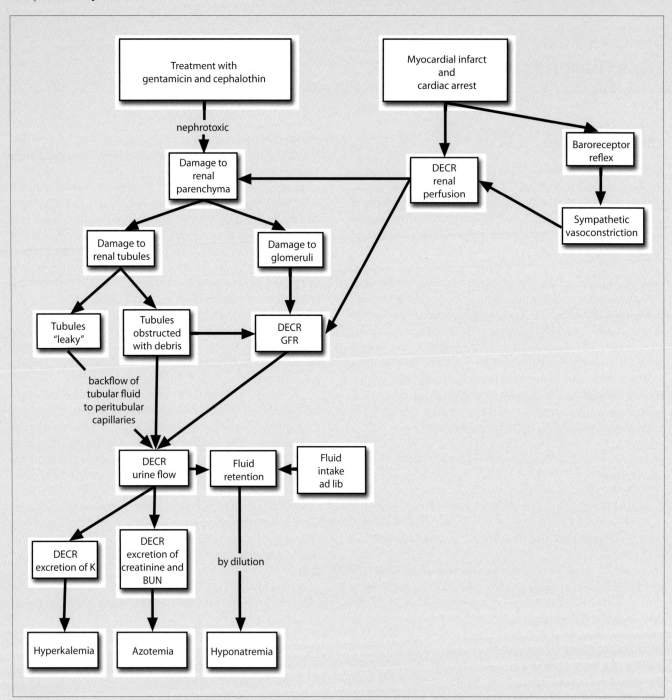

Fig. VII.1 Reverend Fisher's Kidneys have been subjected to two insults, the nephrotoxic effects of the antibiotics with which he was treated and reduced renal perfusion as a consequence of his heart attack.

Section VIII | Gastrointestinal System and Nutrition

Overview

Case Presentation

Chapters

Answers to Applying What You Know

Case Analysis

Overview

All cells in the body must obtain substrates from which they can generate the energy needed to power all of their functions. In addition, the cells must obtain the molecular building blocks from which to synthesize the compounds that make up their structure. The gastrointestinal (GI) system takes in food from the environment, breaks it down into smaller, absorbable molecules, then transports these molecules into the vascular compartment for transport to every cell in the body.

To accomplish these steps requires the coordinated function of several organs. The functions include the movement of ingested food through the GI tract (motility), the production of the substances that play a role in digestion, such as gastric acid and pancreatic enzymes (secretion), the breaking down of food into smaller molecules (digestion), and, finally, the transport of the products of digestion into the vascular compartment (absorption).

The coordination of the organs involved and these functions is brought about by the enteric nervous system and a set of hormones secreted in the GI system. The central nervous system also provides important inputs.

Chief Complaint

Mrs. Schilling has a 4-month history of diarrhea and has lost 20 pounds in the last month.

History of Present Illness

Mary Schilling is a 5'9", 58-year-old woman who presents with gastrointestinal problems that include 4 months of frequent stools and intermittent diarrhea, along with an increase in the volume of her stools. Over the same period, she complains of increasing lethargy and hypersomnolence.

Mrs. Schilling reports abdominal distention, bloating, and occasional nausea that she believes began ~2 months ago and has increased in intensity and frequency in the last month. She has had four to six bowel movements a day, usually within an hour of eating. Her stool is foul-smelling and floats on top of the toilet water. She also describes frequent flatulence. She reports cramping after some meals, especially those with high fat content. She occasionally has abdominal pain. The pain is epigastric, sharp and severe, shooting to her back.

Her appetite was normal until about 3 weeks ago, when she lost interest in eating. Over the last month, she has lost 20 pounds. She diligently checks her weight every morning before showering. One month ago, she was 150 pounds (body mass index [BMI] of 22.1), and today she weighs 130 pounds (BMI of 19.2).

She tried Imodium AD (a drug that slows peristalsis; McNeil Consumer Healthcare, Fort Washington, PA) for the diarrhea, but it did not help, and she has stopped taking it.

Medications

Calcium supplements

Allergies

She has no known allergies.

Past Medical History

She has had intermittent elevated blood pressure readings but has never been on antihypertensive drugs. In the past decade, she has a history of two previous presentations to the emergency room (ER) for abdominal pain. The first was 10 years ago, and she was given the diagnosis of dyspepsia and started on a trial of H2 blockers. She was lost to follow-up at that time. She presented to the ER again ~3 years ago complaining of severe right upper quadrant pain. She was hospitalized for 2 days and was found to have a gallstone in the common bile duct that was removed by an endoscopic procedure.

She has had no other surgeries.

Family History

- Maternal aunt: some kind of intestinal disorder.
- Paternal grandmother: diabetes (developed in adulthood), breast cancer at age 45, and a history of "nervous breakdowns."
- Children: all generally healthy except her 23-year-old daughter, who has asthma.

Social History

Mrs. Schilling is married with four children, ages 20, 23, 27, and 29. She denies tobacco use. She drinks alcohol "only on special occasions." She denies drug use. She works as a physical education teacher in a grammar school.

Physical Examination

- *General appearance* | Mrs. Schilling is in no apparent distress. She appears quite thin. She is comfortable, sitting quietly on the exam table.
- *Vital signs*
  - Temperature: 98.4°F (oral)
  - Blood pressure: 140/90 mm Hg
  - Radial pulse: 68/minute
  - Respiratory rate: 16 /minute (in a comfortable pattern)
- *Skin* | Scattered small bruises on both upper arms
- *HEENT (head, eyes, ears, nose, throat* | Normal
- *Lymph nodes* | Normal
- *Neck* | Thyromegaly (enlarged thyroid gland)
- *Lungs* | Clear to auscultation and percussion
- *Cardiovascular* | Normal S_1, S_2; no murmurs; peripheral pulses are normal
- *Abdomen* | Abdomen is slightly distended. Bowel sounds are hyperactive. Some lower abdominal tenderness is elicited with deep palpation. There is mild tenderness in the epigastric region. Liver span is 10 cm by percussion. No splenomegaly, no guarding, no rebound tenderness, no masses or hepatosplenomegaly. Rectal exam reveals yellow, foul-smelling stool in vault, with no occult blood.
- *Breasts* | No masses or discharges
- *Genital and pelvic exam* | Normal
- *Extremities* | Normal
- *Neurologic exam*
  - Mental status: alert and oriented to time, place, and person
  - Cranial nerves: normal
  - Motor function: 5/5 strength
  - Deep tendon reflexes (DTRs): normal
  - Sensation: normal

Laboratory Results

	Value	Normal Range
Hemoglobin	10 g/dL	12.0–16.0
MCV	109 fL	80–100
Prothrombin time	18.4 sec	9–13
INR	2.1	1.0
APTT	35 sec	25–35
Glucose	60 mg/dL	60–109
Protein	5.7 g/dL	6.0–8.2
Albumin	2.7 g/dL	3.5–5.0
Cholesterol	110 mg/dL	0–200

Abbreviations: APTT, activated partial thromboplastin time; INR, international normalized ratio; MCV, mean corpuscular volume.

KUB (an x-ray to examine the kidneys, ureters, and bladder)

Calcifications in upper abdomen

Abdominal Computed Tomography

- Pancreatic scarring and atrophy
- Liver appears normal
- There is no splenomegaly

GI Test Results

- 72-hour quantitative fecal fat analysis: 25 g (normal < 21 g)
- Xylose absorption test (patient drinks 500 mL of a solution of 25 g xylose, a monosaccharide, and urine is collected for 5 hours): 3 g of xylose in the urine (normal ≥ 4 g)

Small Intestine X-ray

The mucosa looks normal, but the jejunal lumen is dilated to 30 mm.

Biopsy

A biopsy of the small intestine is performed via endoscopy and reveals a flat mucosal surface (flattening of villi) with plasmocytic infiltration of the subepithelial region.

Diagnosis

Mrs. Schilling is suffering from celiac sprue, a malabsorption disorder resulting from damage to her intestinal mucosa.

Management

Therapy is begun with a gluten-free diet (no wheat, barley, oats, rye, or their flour; no beer, ale, vodka, or whiskey; no gluten-containing ice cream; other dairy products; or chewing gum). Mrs. Schilling's symptoms improve within the first week of the new diet. A repeat quantitative fecal fat analysis is normal after 2 weeks on the diet.

Some Things to Think About

1. Mrs. Schilling has fat in her stool (steatorrhea). What changes to normal function will impact the digestion and absorption of fats?

2. Mrs. Schilling's weight loss suggests she is not absorbing other nutrients as well, in particular carbohydrates. By what mechanisms are carbohydrates digested and absorbed?

3. Some of Mrs. Schilling's symptoms result from the failure to absorb micronutrients. What are these, and by what mechanism(s) are they absorbed?

4. Mrs. Schilling has signs and symptoms suggestive of intestinal hypermotility. What determines the motility of the gastrointestinal tract? How does Imodium affect motility?

The food that we eat is the ultimate source of the energy used by our cells to do everything that cells do. That food is also the ultimate source of the materials with which the cells build themselves and hence build the body. There are a great many nutrients required by the human body, and we will be describing them in this chapter. In the chapters that follow, we will discuss the functions of the gastrointestinal (GI) system that convert the food that is ingested into chemical forms that can be absorbed into the body and used by cells for energy and building cell structures.

General Model: Energy

All biologic organisms are open systems that must obtain material from the external environment to grow, develop, and survive. In particular, animals must obtain food from which they can derive the energy needed to power all their functions and from which they can build their structure.

Macronutrients

The bulk of a diet is comprised of proteins, carbohydrates, and fats (see Appendix B); these are called *macronutrients*. Macronutrients provide energy and the substrates needed to build the structures of the body; they are consumed in much larger quantities than other nutrients, such as vitamins and minerals, which are called *micronutrients*.

Fat

Fat is a high-energy nutrient that is stored in adipose cells and can be used by most, but not all, cells to power their metabolism. It provides the constituent molecules for cell membranes. Fat makes food rich and tasty and is physiologically important for generating the feeling of satiety. Fat is required for the absorption of fat-soluble vitamins. More than 90% of dietary fat is in the form of triacylglycerols (triglycerides), which supply the essential fatty acids required by the body. Triacylglycerols obtained from plants are generally richer in unsaturated fatty acids than those from animals. Salient exceptions are coconut and palm oils, which are rich in saturated fat, and fish, which is rich in unsaturated fats. The unsaturated fatty acids may be monounsaturated (olive oil) or polyunsaturated (corn and soybean oils).

Essential fatty acids are required for fluidity of membrane structure (see Chapter 2) and for synthesis of prostaglandins, prostacyclins, thromboxanes, and leukotrienes (Chapter 37). Dietary fat provides the essential fatty acids: linoleic and linolenic acids. Arachidonic acid becomes essential if linolenic acid, from which it is produced, is absent in the diet. A deficiency of essential fatty acids is characterized by scaly dermatitis, hair loss, and poor wound healing. Because fats are widely distributed in nature, a deficiency is rare.

Cholesterol is an essential component of cell membranes and serves as a precursor of bile acids, steroid hormones, and vitamin D. However, elevated levels of cholesterol increase the risk of coronary heart disease due to the formation of atherosclerotic plaque in coronary vessels. Plasma cholesterol level is moderately decreased when low-cholesterol diets are consumed. Egg yolk and meat are very rich in cholesterol, which is found only in animal products. Plant products, including margarine and vegetable oils, contain no cholesterol.

Saturated fatty acids are present mainly in dairy and meat products and some vegetable oils, such as coconut and palm oils. They tend to raise the total plasma cholesterol and the cholesterol in low-density lipoproteins (LDL), resulting in increased risk of coronary artery disease.

n-6 (ω-6, omega-6) Polyunsaturated fatty acids like linoleic acid are found in corn, safflower, soybean, and sunflower oils. Consumption of these fatty acids (with a double bond located six carbons from the methyl-group end) lowers plasma cholesterol. They lower plasma LDL, but also lower the high-density lipoprotein (HDL), which is considered healthier.

n-3 (ω-3, omega-3) Polyunsaturated fatty acids are found in oily fish and soybean. Diets rich in these fatty acids (with a double bond three carbons from the methyl-group end) reduce plasma triacylglycerols and decrease the risk of heart disease. They inhibit the conversion of arachidonic acid to thromboxane A_2 (TXA_2) by platelets and are themselves converted to TXA_3, which is less thrombogenic than TXA_2. Thus, they decrease platelet aggregation and are antithrombogenic.

Monounsaturated fats are as effective as polyunsaturated fats in lowering blood cholesterol when substituted for saturated fatty acids. In contrast to the effect of n-6 polyunsaturated fats, monounsaturated fats do not lower HDL.

Trans fatty acids do not occur naturally in significant amounts, but are formed during the hydrogenation of liquid vegetable oils into margarine. These fatty acids, unlike the naturally occurring cis isomers, raise plasma cholesterol levels.

Carbohydrates

Carbohydrates are the major source of biologic energy used by the organism, and all cells can use carbohydrates (usually in the form of glucose). Carbohydrates (glucose) can be stored as glycogen and converted into lipids for storage in adipose cells. With low intake of carbohydrates, the carbon skeletons formed by deamination of amino acids can release energy or can be converted into glucose. However, the breakdown of dietary proteins for energy release is wasteful because high-protein food is much more "expensive" than high-carbohydrate food. Carbohydrates are thus "protein-sparing" because they allow amino acids to be used for repair and maintenance of tissue protein rather than for gluconeogenesis. However, if carbohydrates are totally excluded from the diet, the energy released by proteins and fats decreases drastically, and they are converted mostly into ketone bodies. Even the glucose formed from the carbon skeletons of amino acids are not oxidized completely and form ketone bodies. These facts are summed up by the adage "Fats burn in the flame of carbohydrates" and explain not only the ketogenic effect of the Atkins diet (a zero-carbohydrate diet with no restrictions on proteins and fats), but also its weight-reducing effect despite the liberal intake of fats and proteins.

Carbohydrates in the normal diet are either monosaccharides and disaccharides (simple sugars) or polysaccharides (complex sugars). Glucose and fructose are the principal monosaccharides found in food and are abundant in fruits and honey. The most abundant disaccharides are sucrose (glucose + fructose), lactose (glucose + galactose), and maltose (glucose + glucose). Ordinary table sugar is sucrose, which is abundant in sugarcane. Lactose is the principal sugar found in milk. Maltose is a product of enzymatic digestion of polysaccharides. It is found in significant quantities in beer and liquors produced from barley. Polysaccharides are mostly polymers of glucose and do not have a sweet taste. Starch is a polysaccharide that is abundant in plants. Common sources of starch include wheat and other grains, potatoes, peas, beans, and vegetables.

Protein

Protein is required for repair and maintenance of tissue proteins and for growth in general. Protein consumed in excess of the body's needs is deaminated into carbon skeletons, which are metabolized to provide energy or to synthesize fatty acids. Proteins are made of different combinations of up to 20 different types of amino acids (see Appendix B). Like the amino acids that constitute them, one end of the protein molecule has an NH_2 group (the N terminal), and the other end has a COOH group (the C terminal). Ten of the amino acids are nutritionally essential because they cannot be synthesized in the body in adequate amounts. The essential amino acids are valine, leucine, isoleucine, threonine, methionine, arginine, lysine, histidine, phenylalanine, and tryptophan. Of these, arginine and histidine are required only during periods of rapid tissue growth characteristic of childhood or recovery from illness.

The ability to provide the essential amino acids required for tissue maintenance determines the biologic value of a dietary protein. The nutritive quality of a protein—its biologic value—is measured on a relative scale, with whole egg protein or egg albumin scored at 100. Proteins from animal sources (meat, poultry, milk, fish) have a high biologic value because they contain all the essential amino acids in proportions similar to those required for synthesis of human tissue proteins. Proteins from wheat, corn, rice, and beans have a lower biologic value than animal proteins.

Protein–Energy Malnutrition (PEM)

Insufficient intake of protein or energy-yielding food causes loss of both body mass and adipose tissue. There are two syndromes of PEM, marasmus and kwashiorkor, which result from a reduction in the consumption of protein and/or the total caloric intake (**Table 66.1**).

Marasmus results from catabolism and depletion of the somatic protein compartment represented by the skeletal

Table 66.1 Comparison of Kwashiorkor and Marasmus

Kwashiorkor	Marasmus
Similarities	
Both occur due to insufficient intake of protein and/or calories	
Both sets of patients show apathy, inactivity, and irritability	
Both sets of patients show growth retardation	
Differences	
Usually seen in recently weaned infants	Usually seen in children who have been weaned early or have never been breast-fed
Visceral protein compartment (liver) is depleted	Somatic protein compartment (muscle) is depleted
Hypoalbuminemia present	Serum albumin normal or slightly decreased
Edema is characteristically present	Edema is not present
Body weight remains normal	Severe wasting is present
Face puffy and moon-shaped	Face shriveled and monkey-like
Impaired appetite	Voracious appetite

muscles. The visceral protein compartment is depleted only marginally. It is for this reason that serum albumin levels remain normal or only slightly decreased. Subcutaneous fat is mobilized, resulting in emaciated extremities and monkey-like facies. The skin appears dry and inelastic. In comparison, the head appears too large for the body. The main brunt of the disease process falls on weight gain.

In **kwashiorkor,** protein deprivation is relatively greater than reduction in total calories. Unlike marasmus, marked protein deprivation is associated with severe loss of the visceral protein compartment represented mainly by protein stores in the liver. This leads to hypoalbuminemia and edema. Compromised weight-for-age may be masked by fluid retention and relative sparing of subcutaneous fat and muscle mass. Fatty liver is often present. Hairs are sparse, brittle, and depigmented. Many of these changes are due to damage by free radicals, which are present in excessive amounts in kwashiorkor.

Micronutrients

Vitamins

Vitamins are physiologically important substances that are required in small quantities in the diet. Unlike the major nutrients, they do not generate metabolic energy, but serve other specialized functions in the body. Their deficiency can result in serious symptoms and even death (**Table 66.2**). Vitamins have been categorized on the basis of their solubility as the fat-soluble vitamins (vitamin A, D, E, and K) and the water-soluble vitamins (vitamin B_1, B_2, B_3, B_5, B_6, B_{12}, folate, and vitamin C).

Table 66.2 Vitamins, Their Physiologic Role, Dietary Sources, and Deficiency Signs and Symptoms

Vitamin	Functions	Dietary Sources	Causes and Features of Deficiency Disease
Water-soluble Vitamins			
Thiamine Vitamin B₁	Thiamine is converted in tissues to thiamine pyrophosphate (TPP), which serves as a coenzyme for the oxidative decarboxylation of ketoacids and transketolase reaction in the hexose monophosphate shunt pathway.	Legumes, pork, liver, nuts, the germ of cereals, yeast, and outer layers of seeds	Deficiency is uncommon except in chronic alcoholics because of poor intestinal absorption and inadequate dietary intake. Thiamine deficiency causes beriberi, which has two forms. In *dry beriberi*, neuromuscular symptoms predominate, with demyelination of somatic nerves and wasting of muscles. *Wet beriberi* occurs in severe thiamine deficiency. It is associated with edema due to cardiac insufficiency, which, in turn, is probably due to inadequate metabolism and accumulation of pyruvic acid and lactic acid. In alcoholics, thiamine deficiency results in Wernicke-Korsakoff syndrome. The acute stage of this disease is known as Wernicke encephalopathy, which is characterized by delirium and ataxia. In the chronic stage, there is Korsakoff psychosis.
Riboflavin Vitamin B₂	Riboflavin is converted to flavin mononucleotide (FMN) in intestinal mucosa and to flavin adenine dinucleotide (FAD) in liver. The flavin nucleotides serve as coenzymes for the flavin dehydrogenases in the redox reactions of the electron transport chain.	Milk, eggs, liver, and green leafy vegetables	Ariboflavinosis is rare. It is associated with glossitis, stomatitis, cheilosis (reddening of the mucous membranes of the lips), and dermatitis. The dermal lesions occur especially around the nasolabial and scrotal areas.
Niacin Vitamin B₃	Niacin is converted to the coenzymes NAD⁺ (nicotinamide adenine dinucleotide) and NADP (nicotinamide adenine dinucleotide phosphate). NADH⁺H⁺ and NADPH⁺H⁺ are essential for anabolic redox reactions such as cholesterogenesis and lipogenesis in the extramitochondrial compartments of the cell; NAD⁺ and NADP are used in the catabolic redox reactions in the mitochondrial matrix.	Unrefined grains, yeast, liver, legumes, and lean meats	Limited amount of niacin can be synthesized in the body from tryptophan. Niacin deficiency is endemic among poor people who subsist chiefly on maize, which is deficient in tryptophan. Pellagra (meaning "rough skin") affects the gastrointestinal tract, skin, and central nervous system. It causes the three Ds: diarrhea, dermatitis, and dementia.
Pantothenic acid Vitamin B₅	Pantothenic acid is converted into coenzyme A, which plays a key role in several reactions. An example is conversion of succinate to succinyl CoA, which is a precursor for heme.	Yeast, liver, and eggs	Rare
Pyridoxine Vitamin B₆	Pyridoxine is converted into pyridoxal phosphate, which acts as a coenzyme for aminotransferases.	Whole-grain cereals, wheat, corn, nuts, muscle meats, liver, and fish	Rare, except in alcoholics, in women taking oral contraceptives, in infants fed formula diet low in this vitamin, and in patients receiving isoniazid for the treatment of tuberculosis. Isoniazid binds with pyridoxal, and the pyridoxal-hydrazone complex is rapidly excreted in urine. Clinical symptoms include neuronal dysfunctions, which may be due to impaired synthesis of neurotransmitters, such as norepinephrine and serotonin, and anemia due to impaired heme biosynthesis. Sideroblastic anemia and personality changes are seen in severe deficiency.
Biotin	Biotin serves as the prosthetic group for the carboxylases, transferring CO₂ to acceptor molecules (carboxylation reactions).	Liver, kidney, milk, egg yolk, corn, and soya milk	Intestinal microorganisms synthesize biotin. Hence, biotin deficiency is caused by (1) antibiotics that inhibit growth of intestinal microorganisms and (2) consumption of excess raw egg. Egg white contains the protein avidin, which binds biotin tightly and prevents its utilization in the diet. Biotin deficiency causes seborrheic dermatitis, anorexia, nausea, and muscular pain. Children with biotin deficiency have immunodeficiency.

(continued on page 422)

Table 66.2 *(Continued)* **Vitamins, Their Physiologic Role, Dietary Sources, and Deficiency Signs and Symptoms**

Vitamin	Functions	Dietary Sources	Causes and Features of Deficiency Disease
Water-soluble Vitamins			
Folic acid	Folic acid is converted into tetrahydrofolic acid (THF), which is essential for transmethylation reactions in DNA synthesis.	Leafy green vegetables, yeast, pulses, and liver	Folate deficiency occurs due to (1) inadequate intake, which is not uncommon in alcoholics, teenagers, and infants; (2) increased requirements, as in pregnancy, infancy, malignancy, and increased hematopoiesis (chronic hemolytic anemias); and (3) malabsorption. Folate deficiency affects rapidly multiplying cells, such as hemopoietic cells, resulting in megaloblastic anemia.
Cobalamin Vitamin B$_{12}$	Vitamin B$_{12}$ is required for recovery of THF from methyl trap and formation of SAM (S-adenyl methionine), which is important for myelination of neurons.	Animal products (meat, liver, kidney, fish, egg) and milk	Vitamin B$_{12}$ deficiency occurs mostly due to a reduction in its intestinal absorption, the causes of which could be (1) inadequate production of intrinsic factor (IF), as occurs in pernicious anemia and gastrectomy, and (2) diseases or resection of terminal ileum. Deficiency can also occur if (3) the vitamin is consumed in the intestine by bacteria, as in the blind-loop syndrome or by fish tapeworm. Vitamin B$_{12}$ deficiency results in megaloblastic anemia and neurologic signs and symptoms.
Ascorbic acid Vitamin C	Vitamin C is a reducing agent and functions as a coenzyme in hydroxylation reactions. It is important for the synthesis of collagen, epinephrine, bile acid, and steroids. It is also required for absorption of iron, bone mineral formation, and degradation of tyrosine. It is one of the three nutrients with antioxidant properties; the other two are vitamin E and β-carotene. Hence, it provides protection against the free radicals and is thought to prevent atherosclerosis, coronary artery disease, and cancer.	Citrus fruits, potatoes (particularly their skins), green vegetables, and tomatoes. *Embelia officinalis* (amla, Indian gooseberry) is the richest source.	Vitamin C deficiency occurs due to decreased dietary intake, which is uncommon. It can occur in infants on processed milk formulas unsupplemented by citrus fruits and vegetables. Vitamin C deficiency causes scurvy, characterized by sore, spongy gums, fragile blood vessels, swollen joints, and anemia. There is impairment of wound healing and bone formation, which may lead to osteoporosis. Integrity of the blood vessels is decreased because of decreased collagen strength of the vessel walls. It leads to frequent rupture of blood vessels. There is reduction in immunity.
Fat-soluble Vitamins			
Vitamin A Retinol	Retinol derivatives (retinoids) are essential for vision, which is mediated by retinal. Another retinol derivative, retinoic acid, is essential for growth, reproduction, and maintenance of epithelial tissues, serving as a transcriptional regulator like other group I hormones.	Liver, kidney, butter fat, oils, egg yolk, green leafy vegetables, fruits	Causes of vitamin A deficiency include (1) decreased dietary intake of the vitamin or the carotene provitamin; (2) malabsorption of fats, as in obstructive jaundice; and (3) increased excretion, as in proteinuria. In blood, vitamin A is bound to plasma proteins. Night blindness is the earliest symptom, followed by retinal degeneration. The bulbar conjunctiva becomes dry (xerosis), and small gray plaques with foamy surfaces develop (Bitot's spots). There is ulceration of the cornea (keratomalacia) and dryness and hyperkeratosis of the skin.
Vitamin D Calciferol	The active form of vitamin D is DHCC (dihydrocholecalciferol). On bone, DHCC has an antirachitic effect. In the kidney and intestine, DHCC stimulates the absorption of Ca^{2+} and phosphates by inducing the synthesis of carrier proteins.	Liver, egg yolk, and butter	Causes of vitamin D deficiency include decreased dietary intake of the vitamin or the carotene provitamin, malabsorption of fats, as in obstructive jaundice, and increased losses, as in nephrotic syndrome. In blood, vitamin D is bound to plasma proteins. Vitamin deficiency results in rickets in children and osteomalacia in adults.
Vitamin E Tocopherol	Vitamin E is the most potent fat-soluble antioxidant and scavenger of free radicals. Vitamin E delays aging and cataract formation and improves athletic performance. There is an inverse relationship between vitamin E intake and risk of coronary artery diseases.	Vegetable seed oils, liver, and eggs	Absorption of vitamin E is dependent on appropriate intestinal fat absorption, which requires bile salts. Vitamin E deficiency is rare, but it is associated with liver atrophy, neurologic disorders, and red blood cell hemolysis due to decreased protection for red blood cells against peroxides.
Vitamin K Quinone	Reduced hydroquinone, which is the active form of vitamin KH$_2$, acts as a cofactor for the carboxylation reactions in the synthesis of coagulation factors 2, 7, 9, and 10.	Green leafy vegetables, egg yolk, and liver	The main causes of vitamin K deficiency are (1) inadequate dietary intake; (2) malabsorption of fats, as in obstructive jaundice; (3) hepatocellular disease; and (4) antibiotics that kill gut microflora. Vitamin K deficiency impairs blood coagulation, resulting in prolonged bleeding time.

Water-soluble vitamins are precursors of coenzymes (**Fig. 66.1**). The fat-soluble vitamins A and D act more like hormones. For example, vitamin A is important in visual transduction in the retina, whereas vitamin D is an important hormone that plays a role in calcium homeostasis. Vitamin K is a coenzyme. Vitamins C and E and β-carotenes have antioxidant properties. They inactivate oxygen radicals, which are harmful to the body.

Vitamins cannot be synthesized in the human body and so must be obtained from food. An exception is vitamin D, which can be photosynthesized in the skin (Chapter 78). Some vitamins can be synthesized by the intestinal microorganisms, but with the exception of biotin, the quantity synthesized by intestinal microflora is not sufficient to meet the daily requirement.

Fat-soluble vitamins (A, D, E, and K, or their precursor provitamins) are not easily absorbed from the diet, but ample reserves are stored in tissues. Vitamin E is stored in adipose tissue; other fat-soluble vitamins are stored in the liver. For the same reason, fat-soluble vitamins can accumulate and reach toxic levels. The water-soluble vitamins are easily absorbed from the intestine, transported to the tissues, and readily eliminated from the body in urine so that they are neither stored in the body nor accumulate easily to toxic levels.

Mineral Nutrients

Mineral nutrients are divided into *macrominerals* (ions of sodium, calcium, potassium, chlorine, sulfur, and magnesium) that are required in quantities of more than 100 mg/day and *microminerals* or *trace minerals* (ions of chromium, cobalt, copper, iodine, iron, manganese, molybdenum, selenium, zinc, and several others) that are required in much smaller quantities in the diet. Macrominerals are major components of the body's fluids and the inorganic matrix of bone. The microminerals are mostly important components of enzymes, hormones (in the case of iodine), and hemoglobin (in the case of iron). Deficiencies of trace metals are relatively uncommon, although the lack of iodine or iron does occur for a variety of reasons and have obvious consequences.

Intestinal absorption of dietary minerals requires specific carrier proteins (see Mechanism of Iron Absorption subsection, Chapter 24). Synthesis of these carrier proteins serves as an important mechanism for control of mineral levels in the body. Excretion of minerals occurs through the renal or the hepatobiliary route. The minerals are transported in blood as complexes with carrier proteins. For example, iron is bound to transferrin in plasma. Apoceruloplasmin, a glycoprotein, is synthesized in the liver and binds with six copper atoms to form ceruloplasmin. Ninety percent of the copper in the body is tightly bound in ceruloplasmin, and the rest is loosely bound to albumin. Because ceruloplasmin, binds very tightly to copper, it refuses to deliver copper to tissues easily and is of less use as a transport protein than albumin.

Metallothioneins The tissue levels of certain metals are partly regulated by metallothioneins, a group of small proteins found in the cytosol of liver, kidney, and intestine. Metallothioneins have a high content of cysteine, and the SH group of cysteine binds to such metals as copper, zinc, cadmium, and mercury. A sudden rise in the concentration of these minerals induces the synthesis of metallothioneins, which suggests that metallothioneins have a protective role against the toxic effects of these minerals. The fact that an excessive amount of dietary zinc causes copper deficiency is explained by the higher binding affinity of metallothioneins for copper. Excess dietary zinc induces synthesis of metallothioneins, which trap copper within the intestinal mucosal cell. Copper is subsequently lost with mucosal cell exfoliation.

Wilson disease (hepatolenticular degeneration) is a rare autosomal, recessively inherited disorder in which the biliary excretion of copper is impaired. It leads to copper accumulation, initially in the liver and subsequently in other organs, including the brain. This results in hemolytic anemia, liver damage, and neurologic dysfunction.

The increase of copper in liver cells inhibits the coupling of copper to apoceruloplasmin and leads to low levels of

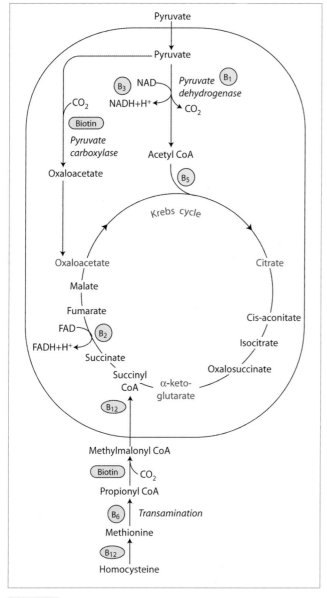

Fig. 66.1 Vitamins and their role in metabolic reactions.

plasma ceruloplasmin. The disease is treated by administration of D-penicillamine, a copper chelator, which permits urinary excretion by forming a water-soluble copper complex.

Dietary Fibers

Dietary fibers are plant carbohydrates (with the exception of lignin) in our diet that are resistant to digestion in the gut. They consist of insoluble fibers, such as celluloses and lignin, and soluble fibers, such as hemicelluloses, gums, mucilages, and pectin. Whole-grain cereals, fruits, vegetables, and pulses provide a good natural source of both soluble and insoluble fibers. Wheat bran and other whole grains are rich in insoluble fiber, whereas oat bran, peas, and beans are rich in soluble fiber.

Physiologic effects | Dietary fiber provides no energy but has several beneficial effects. Fiber absorbs up to 15 times its own weight in water and swells up, increasing the bulk of fecal matter. Increased bulk of stool increases colonic motility and hastens the intestinal transit of chyme. Anaerobic bacterial fermentation of fiber in the colon results in the formation of water, carbon dioxide, hydrogen, and short-chain fatty acids such as acetic, propionic, and butyric acids. The short-chain fatty acids are well absorbed by the colon and have a trophic effect on the colonic mucosa. They also promote the absorption of water, sodium, and chloride.

If the amount of dietary fiber is small, the diet is said to lack bulk. When the bulk of fecal matter in the colon is small, the colon is inactive, and bowel movements are infrequent. Starvation and parenteral nutrition lead to atrophy of the mucosa of the colon. The atrophy is reversed if fibers like pectin are present in the colon.

Therapeutic role | The recommended intake of fiber is 25 to 35 g/day. In constipation, fibers act as *bulk laxatives,* providing a larger volume of indigestible material to the colon and making the stool softer. In diarrhea, restricting the amount of dietary fiber slows intestinal transit and therefore decreases the frequency and volume of stool. Fibers bind to toxic compounds, including certain carcinogens, decreasing their absorption. Fibers also bind to carcinomatous foci on the colonic mucosa and wash them away. Consumption of a high-fiber diet is said to lower the serum cholesterol and result in a low incidence of constipation, hemorrhoids, diverticulosis, cancer of the colon, diabetes mellitus, and coronary artery disease.

High-fiber supplements available are commonly methyl cellulose preparations. Patients should drink large amounts of water along with the fiber to enable it to swell and retain water.

Overenthusiastic consumption of high-fiber dietary supplements should be avoided. Large amounts of fiber can impair the absorption of iron, calcium, and fat-soluble vitamins. Swollen fibers can form a solid mass inside the esophagus called *bezoar;* these supplements are best avoided in people with disorders of esophageal motility.

Summary

- The fats, carbohydrates, and proteins in our diets are macronutrients that are required in large amounts.

- Macronutrients are used to produce energy (ATP) to power all of the organism's functions and to build the constituent parts of the organism.

- Vitamins and minerals are considered micronutrients and are required in much smaller quantities.

- Vitamins have important functions as coenzymes, whereas minerals make up the bulk of the solutes in intracellular and extracellular fluid and bone.

Applying What You Know

66.1. Mrs. Schilling has been losing weight over the past month. What condition *must* be present if she is losing weight?

66.2. Mrs. Schilling's lethargy is most likely the result of her having too low quantities of which macronutrient available for use by the body? Explain.

Structure of the Alimentary Canal

The functions of the different parts of the gastrointestinal (GI) tract—the esophagus, stomach, duodenum, small intestine, and colon—are discussed separately in the following chapters. It is worth noting that the term *digestion* is frequently used in two different ways. In the general sense, the term *digestion* is used to describe all of the processes that are involved in the body's obtaining nutrients from the food we eat. However, digestion also specifically refers to the process by which the ingested food is broken down into small molecules that can be absorbed into the body.

The GI organs show certain common structural features that are discussed here briefly.

The wall of the alimentary canal is made of four layers (**Fig. 67.1**). From inside out, these layers are the mucosa, the submucosa, the tunica muscularis, and the serosa. The mucosa is further made up of three layers: the lining epithelium, a highly vascular connective tissue called the lamina propria, and a narrow layer of muscle fibers called the muscularis mucosae. Contraction of the muscularis mucosae can relieve the tension on the mucosal surface even as the outer muscle layers remain relaxed. This enables the mucosal glands to function normally.

The tunica muscularis is made of two layers, the inner circular muscle layer and the outer longitudinal muscle layer. A third layer, the oblique muscle layer, is found only in the gastric fundus, internal to the circular muscle layer. The circular muscle layer is thickened to form the GI sphincters. Striated muscle makes up the walls of the pharynx and the proximal one-third of the esophagus. Striated muscle also makes up the external anal sphincter.

Intramural nerves (i.e., nerves in the wall) of the GI tract form two *plexuses* of the gut: the submucous (Meissner's) plexus, which is present in the submucosa, and the myenteric (Auerbach's) plexus, which is present between the circular and longitudinal muscle layers. Both contain ganglia that are formed by the cell bodies of the intramural nerves. These intrinsic nerves constitute the *enteric nervous system*.

Extrinsic nerves | The ganglion cells of the intramural plexus are innervated by postganglionic sympathetic fibers and preganglionic parasympathetic fibers. The parasympathetic control is exerted through the vagus nerve, which controls the distal esophagus, stomach, liver, pancreas, small intestine, and probably the proximal colon, and the pelvic splanchnic nerve (S2–S4), which controls the distal colon and rectum. The parasympathetic fibers constitute less than 10% of vagal fibers. Ninety percent of the vagal fibers are afferents. The vagus also contains somatic motor nerves to the striated muscle of the proximal esophagus and sympathetic fibers that enter the vagus from the cervical sympathetic ganglia.

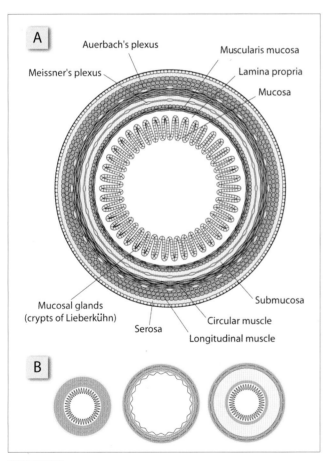

Fig. 67.1 **(A)** Transverse section of the alimentary canal, showing its four layers. Also shown are the ganglionated and aganglionic nerve plexuses. **(B)** Changes in the muscularis mucosa during gastrointestinal activity. (*Below left*) Normal lumen with the mucosa thrown into folds. (*Below middle*) Dilatation of the lumen stretches out the mucosal folds. (*Below right*) Contraction of the muscularis mucosa relieves the tension on the mucosa and restores the folds.

General Models: Communications and Homeostasis

Like all physiologic systems, neural and endocrine information must be passed from cell to cell for the coordinated functions of the GI system to occur. However, the GI system is nearly unique in that this information is not used to maintain a state of homeostasis (basically, the GI system processes everything presented to it in the diet).

Motor Functions

Mastication

Mastication involves movements of the jaws, action of the teeth, and coordinated movements of the tongue and other muscles of the oral cavity. The masticatory muscles (masseter, temporalis, and pterygoids) and the tongue show automatic coordinated movements that are controlled by a brainstem center. Mastication is aided by the secretion of saliva, which acts as a lubricant.

Deglutition

The coordination center of swallowing (deglutition) is located in the brainstem. The afferent arc comprises the trigeminal, glossopharyngeal, and vagus nerves. The efferent arc reaches the pharyngeal musculature and the tongue through the trigeminal, facial, and hypoglossal nerves. Swallowing has three phases: the oral phase, the pharyngeal phase, and the esophageal phase.

The **oral phase** is the voluntary phase in which the bolus is squeezed out of the oral cavity into the pharynx. This squeezing is made possible through the following steps. (1) The jaws are shut, and the lips are closed. (2) The tongue brings the bolus into the midline between the anterior portion of the tongue and the hard palate. The tip of the tongue then presses firmly against the roof of the hard palate and limits the bolus anteriorly. (3) The voluntary contraction of the mylohyoid muscle pushes the bolus toward the posterior pharyngeal wall.

In the **pharyngeal phase,** the bolus enters the pharynx and stimulates the sensory endings of the glossopharyngeal nerve in the posterior pharyngeal wall, soft palate, and epiglottis. This initiates the deglutition (swallowing) reflex. The *deglutition center* is located in the medulla.

The deglutition reflex coordinates the sequential occurrence of the following steps (**Fig. 67.2**). (1) The oral cavity is shut off from the pharynx by the approximation of the palatopharyngeal arch. (2) The nasopharynx is shut off from the pharynx by the elevation of the soft palate. (3) The glottis is shut off from the pharynx by the approximation of the vocal cords. (4) The hyoid is raised by the contraction of the digastric and the geniohyoid. The larynx rises with the hyoid and brings the epiglottis in the path of the bolus. (5) The bolus tilts

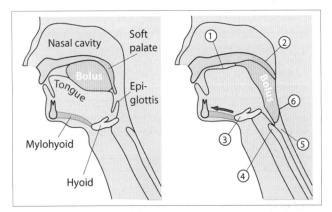

Fig. 67.2 Stages of swallowing. (1) The tongue rises, closing the oropharynx. (2) The soft palate rises, shutting off the nasopharynx. (3) The hyoid rises and moves forward. (4) The anterior wall of the esophagus is drawn forward by the hyoid. (5) The esophageal lumen is pulled open. (6) The epiglottis tilts backward to shut off the glottis.

the epiglottis backward over the closed glottis. The lumen of the esophagus is pulled open by the forward movement of the larynx and trachea, the posterior walls of which are attached to the anterior walls of the pharynx and the esophagus, respectively. (6) Breathing is arrested. (7) The upper esophageal (hypopharyngeal) sphincter (formed by the cricopharyngeus muscle, which guards the upper end of the esophagus, briefly relaxes, and the bolus enters the upper esophagus. (8) The cricopharyngeus contracts, the glottis reopens, and breathing resumes.

Esophageal Phase

Once the bolus enters the esophagus, it is propelled by peristalsis at a velocity of 2 to 3 cm/s. The movement of the bolus is aided by gravity, and therefore food travels through the esophagus faster in the standing rather than in the supine position. However, peristaltic waves are strong enough to propel food against gravity; hence, swallowing is possible even when a person is standing on his head.

There are two types of peristaltic waves in the esophagus. *Primary peristaltic waves* originate in the pharynx during the pharyngeal phase of swallowing and travel down the esophagus. The contraction of the esophageal wall begins at the upper esophageal sphincter when the bolus enters the esophagus and travels down the lower esophageal sphincter. Primary peristalsis thus ensures that the lower sphincter relaxes in synchrony with the relaxation of the upper esophageal sphincter.

Secondary peristaltic waves originate in the esophagus itself when the esophageal wall is stretched by the bolus. Secondary waves continue to be produced until the bolus is dislodged from the esophagus into the stomach. They begin above the bolus and push the bolus down. The propulsive force produced is proportional to the bolus size.

Prevention of Esophageal Reflux

Anatomically, the *lower esophageal sphincter* is only vaguely identifiable as a slight thickening of the muscle coat of the esophageal wall. It is ~5 cm in length, of which 3 cm lie below the diaphragm and 2 cm above it. Part of the ability of the esophagus to resist reflux depends upon the segment that lies below the diaphragm. Any rise in the intra-abdominal pressure squeezes not only the stomach but also the intra-abdominal part of the esophagus, occluding its lumen so that the reflux is prevented. In pregnancy, the enlarged uterus pushes the stomach up and pushes the intra-abdominal portion of the esophagus into the thorax. Hence, reflux is common in pregnancy. Another cause of the reflux is the high progesterone level in pregnancy, which reduces the tone of the lower esophageal sphincter.

Reflux is also prevented by the oblique angle of entry of the esophagus into the stomach, which is called the *angle of His* (**Fig. 67.3**). Any increase in intragastric pressure tends to push the stomach upward and to the right, and thereby compresses and closes the end of the esophagus. The angle of His is almost nonexistent in many infants, and the esophagus tends to form a straight line with the stomach. Hence, reflux is quite common in infants.

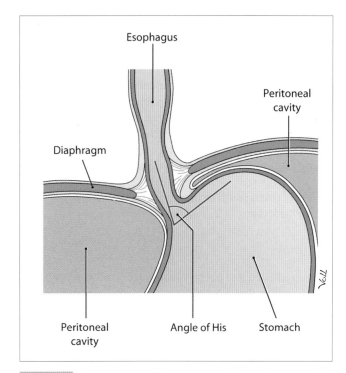

Fig. 67.3 The geometry of the junction of the esophagus and the stomach (the angle of His) helps to prevent reflux of the contents of the stomach. Because of this geometry, expansion of the stomach tends to compress the esophagus, thus closing it.

The tone of the lower esophageal sphincter is mainly under vagal (cholinergic) control. Hence, parasympatholytic agents like atropine should not be given to a patient with reflux esophagitis. When reflux does occur, it stimulates secondary peristaltic waves that sweep the offending material back down into the stomach.

Secretory Functions

The principal secretory event in the mouth is the secretion of the saliva. About 1 L of saliva is secreted each day by the three salivary glands: 250 mL is secreted by the parotid, 700 mL by the submandibular, and 50 mL by the sublingual glands. Depending on the type of secretion, salivary acini are categorized into two types: serous and mucous. Serous acini secrete the watery saliva containing more than 90% water, and mucous acini secrete a more viscous fluid containing the glycoprotein mucin, which makes the saliva sticky and viscous. The parotid gland is purely serous, the sublingual gland is largely mucous, whereas the submandibular is a mixed gland (**Fig. 67.4**).

Saliva has the following functions: (1) It keeps the mouth moist and clean and protects the tooth enamel. (2) It acts as a lubricant and thereby aids in speech, chewing, and swallowing. (3) It helps in bolus formation by acting as a glue. (4) It dissolves food particles and is therefore necessary for taste. (Taste receptors respond only to dissolved substances.) (5) It is alkaline and therefore helps to neutralize the gastric

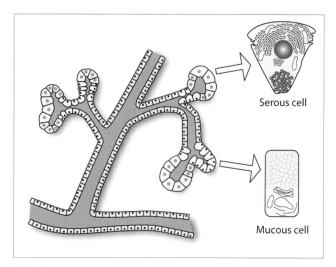

Fig. 67.4 Salivary acini and ducts. Insets show the serous and mucous cells.

juices that might regurgitate into the esophagus. (6) It contains amylase, which initiates digestion of carbohydrates, and lipase, which contributes to fat digestion. (6) It contains lysozyme and lactoferrin, which have antibacterial action.

Composition of Saliva

Saliva is composed of water, electrolytes, enzymes, glycoproteins, and growth factors. The composition of saliva depends on the particular salivary gland, the stimulus, and the rate of flow. The composition of saliva at basal flow rates is given in **Table 67.1**.

The organic components of saliva are secreted by the duct cells of the salivary gland. The salivary fluid is formed by transudation of plasma and therefore is isotonic when freshly formed. During its transit through salivary ducts, sodium (Na^+) and chloride (Cl^-) are reabsorbed from it; potassium (K^+) and bicarbonate (HCO_3^-) are secreted into it. Because the absorption of NaCl is more rapid than the secretion of $KHCO_3$, and because the duct epithelium is not freely permeable to water, the saliva becomes hypotonic. Aldosterone promotes Na^+ reabsorption and K^+ secretion in the salivary ducts. The slower the salivary flow rate, the greater is the change in the ionic composition of saliva in the ducts. Despite the secretion of

Table 67.1 Characteristics of Saliva

Tonicity	Hypotonic
pH	7.0–8.0
Na^+ and Cl^-	Lower than in plasma
K^+ and HCO_3^-	Higher than in plasma
Other ions	Ca^{2+}, Mg^{2+}, PO_4^{3-}
Organic contents	Proteins (e.g., amylase) and glycoproteins (e.g., mucin)

bicarbonates into the saliva, the salivary pH at low flow rates is ~7.0 because some amount of Na^+ is reabsorbed from the ducts through Na^+–H^+ antiport.

Control of Salivary Secretion

Salivary secretion is exclusively under neural control (**Fig. 67.5**). The salivary glands are innervated by both parasympathetic cholinergic nerves and sympathetic adrenergic nerves.

The *preganglionic parasympathetic fibers* to the salivary gland originate in the salivatory nuclei of the brainstem. They reach the submandibular and lingual glands through the facial nerve and the parotid gland through the glossopharyngeal nerve. Parasympathetic postganglionic cholinergic nerve fibers secrete acetylcholine and vasoactive intestinal peptide (VIP). These nerves may be stimulated (1) through *unconditioned reflex,* by the presence of food (especially dry or sour food) in the mouth, or (2) through *conditioned reflex,* the smell or even the thought of good food.

Parasympathetic stimulation causes profuse secretion of watery saliva. The secretion of amylase is also increased. However, due to the large increase in watery secretion, the amylase concentration in the saliva decreases. The local vasodilation required for increased salivary secretion is caused by VIP, which is a cotransmitter with acetylcholine in some of the postganglionic parasympathetic neurons. The tissue kallikrein secreted by the actively secreting salivary cells contributes to the hyperemia (see **Fig. 37.2**).

Sympathetic discharge causes vasoconstriction and inhibits the secretion of serous saliva, but increases the enzyme concentration in saliva. The sympathetic discharge associated with fear and excitement makes the mouth dry. Cholinergic and α-adrenergic agonists act through the group IIA hormonal mechanism; β-adrenergic agonists act through the group IIC hormonal mechanism (see Chapter 75).

Reflex salivary secretion occurs when mechanoreceptors and chemoreceptors in the oral cavity respond to the texture of food and its chemical composition. They are also stimulated by dryness of the mouth. The afferent impulses are integrated in the *salivation center* (distinct from the salivary nucleus) in the medulla. This center is near the centers regulating respiration and vomiting. The salivation center also receives inputs from the cerebral cortex, amygdala, and hypothalamus.

Digestive Functions

Digestive events in the mouth include the actions of two enzymes, an amylase and a lipase. *Salivary amylase* is an α-amylase (also called ptyalin) with an optimum pH of 6.7. It breaks down the starches by hydrolyzing the 1:4α linkages (see **Fig. 69.8**). Its action is very short-lasting because it is inactivated by the acidic gastric pH shortly after entering the stomach.

Lingual lipase is secreted by Ebner's glands on the dorsal surface of the tongue. The lipase remains active in the stomach and contributes to fat digestion in the stomach.

Summary

- The walls of the GI tract are made up of four layers (mucosa, submucosa, tunica muscularis, and serosa), with two neural plexus (submucosal and myenteric) between the layers.

- The GI tract is innervated by the sympathetic and parasympathetic portions of the autonomic nervous system.

- The motor function of chewing and swallowing convey the ingested food to the stomach.

- Salivary secretion lubricates the chewed food and aids in its passage to the stomach.

- Salivary secretions contain two enzymes that begin the digestion of food (but are not essential for it).

Applying What You Know

67.1. Mrs. Schilling has in the past taken several different pills (Imodium, calcium supplements). Is the mechanism involved in swallowing a pill a voluntary one, or is it a reflex? Explain.

67.2. Mrs. Schilling's saliva is tested to determine whether it is normal. Its pH is found to be 6.9 due to the bicarbonate that is present in it. Why is the maintenance of a slightly alkaline pH important for saliva function?

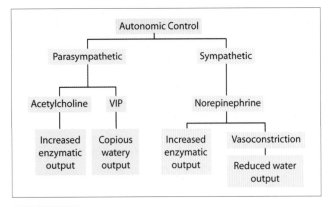

Fig. 67.5 Effect of autonomic nerve stimulation on salivary secretion. VIP, vasoactive intestinal peptide.

68 Functions of the Stomach

The stomach is divided into the cardia, fundus, corpus (body), antrum, and pylorus (**Fig. 68.1A**). Movement of food in and out of the stomach is controlled by two sphincters, the cardiac and the pyloric. The gastric mucosa forms prominent folds, called rugal folds, that increase its surface area (**Fig. 68.1B**).

The stomach has motor, secretory, and digestive functions. (1) The stomach acts as a reservoir able to relax to accommodate large volumes of food with only small increases in pressure. (2) It grinds food to optimum-sized particles. (3) It mixes the bolus with the gastric juice and converts the bolus into a chyme. (4) It controls its own emptying, retaining the solid portion of the meal until most of the liquid has emptied. (5) It sieves the food, retaining larger particles, permitting more time for their further breakdown. (6) It regulates the rate at which chyme is delivered to the intestine. (7) It secretes hydrochloric acid, which kills bacteria that enter with the food. (8) It secretes pepsin, which begins the digestion of proteins.

Motor Functions

Motility of the Empty Stomach

Migrating motor complexes (MMCs) are the contraction waves produced by the electrical activity of the single-unit smooth muscle of the gastrointestinal (GI) tract. The electrical activity is called the *basal electrical rhythm* (BER). It originates in pacemaker cells located in the outer circular muscle layer near the myenteric plexus. The pacemaker cells are star-shaped mesenchymal cells (the interstitial cells of Cajal) whose processes make synaptic contacts (electrical synapses) with the smooth muscle cells. When there are no MMCs, the BER consists of rhythmic oscillation of the resting potential between –65 and –45 mV. The oscillations occur due to rhythmic changes in calcium (Ca^{2+}) and potassium (K^+) permeabilities. The MMCs occur when the electrical oscillations generate spikes (action potentials).

MMCs occur in a cyclical pattern, each cycle lasting 90 minutes (**Fig. 68.2**). It occurs in three phases. *Phase I* is the phase of quiescence in which there are no contractions and no spike potentials on the underlying BER. It is the longest phase, lasting ~80 minutes. *Phase II* is associated with irregular spikes on the BER and irregular contractions. It lasts ~6 minutes. *Phase III* is associated with regular contractions and regular spike potentials on the BER. It lasts ~3 minutes. It is associated with a rise in plasma motilin, a GI hormone. Phase III MMCs originate in the stomach or the duodenum. Those originating in the stomach have a frequency of 3/min; those originating in the duodenum have a frequency of 11/min. Most MMCs pass along the entire bowel to the terminal ileum with a velocity of 5 cm/min.

During phase II and phase III MMCs, there is an increase in the secretion of gastric, bile, and pancreatic juices. They may clear the stomach and small intestine of luminal contents in preparation for the next meal: they have been called the

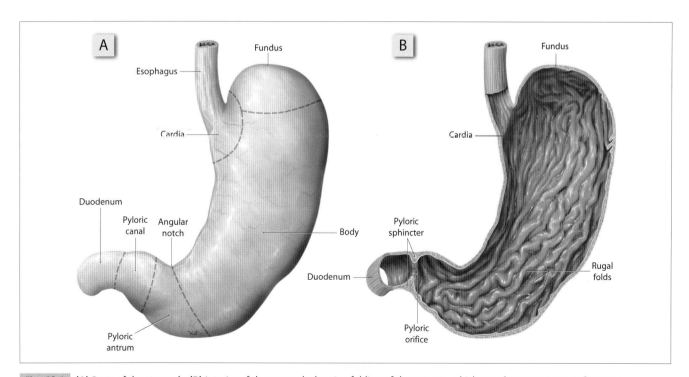

Fig. 68.1 **(A)** Parts of the stomach. **(B)** Interior of the stomach showing folding of the mucosa, which greatly increases its surface area.

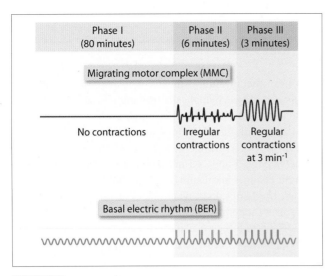

Fig. 68.2 Migrating motor complex and basal electric rhythm.

"interdigestive housekeepers." MMCs are probably responsible for the hunger contractions.

Motility of the Fed Stomach

When food enters the stomach, the fundus and upper part of its body relax to accommodate the food with little increase in pressure. This is called *receptive relaxation*. Receptive relaxation is vagally mediated and is synchronized with the primary peristaltic waves in the esophagus.

After food enters the stomach, the interdigestive MMCs are replaced by gastric peristalsis. Cinefluoroscopic studies show that the gastric peristalsis is characterized by two successive contraction rings moving down the gastric body—a minor ring followed 2 to 3 seconds later by a major ring that occludes the gastric lumen. The minor ring does not occlude the lumen, but the pylorus closes when the ring reaches it. Gastric emptying occurs only until the minor ring reaches the pylorus. By then, the major ring has reached the midantrum, and as it progresses toward the distal antrum, the food grinds against the closed antrum and then squirts back into the proximal stomach, churning and mixing the food in the process. The latency between the two contraction rings is determined by the action potential. The initial spike triggers the minor ring; its plateau triggers the major ring.

The peristaltic waves begin near the middle of the body of the stomach and sweep downward toward the pyloric sphincter (antral peristalsis). As the wave approaches the pylorus, the sphincter closes. Hence, only a small amount of liquefied chyme squirts through the sphincter into the duodenum. The more solid chyme cannot pass through the closed sphincter.

Control of Gastric Emptying

The gastric emptying time is ~4 hours. The rate of gastric emptying is proportional to the volume of the gastric contents. Gastric distention stimulates stretch receptors in the gastric wall and results in reflex gastric contraction, partly through increased vagal discharge to the stomach, and partly through the release of gastrin. Vagotomy slows gastric emptying and causes gastric atony and distention. Liquids leave the stomach much faster, flowing around the solid food in the stomach. Smaller particles leave the stomach faster than larger particles.

Enterogastric reflexes | Gastric emptying is regulated mainly from the duodenum through the enterogastric reflexes, which ensure that the gastric chyme does not enter the duodenum too fast. These reflexes are mostly mediated by GI hormones (see **Table 72.1**). (1) *Acid in the duodenum* stimulates the release of secretin, which reduces gastric motility and increases pyloric sphincteric tone. (2) Products of fat digestion stimulate the release of several GI hormones, such as cholecystokinin, gastric inhibitory polypeptide (GIP), vasoactive intestinal peptide (VIP), and peptide YY, all of which reduce gastric motility. Even before these hormones were identified, the presence of a hormonal mediator was suspected and was provisionally named enterogastrone, a term that is obsolete today. Fats are very effective in inhibiting gastric emptying. Some people consume fats before consuming alcoholic drinks. The fat keeps the alcohol in the stomach longer, slowing its absorption and reducing the chances of intoxication. (3) Products of protein digestion stimulate the release of gastrin, cholecystokinin, and GIP, all of which slow gastric emptying.

The enterogastric reflexes are also mediated by local neural circuits. (1) Entry of hyperosmolar chyme into the duodenum reflexly slows gastric emptying by stimulating the duodenal osmoreceptors and chemoreceptors. (2) Mechanical distention of duodenum reflexly retards gastric emptying by stimulating duodenal stretch receptors.

General Models: Communications and Homeostasis

Gastric emptying is a process that must be controlled by information arising in both the stomach itself and the duodenum. This information is carried by both neural and humoral mechanisms. However, the negative feedback that is present does not homeostatically regulate the system; it simply prevents emptying from occurring too quickly for the duodenum to cope with the load being presented to it.

Secretory Functions

The gastric mucosa (**Fig. 68.3**) contains several gastric glands. Several of these glands open in a common chamber (gastric pit) that opens on the surface of the gastric mucosa. In the pyloric and cardiac regions, the gastric glands secrete mucus only. In the body and fundus of the stomach, the glands contain parietal cells (oxyntic cells) that secrete hydrochloric acid and intrinsic factor, and chief cells (zymogen cells or peptic cells) that secrete pepsinogens. These secretions mix with mucus secreted by the cells in the neck of the glands. The gastric gland also contains G cells that secrete gastrin, D cells that secrete somatostatin, and ECL cells that secrete histamine.

Gastric mucus is an important component of the mucosal barrier that protects the gastric mucosa from autodigesti-

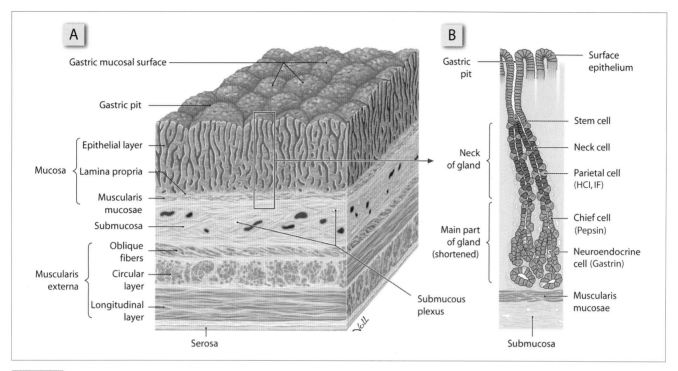

Fig. 68.3 **(A)** Gastric mucosa and **(B)** the cells of a gastric gland. There are three kinds of secretory cells in the gastric gland, each producing different products. IF, intrinsic factor.

on. The mucus protects the gastric mucosa from mechanical and chemical damage. The bicarbonate ions (HCO_3^-) secreted by mucus cells become trapped in the mucus gel, increasing the pH and thereby reducing the corrosive action of gastric acid. The acid secreted by the gastric glands does not disrupt the entire mucus layer, but crosses it by creating fine channels through it. Certain acid-resistant peptides in the mucosa called trefoil peptides contribute to the mucosal barrier. The tight junctions between the mucosal cells are also part of the mucosal barrier. Breakdown of the mucosal barrier can result in gastric ulcers.

Mechanism of Gastric Acid Secretion

Gastric acid secretion (**Fig. 68.4**) can be understood in two steps: the secretion of hydrogen (H^+) and the secretion of chloride (Cl^-).

Secretion of hydrogen ions | (1) H^+ ions are produced inside the cell through the reaction of CO_2 (produced by the metabolism) with water. The reaction is catalyzed by the enzyme carbonic anhydrase that is present in the parietal cells in large amounts. (2) The H^+ ions are secreted by the parietal cell through its apical membrane by a primary active transport (requiring adenosine triphosphate [ATP]) with coupled antiport of K^+ ions. The H^+–K^+ exchanger is electroneutral. (3) The HCO_3^- produced are transported out of the parietal cell at the basolateral border with a coupled antiport of Cl^- into the cell. The movement of these ions is passive, but it is the activity of the Na^+–K^+ pump that creates the electrical potential gradient that moves Cl^- out of the cell across the apical membrane. The HCO_3^-–Cl^- exchange is again electroneutral. The HCO_3^- transported out of the parietal cells enters the bloodstream and

increases the blood pH. Therefore, after a meal, there is a rise in blood pH called the postprandial *alkaline tide*.

General Model: Energy

The production of hydrochloric acid, HCl, is clearly an energy-dependent process. One consequence of this is the need for adequate perfusion of the stomach to supply the oxygen and glucose needed to produce ATP.

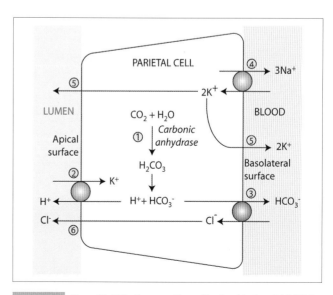

Fig. 68.4 Steps (1–6) in the secretion of hydrochloric acid (HCl) by the parietal cell of the gastric gland (see the text for an explanation).

Secretion of chloride ions | (4) The Na$^+$–K$^+$ pump located on the basolateral membrane of the parietal cell pumps out three Na$^+$ ions for every two K$^+$ ions pumped in. The interior of the parietal cell therefore becomes negative. (5) The K$^+$ ions that are pumped in diffuse out through the K$^+$ channels present on the basolateral as well as apical membranes. This diffusion further increases the intracellular negativity of the parietal cell. (6) The high intracellular negativity forces out Cl$^-$ ions through the Cl$^-$ channels located on the apical membrane.

Control of Gastric Acid Secretion

In an unstimulated parietal cell, considerable amounts of inactive H$^+$–K$^+$ ATPase are stored inside the cells on the membranes of the endoplasmic reticulum. When the parietal cell is stimulated, these H$^+$–K$^+$ ATPase-bearing membranes fuse with the apical membrane of the cell, greatly increasing its surface area and delivering the H$^+$–K$^+$ ATPase to the site where it can pump out H$^+$. On removal of the stimulus, the apical cell membrane is internalized into the cell to reform the cytoplasmic tubulovesicular membrane system and storing the H$^+$–K$^+$ ATPase. The fusion of the cytoplasmic tubulovesicular membranes with the apical cell membrane requires high concentrations of Ca^{2+}, which is brought about by neurohormonal mediators.

There are five well-known neurohormonal mediators (**Table 68.1** and **Fig. 68.5**) of gastric acid secretion. Three of these

Table 68.1 Neurohormonal Controllers of Gastric Acid Secretion

Neurohormone	Mechanism*	Action
Acetylcholine (muscarinic)	Group IIC	Stimulatory
Gastrin	Group IIC	Stimulatory
Histamine	Group IIA (Gs)	Stimulatory
Prostaglandin E$_2$	Group IIA (Gi)	Inhibitory
Somatostatin	Group IIA (Gi)	Inhibitory

*See Chapter 75 for details.

are stimulatory, and two are inhibitory. Receptors for each of these mediators are present on the membrane of the parietal cell. These mediators are secreted mainly by three types of paracrine cells.

G cells are located at the base of the gastric glands and are especially abundant in the pyloric gastric glands. They secrete gastrin, which stimulates HCl secretion. Gastrin secretion is stimulated by GRP (gastrin-releasing peptide) and inhibited by somatostatin and prostaglandin E$_2$ (PGE$_2$).

D cells are located adjacent to the G cells and parietal cells. They secrete somatostatin that inhibits HCl secretion in two ways; directly, by inhibiting the parietal cells, and indirectly,

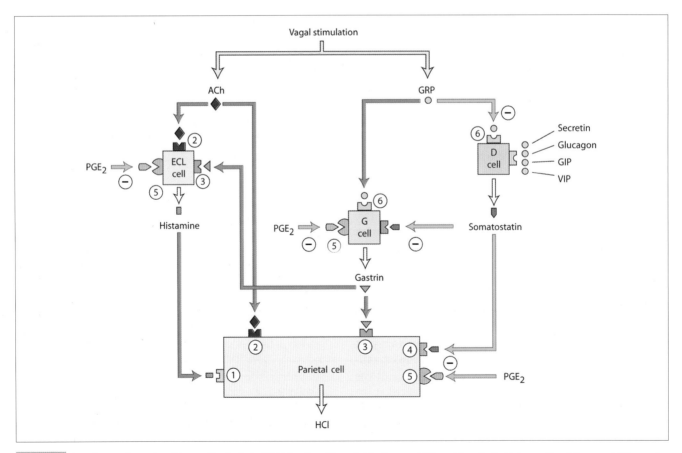

Fig. 68.5 Regulators of gastric acid secretion include (1) histamine, (2) acetylcholine, and (3) gastrin, all of which are stimulatory, and (4) somatostatin and (5) prostaglandin E$_2$, which are inhibitory. (6) GRP is gastrin-releasing peptide. The red arrows represent stimulatory influences, and the blue arrows represent inhibitory influences. ECL, enterochromaffin-like; GIP, gastric inhibitory polypeptide; VIP, vasoactive intestinal peptide.

by inhibiting the G cells. GRP stimulates acid secretion by inhibiting somatostatin release (see **Fig. 81.7**). On the other hand, secretin, enteroglucagon, GIP, and VIP inhibit gastric secretion by stimulating somatostatin release.

Enterochromaffin-like (ECL) cells are found in the corpus of the stomach, in the base of the gastric gland. They secrete histamine that stimulates HCl secretion from parietal cells. ECL cells have gastrin, acetylcholine (ACh), and PGE_2 receptors. They release histamine in response to both circulating gastrin and the ACh released by vagal fibers. Stimulation of ECL cells seems to be an important mechanism through which gastrin stimulates acid secretion.

Effect of the Vagus Nerve on Gastric Secretion

Vagal fibers to the stomach have two neurotransmitters, GRP and ACh. The GRP increases gastrin secretion from G cells with consequent increase in acid secretion. The GRP also inhibits somatostatin secretion from D cells and thereby disinhibits HCl secretion from parietal cells. Acetylcholine increases the secretion of gastric acid, pepsin, and mucus. Part of the acid secretion is mediated by ECL cells that secrete histamine. Hypoglycemia increases acid and pepsin section by stimulating central vagal discharge.

Phases of Gastric Acid Secretion

Interdigestive phase (basal acid secretion) | Acid is continuously secreted by the stomach even between meals and during sleep. A circadian rhythm is seen, with basal secretion reaching its peak around midnight and its trough around 7:00 AM. Because most of the basal secretion is abolished by vagotomy, it is believed that the interdigestive phase of gastric acid secretion is vagally mediated. Like the cephalic phase, the basal acid secretion is influenced by psychic factors.

The **cephalic phase** of gastric secretion (**Fig. 68.6**) accounts for up to 50% of the acid secreted in response to a normal meal. It is vagally mediated and is easily conditioned. The unconditioned stimulus is the presence of food in the mouth. Conditioned stimuli, the sight, smell, or thought of food, increase gastric secretion. The cephalic phase of gastric secretion is also influenced by psychic states: it is increased with anger and hostility and is reduced with fear and depression.

The **gastric phase** of acid secretion (**Fig. 68.6**) comes into play when food makes contact with the gastric mucosa. It accounts for up to 50% of the acid secretion in response to a meal. Acid secretion in this phase is brought about by two factors: (1) gastrin secretion, which in turn is stimulated by two factors, a reduction in antral acidity due to the buffering effect of the meal, and the stimulatory effect of small peptides, amino acids, alcohol, and caffeine; and (2) the stretch of the stomach wall, which activates a vagovagal reflex as well as a local intragastric reflex.

Intestinal phase | When food enters the intestine, gastric secretion is inhibited by the same intestinal factors that reduce gastric motility through the enterogastric reflex (see above). Briefly, they are (1) acid in the duodenum, (2) products of fat digestion, (3) osmolarity of the duodenal chyme, and (4) mechanical distention of the duodenum. Products of

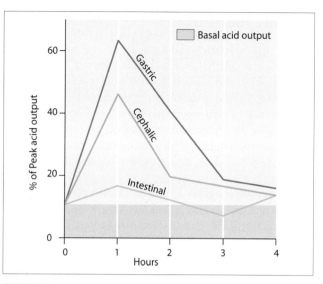

Fig. 68.6 Phases of gastric acid secretion.

protein digestion, however, have a slight stimulatory effect on gastric acid secretion (**Fig. 68.6**). It accounts for about 5% of the total gastric acid secretion that occurs following a meal. The hormone enterogastrone was thought to mediate the inhibition of gastric secretion in the intestinal phase.

Gastric Acid Output

Measurement of gastric acid output has considerable clinical importance. Gastric acid secretion is increased in duodenal ulcer, gastric ulcer, and Zollinger–Ellison syndrome; it is reduced after vagotomy and in pernicious anemia.

Basal acid output (BAO) is the rate of acid secretion in the absence of all avoidable stimulations. In the night-fasting secretion test, continuous gastric suction is performed through an indwelling nasogastric catheter from 9:00 PM to 9:00 AM. The room is kept devoid of food and even its odor. Normally, ~400 mL of gastric juice is collected overnight. The HCl concentration in the juice collected gives the basal acid output. The normal BAO is < 10 mM/h.

Maximal acid output (MAO) is the gastric acid secretion produced by stimulants such as pentagastrin and histamine. The acid output is measured every 15 minutes for 1 hour. MAO represents the total acid output over 1 hour and is normally < 50 mmol/h. The *peak acid output* (PAO) is calculated by totaling the two highest consecutive 15-minute outputs and multiplying by 2.

The **Hollander insulin test** is performed after surgically interrupting the vagal nerve supply to the stomach (an operation performed as a surgical remedy of peptic ulcer) to test the completeness of the vagotomy performed. The vagus is stimulated by insulin-induced hypoglycemia. The gastric juice is collected and analyzed for its acid content.

Regulation of Pepsinogen Secretion

The regulation of pepsinogen secretion is not well understood. In general, acid secretion and pepsinogen secretion are similarly affected by most stimuli. However, pepsinogen secretion does not show distinct phases (cephalic, gastric, and intestinal).

Digestive Functions

Gastric (hydrochloric) acid has a pH of ~1.0 and serves the following functions. (1) It acts as a good solvent that dissolves foodstuffs insoluble in water. Gastric acid is necessary for iron absorption because it dissolves the insoluble ferric salts and complexes. It is also necessary for vitamin B_{12} absorption. (2) Its acidic pH is required for activation of pepsin. (3) It is a strong disinfectant, killing bacteria and other microorganisms in the ingested food. (4) It stimulates the duodenum to secrete secretin.

The **gastric enzymes** are pepsin, which digests proteins, and gastric lipase, which digests fats. Gastric lipase is of little importance in fat digestion except in cases of pancreatic insufficiency. Pepsin cleaves food proteins, forming small peptides. When secreted by the chief cells, pepsin is in its inactive form, a larger protein called pepsinogen. Acid in the lumen converts pepsinogen to pepsin. Pepsin once formed also attacks pepsinogen, producing more pepsin molecules (*autocatalysis*).

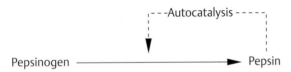

Nevertheless, the amount of protein digestion that occurs in the stomach is relatively small, and the absence of gastric digestion does not materially affect the ability of the GI tract to digest and absorb proteins in the diet.

Summary

- The basal electrical rhythm of the stomach drives the patterns of motor activity that are present.

- Peristaltic contractions move the contents of the stomach toward the pylorus.

- The emptying of the stomach into the duodenum is controlled by hormonal and endocrine signals from the duodenum to the stomach.

- The secretion of gastric acid involves the active transport of H^+ ions into the lumen of the stomach and the active and passive transport of other electrolytes.

- Physiologic control of gastric acid secretion is exerted by the vagus nerve and by gastrin.

- Little digestion of food occurs in the stomach.

Applying What You Know

68.1. Mrs. Schilling was prescribed an H_2 (histamine receptor) blocker to control her dyspepsia. What other kind of drug might be used to reduce HCl production?

68.2. Mrs. Schilling begins suffering from abdominal distress within an hour or so of eating a meal. What effect might this have on her production of HCl?

Secretory Functions

Duodenal secretions are derived from two main sources: the liver produces bile juice (some is stored in the gallbladder), and the pancreas produces an exocrine secretion. In addition to the above, the Brunner glands in the duodenal mucosa secrete thick alkaline mucus that protects the duodenal mucosa from the gastric acid. There is also an appreciable secretion of HCO_3^- that is independent of Brunner glands.

Hepatic Bile Juice Production

The bile juice is secreted continuously by the liver into the bile canaliculi that drain into the right and left hepatic ducts (**Fig. 69.1**). The two hepatic ducts join to form the common hepatic duct. Shortly after its formation, the common hepatic duct joins with the cystic duct of the gallbladder to form the common bile duct. Shortly before draining into the duodenum through the duodenal papilla, the common bile duct joins the pancreatic duct to form the ampulla of Vater. The duodenal papilla is guarded by a sphincter called the sphincter of Oddi that opens only when fatty food is being digested in the duodenum. At other times it remains closed so that the bile secreted by the liver is diverted through the cystic duct to the gallbladder where up to 50 mL of bile is stored. When stimulated by the digestion of fatty food, the gallbladder contracts with simultaneous relaxation of the sphincter of Oddi, emptying its stored bile into the duodenum.

The major **constituents of the bile juice** are bile salts (mainly, taurocholates and glycocholates), bile pigments (bilirubin and biliverdin), lipids (cholesterol, lecithin, fatty acids, and triglycerides), and electrolytes (**Fig. 69.2**). Cholesterol is present in a concentration of 60 to 170 mg/L. Higher concentrations of cholesterol in bile predispose to gallstones. The cations sodium (Na^+), potassium (K^+), and calcium (Ca^{2+}) are all present in concentrations ~20% greater than in the plasma. The two major anions are chloride (Cl^-) and bicarbonate (HCO_3^-). Cl^- is present in concentrations less than in plasma, whereas HCO_3^- concentration is much more than in plasma, which makes the bile juice alkaline (pH 7.0–7.4).

Of all the constituents of bile, only the bile salts are of importance to the digestive system. Bile salts, such as phospholipids, are amphipathic molecules because the steroid nucleus (hydrophobic) lies in a single plane, whereas the polar (hydrophilic) groups, for example, the hydroxyl and carboxyl groups, as well as the peptide bond, project on one side (**Fig. 69.3**). The amphipathic property makes bile salts important for fat emulsification and micelle formation. They also have a choleretic action.

The enterohepatic circulation ensures that all of the bile salts delivered to the duodenum do not leave the body in the feces. Active transporters in the ileum reabsorb bile salts and return them to the hepatic portal vein, which returns them to the liver for reuse (**Fig. 69.4**). Consequently, only a small percentage of the bile salts is lost.

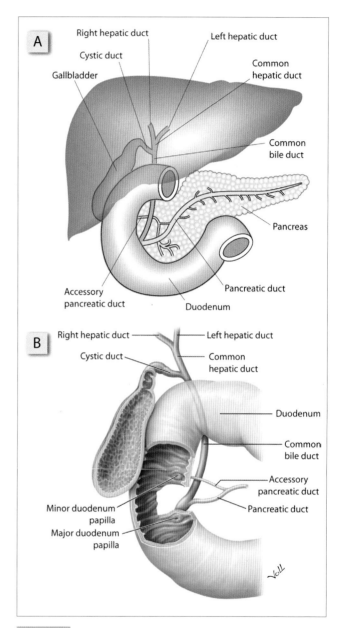

Fig. 69.1 **(A)** The bile and pancreatic ducts and the associated organs. **(B)** The opening of the ducts inside the duodenum.

Control of biliary secretion | The entry of bile into the duodenum increases either when the liver cells increase their bile secretion or when the gallbladder empties its stored bile.

Substances that increase hepatic bile secretion are called *choleretics*. Examples of choleretics are secretin and bile salts. Vagal stimulation also increases bile secretion. Bile salts increase the hepatic secretion of bile but inhibit the synthesis of new bile salts. Despite the inhibition of fresh bile salt synthesis, the amount of bile salts in the bile does not decrease. This is because the bile salts secreted into the duodenum are

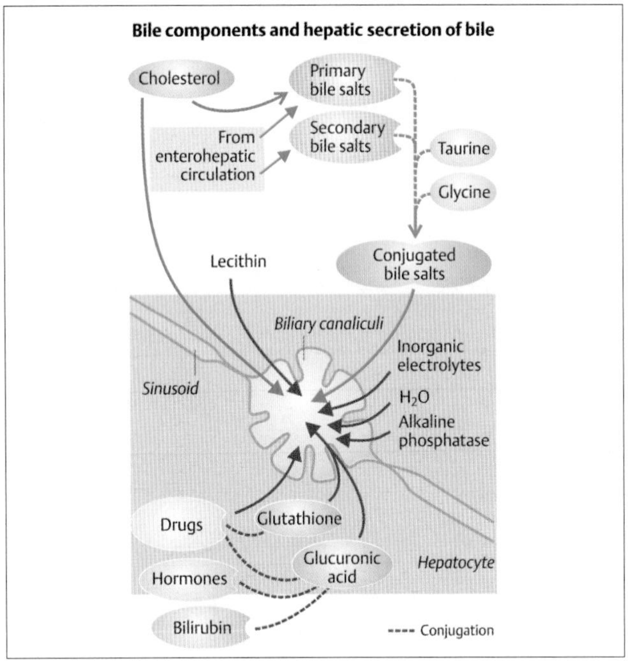

Bile components and hepatic secretion of bile
Cholesterol
Primary bile salts
From enterohepatic circulation
Secondary bile salts
Taurine
Glycine
Lecithin
Conjugated bile salts
Biliary canaliculi
Sinusoid
Inorganic electrolytes
H_2O
Alkaline phosphatase
Drugs
Glutathione
Glucuronic acid
Hepatocyte
Hormones
Bilirubin
Conjugation

Fig. 69.2 The hepatic production of bile.

reabsorbed from the intestine and resecreted into the bile juice (enterohepatic circulation). Drugs that stimulate the liver to increase the output of bile of low specific gravity are called *hydrocholeretics.*

Substances that cause gallbladder contraction are called cholagogues. A well-known cholagogue is cholecystokinin (CCK). Fatty acids and amino acids (products of digestion) in the duodenum stimulate the release of CCK, which causes gallbladder contraction and opens the sphincter of Oddi. CCK also stimulates vagal nerve endings, bringing about the release of acetylcholine (ACh), which also stimulates the gallbladder.

General Model: Communications

Information about the presence of fats in the duodenum is used to prepare for the digestion of fats that must occur. This information is carried by humoral and neural signaling mechanisms.

Pancreatic Juice

The portion of the pancreas that secretes the pancreatic juice is called the exocrine pancreas to distinguish it from the endocrine pancreas (islets of Langerhans) that secrete insulin and other hormones. Structurally, it is quite similar to the salivary glands. The smaller pancreatic canaliculi coalesce into a single duct called the duct of Wirsung and occasionally, another accessory duct called the duct of Santorini. The duct of Wirsung joins the common bile duct to form the ampulla of Vater. The duct of Santorini, when present, opens either into the duct of Wirsung or directly into the duodenum through a separate opening.

The pancreatic juice is the major source of digestive enzymes that digest all components of the food—proteins, carbohydrates, fats, and nucleic acid. Its highly alkaline pH neutralizes the gastric HCl in the chyme that enters the duodenum. The volume of pancreatic juice secreted per day is ~500 to 1500 mL. It is highly alkaline (pH 8.4) due to its high HCO_3^- concentration, which is 2 to 5 times higher than the plasma concentration. As the flow rate of pancreatic juice increases, its HCO_3^- concentration increases, and Cl^- concentration decreases (**Fig. 69.5**). The reciprocal relationship with flow rate occurs because HCO_3^- is secreted in the small ducts but is reabsorbed in the large ducts in exchange for Cl^-. The exchange decreases at higher flow rates. The Na^+ and K^+ concentrations are similar to those of plasma and do not change with flow rate.

Control of pancreatic secretion | Pancreatic juice secretion has a cephalic phase that is neurally mediated and an intestinal phase that is hormonally mediated. There is no well-defined gastric phase of pancreatic secretion.

A
OH
NH—CH2—C—O—Na
O
O
HO
OH
B
OH
OH
OH
N
Na

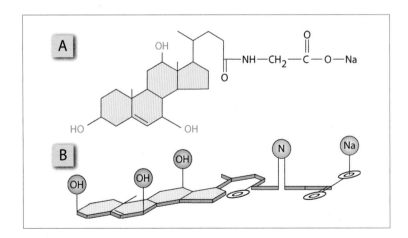

Fig. 69.3 **(A)** Chemical structure of bile salt sodium glycocholate. **(B)** Chemical structure of bile salt redrawn to show that the hydrophilic radicals project outside the plane of the steroid ring.

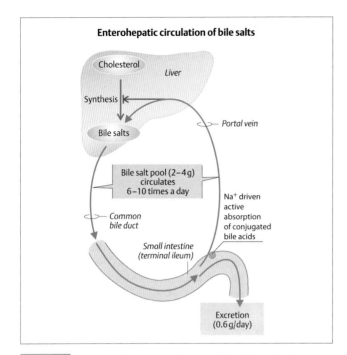

Fig. 69.4 The enterohepatic circulation of bile salts. Bile salts are actively reabsorbed in the ileum and transported into the hepatic portal vein, which returns them to the liver; as a consequence, only a small fraction of the bile salts produced is lost from the body in the feces.

The *cephalic phase* of pancreatic secretion is vagally mediated and is initiated by conditioned reflex in response to the sight or smell of food. The pancreatic juice produced is small in amount but rich in enzymes. The vagal effect is mediated not only by ACh, but by other neurotransmitters, such as vasoactive intestinal peptide (VIP) and glomerular filtration rate (GFR), that are also released by the vagal endings.

The *intestinal phase* of pancreatic secretion is controlled by two hormones: CCK and secretin. Secretin acts on the pancreatic ducts to cause secretion of large amounts of a very alkaline pancreatic juice that is rich in bicarbonates and poor in enzymes. CCK acts on the acinar cells to cause the release of zymogen granules and production of a concentrated pancreatic juice that is rich in enzymes.

Cells secreting secretin and CCK are found at several sites but notably, in the mucosa of the upper intestine. Both of these hormones are secreted just when they are needed—when food reaches the duodenum. The secretions of both are stimulated by the contact of the intestinal mucosa with the acid, peptides, and amino acids present in the chyme. CCK secretion is additionally stimulated by the presence of long chain fatty acids in the duodenum. Thus, both CCK and secretin mediate a physiologic reflex wherein the food itself stimulates the secretion of the digestive juice required to digest it.

Insulin, it is now believed, has long-term effects on the regulation of pancreatic enzyme synthesis. The venous blood from the islets of Langerhans passes through the pancreatic acini before returning to the systemic circulation. This exposes the pancreatic acini to high concentrations of insulin, which influences the synthesis of pancreatic enzymes.

Digestive Functions

Action of Bile Salts

The role of bile salts in fat digestion is threefold: (1) emulsification of fats; (2) formation of micelles; and (3) activation of an enzyme called bile salt-activated lipase, which is present in milk.

Emulsification is the division of large lipid droplets into smaller droplets ~1 mm in diameter (**Fig. 69.6A**). Emulsification increases the surface to volume ratio of the lipid droplets, facilitating the action of lipases. The process of emulsification requires churning of the fat (done by the pyloric antrum) and the presence of detergents in the form of bile salts (in bile juice) and phospholipids (in bile juice as well as in the food). Churning breaks up large lipid droplets into smaller ones; the detergents prevent the reaggregation of the smaller droplets into larger ones. Detergents form a coating on the small lipid droplets with their polar residues facing outward. These polar residues on small lipid droplets repel each other, preventing the reaggregation into larger droplets.

Formation of micelles | Micelles are much smaller than emulsified droplets, ~5 nm in diameter, and are cylindrical in shape (**Fig. 69.6B**). Most of the lipid content is in the form of fats that have already been digested and are therefore absorbable. The main function of micelles is to assist in the absorption of fats. The composition of micelles is similar, but not identical, to that of emulsified droplets. Each micelle contains detergents (bile salts and phospholipids) and absorbable fats (fatty acids, monoglycerides, and cholesterol). The detergents are located on the micellar surface. The absorbable fats are present in the hydrophobic center of the micelle.

Actions of Pancreatic Enzymes

Digestion of proteins | The pancreatic juice contains three endopeptidases (trypsin, chymotrypsin, and elastase) and two exopeptidases (carboxypeptidase A and B) that cleave proteins at different sites (**Fig. 69.7**). Endopeptidases break the pep-

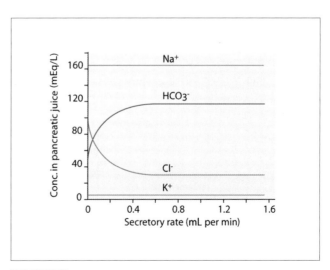

Fig. 69.5 Effect of secretory rate on the concentration of ions in pancreatic juice.

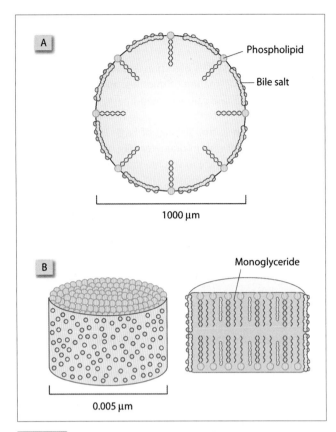

Fig. 69.6 **(A)** An emulsified lipid droplet. **(B,** *left***)** A micelle. **(B,** *right***)** Structure of a micelle sectioned along its axis. Note that the lipid droplets are 100,000 times larger than the micelles.

tides somewhere in the middle. Exopeptidases break the peptide chain near its end, releasing single amino acids.

All the above enzymes are secreted from the pancreas as inactive precursors (zymogens). Chymotrypsinogen, proelas-

tase, and procarboxypeptidases are converted into their active forms by the action of trypsin. Trypsin itself is activated from trypsinogen by the action of enteropeptidase (enterokinase) secreted by the intestinal mucosa. Once activated, trypsin activates a large number of proenzymes: chymotrypsinogen, proelastase, procarboxypeptidase, prophospholipase A_2, and procolipase. Trypsin also autoactivates itself by acting on trypsinogen.

Digestion of carbohydrates | The pancreatic juice contains pancreatic α-amylase, which digests starch, hydrolyzing the 1:4α linkages but sparing the 1:6α linkages, the terminal 1:4α linkages, and the 1:4α linkages next to branching points (**Fig. 69.8**). Consequently, the end products of α-amylase digestion are mostly the disaccharide maltose (two α-glucose residues linked by 1:4α bonds), the trisaccharide maltotriose (three α-glucose residues linked by 1:4α bonds), oligosaccharides (several glucose residues linked by 1:4α bonds), and α-limit dextrins (polymers of glucose containing an average of about eight glucose molecules with 1:6α linkages).

Digestion of fats (**Fig. 69.9**) is brought about by the following pancreatic enzymes. (1) Pancreatic lipase hydrolyzes primary ester linkages at positions 1 and 3 of triacylglycerols, yielding mostly free fatty acids and 2-monoglycerides. Pancreatic lipase is inhibited by bile salts. (2) Colipase helps overcome the inhibition of lipase by bile salts. (3) Bile salt-activated lipase breaks down triacylglycerol completely into glycerol and fatty acids. It also catalyzes the hydrolysis of cholesteryl esters, esters of fat-soluble vitamins, and phospholipids. Human milk contains an enzyme that is very similar to bile salt-activated lipase. It ensures complete digestion of milk fat and is of particular importance in premature infants whose pancreatic secretions are not fully operational. (4) Cholesteryl ester hydrolase acts on cholesteryl esters, releasing cholesterol in nonesterified free form. (5) Phospholipase A_2 hydrolyzes the

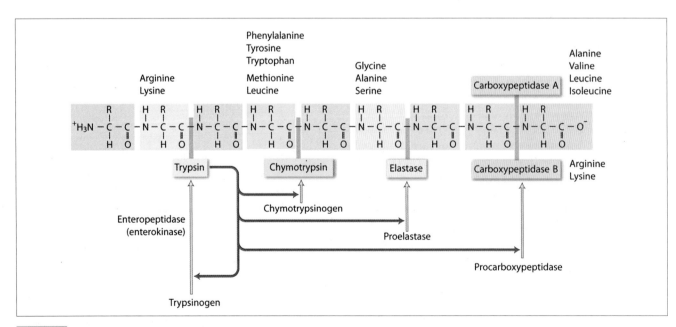

Fig. 69.7 Action of pancreatic enzymes on proteins. Each enzyme cleaves peptide bonds that are adjacent to specific amino acids.

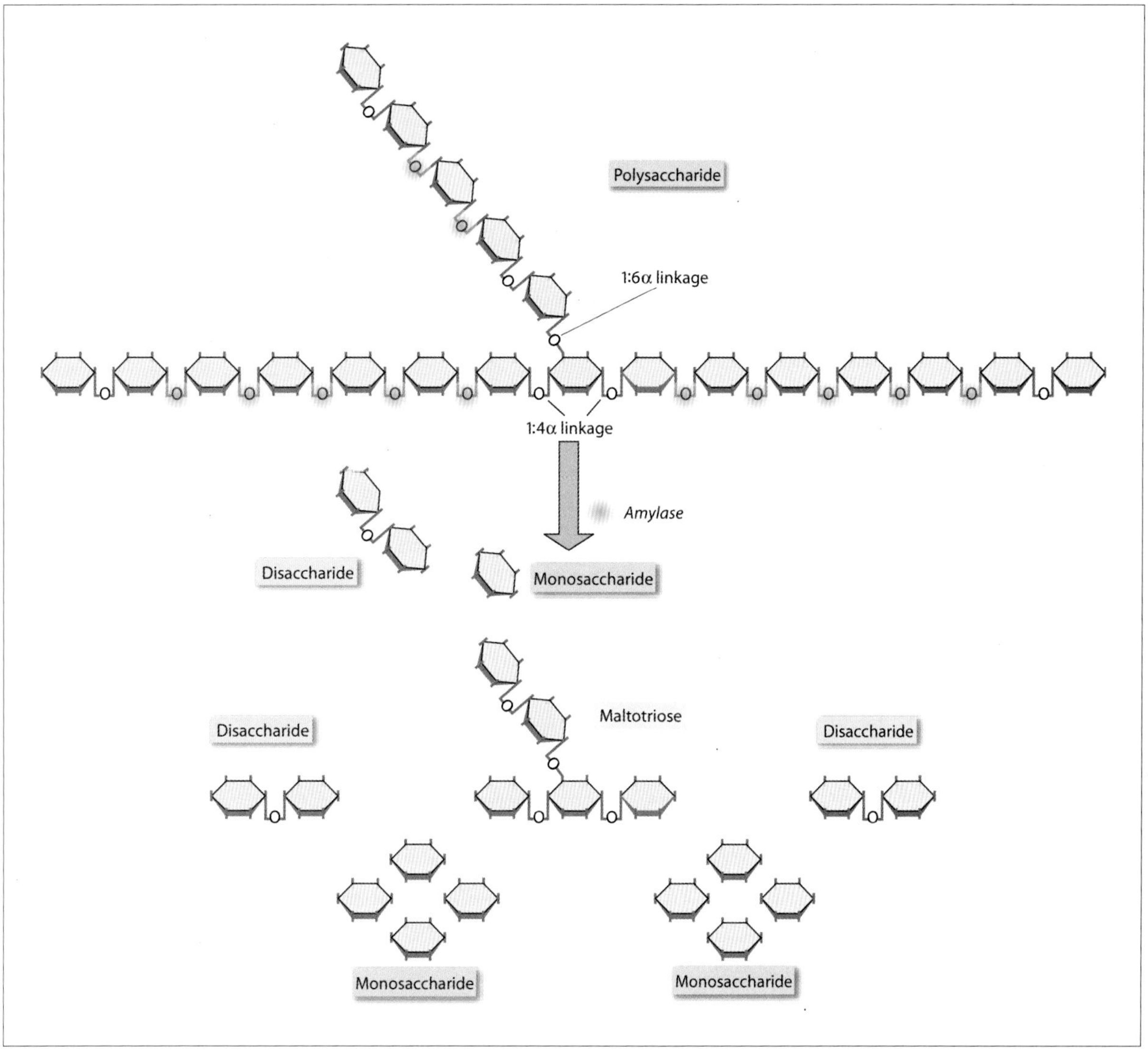

Fig. 69.8 Digestion of carbohydrates (polysaccharides) into disaccharides and monosaccharides.

ester bond in the 2-position of glycerophospholipids to form lysophospholipids, which, being detergents, aid emulsification and digestion of lipids.

Digestion of nucleic acids is brought about by ribonuclease and deoxyribonuclease.

Absorptive Functions

Significant amounts of absorption occur in the duodenum. In general, the absorptive pattern in the duodenum resembles that in the jejunum. For example, the duodenum and upper jejunum have the highest capacity to absorb sugars, dipeptides and tripeptides, and fats. Calcium and phosphate absorptions are especially high in the duodenum and ileum. The duodenum is also the principal site of absorption of nonheme iron.

Water may move either into or out of the duodenum depending on the tonicity of the chyme across the duodenal mucosa. Usually, the semisolid chyme extracts water into the duodenum lumen. However, when the chyme is watery, wa-ter may be reabsorbed from the duodenum. Sodium ion reabsorption occurs throughout the intestine, beginning in the duodenum. Bicarbonates are secreted into the duodenal lumen. Lower down in the ileum, bicarbonates are reabsorbed.

> **General Models: Flow and Energy**
>
> The movement (flow) of water is always passive. That is to say, water moves down its own concentration gradient. In the duodenum and elsewhere, osmotic gradients are produced by the active (energy requiring) pumping of solutes, particularly Na^+.

Pancreatic Function Tests

Analysis of Pancreatic Juices
The pancreatic secretions are collected by passing a double-lumen radiopaque (Dreiling) tube into the alimentary canal in such a way that one lumen drains the stomach, and the other

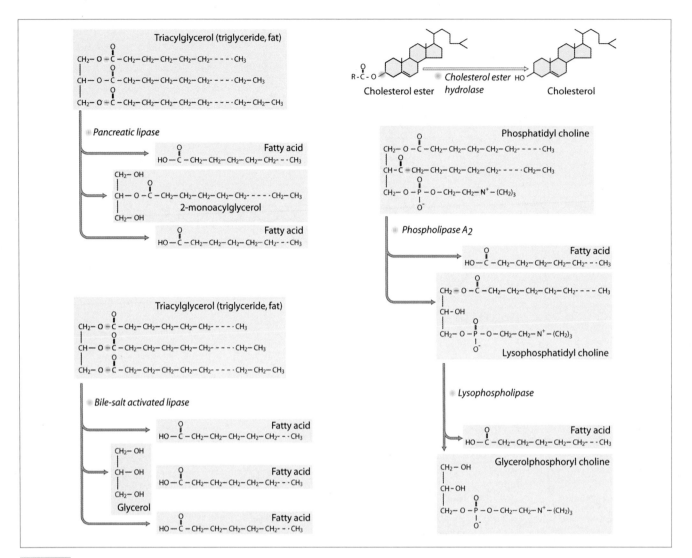

Fig. 69.9 Digestion of fats into fatty acids.

drains the duodenum. In this way, the duodenal contents are collected free from gastric contamination. The pancreatic juice secretion can be stimulated either directly by injecting secretin or cholecystokinin or by consuming a standardized test meal. The secretin test measures the secretory capacity of the pancreatic duct. It is decreased in chronic pancreatitis. In the combined secretin-CCK test or following a test meal, both bicarbonate and enzyme output are stimulated in normal subjects. With mild pancreatic damage, only the bicarbonate output is affected. With advanced damage, both are affected. However, test meals can give false-positive results. For example, the enzyme activity may be low, not due to pancreatic insufficiency, but due to some disease of the intestinal mucosa that results in inadequate release of cholecystokinin.

Analysis of Digestion Products

Stool examination | The stool is examined microscopically for undigested meat fibers and fat, the presence of which indicates a lack of proteolytic and lipolytic enzymes. The test is reliable and simple, but not sensitive enough to detect milder cases of pancreatic insufficiency.

Fecal fat test | The subject is fed a test diet containing adequate amounts of fats. A red carmine dye indicator is ingested before and after the test meal for identifying the stool resulting from the test meal. Normally, fecal fat is < 7% of the dietary intake. Increases in fecal fat occur when fat digestion or absorption is decreased.

The **triolein breath test** involves oral administration of radiolabeled triolein (the triglyceride of oleic acid). Metabolism of the triolein releases radiolabeled carbon dioxide (CO_2), which is exhaled. The amount of radiolabeled CO_2 exhaled is less if the triolein is not digested or not absorbed.

The **tripeptide hydrolysis test** utilizes a synthetic peptide N-benzoyl-l-tyrosyl-p-aminobenzoic acid (Bz-Ty-PABA) for testing chymotrypsin activity. The peptide is cleaved by chymotrypsin into Bz-Ty and PABA. The PABA is rapidly absorbed. If chymotrypsin activity is low, PABA excretion in urine decreases.

The **dual-label Schilling test** is based on the knowledge that trypsin plays a role in vitamin B_{12} absorption. It is known that cobalamin requires intrinsic factor for its absorption. However, before it can bind to the intrinsic factor, the ingested cobalamin is attached to a protein present in the gastric juice called the R protein. In the duodenum, trypsin degrades the R protein, releasing the cobalamin, which can then bind to the intrinsic factor. Hence, in pancreatic insufficiency, there is malabsorption of vitamin B_{12}.

The patient is given to ingest a mixture of ^{57}Co-cobalamin complexed with intrinsic factor, and ^{58}Co-cobalamin complexed with R protein. Normally, both ^{57}Co-cobalamin and ^{58}Co-cobalamin are absorbed and excreted in urine in equal amounts. In pancreatic insufficiency, the urinary excretion of ^{58}Co-cobalamin (which was complexed with R protein) is reduced.

Summary

- The digestion occurring in the duodenum is the result of biliary secretions and secretions from the pancreas.

- The bile salts, produced in the liver, are involved with the digestion of fats. The secretions of the pancreas, the pancreatic enzymes, and bicarbonate solution are involved in the digestion of carbohydrates, fats, and proteins.

- The bile salts emulsify lipid droplets and aid in the formation of micelles, which contain digested lipids.

- The bicarbonate solution secreted by the pancreas increases the pH of the duodenal contents so that the pancreatic enzymes can function.

- Peptidases break proteins into amino acids, amylases break down carbohydrates into simple sugars, and lipases digest fats into glycerol and fatty acids; only the "monomeric" products of digestion can be absorbed.

Applying What You Know

69.1. Mrs. Schilling had a gallstone removed from her common bile duct. What are the effects of a gallstone?

69.2. Mrs. Schilling's abdominal computed tomography scan revealed pancreatic scarring and atrophy. What functions of the pancreas would be affected by these changes?

69.3. If Mrs. Schilling had a Schilling test performed (the names are a coincidence), it would probably show that she has a decreased rate of absorption of vitamin B_{12}. Which of Mrs. Schilling's signs and symptoms are probably related to her vitamin B_{12} deficiency?

Mechanical Functions

Motility Patterns

In the unfed state, motility in the small intestine is characterized by the migrating motor complexes (MMCs) that pass down the stomach and intestines at regular intervals. As in the stomach, the MMCs are replaced following a meal by motility patterns: segmentation and peristalsis. The MMCs are much stronger than the peristaltic waves.

Segmentation contractions are ringlike contractions of the circular smooth muscle of the gut that appear at regular intervals (**Fig. 70.1**). The intestine becomes transiently compartmentalized into several short segments. The contractions disappear after a few seconds, only to reappear as another set of ring contractions in the segments between the previous contractions. They move the chyme to and fro and increase its exposure to the mucosal surface. A variant of the segmentation contractions are the *tonic contractions* that last somewhat longer, isolating one segment of the intestine from another. Segmentation and tonic contractions slow down the transit of chyme in the small intestine. This permits longer contact of the chyme with the enterocytes (cells of the intestinal mucous membrane) and thereby improves absorption.

Peristaltic waves propel the intestinal chyme toward the large intestines. Peristaltic waves are contraction rings of the intestine that travel short distances along the intestine at velocities of 2 to 3 cm/sec. Very intense peristaltic waves called peristaltic rushes are not seen normally, but occur when the intestine is obstructed. Most waves pass regularly in an oral to caudal direction.

Reflexes

Peristaltic reflex is induced by a localized distention of the intestine. It results in peristaltic contraction proximal to the distention and inhibition distal to it. It is unlikely that the peristaltic reflex is of any physiologic significance because the intestine is rarely distended to the degree required to induce the reflex. The peristaltic reflex is not a spinal reflex: it is coordinated by the enteric nervous system of the intestine.

In the **gastroileal reflex,** excessive secretory and motor activity of the stomach brings about a reflex increase in the motility of the terminal part of the ileum and accelerates the movement of material through the ileocecal sphincter. The reflex is vagally mediated.

In the **intestinointestinal reflex,** overdistention of one segment of the intestine relaxes the smooth muscle in the rest of the intestine.

Secretory Functions

The tubular intestinal glands, also known as the crypts of Lieberkühn, secrete an isotonic fluid called the succus entericus. Most of the enzymes usually found in this secretion come from the desquamated mucosal cells. Cell-free succus entericus hardly contains any enzymes. The secretion of succus entericus is stimulated by gastrointestinal hormones, such as vasoactive intestinal peptide (VIP), but is unaffected by vagal stimulation. The mucus secreted by the intestine comes from the enterocytes and the goblet cells in the epithelium.

Digestive Functions

Digestion of all constituents of food is completed in the small intestine. Intestinal digestion occurs at three locations: the intestinal lumen, the brush border, and inside the cells making up the mucosa. Relatively little digestion occurs in the lumen itself. Most of the digestion occurs at the intestinal brush border to which the digestive enzymes are attached. Some dipeptides and tripeptides are actively transported into the intestinal cells and hydrolyzed by intracellular peptidases. The amino acids so formed diffuse out into the bloodstream. The same is true for some lipids.

Carbohydrate digestion | There are five enzymes responsible for carbohydrate digestion at the intestinal brush border. (1) Sucrase breaks down sucrose into glucose and fructose. (2) Maltase (α-glucosidase) breaks the 1:4α linkages and releases glucose. (3) Isomaltase (α-dextrinase) breaks down the 1:6α linkages and releases glucose. (4) Lactase (β–glucosidase) breaks down lactose into glucose and galactose. (5) Trehalase hydrolyzes trehalose, a 1:1α-linked dimer of glucose, into two glucose molecules.

Protein digestion | There are five enzymes responsible for protein digestion at the intestinal brush border. (1) Enteropeptidase (enterokinase) is meant only for activating trypsinogen to trypsin. (2) Aminopeptidase is an exopeptidase that breaks the peptide bonds next to N-terminal amino acids of peptides. (3) Carboxypeptidase is an exopeptidase that breaks the last peptide bond toward the C terminal. (4) Endopeptidases break peptide bonds somewhere in the middle of the polypeptide. (5) Dipeptidase splits dipeptides into amino acids.

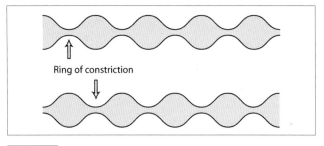

Ring of constriction

Fig. 70.1   Segmentation contractions of the intestine.

About half the protein in the intestine comes from ingested food, and the rest comes from digestive juices and desquamated mucosal cells. Most of the protein is digested in the small intestine. Any undigested protein is digested in the colon by bacterial action. The protein in the stools is not of dietary origin, but comes from bacteria and cellular debris.

Nucleic acid digestion Three intestinal enzymes help in digestion of nucleic acids. (1) Polynucleotidases split nucleic acids into nucleotides. (2) Nucleosidases catalyze the phosphorylation of nucleosides to give the free nitrogen base plus a pentose phosphate. (3) Phosphatase removes the phosphate from pentose phosphate formed as a result of nucleic acid digestion. It also removes the phosphates from organic phosphates in the diet.

Fat digestion in the intestine is brought about mostly by the enzymes in pancreatic juice. However, the intestinal mucosal cells have on them a phospholipase that attacks phospholipids to produce glycerol, fatty acids, phosphoric acid, and bases such as choline.

Absorptive Functions

Absorption of Carbohydrates

Monosaccharides are rapidly absorbed from the intestine before the meal reaches the terminal part of the ileum. Pentoses are absorbed by simple diffusion. Glucose and galactose are absorbed by facilitated diffusion employing sodium-dependent glucose transporter (SGLT) and glucose transporter (GLUT-2). Fructose employs GLUT-5 and GLUT-2 for diffusion across the luminal and basolateral membranes, respectively (**Fig. 70.2A**). When SGLT is congenitally defective, the resulting glucose or galactose malabsorption causes severe diarrhea that is often fatal if glucose and galactose are not promptly removed from the diet.

Insulin has no direct effect on intestinal transport of sugars. In this respect, intestinal absorption resembles glucose reabsorption in the proximal convoluted tubules of the kidneys. Neither of the processes requires phosphorylation. Both are essentially normal in diabetes mellitus but are depressed by the drug phlorhizin.

Absorption of Proteins

Amino acids are absorbed more in the jejunum than in the ileum. Some amino acids are reabsorbed through simple diffusion. However, most amino acids employ transporters, both for entering the enterocytes across the brush border and for diffusing out across the basolateral membrane. There are several transporters specific to individual or groups of amino acids. Some of these involve cotransport with Na⁺; others are Na⁺-independent.

Congenital defects in amino acid transport usually affect both intestinal absorption and renal tubular reabsorption, for example, cystinuria and Hartnup disease, which occur due to impaired transport of basic and neutral amino acids, respectively.

Small peptides Absorption of small peptides is more in the ileum but less in the jejunum. Dipeptides and tripeptides are transported across the brush border through secondary active

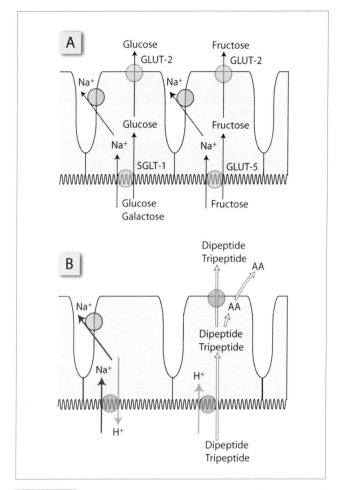

Fig. 70.2 Transport across intestinal mucosa. **(A)** Transport of monosaccharides. **(B)** Transport of small peptides. GLUT, glucose transporter; SGLT, sodium-dependent glucose transporter.

transport (**Fig. 70.2B**). Most of the peptides that enter the enterocyte are cleaved into amino acids inside the cell. The amino acids diffuse out of the basolateral membrane into the portal blood. However, some small peptides are not broken down inside the enterocyte: they diffuse out into the bloodstream unchanged, possibly using a transporter.

Proteins A small amount of protein passes unaltered from the intestine into the blood. The protein is endocytosed by the intestinal epithelium and exocytosed into the bloodstream. The amount of protein absorbed in this way is substantial in infants but declines with age. In infants, the immunoglobulin A (IgA) present in maternal colostrum is thus able to enter the circulation and provide passive immunity.

In adults, certain food proteins may produce an allergic response after being absorbed without being digested. Several bacterial and viral proteins are absorbed by the large microfold (M) cells present on Peyer's patches. The M cells pass the antigens to the lymphoblasts in Peyer's patches. The activated lymphoblasts enter the circulation, only to return to the intestinal mucosa and other epithelia where they secrete IgA in response to subsequent antigenic exposures.

The **purine** and **pyrimidine** bases formed by the digestion of nucleic acids are absorbed by an active transport process.

Absorption of Fats

A barrier to the absorption of fat molecules is the unstirred layer, a stationary layer of luminal fluid that is in contact with the mucosal surface of the intestine. Digested fats must therefore be converted to micellar form for passage across the unstirred layer. The thickness of the unstirred layer increases in certain disease states such as celiac sprue, thereby contributing to malabsorption.

More than 95% of the ingested fat is absorbed in the intestine. The micelles move down their concentration gradient through the unstirred layer to the brush border of the mucosal cells. The lipids diffuse out of the micelles, and a saturated aqueous solution of the lipids is maintained in contact with the brush border of the mucosal cells.

All fatty acids enter the enterocytes by facilitated diffusion (**Fig. 70.3**). Once inside the mucosal cell, short- and long-chain fatty acids are dealt with differently. Short-chain fatty acids (containing < 10 carbon atoms) pass from the mucosal cells directly into the portal blood. Long-chain fatty acids (> 10 carbon atoms) are rapidly reesterified to triglycerides in the mucosal cells, maintaining a favorable diffusion gradient of lipids. Most of the triglyceride is formed by the acylation of the absorbed 2-monoglycerides. The triglycerides are then coated with a layer of protein and phospholipid to form *chylomicrons*. The cholesterol that enters the enterocyte is esterified with fatty acids and incorporated into chylomicrons. The chylomicrons leave the cell and enter the lymphatics. During fat absorption, the lymph in the villi becomes milky due to suspended chylomicrons. The lymphatic channels in the villi are therefore called lacteals, and the lymph they carry is called *chyle*.

Absorption of Water and Electrolytes

Water | The intestines are presented each day with ~2 L of ingested fluid plus 7 L of secretions from the mucosa of the gastrointestinal tract and associated glands (**Fig. 70.4**). All but 200 mL of this amount of fluid is reabsorbed. Depending on the amount of water ingested with meals, the duodenal contents may be hypotonic or hypertonic. Accordingly, water may move out of the duodenum into the plasma or vice versa. In either case, by the time the food enters the jejunum, it is usually isotonic to the plasma across the intestinal wall.

Sodium is actively absorbed throughout the small and large intestines. The active transport of sodium (Na^+) is coupled to the absorption of glucose, amino acids, and certain other substances. Hence, the presence of glucose in the intestinal lumen facilitates the reabsorption of Na^+. For the same reason, glucose is added to the orally administered NaCl solutions in the treatment of Na^+ and water loss in diarrhea.

Potassium | There is bidirectional movement of potassium (K^+) across the intestinal wall, both passive and active. In the jejunum and ileum, there is net absorption of K^+ from the lumen, mainly because of solvent drag associated with water absorption.

Vitamins and Minerals

Water-soluble vitamins B_1, B_2, B_3, B_5, B_6, biotin, and vitamin C are mostly absorbed in the jejunum through Na^+ cotransport. Folic acid and vitamin B_{12} are absorbed in the ileum (see Chapter 24). Fat-soluble vitamins A, D, E, and K are poorly absorbed if fat absorption is depressed. Absorption of iron is discussed

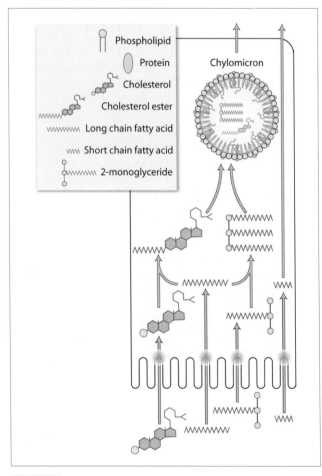

Fig. 70.3 Absorption of fats.

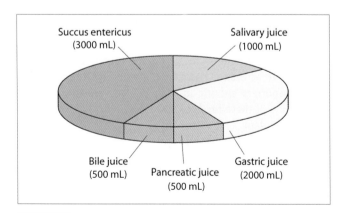

Fig. 70.4 The constituents of the 7 liters of digestive juices that are secreted daily into the gastrointestinal tract.

in detail in relation to hematinic factors (see Chapter 24). Absorption of calcium and phosphate is discussed in relation to bone metabolism (see Chapter 78).

Summary

- When the small intestine is empty, the motor pattern is characterized by migrating motor complexes; when filled with chyme, segmentation and peristalsis occur, mixing and propelling the chyme aborally.

- Absorption of digested food is completed in the small intestine.

Applying What You Know

70.1. Mrs. Schilling tried Imodium to control her diarrhea. This drug slows peristalsis in the intestine. How would this affect her diarrhea?

70.2. Mrs. Schilling is given a solution of xylose to drink, and the appearance of xylose in her urine is measured. What changes in intestinal function would result in reduced renal excretion of xylose? Explain.

70.3. Mrs. Schilling is suffering from steatorrhea, the appearance of large quantities of fat in her stool. What changes in intestinal function could result in this condition? Explain.

70.4. During the physical examination, it is noted that Mrs. Schilling has numerous small bruises on her arms. What would cause this?

The colon is also called the large intestine, as its diameter is greater than that of the ileum, although it is much shorter in length. Its external muscle layer is organized into three longitudinal bands called the teniae coli. The wall of the colon bulges out as haustra through the gaps between the teniae coli. Colonic mucosa does not have villi. Colonic glands secrete mucus only. The nerve supply of the colon is similar to that in the ileum. The sympathetic nerve supply to the internal anal sphincter (made of smooth muscle) is excitatory; the parasympathetic supply is inhibitory. The external anal sphincter (a skeletal muscle) is innervated by the pudendal nerve.

Motor Functions

Colonic motility has been studied through pressure recordings, cineradiography, and recording of transit time, each method providing a different type of information. The movements of the colon are coordinated by the basal electric rhythm (BER) of the colon. The frequency of this wave increases along the colon, from ~9/min at the ileocecal valve to 16/min at the sigmoid.

Pressure Changes in the Colon

Intraluminal pressure recordings are of little use in studying colonic motility because colonic contractions can occur without pressure changes, and conversely, pressure changes can occur due to a distant contraction. Moreover, large shifts of colonic contents can occur with very little intraluminal pressure change. This occurs when the adjacent segments are patent and their resistance is low, as occurs in children or in diarrhea. Conversely, large variations of pressure (70–80 mm Hg) may bring about no transport of feces. This occurs when interhaustral contractions almost occlude the lumen, as occurs in constipation.

General Models: Elasticity and Flow

The elastic properties of the colon clearly play a role in the pressure changes that occur in the colon. The pressure changes that are present and the patency (and hence the resistance) of segments of the colon determine the flow of colonic contents.

Cineradiography of Colonic Motility

Cineradiography indicates the pattern of colonic contractions, as well as the movement of the colonic contents. The following motility patterns can be observed using cineradiography.

Haustral shuttling | is the most common form of colonic motility in which the haustral contents are squirted short distances in both directions by random segmental contraction of the circular muscles. Like the segmentation contractions of the ileum, these contractions are not progressive but slowly knead the fecal mass, facilitating water absorption. Similar contractions in the sigmoid colon are responsible for the shape of well-formed feces.

Segmental propulsion (peristalsis) | causes the contents of a haustrum to be expelled into the next haustrum. The direction of propulsion may be aboral (away from the mouth) or adoral (toward the mouth), but the propulsion predominates over the retropulsion. In irritable bowel syndrome, propulsive movements are increased without any apparent reason, resulting in frequent urge for defecation.

Systolic multihaustral propulsion (mass contraction) | begins in the middle of the transverse colon with several adjacent segments contracting simultaneously and transporting the bowel contents at 2 to 5 cm/min as far as the rectum. Mass movements are quite infrequent, occurring at intervals of several hours. Mass contraction is also produced reflexly by the gastrocolic reflex (see below).

Colonic Transit

Transit time | An ingested meal reaches the cecum in ~4 hours, the hepatic flexure in 6 hours, the splenic flexure in 9 hours, and the sigmoid colon in 12 hours. From the pelvic colon to the anus, the transport is much slower, and as much as a quarter of the residue of a test meal is retained in the rectum for up to 3 days. Complete expulsion of the meal in stool takes more than a week. If beads of three different colors are consumed on 3 consecutive days, beads of all three colors are found in the stool from the third day onward. It indicates that there is a pool, probably in the cecum and sigmoid colon, where residues get mixed. High-fiber diets pass more rapidly through the colon.

Ileocecal transit | The portion of the ileum containing the ileocecal valve projects slightly into the cecum, so that a rise in colonic pressure squeezes it shut, whereas a rise in ileal pressure pushes it open. It is normally closed and prevents reflux of colonic contents into the ileum. Each time a peristaltic wave reaches it, it opens briefly, permitting some of the ileal chyme to squirt into the cecum.

Colonic Reflexes

Defecation reflex | Defecation is a spinal reflex initiated by the distention of the rectum with feces (**Fig. 71.1**). The distention is sensed by mechanoreceptors located in the wall of the anal canal. It brings about reflex contractions of the colon and with it, the desire to defecate. The urge to defecate is first felt when rectal pressure increases to ~18 mm Hg. When the rectal pressure reaches 55 mm Hg, the internal sphincter relaxes reflexly, which is called the rectoanal inhibitory reflex. The relaxation is mediated by cholinergic parasympathetic fibers originating from the sacral spinal cord (S2) and reaching the rectum through the pelvic splanchnic nerve (nervi erigentes). The afferent fibers, too, reach the spinal cord through the pelvic splanchnic nerve.

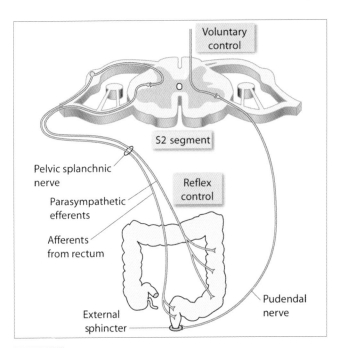

Fig. 71.1 The defecation reflex. Afferent (sensory) information from the colon is passed to the spinal cord, with efferent (motor) returning to the colon. Descending inhibitory controls normally keep the anal sphincter closed unless that inhibition is consciously stopped.

Defecation can be voluntarily inhibited by keeping the external anal sphincter contracted. Defecation can be voluntarily initiated at any time when the rectal pressure is between 18 and 55 mm Hg. This is done by voluntarily relaxing the external sphincter and straining, that is, performing the Valsalva maneuver to increase the intra-abdominal pressure. Voluntary defecation is not possible at lower rectal pressures. Chronic spinal patients have no voluntary control on defecation, and evacuation is entirely by reflex in such individuals.

The **gastrocolic reflex** is the mass contraction of the colon brought about reflexly by the distention of the stomach. The reflex consists of an early neural phase (within 10 minutes of eating), which is abolished by anticholinergic drugs, and a delayed hormonal phase, which coincides with the peak level of gastrin. Because of this reflex, children defecate almost routinely after meals. In adults, bowel training suppresses this reflex.

Absorptive Functions

In the colon, significant amounts of Na$^+$ and water are absorbed. However, humans can survive after total colectomy, as is done in cases of carcinoma of the colon, provided fluid and electrolyte balance is maintained. The colon offers a large surface for absorption that can be utilized for rectal drug administration with suppositories. However, the use of an enema can pose a problem because large amounts of water may be absorbed, causing water intoxication, coma, and death, especially in children.

Sodium and water absorption | Na$^+$ is actively transported out of the colon, generating an osmotic gradient. Water follows

down the osmotic gradient through paracellular pathways. The Na$^+$–K$^+$ pump is located on the basolateral membrane of the colonic epithelial cell. There are at least two different mechanisms of Na$^+$ absorption at the apical surface of the cells in the colon. In the distal colon, Na$^+$ transport occurs through a Na$^+$-unitransporter, which is electrogenic (**Fig. 71.2A**). The channels through which Na$^+$ enters the cell are amiloride-sensitive, and the entire process is similar to the electrogenic Na$^+$-unitransport that occurs in the renal tubule. In the proximal colon, Na$^+$ is reabsorbed mostly through coupled Na$^+$–H$^+$ antiport and HCO$_3^-$–Cl$^-$ antiport (**Fig. 71.2B**), as occurs in the renal tubule (see **Fig. 55.2**). The HCO$_3^-$–Cl$^-$ exchange accounts for the high bicarbonate concentration of colonic secretion. Saline cathartics such as magnesium sulfate are poorly absorbed salts that retain their osmotic equivalent of water in the intestine, thus increasing intestinal volume, which exerts a laxative effect.

General Models: Energy and Flow

Active transport of solutes, principally Na$^+$, establishes an osmotic gradient that drives the flow of water down the osmotic gradient. The availability of oxygen and glucose is thus essential to provide the energy required to move solutes. Blood flow to the gastrointestinal tract increases following a meal to make this possible.

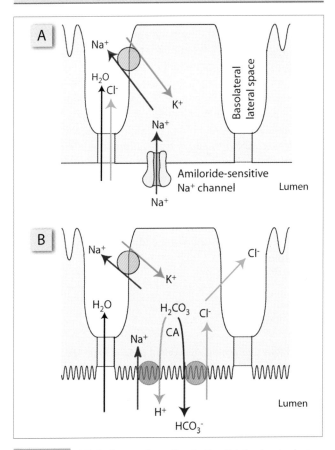

Fig. 71.2 (A) Sodium reabsorption in the distal colon is electrogenic because movement of Na$^+$ contributes to the establishment of the transmembrane potential. (B) Na$^+$ reabsorption in the proximal colon is electroneutral; the transmembrane potential is not affected because countertransport of ions with the same charges is occurring.

Potassium absorption or secretion | Colonic absorption and secretion of K^+ are delicately balanced. When the K^+ concentration of the colonic contents is low, there is net secretion, and when it is high, there is net absorption. Mostly, there is a net secretion of K^+ into the colon, and the loss of colonic fluids can lead to severe hypokalemia.

Feces

The composition of the solid part of feces, which comprises only a quarter of its total weight, is given in **Table 71.1**. Fecal protein and fat are not of dietary origin, but come from bacteria and cellular debris. Hence, fecal composition is relatively unaffected by dietary variations, and appreciable amounts of feces are passed even during prolonged starvation.

The pH of the stool is slightly acidic due to the organic acids formed from carbohydrates by colonic bacteria. The brown color of the stool is due to the presence of urobilin, which is formed by the oxidation of urobilinogen (colorless). Urobilinogens are formed from bilirubin by the action of colonic bacteria. Darkening of feces upon standing in air is due to the oxidation of residual urobilinogens to urobilins.

Intestinal Bacteria

The colon is sterile at birth but soon becomes colonized by bacteria. The bacterial count is less in the ileum and jejunum, and nearly absent in the stomach and duodenum due to the inhibitory action of HCl. Colonic bacteria can be symbionts (sharing a mutually beneficial relationship with the host), pathogens (harmful to the host), or commensals (neither beneficial nor harmful). In immunosuppressed individuals, pathogenic colonic bacteria enter the bloodstream in large numbers, producing fatal septicemia. Even in normal subjects, the spread of *Escherichia coli* to the urinary tract causes severe infection.

Beneficial bacterial reactions | Symbiotic colonic bacteria synthesize vitamin K, B group vitamins, and folic acid. Some of these are absorbed in significant amounts and supplement dietary intake. Unabsorbed lactose is converted to short-chain fatty acids by colonic bacteria. These fatty acids enhance colonic absorption of Na^+ and water and also have a trophic effect on the colonic mucosa.

Detrimental bacterial reactions | Nutrients such as vitamin C, vitamin B_{12}, and choline are consumed by some bacteria and lead to deficiency symptoms unless these are supplemented in the diet. Colonic bacteria also produce ammonia, which is absorbed by blood but is quickly detoxified in the liver. Hence, liver dysfunction results in hyperammonemia, causing neurologic symptoms (hepatic encephalopathy). The condition is treated with osmotic cathartics such as lactulose, which reduces the colonic load of ammonia-forming proteins and also acidifies the colonic contents, promoting the growth of bacteria that do not form ammonia. Colonic bacterial activity is associated with higher plasma low-density lipoprotein (LDL) and cholesterol levels. Poorly absorbed antibiotics (luminal antibiotics), such as neomycin, that modify the intestinal flora, lower LDL and the plasma cholesterol level.

Indifferent bacterial reactions | Commensal colonic bacteria convert primary bile acids (cholic acid and chenodeoxycholic acid) into secondary bile acids (deoxycholic acid and lithocholic acid). Colonic bacteria synthesize indole, skatole, mercaptans, and hydrogen sulfide, which contribute to the fecal odor. Even methane is formed in some individuals. Commensals also form hydrogen from unabsorbed carbohydrates. The hydrogen is absorbed and expired in breath. In *lactose intolerance*, breath hydrogen increases following a dietary load of lactose and is used as a diagnostic test called the *hydrogen breath test*. Some colonic bacteria synthesize potentially toxic amines such as histamine and tyramine, which were thought to produce autointoxication in constipated patients, but are now known to be harmless.

Summary

- Motility in the colon comprises haustral shuttling, peristalsis, and mass contractions.

- The defecation reflex, relaxation of the internal anal sphincter, occurs when the pressure in the rectum gets high enough. However, voluntary control of the external anal sphincter can keep defecation from occurring.

- The major absorptive function of the colon is absorption of NaCl, with water moving passively down the osmotic gradient that is established.

Applying What You Know

71.1. Mrs. Schilling's frequent bouts of diarrhea could cause dehydration. Oral rehydration fluids contain both glucose and electrolytes, particularly sodium. Explain the mechanism by which this therapy works.

Table 71.1 Composition by Weight of Solid Fecal Matter

Constituent	Weight %
Dead bacteria	30
Undigested roughage, sloughed epithelial cells, and the solid constituents of gastrointestinal secretions (e.g., bile pigments)	30
Fats	10–20
Inorganic matter	10–20
Proteins	2–3

Gastrointestinal (GI) hormones are secreted by endocrine cells located in the GI mucosa. They often act in a paracrine fashion, but they also enter the circulation. They play an important role in the regulation of GI secretion and motility. Structurally, and to a lesser extent functionally, these hormones are of two types: the *gastrin family,* which includes gastrin and cholecystokinin (CCK); and the *secretin family,* which includes secretin, glucagon, glicentin, vasoactive intestinal polypeptide (VIP), and gastric inhibitory polypeptide (GIP). Because gastrin and CCK belong to the same family, their actions are similar but differ in strength. For example, both gastrin and CCK stimulate gastric secretion and gallbladder contraction, but gastrin's effect on gastric secretion is much greater than CCK's effect, and CCK's action on the gallbladder is much greater than gastrin's. A comparison of gastrin, CCK, and secretin is given in **Table 72.1**.

Many of these GI hormones are also found in the brain and peripheral nerves. For example, CCK, which stimulates gallbladder contraction, is also found in the brain, where it is involved in the regulation of food intake and in the production of anxiety and analgesia. This dual presence has been called the *gastrocephalic axis.* Cells secreting GI hormones can form tumors. Most of these tumors are either *gastrinomas* or *glucagonomas.*

General Model: Communications and Homeostasis

The GI hormones behave like other hormones (see Section IX), and they transmit information cell to cell, whether locally or via the circulation. Their effects on the GI system are to coordinate the function of the many components of the system. The major function of absorption of nutrients is not homeostatically controlled; with the exception of a few inorganic solutes, the GI system absorbs all of the nutrients presented to it.

Gastrin

Gastrin is produced by the G cells located in antral gastric glands (see **Fig. 68.3**). G cells belong to a larger family of cells called the APUD cells (amine precursor uptake and decarboxylation). Gastrin-secreting cells are also found in the pituitary gland, brain, and nerves, as well as the fetal pancreatic islets. Gastrin-secreting tumors (gastrinomas) are most common in the pancreas.

Structurally, gastrin shows both macroheterogeneity (variable length of the polypeptide) and microheterogeneity (minor differences in amino acid sequence). The principal form of gastrin-causing gastric acid secretion is G_{17}, which has 17 amino acid residues. All forms of gastrin have an identical sequence of five amino acids at their C terminal. The prohormone preprogastrin is cleaved to produce active C-terminal regions of varying sizes, such as mini gastrin, with 14 amino acids (G_{14}), little gastrin (G_{17}), big gastrin (G_{34}), or the "big big" gastrin, with more than 34 amino acids. Most of the gastrin is either G_{17} or G_{34}. Both are equally potent in stimulating acid secretion. Each form is best suited for a particular action of gastrin.

Gastrin secretion is increased by the presence of the products of protein digestion in the stomach, particularly phenylalanine and tryptophan, which act directly on the G cells. It is also stimulated by distention of the stomach and vagal stimulation. Postganglionic vagal fibers innervating the G cells have gastrin-releasing polypeptide (GRP), and not acetylcholine (ACh), as their neurotransmitter; therefore, atropine does not inhibit the gastrin response to a test meal. Acid in the duodenum inhibits gastrin secretion, partly by a direct action on G cells and partly by release of somatostatin, which inhibits gastrin secretion.

Gastrin acts through the group IIC mechanism (see **Fig. 75.6**). The main actions of gastrin are stimulation of gastric acid and pepsin secretion, stimulation of gastric motility, and stimulation of growth of the mucosa of the stomach, ileum, and colon (the *trophic effect*). Gastrin stimulates both insulin and glucagon secretion. After a protein meal, gastrin is secreted in sufficient amounts to increase insulin secretion. Gastrin plays a role in the pathophysiology of duodenal ulcers.

Cholecystokinin–Pancreozymin

CCK and pancreozymin (PZ) were earlier thought to be two different hormones—one (CCK) stimulating gallbladder contraction, and the other (PZ) stimulating enzyme-rich pancreatic secretion. It is now known that the two are the same, and have been named CCK-PZ, or simply CCK. Like gastrin, CCK shows both macroheterogeneity and microheterogeneity. There are two types of CCK receptors: CCK-A and CCK-B. Both types of receptors are found in the brain, but the GI tract contains only CCK-A receptors. In the brain, CCK receptors are present in the area postrema.

CCK secretion is stimulated by contact of the intestinal mucosa with the products of digestion, particularly peptides and amino acids, and also by the presence in the duodenum of fatty acids containing more than 10 carbon atoms.

CCK acts through the group IIC hormonal mechanism (see **Fig. 75.6**) and has the following functions. (1) It causes contraction of the gallbladder. (2) It causes the secretion of enzyme-rich pancreatic juice. (3) It potentiates the action of secretin on the pancreas. (4) It inhibits gastric emptying. It also augments the contraction of the pyloric sphincter, thus preventing the reflux of duodenal contents into the stomach. (5) It increases the motility of the small intestine and colon. (6) It exerts a trophic effect on the pancreas. (7) It increases the secretion of enterokinase. (8) It stimulates both insulin and glucagon secretion. (9) It produces satiety.

Secretin

Secretin is secreted by the S cells located deep in the jejunal glands. Its secretion is increased when acid and the products of protein digestion come in contact with the jejunal mucosa.

Secretin acts through the group IIA hormonal mechanism (see **Fig. 75.5**). The following are the functions of secretin. (1) It stimulates the secretion of a watery, alkaline (bicarbonate-rich) pancreatic juice. (2) It potentiates the action of CCK on the pancreas. (3) It increases the hepatic secretion of bile; it is a choleretic. (4) It decreases gastric acid secretion. (5) It increases the tone of the pyloric sphincter.

Other Gastrointestinal Hormones

Gastric inhibitory peptide (GIP) is so called because it inhibits gastric secretion and motility. It also stimulates insulin secretion. GIP secretion is stimulated by glucose and fat in the duodenum; therefore, GIP qualifies as enterogastrone (see below), but it is not potent enough, and there are better candidates. GIP is secreted by the K cells in the duodenal and intestinal mucosa.

Vasoactive intestinal peptide (VIP) is so named because it dilates peripheral blood vessels and relaxes intestinal smooth muscles. Thus, it causes a marked increase in watery intestinal secretions. VIP also inhibits gastric acid secretion. VIP-secreting tumors are called VIPomas and result in severe diarrhea. VIP is also found as a cotransmitter with ACh in brain and autonomic nerves. VIP potentiates the effect of ACh on salivary secretion.

Peptide YY is an effective inhibitor of gastrin-mediated acid secretion. Also, its release from the jejunal mucosa is stimulated by the presence of fats in the lumen. Peptide YY is the best qualified as an enterogastrone.

Motilin is secreted by cells in the duodenal mucosa and causes contraction of intestinal smooth muscle. Motilin is a regulator of the "housekeeper waves" of the intestines (see Migrating Motor Complexes subsection, Chapter 68).

Neurotensin is abundant in the mucosa of the ileum. Its release is stimulated by fatty acids. It inhibits GI motility and increases ileal blood flow.

Gastrin-releasing polypeptide (GRP) is the neurotransmitter in the vagal endings innervating G cells. It increases gastrin secretion. It enters the circulation when secreted in very large amounts.

Somatostatin and **glucagon** are discussed in Chapter 81.

Guanylin is secreted by cells of the intestinal mucosa. It causes increased chloride secretion into the intestine through the group IIB hormonal mechanism. The enterotoxin of certain strains of *Escherichia coli* has a structure similar to guanylin and causes diarrhea by increasing intestinal chloride secretion.

Hormonal Feedback Controls

Gastrointestinal hormones exert feedback control on several GI functions. One example is the control of acidity in the

duodenum (**Fig. 72.1A**). When the acid enters the duodenum, it inhibits gastrin secretion and stomach motility, both of which reduce the entry of the acidic chyme into the duodenum. Hence, gastrin secretion is elevated in achlorhydria. At

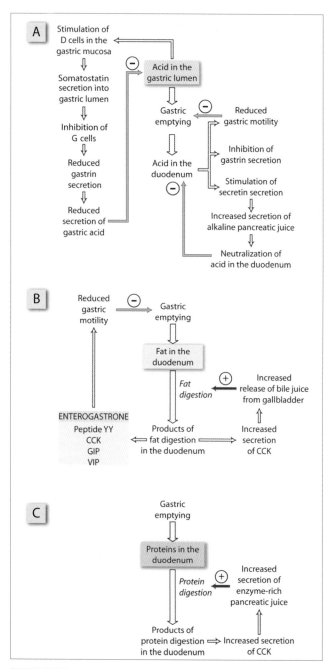

Fig. 72.1 Feedback control of gastrointestinal (GI) functions that are mediated through GI hormones. **(A)** Negative feedback control of duodenal acidity. **(B)** Positive and **(C)** negative feedback stimulated by the presence of food in the duodenum control the digestion of fats and proteins. *Red arrows* represent stimulatory effects; *blue arrows* represent inhibitory effects. CCK, cholecystokinin; GIP, gastric inhibitory polypeptide; VIP, vasoactive intestinal peptide.

Table 72.1 Summary of the Properties of Gastrin, Cholecystokinin, and Secretin

	Gastrin	Cholecystokinin	Secretin
Secreted by	G cells in antral and duodenal mucosa	Mucosa of upper intestine	S cells in ileal mucosal glands
	TG cells in stomach and ileum	Brain and nerves	
	Pancreatic islets in fetus		
	Pituitary		
	Brain and nerves		
Stimulated by	Peptides and amino acids in stomach and duodenum	Peptides and amino acids in small intestine	Peptides and amino acids in small intestine
	Distention of stomach	Fatty acids (> 10 carbons) in duodenum	Acid in small intestine
	Vagal neurotransmitter GRP		
	Epinephrine		
Inhibited by	Acid in duodenum		
	Secretin, GIP, VIP, CCK		
	Glucagon		
	Calcitonin		
Mode of action	Group IIC hormone	Group IIC hormone	Group IIA hormone
Effects on exocrine secretions	Gastric acid (+)	Pancreatic enzymes (+)	Pancreatic HCO_3^- (+)
	Pepsin (+)	Enterokinase (+)	Hepatic bile (+)
			Gastric acid (−)
Effects on endocrine secretions	Insulin (+)	Insulin (+)	Glucagon (−)
	Glucagon (+)	Glucagon (+)	Potentiates CCK
		Potentiates secretin	
Effects on gastrointestinal motility	Gastric motility (+)	Pyloric sphincter tone (+)	Pyloric sphincter tone (+)
		Gastric emptying (−)	
		Gallbladder contraction (+)	
		Small intestine, colon motility (+)	
Other effects	Trophic effect on the mucosa of stomach, ileum, and colon	Trophic effect on pancreas	
		Satiety	

Abbreviations: CCK, cholecystokinin; GIP, gastric inhibitory polypeptide; GRP, gastrin-releasing polypeptide; VIP, vasoactive intestinal peptide.

the same time, the release of secretin by acid exerts another feedback control on acidity. Secretin causes copious secretion of alkaline pancreatic juice into the duodenum, neutralizing the acid from the stomach.

Similarly, the digestion of fats (**Fig. 72.1B**) and protein (**Fig. 72.1C**) is controlled by feedback involving CCK. Bile and pancreatic juice promote the digestion of fat and protein, respectively. The products of this digestion stimulate further CCK secretion and secretion of other hormones, thus resulting in a positive feedback that stops only when the products of digestion move farther down the GI tract.

Anticipatory Secretion of Insulin and Glucagon

Glucose absorbed from the intestine stimulates the pancreas to secrete insulin, which prevents hyperglycemia. Amino acids absorbed from the intestine stimulate the release of both insulin and glucagon from the pancreas. This ensures that a protein-rich zero-carbohydrate diet does not produce hypoglycemia due to insulin secretion alone.

There is also an anticipatory increase in the secretion of insulin and glucagon even before the glucose and amino acids are absorbed. This anticipatory increase is mediated by GI hormones (**Fig. 72.2**).

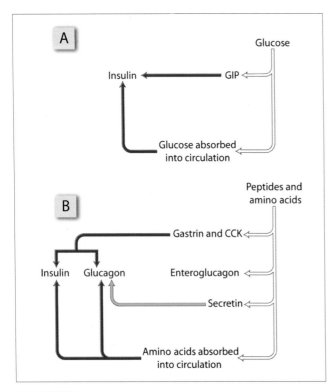

Fig. 72.2 Gastrointestinal hormones mediating an anticipatory secretion of insulin in response to **(A)** glucose and **(B)** insulin and glucagon in response to the presence of peptides and amino acids in the intestine. *Red arrows* represent stimulatory effect; *blue arrows* represent inhibitory effects. CCK, cholecystokinin; GIP, gastric inhibitory polypeptide.

Summary

- The three major gastrointestinal hormones are gastrin, CCK–pancreozymin, and secretin.

- Gastrin is released by G cells in the antrum of the stomach and in the duodenum. The stimuli for release include amino acids, distention of the stomach, and vagal activity. Gastrin stimulates gastric acid secretion and gastric motility. CCK is secreted in the duodenum stimulated by products of digestion. CCK causes contraction of the gallbladder and the opening of the sphincter of Oddi.

- Secretin is secreted by cells in the jejunum stimulated by H⁺ ions and the products of protein digestion. One major function is the stimulation of a bicarbonate-rich pancreatic juice.

Applying What You Know

72.1. Mrs. Schilling has steatorrhea, fat in her stool. Blocking the action of which of the gastrointestinal hormones would make this problem worse? Explain the mechanism.

Upper Gastrointestinal Disorders

Disorders of the Lower Esophageal Sphincter

Achalasia is a condition in which the lower esophageal sphincter (LES) has a high basal tone and relaxes incompletely on swallowing. The esophagus becomes massively dilated due to accumulation of food in it (**Fig. 73.1**). The condition is treated by pneumatic dilation of the sphincter or incision of the esophageal muscle (myotomy). Injection of botulinum toxin into the LES inhibits release of acetylcholine (ACh) from vagal endings in the LES, producing lasting relief.

Gastroesophageal reflux occurs due to the incompetence of the LES, allowing the acidic gastric contents to regurgitate into the esophagus. It causes esophagitis, ulceration, scarring, and stricture of the esophagus. The condition is treated by inhibition of acid secretion with histamine (H2) receptor blockers. It can also be controlled surgically by fundoplication, which is wrapping a portion of the fundus of the stomach around the lower esophagus so that the LES is inside a short tunnel of stomach.

Vomiting (Emesis)

Vomiting is the rapid ejection of gastric contents caused by reversed peristalsis in the intestine aided by simultaneous contraction of abdominal muscles and diaphragm. The sequence of events during vomiting is as follows. (1) The breath is held in midinspiration followed by closure of the glottis. This prevents the aspiration of vomitus. (2) The hyoid moves upward and forward, resulting in the pulling open of the upper esophageal sphincter. (3) A reverse peristaltic wave originating in the middle of the intestine propels the chyme into the duodenum. The stomach and its pyloric sphincter relax to receive the duodenal contents. (4) An increase in the abdominal pressure forces the chyme into the esophagus and out of the mouth.

The coordinated response is controlled by a vomiting center in the reticular formation of the medulla. The center lies close to the nucleus of tractus solitarius (NTS) in the medulla. It controls the peripheral components of the vomiting act through cranial nerves (CNs) V, VII, IX, X, and XII (**Fig. 73.2**). Vomiting is often preceded by retching, which involves all the sequences of vomiting, but produces no vomitus. The chyme is not ejected because the abdominal pressure is not strong enough to overcome the resistance of the upper esophageal sphincter.

There are different ways in which the vomiting center is stimulated. (1) Irritation of upper gastrointestinal (GI) mucosa is a common cause of vomiting. Vomiting can also be initiated through the gag reflex by physical stimulation of the back of the throat. These afferent impulses reach the vomiting center through CN IX and CN X. (2) Emetic drugs such as apomorphine and ipecac can trigger vomiting. These stimulate the chemoreceptor trigger zone located in or near the area postrema.

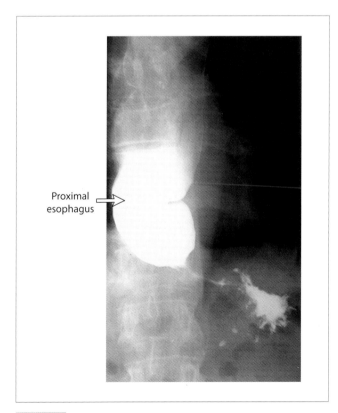

Fig. 73.1 Achalasia. The grossly dilated proximal esophagus and the narrow ganglion depleted segment are outlined radiographically after the administration of oral contrast medium.

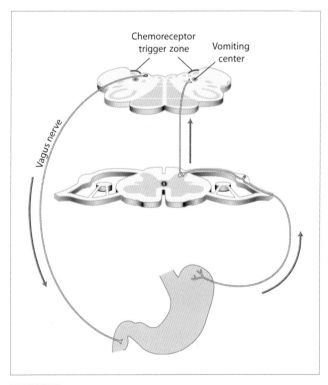

Fig. 73.2 The anatomic pathway underlying the vomiting reflex.

Impulses from the chemoreceptor trigger zone are relayed to the vomiting center. The neurons in the chemoreceptor trigger zone appear to be dopaminergic and serotonergic. Dopamine and serotonin antagonists are therefore effective antiemetic drugs. The vomiting that occurs in uremia and in radiation sickness is also mediated through the chemoreceptor trigger zone and occurs due to the endogenous production of emetic substances. (3) Motion sickness is associated with vomiting. The stimulus causing such vomiting originates in the vestibular apparatus (inner ear). The afferent impulses relay in the vestibular nuclei and then in the chemoreceptor trigger zone before finally reaching the vomiting center. (4) Raised intracranial tension stimulates the vomiting center directly, causing *projectile vomiting*—a rapid, forceful vomiting not accompanied by nausea. (5) Psychic stimuli, such as sickening sights and foul odors, cause vomiting. The neural pathways involved in such vomiting reach the vomiting center from the limbic system. (6) Severe visceral pain of any kind is known to cause vomiting even when the pain does not involve the GI tract. Thus, the severe pain associated with testicular torsion can produce vomiting.

Peptic Ulcer

Peptic ulcers result from an imbalance between the gastroduodenal mucosal defense mechanisms and the damaging forces that tend to breach the mucosal barrier. The factors that are damaging to the mucosal barrier are as follows. (1) The damaging effect of excessive acid-pepsin secretion is obvious in Zollinger-Ellison syndrome in which there are multiple peptic ulcerations due to excessive acid production by gastrinomas. On the other hand, the role of the acid is put into doubt by the fact that few patients with duodenal ulcers and fewer patients with gastric ulcers show hypersecretion of acid. When present, the hypersecretion of acid is due to increased parietal cell mass, increased sensitivity to secretory stimuli, or impaired inhibition of gastrin release. In some patients with duodenal ulcers, a very rapid gastric emptying into the duodenum may be responsible for damaging the duodenal mucosa by exposing it to excessive acid load. (2) *Helicobacter pylori* infection is present in more than 90% of patients with duodenal ulcers and 70% of those with gastric ulcers. *H. pylori* releases urease, which generates ammonia, and protease, which damages the mucosa. (3) Smoking impairs healing and favors recurrence of ulcers, possibly because it suppresses mucosal prostaglandin synthesis. Alcohol predisposes to ulcers, but the mechanism is not known. (4) Nonsteroidal antiinflammatory drugs (NSAIDs) such as aspirin have a direct irritative effect on the mucosa. They also suppress the synthesis of prostaglandin, which is a physiologic stimulator of mucus secretion. (5) Psychologic stress predisposes to ulcers because stress is associated with chronically elevated plasma levels of epinephrine, which inhibits bicarbonate secretion.

Lower Gastrointestinal Disorders

Disorders of Intestinal Transit

Dumping syndrome | In gastrectomized patients, there is rapid and unregulated dumping of the chyme into the intestine. This has two consequences; one immediately after a meal (the early dumping syndrome) and the other about 2 hours after meals (the late dumping syndrome). In both cases, the attacks last for about a half hour. Early dumping syndrome is associated with hypovolemia and hypotension because the hyperosmotic chyme entering the duodenum results in large amounts of fluid moving from the circulation into the intestinal lumen. Late dumping syndrome occurs due to hypoglycemia. It occurs because the rapid entry of the chyme into the intestine results in rapid absorption of glucose from the intestine. The sudden hyperglycemia induces an abrupt rise in insulin (see Chapter 81) secretion, which overcorrects the hyperglycemia, causing hypoglycemia. The symptoms include weakness, dizziness, and sweating after meals. Apart from dumping syndrome, gastrectomy is also associated with intrinsic factor deficiency, which must be corrected by parenteral injection of cyanocobalamin.

Adynamic ileus | Peritonitis inhibits intestinal motility through reflex stimulation of sympathetic discharge. Intestinal motility is also reduced following mechanical injury to the intestine. In either case, the result is paralytic (adynamic) ileus. In adynamic ileus, the intestinal contents do not move into the colon due to reduced motility, and the intestine becomes irregularly distended by alternate pockets of fluids and gases that appear as multiple air-fluid levels in a radiograph. Fluid levels are not seen normally because the peristaltic churning of fluids with detergents (bile salts) makes the intestinal contents frothy. Adynamic ileus can be relieved by passing a tube through the nose down to the small intestine and aspirating the fluid and gas for a few days until peristalsis returns. Adynamic ileus is commonly seen after abdominal operations. Intestinal peristalsis normally returns 6 to 8 hours after an operation followed by gastric peristalsis, but colonic activity takes 2 to 3 days to return. Passing of flatus by a postoperative patient signifies the resumption of his colonic activity.

Intestinal obstruction | The radiographic appearance of multiple air-fluid levels is also observed in mechanical obstruction of the intestine. However, unlike adynamic ileus, which is usually painless, mechanical obstruction causes severe cramping pain. Proximal to the obstruction, the luminal pressure rises, and the blood vessels in the intestinal wall are compressed, causing ischemia. The intestinal distention aggravates the internal fluid losses by stimulating intestinal secretion. Stimulation of the afferent nerve fibers from the distended segment causes sweating, severe vomiting, and hypotension. The overstretched intestinal wall above the level of the obstruction loses its contractility and becomes completely paralyzed. Patches of necrosis develop on the intestinal wall, leading to perforation. When luminal obstruction is associated with venous obstruction, there is intense capillary engorgement. The peritoneum and the gut lumen fill with plasma exudate. Microbes proliferate in the bowel, liberating toxins. Unrelieved obstruction is fatal.

Several effects of intestinal obstruction depend on the site of obstruction. In high small-intestine obstruction (obstruction occurring in the proximal parts of the small intestine), the absorption of food, water, and digestive juices is impaired. These fluids accumulate above the block and distend the bowel, setting up powerful, colicky peristaltic movements and profuse vomiting. The fluid lost is isosmotic, and its pH is neutral or slightly acidic. The loss of fluids results in dehydration; the loss of acids results in alkalosis. In low small intestine obstruction, symptoms develop more gradually and are less severe as there is a longer segment of normal intestine above the block that can absorb water and solutes.

Malabsorption syndrome | The term *malabsorption syndrome* encompasses several different types of disorders that impair the process of absorption. Generally, the causes of malabsorption syndrome are as follows.

Inadequate digestion is commonly caused by exocrine pancreatic insufficiency. Pancreatic lipase is the principal enzyme that digests fats. In its absence, not only are fats not digested, but the digestion of other foods also suffers. This is because undigested fat forms a coating over the chyme and prevents the penetration of the chyme by enzymes digesting proteins and carbohydrates. The absorption of fat-soluble vitamins (A, D, E, and K) also suffers. Due to reduced fat absorption, the stools become bulky, pale, foul-smelling, and greasy (steatorrhea).

Malabsorption is also caused by deficiency of oligosaccharidases (i.e., lactase) normally present on the intestinal brush border. In such patients, ingestion of sugar causes diarrhea, bloating, and flatulence. The diarrhea is due to the increased number of osmotically active oligosaccharide molecules that remain in the intestinal lumen, resulting in osmotic swelling of the intestinal contents. In the colon, bacteria break down some of the oligosaccharides, further increasing the number of osmotically active particles. The bloating and flatulence are due to the bacterial production of gas (carbon dioxide and hydrogen) from disaccharide residues in the lower ileum and colon.

About 50% of the world's population is lactose intolerant due to low intestinal lactose activity; these individuals suffer from osmotic diarrhea on milk consumption. Yogurt is better tolerated than milk because it contains only bacterial lactose. Lactose intolerance can be treated by an administration of commercial lactose preparations.

Low intestinal bile salt concentration in the intestine, as occurs in liver diseases, reduces fat absorption by impairing micelle formation. Impaired absorption of fats results in steatorrhea. Patients of gastrinoma (gastrin-secreting tumor) who secrete large amounts of gastric acid, often have steatorrhea. The acid enters the duodenum in large amounts and inactivates pancreatic lipase. The acid also precipitates some bile salts. Both contribute to steatorrhea.

Blind loop syndrome | Overgrowth of bacteria within the intestinal lumen can cause steatorrhea due to excessive hydrolysis of conjugated bile salts by the bacteria, and deficiency of vitamin B_{12} due to its consumption by the bacteria. Such overgrowth occurs when there is stasis of ileal contents. It has been named the blind loop syndrome because the condition is common in patients with surgically created blind loops of small intestine. However, it can occur in any condition that promotes massive bacterial contamination of the small intestine.

Inadequate absorptive surface | Removal of short segments of the small intestine generally does not cause severe symptoms because there is compensatory hypertrophy and hyperplasia of the remaining mucosa with gradual normalization of absorptive function (intestinal adaptation). When more than half the small intestine is resected or affected by disease, the absorption of nutrients is compromised, resulting in malnutrition (short bowel syndrome). Because the jejunum has less adaptive capacity than the ileum, distal small bowel resection causes greater malabsorption than removal of a comparable length of proximal small bowel. Intestinal resection also interrupts the enterohepatic circulation of bile salts and thereby aggravates the malabsorption.

Mucosal absorptive defects | An example of a mucosal absorptive defect is gluten-induced enteropathy, also known as celiac sprue or nontropical sprue. Gluten and the related substance gliadin are high-molecular-weight proteins found in wheat primarily, but also in other grains. There is good reason to believe that gliadin triggers an immunologic reaction in the intestinal mucosa that causes damage to the cells and their functions. Another related mucosal absorptive disorder is tropical sprue, which occurs in tropical countries. It is associated with damage to the jejunal mucosa. Its cause is unknown.

Lymphatic obstruction | Because substances absorbed from the intestine must first pass through the lymphatics before entering the veins, lymphatic obstruction causes malabsorption.

Constipation

Constipation and diarrhea are two disorders that are associated with changes in the frequency of bowel movements. Although the two terms are often used as antonyms, their mechanisms are considerably different. Defects in GI motility often underlie constipation but are an uncommon cause of diarrhea. Constipation is difficult to define in terms of the number of bowel movements per day. Many normal humans defecate as infrequently as once every 2 to 3 days or as often as thrice a day. The only symptoms caused by constipation are slight anorexia and mild abdominal discomfort and distention. These symptoms are not due to absorption of toxic substances as was thought earlier because they are promptly relieved by evacuating the rectum and can be reproduced by distending the rectum with inert material. One of the known causes of constipation is Hirschsprung disease. In many patients, the precise cause of the constipation remains unknown and is therefore designated as idiopathic constipation.

Hirschsprung disease is also called aganglionic megacolon. It occurs in children due to congenital absence of the ganglion cells in the myenteric and submucous plexuses of a segment of the distal colon. It results from a failure of the normal cranial-to-caudal migration of neuroblasts during embryonic development. This migration requires the action of endothelins, and the migration fails when there is a mutation in the endothelin B receptor gene.

The absence of peristalsis causes feces to pass the aganglionic colonic segment with difficulty and the afflicted child may defecate as infrequently as once every 3 weeks. The clinical features include abdominal distention and anorexia. The condition can be relieved if the aganglionic segment of the colon is resected, and the segment of the colon above it is anastomosed to the rectum.

Idiopathic constipation is defined as infrequent defecation (less than two bowel movements weekly) due to unestablished cause. It has long been thought to be related to decreased dietary fiber intake, decreased water intake, decreased physical activity, increased serum progesterone levels in women, failure to respond to the urge to defecate, or damage to colonic nerves induced by chronic ingestion of stimulant laxatives. None of these theories is supported by available scientific information. Although insufficient dietary fiber is still considered a major cause of constipation, fiber supplementation does not normalize stool output and frequency in patients with idiopathic constipation.

Constipation in aged patients may be due to colonic spasm caused by a decrease in the vasoactive intestinal peptide- (VIP-) containing inhibitory neurons in colonic myenteric plexus. Idiopathic constipation can also occur in patients who are unable to expel stool from the rectum due to spastic contraction of the pelvic floor musculature (*anismus or spastic pelvic floor syndrome*).

Diarrhea

Diarrhea is both a symptom (what the patient complains of) and a sign (what the physician observes). As a symptom, the term *diarrhea* means an increase in stool frequency or volume or decreased stool consistency. As a sign, diarrhea is defined as an increase in stool weight of more than 250 g/day. About 9 L of fluids (2 L from the diet and 7 L representing secretions from the gut and pancreas) enters the GI tract each day. All but 100 to 200 mL of this fluid is reabsorbed. Diarrhea results when there is an imbalance between absorption and secretion in the intestine.

Osmotic diarrhea | Inadequate digestion of dietary carbohydrates leads to impaired absorption, causing luminal hyperosmolarity and the movement of water into the intestines from the vascular compartment. The resulting diarrhea, called osmotic diarrhea, stops when the individual stops eating.

Diarrhea due to decreased absorption is uncommon and is mostly due to congenital absence of specific transporters. For example, congenital chloridorrhea represents an inability to absorb chloride (Cl^-) due to the lack of Cl^-–HCO_3^- exchange in ileal and colonic mucosa. Antibiotics produce diarrhea by suppressing colonic flora, reducing short-chain fatty acid production and thereby diminishing absorption of fluid and electrolytes.

Diarrhea due to intestinal hypermotility is uncommon and is usually associated with secretory diarrhea (see below). The offending agent stimulates both epithelial cells (causing increased fluid secretion) and smooth muscle cells (causing increased motility).

Secretory diarrhea is produced by secretagogues (agents that induce net fluid and electrolyte secretion in the intestine), such as bacterial enterotoxins and neurohumoral agents. When bound to the intestinal epithelial cells, enterotoxins cause diarrhea by stimulating intracellular second messenger systems.

The classical example of enterotoxin-induced diarrhea is cholera. Its causative agent, *Vibrio cholerae*, does not invade the mucosa, but produces an enterotoxin that binds to receptors on the brush border membrane. The enterotoxin activates the group IIA hormonal mechanism (see **Fig. 75.5**), which reduces the absorption of sodium (Na^+) and Cl^-, leading to reduced water reabsorption and diarrhea. Although it inhibits NaCl absorption by the villus cells, enterotoxin does not affect Na^+–glucose cotransport activity. This is important clinically because glucose–electrolyte solutions given orally are absorbed normally and can entirely replace the need for lifesaving intravenous fluids in patients with cholera.

Neurohumoral agents that regulate intestinal fluid and electrolyte transport cause diarrhea when present in excess. For example, excess VIP causes *watery diarrhea syndrome*, and excess serotonin produces diarrhea in *carcinoid syndrome*. The diarrhea of hyperthyroidism is also an example of secretory diarrhea.

Protein-losing Enteropathy

Small amounts of protein normally filter out of the capillaries into the intestinal lumen. However, when inflammation is present, large amounts of proteins can filter into the intestinal lumen, often resulting in hypoproteinemia.

Disorders of Gastrointestinal-associated Organs

Xerostomia

Temporary inhibition of salivary gland secretion may be caused by infections or anticholinergic agents. More permanent inhibition of secretion results with damage that occurs when head or neck tumors are irradiated. Permanent damage to salivary glands also occurs with Sjögren syndrome, an autoimmune disorder. These disorders lead to dryness of the mouth (xerostomia), difficulty with speech and swallowing, extensive dental caries, and disturbances of taste.

Gallstones

Gallstones afflict up to 20% of the population (although only a fraction of the individuals with gallstones will develop symptoms). Women are much more likely than men to develop gallstones, apparently because of the effects of estrogen on cholesterol metabolism. This means that women who have had children or taken birth control pills are at a higher risk. Increasing age is also a factor.

Gallstones are most commonly made of cholesterol (cholesterol gallstones); others are made of bilirubin calcium salts (pigment gallstones). The most prominent symptom of gallstones is an excruciating biliary pain. When gallstones obstruct the bile duct, it results in obstructive jaundice, steatorrhea, and bleeding tendencies due to defective absorption of vitamin K.

Cholesterol gallstones | Cholesterol is normally rendered soluble in bile by aggregation with water-soluble bile salts and water-insoluble lecithin. When cholesterol concentration exceeds the solubilizing capacity of bile (supersaturation), it starts forming crystals of cholesterol monohydrate (**Fig. 73.3**). This process is called nucleation and is promoted by the

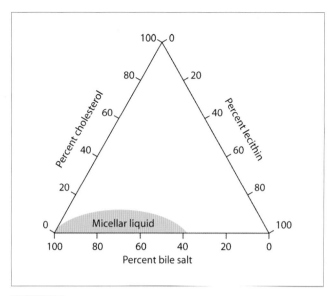

Fig. 73.3 Cholesterol solubility in bile as a function of the proportions of lecithin, bile salts, and cholesterol. If the bile has a composition described by any point in the deeply shaded area, its cholesterol is entirely in micellar solution. Points outside the deeply shaded area describe bile in which there are cholesterol crystals as well.

presence of microprecipitates of calcium salts, which may serve as nucleation sites for cholesterol stones.

If the bile stays longer in the gallbladder, it becomes concentrated and supersaturated with cholesterol, predisposing to gallstones. Prolonged fasting causes infrequent gallbladder contraction and thereby promotes gallstone formation. Pregnancy promotes gallstones because progesterone reduces gallbladder smooth muscle tone and therefore causes bile stasis. Bile stasis can also be due to defective gallbladder motility or diminished responsiveness to cholecystokinin.

Pigment gallstones are formed by the precipitation of calcium salts of unconjugated bilirubin. Bile contains mostly conjugated bilirubin, ~1% of which normally becomes deconjugated in the biliary tract. In hemolytic anemias, there is a rise in bile excretion, and with it, there is a rise in the deconjugated bilirubin, predisposing to pigment stones. Infection of the biliary tract, as with *Escherichia coli,* roundworm, or liver fluke causes deconjugation of conjugated bilirubin, predisposing to gallstones.

Summary

- Disorders of the upper GI system include achalasia (esophageal dilation), gastroesophageal reflux (movement of gastric acid into the esophagus), vomiting, and peptic ulcers.

- Lower GI disorders include disturbances of motility (dumping syndrome, ileus, intestinal obstruction), malabsorption (e.g., celiac sprue), constipation, and diarrhea.

- Disorders of associated digestive organs include xerostomia (inhibition of salivary secretion) and gallstones.

Answers to Applying What You Know

Chapter 66

1 Mrs. Schilling has been losing weight over the past month. What condition must be present if she is losing weight?

To lose weight, the number of calories "burned" by the body must be greater than the number of calories that are consumed and enter the body. If this is the case, regardless of how this imbalance is achieved (i.e., it does not matter what "diet" is being followed), then the body's expenditure of energy requires the use of already stored energy (fats in adipose cells); hence the loss of weight.

2 Mrs. Schilling's lethargy is most likely the result of her having too low quantities of which macronutrient available for use by the body? Explain.

All cells in the body can use carbohydrates (mostly in the form of glucose) as a source of energy production (adenosine triphosphate [ATP]). The body's store of glucose (or glycogen, a storage form) is relatively small and readily mobilized. Fats are stored in adipose cells, and though they can be used by some cells, this is not true of all cells. The most likely source of Mrs. Schilling's tiredness is a lack of available glucose.

Chapter 67

1 Mrs. Schilling has in the past taken several different pills (Imodium, calcium supplements). Is the mechanism involved in swallowing a pill a voluntary one, or is it a reflex? Explain.

Swallowing involves both a voluntary mechanism and a reflex mechanism. The voluntary component includes the elevation of the tongue followed by the contraction of the mylohyoid muscle. These voluntary actions force the pill being swallowed back to the wall of the pharynx. When the pill is pushed against the wall of the pharynx, sensory receptors in the wall are stimulated, giving rise to a reflex response, which delivers the pill to the upper esophagus without allowing it to enter the trachea. So, swallowing is both voluntary and a reflex.

2 Mrs. Schilling's saliva is tested to determine whether it is normal. Its pH is found to be 6.9 due to the bicarbonate that is present in it. Why is the maintenance of a slightly alkaline pH important for saliva function?

Saliva contains the enzyme amylase that begins the digestion of starches into sugars. Every enzyme operates with maximum effectiveness at some particular pH. Salivary amylase loses its effectiveness at acidic pH, and the bicarbonate secreted into saliva maintains the pH near its optimum value. When the chewed bolus of food (containing salivary amylase) reaches the stomach where the pH is very low, the enzyme is inactivated.

Chapter 68

1 Mrs. Schilling was prescribed an H_2 (histamine receptor) blocker to control her dyspepsia. What other kind of drug might be used to reduce hydrochloric acid (HCl) production?

Gastric acid secretion can be reduced by blocking any of the key steps illustrated in **Fig. 68.4**. For example, inactivating the carbonic anhydrase (CA) that is present in the parietal cells would block the production of H^+ ions. However, a pharmacologic blocking agent would have to be specific for parietal cell CA because CA plays a key role in the renal tubules and red blood cells. Blocking hydrogen carbonate ion (HCO_3^-) transport across the basolateral membrane would also inhibit H^+ formation by mass action. The most direct approach is to inhibit the hydrogen–potassium (H^+–K^+) exchanger (the "proton pump") at the luminal membrane, and there are several available drugs that do this. An H_2 blocker reduces acid secretion by blocking the receptor for histamine (see **Fig. 68.5**), a powerful stimulator of the parietal cell production of acid.

2 Mrs. Schilling begins suffering from abdominal distress within an hour or so of eating a meal. What effect might this have on her production of HCl?

Just as increased gastric acid secretion can be conditioned by the sight or smell of food, repeated bouts of abdominal distress after eating could decrease HCl production. The anticipated reaction, pain and/or discomfort, could result in *decreased* vagal activity and hence decreased acid production.

Chapter 69

1 Mrs. Schilling had a gallstone removed from her common bile duct. What are the effects of a gallstone?

A gallstone obstructs flow in the bile duct in which it is located. Therefore, bile juice accumulates behind the stone and stretches the wall of the duct. This stretch stimulates sensory endings and causes great pain. The obstruction also prevents bile juice from entering the duodenum and thus makes fat digestion more difficult.

2 Mrs. Schilling's abdominal computed tomography scan revealed pancreatic scarring and atrophy. What functions of the pancreas would be affected by these changes?

The pancreas has two important functions related to utilization of the food eaten. Exocrine glands produce pancreatic juice, a solution of bicarbonate and pancreatic enzymes. Both are required for normal digestion of ingested food, and hence absorption of nutrients (glucose, amino acids, lipids) in the intestine. The pancreas is also an endocrine gland secreting two hormones that play a major role in controlling metabolism, insulin, and glucagon (see Chapter 81). Damage to the pancreas can affect either or both of these important physiologic functions.

3 If Mrs. Schilling had a Schilling test performed (the names are a coincidence), it would probably show that she has a decreased rate of absorption of vitamin B_{12}. Which of Mrs. Schilling's signs and symptoms are probably related to her vitamin B_{12} deficiency?

Vitamin B_{12} plays an important role in the formation of hemoglobin and red blood cells. Lack of vitamin B_{12} can result in an anemia. Note that Mrs. Schillings' hemoglobin concentration is low. This condition could also be contributing to her lethargy because oxygen delivery to her tissues will be compromised by the reduced hemoglobin.

Chapter 70

1 Mrs. Schilling tried Imodium to control her diarrhea. This drug slows peristalsis in the intestine. How would this affect her diarrhea?

Slowing peristalsis will slow the movement of chyme from the intestine to the colon. There is thus more time for the transport processes in the walls of the intestine to absorb sodium and other substances. Because water moves with sodium, this will increase the absorption of water and reduce diarrhea.

2 Mrs. Schilling is given a solution of xylose to drink, and the appearance of xylose in her urine is measured. What changes in intestinal function would result in reduced renal excretion of xylose? Explain.

Xylose is a monosaccharide; therefore, it does not have to be enzymatically digested. Thus, the activity of amylases (their rate of production in the pancreas or the pH in the intestine) will have no effect of the rate of absorption. However, any damage or change to the villi and microvilli will affect the rate at which the xylose can be transported into the blood. A reduced rate of urinary excretion of xylose suggests a reduced rate of intestinal absorption and hence some problem with the transport mechanisms or structures involved.

3 Mrs. Schilling is suffering from steatorrhea, the appearance of large quantities of fat in her stool. What changes in intestinal function could result in this condition? Explain.

Fats are digested in the intestine by pancreatic lipases. These enzymes require an alkaline environment for optimal functioning. Thus, a reduction in the rate of production of lipases in the pancreas, or a decrease in bicarbonate production, will ad-

versely affect fat digestion. The brush border does not contain lipases. In addition, any reduction in the surface area available for absorption will result in increased fat in the stool.

4 During the physical examination, it is noted that Mrs. Schilling has numerous small bruises on her arms. What would cause this?

Mrs. Schilling's bruises are the consequence of impaired absorption of vitamin K, an essential component of the clotting mechanism. Because vitamin K is fat soluble, impaired fat absorption will also limit vitamin K absorption.

Chapter 71

1 Mrs. Schilling's frequent bouts of diarrhea could cause dehydration. Oral rehydration fluids contain both glucose and electrolytes, particularly sodium. Explain the mechanism by which this therapy works.

Absorption of water in the gastrointestinal tract is driven by an osmotic gradient across the walls of the intestine created by the active absorption of sodium. Sodium crosses the luminal membrane of the enterocytes coupled to the cotransport of glucose. Thus, rehydration fluids containing both sodium and glucose are most effective at promoting the absorption of water.

Chapter 72

1 Mrs. Schilling has steatorrhea, fat in her stool. Blocking the action of which of the gastrointestinal hormones would make this problem worse? Explain the mechanism.

The proper digestion of fat requires the presence of bile in the duodenum. Bile release from the gallbladder is stimulated by cholecystokinin (CCK) released from the duodenum when the secretory cells are stimulated by the products of fat digestion there. In addition, CCK reduces gastric motility and hence slows gastric emptying. This is important because it gives the duodenum the time needed to properly digest the fats present in the ingested food.

Thus, anything that blocks the action of CCK will speed up gastric emptying and reduce the amount of bile present. Fat digestion will be less complete, resulting in even more fat in Mrs. Schilling's stool.

Clinical Overview

Review of patient condition | Mrs. Schilling is suffering from celiac (nontropical) sprue, a disease in which intestinal digestion and absorption of food is reduced. The pathophysiology present arises from an immunologic response of her intestinal villi to gluten, a protein present in many grains.

Etiology | Celiac disease results from an immunologic response to a protein, gliadin (one form of gluten), found in certain grains, including wheat, barley, and rye. Antibodies to gliadin are formed as well as autoantibodies (that react with the body's own tissues), which cause in an inflammatory process that damages the mucosa of the small intestine.

Prevalence | This disease is undoubtedly underdiagnosed for a variety of reasons, but it is thought that more than 1% of Americans suffer from celiac sprue. Its prevalence varies considerably around the world. There is a genetic component to the disease, and relatives of a patient diagnosed with celiac sprue are much more likely to have the disease than an individual without that genetic background.

Diagnosis | The initial diagnosis is usually made from the patient's signs and symptoms. There are a variety of tests that can contribute to the diagnosis, including the xylose absorption test and the 24-hour fecal fat measurement. Radiologic studies can demonstrate abnormalities in the small intestine. Intestinal biopsy can directly demonstrate destruction of the villi and microvilli. Tests for the presence of the antibodies involved (immunoglobulins) have a high sensitivity and specificity and can confirm a diagnosis.

Treatment | Treatment consists of removing all gluten from the patient's diet. Although this is not easy to implement because wheat and other gluten-containing grains are present in a great many foods, it is becoming easier to accomplish, as the prevalence of the disease becomes better known, and manufacturers are beginning to produce gluten-free products. Reversal of symptoms can occur within a few weeks of removing gluten from the diet.

Understanding the Physiology

The intestinal brush border is essential for both digestion and absorption. It contains enzymes for the digestion of carbohydrates and proteins, and in their absence digestion of these two classes of nutrients is incomplete. The microvilli are also the site at which absorption of the products of digestion of carbohydrates, proteins, and fats occur. In a patient with celiac sprue, not only is digestion impaired, but the products of digestion cannot be absorbed.

There are several important consequences of this. The undigested chyme is hyperosmolar and pulls water into the intestine from the vascular compartment. This results in bloating and diarrhea. The volume of diarrheal fluid lost can contribute to electrolyte depletion. The stool produced contains a great deal of undigested dietary fat.

The failure to absorb nutrients leads to weight loss, particularly if the many gastrointestinal symptoms result in a reduced appetite.

The inability to absorb vitamins has other consequences. Anemia can result from the lack of folate and iron (her hemoglobin concentration is below normal). Coagulation time increases (her prothrombin time and international normalized ratio [INR] are too high) due to a lack of vitamin K. This, in turn, can result in easy bruising (seen on her upper arms). The failure to absorb amino acids results in reduced concentration of plasma proteins and albumin. The results can be edema formation due to decreased plasma oncotic pressure.

A flow chart (**Fig. VIII.1**) illustrating the mechanisms described here follows.

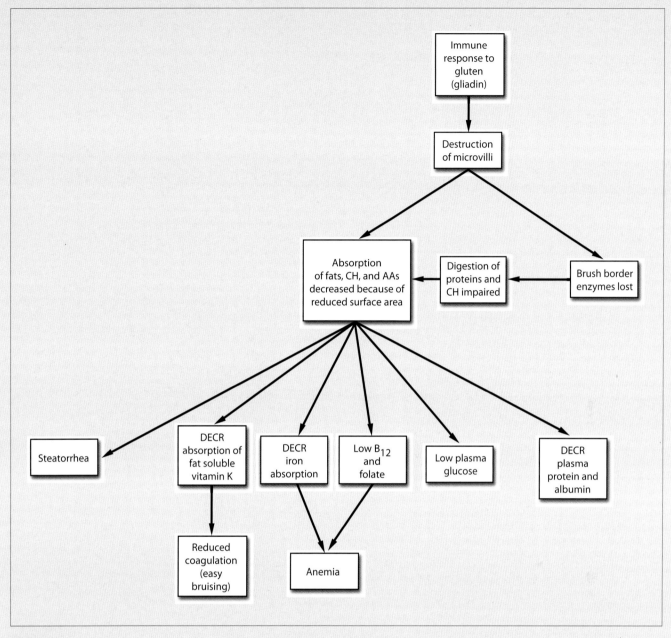

Fig. VIII.1 Mrs. Schilling's many problems begin with an inability to absorb macro- and micro-nutrients because of damage to her intestinal mucosa.

Section IX | Endocrine System

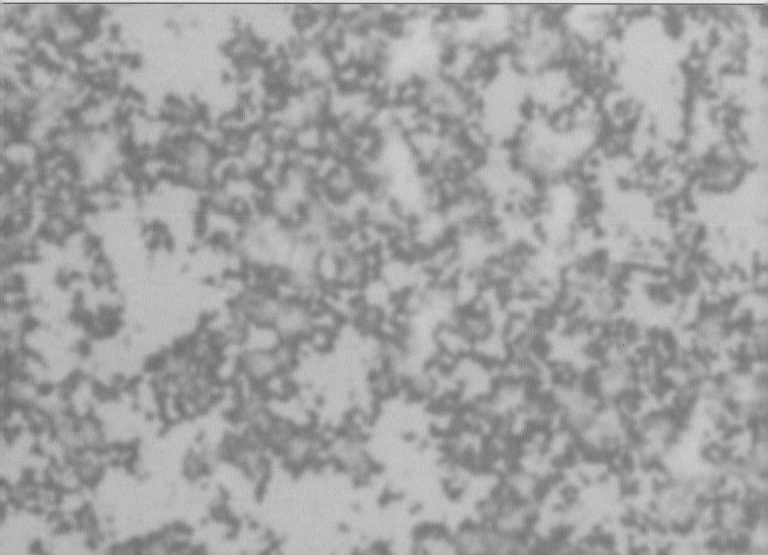

Overview

The endocrine system is one of the two major information processing systems of the body. We have already discussed the basic principles of neural information processing systems: generation and conduction of the action potential and synaptic transmission between neurons and neurons and effectors. The endocrine system also employs chemical signals to carry information throughout the body, although the mechanisms are somewhat different. The signal molecules are hormones that are produced in specialized cells in endocrine organs. The hormones are released into the extracellular space, where they diffuse into capillaries to be carried to every tissue, or the hormone molecules diffuse a short distance to affect neighboring cells.

Hormones must bind to a specific receptor to affect a cell's function. These receptors may be found on the cell membrane or inside the cell in the cytoplasm or in the nucleus. Every cell that has a receptor for a particular hormone will respond to the binding of that hormone to a receptor.

Hormones affect cell function by altering the activity of the enzymes that produce the metabolism of the cell. There are several different mechanisms by which the binding of a hormone molecule to a receptor brings about changes in enzyme activity.

Hormones are involved in maintaining water and electrolyte balance, regulating the metabolism of carbohydrates, proteins, and fats, regulating growth and development, and, as we will see in the final section, generating reproductive phenomena.

Section IX Case Presentation:
Mrs. Omaya has been tired since giving birth.

Chief Complaint

Roberta Omaya, a 27-year old woman, presents to you complaining of fatigue ever since she had a baby 9 months ago.

History of Present Illness

She had been in good health up to and throughout the pregnancy (her second). She recalls being told that she was mildly anemic, but she took vitamins and iron supplementation as prescribed.

Mrs. Omaya was able to nurse for only 1 month because her milk production was scant. She has not begun menstruating again since the delivery. She has been unable to lose the weight she gained during her pregnancy. She also notes that her skin has become rough and her voice deeper since the birth of her son.

Past Medical History

Mrs. Omaya has a 2-year-old child delivered by normal spontaneous vaginal delivery. She has had no significant medical problems, and her second pregnancy was easier than her first.

Physical Examination

- *General appearance* | Well-developed, well-nourished woman in no apparent distress
- *Vital signs*
  - Temperature: 98.6°F (oral)
  - Blood pressure: 100/70 mm Hg (sitting), 90/65 mm Hg (standing)
  - Pulse: 60/min (sitting), 80/min (standing)
- *Skin* | Coarse texture present
- *Lymph nodes* | No lymphadenopathy
- *HEENT (head, eyes, ears, nose, throat)* | Normal
- *Neck* | No masses or adenopathy
- *Lungs* | Clear to auscultation and percussion bilaterally
- *Cardiovascular* | Normal heart sounds without murmurs; pulses strong and symmetric
- *Abdomen* | Normal bowel sounds; soft, obese, nondistended, nontender, no organomegaly or masses
- *Extremities* | No cyanosis, clubbing, or edema
- *Neurological exam* | Normal except for deep tendon reflexes that are symmetric with slowed recovery throughout

Laboratory Tests

Plasma Concentration	Value	Normal Range (Female)
Sodium	128 mmol/L	137–147
Potassium	5.5 mmol/L	3.5–5.3
Chloride	102 mmol/L	99–108
CO_2	25 mmol/L	22–28
Glucose (fasting)	62 mq/dL	60–109

Past Medical History (Continued)

Following examination of the laboratory report, you continue questioning her about her pregnancy. Mrs. Omaya reports that her labor was uncomplicated and that she had a normal spontaneous vaginal delivery. However, there was some postpartum hemorrhage, and the placenta was retained. It was finally expressed 30 minutes after delivery, and it was followed by a huge blood clot. She was told that her blood pressure had dropped precipitously and that she had required a transfusion with 6 units of whole blood. Thereafter, her recovery was uneventful, and she was discharged 5 days later.

You order some additional tests.

Endocrine Laboratory Tests

	Value	Normal Range
Cortisol (8 AM)	3.0 µg/dL	5–25
Cortisol (4 PM)	2.9 µg/dL	3–15
Free T_4	0.4 µg/dL	0.6–1.7
Insulin-like growth factor (IGF-1)	64 ng/mL	90–360
Thyroid-stimulating hormone (TSH)	< 1.0 µU/mL	1–10
Prolactin (PRL)	3.6 ng/mL	5–25
Luteinizing hormone (LH)	2.8 mU/mL	5–30
Follicle-stimulating hormone (FSH)	2.3 mU/mL	5–16
Growth hormone (GH)	< 0.25 ng/mL	0–10

Diagnosis

Mrs. Omaya had experienced ischemic damage to the pituitary as a result of the hemorrhage that occurred during delivery. This damage resulted in hyposecretion of the anterior pituitary hormones.

Some Things to Think About

1. Mrs. Omaya's problems are the consequence of damage to her anterior pituitary. What differences between the two parts of the pituitary account for the fact that her posterior pituitary is normal?

2. Mrs. Omaya has reduced levels of many hormones. Which ones will need to be replaced or supplemented, and why?

3. Mrs. Omaya's fasting glucose level is at the low end of normal, although there is no reason to believe that her pancreas has been damaged. What hormones contribute to blood glucose regulation?

4. Mrs. Omaya's many symptoms are the result of deficiencies of certain hormones: some steroid hormones, and other protein or peptide hormones. By what mechanisms do these different hormones act?

Hormones alter cell function by altering the activity of enzymes and thus altering the cell's metabolism. Some of the important metabolic pathways involving carbohydrates, lipids, and proteins that are targets for hormone action are described here.

General Models: Energy and Homeostasis

The transformation and transfer of matter and the energy derived from it, in cells and between cells, are essential functions that must be performed in the living organism. The endocrine system plays a major role in controlling these metabolic pathways. The plasma concentration of glucose, an important component in these pathways, is homeostatically regulated.

Catabolism of Acetyl CoA

Acetyl coenzyme A (acetyl CoA) is formed by the catabolism (breakdown) of the three macronutrients—proteins, carbohydrates, and fats—and it represents the substrate for the final common catabolic pathway. Each molecule of acetyl CoA yields 12 molecules of adenosine triphosphate (ATP) when completely oxidized by passing through the Krebs cycle and the electron transport chain.

Krebs Cycle

The Krebs cycle is a cyclical metabolic pathway that begins with the formation of citric acid from oxaloacetic acid (a constituent of the cycle and acetyl CoA (derived from the breakdown of glucose and fatty acids). The cycle takes citric acid through a series of intermediates, finally regenerating the oxaloacetic acid. As citric acid is oxidized, nicotinamide adenine dinucleotide (NAD^+) is reduced to $NADH+H^+$, carbon dioxide (CO_2) is produced, and energy is released. The energy released is harnessed in ATP molecules (**Fig. 74.1**).

$$\text{Oxaloacetic acid} + \text{Acetyl CoA} + H_2O \rightarrow \text{Citric acid} + \text{Coenzyme A}$$

$$\text{Citric acid} + \text{ADP} + FAD^+ + 4NAD^+ \rightarrow \text{Oxaloacetic acid} + 2CO_2 + H_2O + \text{ATP} + FADH+H^+ + 4NADH+H^+$$

The net result is

$$\text{Acetyl CoA} + \text{ADP} + FAD^+ + 4NAD^+ \rightarrow \text{Coenzyme A} + 2CO_2 + \text{ATP} + FADH+H^+ + 4NADH+H^+$$

Although oxaloacetate is regenerated in the Krebs cycle, some amount of oxaloacetate is still lost and must be replenished regularly. The replenishment of oxaloacetate is provided by glycolysis (**Fig. 74.2**), and in the absence of the replenishment,

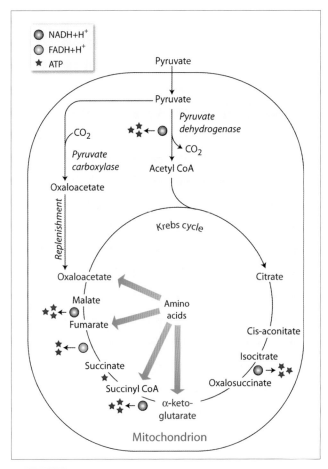

Fig. 74.1   The Krebs cycle is an important producer of adenosine triphosphate (ATP) used by cells to power all their activity. It begins with acetyl CoA combining with oxaloacetate, which is regenerated as the cycle proceeds. Some oxaloacetate is lost and is replaced by glycolysis.

the Krebs cycle slows down markedly. The fact that glycolysis is required for keeping the Krebs cycle running is important for understanding ketogenesis.

The $NADH+H^+$ produced (**Fig. 74.2**) is oxidized through the electron transport chain (**Fig. 74.3**) with the formation of more molecules of ATP and equally important, the regeneration of NAD^+ for reuse. The oxidation of $NADH+H^+$ is possible only when there is a sufficient availability of oxygen, which is during aerobic metabolism. In the absence of oxygen, NAD^+ is not regenerated and remains in its reduced $NADH+H^+$ form. The absence of NAD^+ has two important consequences. First, the Krebs cycle comes to a halt, resulting in substantial loss of ATP generation. Second, the pyruvate formed through glycolysis is not converted into acetyl CoA. Instead, it is reduced to lactate by $NADH+H^+$.

Each molecule of pyruvate fed into the Krebs cycle produces 1 ATP, 1 $FADH+H^+$, and 4 $NADH+H^+$. When the ATP yield of $FADH+H^+$ and $NADH+H^+$ are also considered, the Krebs cycle

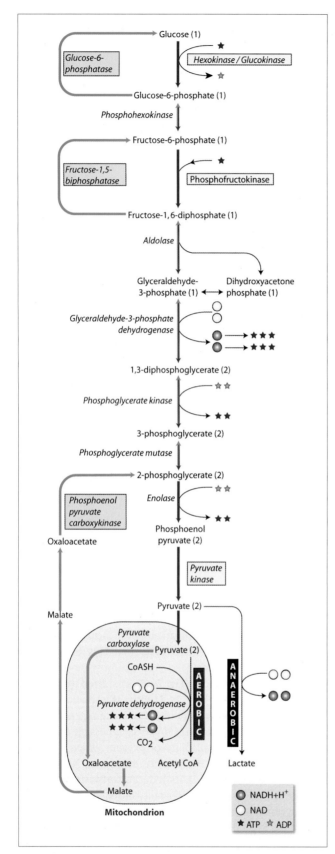

Fig. 74.2 Glycolytic and gluconeogenic pathways. Note that the metabolic steps in the middle can run in either direction. When the reactions run from top to bottom, glycolysis occurs; when they run from bottom to top, gluconeogenesis occurs.

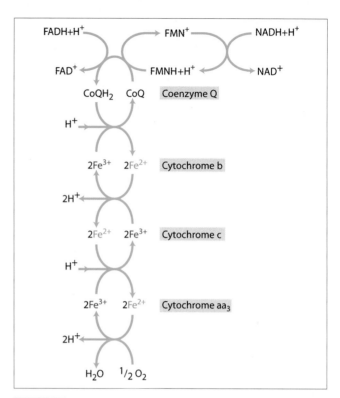

Fig. 74.3 Electron transport chain. The hydrogen (H^+) ions that are produced drive the activity of adenosine triphosphate (ATP) synthase molecules that make ATP.

produces 15 ATP molecules per pyruvate molecule. Because 1 molecule of glucose produces 2 molecules of pyruvate, the net yield from the Krebs cycle per molecule of glucose is 30 ATP molecules.

Electron Transport Chain

The catabolism of carbohydrates, fats, and proteins not only releases energy that is harnessed in ATP molecules, but also yields reduced coenzymes like $NADH+H^+$ and $FADH+H^+$ that are excellent fuels for oxidation and energy release. These must react with oxygen for maximum release of energy. However, transfer of the hydrogen atoms directly to oxygen would result in an extremely wasteful reaction. To avoid this, the reduced coenzymes are made to undergo oxidation (i.e., loss of an electron) in small steps, each of which releases a small amount of energy that is captured in ATP. Each step transfers the electron to a substrate with a slightly lower redox potential. These substrates constitute the electron transport chain (**Fig. 74.3**) or the respiratory chain. Each molecule of $NADH+H^+$ and $FADH+H^+$, when oxidized completely through the electron transport chain, results in the formation of three and two molecules of ATP, respectively.

Carbohydrate Metabolism

Glycolysis

Embden-Meyerhof pathway | Glycolysis is the major pathway for glucose utilization in all cells. It can work under both

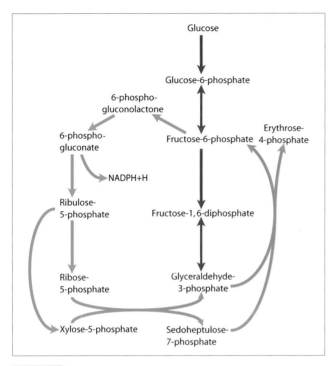

Fig. 74.4 Hexose monophosphate (HMP) shunt pathway.

aerobic and anaerobic conditions. In glycolysis, one molecule of glucose is oxidized to two molecules of pyruvate. In the process, there is a net gain of two ATP molecules (two are consumed, while four are produced). In addition, two molecules of NADH+H$^+$ are generated. These are oxidized through the electron transport chain, generating six molecules of ATP. The total yield of glycolysis under aerobic conditions is therefore eight molecules of ATP.

$$\text{Glucose} + 2\text{ATP} \rightarrow 2\text{Pyruvate} + 2\text{NADH+H}^+ (= 6\text{ATP}) + 4\text{ATP}$$

The pyruvate molecule can undergo two different reactions. Under *aerobic conditions,* it mostly diffuses into the mitochondria, is decarboxylated into acetyl CoA, and enters the Krebs cycle.

$$\text{Pyruvate} + \text{NAD}^+ + \text{CoA} \rightarrow \text{Acetyl CoA} + \text{NADH+H}^+ + \text{CO}_2$$

Under *anaerobic conditions,* the NADH+H$^+$ produced by glycolysis reduces the pyruvate to lactic acid. The reduction of pyruvate regenerates the NAD$^+$ from NADH+H$^+$, allowing the glycolysis to continue. However, because the two molecules of NADH+H$^+$ are spent in reduction of two molecules of pyruvate and not in ATP production, the net yield of glycolysis per molecule of glucose falls to two ATP molecules only.

$$\text{Pyruvate} + \text{NADH+H}^+ \rightarrow \text{Lactate} + \text{NAD}^+$$

HMP shunt pathway | Between glucose-6-phosphate and glyceraldehyde-3-phosphate, there is an alternate pathway for glycolysis called the *pentose phosphate pathway* or the *hexose monophosphate (HMP) shunt pathway* (**Fig. 74.4**). No ATPs are consumed or generated in this pathway. Its importance lies in the fact that (1) it produces ribose sugar that is essential for nucleic acid synthesis, and (2) it generates NADPH+H$^+$ (instead of NADH+H$^+$), which is essential for fatty acid and steroid biosynthesis. NADPH+H$^+$ is also required by the liver microsomal enzyme system that hydroxylates steroids, alcohols, and several drugs. NADPH+H$^+$ is required for antioxidant reactions and for the respiratory burst in phagocytes.

Glucose-sorbitol-fructose pathway | Glucose is also converted into fructose by way of sorbitol (**Fig. 74.5**). The pathway is present in sperm, where fructose is the preferred source of energy. The pathway is also present in liver cells, providing the cells with a mechanism through which dietary sorbitol can be fed into the glycolytic or gluconeogenic pathway.

The cells of the retina, lens, kidney, and nerves contain aldose reductase but not sorbitol dehydrogenase. Hence, these cells convert glucose into sorbitol but do not convert it further to fructose. When there is hyperglycemia, a large amount of glucose enters these cells and is converted into sorbitol. The accumulated sorbitol holds water, and the cell swells up due to osmosis. The retinopathy, cataract, nephropathy, and neuropathy of diabetes mellitus have been attributed partially to this osmotic swelling of the cells.

Gluconeogenesis

Gluconeogenesis (**Fig. 74.2**) is the synthesis of glucose from noncarbohydrate sources. It ensures a continuous supply of glucose (necessary for organs like the brain, exercising muscles, erythrocytes, cornea, and testes) even during starvation when there is no carbohydrate intake, and body glycogen stores are

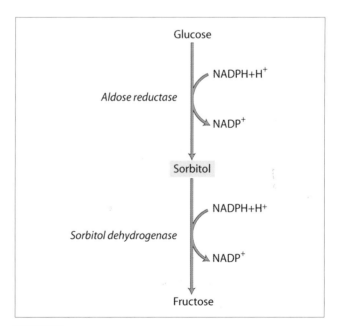

Fig. 74.5 Glucose-sorbitol-fructose pathway.

depleted. Ninety percent of the gluconeogenesis occurs in the liver, and 10% occurs in the kidneys. Gluconeogenesis is made possible by three key gluconeogenic enzymes that drive the glycolytic pathway in reverse gear, resulting in the formation of glucose from acetyl CoA. These three enzymes are *phosphoenol pyruvate kinase, fructose-1,5-biphosphatase,* and *glucose-6-phosphatase.*

Gluconeogenesis makes it possible to convert pyruvic acid to glucose. However, it cannot convert acetyl CoA to glucose due to the irreversibility of the reaction in which pyruvate is converted to acetyl CoA. It can be argued that because acetyl CoA is converted to oxaloacetate through the Krebs cycle, it should be convertible to glucose as well. That, however, is not so because when a molecule of acetyl CoA enters the Krebs cycle, it actually consumes a molecule of oxaloacetate rather than producing one. Hence, the molecule of oxaloacetate formed later in the cycle is only a regeneration of the molecule consumed earlier and therefore cannot result in a net glucose gain.

The irreversibility of the pyruvate-to-acetyl CoA conversion explains why fat, which yields acetyl CoA on hydrolysis, results in ketogenesis and not gluconeogenesis. For the same reason, leucine and lysine, which yield acetyl CoA on deamination, are called *ketogenic amino acids.* Amino acids that yield pyruvate are called *glucogenic amino acids.* Amino acids that yield oxaloacetate or any of its precursors in the Krebs cycle are also glucogenic (**Fig. 74.6**).

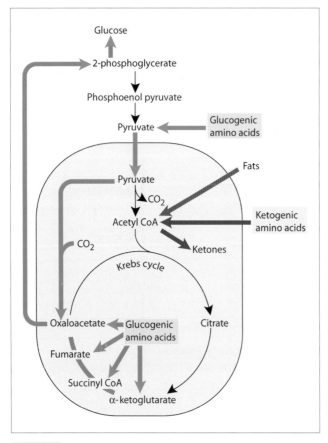

Fig. 74.6   Glucogenic and ketogenic amino acids.

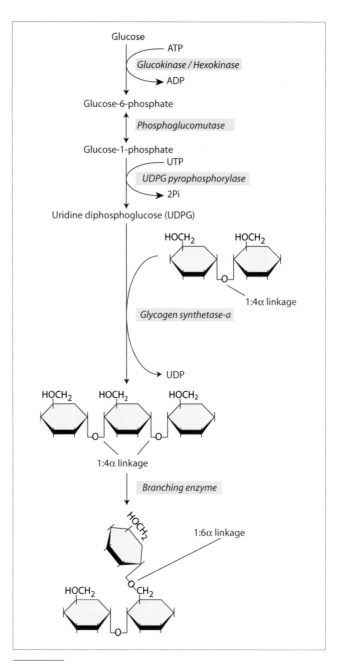

Fig. 74.7   Glycogenesis.

Glycogenesis

Glycogenesis (**Fig. 74.7**), or the synthesis of glycogen from glucose, occurs mainly in the organs that store glycogen: muscle and liver. Glycogenesis begins with the phosphorylation of glucose to glucose-6-phosphate. The reaction is catalyzed by *hexokinase* in muscle and *glucokinase* in liver. The glucose-6-phosphate isomerizes to glucose-1-phosphate and reacts with uridine triphosphate (UTP) to form uridine diphosphoglucose (UDPG). The UDPG molecules are the building blocks of glycogen. They bind to each other through 1:4α linkages in the presence of the enzyme *glycogen synthetase-a* to form long straight chains of glycogen. A *branching enzyme* brings ~1:6α linkages between UDPG molecules, resulting in the formation of branched glycogen molecules.

Glycogenolysis

Glycogenolysis (**Fig. 74.8**) is the breaking down of glycogen into glucose molecules. It involves delinking of single glucose molecules from glycogen by the enzyme *phosphorylase,* which breaks the 1:4α linkages, and the *debranching enzyme,* which breaks the 1:6α linkages. Because the linkages are phosphorylated before they are broken, the product of glycogenolysis is glucose-6-phosphate (and not glucose). In the liver, glucose-6-phosphate is dephosphorylated to glucose and released in blood. In the muscle, the glucose-6-phosphate produced is consumed by the muscle itself through glycolysis.

Glycogenesis and glycogenolysis are under hormonal control. The control, which is exerted through the enzymes glycogen synthetase and phosphorylase, is reciprocal: when one is stimulated, the other is inhibited (**Fig. 74.9**).

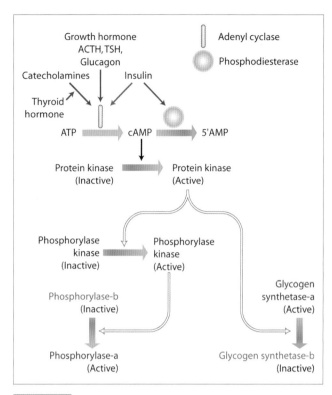

Fig. 74.9 Hormonal control of glycogenesis and glycogenolysis. Note the indicated changes from inactive states (*pink*) to active states (*blue*). ACTH, adrenocorticotrophic hormone; AMP, adenosine monophosphate; ATP, adenosine triphosphate; cAMP, cyclic adenosine monophosphate TSH, thyroid-stimulating hormone.

Fat Metabolism

Fatty Acid Synthesis

Fatty acid synthesis (**Fig. 74.10**) occurs primarily in liver and lactating mammary glands, and to a lesser extent, in adipose tissue and kidney. Fatty acids that occur in natural fats are straight chain derivatives and contain an even number of carbon atoms because the building units from which they are synthesized are the molecules of acetyl CoA, which have two carbon atoms each. Acetyl CoA is produced inside the mitochondria from various metabolic pathways. From there, it must enter the endoplasmic reticulum, where the biosynthesis of fatty acids takes place. Acetyl CoA cannot diffuse across the mitochondrial membrane. Hence, it is converted into citric acid and then reconverted into acetyl CoA after crossing the mitochondrial membrane and entering the cytosol. Once inside the endoplasmic reticulum, the enzyme *fatty acid elongase* condenses several molecules of acetyl CoA together into a growing chain of fatty acid. One by one, molecules of acetyl CoA are transferred from malonyl CoA to the growing chain. Malonyl CoA itself is formed by the carboxylation of acetyl CoA. Fatty acid biosynthesis requires NADPH+H$^+$ (instead of NADH+H$^+$), which comes from the HMP shunt pathway.

β-Oxidation of Fatty Acids

The β-oxidation of fatty acids (**Fig. 74.11**) occurs in all cells except neurons, erythrocytes, and adrenal medulla. In β-oxidation

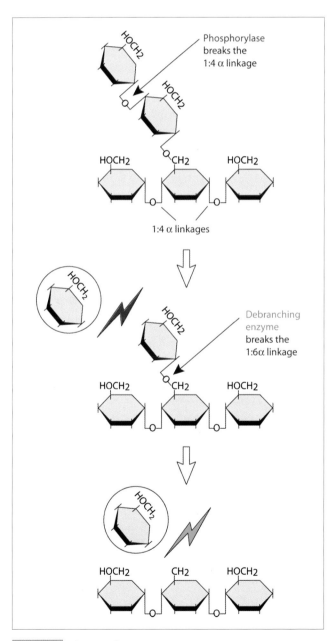

Fig. 74.8 Glycogenolysis.

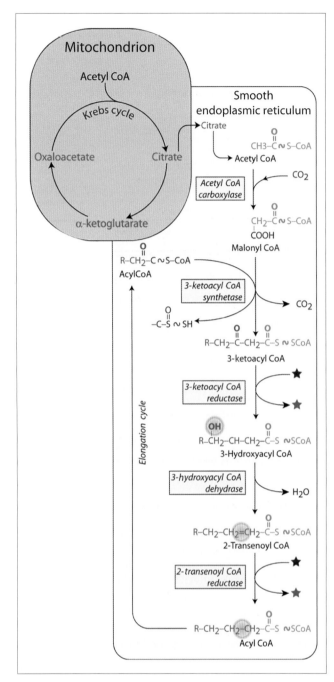

Fig. 74.10 Fatty acid synthesis.

through facilitated diffusion employing the membrane-bound carrier palmityl transferase. Once inside, the acyl CoA is converted to ketoacyl CoA through three intermediate steps that generate one molecule each of FADH+H⁺ and NADH+H⁺. In the final step, a molecule of acetyl CoA is split off from the acyl CoA molecule by the enzyme thiolase. The process repeats itself until the chain is broken down into acetyl CoA molecules.

A large number of ATP molecules are formed in the process. For example, in the case of a molecule of palmitate, 5 molecules of ATP are produced for each of the 7 molecules of acetyl CoA that are split off, giving a total of 35 ATP molecules. Each of the 8 molecules of acetyl CoA formed yields 12 molecules of ATP when fed into the Krebs cycle, giving a total of 96 ATP molecules. Subtracting the 2 molecules of ATP that are consumed for regenerating from AMP the single molecule of ATP consumed during the initial activation of fatty acid, the net gain from P-oxidation of one molecule of palmitate is 129 molecules of ATP.

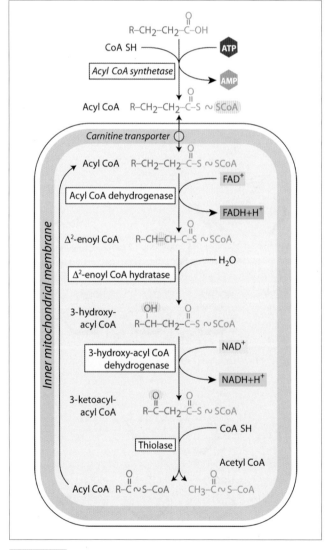

Fig. 74.11 β-oxidation of fatty acids.

of fatty acids, two carbon atoms are cleaved at a time from the acyl CoA molecule, starting at the carboxyl end. The chain is broken between the C-2 (earlier called α-carbon) and C-3 (earlier called β-carbon); hence the name. Much smaller amounts of α-oxidation, that is, removal of one carbon atom at a time, occur in the brain.

In β-oxidation, the fatty acid is first activated with a molecule of ATP. Further oxidation occurs in the mitochondria. The smaller acyl CoA molecules (e.g., acetyl CoA) enter the mitochondria easily, but the larger ones (e.g., palmitoyl CoA) must be transported across the inner mitochondria membrane

Ketogenesis

Ketone bodies, acetone and β-hydroxy butyric acid (**Fig. 74.12**), are formed in the mitochondria of hepatocytes by the condensation of two molecules of acetyl CoA. The liver constantly produces ketone bodies at a low rate. However, during starvation, large amounts of ketone bodies are formed by the liver. These are released into the bloodstream and transported to peripheral tissues for energy release. The heart prefers ketone bodies to glucose as a fuel. The brain can utilize ketone bodies only when their concentration in the blood is high. Erythrocytes cannot utilize ketone bodies at all.

The two prerequisites for ketone body formation are (1) reduction in the amount of glycolysis, and (2) production of large amounts of acetyl CoA from other sources, such as the oxidation of fatty acids and deamination of ketogenic amino acids. Both occur during starvation and in diabetes mellitus. The reason is as follows. During glycolysis, some of the pyruvate is converted into oxaloacetate. The oxaloacetate produced through glycolysis is important for replenishing the oxaloacetate lost from the Krebs cycle. Thus, if glycolysis is impaired or carbohydrates are completely removed from the diet, the Krebs cycle comes to a halt. The acetyl CoA molecules that are formed from proteins and fats are therefore unable to enter the Krebs cycle and instead, are converted into ketone bodies.

Lipogenesis

Lipogenesis (**Fig. 74.13**) is the production of lipids (triacylglycerol) from fatty acids and glycerol. It occurs in the liver and adipose tissues. Adipose tissue stores the synthesized lipids within itself, while the liver releases it into the bloodstream in the form of VLDL. As mentioned earlier, only small amounts of de novo fatty acid synthesis occur in adipose tissue.

Most of the fatty acids for lipogenesis in adipocytes come from dietary fat (in the form of chylomicrons) and a lesser amount from the liver as VLDL. For the reaction to occur, fatty acid must first be activated into acyl CoA by the enzyme acyl CoA synthetase, and glycerol must be phosphorylated by the

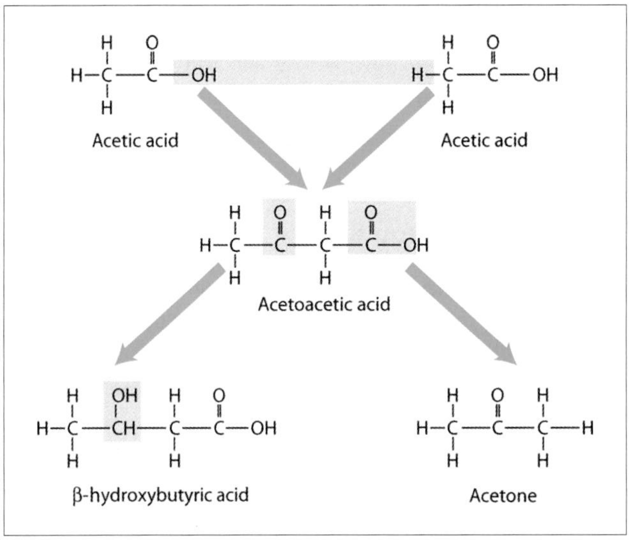

Fig. 74.12 Structure and formation of ketone bodies.

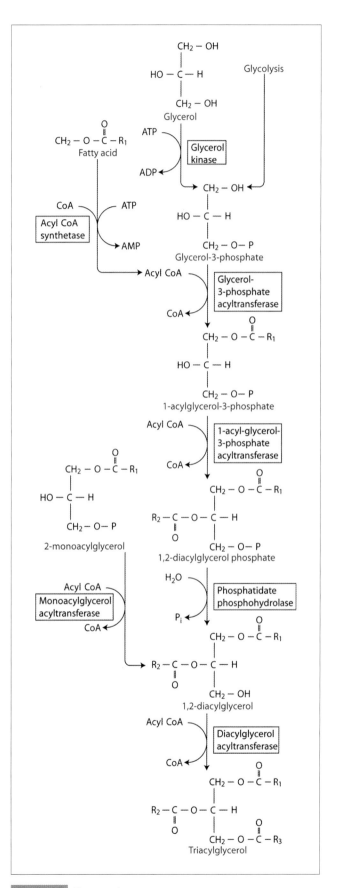

Fig. 74.13 Lipogenesis.

enzyme glycerol kinase. Glycerol kinase is absent in adipose tissue. However, the presence of glycerol kinase is not essential for lipogenesis because glycerol phosphate (phosphoglycerate, see **Fig. 74.2**) is also produced, in the liver as well as in adipose tissue, during glycolysis. Formation of triacylglycerol from acyl CoA and glycerol phosphate proceeds through four steps, as shown in **Fig. 74.13**.

Lipolysis

Lipids are stored only in adipose tissue; therefore, lipolysis occurs only in adipose tissue (**Fig. 74.14**). The triacylglycerol is hydrolyzed by the action of hormone-sensitive lipase into fatty acids and glycerol. The enzyme is activated by circulating catecholamines.

Protein Metabolism

About 1 to 2% of the total body protein, mostly muscle protein, is broken down daily into amino acids. Nearly 25% of these amino acids are deaminated; the rest are reutilized for protein synthesis. The breakdown of amino acids occurs in two steps.

In the first step, the amino acid that is to be degraded undergoes transamination. It transfers its NH_2 group to a keto acid called ketoglutarate, resulting in the formation of glutamate, an amino acid (**Fig. 74.15A**). The degraded amino acid itself changes to the corresponding keto acid and enters the Krebs cycle. Glutamate therefore represents the by-product of deamination of various amino acids.

In the second step, the NH_2 group of glutamate reacts with CO_2 to form urea, which is excreted as a nontoxic waste product. The formation of urea involves intermediates such as ornithine, citrulline, arginosuccinate, and arginine, all of which are regenerated and form the urea cycle (**Fig. 74.15B**).

Glutamate also rapidly mops up the NH_3 that is formed by enteric bacteria and that enters the liver through portal blood.

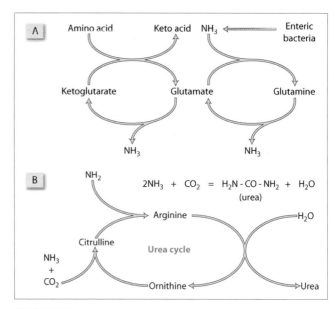

Fig. 74.15 **(A)** Amino acid catabolism and detoxification of ammonia. **(B)** Urea cycle.

The product of glutamate and NH_3 is glutamine. The glutamate is later regenerated when the NH_3 is removed from glutamine to form urea.

Summary

- Acetyl CoA, the precursor for the common energy-yielding pathway, can be derived from the breakdown of carbohydrates, fats, and, to a lesser extent, proteins.

- The Krebs cycle is a particularly efficient source of ATP.

- Glycolysis, the catabolism of glucose, is the primary source of ATP for all cells.

- The β-oxidation of fatty acids is an important source of ATP.

- Proteins are broken down into amino acids, a fraction of which enter energy (ATP) producing pathways, with the remainder being reutilized in protein synthesis.

Applying What You Know

74.1. Mrs. Omaya complains about suffering from fatigue since giving birth. How might her low blood glucose contribute to that symptom?

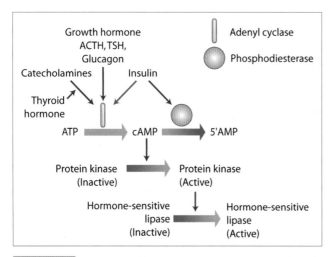

Fig. 74.14 Activation of hormone-sensitive lipase. Note the indicated changes from inactive states (*pink*) to active states (*blue*). ACTH, adrenocorticotrophic hormone; AMP, adenosine monophosphate; ATP, adenosine triphosphate; cAMP, cyclic adenosine monophosphate. TSH, thyroid stimulating hormone.

Hormones are chemical messengers controlling cellular functions. They are secreted into the circulation by ductless endocrine glands and thereby exert widespread actions. Endocrine systems and their hormones are involved in controlling many functions and in regulating many aspects of the internal environment.

General Models: Communications and Homeostasis

Endocrine systems are chemical or humoral cell–cell processing systems, and as will be discussed later, they interact with the nervous system. This information processing is an essential feature of all of the systems that maintain homeostasis.

Several hormones act in a *paracrine way*—they exert their effect on neighboring target cells, for example, the effect of gastrin on D cells secreting somatostatin (see **Fig. 81.7**) or the effect of testosterone on spermatogenesis.

Sometimes, a hormone acts in an *autocrine way*—it acts on the cell from which it is secreted. The term *cytokine* is a general name for small proteins that act in an autocrine or paracrine manner. Some cytokines have systemic effects as well. For example, interleukin-1 (IL-1) and IL-3 produce fever. Cytokines are secreted mostly by lymphocytes and macrophages, but also by endothelial cells, neurons, and glial cells.

Cellular functions are also controlled by neurotransmitters released by neurons. Neural effects are much more localized and much faster than hormonal effects. The distinction between hormones and neurotransmitters is, however, becoming blurred, as evident from terms like *neurohormone* and *neurosecretion* that are applicable, for example, to posterior pituitary hormones. Another example is cholecystokinin, which is secreted by S cells in the mucosal glands and also by neurons in the brain.

Hormones control cellular activity by modifying the activity of enzymes and hence the flow of substrates within the cell. All hormones act through specific receptors present on hormone-sensitive target cells. Hormones bind to their receptors with high specificity and affinity. Receptors have two functional domains: a *recognition domain* that binds the hormone and a *coupling domain* that generates a signal that couples hormone recognition to some intracellular function. Based on their mechanism of action, hormones have been classified as shown in **Table 75.1**. Group I hormones are lipid soluble and enter the cell and the nucleus, where they bind to receptors. Group II hormones are water soluble and bind to receptors located on the cell membrane.

Group I Hormones

Group I hormones (steroid/retinoid/thyroid hormones), examples of which are listed in **Table 75.1**, are lipid soluble and easily diffuse across the cell membrane. Inside the cell, they bind to intracellular receptors (in the cytoplasm and the nucleus) and affect gene expression. Typically, the products of stimulated gene expression are enzymes. This mechanism is illustrated in **Fig. 75.1**.

There is increasing evidence that at least some group I hormones, after binding to cytoplasmic receptors, activate second messenger signaling pathways, producing what are called non-nuclear effects. These occur significantly sooner than the effects resulting from alteration of gene expression.

Group II Hormones

Group II hormones are water-soluble peptide hormones that cannot enter the cell. They act by binding to the receptors on target cell membranes and initiating a chain of reactions within the cell membrane and inside the cell. In doing so, they activate a series of messengers and enzymes. Depending upon the type of second messenger (the hormone itself is the first messenger), the group II hormones are classified into four subgroups called IIA, IIB, IIC, and IID (**Tables 75.1** and **75.2**). All group II hormones bind to a specific receptor, a G protein (guanosine triphosphate [GTP]–dependent protein). The hormone-receptor complex then activates a membrane-located enzyme, or in some cases, an ion channel. Second messenger signaling systems are activated, and some of the cell's metabolic pathways are altered (producing the biologic effect) by changes in the activity of the involved enzymes. **Figure 75.2** illustrates the pieces that make up this action "kit."

Hormonal receptors are integral proteins present in the cell membrane (**Fig. 75.3**). Receptors coupled to G proteins have seven membrane-spanning domains. The G protein is a complex of three subunits (α, β, and γ) that are anchored to the plasma membrane. In the absence of hormone, an inactive molecule of guanosine diphosphate (GDP) is bound to its α subunit, which has intrinsic GTPase activity. When the hormone binds to the receptor, the receptor undergoes a conformational change and activates the G protein. Activation of the G protein is associated with the replacement of the GDP molecule on its α subunit by GTP. The GDP-GTP exchange on the G protein leads to the separation of its α subunit bound to GTP from its β and γ subunits. The α-GTP complex binds to a membrane-located enzyme and activates it. The activation is terminated only when the GTP is split by the intrinsic GTPase activity of the α subunit.

The membrane-located enzyme may be adenylyl cyclase, guanylyl cyclase, or phospholipase C. Instead of an activating enzyme, there can be a membrane-located ionic channel that becomes activated through phosphorylation (**Fig. 75.4**). This permits the movement of ions across the membrane. The second messenger may be cyclic adenosine monophosphate (cAMP), cyclic guanosine monophosphate (cGMP), or diacylglycerol (DAG) and inositol triphosphate (IP$_3$). Group IID hormones do not have a separate membrane-located enzyme or a second messenger. Rather, the receptor itself has the enzymatic activity for activating target enzymes (**Table 75.2**).

Table 75.1 Examples of Group I and Group II Hormones

Location (or Function)	Group I	Group IIA	Group IIB	Group IIC	Group IID
Hypothalamic		Corticotropin-releasing hormone (CRH)			
		Gonadotropin-releasing hormone (GnRH)		Thyrotropin-releasing hormone (TRH)	
Pituitary, anterior		Thyroid-stimulating hormone (TSH)			Growth hormone (GH)
		Adrenocorticotrophic hormone (ACTH)			Prolactin
		Melanocyte-stimulating hormone (MSH)			
		Follicle-stimulating hormone (FSH)			
		Luteinizing hormone (LH)			
Pituitary, posterior		Antidiuretic hormone (ADH)		Oxytoxin	
Thyroid	Thyroid hormone (TH)				
Calcium regulating	Dihydrocholecalciferol (DHCC)	Parathyroid hormone (PTH)			
		Calcitonin			
Adrenal cortex	Cortiosl				
	Aldosterone				
Adrenal medulla		Epinephrine (via α$_2$ receptors)		Epinephrine (via α$_1$ receptors)	
Pancreas		Glucagon			Insulin
		Somatostatin			
Reproductive (gonads)	Estrogen				
	Progesterone				
	Testosterone				
Placenta		Human chorionic gonadotropin (hCG)			Human chorionic somatomammotropin (hCS)
GI tract		Secretin		Gastrin	
				Cholecystokinin (CCK)	Insulin
Other	Retinoic acid		Atrial naturetic protein (ANP)	Acetylcholine	Erythropoietin
	Angiotensin II		Nitric oxide (NO)		Insulin-like growth factor (IGF)

Abbreviations: CRH, human corticotropin-releasing hormone; TRH, thyrotropin-releasing hormone; GnRH, gonadotrophin-releasing hormone; TSH, thyroid-stimulating hormone; ACTH, adrenocorticotropic hormone; MSH, melanocyte-stimulating hormone; FSH, follicle-stimulating hormone; LH, luteinizing hormone; HCG, human chorionic gonadotropin; HCS, human chorionic somatotropin; GH, growth hormone; IGF, insulin-like growth factor; TH, thyroid hormone; ADH, antidiuretic hormone; PTH, parathyroid hormone; DHCC, dehydroxycholecalciferol; CCK, cholecystokinin; ANP, atrial natriuretic peptide; NO, nitric oxide.

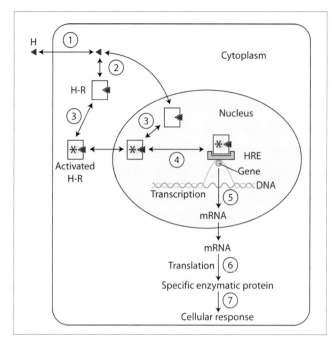

Fig. 75.1 Mechanism of group I hormonal action. Hormone (H) diffuses across the plasma membrane (1) and binds to its specific receptor (R) protein (2), either in the cytoplasm or in the nucleus, to form the hormone-receptor complex (H-R). The binding brings about a conformational change in the receptor, which now becomes activated (3). The activated H-R complex binds to specific regulatory regions of the deoxyribonucleic acid (DNA) called the hormone response element, or HRE (4). This binding facilitates transcription of the adjacent gene(s) by ribonucleic acid (RNA) polymerase, thereby increasing the rate of messenger RNA (mRNA) formation (5). The newly synthesized protein (6), usually an enzyme, induces cellular response (7).

The effector enzymes are mostly the different types of kinases (e.g., cAMP-dependent protein kinase, cGMP-dependent protein kinase, and protein kinase C, etc.) that activate various protein enzymes by phosphorylating them. Thus, glycogenolysis and glycogenesis are regulated by controlling the activity of glycogen synthetase (see **Fig. 74.9**), and lipolysis is regulated by controlling the activity of hormone-sensitive lipase (see **Fig. 74.14**).

Group IIA Hormones

The second messenger for group IIA hormones (**Fig. 75.5A**) is cyclic AMP, and the enzyme that catalyzes its formation is adenylyl cyclase. The protein kinase involved is called cAMP-dependent protein kinase. The G protein may either stimulate or inhibit adenylyl cyclase and is accordingly called stimulatory G protein (G_s) or inhibitory G protein (G_i). The actions of G_s or G_i are attributable to their a_s and a_i fractions, respectively. a_s and a_i have other actions in addition to their effect on adenylyl cyclase. For example, a_i stimulates channels and inhibits Ca^{2+} channels, whereas α_s does the opposite. The activation of cAMP protein kinase by a group IIA hormone is shown in **Fig. 75.5A**.

The cAMP is hydrolyzed to 5′AMP by the enzyme phosphodiesterase. Inhibitors of phosphodiesterases such as methylated xanthine derivatives (caffeine) increase intracellular cAMP

and thereby prolong the action of hormones. In intestinal epithelial cells, cholera toxin irreversibly inactivates the GTPase activity of G_s. The adenylyl cyclase therefore remains in a perpetual state of activation. This results in continuous formation of cAMP. The cAMP activates protein kinase and phosphorylates various membrane transport proteins, resulting in the active transport of electrolytes into the intestinal lumen. Water follows passively, causing life-threatening diarrhea.

Group IIB Hormone

In group IIB hormones (**Fig. 75.5B**), cyclic GMP acts as a second messenger, and the enzyme that catalyzes its formation is guanylyl cyclase. Guanylyl cyclase has two isomers, one of which is present in the membrane as an integral protein. The other is present in the cytosol. The membrane isozyme of guanylyl cyclase is activated by the hormone atrial natriuretic peptide (ANP). The cytosolic guanylyl cyclase is activated by nitric oxide (NO).

cGMP activates cGMP-dependent protein kinase (also called protein kinase G). The kinase phosphorylates the myosin light chain of smooth muscle, thereby causing its relaxation. Thus, ANP acts by relaxing afferent arterioles and mesangial cells. NO mediates the hypotensive action of nitroprusside. Inhibitors of cGMP phosphodiesterase such as sildenafil (Viagra; Pfizer Pharmaceuticals, New York, NY) enhance and prolong these responses.

Group IIC Hormones

The second messengers in group IIC hormones (**Fig. 75.6A**) are diacylglycerol (DAG) and inositol-1,4,5-triphosphate (IP_3), which are produced from phosphatidylinositol-4,5-biphosphate (PIP_2) by the action of phospholipase C (PLC). PIP_2 is a membrane phospholipid. DAG activates the enzyme protein kinase C. IP_3 acts on the endoplasmic reticulum, releasing calcium (Ca^{2+}) from it. The increase in cytosolic Ca^{2+} activates calmodulin-dependent protein kinase. The protein kinases phosphorylate enzymatic proteins into their physiologically active forms and thereby mediate hormonal actions.

Table 75.2 Classification of Hormones

Class	Membrane-located Enzyme	Second Messenger	Kinase
IIA	Adenylyl cyclase	cAMP	cAMP-dependent protein kinase
IIB	Guanylyl cyclase	cGMP	cGMP-dependent protein kinase
IIC	Phospholipase C	DAG and IP_3	Protein kinase C, calmodulin-dependent protein kinase
IID	–	–	Serine or threonine kinase (present as part of the receptor)

Abbreviations: cAMP, cyclic adenosine monophosphate; cGMP, cyclic guanosine monophosphate; DAG, diacylglycerol; IP_3, inositol-1,4,5-triphosphate.

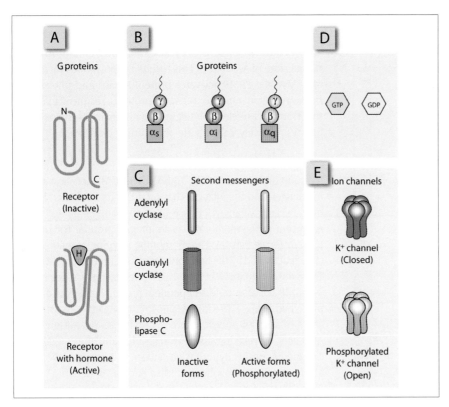

Fig. 75.2 The hormone action "kit." The shapes and colors used here are the same in all figures of this chapter. **(A)** When a receptor (a membrane-spanning protein with an N terminal outside the cell and a C terminal inside) binds a molecule of the hormone, it undergoes a conformational change that "activates" it. **(B)** G proteins are trimeres with identical γ and β subunits and three different possible α units. **(C)** Three second messenger molecules that can be either activated or inactivated. **(D)** Guanosine triphosphate (GTP) and guanosine diphosphate (GDP). **(E)** Phosphorylating a K channel activates or opens it.

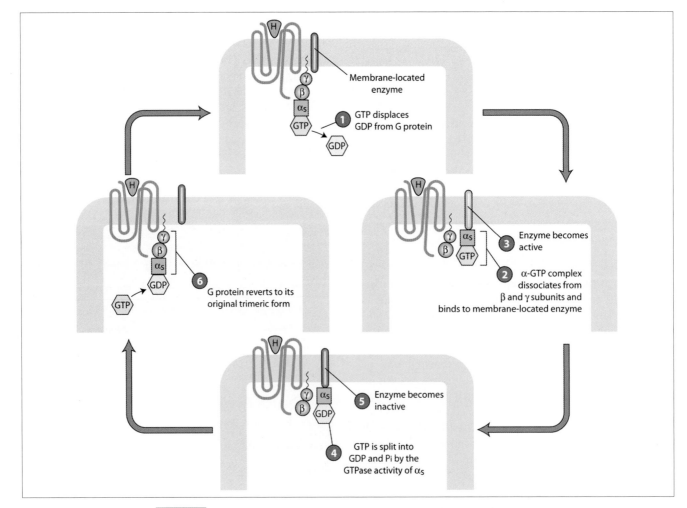

Fig. 75.3 Activation of membrane-located signaling enzymes by group II hormones.

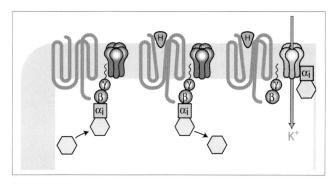

Fig. 75.4 Opening (activation) of a potassium channel by G_i.

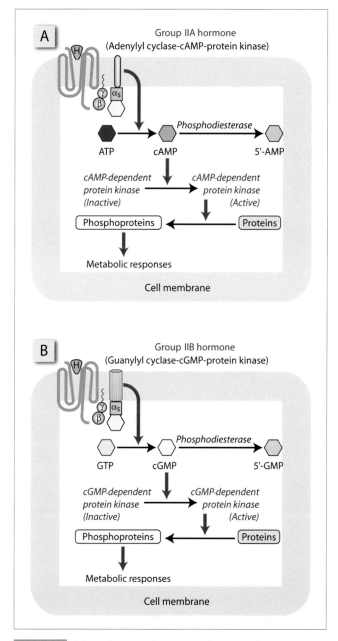

Fig. 75.5 **(A)** Mechanism of a group IIA hormone that activates G. Activation of G_s results in the formation of cyclic adenosine monophosphate (cAMP) as the second messenger. The cAMP, in turn, activates a specific type of protein kinase. **(B)** Mechanism of action of group IIB hormones. The second messenger is cyclic guanosine monophosphate (cGMP). ATP, adenosine triphosphate; GTP, guanosine triphosphate.

Group IID Hormones

These hormones (insulin, growth hormone, prolactin, and insulin-like growth factor) act through a protein kinase cascade (**Fig. 75.6B**). Receptors for these hormones have intrinsic tyrosine kinase activity. The insulin receptor consists of two α chains located on the outer surface of the plasma membrane and two β chains that span the entire membrane thickness and protrude into the cytosol. The α chains contain the insulin-

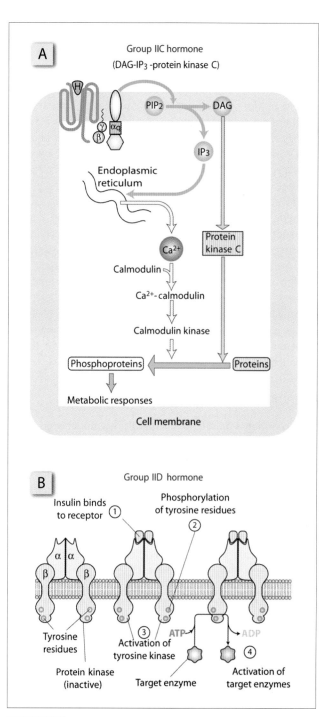

Fig. 75.6 **(A)** Mechanism of group IIC hormones. Note that the hormone produces two second messengers, diacylglycerol (DAG) and inositol-1,4,5-triphosphate (IP_3), which activate protein kinase C and calmodulin kinase, respectively. **(B)** Mechanism of group ID hormones. Note that the enzyme protein kinase forms a part of the receptor molecule. ATP, adenosine triphosphate; ADP, adenosine diphosphate.

binding domain, and the β chains have the tyrosine kinase domain. Binding of insulin to the α chain activates the tyrosine kinase of the β chains. Tyrosine kinase autophosphorylates itself at its tyrosine residues in the chain. The phosphorylated β chain acquires an enzymatic property and activates a second protein kinase, which may then activate a third serine or threonine kinase. Eventually, phosphorylation of serine or threonine residues alters the activity of enzymes crucial to certain cellular functions.

Hormone Receptors on Cells

Every cell has many receptors that allow it to respond to a large number of different hormones. Thus, hormones can elicit a large number of different biologic responses from any cell. Furthermore, hormones interact with one another in a variety of ways. Two hormones can inhibit the action of one another; that is, they can act antagonistically. Two other hormones can act synergistically, with the magnitude of the response elicited by the two hormones present simultaneously being greater than would be the sum of their separate responses.

In the case of hormones whose biologic responses oppose one another, both hormones act through the same set of metabolic pathways. For example, both insulin and glucagon affect blood glucose concentration by their action on muscle cells. Insulin promotes the conversion of glucose into glycogen while at the same time inhibiting the breakdown of glycogen into glucose. Glucagon has exactly the opposite effects: it promotes glycogenolysis and inhibits glycogenesis. When more than one hormone acts on a metabolic pathway, it is essential to understand where the balance of the effects occurs.

Summary

- All hormones must bind to a specific receptor in or on a cell for the cell to respond.

- All hormones alter target cell function by changing the activity of enzymes and/or altering the state of membrane channels.

- Group I hormones are lipid soluble and bind to intracellular (in some case, intranuclear) receptors and alter gene expression (the production of enzymes).

- Group II hormones (all subtypes) bind to receptors in the cell membrane and activate a cascade of effects that result in altered enzyme activity. There are several different intracellular signaling systems that are employed.

Applying What You Know

75.1. Mrs. Omaya has a very low thyroid hormone (T_4) level. How does the thyroid hormone that is available exert its effect on its target cells?

75.2. Mrs. Omaya's posterior pituitary appears to be normal, which means she has appropriate levels of antidiuretic hormone (ADH). What are the target cells for ADH, and how does ADH affect their function?

Hypothalamic Hormones

A major function of the endocrine system is to maintain homeostasis of the internal environment, which explains why much of the endocrine system is ultimately under the control of the hypothalamus, the part of the brain that controls visceral functions of the body.

Hypothalamic control of hormone release (**Fig. 76.1**) involves the longest pathway in the case of insulin secretion by the pancreatic islets (but note that this neural control of insulin release is *not* the primary controller of insulin secretion; see Chapter 81). The islets are innervated by postganglionic autonomic fibers that are ultimately under hypothalamic control. The hypothalamic control pathway is shorter for the adrenal medulla, which is innervated by the preganglionic sympathetic neurons. The hypothalamic control pathway is shorter still for the posterior pituitary in which the axons of the hypothalamic neurons directly reach the posterior pituitary and secrete the hormones (oxytocin and antidiuretic hormone [ADH]). The

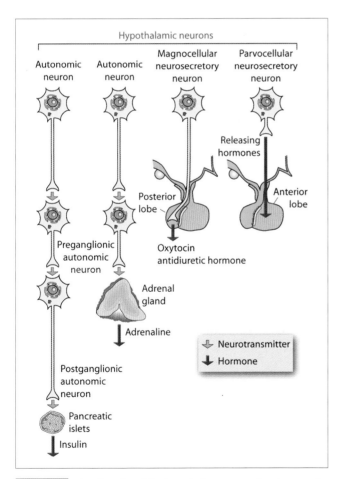

Fig. 76.1 The "length" of the hypothalamic control pathways. The pathway is longest for control of insulin secretion (but note that insulin release is most significantly stimulated by increases in blood glucose) and shortest for anterior pituitary hormones.

shortest control pathway is represented by the hypothalamic control of the anterior pituitary in which the hypothalamic neurons do not send axons far out, but simply release their secretions (releasing hormones) into the bloodstream.

General Model: Communications

The hypothalamus–pituitary system is the site of integration between neural and hormonal information processing systems. The mechanisms involved, which will be discussed below, are all examples of cell–cell communications.

Two facts are obvious from the above examples. First, the longer the control arm, the more localized is the domain of control; and second, the difference between a neurotransmitter and a neurosecretion lies in the extent of their effect. Though both are secreted by a neuron, the effect of a neurotransmitter is localized to the postsynaptic membrane, whereas that of a neurosecretion is more widespread. Neurosecretions are mostly peptides, except dopamine, which controls prolactin secretion (see Chapter 88).

Magnocellular and Parvocellular Systems

The magnocellular neurosecretory system refers to the neurosecretory neurons of the supraoptic and paraventricular nuclei, which make the neurohormones ADH and oxytocin and release them from their axon terminals.

The *parvocellular neurosecretory system* refers to the neurosecretory neurons originating in the arcuate nucleus and terminating directly on the capillaries in the median eminence. These neurons secrete the hypophysiotropic hormones (releasing or inhibiting hormones), which reach the anterior pituitary through the hypothalamo-hypophysial portal system and stimulate or inhibit its hormonal secretion. Examples of hypophysiotropic hormones are the somatotropin-releasing hormone (SRH), prolactin-inhibiting hormone (PIH, now known to be dopamine), thyrotropin-releasing hormone (TRH), corticotropin-releasing hormone (CRH), and gonadotropin-releasing hormone (GnRH). These hypophysiotropic hormones are discussed separately with the hormones they control.

Hypothalamo-hypophysial axis | The secretory activity of the anterior lobe of the pituitary gland is controlled by hypothalamic hormones that reach the pituitary (hypophysis) through the hypothalamic–hypophysial portal system. Under the influence of the hypothalamic-releasing hormones, the anterior lobe of the pituitary releases a set of hormones called the *hypophysiotropic hormones*, which increase the secretory activity of the target glands, such as the thyroid gland, adrenal cortex, and gonads. The hormones produced by target endocrine organs inhibit the hypothalamus and the pituitary, causing a decrease in the secretion of their tropic hormones. This is called *negative feedback control* and is an important mechanism regulating hormone synthesis and secretion (**Fig. 76.2**). Many hormones (the parathyroid hormone, calcitonin, insulin, and glucagon are examples) are not under hypothalamo-hypophysial control, but have their own regulatory mechanisms.

The negative feedback control occurs in three ways. In *long loop feedback,* the target organ hormones (or the substrates produced through their action) inhibit both the hypothalamus and the anterior lobe of the pituitary gland. *Short loop feedback* is a negative feedback exerted by the anterior pituitary tropic hormones on the hypothalamus, decreasing its secretion of hypophysiotropic hormones. In *ultrashort loop feedback,* the hypophysiotropic hormones inhibit their own secretion.

Pituitary Gland

The pituitary gland (see **Fig. 76.3**) lies in a bony walled cavity, the sella turcica of the sphenoid bone at the base of the skull, and is closely associated with the hypothalamus of the brain. The infundibular stem (neural stalk) of the posterior lobe arises in the median eminence of the hypothalamus.

The pituitary gland (hypophysis) originates in early embryonic life from two sources. The *adenohypophysis* (anterior lobe of the pituitary or the anterior pituitary) is formed by an upward evagination of Rathke's pouch (ectoderm) and grows dorsally toward the infundibulum, where it meets the *neurohypophysis* (posterior lobe of the pituitary or the posterior pituitary), which is derived from a downward outgrowth of the infundibular process from the diencephalon. The posterior pituitary, therefore, represents an extension of the brain.

Hypothalamo-hypophysial portal system | The adenohypophysis receives 90% of its blood supply from the long portal veins and the remaining 10% from the short portal vein

(**Fig. 76.3B**). The long *portal veins* drain the capillary bed of the superior hypophysial artery, which is located in the median eminence and infundibular stalk. This hypothalamo-hypophysial portal system is important for the transport of the hypophysiotropic hormones from the hypothalamus to the pituitary. The *short portal vein* drains the capillary bed of the inferior hypophysial artery, which is located in the neurohypophysis.

Anterior Pituitary (Adenohypophysis)

The anterior pituitary has three parts (**Figs. 76.3** and **76.4**). The *pars distalis* represents the bulk of the anterior lobe in humans and is the source of the pituitary tropic hormones. The *pars tuberalis* surrounds the infundibular stem. It does not secrete any hormone. Between these two parts is the *pars intermedia,* which is almost nonexistent in humans.

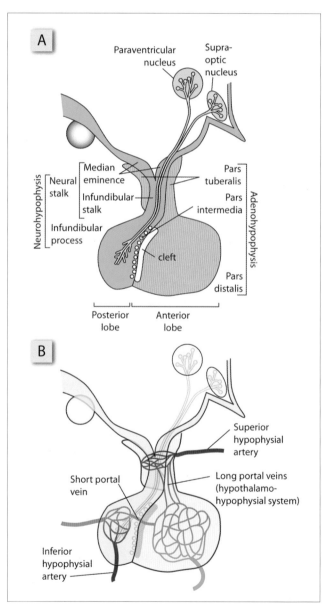

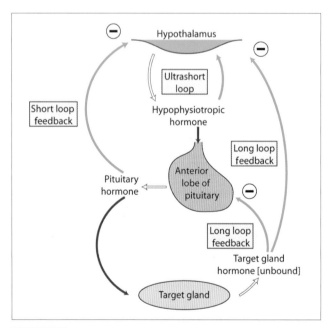

Fig. 76.2 The hypothalamo-hypophysial control of a target gland. Several negative feedback pathways (in *blue*) are built into the control system.

Fig. 76.3 (A) Parts of the pituitary gland. Also shown are the connections of the posterior pituitary with the hypothalamic nuclei. (B) The hypothalamo-hypophysial portal system.

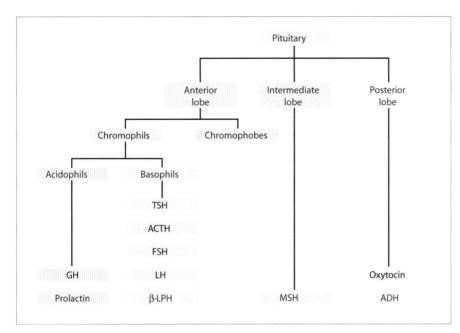

Fig. 76.4 Hormones secreted by the anterior, intermediate, and posterior lobes of the pituitary gland. GH, growth hormone; TSH, thyroid-stimulating hormone; ACTH, adrenocorticotropic hormone; FSH, follicle-stimulating hormone; LH, luteinizing hormone; β-LPH, beta-lipotrophic hormone; MSH, melanocyte-stimulating hormone; ADH, antidiuretic hormone.

The pars distalis of the anterior lobe contains two types of cells: the chromophobes and the chromophils. The *chromophobes* do not have any physiologic significance. The *chromophils* exist in two forms: the acidophils (80%) and basophils (20%). *Acidophils* secrete prolactin and growth hormone (GH). GH-secreting acidophils are called somatotropes, and prolactin-secreting acidophils are called mammotropes. Some acidophils secrete both GH and prolactin. These cells are called somatomammotropes.

Basophils secrete tropic hormones that stimulate other endocrine glands, namely, thyroid-stimulating hormone (TSH), adrenocorticotropic hormone (ACTH), luteinizing hormone (LH), follicle-stimulating hormone (FSH), and β-lipotropic hormone (β-LPH).

Growth hormone is discussed below. The other tropic hormones (TSH, ACTH, LH, and FSH) are discussed in later chapters in this section.

Intermediate Lobe of the Pituitary
The intermediate lobe of the pituitary secretes the melanocyte-stimulating hormone (MSH), a peptide hormone that is structurally similar to ACTH. Both MSH and ACTH are derived from a larger molecule called the pro-opiomelanocortin (POMC). MSH, ACTH, and other POMC derivatives (**Fig. 76.5**) have similar actions: they increase skin pigmentation (due to increased melanin synthesis), stimulate adrenal glucocorticoid production, and reduce food intake.

Melanin is the pigment that lends color to the hair and skin. The organelles containing melanin are called melanosomes, which are present in cells called melanocytes. Melanocytes are different from the melanophores present in fish, reptiles, and amphibians. Melanophores can quickly change color through a redistribution of their colored and refractile granules that is controlled by MSH. Melanocytes cannot change their color quickly; therefore, the role of MSH in humans remains unknown.

Albinism is a congenital condition in which there is a genetic inability to synthesize melanin. In *piebaldism*, there is patchy depigmentation of the skin due to impaired migration of pigment cell precursors from the neural crest during embryonic development. The condition is congenital, and even the pattern of depigmentation is inherited. In *vitiligo*, the patchy depigmentation develops after birth and is progressive.

Posterior Pituitary (Neurohypophysis)
The posterior pituitary (see **Figs. 76.1** and **76.3**) is made of neurosecretory neurons originating from the magnocellular neurosecretory system of the hypothalamus. These unmyelinated nerve fibers arise from the supraoptic and paraventricular

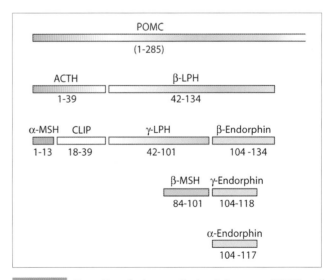

Fig. 76.5 Formation of adrenocorticotropic hormone (ACTH) and β-melanocyte-stimulating hormone (β-MSH) from proopiomelanocortin (POMC). LPH, lipotrophic hormone.

nuclei and descend through the infundibulum to terminate in the posterior lobe. The oxytocin and antidiuretic hormone released from the posterior lobe into the circulation are the neurosecretions of these nerve fibers. The posterior pituitary does not have secretory cells of its own.

Growth Hormone

Growth hormone (GH) is also known as somatotropin. It is a polypeptide synthesized and secreted by somatotropes, which are a subpopulation of the acidophils present in the adenohypophysis. GH is stored in very large amounts in the pituitary and is secreted episodically at 2-hour intervals. About half of the plasma GH is bound to a GH-binding protein.

Control of Growth Hormone Secretion
GH secretion is controlled by two hypothalamic hormones: somatotropin-releasing hormone (SRH) which increases GH secretion, and somatostatin which decreases GH secretion. GH exerts a negative feedback (short loop) on the secretion of SRH. Also, SRH inhibits its own release via an ultrashort feedback loop (**Fig. 76.6**).

GH increases the synthesis of somatomedin in liver. Somatomedin reduces GH secretion by inhibiting SRH secretion (long loop negative feedback) and stimulating somatostatin secretion.

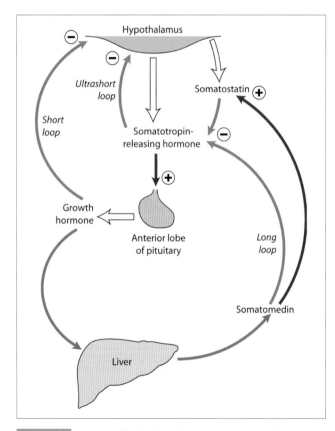

Fig. 76.6 Negative feedback (in *blue*) control of growth hormone secretion. Growth hormone has many effects on cellular metabolism. The effect of growth hormone on the processes of growth is actually mediated by somatomedin.

GH secretion is increased in hypoglycemia or when hypoglycemia is imminent, as in fasting, and decreases in obesity. It also increases in stressful situations like fever or emotional trauma. The physiologic significance of this is explained below. There are, however, several other stimuli for GH secretion whose physiologic significance is not understood. For example, GH secretion increases during deep sleep and decreases during rapid-eye movement (REM) sleep. Dopamine agonists like bromocriptine stimulate GH secretion and have been used in the treatment of GH deficiency. Certain amino acids, like arginine and lysine, also increase GH secretion. Estrogens increase but progesterone decreases GH secretion, which is the reason why a decline in GH secretion is observed in late pregnancy. Glucocorticoids decrease GH secretion, but their predominant effect is the interference with the metabolic actions of GH.

Physiologic Effects of Growth Hormone
Skeletal growth | The effect of GH on skeletal growth is mediated by somatomedins, a family of polypeptides also called insulin-like growth factors (IGFs). They are synthesized in the liver and in the bone itself. The growth-promoting action of somatomedins is helped by their insulin-like actions (see below).

Somatomedin (whose release is stimulated by GH), stimulates proliferation of chondrocytes and osteocytes resulting in increased deposition of cartilage and increased ossification of the newly formed cartilage. Before the closure of epiphyseal plates, the increase in chondrogenesis exceeds its ossification, resulting in the widening of the cartilaginous epiphyseal plate. The bones grow longer, resulting in a rapid increase in height. After epiphyseal closure, chondrogenesis does not occur; only subperiosteal bone deposition occurs due to increased activity of the osteocytes. Hence, there is no increase in bone length, but bone thickening continues through subperiosteal bone deposition. Osteocytic activity, as explained in Chapter 78, is associated with both deposition as well as resorption of bone and therefore, is associated with increased urinary excretion of hydroxyproline. It is this growth that accounts for the changes seen in acromegaly (see below). GH promotes renal reabsorption of calcium (Ca^{2+}) and phosphate (PO_4^{3-}), which are important for bone growth.

Protein metabolism | GH has predominantly anabolic effects on skeletal and cardiac muscle where it promotes amino acid transport into cells and increases protein synthesis. GH causes positive nitrogen balance—it promotes protein anabolism and reduces the plasma concentration and urinary excretion of nitrogenous products of protein catabolism like amino acids and urea. GH also promotes renal reabsorption of Na^+, K^+, and Cl^-.

Carbohydrate and fat metabolism | The effects of GH on carbohydrate and fat metabolism are complicated by the fact that though GH itself has antiinsulin effects, the somatomedins it produces have insulin-like effects.

The *antiinsulin effect* of GH is primarily its lipolytic effect on the adipose tissues, which results in the mobilization of large amounts of free fatty acid (FFA) and glycerol. The FFA is oxidized to acetyl CoA. There is suppression of glycolysis and stimulation of gluconeogenesis, converting the large amounts of acetyl CoA into glucose, which accumulates intracellularly. Excess acetyl CoA is converted into ketone bodies. The entire sequence takes ~2 hours to manifest. The large amounts of glucose formed through gluconeogenesis and the inhibition of glycolysis lead to hyperglycemia, which has been called *pituitary hyperglycemia* to differentiate if from diabetic hyperglycemia. In the long run, however, pituitary hyperglycemia stimulates excessive insulin secretion from the pancreas, leading to B cell exhaustion and frank diabetes mellitus.

The *insulin-like effects* of GH are attributable to the formation of somatomedins and are relatively quicker, appearing in ~30 minutes. Somatomedins bind to insulin receptors and induce most of the metabolic effects of insulin, although to a lesser degree.

A further complication of the metabolic effects of GH is the fact that the induction of somatomedins by GH requires a high insulin level along with adequate nutrients. When the insulin level is high, the GH level is low, but the amount of somatomedin formed from it increases. Thus, in the *well-fed state* when the insulin level is high, somatomedin level is also high, and it brings about increased growth. Conversely, in the *fasting state*, the low insulin level reduces somatomedin formation; therefore, growth is suppressed, while the high, GH level prevents hypoglycemia. In diabetes mellitus, reduced somatomedin formation retards growth, and the high GH level aggravates the diabetes through its anti-insulin metabolic effects.

General Model: Energy

Growth hormone is a good example of the mechanisms that hormones use to regulate and control physiologic functions; GH can bring about many different changes to the cell's machinery for transforming matter and energy (mobilizing stored substrates for energy production).

Growth Hormone Disorders

Hyposecretion of GH causes dwarfism. Hypersecretion of GH causes gigantism and acromegaly. In some cases of GH hypersecretion, growth retardation can occur if the somatomedin levels are depressed, for example, in kwashiorkor. Both GH and somatomedin levels are normal in the African pygmies.

Gigantism and Acromegaly

Gigantism and acromegaly occur due to hypersecretion of GH. Tumors of somatotropes secrete large amounts of GH. Tumors of somatomammotropes secrete both GH and prolactin.

Overproduction of GH during adolescence results in gigantism, which is characterized by excessive growth of the long bones. Patients may grow to heights of as much as 8 feet. Excessive GH secretion during adulthood, that is, after the epiphyseal (growth) plates of long bones have fused, causes growth in those areas where cartilage persists. This leads to acromegaly.

In acromegaly, increased growth hormone secretion results in enlargement of the hands and feet (*acro*: extremities) and soft tissue hypertrophy (e.g., cardiomegaly, hepatosplenomegaly, and renomegaly). The protrusion of the lower jaw (mandibular prognathism) together with the prominent brow, cheek bone, and other facial bones produce the coarse facial features called acromegalic facies. Body hair is increased. About a quarter of the patients have abnormal glucose tolerance tests, and a few develop lactation in the absence of pregnancy.

Signs of acromegaly that are related to the local effects of the tumor include enlargement of the sella turcica, headache, and visual disturbances, such as bitemporal hemianopia.

Acromegaly is treated by selective surgical excision of the pituitary adenoma. Bromocriptine, a stimulator of GH secretion in normal individuals, is effective in suppressing GH levels in many acromegalic patients.

Pituitary Dwarfism

Decreased GH secretion in children leads to stunted growth or dwarfism. It is characterized by maxillary prognathism in contrast to the mandibular prognathism that characterizes acromegaly. Hair growth is impaired, and hypoglycemia may be present. Unlike individuals with congenital hypothyroidism, the body proportions of the pituitary dwarf are not infantile but are like those of an adult.

GH deficiency may be part of an overall lack of anterior pituitary hormones (panhypopituitarism) or from an isolated genetic deficiency, which is rare in adults. Dwarfism due to GH deficiency can be treated with human GH. Genetic defects usually affect the GH receptors rather than GH secretion. In *Laron-type dwarfs*, the hepatic synthesis of somatomedin is impaired because the GH receptors in the liver are resistant to the action of GH. In *pygmies*, even the GH receptors are normal, suggesting that the defect lies in the mechanisms subsequent to the receptor binding of the hormone.

Summary

- The hypothalamus is the major site at which the nervous system and the endocrine system interact with one another.

- The hypothalamic–pituitary–target organ axis controls the release of many hormones.

- The anterior pituitary is the source of releasing hormones that control the secretion of peripheral hormones.

- The posterior pituitary releases oxytocin and antidiuretic hormone. Both are synthesized in the hypothalamus, transported to the pituitary, and released into the circulation there.

- Growth hormone, released from the anterior pituitary, has widespread actions on the body's metabolism.

- Growth hormone stimulates the secretion of somatomedin (insulin-like growth factor) from the liver; it is IGF that directly stimulates bone growth.

Applying What You Know

76.1. Mrs. Omaya has low levels of several anterior pituitary hormones (TSH, PRL, LH, FSH). At what location would a single discrete lesion give rise to these findings? Explain.

76.2. Mrs. Omaya experienced some insult (probably ischemic) to her anterior pituitary, yet there is nothing to suggest that her posterior pituitary was affected. Given that both parts of the pituitary are in close proximity to one another in a confined space, how can you account for this?

76.3. What needs to be done to help Mrs. Omaya? How would this be accomplished?

The functional unit of the thyroid gland (**Fig. 77.1**) is the follicle (acinus) enclosed by a single layer of cuboidal cells (follicular epithelium). The follicle is surrounded by a rich capillary plexus. The lumen of the follicle is filled with a colloidal fluid containing a protein called thyroglobulin. Microvilli extend into the colloid from the apical border of the follicular cells (**Fig. 77.2**).

A thyroid follicle that is actively secreting thyroid hormones looks somewhat different from one that is inactive. An inactive follicle is large, lined by flat cells, and contains abundant colloid. In contrast, an active follicle is smaller, is lined with columnar cells, and contains less colloid. The colloid is scooped out at the tip of the follicular cell forming the reabsorption lacunae (**Fig. 77.2**). The parafollicular (C) cells, which secrete calcitonin, do not communicate with the follicular lumen.

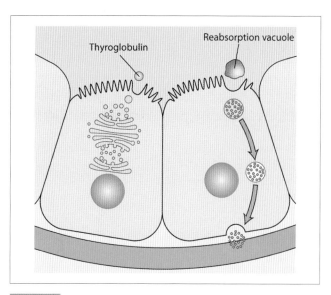

Fig. 77.2 Secretion and reabsorption of thyroglobulin by the follicular cells of the thyroid gland.

Thyroid Hormone

The thyroid gland secretes iodothyronines, iodine derivatives of the amino acid tyrosine. The major thyroid hormones are 3,5,3',5'-tetraiodothyronine (thyroxine), which is abbreviated as T_4 to denote the four iodine atoms, and 3,5,3'-triiodothyronine, or T_3. A third iodothyronine called the reverse 3,3',5'-triiodothyronine (rT_3) is biologically inactive and is formed by peripheral conversion of T_4 catalyzed by the enzyme 5-deiodinase. The term *thyroid hormone* (TH) denotes both thyroxine (T_4) and triiodothyronine (T_3). Both T_4 and T_3 have similar physiologic actions, although there are important quantitative differences (concentration, level of biologic activity) between them. T_4 is often considered to be the prohormone of T_3 (**Table 77.1**).

The thyroid cell also synthesizes a soluble protein substrate called thyroglobulin. This glycoprotein provides the tyrosine residues for the synthesis of T_4 and T_3. It also represents the storage form of thyroid hormones. Both T_4 and T_3 are bound to thyroglobulin until they are finally secreted into the bloodstream.

The role of the follicular cell in hormone synthesis is threefold. (1) It takes up iodide (I^-) from blood and oxidizes it to I^+. (2) It synthesizes thyroglobulin and thyroxine peroxidase and secretes them into the follicular lumen. (3) The follicular cell reabsorbs the colloid bound to thyroid hormones, digests the thyroglobulin, and releases the thyroid hormones into circulation.

Biosynthesis and Secretion

Thyroid hormone biosynthesis requires iodide, adequate amounts of which must be provided in the diet. The steps of thyroid hormone biosynthesis can be seen in **Fig. 77.3**.

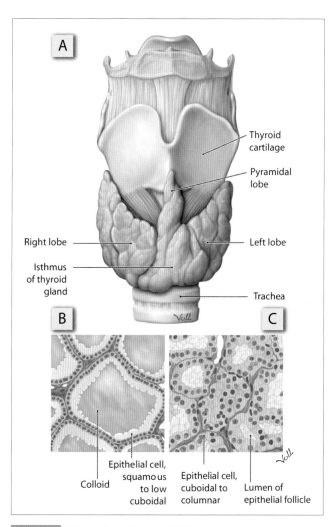

Fig. 77.1 **(A)** The thyroid gland. **(B)** The difference between inactive follicles and **(C)** active thyroid follicles.

Table 77.1 Comparison of Triiodothyronine (T₃) and Tetra-iodothyronine (T₄)

- T₄ is secreted in much larger amounts (80 µg/day) by the thyroid as compared with T₃ (6 µg/day).
- Most of the T₄ secreted by the thyroid is converted in the liver, kidney, and pituitary to T₃ by the action of 5′-deiodinase.
- T₄ is more stable, being bound to plasma protein in greater proportion and more avidly. Proportion of free T₄ is 0.02%, and that of free T₃ is 0.2%. Hence, although T₄ is secreted in much greater amounts, the plasma concentration of free T₄ is only twice that of free T₃.
- T₄ remains mostly extracellular, whereas T₃ penetrates cells readily. T₃ binds much more avidly to the hormone receptors in the nucleus. Hence, nearly all the nuclear receptors are found bound to T₃ and not T₄.
- T₃ is 10 times more potent than T₄ in all hormonal actions including the feedback inhibition of thyroid-stimulating hormone release.

General Models: Energy and Flow

The uptake (flow) of iodine into the thyroid cells for incorporation into thyroid hormones requires the use of energy to power the pump that is required; iodine can only flow against its electrical potential and concentration gradient if work is done by the pump.

Iodide uptake | The thyroid cell takes up iodide through secondary active transport. It employs a Na⁺–I⁻ symporter on its basal membrane, which derives its energy from the Na⁺–K⁺ ATPase pump. Because iodide has a negative charge, and the thyroid cell has an intracellular potential of –50 mV, iodide pumping occurs against an electrical gradient. As iodide accumulates inside the cell, the pumping has to occur against a concentration gradient as well.

Oxidation of iodide | Once inside the thyroid cell, I⁻ is rapidly oxidized to I⁺ by the enzyme thyroperoxidase located on the luminal surface of the follicular cell. The conversion of I⁻ into I⁺ prevents the back-diffusion of iodide into circulation (iodide trapping). Despite rapid oxidation, I⁻ concentration inside the thyroid cell remains higher than its plasma concentration.

Iodination of thyroglobulin | I⁺ diffuses into the lumen of the thyroid follicle and binds to the tyrosyl residues of thyroglobulin in the presence of thyroperoxidase. The iodination of thyroglobulin results in the formation of monoiodotyrosine (MIT) and diiodotyrosine (DIT) (**Fig. 77.4**).

Coupling (condensation) of iodotyrosines | Two molecules of the iodotyrosines react in the presence of thyroperoxidase to form T₃ and T₄ (iodothyronines). T₄ is produced by the coupling of two DIT molecules; T₃ is produced by the coupling of MIT with DIT.

Secretion | The thyroglobulin molecules, along with the T₃ and T₄ molecules attached to it, are endocytosed by the thyroid cell. The endocytotic vesicles containing colloid droplets fuse with lysosomes and migrate to the base of the cell (**Fig. 77.2**).

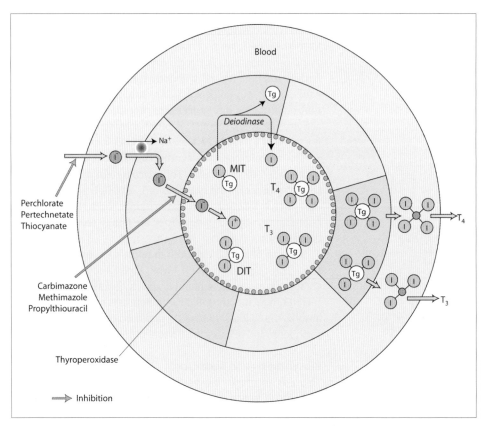

Fig. 77.3 Uptake, oxidation, and organification of iodine and the release of thyroid hormones. DIT, diiodotyrosine; MIT, monoiodotyrosine.

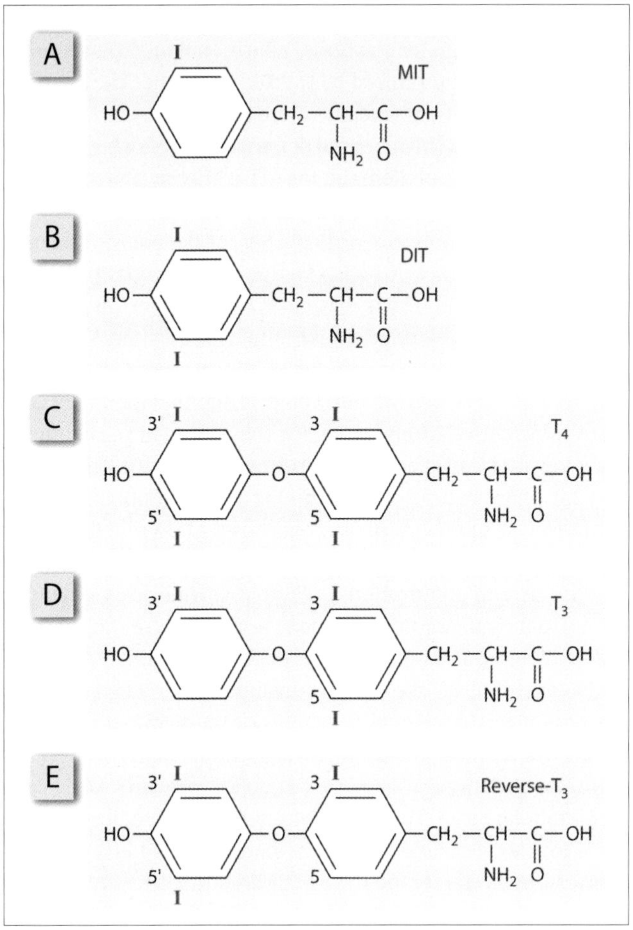

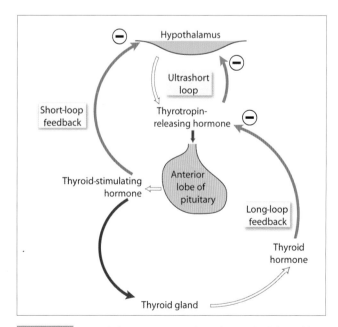

Fig. 77.4 The structure of **(A,B)** the precursors of thyroid hormone and **(C–E)** the three thyroid hormones. Reverse-T_3 has no biological activity.

more of it binds to plasma protein); this results in thyroid-stimulating hormone (TSH) secretion from the pituitary. TSH stimulates greater TH secretion from the thyroid and thereby restores the plasma TH concentration toward its normal level.

Thyroid hormone is metabolized in the liver by deiodination, deamination, and, finally, conjugation with glucuronic acid. The glucuronide conjugate is secreted through the bile duct into the intestine and excreted in the feces.

Control of Thyroid Function

Hypothalamic–hypophysial–thyroid axis | The activity of the thyroid gland is controlled by the TSH secreted by the basophils (thyrotropes) in the anterior pituitary (**Fig. 77.5**). TSH stimulates all the steps of TH biosynthesis. TSH secretion is inhibited by plasma T_3. Although T_4 does not inhibit TSH secretion directly, it does so indirectly through its conversion to T_3 within the pituitary. When plasma concentration of TH falls, TSH secretion is stimulated (disinhibited), and the thyroid gland secretion increases to restore the plasma level of thyroid hormones. TSH secretion is stimulated by thyrotropin-releasing hormone (TRH), a tripeptide synthesized by the hypothalamus. Like TSH, TRH secretion is inhibited by T_3. The secretion of TH also decreases in stressful conditions like burns, trauma, fever, and starvation.

The **effect of iodine** on thyroid functions is quite complex. The most obvious effect of administering a high dose of iodine is a decrease in the release of thyroid hormones. This effect is very prompt and is quicker than the action of antithyroid drugs. Hence, iodine was used in the treatment of thyrotoxicosis and is still used in preparing patients for thyroid surgery. However, the effect is not observed on repeated administration of iodine, a phenomenon called *iodine escape*, the mechanism of which is not understood.

Administration of a high dose of iodine (2 mg or more) has a triphasic response on the organification of iodine. Initially,

Release | The lysosomal proteases digest the thyroglobulin and release the iodotyrosines (MIT, DIT) and iodothyronines (T_3, T_4). Only T_3 and T_4 diffuse out into the circulation. MIT and DIT are stripped off their iodine residues by the action of an intracellular enzyme called iodotyrosine deiodinase. The iodide released exceeds the iodide taken up from circulation and is utilized for new hormone synthesis.

Transport, Metabolism, and Excretion

Most of the circulating thyroid hormone is protein bound, leaving only 0.02% T_4 and ~0.2% T_3 unbound or free. There are three thyroid hormone-binding plasma proteins: thyroxine-binding globulin (TBG), thyroxine-binding prealbumin (TBPA), and thyroxine-binding albumin (TBA). Whenever the concentration of unbound thyroid hormone falls, it is partly restored by the dissociation of the protein-bound thyroid hormone. The reverse occurs when the free hormone level rises. Hence, the hormone-binding proteins buffer fluctuations in plasma hormonal level. Changes in the plasma protein concentration do not normally produce sustained changes in the free hormone level. When the plasma protein concentration increases, as in pregnancy, there is a temporary fall in the free TH level (as

Fig. 77.5 Hypothalamic–pituitary–thyroid control of thyroid hormone release. Negative feedback pathways are shown as blue arrows.

there is a brief increase in iodine uptake in the thyroid gland (more iodine is available to the pump) and an increase in thyroid hormone production. Shortly thereafter, the high intrathyroid iodide concentration inhibits hormone production, an effect known as the *Wolff-Chaikoff effect.* Prolonged administration of a high dose of iodine, however, produces an "escape" from the Wolff-Chaikoff effect. The Na^+–I^- symporter is downregulated, and the intrathyroid iodide concentration is therefore reduced, and with it, the Wolff-Chaikoff effect subsides. If, however, the autoregulation is absent due to thyroid dysfunction, the Wolff-Chaikoff effect will persist and keep the iodine organification suppressed. The effect is known as the *Jod-Basedow effect*, and it explains the cause of hypothyroid iodide goiter (**Fig. 77.6**).

Goitrogens are antithyroid substances that inhibit the synthesis of thyroid hormone, causing thyroid enlargement (goiter). Certain vegetables, such as plants of the Brassica family (cabbages), contain progoitrin as well as a goitrin activator that converts the progoitrin into goitrin. Goitrin activators present in vegetables are destroyed by cooking, but goitrin activators are also synthesized by intestinal bacteria. Hence, excessive consumption of vegetables like cabbage produces goiter (cabbage goiter).

Physiologic Effects of Thyroid Hormone

The physiologic actions of thyroid hormone can be summarized as twofold: morphogenesis (growth and differentiation) and calorigenesis (energy production). These actions are mediated by thyroid hormone receptors in the nucleus of the target cells (group I hormonal mechanism) to increase messenger ribonucleic acid (mRNA) transcription and protein synthesis. The proteins synthesized not only are structural proteins that contribute to morphogenesis, but also include an enormous number of enzymes (which are proteins), membrane transporter proteins (e.g., glucose transporters), and membrane pumps (e.g., Na^+–K^+ adenosinetriphosphatase [ATPase] and Ca^{2+} AT-

Pase). These enzymes of intermediary metabolism promote anabolic and catabolic reactions, which explains the complex metabolic picture produced by thyroid hormone. The increase in metabolic reactions and the increase in the activity of the Na^+–K^+ pump result in increased demand for adenosine triphosphate (ATP). This high demand for ATP is met by an increase in cellular respiration inside the mitochondria, which increases its oxygen consumption. Normally, 68% of the energy released in the mitochondria through oxidative phosphorylation is captured into ATP, and 32% is wasted as heat. Hence, an increase in oxidative phosphorylation not only increases the ATP yield, but also increases the heat produced (thermogenesis). Earlier it was believed that thyroid hormone caused uncoupling of oxidative phosphorylation: it reduced the ATP yield so that more energy was released as heat. It is now known that this is true only for pharmacologic doses (higher than physiologic levels) of thyroid hormones. At physiologic doses of thyroid hormone, the ratio of ATP to heat output remains unaltered.

Growth and maturation | Thyroid hormone is essential for normal ossification of cartilage and bone growth, normal erythropoiesis, and normal onset of puberty and lactation. TH is also essential for the normal myelination and synaptic development in the central nervous system (CNS); its absence during the critical developmental period results in serious mental retardation.

Metabolic rate | Thyroid hormone seems to adjust the set point for the metabolic rate of the body. Thyroid hormone increases the basal metabolic rate (BMR) and also increases the body temperature. Note, however, that the thyroid plays no direct role in temperature regulation (Chapter 43). Calorigenesis is the most striking effect of thyroid hormones.

General Model: Energy

The control of the basal metabolic rate plays an important role in determining the body's utilization of energy, and increased or decreased levels of thyroid hormone have profound, widespread effects on many physiologic functions.

Carbohydrate metabolism | Thyroid hormone has both hypoglycemic and hyperglycemic effects. The hypoglycemic effect is the increased glycolysis. The hyperglycemic effects are stimulation of glycogenolysis and gluconeogenesis and enhanced intestinal glucose absorption due to increased activity of glucose transporters and increase in gastrointestinal motility. The net effect is hyperglycemia and depletion of liver glycogen. There is increase in food intake in response to the increased glucose utilization.

Protein metabolism | Thyroid hormone has a potent protein anabolic effect; however, in large doses, it has a protein catabolic effect. Thyroid hormone inhibits synthesis of glycosaminoglycans and fibronectin in fibroblasts.

Fat metabolism | Thyroid hormone stimulates both lipogenesis and lipolysis. The lipolysis exceeds lipogenesis. Hormone-sensitive lipase mobilizes fat from adipose tissues, increasing the plasma concentrations of free fatty acid (FFA)

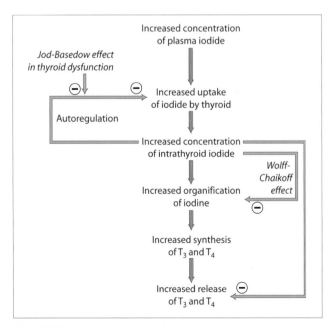

Fig. 77.6 Effect of iodine on thyroid functions.

and glycerol. The elevated levels of FFA and glycerol promote hepatic triglyceride synthesis. However, when the triglycerides synthesized in the liver are released into the circulation, they are again broken down into FFA and glycerol by lipoprotein lipase. Thyroid hormone also enhances de novo cholesterol synthesis as well as bile acid synthesis. Yet plasma cholesterol decreases due to increased low-density lipoprotein (LDL) receptor formation in the liver and the consequent increase in the removal of cholesterol from the circulation. Overall, there is an increase in the plasma FFAs and glycerol and a decrease in the plasma triglycerides, phospholipids, and cholesterol.

Vitamin metabolism | Thyroid hormone is required for the hepatic conversion of carotene to vitamin A. In hypothyroid states, the serum carotene is elevated, and the skin becomes yellow. The color of the sclera of the eye is not affected in carotenemia, which distinguishes it from jaundice in which the sclera, too, is stained yellow.

Cardiovascular effects | The increase in metabolic rate and body temperature imposes greater demands on the cardiorespiratory system. The rise in body temperature is associated with increased cutaneous vasodilatation and sweating. Also, the increase in metabolic rate imposes a greater oxygen demand, which produces autoregulatory vasodilatation in the muscle bed. Vasodilatation lowers the diastolic blood pressure. The fall in blood pressure results in a compensatory increase in blood volume through renal mechanisms. The vasodilatation and hypervolemia result in a rise in central venous pressure (CVP) and with it, a rise in cardiac output. The increase in cardiac output tends to lower the CVP. However, when the CVP is very high, it remains elevated despite the increase in cardiac output, resulting in high-output cardiac failure.

The increase in cardiac output is also attributable to a direct effect of thyroid hormone on cardiac contractility. In part, this is because it increases the synthesis of β-adrenergic receptors, which potentiates the cardiac effect of catecholamines, and increases the synthesis of an isoform of the myosin heavy chain, which has greater ATPase activity than the β isoform.

Thyroid Disorders

Goiter

A prominent enlargement of the thyroid gland is called a goiter. Thyroid enlargement does not necessarily mean that the thyroid is functionally overactive. A goiter may be associated with a hypothyroid, hyperthyroid, or euthyroid state. A euthyroid goiter, for example, can occur if thyroid hormone synthesis is impaired by goitrogens and is subsequently restored to normal by increased TSH secretion through hypothalamo–hypophysial feedback.

The recommended minimum intake of iodine is 150 μg/day, which is equal to the amount of iodine taken up daily by a normal thyroid gland. During pregnancy, the recommended intake is 200 μg/day. Goiter occurs when the intake decreases to less than half of the recommended amount. Iodide is added to commercial preparations of salt and bread to prevent the occurrence of goiter.

Hypothyroidism

Although mild iodine deficiency causes a euthyroid goiter, as explained above, severe iodine deficiency is the most common cause of hypothyroid goiter. Less common causes of hypothyroidism are diseased or maldeveloped thyroid, genetic enzyme deficiency, antithyroid therapy, and goitrogens in the diet.

The signs and symptoms of hypothyroidism include fatigue, lethargy, sleepiness, muscular weakness, bradycardia, decreased cardiac output, hypovolemia, weight gain, constipation, mental sluggishness, sparse and coarse hair, characteristic facies, scaly skin, husky voice, and in severe cases, an edematous appearance throughout the body called *myxedema.* Myxedema is not due to fluid retention, but to the deposition in the interstitial fluid of large quantities of gel-like substances (proteins mixed with hyaluronic acid and chondroitin sulfate). Hence, instead of the usual pitting edema that occurs due to an increase in interstitial volume, myxedema results in nonpitting edema. The huskiness of voice is common enough in hypothyroidism to justify the claim that myxedema can be diagnosed just by talking to the patient. Finally, the mental sluggishness can progress to myxedema "madness" in severe cases of hypothyroidism. Hypothyroidism is associated with a rise in blood cholesterol, predisposing to atherosclerosis with all its complications: peripheral vascular disease, coronary artery disease, and deafness.

The laboratory diagnosis of hypothyroidism includes the estimation of plasma concentration of thyroid hormones (lowered), the BMR (reduced), and the systolic ejection time (prolonged).

Congenital hypothyroidism | When thyroid deficiency occurs during fetal life, infancy, or childhood, the result is a characteristic change to many developmental processes. Skeletal growth is inhibited more than the soft tissue growth. Therefore, soft tissues enlarge excessively, producing the characteristic appearance of these individuals, which includes a pot belly and a large protruding tongue. The ratio of the upper part (iliac crest to the crown of the head) to the lower part (iliac crest to the heel) of the body is ~1.7:1 at birth and reduces to 1:1 by the age of 7 to 9 years. In these individuals, however, the infantile proportions persist so that the upper part of the body is taller than the lower part.

Development of the fetus is dependent on the maternal T$_4$ that reaches it through the placenta; therefore, maternal hypothyroidism results in neonatal hypothyroidism. It is important to treat neonatal hypothyroidism immediately at birth. If left untreated until 2 years of age, there is a marked decrease in the myelination and arborization of neurons in the brain, which is dependent on thyroid hormone for its early development. These changes are irreversible after 2 years of age and result in serious mental retardation.

Hyperthyroidism

The most common cause of hyperthyroidism is Graves disease, an autoimmune disease in which autoantibodies are formed against TSH receptors. The TSH receptors are activated by the autoantibodies, resulting in hypersecretion of thyroid hormone. Hyperthyroidism can also occur due to a TSH-secreting tumor of the anterior pituitary.

Clinical features of hyperthyroidism include intolerance to heat, excessive sweating, and weight loss (due to the high metabolic rate), muscle weakness (thyrotoxic myopathy, due to increased breakdown of muscle proteins), diarrhea (due to increased gastrointestinal motility), nervousness and psychic disorders, inability to sleep, and tremors of the hands. Palpitations and arrhythmias occur due to increased cardiac response to circulating catecholamines, and the pulse pressure is high. High output cardiac failure may develop in severe cases. The BMR rises, and the systolic ejection time shortens.

Patients of Graves disease develop *exophthalmos*—proptosis of the eyeballs. In this condition, the eyelids do not close completely when the person blinks or is asleep. It is caused by the accumulation of fluid and cells in retrobulbar tissues and a varying degree of spasm of the upper eyelid.

Severe exacerbation of hyperthyroidism is called *thyroid storm* or *thyrotoxic crisis*. In the past, it was seen postoperatively in patients poorly prepared for surgery. Its incidence has decreased now with preoperative use of antithyroid drugs and iodide.

The treatment of hyperthyroidism includes surgical removal of the thyroid and use of antithyroid drugs.

Thyroid Function Tests

Thyroid dysfunction should be suspected if the BMR, serum cholesterol, and systolic ejection time are outside their respective normal ranges. The following tests are necessary for confirming a thyroid dysfunction.

Tests of thyroid activity | The normal serum T_4 is ~8 µg/dL, and normal serum T_3 is 0.15 µg/dL. They are measured by radioimmunoassay. Higher or lower values are suggestive of hyperthyroidism or hypothyroidism, respectively.

Radioactive iodide uptake by the thyroid gland indicates the functional status of the thyroid gland. A 24-hour uptake normally ranges between 5 and 35% of the administered dose of I^{131}, a β emitter. The uptake increases in hyperthyroidism and decreases in hypothyroidism.

Scintiscanning localizes the sites of accumulation of the radionuclides and thereby detects localized areas of thyroid hyperactivity or hypoactivity. Technetium 99m, a gamma emitter, is used for radioimaging of the thyroid because it is transported into the thyroid, but unlike iodide, it is not organified and therefore diffuses back into the circulation.

Tests for hormonal feedback control | The basal concentration of serum TSH is 7 µU/mL. It increases on TRH administration and decreases on TH administration.

The *TRH stimulation test* is helpful in diagnosing mild abnormalities of thyroid function. The thyroid hormone feedback at the level of the pituitary reduces the TRH receptors on the pituitary and also inhibits the transcription of TSH. In hyperthyroidism of thyroid origin, the high level of circulating TH renders the pituitary insensitive to TRH. Stimulation by TRH therefore elicits little TSH secretion from the pituitary.

Conversely, there is an exaggerated TSH secretion in response to TRH administration in hypothyroidism of thyroid origin.

In the *thyroid suppression test*, TH is administered to suppress the pituitary secretion of TSH. Suppression of TSH secretion reduces the radioactive iodine uptake to 50% of normal. Lack of suppression indicates autonomous production of TH.

Tests of thyroid damage | These tests detect actual or potential damage to the thyroid gland. In carcinoma of the thyroid, thyroglobulin is released into the bloodstream. The presence of autoantibodies to the thyroid gland indicates thyroid disorders. For example, antimicrosomal antibody suggests Hashimoto disease, and antithyroglobulin antibody suggests Graves disease.

Antithyroid Drugs

Drugs that inhibit thyroid hormone synthesis are used in the treatment of hyperthyroidism. Antithyroid drugs are grouped into two classes: agents that block iodide transport and agents that inhibit the coupling of iodotyrosyl residues in thyroglobulin.

Drugs that block iodide uptake include pertechnetate (TcO_4^-), perchlorate (ClO_4^-), thiocyanate (SCN^-), and nitrate (NO_3^-). These monovalent anions are competitive inhibitors of iodide transport. ClO_4^- and SCN^- are no longer used because of their toxicity.

Drugs preventing iodotyrosine formation are the thioamides (propylthiouracil, methimazole, and carbimazole), which are competitive inhibitors of thyroxine peroxidase. Thioamides also inhibit the coupling reactions mediated by thyroxine peroxidase. Propylthiouracil additionally inhibits 5′-deiodinase, leading to a reduction in the extrathyroidal synthesis of T_3.

Some other drugs that inhibit thyroid function are radioiodine I^{131}, which is used in the treatment of Graves disease, and lithium carbonate, which inhibits the iodination of thyroglobulin. The radiation from I^{131} destroys the thyroid tissues.

Summary

● Thyroid hormone is an iodinated tyrosine molecule present in two biologic active forms, T_3 containing three iodine ions and T_4 containing four.

● Release of thyroid hormone is controlled by thyroid-stimulating hormone from the pituitary gland.

● Thyroid hormone acts by binding to intracellular receptors and altering gene transcription.

● Thyroid hormone affects growth and development in neonates and children and the basal metabolic rate in all individuals.

Applying What You Know

77.1. Mrs. Omaya's laboratory reports show that she has low T_4 and low TSH. Where in her endocrine system could dysfunction give rise to these two abnormalities? Explain.

77.2. Which of Mrs. Omaya's findings on the physical examination suggests that she is in a hypothyroid state? Which finding would preclude her problem being a dietary one?

77.3. Mrs. Schilling was found to have an enlarged thyroid gland on physical examination. How would you explain the mechanism resulting in this hypertrophied state?

Calcium (Ca^{2+}) is an electrolyte that plays key roles in a large number of physiologic processes: (1) contraction of muscle, (2) release of neurotransmitters from axon terminals and hormones and hormones from gland cells, and (3) determination of the activity of enzymes. Thus, it is essential that the concentration of calcium be homeostatically regulated.

There are three hormones that contribute to regulating calcium balance: parathyroid hormone, calcitonin, and calcitriol. These hormones control the calcium balance of the body by acting on three tissues: bone, intestine, and kidney. Before discussing these hormones, it is necessary to understand the physiology of bone tissue and its role in body calcium balance; bone is, after all, the site at which most of the calcium in the body is stored.

Bone Tissue

Bone Chemistry
Bone consists of bone cells and an extracellular matrix. One-third of the matrix is made of organic components called the osteoid, and two-thirds is made of inorganic mineral crystals. The osteoid is made of collagen and glycosaminoglycans and is deposited by the bone cells around themselves. The inorganic minerals are the hydroxyapatite and fluorapatite crystals. The chemical formula for hydroxyapatite crystal is

$$[(Ca_3(PO_4)_2]_3 \cdot Ca(OH)_2$$

and for fluorapatite crystal

$$[(Ca_3(PO_4)_2]_3 \cdot CaF_2$$

The Ca^{2+}: P ratio in bone is ~1.7:1. Amorphous $Ca_3(PO_4)_2$ is deposited in the matrix when a certain critical value called the *solubility product* is exceeded. It is slowly converted to hydroxyapatite and fluorapatite crystals through the addition of hydroxides and fluorides. When the solubility product exceeds 60, there is *metastatic calcification*—deposition of $Ca_3(PO_4)_2$ in tissues other than the bone.

Bone Histophysiology
New bone is always formed in thin layers. These layers may form concentric lamellae, as in cortical (compact) bone, or a meshwork of bone spicules, as in trabecular (spongy) bone. The concentric lamellae of cortical bone are arranged around a central channel (haversian canal) that contains the capillary blood supply (**Fig. 78.1**). The entire structure is called the osteon and constitutes the basic unit of cortical bone. Present in the bone tissue are three types of cells: the osteoblasts, the

osteocytes, and the osteoclasts. The osteoblasts and osteocytes develop from the osteoprogenitor stem cells; the osteoclasts belong to the monocyte–macrophage system.

Osteoblasts are bone-forming cells present on bone surfaces. They secrete matrix constituents: collagen, other noncollagenous proteins such as osteocalcin and osteonectin, and ground substance. They also contain abundant alkaline phosphatase that hydrolyzes phosphate esters. The phosphate liberated by active osteoblasts raises the local phosphate concentration to the point where the solubility product is exceeded, and mineral crystals precipitate. Although primarily concerned with bone accretion, osteoblasts also facilitate bone resorption, ensuring that there is continuous bone remodeling (see below).

Osteocytes are osteoblasts that have been buried in the bone matrix. Each cell is surrounded by its own lacuna, but an extensive canalicular system connects the osteocytes to the osteoblasts present on the bone surface. The long cell processes of osteocytes are connected through gap junctions to other osteocytes and to the surface osteoblasts, forming a functional syncytium. To survive, osteocytes must ensure that the canalicular system is not obliterated completely. Hence, osteocytes promptly break down any freshly formed mineral crystals (*osteocytic osteolysis*) and transport the calcium released to the exterior. Osteocytic osteolysis should not be confused with bone resorption (see below), which involves the complete breakdown of the bone matrix as well.

Osteoclasts are giant, multinucleated cells formed by the fusion of several precursor cells. Like osteoblasts, they are present on the bone surface. They attach to the bone surface through integrins, sealing off a small enclosed area (**Fig. 78.2A**). The part of the cell membrane that faces the bone surface becomes ruffled and is called the ruffled border. Collagenase, acid phosphatase, lysosomal enzymes, and H^+ are secreted across the ruffled border into the enclosed space, causing bone resorption in the underlying bone surface. H^+ dissolves the bone minerals; enzymes digest the organic bone matrix.

Bone Turnover
Throughout life, a significant fraction of bone is continuously replaced by new bone. This process is called bone turnover (or bone remodeling) and involves both bone accretion and bone resorption. Most of the bone turnover occurs at bone surfaces. In compact bone, bone turnover occurs both at the endosteal surface adjoining the marrow cavity and at the subperiosteal surface. Trabecular bone presents with a very large surface area and therefore has a much greater bone turnover.

Bone turnover is brought about by osteoblasts (causing bone accretion) and osteoclasts (causing bone resorption) working in tandem. Activated osteoblasts secrete an osteoclast-stimulating factor that activates osteoclasts. Osteoblasts also secrete the enzyme procollagenase and plasminogen activator. Plasminogen activator catalyzes the conversion of serum plasminogen to plasmin. This, in turn, releases collagenase from

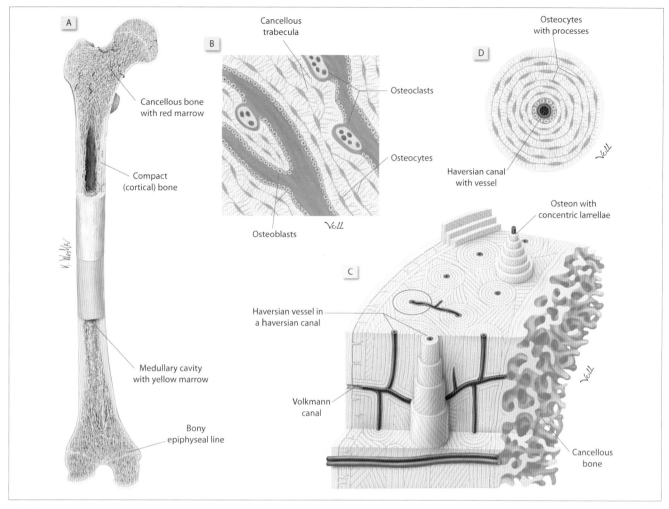

Fig. 78.1 **(A)** A coronal section through parts of a femur, showing compact and cancellous bone. **(B)** Cancellous trabecula and bone cells. **(C)** Three-dimensional presentation of the structure of compact bone, showing the haversian canals and Volkmann canals. **(D)** Microstructure of an osteon.

its proenzyme procollagenase. Collagenase depolymerizes collagen, softening the matrix and making it accessible to the activated osteoclasts (**Fig. 78.2B**).

The extent of bone accretion, bone resorption, and bone turnover (both bone accretion and resorption) are indicated by the serum level of certain enzymes. *Alkaline phosphatase* is secreted by active osteoblasts; therefore, its serum concentration increases during bone accretion. *Hydroxyproline,* the major metabolite of collagen, is produced during bone resorption; therefore, its urinary level provides an index of bone resorption. *Osteocalcin* (a protein) is released from osteoblasts during bone accretion and from the bone matrix during bone resorption. Hence, its serum level is an index of bone turnover.

Bone Disorders

Osteoporosis is associated with a loss of bone matrix and occurs whenever osteoclastic activity exceeds osteoblastic activity. It is associated with a reduction in bone mass per unit volume with a normal ratio of mineral-to-organic matrix. Osteoporosis and fractures are more common in bones containing

a higher proportion of trabecular bone, for example, the distal forearm (Colles fracture), vertebral bodies (kyphosis), and hip bone.

Osteoporosis is observed normally after the age of 35 years (involutional osteoporosis) and is more marked in postmenopausal women. Estrogen has a protective action against osteoporosis because it stimulates the secretion of cytokines that inhibit the development of osteoclasts and also increases the rate of apoptosis of osteoclasts. Osteoporosis also occurs following prolonged immobilization (disuse osteoporosis). Calcitonin and bisphosphonates (e.g., etidronate) inhibit osteoclastic activity and have been used in the treatment of osteoporosis.

Osteomalacia and **rickets** occur due to inadequate mineralization of the bones (**Fig. 78.3A**). Failure of the organic matrix (osteoid) to mineralize normally results in an excess of unmineralized bone. Osteomalacia occurs in adults; rickets occurs in children prior to the closure of the epiphyses. Hence, it affects the mineralization of not only the osteoid, but also the epiphyseal cartilages, which increase in thickness. Moreover, rickets is associated with bony deformities

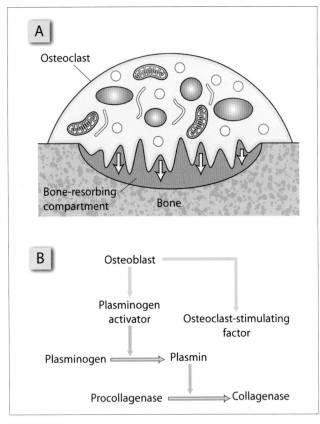

Fig. 78.2 **(A)** Bone resorption by an osteoclast. **(B)** Bone resorptive mechanism of an osteoblast.

such as bow legs. In osteomalacia, gross bony deformities are uncommon. Both rickets and osteomalacia are associated with hypocalcemia.

Osteitis fibrosa cystica is characterized by osteoclastic bone resorption, which results in subperiosteal erosions, especially in phalanges, long bones, and distal ends of clavicles.

The endosteal surface shows fewer trabeculae, and the bone marrow becomes fibrous.

In **osteosclerosis** there is enhanced bone density in the upper and lower margins of vertebrae. It is seen in calcium deficiency and occurs mainly due to bone remodeling and redistribution of bone minerals. *Osteopetrosis* (**Fig. 78.3B**) is a congenital form of osteosclerosis in which the osteoclasts are defective. The unopposed action of osteoblasts results in an increase in bone density.

Body Calcium Pools

The total body calcium content (**Fig. 78.4**) of ~1 kg is distributed in two major pools: the extracellular fluid (ECF) pool and the bone pool. The ECF calcium pool contains only ~1.2 g of calcium; the rest is present in the bone pool. There is continuous exchange of calcium between the two pools. Within the bone calcium pool, there is a smaller *rapidly exchangeable* bone calcium pool of ~4 g. The calcium in this pool rapidly exchanges with the calcium in the ECF. The remaining bone calcium pool is called the *slowly exchangeable* bone calcium pool that requires parathyroid hormone for its mobilization. The calcium in this pool enters the ECF only when the bone tissue is broken down (bone resorption). Conversely, ECF Ca^{2+} enters this pool only when new bone is deposited (bone accretion). The total size of the body calcium pool remains constant because the amount lost daily in urine (0.1 g) is replenished by an equal amount of dietary Ca^{2+} absorbed from the gastrointestinal tract.

The plasma concentration of total Ca^{2+} is ~10 mg/dL. About 45% is *ionized* or free Ca^{2+}, which is freely diffusible and brings about the physiologic effects of Ca^{2+}. Another 10% is present as *poorly ionizable* Ca^{2+} salts of phosphate, bicarbonate, and citrate, which are freely diffusible and provide an immediate reserve of Ca^{2+} during sudden hypocalcemia. The remaining 45% of the Ca^{2+} is *nondiffusible*, being bound to albumin. The albumin releases Ca^{2+} slowly when plasma Ca^{2+} concentration decreases.

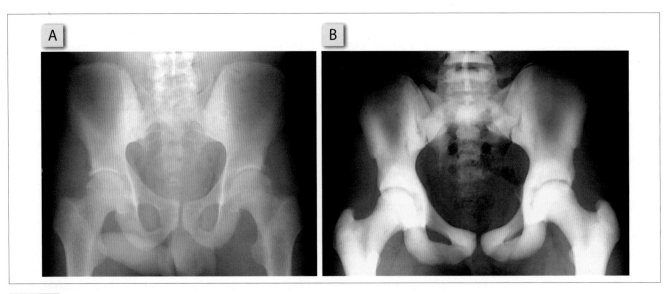

Fig. 78.3 **(A)** Reduced bone density in osteomalacia. **(B)** Increased bone density in osteopetrosis.

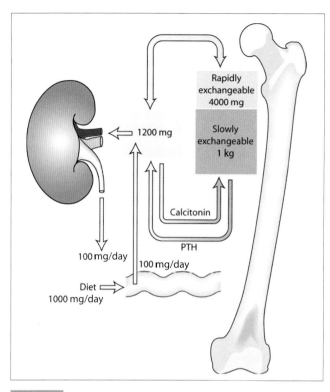

Fig. 78.4 Body calcium compartments. In a normal individual, the gains and loses of calcium are equal. PTH, parathyroid hormone.

> **General Model: Reservoir**
>
> The plasma compartment is a reservoir for calcium, and to understand the effects of calcium-regulating hormones requires keeping track of the various inputs to and outputs from the sites involved.

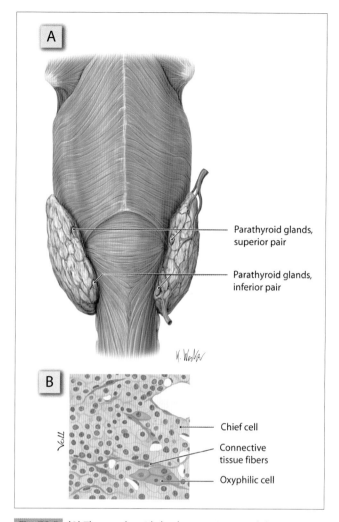

Fig. 78.5 **(A)** The parathyroid glands, posterior view. **(B)** Microscopic structure of parathyroid gland.

Calcium-regulating Hormones

Parathyroid Hormone

Parathyroid hormone (PTH) is a group IIA polypeptide hormone secreted by the chief cells of the parathyroid glands (**Fig. 78.5**). It increases bone remodeling by directly stimulating osteoblasts and indirectly stimulating osteoclasts through the osteoclast-stimulating factor. However, the bone resorption exceeds bone accretion; therefore, PTH causes a net bone resorption. It also stimulates the synthesis of activated vitamin D_3 and thereby stimulates the absorption of calcium in the small intestine.

Calcium homeostasis | When plasma Ca^{2+} falls, PTH secretion increases. PTH raises plasma Ca^{2+} in three ways. (1) It mobilizes bone Ca^{2+} by increasing bone resorption. (2) It increases the gastrointestinal absorption of Ca^{2+} by increasing activated vitamin D synthesis: PTH increases vitamin D formation by stimulating 1α-hydroxylase activity in the proximal tubular cells of the kidney. (3) It increases Ca^{2+} reabsorption in the distal nephron. However, because it also produces hypercalcemia, the large amounts of Ca^{2+} filtered into the tubules result

in hypercalcuria despite the enhanced tubular reabsorption. Interestingly, a parathyroid hormone-related protein (PTHrP) can bind to PTH receptor and mimic its actions. PTHrP is the major cause of hypercalcemia in cancer.

The PTH-induced dissolution of the hydroxyapatite crystals in the bone is also associated with bicarbonate release, which tends to produce metabolic alkalosis. However, the simultaneous bicarbonaturia produced by the tubular action of PTH minimizes the alkalosis produced by the dissolution of hydroxyapatite crystals.

Bone resorption releases both Ca^{2+} and phosphates into plasma. A simultaneous elevation of phosphates along with Ca^{2+} would cause precipitation of $Ca_3(PO_4)_2$ in tissues and a lowering of plasma ionized calcium. PTH prevents such precipitation of $Ca_3(PO_4)_2$ through its *phosphaturic effect,* which lowers the plasma phosphate levels. The phosphaturia occurs because PTH decreases the proximal tubular reabsorption of phosphate.

Phosphate homeostasis | In an indirect way, PTH also maintains constancy of the plasma phosphate level. An increase in plasma phosphate is associated with increased precipitation of $Ca_3(PO_4)_2$ as the solubility product is exceeded. The resultant decrease in plasma Ca^{2+} stimulates PTH secretion, which, in turn, increases the urinary excretion of phosphates (**Fig. 78.6**).

Calcitonin

Calcitonin is a polypeptide hormone secreted by the parafollicular (C) cells of the thyroid gland. Its secretion is stimulated by hypercalcemia (**Fig. 78.7**). Calcitonin secretion is also influenced by gastrointestinal hormones such as gastrin and glucagon (stimulators) and somatostatin (inhibitor). Calcitonin produces hypocalcemia and hypophosphatemia by inhibiting osteoclastic bone resorption and also by increasing the urinary excretion of calcium and phosphate ions. Osteoclasts have receptors for calcitonin on them.

Calcitonin deficiency causes few problems so long as the parathyroid gland functions normally. Calcitonin may be important during pregnancy and lactation when the calcium demand of the body rises considerably. The excess calcium demand can be met either by higher dietary intake or by mobilizing calcium through bone resorption. Calcitonin might be important in preventing excessive bone resorption in such situations.

Activated Vitamin D
Vitamin D (also known as dihydrocholecalciferol) is a lipid-soluble hormone. It acts like a group I (steroid) hormone that interacts with nuclear receptors in target cells. However, it is also hydrophilic, as it contains three hydroxyl groups. Hence, it also acts like a group IIB hormone, acting through membrane

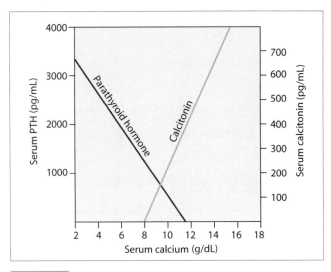

Fig. 78.7 Reciprocal relationship between parathyroid hormone (PTH) and calcitonin secretion. When serum calcium increases, serum PTH decreases, and serum calcitonin increases.

receptors with cyclic guanosine monophosphate (cGMP) as the second messenger.

Calcitriol is synthesized from vitamin D_3 (cholecalciferol) in two steps (**Fig. 78.8**). Vitamin D_3 is first converted in the liver to calcidiol (25-hydroxycholecalciferol) by 25-hydroxylase. Next, it is metabolized in the kidney to calcitriol (1,25-dihydroxycholecalciferol) by 1α-hydroxylase. Calcidiol is the major circulating form of vitamin D_3; calcitriol is the final active form of vitamin D_3. Mole for mole, calcitriol is 100 times more potent than calcidiol and 300 times more potent than vitamin D_3.

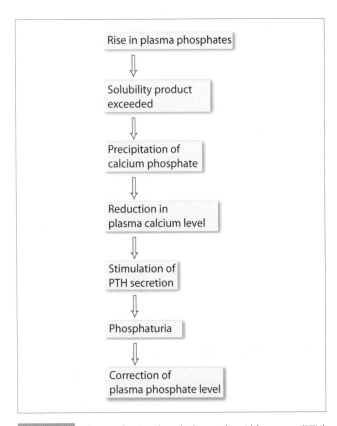

Fig. 78.6 The mechanism by which parathyroid hormone (PTH) maintains phosphate homeostasis.

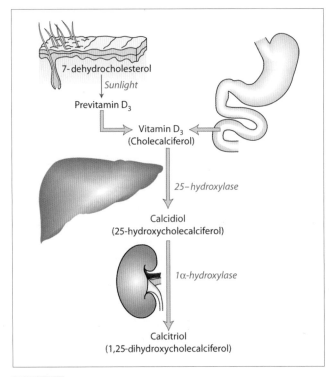

Fig. 78.8 The formation of vitamin D.

Vitamin D$_3$ is synthesized in skin and is also present in the diet. The keratinocytes of the stratum corneum of the epidermis contain 7-dehydrocholesterol, which is converted into previtamin D$_3$ through photoactivation by solar ultraviolet radiation in the wavelength of 290 to 315 nm. Previtamin D$_3$ is then slowly converted into vitamin D$_3$ (cholecalciferol). Fatty fish and cod liver oil are rich dietary sources of vitamin D$_3$. Absorption of dietary vitamin D$_3$ occurs mainly in the ileum and requires bile salts.

Calcitriol production is increased by PTH and hypophosphatemia (**Fig. 78.9A**). PTH activates renal 1α-hydroxylase, which catalyzes the conversion of 25-hydroxycholecalciferol to 1,25-dihydroxycholecalciferol. In its turn, calcitriol exerts a negative feedback on PTH secretion. Hypophosphatemia increases calcitriol by directly activating renal 1α-hydroxylase. Hypocalcemia increases calcitriol synthesis indirectly through its stimulation of PTH secretion.

Effect on bone | Calcitriol, like PTH, has the opposite effects on bone, increasing both bone deposition and bone resorption. However, its net effect is increased mineralization of the bone. Calcitriol stimulates osteoblasts to lay down osteoid (osteoblasts and their precursors have nuclear receptors for calcitriol) and further promotes the mineralization of the osteoid by maintaining adequate concentrations of extracellular Ca^{2+} and phosphates. Activated osteoblasts secrete osteoclast-stimulating factor, which induces the development of osteoclasts from their precursors. (Osteoclasts themselves do not have any calcitriol receptor.) Osteoclastic activation promotes bone resorption.

Effect on intestine | Calcitriol promotes intestinal absorption of Ca^{2+} and phosphate, which contributes to increased bone mineralization. Ca^{2+} absorption occurs principally in the duodenum; phosphates are absorbed mostly from the jejunum and ileum. Both are absorbed through secondary active transport. Ca^{2+} is extruded across the basolateral membrane of duodenal enterocytes by a Ca^{2+}–adenosinetriphosphatase (ATPase) pump (**Fig. 78.9B**). Calcitriol induces the synthesis of this pump protein. Increased activity of the Ca^{2+}–ATPase pump lowers the intracellular Ca^{2+}, which promotes the facilitated diffusion of Ca^{2+} at the brush border membrane of intestinal microvilli. Calcitriol also induces the synthesis of a calcium-binding protein called calbindin. The exact role of calbindin in calcium absorption is not known. Calcitriol stimulates intestinal phosphate uptake via a Na$^+$–phosphate symporter.

Effect on kidney | In the kidney, calcitriol stimulates reabsorption of phosphate in the proximal tubule and reabsorption of Ca^{2+} in the distal tubule. As in enterocytes, calbindin is present in renal tubular cells and probably has a role in increasing Ca^{2+} absorption.

General Models: Balance of Forces and Homeostasis

It is essential to recognize that there is a critically important balance of forces determining the concentration of calcium that is present in the blood. The hormones homeostatically regulating calcium concentration act in concert to keep calcium at an appropriate concentration.

Calcium Balance Disorders

Hypoparathyroidism

Primary hypoparathyroidism | When the parathyroid glands secrete inadequate amounts of PTH, it is called primary hypoparathyroidism. The reduced secretion may be due either to a deficiency in PTH secretion or to the accidental removal of parathyroid tissue during thyroid surgery. It results in hypocalcemia and hyperphosphatemia. Soft tissue calcification is also common, especially in the basal ganglia, and is probably due to the hyperphosphatemia and the precipitation of calcium phosphate salts.

If the hypocalcemia is severe enough, it results in tetany, a condition associated with spontaneous excitability of nerves leading to muscle spasms. The spasms mostly involve the extremities and the larynx. Laryngeal spasm can be fatal. Latent tetany can be diagnosed by eliciting Chvostek's and Trousseau's signs. *Chvostek's sign* is the ipsilateral contraction of the facial muscles elicited by the percussion of the facial nerve just anterior to the earlobe. *Trousseau's sign* is the carpopedal spasm elicited by application of occlusive pressure (with a blood pressure cuff) on the arm. The carpopedal spasm appears as thumb adduction, metacarpophalangeal joint flexion, and interphalangeal joint extension.

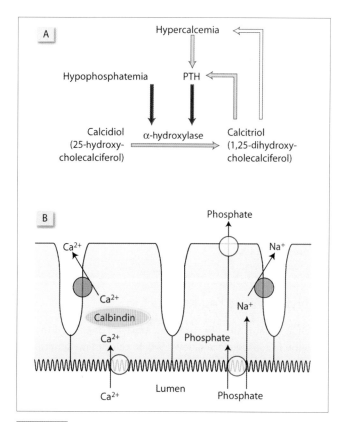

Fig. 78.9 (A) Control of vitamin D production. (B) Effect of vitamin D on calcium absorption in the intestine. Inhibitory effects are shown in blue.

Secondary hypoparathyroidism is caused by the feedback suppression of PTH secretion by increased plasma Ca^{2+} concentration, for example, by excessive intake of vitamin D.

In **pseudohypoparathyroidism,** PTH receptors are resistant to the action of PTH. Hence, hypocalcemia and hyperphosphatemia are present, but PTH secretion is elevated due to feedback stimulation of the parathyroid by hypocalcemia (**Table 78.1**).

Hyperparathyroidism

Primary hyperparathyroidism | When the excessive secretion of PTH is caused by a tumor of the parathyroid gland or by ectopic parathyroid tissue, it is called primary hyperparathyroidism. Excess PTH leads to hypercalcemia and hypophosphatemia with increased urinary excretion of Ca^{2+}, phosphates, and hydroxyproline. Nephrolithiasis (kidney stones) is common. The stones are composed of calcium oxalate or calcium phosphate. Bones show osteopenia (reduction in bone mass) and may develop osteitis fibrosa cystica.

Secondary hyperparathyroidism | If the excessive PTH secretion is secondary to hypocalcemia, it is called secondary hyperparathyroidism. Such hypocalcemia can occur if vitamin D is deficient in diet, is poorly absorbed due to malabsorption of fats, or is not converted to calcitriol due to renal disease. Secondary hyperparathyroidism can also occur when there is an increased demand for Ca^{2+}, as during pregnancy and lactation.

Hypovitaminosis D

Hypovitaminosis D results in rickets or osteomalacia, moderate hypocalcemia, severe hypophosphatemia, and secondary hyperparathyroidism. The secondary hyperparathyroidism minimizes the hypocalcemia but aggravates the hypophosphatemia and bone changes.

Hypervitaminosis D

Hypervitaminosis D occurs following ingestion of excess vitamin D. Hypervitaminosis D results in hypercalcemia and hypercalciuria. In severe cases, there is widespread ectopic calcification.

Although sunlight stimulates vitamin D production, excessive exposure to sunlight does not cause vitamin D toxicity because of the slow release of the freshly synthesized vitamin D_3 from the skin. Moreover, calcitriol inhibits the proliferation of the keratinocytes, which constitutes another regulatory mechanism for preventing excessive synthesis of vitamin D_3 by the skin (**Fig. 78.10**).

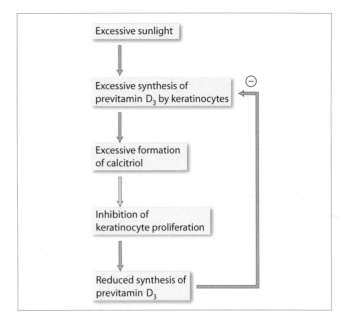

Fig. 78.10 Regulatory mechanism preventing hypervitaminosis on exposure to sunlight.

Summary

- Bone is the major storage site for calcium, and the physiologic processes underlying bone growth and remodeling contribute to calcium regulation.

- The three hormones that together maintain calcium homeostasis are parathyroid hormone (PTH), calcitonin, and vitamin D.

- PTH increases plasma calcium by releasing calcium from bone, increasing renal reabsorption of calcium, and stimulating the production of vitamin D.

- Calcitonin reduces calcium levels by promoting increased incorporation of calcium into bone and by increasing the excretion of calcium.

- Vitamin D increases the absorption of calcium in the gastrointestinal tract.

Applying What You Know

78.1. What is the effect of Mrs. Omaya's depressed thyroid function (a consequence of low TSH) on calcium metabolism?

Table 78.1 Comparison of Different Types of Hypoparathyroidism

	PTH Secretion	Plasma Calcium
Primary hypoparathyroidism	Reduced	Reduced
Secondary hypoparathyroidism	Reduced	Increased
Pseudohypoparathyroidism	Increased	Reduced

Abbreviation: PTH, parathyroid hormone.

The adrenal glands are paired structures situated above the kidneys (**Fig. 79.1A**). The adrenal gland consists of an outer cortex and an inner medulla (**Fig. 79.1B**). The hormones secreted by the adrenal cortex are called corticosteroids, which are classified as glucocorticoids, mineralocorticoids, and androgens.

The fetal adrenal cortex is much larger than the medulla. By the third year of life, three distinct zones of cells have formed in the adrenal cortex (**Fig. 79.1C**). The zona glomerulosa is the outermost layer and is the site of mineralocorticoid synthesis. The wider middle zone is the zona fasciculata, and the innermost layer is the zona reticularis. The middle and inner zones of the adrenal cortex synthesize and secrete glucocorticoids and androgens. The middle zone secretes more glucocorticoids, and the inner zone secretes more androgens. The adrenal cortex is essential for life, although the adrenal medulla is not. Following adrenalectomy, the mineralocorticoid deficiency results in hypotension, circulatory insufficiency, and eventually fatal shock.

The adrenal cortex receives a very large blood flow per gram of tissue. It is perfused by a dense network of capillaries fed by short cortical arteries. Some of the capillaries drain into the adrenal medulla, providing the medulla with a portal circulation.

Corticosteroids

Corticosteroids with predominantly *glucocorticoid* activity are cortisol, corticosterone, and 11-dehydrocorticosterone. Corticosteroids with predominantly *mineralocorticoid* activity are aldosterone and 11-deoxycorticosterone. In addition, cortisol has some significant mineralocorticoid activity, and aldosterone has some mineralocorticoid activity. Corticosteroids with *androgenic* activity are dehydroepiandrosterone (DHEA), dehydroepiandrosterone sulfate (DHEAS), and androstenedione.

The adrenal cortex also secretes testosterone and estrogens, but the amounts secreted are too small to be effective physiologically. In addition, the androgenic activities of androstenedione, DHEA, and DHEAS are too weak to be physiologically important. However, DHEA is converted in adipose tissues to potent androgens, such as testosterone and dihydrotestosterone, as well as estrogens, mainly estrone. The peripheral conversion of DHEA to potent androgens is of little significance in men but is of significance in women, as they cause axillary and pubic hair growth and stimulate libido. The peripheral conversion of DHEA to estrogens is important in both men and women, as explained below.

In *men,* the principal source of the estrogen that is present is the peripheral conversion of adrenal DHEA, with much

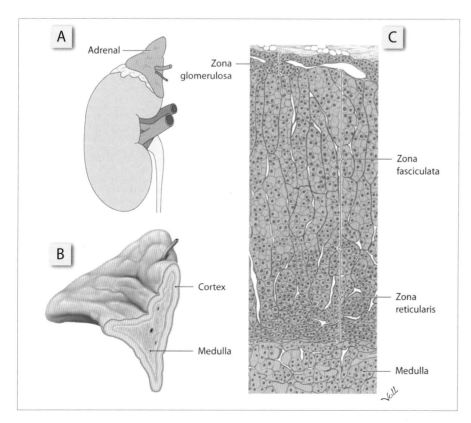

Fig. 79.1 **(A)** Location of the adrenal gland. **(B)** Right adrenal gland cut open. **(C)** Histologic section from an adrenal gland.

smaller amounts coming from the testes. Estrogens hasten the closure of epiphyses, enhance the secretion of growth hormone at puberty, mediate the inhibition of gonadotropin secretion in the pituitary by testosterone, and may regulate the plasma level of high-density lipoproteins. They may be responsible for gynecomastia in the aged due to an imbalance of the testosterone-to-estrogen ratio.

In *premenopausal women,* the principal source of estrogen is estradiol from the ovaries, with much smaller amounts of estrone formed by peripheral conversion of adrenal DHEA. In *postmenopausal women,* the peripheral formation of estrogen predominates. Because adipose tissue is the major site of estrone synthesis from DHEA, the total estrogen in a massively obese postmenopausal woman may be even greater than in a premenopausal woman.

Biosynthesis

The steps in the biosynthesis of corticosteroids are shown in **Fig. 79.2,** and the structures of the hormones are shown in **Fig. 79.3**. Some of the enzymes in the biosynthetic pathway are located in the mitochondria, and others are located on the smooth endoplasmic reticulum. Hence, during steroid synthesis, the substrates must move in and out of the mitochondria for the appropriate reactions to occur.

Corticosteroid synthesis begins with the uptake of cholesterol, side-chain cleavage of cholesterol, and formation of pregnenolone. Although the adrenal cortex can synthesize its own cholesterol from acetyl CoA, most of the cholesterol for its steroid synthesis is provided by plasma low-density lipoproteins (LDLs). The adrenal cortex stores cholesterol in the form of esters and deesterifies it during steroid synthesis. Cholesterol is converted to pregnenolone by 20,22-desmolase, a mitochondrial enzyme. It is the rate-limiting step in corticosteroid biosynthesis. Pregnenolone is the common precursor of all steroid hormones, both mineralocorticoids and glucocorticoids.

In the *mineralocorticoid pathway,* pregnenolone is converted to progesterone by the enzyme 3β-hydroxy dehydrogenase.

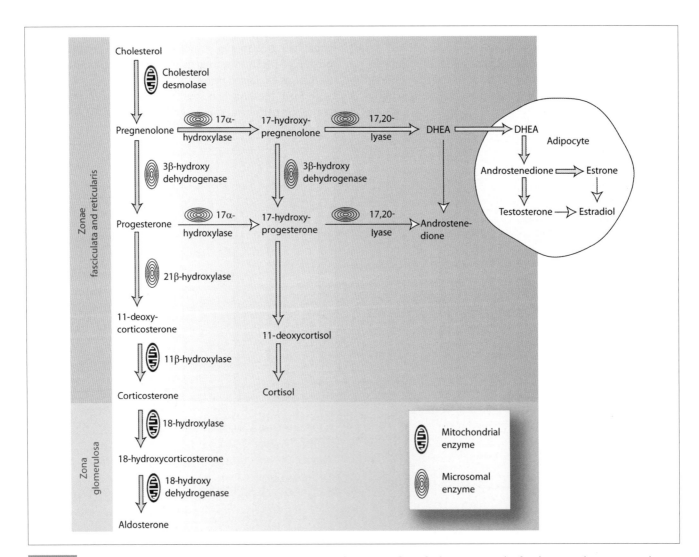

Fig. 79.2 Biosynthesis of steroid hormones. The *thick yellow arrows* indicate major flow of substrates. Details of androgen and estrogen production are shown in **Fig. 82.1**. DHEA, dehydroepiandrosterone.

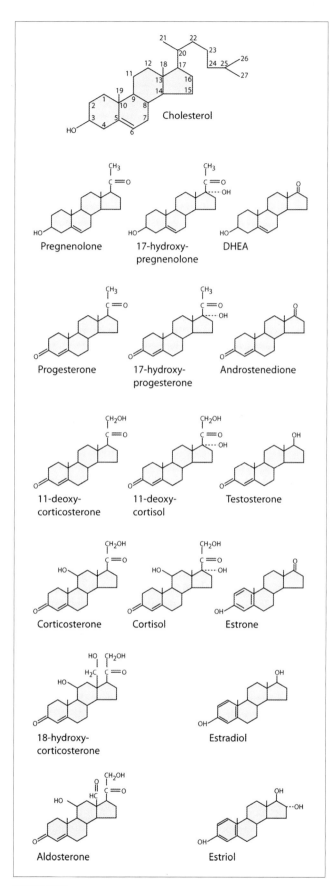

Fig. 79.3 Chemical structures of the steroid hormones. DHEA, dehydroepiandrosterone.

Progesterone is then sequentially hydroxylated at the C-21, C-11, and C-18 positions to form 18-hydroxycorticosterone (**Fig. 79.3**). 18-hydroxycorticosterone is converted to aldosterone by the mitochondrial enzyme 18-hydroxy dehydrogenase, which is found only in the zona glomerulosa.

In the *glucocorticoid pathway*, pregnenolone is sequentially hydroxylated at the C-17, C-21, and C-11 positions to form cortisol. The zona glomerulosa cannot synthesize cortisol, as it lacks 17α-hydroxylase.

In the *androgenic pathway*, DHEA and androstenedione are produced, respectively, from 17α-hydroxypregnenolone and 17α-hydroxyprogesterone by the action of 17,20-lyase.

Biosynthetic Defects

Genetic deficiency of the enzymes necessary for corticosteroid biosynthesis results in reduction in cortisol synthesis (**Fig. 79.4**). Low plasma cortisol causes feedback stimulation of andrenocorticotropic hormone (ACTH) secretion, leading to hyperplasia of the adrenal cortex, giving it the name *congenital adrenal hyperplasia* (CAH). Hypersecretion of ACTH results in excessive production of those substrates that are proximal to the deficient enzymes, leading to various clinical manifestations (**Table 79.1**). For example, the production of sex hormones is affected, resulting in genital abnormalities. Hence, the condition is also known as the *adrenogenital syndrome*.

21β-hydroxylase deficiency (**Fig. 79.4A**) results in deficient production of both glucocorticoids and mineralocorticoids. Mineralocorticoid deficiency results in excessive loss of body salt and water, and the condition is called the *salt-losing form of CAH*. Most of the substrates are diverted to the androgenic pathway, resulting in the production of large amounts of DHEA, which is a weak androgen and contributes to the increased urinary level of 17-ketosteroids. Outside the adrenal gland, DHEA is metabolized to testosterone, estrone, and estradiol. In girls, this enzyme deficiency results in female pseudohermaphroditism and virilization.

11β-hydroxylase deficiency (**Fig. 79.4B**) results in impaired production of corticosterone and aldosterone, but excessive production of 11-deoxycorticosterone, which has ~3% of the activity of aldosterone. This results in sodium and water retention, hypertension, and hypokalemia, and the condition is called the *hypertensive form of CAH*. There is reduced cortisol production, but the production of 11-deoxycortisol, which is not bioactive, is increased. There is also an excessive secretion of DHEA with all its consequences.

17α-hydroxylase deficiency (**Fig. 79.4C**) occurs in both the adrenal cortex and gonads. A deficiency of 17α-hydroxylase results in impaired synthesis of cortisol, androgens, and estrogens. Most of the substrates enter the mineralocorticoid pathway, causing hypertension and disturbances of water, electrolyte, and pH balance. Although cortisol production decreases, the excessive production of corticosterone, a weak glucocorticoid, prevents the symptoms of glucocorticoid deficiency. In women, the low estradiol levels result in sexual infantilism. In men, the low testosterone level is associated with feminization and male pseudohermaphroditism.

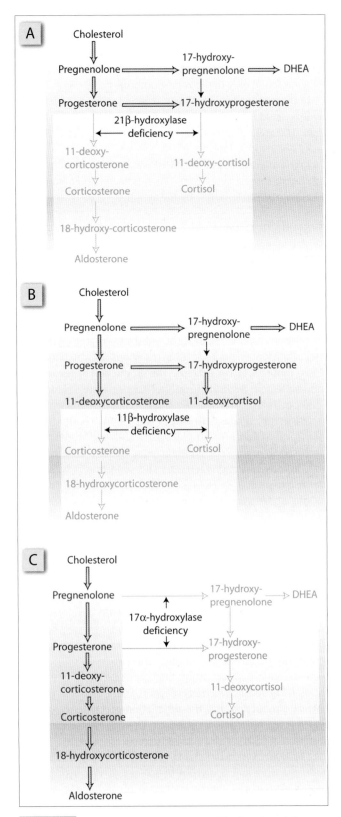

Fig. 79.4 **(A)** Steroid biosynthesis in 21β-hydroxylase deficiency, **(B)** 11β-hydroxylase deficiency, and **(C)** 17α-hydroxylase deficiency. DHEA, dehydroepiandrosterone.

Table 79.1 Effects of Different Enzyme Defects in Congenital Adrenal Hyperplasia

	Glucocorticoid Effect	Mineralocorticoid Effect	Androgenic Effect
21β-hydroxylase	Low	Low: salt-losing	High: virilizing
11β-hydroxylase	Low	Moderate: hypertensive	High: virilizing
17α-hydroxylase	Low	Excess: hypertensive	Low: feminizing

Transport and Metabolism

About 90% of the plasma cortisol is bound to cortisol-binding globulin (CBG, or transcortin), which is an α-globulin, and ~6% of the plasma cortisol is bound to plasma albumin. About 4% is unbound and represents the physiologically active steroid. The bound cortisol represents a reservoir from which the hormone is released as plasma levels fall (when hormone binds to receptors).

Cortisol is inactivated in the liver to dihydrocortisol and tetrahydrocortisol and conjugated with glucuronic acid and sulfates to form water-soluble metabolites that are readily excreted by the kidney. Aldosterone is excreted in urine as a glucuronide conjugate. Androgens are excreted in urine after conversion to androsterone, etiocholanolone, and several other metabolites that are collectively called urinary 17-ketosteroids.

Glucocorticoids

Control of Glucocorticoid Secretion

The adrenal cortex is under the control of the hypothalamo–hypophysial axis (**Fig. 79.5**). The corticotropin-releasing hormone (CRH) released from the hypothalamus stimulates ACTH secretion from the anterior pituitary. ACTH stimulates the output of glucocorticoids and, to a lesser extent (and only when the concentration of ACTH is high), aldosterone.

The hypothalamo–hypophysial axis exhibits feedback control by cortisol. Thus, a fall in cortisol level stimulates ACTH and CRH secretions (long-loop feedback), resulting in the restoration of cortisol levels. Short-loop feedback (ACTH-inhibiting CRH) and ultrashort-loop feedback (CRH regulating its own output) also occur. The integrity of this feedback control system can be determined by the dexamethasone suppression test. Dexamethasone, a synthetic glucocorticoid, is a potent inhibitor of ACTH and CRH secretion. If administration of dexamethasone reduces cortisol secretion, it indicates that the pituitary is responsive to CRH and that the adrenal cortex is responsive to ACTH.

Glucocorticoid secretion shows a diurnal variation (**Fig. 79.6**) and increases sharply in response to stress. These responses are mediated by diurnal release of CRH from the hypothalamus.

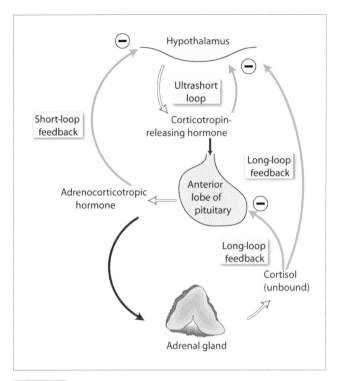

Fig. 79.5 Hypothalamio–hypophysial control of cortisol secretion. Negative feedback pathways are shown as *blue arrows*.

Physiologic Actions of Glucocorticoids

Effect on blood cells | Cortisol stimulates hemopoiesis and increases the number of circulating erythrocytes, neutrophils, and platelets. Neutrophilia occurs due to excess release from bone marrow, reduced margination, and reduced diapedesis into tissues. Cortisol reduces the number of circulating lymphocytes, monocytes, eosinophils, and basophils by promoting their migration from blood into tissues.

Antiinflammatory effects | Glucocorticoids inhibit inflammatory and allergic reactions in several ways. (1) They stabilize lysosomal membranes, thereby, inhibiting the release of proteolytic enzymes. (2) They decrease capillary permeability, thereby inhibiting leukocytic diapedesis and reducing inflammatory exudations. (3) Cortisol decreases the release of inflammatory mediators such as serotonin, histamine, and hydrolases from granulocytes, mast cells, and macrophages. It also inhibits prostaglandin synthesis.

Anti-immunity effects | Glucocorticoids cause involution of the lymph nodes, thymus, and spleen. In high doses, they suppress both humoral immunity (by reducing B-cell proliferation) and cell-mediated immunity (by inhibiting T-cell proliferation and cytokine release).

Antiallergic effects | The basophilopenia caused by cortisol reduces allergic response due to a decrease in histamine release.

Renal effects | Glucocorticoids facilitate rapid excretion of a water load (increases free-water clearance) and also enhance uric acid excretion. A fall in plasma cortisol is associated with reduction in glomerular filtration rate (GFR) and renal plasma flow. Mineralocorticoids do not have these effects.

Gastric effects | Cortisol increases gastric acid secretion and decreases gastric mucosal cell proliferation. Hence, prolonged cortisol treatment predisposes to peptic ulceration. Stress, which is invariably associated with excessive glucocorticoid secretion, often results in gastric ulcers (*stress ulcers*).

Psychoneural effects | High cortisol levels can cause irritability, depression, insomnia, amnesia, and lower seizure threshold. Low cortisol levels can reduce the synthesis of epinephrine (see **Fig. 80.1**) by inhibiting the activity of the enzyme phenylethanolamine *N*-methyltransferase (PNMT).

Antigrowth effects | Large doses of cortisol reduce Ca^{2+} absorption from the gut (by antagonizing calcitriol), inhibit mitosis of fibroblasts, and cause degradation of collagen. These effects lead to osteoporosis. The breakdown of collagen leads to an increase in urinary hydroxyproline excretion. Cortisol delays wound healing because of the reduction of fibroblast proliferation. Connective tissue is reduced in quantity and strength. Cortisol inhibits the anabolic actions of growth hormone and insulin-like growth factor-1, particularly in bone. Excess cortisol suppresses growth hormone secretion and inhibits somatic growth. In large doses, cortisol causes muscle atrophy and weakness (*steroid myopathy*).

Vascular effect | Cortisol enhances catecholamine synthesis by activating PNMT. In pharmacologic doses, cortisol enhances the vascular responsiveness to norepinephrine (the *permissive action*) and thereby helps in maintaining normal blood pressure and volume. Absence of cortisol results in vasodilatation and hypotension.

Stress adaptation | Any condition that disrupts or threatens to disrupt homeostasis is called a stress. Stress increases ACTH secretion, resulting in increased glucocorticoid secretion. The physiologic significance of this, however, is poorly understood because resistance to stress is not increased by the administration of glucocorticoids.

Stressful situations that increase ACTH secretion include severe physical trauma, pain, surgery, circulatory shock, fever, hypothermia, hypoglycemia, infections, emotional trauma, and severe exercise.

ADH secretion | Cortisol has a negative feedback effect on ADH secretion. The water intoxication caused by cortisol

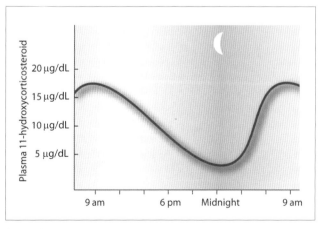

Fig. 79.6 Diurnal variation in glucocorticoid secretion. Peal glucocorticoid levels are present sometime between 8 and 9 AM.

deficiency is largely related to increased release of ADH. Hence, ADH antagonists are able to relieve the water intoxication caused by cortisol deficiency.

The **metabolic effects** of cortisol (**Fig. 79.7**) can be summarized as an overall catabolic effect with an anabolic effect on the liver, where both glycogenesis and gluconeogenesis are stimulated. Cortisol helps the body during starvation by maintaining normal blood glucose and storing up liver glycogen at the expense of breaking down body fats and expendable proteins.

Carbohydrate metabolism (1) Cortisol causes hyperglycemia due to increased gluconeogenesis. It also blocks glucose transport into muscle and adipose tissue, which contribute to the hyperglycemia. These effects result in glucose intolerance and eventually *steroid diabetes.* The hyperglycemia causes a compensatory hyperinsulinemia. (2) Cortisol also promotes hepatic glycogenesis and increases the glycogen content of the liver.

The increase in gluconeogenesis occurs mainly due to two reasons: (1) Cortisol mobilizes amino acids from muscles and bones, making available amino acids for gluconeogenesis. Cortisol also augments the synthesis and activity of key gluconeogenic enzymes, especially, fructose 1,6-bisphosphatase. (2) Cortisol causes lipolysis in adipose tissues, making available free fatty acids and glycerol for gluconeogenesis.

Protein metabolism (1) Cortisol enhances the release of amino acids from proteins in skeletal muscle and bone matrix. The amino acids released, especially alanine, are transported to the liver and deaminated for gluconeogenesis. The deamination leads to an increase in urea synthesis and excretion. (2) Glucocorticoids also have an anti-anabolic effect as they inhibit protein synthesis, probably at the translational level.

Fat metabolism (1) Cortisol causes lipolysis in adipose tissue by stimulating hormone-sensitive lipase. The fatty acids mobilized from adipose tissue are used for gluconeogenesis.

Cortisol also has a permissive (potentiating) action on the lipolytic effects of catecholamines and glucagon. (2) Despite the lipolysis, cortisol increases total body fat and causes a redistribution of fat with characteristic centripetal distribution that is seen in Cushing syndrome. The lipogenic effect is probably due to the hyperinsulinemia produced by cortisol. Other contributory factors could be the stimulation of leptin synthesis in adipocytes and the stimulation of differentiation of preadipocytes to adipocytes.

> **General Model: Communication**
>
> Cortisol provides a good illustration of the anatomic diffuseness of hormonal (cell–cell) information-processing systems. Almost all of the cells in the body have receptors for cortisol, and thus all are affected by changes in cortisol levels.

Mineralocorticoids

Aldosterone is the principal mineralocorticoid secreted by the adrenal gland, although corticosterone is secreted in sufficient amounts to exert a minor mineralocorticoid effect. Deoxycorticosterone, too, has a weak mineralocorticoid activity, but normally it is not secreted in appreciable amounts. A large amount of progesterone also has some mineralocorticoid activity, but it does not have any physiologic role in the control of sodium excretion.

Control of Mineralocorticoid Secretion

Mineralocorticoid secretion is stimulated by hyperkalemia, angiotensin II, ACTH, and hyponatremia, in reducing order of efficacy (**Fig. 79.8**). (1) Aldosterone secretion in response to

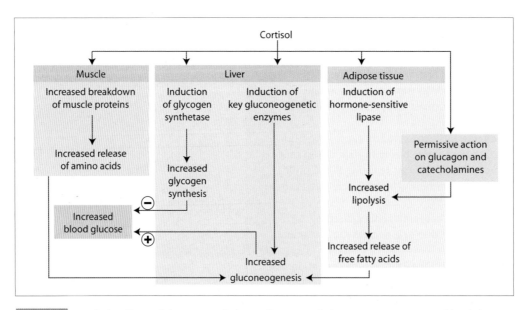

Fig. 79.7 Metabolic effects of glucocorticoids (cortisol). Increased gluconeogenesis increases blood glucose, whereas increased glycogen synthesis will decrease blood glucose.

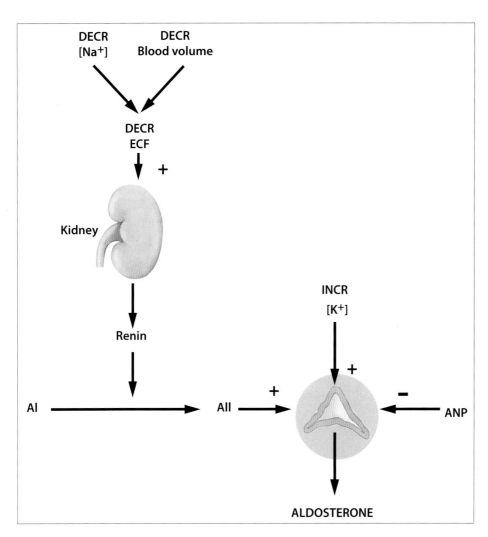

Fig. 79.8 The control of aldosterone secretion. The most potent determinant of secretion is increased [K^+]. Angiotensin II (AII), which results from stimulation of the kidneys by decreased extracellular fluid (ECF) and decreased [Na^+], is also a potent stimulus to aldosterone release. Atrial natriuretic protein (ANP) inhibits aldosterone release.

hyperkalemia forms the basis for renal regulation of body potassium balance. (2) Stimulation of aldosterone secretion by angiotensin II is important for the correction of hypovolemia and hypotension. It also explains why aldosterone secretion increases on prolonged standing. (3) Stimulation of aldosterone secretion by ACTH results in the diurnal variation of aldosterone secretion. It also explains why aldosterone secretion increases in response to stress. ACTH is not an important physiologic regulator of aldosterone secretion. When ACTH tends to increase aldosterone secretion, angiotensin II and potassium ions promptly oppose any change in aldosterone level. However, in an interesting syndrome called *glucocorticoid-remediable aldosteronism*, ACTH exerts a stronger control of aldosterone secretion than angiotensin II or hyperkalemia and therefore results in hyperaldosteronism. It is treated by cortisol administration, which decreases ACTH secretion through negative feedback.

A fall of ~20 mEq/L in plasma Na^+ stimulates aldosterone secretion, but such changes are rare. Physiologically, hyponatremia is a weak stimulator of aldosterone secretion, and fortunately so. We know that excessive water intake results in dilutional hyponatremia and water diuresis. The diuresis would not occur if hyponatremia were a potent stimulus for aldosterone secretion.

Physiologic Actions of Mineralocorticoids

Aldosterone acts mainly on the cortical collecting ducts to increase the reabsorption of Na^+ and the secretion of K^+ and H^+ ions. Aldosterone is a major controller of K^+ homeostasis. It is of secondary importance in regulation of fluid and electrolyte balance despite its effect on Na^+ and water reabsorption. Mineralocorticoids also increase the reabsorption of Na^+ from the sweat and digestive juices as they flow out through the glandular ducts.

Adrenocortical Dysfunctions

Cushing Syndrome

Cushing syndrome results from hypersecretion of cortisol. It can be caused by ACTH-secreting pituitary tumors (ACTH-dependent Cushing syndrome) or cortisol-secreting adrenal or ectopic tumors (ACTH-independent Cushing syndrome). ACTH-independent Cushing syndrome is associated with feedback suppression of ACTH secretion. (Earlier, ACTH-dependent Cushing syndrome was called Cushing "disease"—a practice that caused needless confusion and is better avoided.)

Cushing syndrome has all the features that would be expected from the excessive actions of cortisol, and only the clinically important ones are recapitulated here. (1) The patient has a characteristic appearance due to redistribution of body fat: a moon face, truncal obesity with pendulous abdomen, and a buffalo (or dowager's) hump. (2) Due to a general increase in catabolism, there is osteoporosis of bones, atrophy of muscles, and thinning of skin. The abdomen shows reddish purple striae due to stretching of its skin by excess fat deposition. Telltale signs of easy bruisability (due to skin thinning) and poor wound healing are present. (3) Sex-related problems include amenorrhea and hirsutism (in women), impotency (in men), and decreased libido (in both). Psychological problems range from irritability to severe depression and even psychosis. (4) Investigations reveal hypertension (due to Na$^+$ and water retention), glucose intolerance, hyperlipidemia, hypercholesterolemia, and excessive urinary 17-ketosteroids.

Adrenal Insufficiency

Adrenal insufficiency is called *primary* when the reduced adrenocortical secretion occurs due to a disorder of the adrenal gland itself. It is called *secondary* when it is due to inadequate stimulation of the adrenals by ACTH.

In primary adrenal insufficiency (Addison's disease), there is deficiency of cortisol, aldosterone, and DHEA. Deficiency of cortisol results in hypoglycemia and hyperpigmentation of the skin. The hyperpigmentation is caused by the feedback *hypersecretion of ACTH,* which has β-melanocyte-stimulating hormone (MSH)-like structure and activity. In fact, a part of the ACTH peptide is identical in structure to β-MSH (see **Fig. 76.5**). *Deficiency of aldosterone* causes hyponatremia with hypotension, and hyperkalemia with metabolic acidosis. These electrolyte abnormalities cause gastrointestinal symptoms, such as nausea, vomiting, diarrhea, and abdominal cramps. *Deficiency of androgens* leads to the loss of axillary and pubic hair, reduced muscle mass, and loss of libido in men and women.

Secondary adrenal insufficiency is similar to primary adrenal insufficiency except for two major differences. (1) The secretion of aldosterone remains nearly unaffected; therefore, fluid and electrolyte disturbances do not occur. The hypotension that occurs occasionally is attributable to cortisol deficiency. (2) There is absence of hyperpigmentation because there is no hypersecretion of ACTH.

Hyperaldosteronism

Primary hyperaldosteronism (Conn syndrome) is seen in patients with aldosterone-producing adenoma. Benign adenomas typically exhibit the normal diurnal pattern of aldosterone secretion, which suggests that the aldosterone synthesis is still under the control of ACTH. However, there is an absence of the increase in aldosterone secretion that normally occurs on standing. The absence is attributable to the marked suppression of the renin–angiotensin system by the hypokalemia, which is prominent in Conn syndrome. The hypokalemia also impairs insulin secretion, causing glucose intolerance; depolarizes the muscle membrane, causing muscle weakness; and impairs the urine-concentrating ability of the kidney (hypokalemic nephropathy), causing polyuria.

Hyperaldosteronism also causes *hypernatremia* with reduced Na$^+$ excretion in urine and reduced Na$^+$ secretion in sweat, saliva, and gastrointestinal secretions. The hypernatremia is not severe because of the *mineralocorticoid escape*—an escape from the Na$^+$-retaining effects of chronic aldosteronism. For the same reason and also due to the polyuria associated with hypokalemic nephropathy, edema almost never occurs in Conn syndrome.

Secondary hyperaldosteronism is prominently associated with edema. The movement of Na$^+$ and water out of circulation into interstitial spaces results in hypovolemia, which stimulates aldosterone secretion. The rise in the aldosterone level is unable to correct the hypovolemia because the retained water and electrolytes promptly move out again into the interstitium, aggravating the edema. Hypokalemia is not prominent because the hypovolemia reduces the urinary flow rate through renal tubules, inhibiting tubular II secretion.

Corticosteroid Therapy

Use | Adrenocorticosteroid therapy is often life-saving. (1) Corticosteroids are used for substitution therapy in primary or secondary adrenal insufficiency and also in nonendocrine conditions. (2) Corticosteroids have both antiinflammatory and immunosuppressive effects and therefore are used in the treatment of chronic inflammatory disorders, such as rheumatoid arthritis, and collagen disorders. For the same reason, they are administered to organ transplant recipients for reducing the chances of graft rejection. However, treatment with large doses of glucocorticoids predisposes to infections, making antibiotics a necessary adjunct to steroid therapy. (3) Due to their antiallergic effects, they are used in bronchial asthma and skin diseases. (4) Due to their antilymphocytic effect, they are used in malignancies such as lymphocytic leukemias and lymphomas. In breast cancers that are aggravated by estrogens, corticosteroids are administered for indirectly suppressing estrogen secretion. Corticosteroids suppress adrenocortical activity by feedback inhibition of ACTH secretion so that the adrenal cortex produces less of the androgenic precursors of estrogens. (5) Because corticosteroids reduce edema, they are used in cerebral edema. Patients of cerebral stroke are often administered corticosteroids. The stress associated with the cerebral stroke tends to cause stress ulcers, and the administration of corticosteroids aggravates them. Hence, simultaneously with steroid therapy, these patients are administered antacids. (6) Because glucocorticoids enhance the vascular responsiveness to norepinephrine, they are frequently administered in circulatory shock along with other drugs. However, their efficacy in shock remains debatable.

Because long-term corticosteroid therapy is associated with suppression of the axis, the therapy should not be stopped suddenly. Abrupt cessation of steroid therapy is associated with life-threatening adrenal insufficiency. Hence, the dose of the steroid must be slowly decreased or tapered. Full recovery from hypothalamio–hypophysial–adrenocortical suppression may require as long as 1 year following cessation of all steroid therapy.

Misuse | Steroids are commonly used as antiinflammatory agents, but they only suppress inflammation without eliminating its cause. Application of a cortisone cream alleviates an itchy rash, but the sensitivity to the allergen persists: the next exposure will produce the rash again.

Summary

- The adrenal cortex is composed of three layers of cells, with each layer releasing different hormones. The zona glomerulosa secretes the mineralocorticoid aldosterone, the zona fasciculata secretes predominantly glucocorticoids such as cortisol, and the zona reticularis secretes androgens.

- All of the adrenal cortical hormones are synthesized from a common precursor, cholesterol.

- All of the cortical steroids are transported bound to plasma proteins.

- Cortisol secretion is controlled by the hypothalamic–pituitary–adrenal cortex axis, with the immediate stimulus for secretion of cortisol being ACTH.

- Cortisol has a myriad of effects on metabolism, immune and stress responses, and many organ systems.

- Aldosterone secretion is stimulated by increased plasma $[K^+]$, angiotensin II, and reduced plasma $[Na^+]$.

- Aldosterone acts on the collecting ducts of the kidneys to increase sodium reabsorption and potassium excretion.

Applying What You Know

79.1. Mrs. Omaya has a low concentration of cortisol. What are possible mechanisms that could result in this finding? Explain.

79.2. Mrs. Omaya's laboratory report shows both low $[Na^+]$ and high $[K^+]$. What is the most likely explanation for these findings?

80 Hormones of the Adrenal Medulla

The adrenal medulla represents essentially an enlarged and specialized sympathetic ganglion. It consists of chromaffin cells or pheochromocytes, which are the functional analogues of the sympathetic postganglionic fibers of the autonomic nervous system. The adrenal medulla is the only autonomic neuroeffector organ without a two-neuron sympathetic innervation (see **Fig. 76.1**). It is innervated by long sympathetic preganglionic, cholinergic neurons that form synaptic connections with the chromaffin cells. The secretory vesicles of the chromaffin cells are called chromaffin granules. Approximately 80% of the chromaffin granules in the adrenal medulla synthesize epinephrine, and the remaining 20% synthesize norepinephrine.

The adrenal medulla has a dual blood supply being perfused by (1) long cortical arteries and by (2) vessels draining the cortical capillary bed. Like the adrenal cortex, the adrenal medulla has a high blood flow per gram of tissue. This pattern of circulation ensures a high concentration of corticosteroids in the adrenal medulla and allows the corticosteroids to increase epinephrine secretion through a permissive (potentiating) action.

The adrenal medulla synthesizes and secretes bioactive amines called catecholamines, which are dihydroxylated phenolic amines. The catecholamines secreted by the adrenal medulla are epinephrine and norepinephrine. Most of the circulating epinephrine comes from the adrenal medulla, with moderate contributions from postganglionic sympathetic fibers and the central nervous system.

General Model: Communications

The adrenal medulla is a prime example of the integration of neural and humoral information processing, with chemical signals passed from preganglionic cell to chromaffin cell, and the catecholamines that are released circulating all over the body to affect cell function.

Control of Catecholamine Synthesis

The biosynthesis of catecholamines is shown in **Fig. 80.1**. The following points should be noted. (1) The precursor of all catecholamines is tyrosine, which is derived from the diet or through hepatic hydroxylation of phenylalanine. (2) Tyrosine hydroxylase is the rate-limiting enzyme in the overall biosynthesis of epinephrine. (3) Except dopamine hydroxylase, which is present inside the chromaffin granule, all enzymes in this biosynthetic pathway are cytosolic. Dopamine enters the chromaffin granule, where it is converted to norepinephrine by dopamine β-hydroxylase. (4) Norepinephrine must diffuse back into the cytoplasm for methylation by phenylethanolamine N-methyltransferase (PNMT) to epinephrine. The epinephrine formed reenters the chromaffin granule.

Epinephrine is not secreted in significant amounts by neurons because PNMT is present in significant concentrations

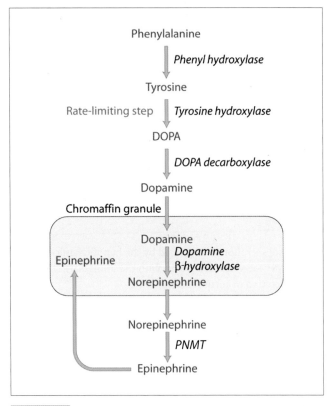

Fig. 80.1 Biosynthesis of catecholamines (epinephrine and norepinephrine). The activity of the enzyme PNMT is facilitated by cortisol. DOPA, 3,4-dihydroxyphenylalanine; PNMT, phenylethanolamine N-methyltransferase.

only in the adrenal medulla. Moreover, PNMT activity is induced by very high local concentration of glucocorticoids, which are found only in the portal blood draining the adrenal cortex.

Control of Catecholamine Secretion

The adrenal medulla is stimulated simultaneously with the sympathetic nervous system in emergency (fight-or-flight) situations. Catecholamines help to prepare the individual to cope with emergencies. Catecholamines are secreted in response to any stressful stimulus. The ratio of norepinephrine to epinephrine secreted varies with the type of stimulus. Catecholamine release is stimulated by acetylcholine from the preganglionic sympathetic nerve endings innervating the chromaffin cells. Epinephrine synthesis is dependent on cortisol, and therefore indirectly dependent on adrenocorticotrophic hormone (ACTH) and corticotropin-releasing hormone.

Inactivation of Circulating Catecholamines

Circulating catecholamines are sequentially metabolized by two enzymes, MAO (monoamine oxidase) and COMT (catechol-O-methyltransferase). Both are widely distributed in tissues, with MAO being particularly abundant in nerve terminals. After both enzymes have acted, the final products are VMA

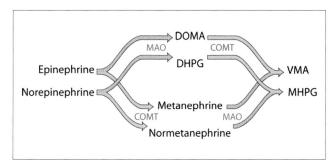

Fig. 80.2 Alternative pathways for the metabolic degradation of catecholamines by monoamine oxidase (MAO) and catechol-*O*-methyltransferase (COMT). DOMA, dihydroxymandelic acid; MHPG, 3-methoxy 4-hydroxyphenylglycol; VMA, vanillyl mandelic acid.

(vanillyl mandelic acid) and MHPG (3-methoxy 4-hydroxy-phenylglycol). However, depending upon which of them acts first, the intermediate metabolites are either DOMA (dihydroxymandelic acid) or metanephrine and normetanephrine (**Fig. 80.2**). Circulating catecholamines are mostly excreted as metanephrine and normetanephrine.

Adrenergic Receptors

Epinephrine and norepinephrine produce different effects owing to the existence of two types of adrenergic receptors: α and β receptors. Stimulation of α-adrenergic receptors results mostly in the contraction of smooth muscles. Stimulation of

β-adrenergic receptors results in inhibition of smooth muscles (through β_2 receptors) and stimulation of the myocardium (through β_1 receptors).

Epinephrine acts equally on both α and β receptors. Norepinephrine acts predominantly on α receptors. The effects of adrenomedullary stimulation and sympathetic nerve stimulation differ due to the fact that sympathetic nerve endings contain norepinephrine, whereas the adrenal medulla secretes mainly epinephrine.

A chronic increase in catecholamine secretion is associated with a decrease in the number of adrenergic receptors in target cells and a decreased responsiveness to catecholamines (*downregulation*). Conversely, a sustained decrease in catecholamine secretion is associated with an increase in the number of adrenergic receptors in target cells and an increased responsiveness to catecholamines (*upregulation*). This relationship may account for the phenomenon of *denervation hypersensitivity* that is observed in target organs following autonomic denervation.

Physiologic Effects

Epinephrine and norepinephrine mainly have cardiovascular and metabolic effects. The cardiovascular effects of epinephrine and norepinephrine are discussed in Chapter 37. The metabolic effects of epinephrine and norepinephrine are discussed below (**Fig. 80.3**). Both act on the central nervous system to increase alertness.

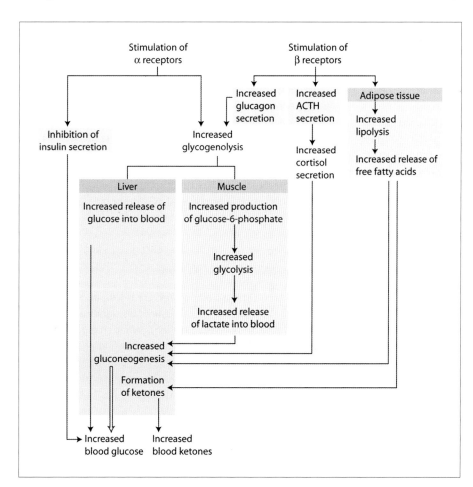

Fig. 80.3 Epinephrine, acting on α and β receptors, has widespread metabolic effects. ACTH, adrenocorticotrophic hormone.

Carbohydrate metabolism | Catecholamines stimulate gluconeogenesis. Stimulation of α-adrenergic receptors increases glycogenolysis in the liver by activating glycogen phosphorylase and inhibiting glycogen synthetase (see **Fig. 74.9**). Liver contains glucose-6-phosphatase; hence, hepatic glycogenolysis results in the release of free glucose into the bloodstream. Stimulation of β-adrenergic receptors increases glycogenolysis in muscle by activating glycogen phosphorylase and inactivating glycogen synthetase activity. Muscle lacks glucose-6-phosphatase; therefore, epinephrine-induced glycogenolysis in muscle does not release free glucose into the bloodstream. Instead, glycogenolysis ends with the formation of glucose-6-phosphate. The glucose-6-phosphate is metabolized to lactate, which is released into the blood. The liver takes up the lactate and converts it back to glucose.

The cause of epinephrine-induced hyperglycemia is twofold: (1) the glycogenolysis induced by α-adrenergic stimulation of the liver and (2) the gluconeogenesis from lactate that occurs as a consequence of β-adrenergic stimulation of muscles. The stores of liver glycogen (~100 g) decrease only transiently after adrenergic stimulation, suggesting that hepatic glycogenolysis is not the main source of hepatic glucose release. Rather, it is the hepatic gluconeogenesis from the lactate derived from muscle glycogen (300 g) that is the major source of the glucose released by the liver following adrenergic stimulation.

The epinephrine-induced β-adrenergic stimulation results in increased glucagon secretion, which, like epinephrine, increases hepatic glycogenolysis and gluconeogenesis. Epinephrine stimulates ACTH secretion, which, in turn, stimulates the secretion of cortisol, a potent gluconeogenic hormone. Epinephrine suppresses insulin secretion (α-adrenergic effect) and inhibits glucose transporter GLUT-4. As a result, the facilitated diffusion of glucose into muscle and adipose tissue is inhibited. The glucose uptake by exercising muscle is not epinephrine-induced but a direct effect of muscle contraction itself. As the exercising muscle consumes more glucose, the intracellular glucose concentration falls, increasing the facilitated diffusion of glucose into the muscle cell despite the inhibitory effect of epinephrine.

Fat metabolism | Epinephrine activates hormone-sensitive lipase by stimulating β-adrenergic receptors on fat cells and thereby increasing lipolysis. Free fatty acids mobilized from adipose tissue are converted in the liver to acetoacetate and β-hydroxybutyrate. These are released in the bloodstream and reach the peripheral tissues, where they are used as energy sources.

Metabolic rate | Catecholamines cause a biphasic (a large, immediate and a small, delayed rise) rise in the metabolic rate and body temperature. The *immediate rise* is due to the increased heat production from muscular activity and the decreased heat loss due to cutaneous vasoconstriction. The *delayed rise* is due to hepatic oxidation of the lactate released during muscle activity.

Potassium balance | Catecholamines cause a biphasic (an initial rise followed by a prolonged fall) change in plasma potassium (K^+). The *initial rise* is possibly due to release of K^+ from

the liver. The *delayed fall* is probably due to increased entry of K^+ into skeletal muscle that is mediated by β-adrenergic receptors. Activation of α receptors opposes the delayed fall in K^+. It is possible that catecholamines have a role in regulating the ratio between extracellular and intracellular K^+.

Adrenal Medulla Dysfunctions

Hyposecretion of catecholamines can occur following adrenalectomy or destruction of the adrenal glands due to diseases. Such hyposecretion produces no clinical symptoms because the catecholamine production from the sympathetic nerve endings is adequate for normal biologic requirements.

Pheochromocytoma is a chromaffin cell tumor that secretes large amounts of catecholamines, usually predominantly norepinephrine. Ninety percent of pheochromocytomas are benign and are treated by surgical removal of the tumor. Pheochromocytoma patients have hypertension and are prone to orthostatic hypotension. The hypersecretion of catecholamines is also associated with severe headache, sweating (cold sweating or adrenergic sweating), palpitations, chest pain, extreme anxiety, pallor of the skin caused by vasoconstriction, and blurred vision. If epinephrine is secreted predominantly, the heart rate is increased. If norepinephrine is the predominant hormone, the heart rate decreases reflexly in response to marked hypertension (see **Fig. 37.4**). The urinary excretion of catecholamines, metanephrines, and VMA are increased.

Summary

- The adrenal medulla is a modified sympathetic ganglion; neural activity in the preganglionic pathway causes release of epinephrine and norepinephrine from medullary chromaffin cells.

- Epinephrine and norepinephrine affect cell functions via α-adrenergic and β-adrenergic receptors.

- The catecholamines have important roles in regulating the body's metabolism as well as widespread sympathetic effects.

Applying What You Know

80.1. Mrs. Omaya's blood pressure is low, and she exhibits orthostatic hypotension (her pressure falls significantly in going from a supine to an erect position). What changes in her endocrine function might contribute to this finding? Explain the mechanism at work.

The role of the endocrine pancreas is to regulate blood glucose concentration. This is important for two reasons. (1) Every physiologic process requires the availability of energy, which ultimately comes from the metabolism of nutrients, particularly glucose. Some cells (e.g., neurons in the central nervous system [CNS]) are particulary sensitive to the lack of glucose. Furthermore the need for glucose and the availability of glucose fluctuate throughout the day. Hence, it is essential that glucose be prevented from falling to too low a level. A blood glucose level of less than 60 mg/dL is considered to be hypoglycemic. (2) Hyperglycemia (elevated blood glucose) has serious short-term physiologic consequences, and over the long term (years), a large number of severe pathologic responses result. Hence, blood glucose must not be allowed to get too high. An individual is said to be hyperglycemic when the blood glucose level exceeds 125 mg/dL.

Blood glucose levels in a normal individual are regulated between 80 and 120 mg/dL.

General Model: Homeostasis

Maintenance of a more or less constant blood glucose concentration is, of course, another example of the homeostatic regulation of a critical parameter of the internal environment. You should look for all of the components of a negative feedback that were described in Chapter 4 and revisited in the description of other homeostatic mechanisms.

The tail of the pancreas has about a million pancreatic islets (of Langerhans) that constitute the endocrine pancreas (**Fig. 81.1**). Each islet consists of ~3000 cells of four different types. Twenty-five percent of the islet cells are the α cells that secrete glucagon, 60% are the β cells that secrete insulin, 10% are the D cells that secrete somatostatin, and the remaining 5% are the F cells that secrete a small polypeptide molecule called the pancreatic polypeptide. The islet cells are innervated by both sympathetic and parasympathetic nerve fibers.

Insulin

Insulin (**Fig. 81.2**) is formed in the β cells by the cleavage of proinsulin into insulin and the connecting peptide or C peptide. The C peptide and a small amount of unsplit proinsulin are secreted with insulin and exert a weak insulin-like effect. Insulin is stored in the β cell granules as a crystalline hexamer complex with two atoms of zinc per hexamer. In plasma, insulin is transported as a monomer.

Control of Insulin Secretion

Increased glucose is the principal stimulus for insulin release. As the blood glucose level rises above 80 mg/dL, it stimulates the synthesis and release of insulin. Insulin secretion is also

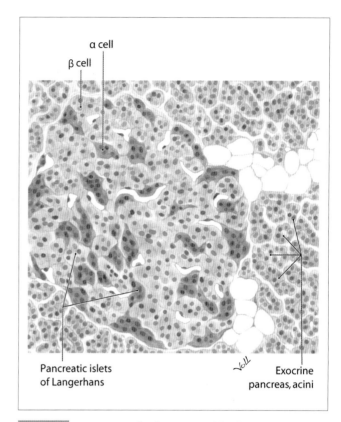

Fig. 81.1 A pancreatic islet showing α and β cells.

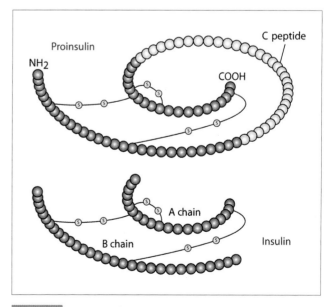

Fig. 81.2 Structure of insulin. The C peptide of proinsulin is cleaved off, leaving insulin composed of two polypeptide chains joined by two disulfide bonds.

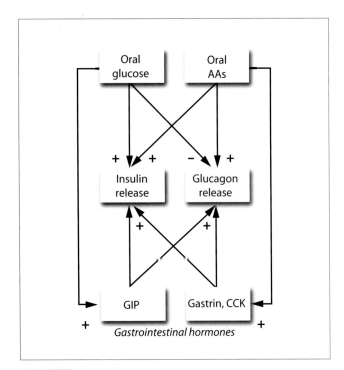

Fig. 81.3 Control of insulin secretion by gastrointestinal hormones. AA, amino acid; CCK, cholesystokinin; GIP, gastric inhibitory polypeptide.

stimulated by essential amino acids, such as arginine, lysine, and phenylalanine.

Gastrointestinal hormones, such as gastric inhibitory polypeptide (GIP), gastrin, and cholecystokinin (CCK), stimulate insulin secretion (**Fig. 81.3**) and account for the higher plasma concentration of insulin after ingestion of glucose or amino acids than after their intravenous administration. Glucagon and growth hormone directly stimulate insulin secretion; somatostatin directly inhibits insulin secretion. Hormones like corticosteroids, estrogens, and progesterone have an anti-insulin effect (they tend to raise blood glucose) and hence induce a compensatory increase in insulin secretion.

Circulating catecholamines, too, raise blood glucose and therefore should stimulate insulin secretion. However, this indirect stimulatory effect on insulin secretion is overridden by the direct suppressive effect of catecholamines on insulin secretion. The β cells have both α- and β-adrenergic receptors, but the α-adrenergic action (inhibition of insulin secretion) predominates the β-adrenergic action (stimulation of insulin secretion). Sympathetic nerves release norepinephrine; therefore, sympathetic discharge inhibits insulin release. Even epinephrine, which stimulates both α and β receptors, inhibits insulin secretion. Vagal stimulation increases insulin secretion.

Hyperkalemia stimulates insulin secretion, and hypokalemia leads to glucose intolerance.

Actions of Insulin

Insulin modifies the activity of several enzymes and increases the number of glucose and amino acid transporters on the cell membrane. The events triggered by the changes in enzymatic activity and cellular transport are numerous (**Fig. 81.4**), but their results are broadly threefold: (1) glycolysis increases in all cells of the body, (2) glycogen accumulates in muscle and liver, and (3) fats accumulate in adipose tissues. The increased glycolysis caused by insulin is important, not for increasing energy yield but for generating substrates for lipogenesis, such as glycerol 3-phosphate and acetyl CoA. Glycolysis also produces the adenosine triphosphate (ATP) and reduced form of nicotinamide adenine dinucleotide (NADH) molecules required for glycogenesis and lipogenesis.

Carbohydrate metabolism | Insulin is the predominant hormone decreasing blood glucose, the others being the insulin-like growth factors (IGFs). Insulin stimulates the uptake of glucose by myocytes, hepatocytes, and adipocytes, and thereby lowers blood glucose. Tissues that do not depend on

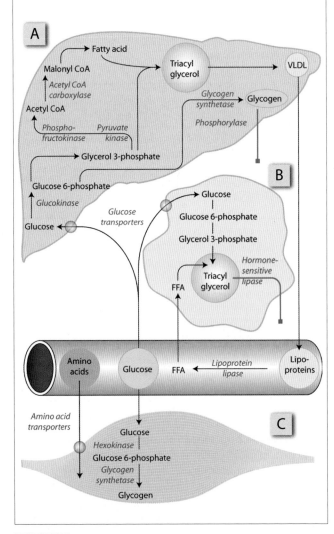

Fig. 81.4 Metabolic actions of insulin on **(A)** the liver, **(B)** adipose cells, and **(C)** muscle cells. Blood glucose is reduced by the uptake and storage of glucose in each of the three organs. Insulin inhibits glycogenolysis in the liver **(A)** and lipolysis in adipose cells **(B)**. Insulin lowers blood glucose concentration. FFA, free fatty acid; VLDL, very-low-density lipoprotein.

insulin for glucose uptake include the brain, erythrocytes, liver, and the epithelial cells of kidney and intestine.

The mechanism through which insulin increases glucose uptake is different in different tissues. In *muscle and adipose tissues,* the rate-limiting step in glucose uptake is facilitated diffusion. Insulin increases facilitated diffusion by increasing the number of glucose transporters (GLUT-4) on the cell membrane. Glucose transporters are present not only on the membrane surface, but also inside the cells as an intracellular pool. Insulin stimulates the translocation of glucose transporters from the intracellular pool to the membrane. GLUT-4 increases in muscles during exercise, but this increase is not dependent on insulin action.

In the *liver,* the rate-limiting step in glucose uptake is the conversion of intracellular glucose into glucose 6-phosphate by the enzyme glucokinase. Insulin increases glucose uptake mainly through the induction of glucokinase so that the glucose entering the liver cells is promptly converted to glucose 6-phosphate (glucose trapping). This keeps the intracellular glucose concentration low and favors entry of glucose into the liver cell. The glucose transporter in the liver cell is GLUT-2, and its presence in the membrane is not insulin dependent.

Increased glucose uptake into liver cells results in increased glycolysis. Glycolysis is stimulated due to the induction of the key glycolytic enzymes, glucokinase, phosphofructokinase, and pyruvate kinase. In the liver, insulin also inhibits phosphoenol pyruvate carboxykinase, a key gluconeogenetic enzyme. Inhibition of gluconeogenesis ensures that products of glycolysis are not converted back into glucose.

In muscle and liver, any surplus glucose that is taken up is converted to glycogen. Insulin induces the enzyme glycogen synthetase, which stimulates glycogenesis. The energy required for the conversion comes from the ATP and NADH produced through glycolysis. Insulin also inhibits the enzyme phosphorylase, which ensures that the glycogen is not broken down again into glucose (see **Fig. 74.9**).

Fat metabolism | After the liver has stored glycogen to its capacity, it converts any surplus glucose into fats. The acetyl CoA produced through glycolysis provides the substrate for de novo synthesis of fatty acids, which is further facilitated by the induction of acetyl CoA carboxylase. Glycolysis also provides glycerol 3-phosphate, which is one of the substrates for lipogenesis. The fats synthesized in the liver are converted into VLDL and released into the bloodstream. Insulin also stimulates lipoprotein lipase, which acts on the circulating VLDL to release fatty acids. The fatty acids are taken up by adipocytes and reconverted into fats. As in the liver, glycolysis provides glycerol 3-phosphate for lipogenesis in the adipose tissue. Insulin also inhibits hormone-sensitive lipase so that the fat synthesized in adipose tissues is not broken down. Thus, insulin is a lipogenic and an antilipolytic hormone.

Protein metabolism | Insulin promotes protein anabolism by stimulating the cellular uptake of neutral amino acids (by all cells except hepatocytes) and increasing messenger ribonucleic acid (mRNA) translation. Insulin also decreases catabolism of amino acids by reducing their hepatic uptake.

> **General Models: Reservoir and Balance of Forces**
>
> The blood is a reservoir into which all nutrients are dumped (particularly glucose) and from which all cells obtain their nutrients. Because hormones have multiple roles in stimulating or blocking uptake, there is a balance of forces that must always be considered in attempting to understand the changes in blood glucose concentrations that occur throughout the day.

Electrolyte balance | Insulin lowers serum potassium (K^+) concentration and also has an antinatriuretic effect. The hypokalemic action of insulin is caused by stimulation of K^+ uptake by muscle and hepatic tissue. Diabetic patients tend to develop hyperkalemia as K^+ moves out of the cells into the extracellular fluid (ECF).

Membrane hyperpolarization | Insulin decreases membrane permeability to both sodium (Na^+) and K^+, but it decreases Na^+ permeability to a greater extent, causing hyperpolarization of the muscle membrane. The membrane hyperpolarization produced by insulin causes movement of K^+ from the extracellular to the intracellular space.

Glucagon

Control of Glucagon Secretion

The three main controllers of glucagon release are glucose, amino acids, and epinephrine. Hypoglycemia stimulates glucagon release. Amino acids absorbed from the intestine stimulate the release of both insulin and glucagon. This ensures that a protein-rich zero-carbohydrate diet does not produce hypoglycemia due to insulin secretion alone. Fatty acids inhibit glucagon release. Gastrointestinal hormones, CCK, gastrin, and GIP mediate the stimulation of glucagon secretion that follows the ingestion of a protein meal (**Fig. 81.3**). Secretin decreases glucagon secretion. The β-adrenergic stimulation by circulating epinephrine or by sympathetic discharge increases glucagon secretion. Both epinephrine and glucagon have similar actions, and they act in synergy.

Actions of Glucagon

The major site of action of glucagon is the liver, with adipose cells also responding. In general, the actions of glucagon (**Fig. 81.5**) are exactly opposite those of insulin.

Protein metabolism | Glucagon increases the hepatic uptake and oxidative deamination of amino acids. In addition to its protein catabolic effect, glucagon has an anti-anabolic effect: it inhibits protein synthesis.

Carbohydrate metabolism | Glucagon causes hyperglycemia due to increased hepatic glycogenolysis (due to stimulation of phosphorylase and inhibition of glycogen synthetase) and gluconeogenesis (due to increased availability of carbon skeletons from deaminated amino acids). Glucagon *does not* stimulate glycogenolysis in muscle.

Fat metabolism | Glucagon stimulates lipolysis by activating hormone-sensitive lipase in adipose tissue. Lipolysis raises the plasma level of fatty acids and glycerol. Glycerol is utilized

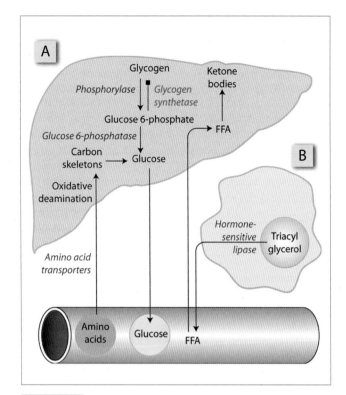

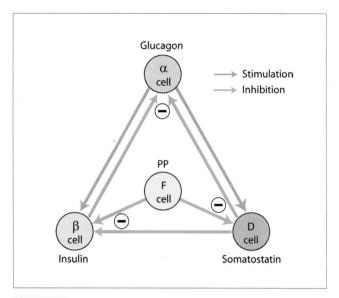

Fig. 81.6 Interrelationship between insulin, glucagon, and somatostatin secretion. PP, pancreatic polypeptide.

Fig. 81.5 Metabolic actions of glucagon on (A) the liver and (B) adipose cells. Glucagon has no effect on skeletal muscle. The actions of glucagon increase blood glucose. FFA, free fatty acid.

as a gluconeogenic substrate in the liver. Glucagon increases the oxidation of fatty acids and therefore has a glucose-sparing effect.

Somatostatin

Somatostatin is a small polypeptide secreted by the D cells of the pancreatic islets and by the parvocellular neurosecretory neurons in the median eminence of the hypothalamus. It is also found in other parts of the brain and in the gastrointestinal tract. Stimuli (e.g., glucose, amino acids, and epinephrine)

that increase insulin secretion also increase the secretion of somatostatin.

Somatostatin inhibits the secretion of growth hormone (GH) and thyroid-stimulating hormone (TSH). It inhibits the secretion of both glucagon and insulin (**Fig. 81.6**), and also inhibits the intestinal absorption of glucose. The net result is hypoglycemia that occurs mainly due to the suppression of glucagon secretion with the consequent fall in hepatic glucose production. Because type 1 diabetes mellitus results from insulin deficiency and the unopposed action of glucagon, somatostatin might prove to be useful in suppressing glucagon while supplementing the insulin through injections. The role of somatostatin in the paracrine regulation of gastric acidity (**Fig. 81.7**) through the inhibition of gastrin has been discussed in Chapter 68. Somatostatin inhibits other hormones and several other gastrointestinal functions, the physiologic significance of which is not understood.

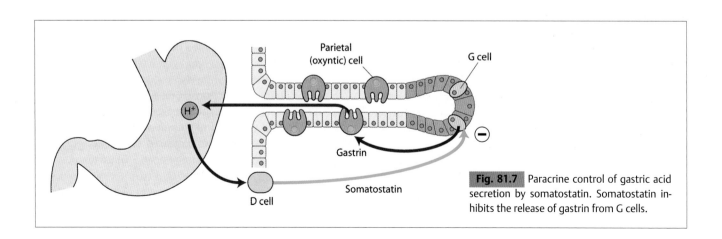

Fig. 81.7 Paracrine control of gastric acid secretion by somatostatin. Somatostatin inhibits the release of gastrin from G cells.

Pancreatic Polypeptide

Pancreatic polypeptide (PP) is secreted mainly by the PP cells (sometimes called F cells) of the pancreas. The secretion of PP is stimulated by ingested proteins and fats largely under the control of cholinergic stimulation by the vagus. Obesity decreases plasma PP levels. Type 1 diabetes is associated with an increased plasma concentration of PP.

Pancreatic polypeptide acts on the endocrine pancreas to inhibit the secretion of insulin and somatostatin. It also acts on the exocrine pancreas to inhibit enzyme and bicarbonate secretion, on the gallbladder to decrease its contractility, on the stomach to inhibit gastric acid secretion, and on the entire gastrointestinal tract to reduce its motility. In general, PP slows down digestive processes.

Disturbances of Blood Glucose

The Absorptive State

The absorptive state lasts up to 4 hours following ingestion of food; during this period, digested food is absorbed, and the monosaccharides, amino acids, and chylomicrons enter the bloodstream in large amounts. The high levels of glucose and amino acids in the blood stimulate insulin secretion and inhibit glucagon secretion. Many of the subsequent metabolic events are under the control of insulin.

Carbohydrates | Most of the surplus glucose is taken up by the liver and muscles, where it is trapped as glucose-6-phosphate, converted to glycogen, and stored. The increased glucose uptake by muscle and liver cells occurs under the influence of plasma insulin, which increases in the absorptive state. In the liver, the stimulation of glycolysis produces acetyl CoA that is used for fatty acid synthesis (**Fig. 81.8**).

Proteins | The surge of amino acids in the blood during the absorptive period briefly stimulates protein synthesis in all cells, resulting in the replacement of the proteins that were degraded after the preceding postabsorptive period. In liver, too, the synthesis of plasma proteins increases. Surplus amino acids are taken up by the liver and the kidney, are deaminated, and converted either to glucose (for storage as glycogen) or to fatty acids (**Fig. 81.9**).

Fats | The chylomicrons released from the intestine (nascent chylomicrons) rapidly lose their triacylglycerol content due to the action of lipoprotein lipase present on the surface of capillary endothelial cells in various tissues of the body (especially adipose tissue and striated muscle), with the notable exception of the liver. None of these organs takes up chylomicrons: they hydrolyze the triglyceride content of chylomicrons passing through them (**Fig. 81.10**). After its triglyceride content has been hydrolyzed, whatever remains of the chylomicron is called the *chylomicron remnant.*

The chylomicron remnants are taken up by the liver and degraded, releasing cholesterol, fatty acids, and amino acids. The fatty acids derived from chylomicron remnants as well as those synthesized de novo are converted into triacylglycerol, incorporated into lipoproteins and released into the bloodstream as VLDL (very-low-density lipoprotein) for transport to all tissues. The adipose tissues synthesize triacylglycerol from glycerol-3-phosphate (derived from glycolysis) and fatty acids (derived mainly from chylomicrons and partly VLDL). The high levels of insulin (which stimulates lipoprotein lipase) and glucose in the postabsorptive state favor lipogenesis in adipocytes. Insulin also inhibits hormone-sensitive lipase and thereby inhibits lipolysis (**Fig. 81.11**).

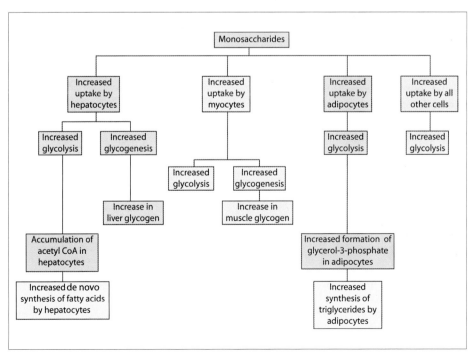

Fig. 81.8 Carbohydrate metabolism in the absorptive phase. These changes are stimulated by the increased insulin that is present.

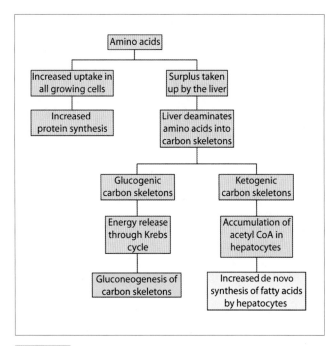

Fig. 81.9 Protein metabolism in the absorptive phase. Here, too, increased insulin is the stimulus for the changes that occur.

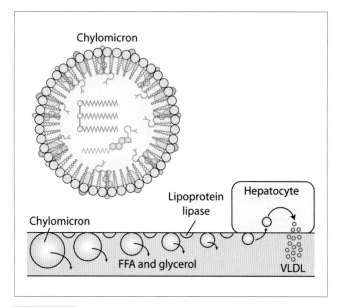

Fig. 81.10 Removal of triglycerides from a chylomicron during its passage through a capillary and the uptake of a chylomicron remnant by the liver. FFA, free fatty acid; VLDL, very-low-density lipoprotein.

General Model: Homeostasis

Following absorption of the digested meal, the concentration of glucose in the blood becomes quite high. The increase in insulin release and decrease in glucagon release act together to ensure that this glucose is taken up by muscle and adipose cells, thus returning blood glucose concentration to the normal level. Allowing blood glucose to get too high or too low has serious consequences; thus, it is important that blood glucose levels be homeostatically regulated.

The Postabsorptive State

After the ingested meal has been digested and absorbed, there is no further entry of nutrients into the blood. To maintain the availability of glucose for use by the cells, the substrates that have been stored in liver, muscle, and adipose cells must be mobilized.

The blood glucose concentration is now falling, thus reducing the release of insulin and increasing the release of glucagon. This change in the concentration of the pancreatic hormones essentially reverses the process that occurred during the absorptive period.

Glycogenolysis and gluconeogenesis in the liver generate large amounts of glucose that enter the circulation. Skeletal muscle breaks down stored glycogen to lactate and pyruvate, and the breaks down of proteins yields amino acids, particularly alanine. All of these products of muscle catabolism are used by the liver for gluconeogenesis. In adipose cells, lipolysis yields free fatty acids (FFAs) and glycerol. Glycerol is used by

the liver to make glucose, and FFAs are used to make ketones (which many cells can utilize as a source of energy).

Typically, the postabsorptive period lasts no more than 8 to 10 hours before another meal is consumed, and the body returns to an absorptive state.

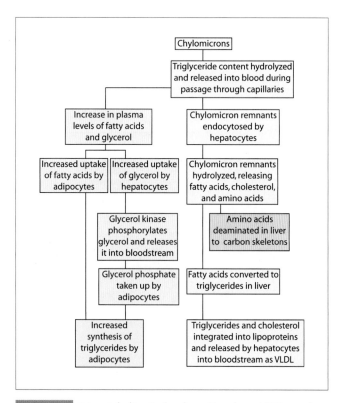

Fig. 81.11 Fat metabolism in the absorptive phase. VLDL, very-low-density lipoprotein.

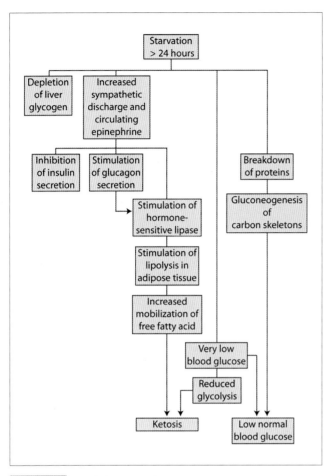

Fig. 81.12 Metabolic events during starvation.

Starvation

Starvation is a form of stress (see **Fig. 79.7**); therefore, it is associated with increased sympathetic discharge and epinephrine secretion. As in the case of exercise, some of the metabolic consequences of starvation are brought about by sympathetic activity and circulating epinephrine, which stimulate glucagon secretion.

Epinephrine and glucagon stimulate glycogenolysis, and within 24 hours of starvation, the liver is depleted of its stored glycogen, which is only ~100 g (**Fig. 81.12**). Thereafter, energy is obtained mostly by the oxidation of fatty acids and amino acids. The breakdown of proteins and fats occurs in a ratio of roughly 1:2. Amino acids are mobilized by the breakdown of proteins. Proteins of the brain and heart are largely spared, and most of the protein that is broken down comes from the spleen, liver, and muscles, in decreasing order. The excess protein breakdown is reflected in increased urinary urea excretion. Adequate blood glucose is necessary for the brain, nerves, erythrocytes, and adrenal medulla that cannot metabolize fatty acids. Until the very end, the liver is able to maintain nearly normal blood glucose levels through gluconeogenesis, using the carbon skeletons of deaminated glucogenic amino acids and the glycerol obtained from lipolysis.

The sympathetic discharge and the circulating epinephrine and glucagon stimulate hormone-sensitive lipase, which hydrolyzes neutral fats present in adipose tissue. In the absence of adequate glycolysis, the fatty acids mobilized from adipose fats are converted into ketone bodies, resulting in ketoacidosis. The formation of ketone bodies by the liver is beneficial because they are released into the blood and transported to tissues such as striated muscles and the renal cortex, which can metabolize them for energy production. Even the brain can utilize ketone bodies when their concentration in the blood is sufficiently high. Complex lipids that form part of the cell membranes and organelles are spared until the very end.

Exercise

Sustained exercise imposes a great demand for energy to power the exercising muscles. This requirement is met through the operation of several mechanisms.

Exercise (**Fig. 81.13**) is associated with increased sympathetic discharge and increased plasma levels of circulating epinephrine, which act directly on the pancreatic islets to inhibit insulin secretion and stimulate glucagon secretion. Although resting muscle cells require insulin for glucose uptake, the inhibition of insulin secretion in exercise does not affect glucose uptake by the exercising muscle cells, which now take up glucose independently of insulin. Both epinephrine and glucagon stimulate glycogenolysis and lipolysis. Lipolysis in adipose tissue releases fatty acids and glycerol, which are taken up by skeletal muscles for oxidation.

Glycogenolysis in the liver results in the release of glucose into the blood. Glycogenolysis in muscles produces glucose-6-phosphate, which is consumed by the muscle itself through glycolysis. Glycolysis converts glucose to pyruvate. Under aerobic conditions, the pyruvate is completely oxidized through the Krebs cycle with the release of large amounts of energy. Under anaerobic conditions, as is commonly seen in severely exercising muscles, the pyruvate is reduced to lactate

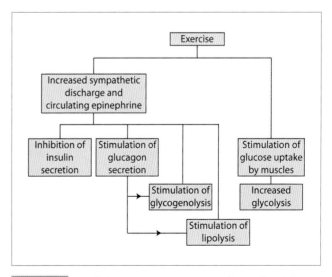

Fig. 81.13 Metabolic events during exercise. The uptake of glucose in exercising muscle is not dependent on the availability of insulin.

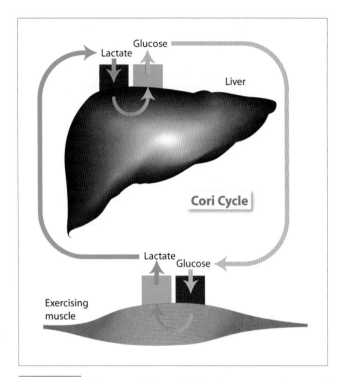

Fig. 81.14 The Cori cycle by which the liver converts lactic acid produced in exercising muscles into glucose for use by the exercising muscle.

Table 81.1 Comparison of Type 1 and Type 2 Diabetes Mellitus

Characteristic	Type 1 (IDDM)	Type 2 (NIDDM)
Synonym	Juvenile-onset diabetes	Adult-onset diabetes
Genetic predisposition	Moderate	Very strong
Defect	β cells destroyed	Insulin resistance and inadequate compensatory increase in insulin secretion
Age at onset	Usually < 30 years	Usually > 40 years
Mode of onset	Abrupt	More gradual
Body weight	Nonobese	Obese
Circulating insulin levels	Low to absent	Normal or elevated
Acute metabolic complications	Ketoacidosis	Hyperosmolar coma
Treatment with Insulin	Essential and always responds	Resistant and usually not required
Response to oral hypoglycemic drugs	Unresponsive	Responsive

Abbreviations: IDDM, insulin-dependent diabetes mellitus; NIDDM, noninsulin-dependent diabetes mellitus.

and released into the bloodstream. The liver takes up the lactate and converts it back to glucose or glycogen. This exchange of lactate between muscle and liver is called the Cori cycle (**Fig. 81.14**).

Diabetes Mellitus

Diabetes mellitus results from a relative or absolute deficiency of insulin together with a relative or absolute excess of glucagon. It is characterized by alterations in carbohydrate, lipid, and protein metabolism, and is clinically diagnosed when the blood glucose exceeds 140 mg/dL. Approximately 10% of all diabetics have type 1 diabetes; the rest have type 2 diabetes. The differences between the two types of diabetes are explained below and are summarized in **Table 81.1**.

Type 1 diabetes (also called insulin-dependent diabetes mellitus, or IDDM) includes patients with severe insulin deficiency. It is called type 1A if the deficiency is due to autoimmune destruction of pancreatic islets, which might be triggered by a viral infection. The nonimmune form of the diabetes is called type 1B. The symptoms of type 1 diabetes appear when more than 80% of the islets are destroyed, and they manifest abruptly as the classic triad of polyuria (excessive passage of urine), polydipsia (excessive thirst), and polyphagia (excessive eating).

Type 2 diabetes (also called noninsulin-dependent diabetes mellitus, or NIDDM) occurs due to a resistance to the action of insulin on cells. The resistance to insulin action can be due to several causes, including an abnormality in insulin structure, abnormality of insulin receptors, downregulation of insulin

receptors, or defects in glucose transporters. Quite often, these patients have a higher-than-normal level of insulin that tries to overcome the insulin resistance. Diabetes occurs only when the compensatory rise in insulin level is inadequate. For example, obese individuals tend to have higher insulin levels due to downregulation of insulin receptors. However, they develop type 2 diabetes only when the rise in insulin proves to be inadequate for overcoming the insulin resistance.

Metabolic Consequences of Diabetes Mellitus
The classic triad of polyuria, polydipsia, and polyphagia is an inadequate summary of the complex clinical picture of diabetes mellitus. The metabolic consequences of diabetes mellitus result not just from the deficiency of insulin but equally important, from the unopposed action of glucagon. Quite often, diabetes mellitus is associated with higher than normal plasma levels of glucagon. The combination of insulin deficiency and glucagon excess has four major metabolic consequences: (1) hyperglycemia and its consequences, (2) polyphagia despite the hyperglycemia, (3) hyperlipidemia and its consequences, and (4) ketoacidosis and its consequences. A somewhat similar metabolic picture is seen in starvation (see **Fig. 81.12**) except that there is no hyperglycemia. Hence, diabetes mellitus has been described as starvation in the midst of plenty.

Hyperglycemia and its consequences The events that lead to hyperglycemia are shown in **Fig. 81.15**. Briefly, the hyper-

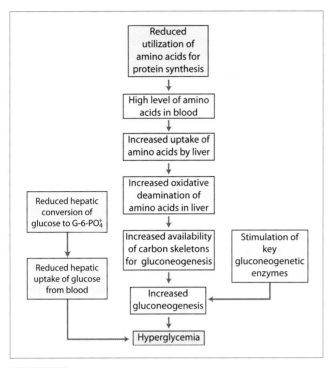

Fig. 81.15 Causes of hyperglycemia in diabetes mellitus.

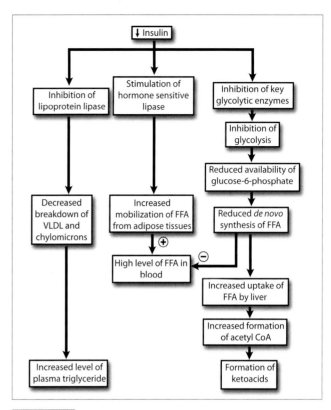

Fig. 81.16 Pathophysiology of hyperlipidemia and ketosis in untreated diabetes mellitus. VLDL, very low-density lipoprotein; FFA, free fatty acid.

glycemia is due to a reduction of glucose uptake by liver cells (because the conversion of glucose to glucose-6-phosphate is inhibited) and the stimulation of gluconeogenesis. Because a lack of insulin reduces protein synthesis, large quantities of amino acids are available for gluconeogenesis.

When the hyperglycemia exceeds the renal threshold of glucose, it results in glycosuria. The glucose in urine acts as an osmotic diuretic that results in polyuria, the passage of large volumes of urine. The polyuria results in dehydration and polydipsia. Severe dehydration leads to coma. Coma can also occur if the hyperglycemia is very high; it is then called hyperosmolar coma. The dehydration is usually not severe enough to cause peripheral circulatory failure or renal failure.

Hyperglycemia results in increased uptake of glucose by various cells even if the number of GLUT- 4 transporters is reduced. This extra glucose that enters the cell is metabolized through the sorbitol pathway (see **Fig. 74.5**). In the cells of the retina, lens, kidney, and nerves, the sorbitol accumulates, leading to osmotic swelling and contributing to the retinopathy, cataract, nephropathy, and neuropathy of diabetes mellitus.

Polyphagia despite hyperglycemia | Normally, a high level of blood glucose should produce satiety. In diabetes, there is polyphagia despite the hyperglycemia. The catch in this paradox is that hunger is actually related to the glucose utilization by the cells of the satiety center in the brain and not to the blood glucose level. In diabetes mellitus, the glucose utilization is reduced in the cells of the satiety center, which therefore signals a glucose deficiency to the feeding center. As a result, hunger is perceived, and food intake increases.

Hyperlipidemia and its consequences | The events that lead to hyperlipidemia are shown in **Fig. 81.16**. The increase in plasma triglyceride occurs mainly due to the reduced breakdown of the VLDL secreted by the liver and the chylomicrons released into blood from the intestine. The FFA level in the blood rises, too, because of lipolysis in adipose tissues. The rise occurs despite a decrease in the hepatic synthesis of fatty acids. The hyperlipidemia and related hypercholesterolemia results in hypertension and coronary heart disease in the long run.

Ketosis and its consequences | Due to the presence of excess free fatty acid in blood, there is increased uptake and oxidation of FFA by the cells. In the liver, increased oxidation of FFA results in accumulation of excess acetyl CoA. Because glycolysis is inhibited in diabetes mellitus, the excess acetyl CoA forms ketoacids (see **Fig. 74.12**). The hydrogen (H^+) of the ketoacids is buffered by the blood buffers. However, when the production of ketoacids exceeds the buffering capacity of the blood, it results in metabolic acidosis with all its complications (see Chapter 63). A characteristic clinical feature of the acidosis is Kussmaul breathing, a form of hyperventilation associated with increased tidal volume and a lesser increase in frequency. Vomiting is another complication of ketoacidosis. The vomiting causes dehydration, and if it is followed by ingestion of plain water instead of an electrolyte solution, hyponatremia

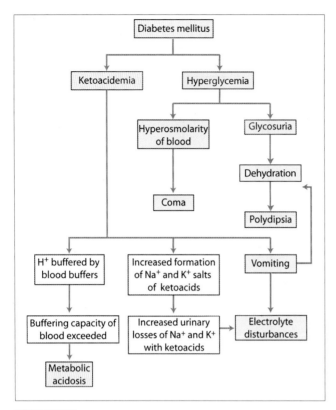

Fig. 81.17 Clinical consequences of ketoacidemia and hyperglycemia in untreated diabetes mellitus.

results (**Fig. 81.17**). Following their buffering by blood buffers, the ketoacids become organic anions. For example, buffering of acetoacetic acid produces acetoacetate. These organic anions increase the plasma anion gap. When excreted in urine, these organic anions carry with them an equal number of cations, mainly Na^+ and K^+. However significant hyponatremia occurs only due to vomiting, as explained above.

Hyperkalemia with intracellular depletion of potassium stores is an important feature of diabetes mellitus. Insulin causes K^+ to move into the cells; therefore, insulin deficiency results in the movement of K^+ from intracellular fluid (ICF) to ECF. The hyperkalemia is associated with kaliuresis, resulting in the depletion of body K^+ stores.

Diagnosis of Diabetes Mellitus

A patient having the classic signs and symptoms of diabetes mellitus is confirmed to be a diabetic if the random plasma glucose is ≥ 200 mg/dL. In the absence of the classic signs, the fasting plasma glucose must be ≥ 126 mg/dL for the diagnosis of diabetes. Those with fasting plasma glucose between 110 and 126 are diagnosed as impaired fasting glucose (IFG), and if the 2-hour postprandial plasma glucose is ≥ 200 mg/dL, the patient is diagnosed as having impaired glucose tolerance (IGT).

The glucose tolerance test (GTT) is no longer considered necessary for diagnosing diabetes mellitus. In the GTT, half-hourly samples of blood and urine were tested for their glucose concentration after administering an oral glucose load of 75 g to the patient. The test remains useful for diagnosing renal glycosuria (see **Fig. 64.1**).

Treatment of Diabetes Mellitus

The treatment of both type 1 and type 2 diabetes includes healthy eating habits, regular exercise, and stopping smoking. Weight reduction is important in type 2 diabetics, nearly 80% of whom are obese. The exercise can be in the form of walking daily for 30 to 60 minutes, or preferably more. The diet should be low in fat (< 30%) and high in carbohydrates (> 55%), preferably high-fiber carbohydrates. Sucrose should be limited to < 50 g per day. Saturated fats should be < 10% of the total energy intake. Cholesterol intake should be limited to < 250 mg per day. Monounsaturated fats like olive oil and rapeseed oil should be encouraged. Proteins should constitute 10 to 15% of the diet.

Insulin therapy is necessary for controlling type 1 diabetes mellitus. On the other hand, up to 20% of type 2 diabetes can be controlled by diet and exercise alone. Other cases of type 2 diabetes are treated with oral hypoglycemic drugs, such as the sulphonylureas that stimulate insulin secretion and the biguanides that increase insulin action and inhibit liver gluconeogenesis. Oral agents may fail to control blood glucose level after a period of apparent success due to worsening B cell function. Most of these patients of "secondary failure" ultimately require insulin.

Summary

- Insulin is released from pancreatic β cells stimulated by increased blood glucose concentrations.

- Insulin decreases blood glucose by increasing glucose uptake in muscle and adipose cells, increasing glycogen formation in the liver (thus promoting glucose uptake). Insulin also stimulates lipid formation in adipose cells and protein formation in muscle cells.

- Glucagon is released from pancreatic α cells stimulated by falling blood glucose levels.

- Glucagon increases blood glucose levels by promoting gluconeogenesis and glycogenolysis in the liver and lipolysis in adipose cells.

- Types 1 and 2 diabetes mellitus are both diseases in which the body's handling of nutrients, particularly glucose, is defective, resulting in short-term metabolic derangements and long-term pathologic changes.

Applying What You Know

81.1. Reverend Wright, the patient with kidney failure, has a fasting blood glucose of 111 mg/dL and no glucose in his urine.

What is the role of insulin in determining the kidney's handling of glucose? Under what conditions will glucose appear in the urine? Explain.

81.2. Mrs. Omaya has a fasting blood glucose level that is at the low end of normal (62 mg/dL). During an overnight "fast," what mechanisms help to prevent hypoglycemia from developing?

81.3. Mr. Lundquist, the patient with pernicious anemia, is a tennis player. While exercising, his muscles are using glucose at an increased rate. Where does this glucose come from? What is the role of the endocrine pancreas? Explain.

Answers to Applying What You Know

Chapter 74

1 Mrs. Omaya complains about suffering from fatigue since giving birth. How might her low blood glucose contribute to that symptom?

All cells produce adenosine triphosphate (ATP) with which to power all of their functions, and the metabolism of glucose is generally the source of that ATP. Thus, lack of glucose will require that cells produce ATP from other precursors, usually fats. Although these compounds yield large amounts of ATP (they are energy-rich), they are not as readily available. Thus, with low blood glucose and limited fat availability, reduced ATP (particularly in muscles) could contribute to Mrs. Omaya's fatigue.

Chapter 75

1 Mrs. Omaya has a very low thyroid hormone (T_4) level. How does the thyroid hormone that is available exert its effect on its target cells?

Thyroid hormone is a group I hormone whose receptors are located in the nucleus. When it binds to these nuclear receptors, changes in gene expression occur, altering the availability and activity of enzymes in the cytoplasm. The metabolic changes that occur represent the biologic response to thyroid hormone.

2 Mrs. Omaya's posterior pituitary appears to be normal, which means she has appropriate levels of antidiuretic hormone (ADH). What are the target cells for ADH, and how does ADH affect their function?

ADH acts on the collecting ducts of the renal tubules to alter their permeability to water. This action makes it possible for the kidneys to produce a concentrated urine. ADH is a group IIA hormone that binds to a receptor on the cell membrane. The result is an increase in cyclic adenosine monophosphate (cAMP) that causes the insertion of aquaporins (channels through which water can move down an osmotic gradient) into the luminal membrane of the collecting duct cells.

Chapter 76

1 Mrs. Omaya has low levels of several anterior pituitary hormones (TSH, PRL, LH, FSH). At what location would a single discrete lesion give rise to these findings? Explain.

Mrs. Omaya's low hormone levels could be the result of a discrete lesion of the anterior pituitary; damage to the cells there would affect release of all anterior pituitary hormones. Furthermore, the pituitary is relatively isolated in a bony cavity, and pathology present there could easily affect all hormones. The neurons in the hypothalamus that produce the hypotha-lamic hormones are scattered fairly widely throughout this region of the central nervous system; it is hard to see how a relatively discrete lesion could affect all of them.

2 Mrs. Omaya experienced some insult (probably ischemic) to her anterior pituitary, yet there is nothing to suggest that her posterior pituitary was affected. Given that both parts of the pituitary are in close proximity to one another in a confined space, how can you account for this?

The anterior and posterior pituitary, although in close proximity to one another, have different embryologic origins and a very different circulation. The anterior pituitary is perfused by a portal circulation, with the first capillary bed located in the median eminence and the second capillary bed in the body of the anterior pituitary. As is typical in portal circulations, the pressure gradient driving flow through the second capillary bed is small. The posterior pituitary is perfused by the more usual circulation with a single capillary bed. A vascular problem, or very low blood pressure resulting from a hemorrhage, could affect one side (the anterior pituitary) and not the other (or at least not to the same extent).

3 What needs to be done to help Mrs. Omaya? How would this be accomplished?

Mrs. Omaya has very low cortisol. This potentially poses a serious risk because cortisol is necessary for the body's response to stressors of all kinds. Obviously, cortisol needs to be supplemented with administration of an appropriate glucocorticoid. Her low thyroid hormone is also easily supplemented. The lack of growth hormone is not a particular problem as long as the other major endocrine regulators of metabolism are able to function. The lack of luteinizing hormone (LH) and follicle-stimulating hormone (FSH) will prevent the normal menstrual cycle and will leave her infertile. However, these hormones are not necessary to maintain health and are both difficult to replace in a way that would restore fertility.

Chapter 77

1 Mrs. Omaya's laboratory reports show that she has low T_4 and low TSH. Where in her endocrine system could dysfunction give rise to these two abnormalities? Explain.

If the primary lesion was in the hypothalamus, this would cause decreased thyrotropin-releasing hormone (TRH), and this would, in turn, result in decreased thyroid-stimulating hormone (TSH) and T_3/T_4.

A primary lesion in the anterior pituitary would cause decreased TSH and hence decreased T_3/T_4. TRH would be increased because of the decreased negative feedback on the hypothalamus.

A primary problem in the thyroid gland would result in decreased T_3/T_4 release, and the reduction in negative feedback would result in increased TRH and TSH. Lack of iodine in the diet would have a similar effect.

Given Mrs. Omaya's many other endocrine problems, it is most likely that her condition is the result of a lesion to the anterior pituitary gland.

2 Which of Mrs. Omaya's findings on the physical examination suggests that she is in a hypothyroid state? Which finding would preclude her problem being a dietary one?

Mrs. Omaya presents with rough skin, slowed deep tendon reflexes, blood pressure that is at the low end of normal, and a significant fall in blood pressure on standing up. All of these are possible consequences of low thyroid hormone. However, Mrs. Omaya does not have a palpable goiter (increased growth of her thyroid gland) because there are no masses reported in the neck. Goiter is most commonly the result of too little iodine in the diet and hence too little thyroid hormone produced.

3 Mrs. Schilling was found to have an enlarged thyroid gland on physical examination. How would you explain the mechanism resulting in this hypertrophied state?

Mrs. Schilling suffers from a serious malabsorption problem with frequent episodes of diarrhea. The rapid transit of the contents of the intestine may be limiting the absorption of iodine. This would, of course, limit the ability of the thyroid gland to make thyroid hormone. One result is decreased negative feedback at the pituitary and the hypothalamus. As a consequence, there are increased levels of TRH and TSH. The TSH then causes hypertrophy of the thyroid gland.

Chapter 78

1 What is the effect of Mrs. Omaya's depressed thyroid function (a consequence of low TSH) on calcium metabolism?

Although the parathyroid glands are anatomically located within the thyroid gland, there is no direct functional connection between them. So altered thyroid function should have no direct effect on parathyroid hormone (PTH) production. It is important to note, however, that surgical or other interventions to deal with thyroid problems must be done carefully to spare the parathyroid glands. PTH is essential for maintenance of calcium balance, and destruction of the parathyroid glands would require hormone replacement therapy.

Chapter 79

1 Mrs. Omaya has a low concentration of cortisol. What are possible mechanisms that could result in this finding? Explain.

If either corticotropin-releasing hormone (CRH) from the hypothalamus or adrenocorticotropic hormone (ACTH) from the anterior pituitary were decreased, there would ultimately be reduced stimulation of the adrenal cortex, and less cortisol would be released.

There are also possible disturbances that would alter the negative feedback mechanisms that determine function in the hypothalamic–anterior pituitary–adrenal system. For example, an increase in the number of cortisol receptors on cells in the hypothalamus would increase the strength of the negative feedback exerted here, and there would thus be less CRH released.

Alternatively, the presence of an autoantibody that binds to the ACTH receptor on cells in the adrenal cortex would prevent ACTH molecules from binding and thus reduce the stimulus to release cortisol; in this case, CRH and ACTH would both be increased.

2 Mrs. Omaya's laboratory report shows both low $[Na^+]$ and high $[K^+]$. What is the most likely explanation for these findings?

When $[Na^+]$ is low and $[K^+]$ is simultaneously high, it suggests that something is happening in the kidneys to the handling of these solutes by the nephrons. Normally, when sodium is reabsorbed (thus raising extracellular fluid $[Na^+]$), potassium is secreted and then excreted (thus lowering extracellular fluid $[K^+]$). The reabsorption of Na^+ and the secretion of K^+ are under the control of aldosterone, a mineralocorticoid released by the adrenal cortex. There is no information about the level of aldosterone that is present. However, we know that cortisol is low. It is also known that cortisol has significant mineralocorticoid activity. So it is possible that the low cortisol is the cause of the changes to sodium and potassium concentrations.

Chapter 80

1 Mrs. Omaya's blood pressure is low, and she exhibits orthostatic hypotension (her pressure falls significantly in going from a supine to an erect position). What changes in her endocrine function might contribute to this finding? Explain the mechanism at work.

When an individual stands up, a baroreceptor reflex response is generated that prevents blood pressure from falling more than a few mm Hg. This is accomplished, to a significant extent, by increased peripheral resistance (due to sympathetic vasoconstriction). The production of epinephrine requires the enzyme phenylethanolamine *N*-methyl transferase (PNMT). The production of this enzyme is promoted by cortisol. So, Mrs. Omaya's low cortisol level results in reduced epinephrine and hence a reduced baroreceptor reflex response.

Chapter 81

1 Reverend Wright, the patient with kidney failure, has a fasting blood glucose of 111 mg/dL and no glucose in his urine. What is the role of insulin in determining the kidneys' handling of glucose? Under what conditions will glucose appear in the urine? Explain.

The kidneys normally reabsorb all of the glucose that is filtered and reaches the proximal tubule. The reabsorptive process involves active transport of Na^+ out of the cell into the interstitium and the cotransport of Na^+ and glucose into the cell from the tubular lumen. The number of cotransporters determines the maximum rate at which glucose can be reabsorbed. That is to say, this process exhibits a transport maximum or T_m. As long as the filtered load of glucose (mg/min) is less than the T_m, all of the filtered glucose is reabsorbed, and there is no glucose in the urine. In a normal individual, the filtered load (that is to say, the blood glucose level) never gets near enough to the T_m to cause glucose to appear in the urine.

The kidneys' handling of glucose is *not* controlled by any hormone. Thus, the elaborate endocrine control of blood glucose level does not involve control of glucose excretion. Glucose will appear in the urine of a diabetic patient (or a normal individual) whenever the filtered load of glucose exceeds the individual's T_m for glucose reabsorption.

2 Mrs. Omaya has a fasting blood glucose level that is at the low end of normal (62 mg/dL). During an overnight "fast," what mechanisms help to prevent hypoglycemia from developing?

Within a few hours of digesting dinner, the endocrine system has succeeded in storing away the glucose; amino acids, and free fatty acids (FFAs) that were absorbed from the gastrointestinal tract. This occurs because the increased blood levels of glucose and amino acids stimulate the release of insulin (and inhibit the release of glucagon).

This means that eventually the fall in blood glucose results in a decrease in insulin secretion and an increase in glucagon secretion. This then begins to mobilize stored energy substrates. Glycogenolysis, principally in the liver, releases glucose. Protein breakdown in muscle yields amino acids, which are used by the liver to make new glucose (gluconeogenesis). Finally, lipolysis in adipose cells results in the release of FFAs, some of which will be used directly by some cells, with the remainder being used by the liver to make ketones that can be used by cells.

These processes prevent blood glucose levels from falling too low (prevent hypoglycemia) during an overnight fast.

3 Mr. Lundquist, the patient with pernicious anemia, is a tennis player. While exercising his muscles are using glucose at an increased rate. Where does this glucose come from? What is the role of the endocrine pancreas? Explain.

During exercise, the use of adenosine triphosphate (ATP) increases. The muscle cells can mobilize stored glycogen to use in producing ATP, but the amount of glycogen available is small and will only power exercise for a few minutes. However, during exercise, the active muscle cells insert glucose transporters into the membrane via a process that is independent of insulin. With glucose use accelerated, there is a steep gradient for transport of glucose into the muscle cells, and this enables the active muscles to produce the additional ATP required to continue contracting.

Section IX Case Analysis:
Mrs. Omaya has been tired since giving birth.

Clinical Overview

Review of patient condition | Roberta Omaya, a 27-year-old woman, has Sheehan syndrome, also known as postpartum hypopituitarism.

Etiology | Mrs. Omaya experienced a significant loss of blood following the delivery of her baby. This resulted in a drop in blood pressure. The anterior pituitary, having undergone some hyperplasia during pregnancy, was dependent on the maintenance of normal blood flow. The anterior pituitary is supplied by a low-pressure portal system and therefore more likely to experience ischemia. The damage to the anterior pituitary results in decreased production of all of the hormones normally released from there.

Prevalence | With improved obstetric care, this condition has become quite rare. However, there are several other causes of panhypopituitarism.

Diagnosis | The patient's medical history and presenting complaints certainly suggest anterior pituitary involvement. Blood tests to measure hormone levels can confirm the diagnosis. A computed tomography (CT) scan of the head can rule out other possible problems.

Treatment | Hormone replacement therapy will be needed. In particular, glucocorticoid and thyroid hormones will have to be supplemented to maintain near normal levels.

Understanding the Physiology

The anterior pituitary is the interface between the hypothalamus (the central nervous system) and a large number of endocrine systems. Releasing and inhibiting hormones released from neurons in the hypothalamus diffuse into the capillary bed of the superior hypophysial artery in the median eminence. The long portal veins then carry them to the anterior pituitary, where they diffuse from the pituitary capillary bed into the tissues stimulated by the endocrine cells located there. The hormones released from the anterior pituitary include growth hormone, prolactin, TSH, ACTH, FSH, and LH.

These anterior pituitary hormones stimulate the release of hormones from distant target glands: T_3 and T_4 from the thyroid gland, cortisol from the adrenal cortex, and estrogen from the ovaries.

Mrs. Omaya suffered a significant blood loss following delivery of her baby. This produced a drop in blood pressure and hence a decrease in perfusion. The anterior pituitary was rendered ischemic for a long enough time that many of the endocrine cells located there were damaged or destroyed. This accounts for the severe decrease in the concentration of cortisol, free T_4, insulin-like growth factor (IGF), TSH, prolactin, LH, FSH, and growth hormone (GH). The lack of these hormones, in turn, accounts for her presenting symptoms: inability to nurse (decreased prolactin), fatigue (decreased thyroid hormone), and failure to resume menstruation (lack of LH and FSH).

There is no evidence that Mrs. Omaya suffered any damage to her posterior pituitary. This is probably due to the fact that the anterior pituitary is perfused by a low-pressure venous portal system whose flow would have been greatly reduced, whereas the posterior pituitary is perfused by a high-pressure arterial system, which probably experienced a smaller fall in pressure.

The accompanying flow chart (**Fig. IX.1**) illustrates the sequence of events that resulted in Mrs. Omaya's many problems.

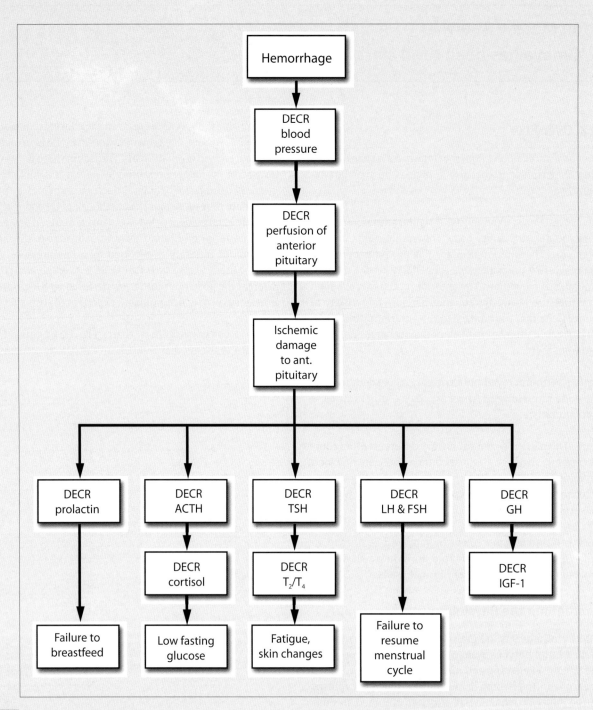

Fig. IX.1 Mrs. Omaya suffers from hypo-pituitarism as a result of ischemic damage to her anterior pituitary.

Section X Reproductive System

Overview

Case Presentation

Chapters

Answers to Applying What You Know

Case Analysis

Overview

The reproductive system and its many processes do not contribute to the maintenance of homeostasis in the individual, and normal functioning of the reproductive system is not essential for the survival of the individual. The functioning of the reproductive system does, of course, play a significant role in directing moods, behavior, and thoughts. Furthermore, reproduction is essential for the perpetuation of the species.

In both men and women, there are three components that make up the reproductive system: the primary reproductive organs (testes and ovaries), the secondary reproductive organs (the various organs of the reproductive tract), and the brain and endocrine system controllers.

Both the male and female reproductive systems carry out two fundamental tasks: production of gametes (sperm and ova) and controlled production of sex hormones. In addition, the female reproductive system must support the development of the fetus, make possible the delivery of the fetus at term, then feed the neonate.

Section X Case Presentation:
Mrs. Anderson is having trouble getting pregnant.

Chief Complaint

Mr. and Mrs. Anderson, both 27 years old, present to the husband's urologist with their concern about Mrs. Anderson's inability to get pregnant over the past 2 years.

History of Present Problem

The couple has been married for 2 years and has been trying to have a child the entire time. This is Mrs. Anderson's second marriage; she has a healthy 3-year-old daughter by her first husband. This is Mr. Anderson's first marriage, and he has not fathered any children.

Past Medical History

Both Andersons are in good health and have been seen by their primary care physicians within the past year. Mrs. Anderson had been taking oral contraceptives prior to her first marriage and stopped after getting married. She became pregnant with her first child within 6 months of her marriage and had an uneventful pregnancy. Labor was induced, and she had a normal vaginal delivery. She breast-fed her daughter for 1 year. Her daughter is a normal, healthy 3-year-old.

Plans for Diagnosing the Problem

Although Mrs. Anderson has had one successful pregnancy, she is advised to see her gynecologist for an examination.

The urologist will test Mr. Anderson to determine whether he has a problem that is impacting their getting pregnant.

Report from the Gynecologist

Mrs. Anderson's gynecologist reports that Mrs. Anderson has had no history of pelvic inflammatory disease and that there are no obvious structural defects that would affect her becoming pregnant. Charting of Mrs. Anderson's basal body temperature was normal. Hormone levels were tested, and all were normal (hypothalamic hormones, anterior pituitary hormones, and estrogen).

Testing of Mr. Anderson

- *Semen analysis*
  - After a period of abstinence of 1 week, a sample of semen was collected in a clean container in the urologist's office and sent for several tests.
  - Volume: 2.3 mL (normal > 2 mL)
  - Sperm concentration: 24 million/mL (40–100 million/mL)
  - Sperm motility: 55% with forward progression (normal 60%), 20% with rapid progression within 60 minutes
  - Morphology: 20% with normal form
- *Sperm function tests*
  - Because the semen analysis did not reveal a likely cause for the couple's infertility, further tests of sperm function were undertaken.
  - Sperm penetration assay: 18% of the sperm used in the assay were seen to penetrate the test ova, from which the zona pellucida had been removed.
  - Human sperm–zona pellucida (ZP) binding assay: the tested sperm exhibited a binding of 25% compared with normal fertile sperm.

Diagnosis

Mr. Anderson's sperm was found to be incapable of fertilization. The source of this problem was not determined.

Some Things to Think About

1. Although Mrs. Anderson has already had one successful pregnancy, it remains possible that the couple's infertility arises from a problem with her reproductive system. What are the processes involved in the production of viable fertilizable eggs?

2. Even if Mrs. Anderson produces fertilizable eggs, what other processes are required for a normal pregnancy to occur?

3. Mr. Anderson has never fathered a child, and it is likely that the couple's infertility is due to a problem with his reproductive system. What processes are involved with the production of viable sperm capable of fertilizing an egg?

4. What are the steps involved in the fertilization of Mrs. Anderson's egg (if present and viable) by Mr. Anderson's sperm (if viable), resulting in a normal pregnancy?

Hormones of the Testes

The hormone-secreting cells in the testes are the Leydig cells and Sertoli cells. The Leydig cell secretes all the androgens: dihydrotestosterone (DHT), testosterone, androstenedione, and dehydroepiandrosterone (DHEA). All of them have 19 carbon atoms, and their androgenic potencies are in a ratio of 60:20:2:1, respectively. The amount of testosterone secreted is 100 times more than the other hormones. The Leydig cell also secretes some androgenic precursors, such as pregnenolone and progesterone. The Sertoli cell secretes small amounts of estradiol.

Testosterone is synthesized in the Leydig cell through the same biosynthetic pathway as the adrenocortical steroids (see **Fig. 79.2**). Cholesterol esters, the major precursors for androgen biosynthesis, are stored in the lipid droplets in the Leydig cells. Androgen biosynthesis in the human testes proceeds mostly from pregnenolone to DHEA and then to androstenedione, testosterone, and dihydrotestosterone, via the Δ^4 pathway (**Fig. 82.1**). Only 20% of dihydrotestosterone is synthesized by the testes. The rest is derived from the peripheral conversion of testosterone in the skin and male reproductive tract (epididymis, prostate gland, and seminal vesicles).

Two-thirds of the total plasma testosterone is bound to albumin, and one-third is bound to testosterone-binding globulin, which is also called sex hormone–binding globulin because it binds estradiol as well. Less than 2% of the plasma testosterone is in the free form.

Testosterone and androstenedione are converted to estradiol and estrone, respectively, through the action of aromatase, which is a microsomal enzyme found in the brain, skin, liver, mammary tissues, adipose tissue, and placenta. These active metabolites (having hormonal activity) are further converted into inactive metabolites, such as androsterone and etiocholanolone. The inactive metabolites, are conjugated in the liver and excreted into the urine as 17-ketosteroids. Of the total urinary ketosteroids, only one-third is of testicular origin; the remainder comes from the DHEA produced by the adrenal cortex. Hence, the urinary 17-ketosteroid reflects mainly adrenocortical activity and is not a good index of testicular function.

General Model: Reservoir

The body is a reservoir in which DHT from a variety of sources is found. If DHT is abnormally low in concentration, it is essential to consider all the possible sources to determine where the problem is located.

General Model: Energy

Transformations of matter and energy underlie the complex metabolic pathways that are required for the synthesis of the steroid hormones. Each step along these pathways is potentially a site at which abnormalities could arise. The absence of a particular enzyme will result in too little of the product that is normally formed and too much of the precursor. Both changes can have significant physiologic consequences.

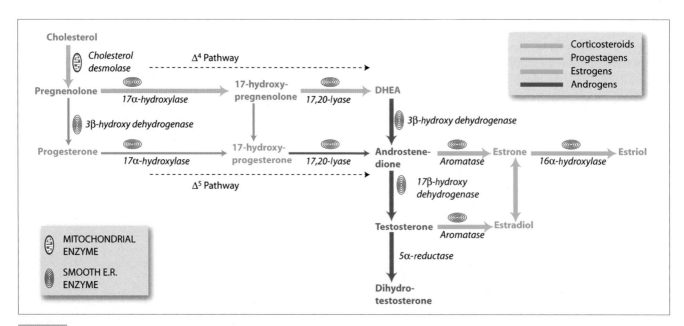

Fig. 82.1 Biosynthesis of sex steroids. Estrogens are shown in green, progesterone in blue, and androgens in red. Note that 17-hydroxy-progesterone has little biologic activity. Note that estrone and estradiol are interconvertible. DHEA, dehydroepiandrosterone.

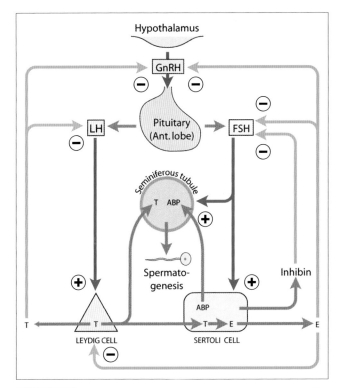

Fig. 82.2 Hormonal control of the testes. Luteinizing hormone (LH) stimulates the secretion of testosterone by Leydig cells. Follicle-stimulating hormone (FSH) stimulates the production of androgen-binding protein (ABP), inhibin, and estradiol. The direct inhibition of testosterone secretion by estradiol is a paracrine effect. Both estradiol and testosterone have inhibitory inputs to the hypothalamus and the anterior pituitary. E, estradiol; GnRH, gonadotropin-releasing hormone; T, testosterone.

Hormonal control of testicular function | Luteinizing hormone (LH) increases testosterone synthesis in the Leydig cells by activating cholesterol desmolase, which is the rate-limiting enzyme for the conversion of cholesterol to pregnenolone (**Fig. 82.1**). In the developing male fetus, the stimulus for testosterone synthesis is HCG (human chorionic gonadotropin), which is structurally and functionally similar to LH.

Follicle-stimulating hormone (FSH) stimulates the Sertoli cells to synthesize androgen-binding protein (ABP), which binds testosterone, increasing its local concentration in the testes and thereby stimulating spermatogenesis. FSH also indirectly increases testosterone synthesis by increasing the number of LH receptors on the Leydig cell. The secretion of FSH and LH from the anterior pituitary is stimulated by gonadotropin-releasing hormone (GnRH), which is secreted by the parvocellular neurosecretory neurons in the hypothalamus. The GnRH secretion is pulsatile and occurs at a frequency of 8 to 14 pulses/day.

General Model: Communications

The control of testosterone secretion involves the processing of many information-bearing chemical (hormonal) signals that are passed from cell to cell.

Consistent with the phenomenon that the secretion of the target hormone inhibits its trophic hormone, testosterone inhibits LH secretion. Estradiol and inhibin inhibit FSH secretion. Inhibin is secreted by Sertoli cells and acts only at the pituitary level; testosterone and estradiol act at both pituitary and hypothalamic levels (**Fig. 82.2**).

Physiologic actions of androgens include the following:

1. *Fetus.* In the fetus, testosterone stimulates the differentiation of the male internal genitalia; dihydrotestosterone stimulates the differentiation of the male external genitalia.
2. *Puberty.* During puberty, androgens stimulate the development of the secondary sexual characteristics, libido, and potency (erectile functions). Most of these are brought about by testosterone. Dihydrotestosterone promotes growth of pubic hair, increased sebum production by sebaceous glands with consequent development of acne, growth of scrotum and prostate, and stimulation of prostatic secretion (**Table 82.1**).
3. *Spermatogenesis.* Testosterone is essential for normal spermatogenesis.
4. *Metabolism.* Testosterone is an anabolic hormone that stimulates cells to make proteins. It stimulates cell division and maturation. In the adolescent, testosterone produces linear skeletal growth and broadens the shoulders; it also causes muscular development (myotrophic effect) and retention of potassium, nitrogen, and phosphorus. Testosterone has a dual effect on skeletal growth because it also accelerates epiphyseal fusion of the long bones and thereby limits linear growth. Treatment with testosterone reduces bone loss and osteoporosis.
5. *Red blood cell production.* Testosterone stimulates erythropoiesis directly as well as erythropoietin secretion in the kidneys.

Table 82.1 Differences between the Actions of Testosterone and Dihydrotestosterone

Testosterone	Dihydrotestosterone
Necessary for the differentiation of the internal genitalia	Necessary for the differentiation of the external genitalia
During puberty, promotes growth of the penis, seminal vesicles, larynx, muscles, and skeleton	During puberty, promotes growth of facial, body, and pubic hair, scrotum, sebaceous glands with increased sebum production and development of acne, and prostate with stimulation of prostatic secretions
Promotes spermatogenesis, increases libido, promotes erythropoiesis, and brings about feedback inhibition of luteinizing hormone	Has none of these effects

Hormones of the Ovary

Endocrine Cells of the Ovary

Three types of ovarian cells (**Fig. 82.3**) are involved in hormone secretion, namely, the granulosa cells, luteal cells, and thecal cells (cells of theca interna). Together they secrete estrogens (estrone, estradiol, and estriol), progesterone, androgens (androstenedione and testosterone), and relaxin.

Thecal cells produce androstenedione and testosterone that are converted in the granulosa cells to estrone and estradiol, respectively, by the enzyme aromatase (**Fig. 82.4**). Thecal cells do not produce appreciable amounts of progesterone because most of the androgens are formed via the Δ^4 and not the Δ^5 pathway (**Fig. 82.1**); therefore, progestogen levels remain low during the follicular phase of the menstrual cycle (see **Fig. 84.2**).

Granulosa cells cannot produce estrogens or progesterone directly from cholesterol because they lack 17α-hydroxylase and 17,20-lyase. Estrogens are synthesized in granulosa cells from the androstenedione obtained from thecal cells. Most of the estrogen produced by granulosa cells is secreted into the follicular fluid; therefore, estrogen levels remain low during the early follicular phase.

Luteal cells are of two types: the theca luteal cells and the granulosa luteal cells formed by the luteinization of thecal and

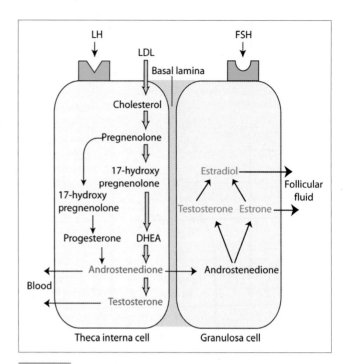

Fig. 82.4 Granulosa cells synthesize estrogens from the androgens provided by the thecal cells. DHEA, dehydroepiandrosterone; FSH, follicle-stimulating hormone; LDL, low-density lipoprotein; LH, luteinizing hormone.

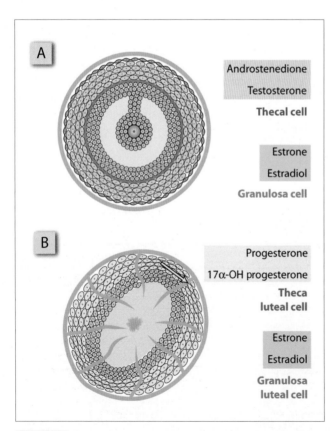

Fig. 82.3 **(A)** Hormones secreted by the granulosa cells and thecal cells in a follicle, and **(B)** luteal cells of the ovary. Note that the theca luteal cells and granulosa luteal cells secrete different hormones. Also note that the granulosa cells secrete estrogens into the follicular fluid, but the granulosa luteal cells secrete estrogens into the blood.

granulosa cells, respectively. Theca luteal cells produce mainly progesterone due to the activation of the Δ^5 pathway of steroid biosynthesis. The granulosa luteal cells secrete estrone and estradiol. These estrogens are secreted directly into the blood capillaries that grow into the corpus luteum; therefore, estrogen levels rise during the luteal phase of the menstrual cycle (see **Fig. 84.2**).

Estrogens

Estradiol (E_2) is the main estrogen secreted by the ovary and is also the most biologically active. Estrone (E_1) is a weak ovarian estrogen. In postmenopausal women, estrone is the dominant plasma estrogen and is mostly formed by the conversion of adrenocortical androstenedione in peripheral tissues, mainly liver and adipose tissue. Estriol (E_3) is not secreted by the ovary. It is formed in small amounts in the liver from estradiol and estrone. Large amounts are secreted only during pregnancy, when it is secreted by the placenta. Note that estr(one) has one hydroxyl group, estra(di)ol has two hydroxyl groups, and es(tri)ol has three hydroxyl groups (see **Fig. 79.3**). Estrone and estradiol are interconvertible (**Fig. 82.1**). The synthesis of estriol by the placenta is described in Chapter 87.

Over 70% of circulating estrogens are bound to sex steroid-binding globulin, and 25% are bound to plasma albumin. Only a small percentage are present in the blood in a free (not bound to plasma proteins) form. Estrogens are metabolized in the liver. Estradiol and estrone are hydroxylated to form estriol and catecholestrogens, which are excreted primarily as glucuronides. Estrone is excreted primarily as a sulfate.

The **physiologic actions** of estrogens can be summarized as follows:

1. *Metabolism.* Estrogens have important protein anabolic effects. They mediate the growth and development of the female reproductive organs, especially that of the gravid uterus. They also promote cellular proliferation in the mucosal linings of these structures.
2. *Endometrium.* Estrogens stimulate the regeneration of the stratum functionalis during the proliferative phase of the endometrial cycle by increasing mitosis. The spiral arterioles of the stratum functionalis grow rapidly under estrogenic influence.
3. *Myometrium.* Estrogens cause hypertrophy of the myometrium and sensitize it to the action of oxytocin, which promotes uterine contractility.
4. *Cervix.* Under the influence of estrogens, the uterine cervix secretes an abundance of copious thin, watery mucus during the preovulatory phase.
5. *Vagina.* The vaginal epithelium cells mature under the effect of estrogen, resulting in the thickening and cornification of the vaginal lining.
6. *Breast.* Estrogens promote the development of the duct and lobuloalveolar system of the mammary gland.
7. *Bone.* Estrogens, like androgens, exert a dual effect on skeletal growth. On the one hand, they cause an increase in osteoblastic activity, resulting in a growth spurt at puberty.

On the other hand, estrogens also hasten bone maturation and promote the closure of the epiphyseal (cartilaginous) plates in the long bones more effectively than does testosterone. Because puberty starts earlier in girls, epiphyseal closure occurs sooner and the female skeleton usually is shorter than the male skeleton. Estrogens, to a lesser degree than testosterone, promote the deposition of bone matrix by causing Ca^{2+} and HPO_4^{2-} retention. Estrogens are responsible for the oval shape of the female pelvic inlet.

8. *Liver.* Estrogens stimulate the hepatic synthesis of the transport globulins, including thyroxine-binding globulin and transcortin. They increase the hepatic synthesis of coagulation factors and therefore predispose to thrombosis. Estrogens also increase the hepatic synthesis of angiotensinogen, leading to retention of Na^+ and water in the body.

Progesterone

Progesterone is secreted mainly by theca luteal cells. It is not bound to sex steroid-binding globulin. Instead, the progesterone is bound primarily to cortisol-binding globulin (transcortin) and albumin. The liver metabolizes progesterone to pregnanediol.

The **physiologic effects** of progesterone are as follows:

1. *Endometrium.* Progesterone promotes secretory changes in the stratum functionalis of the endometrium. The endometrial glands become elongated and coiled and secrete a glycogen-rich fluid. Progesterone is required for the im-

Table 82.2 Differences in the Physiologic Actions of Estradiol and Progesterone

Site of Action	Estradiol	Progesterone
Pituitary-hypothalamus	Inhibits FSH secretion by negative feedback Increases prolactin secretion Inhibits LH secretion by negative feedback in high concentration Stimulates midcycle surge of LH and FSH by positive feedback on pituitary	Inhibits LH secretion by negative feedback
Uterus	Promotes hypertrophy of myometrium Promotes hyperplasia of endometrium Promotes uterine motility	Arrests endometrial mitosis and induces secretory activity Inhibits uterine motility Maintains the decidua and assists in the implantation of blastocyst
Cervix	Causes thinning of cervical mucus	Causes thickening of cervical mucus
Vagina	Causes maturation of vaginal epithelial cells and the thickening and cornification of vaginal mucosa	
Breast	Promotes ductal and lobuloalveolar growth	Promotes lobuloalveolar growth
Kidney	Promotes renal Na^+ retention	Antagonizes the action of aldosterone on the kidneys and promotes the renal excretion of Na^+
Bone	Enhances bone growth, density, and maturation and causes early epiphyseal closure	
Miscellaneous	Promotes development of female secondary sexual characteristics Makes sebaceous secretion more fluid and thus inhibits formation of acne and comedones	Serves as a precursor for steroid hormones Increases basal body temperature Stimulates breathing

Abbreviations: FSH, follicle-stimulating hormone; LH, luteinizing hormone.

plantation of the blastocyst and the maintenance of decidua. Antiprogesterone agents like mifepristone are used for medical termination of pregnancy.

2. *Myometrium.* Progesterone inhibits uterine motility by hyperpolarizing the uterine smooth muscles.

3. *Cervix.* Under the influence of progesterone, the mucus secreted by the cervical glands is reduced in volume and becomes thick and viscid.

4. *Breast.* Progesterone promotes lobuloalveolar growth in the mammary gland.

5. *Kidney.* Progesterone promotes renal excretion of Na^+ (antialdosterone effect). This antagonizes the effects of the elevated aldosterone levels found in pregnancy.

6. *Fetus.* Progesterone contributes to the growth and development of the fetus by acting as a precursor for corticosteroid synthesis by the fetal adrenal cortex.

7. *Brain.* Progesterone stimulates breathing through a direct effect on the brainstem respiratory center.

Differences in the physiologic actions of estrogen and progesterone are described in **Table 82.2**.

Hormonal Control of Ovarian Function

The development of the ovarian follicle is largely under the control of FSH. Ovulation is caused by LH, which also stimulates secretion of progesterone from the corpus luteum. Consistent with the phenomenon of negative feedback in which the secretion of the target hormone inhibits its trophic hormone,

progesterone inhibits LH, and inhibin inhibits FSH secretion. Estradiol, whose secretion is stimulated by LH and FSH, also inhibits both LH and FSH. Progesterone and estrogen act at the hypothalamic and pituitary levels. Inhibin secreted by granulosa cells acts only on the pituitary (**Fig. 82.5**). Under certain conditions, estrogen causes stimulation rather than inhibition of LH, resulting in a positive feedback cycle (see Ovulation, Chapter 84).

General Model: Homeostasis

Although the endocrine mechanisms that control the functions of the gonads (testes and ovaries) have many negative feedback loops, it is important to recognize that these do *not* constitute a homeostatic mechanism. No internal, physiologic parameter is being regulated to maintain a more or less constant concentration of some component of the body.

Summary

- The testes produce testosterone under the control of LH and FSH.

- The physiologic functions of testosterone include the promotion differentiation in the male fetus, the production of the primary and secondary sex characteristics at puberty, and spermatogenesis.

- The ovaries produce estrogen and progesterone under the control of LH and FSH.

- Both estrogen and progesterone are involved in the many changes to the female reproductive tract that result from the ovarian cycle.

Applying What You Know

82.1. Mr. Anderson can only produce sperm if his testosterone level is high enough. What changes in the male reproductive endocrine system could lower his testosterone concentration?

82.2. Mrs. Anderson apparently produces adequate quantities of estrogen and progesterone to maintain normal reproductive function. A decrease in the activity of which enzymes would result in a decrease in both estrogen and progesterone?

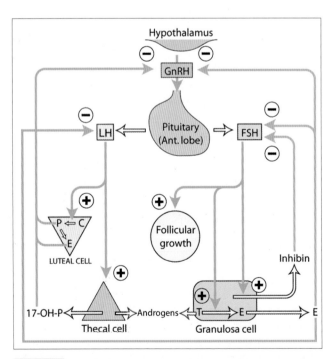

Fig. 82.5 Hormonal control of the ovary during the follicular phase. Progesterone and estradiol both have inhibitory effects on the hypothalamus and the anterior pituitary. Inhibin inhibits only the anterior pituitary. C, cholesterol; E, estradiol; FSH, follicle-stimulating hormone; GnRH, gonadotropin-releasing hormone; LH, luteinizing hormone; P, progesterone; 17-OH-P, 17α-hydroxy progesterone; T, testosterone.

Puberty

Puberty or adolescence is that stage of development when the endocrine and gametogenic functions of the gonads develop for the first time to the point where reproduction is possible. Puberty generally occurs between the ages of 8 and 13 in girls and 9 and 14 in boys. On average, girls begin puberty 1 to 2 years before boys, a phenomenon that has important implications for the growth spurt that occurs as part of puberty (see below). Spermatogenesis in boys and folliculogenesis in girls begin at puberty. They coincide with a surge of sex hormone secretion, resulting in the development of the secondary sexual characteristics.

Secondary Sexual Characteristics

Male secondary sexual characteristics | At puberty, the penis and scrotum increase in size and become pigmented. Rugal folds appear in the scrotal skin. Facial hair develops. The scalp line undergoes temporal recession. Pubic hair develops as a triangle with apex up. Axillary and body hair appear. The pubertal growth spurt occurs. Shoulders broaden. The prostate and seminal vesicles enlarge and start secreting seminal fluid. Sebaceous gland secretion thickens and increases, predisposing to acne. The pitch of the voice becomes lower due to the enlargement of the larynx and the thickening of the vocal cords. The attitude becomes more aggressive, and interest develops in girls. The muscle bulk and strength increases, and there is a positive nitrogen balance.

Female secondary sexual characteristics | In girls, the most striking events associated with the onset of puberty are thelarche (the development of breasts) followed by pubarche (development of axillary and pubic hair) and menarche (the first menstrual period). The initial periods are generally anovulatory: regular ovulation appears about a year later. A less striking event associated with puberty is adrenarche, an increase in the secretion of adrenal androgens that occurs probably because an adrenal androgen-stimulating hormone secreted from the pituitary gland stimulates the enzyme systems in the adrenal glands to channel more pregnenolone to the androgenic pathway. A growth spurt occurs with a characteristic feminine fat deposition. Interest develops in boys.

The pubertal growth spurt | In both boys and girls the increasing levels of sex hormones promotes an increase in the rate of growth of the long bones (the "growth spurt" seen in **Fig. 83.1**). However, these same hormones also accelerate epiphyseal fusion, which causes growth to cease. Because girls start puberty earlier than boys, epiphyseal fusion occurs earlier; thus, they experience less total growth. This accounts for the fact that, on average, adult men are taller than women.

Control of Pubertal Onset

A plausible mechanism of the onset of puberty is that until puberty, the gonadotropin-releasing hormone (GnRH) secretion

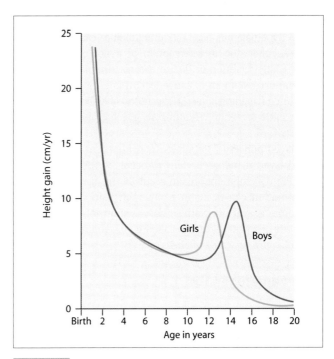

Fig. 83.1   Growth curves (centimeters added each year) for boys (*blue*) and girls (*red*). The female growth spurt occurs earlier than the male growth spurt.

from the hypothalamus is highly sensitive to feedback inhibition by testosterone and estrogens. As a result, the levels of testosterone and estrogen are never able to rise sufficiently high to induce puberty. From birth to puberty, there is a decrease in the sensitivity of the hypothalamus to feedback inhibition by testosterone or estrogens. By puberty, the hypothalamus is no longer sufficiently sensitive to feedback inhibition by testosterone and estrogen; therefore, it secretes adequate amounts of GnRH in its usual pulsatile pattern. In the presence of the normal pulsatile release of GnRH, testosterone and estrogens are secreted in adequate amounts.

Role of leptin | Over the past couple of centuries, the age of pubertal onset has been decreasing at the rate of 1 to 3 months per decade. Such changes are called secular changes and have been attributed to a general improvement in health and nourishment. The link between nourishment and earlier pubertal onset is provided by leptin, a satiety-producing hormone secreted by fat cells. Leptin facilitates the release of GnRH, thereby promoting the onset of puberty. It is observed that young women often stop menstruating when they lose weight and resume menstruation once they regain weight. Therefore, it seems that a critical body weight is required for leptin release and pubertal onset.

Abnormalities of Pubertal Onset

Precocious puberty | Exposure of immature males to androgens or females to estrogens causes early development of secondary sexual characteristics without gametogenesis. This syndrome is called precocious pseudopuberty to distinguish it from true precocious puberty that occurs due to early secretion of pituitary gonadotropins. Hypothalamic diseases are frequently associated with precocious puberty. Lesions of the ventral hypothalamus near the infundibulum cause precocious puberty, either due to interruption of neural pathways that inhibit GnRH secretion or due to chronic stimulation of GnRH secretion originating in irritative foci around the lesion. Sometimes luteinizing hormone (LH) secretion is high despite inadequate GnRH secretion, resulting in *gonadotropin-independent precocity*.

Delayed puberty | Puberty is considered to be pathologically delayed if menarche fails to occur by the age of 17 or testicular development fails to occur by the age of 20. Failure of maturation can occur in panhypopituitarism and Turner syndrome, as well as in some otherwise normal individuals. In males, this clinical picture is called *eunuchoidism*. In females, it is called *primary amenorrhea*.

Male Gametogenesis

Structure of the Testes

Seminiferous tubules | The testes are made of convoluted loops of seminiferous tubules (see **Fig. 85.2**) that drain at both ends into the ducts in the epididymis. Between the coils of seminiferous tubules are the *interstitial cells of Leydig,* which secrete testosterone. The seminiferous tubules contain the male germ cells. The tubule walls are made of Sertoli cells that rest on a basement membrane. The cell membranes of adjacent Sertoli cells are attached through tight junctions, forming a barrier that divides the lumen of the seminiferous tubule into two compartments: a *basal compartment* containing the spermatogonia and the early spermatocytes, and an *adluminal compartment* containing spermatocytes, spermatids, and spermatozoa (**Fig. 83.2**).

The **Sertoli cell** serves numerous functions, which are as follows: (1) It provides nourishment to the developing spermatozoa. (2) The intercellular junctions between adjacent Sertoli cells constitute the blood–testes barrier. (3) It produces inhibin, which suppresses follicle-stimulating hormone (FSH) secretion. (4) It secretes androgen-binding globulin (ABP), which binds testosterone with high affinity and is responsible for the high testosterone concentration in the tubular lumen. (5) It secretes transferrin for transporting iron to tubular cells, ceruloplasmin for transporting copper to the tubular cells, and plasminogen activator, which may mediate proteolytic reactions important for migration of maturing germ cells from the basal compartment to the adluminal compartment. (6) It produces müllerian duct-inhibiting substance (see Chapter 86). (7) It converts the androstenedione and testosterone produced by the Leydig cells to estrone and estradiol, respectively. The small amounts of estrogens secreted inhibit testosterone secretion through a paracrine effect. (8) It absorbs the unnecessary cellular organelles that are cast off from the spermatozoa.

Blood–testes barrier | The blood–testes barrier is formed by tight intracellular junctions between adjacent Sertoli cells

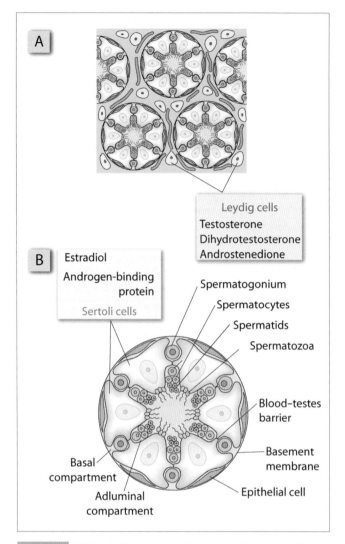

Fig. 83.2 **(A)** Seminiferous tubules in the testis showing Leydig and Sertoli cells. **(B)** A cross section through a seminiferous tubule showing steps in the development of spermatozoa.

in the seminiferous tubule. The barrier separates the basal and adluminal compartments of the seminiferous tubule. Thus, the germ cells too have to cross the barrier as they pass from the basal compartment to the adluminal compartment. The tight junctions between Sertoli cells loosen up to enable the passage of maturing germ cells through the junction, only to tighten up again after they have passed. The blood–testes barrier protects the spermatocytes, spermatids, and spermatozoa from blood-borne toxic substances and circulating antibodies. It also prevents by-products of gametogenesis from entering the circulation and stimulating an autoimmune reaction. Not unexpectedly, the breakdown of the barrier sometimes leads to autoimmune response against the germ cells. Steroids penetrate the barrier with ease. The blood–testes barrier enables the seminiferous tubule to maintain a somewhat different composition of fluid inside its lumen. The fluid in the lumen of the seminiferous tubules contains very little protein and glucose, but is rich in androgens, estrogens, and potassium ions.

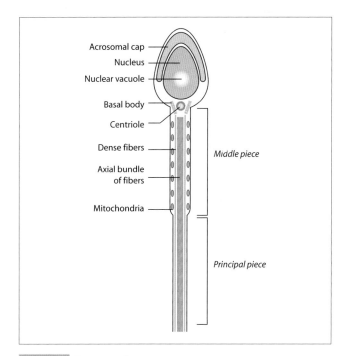

Fig. 83.3 Structure of a sperm.

Sperm (spermatozoon) | Each sperm (**Fig. 83.3**) has a head and a long tail. The head contains an elongated nucleus with highly compact chromatin. Covering the head like a cap is the acrosome, a lysosome-like organelle rich in enzymes involved in sperm penetration of the ovum. The sperm tail is divided into the middle piece, principal piece, the end piece. Through its entire length, the tail has a central axoneme made of two central microtubules surrounded by nine microtubule doublets (see **Fig. 1.4B**). Except in the end piece, the axoneme is surrounded by seven to nine outer dense fibers. The middle piece is surrounded by the spiral mitochondrial sheath made of several mitochondria tightly aligned end to end.

Spermatogenesis

The male gametes or the sperm are formed inside the seminiferous tubules. Male gametogenesis or spermatogenesis is the formation of mature sperm from the primitive germ cells or spermatogonia. Spermatogenesis has three phases (**Fig. 83.4**): the *proliferative phase*, in which there is mitotic multiplication of spermatogonia (stem cells) to form primary spermatocytes; the *meiotic phase,* which leads to the formation of primary spermatids; and the *cytodifferentiative phase*, in which the spermatids differentiate into the primary spermatozoa (spermiogenesis).

The spermatogonia divide and multiply in the basal compartment of the tubules. The spermatocytes formed enter the adluminal compartment, where the remainder of the maturation occurs. Each spermatogonium divides seven times to form 128 primary spermatocytes. The 128 primary spermatocytes undergo the first meiotic division to form 256 secondary spermatocytes, which then complete the second meiotic division to form 512 spermatids. Finally, each spermatid develops into a mature sperm over a span of 74 days.

Spermiogenesis is the transformation of the spermatids into mature spermatocytes or sperm. The spermatids mature into spermatozoa inside the membrane recesses of the Sertoli cells. Mature spermatozoa are released from the Sertoli cells and become free in the lumina of the tubules. The transformation of spermatids into spermatozoa is associated with the following changes. (1) The Golgi apparatus, containing hyaluronidase and other proteases, is transformed to the acrosome, a cap-like structure covering the anterior two-thirds of the sperm head. By releasing its enzyme-rich contents during fertilization, the acrosome penetrates the ovum. (2) The centrioles and mitochondria are transformed into the flagellae (sperm tails). The mitochondria provide energy for the flagellar movement. One centriole is converted into the basal

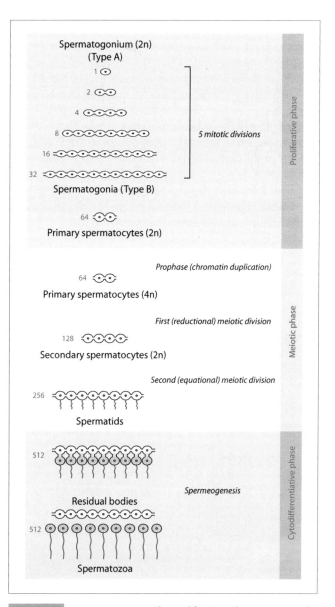

Fig. 83.4 Spermatogenesis. The proliferative phase occurs in the basal compartment of the seminiferous tubule. Due to incomplete cytokinesis, all cells derived from a single spermatogonium remain connected through cytoplasmic bridges. The connections persist until the formation of the spermatozoa.

body from which the dense fibers originate. (3) The nuclear protein histone is replaced by protamine, which surrounds the inactive and highly condensed chromatin in the spermatozoa. The nuclear condensation in the spermatozoa protects the genome from the deleterious effects of mutagens. (4) Unnecessary cellular organelles like ribosomes, lipids, degenerating mitochondria, and Golgi apparatus are cast off from the spermatozoa as residual bodies. The Sertoli cells absorb these bodies. (5) The spermatozoa do not grow or divide any further.

Factors affecting spermatogenesis | The maturation of spermatids to spermatozoa depends on the action of testosterone on the Sertoli cells in which the developing spermatozoa are embedded. Proper spermatogenesis requires that the local concentration of testosterone inside the seminiferous tubule remains high. FSH acts on Sertoli cells to increase their synthesis of ABP and thereby increase the local concentration of testosterone.

The spermatic arteries to the testes run parallel but in the opposite direction to the spermatic veins. This permits a countercurrent exchanger mechanism for conservation of the high local testosterone concentration in the testes (**Fig. 83.5A**). It is to be noted that systemic administration of testosterone inhibits FSH secretion and therefore lowers the local testosterone concentration in the testes.

Spermatogenesis requires a temperature of ~32°C, which is lower than the normal body temperature. This is possible because the testes are located in the scrotum, which is outside the body cavity and is kept cooler by evaporative cooling. Failure of testicular descent (cryptorchidism) results in sterility because of thermal damage to the spermatogonia.

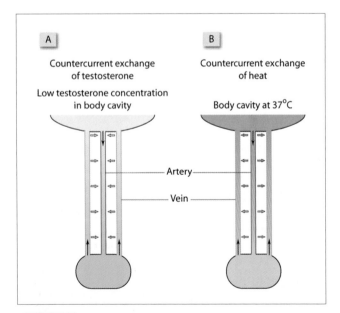

Fig. 83.5 Countercurrent exchanger mechanism for **(A)** maintenance of a high testosterone concentration in the testes and **(B)** the cooling of the testes. The veins leaving the testes contain a high concentration of testosterone, which diffuses into the artery supplying the testes. The result is a high concentration of testosterone maintained in the testes. The warmed blood in the artery loses heat to the neighboring veins, keeping the temperature of the testes lower than that of the body core.

The temperature inside the scrotum is kept low by evaporative cooling. Warm arterial blood at 37°C flowing into the testes tends to increase the testicular temperature. However, this tendency is minimized by the countercurrent heat exchanger mechanism operating between the spermatic arteries and veins (**Fig. 83.5B**). Varicocele (dilatation of veins of the pampiniform plexus) is associated with incompetence of the venous valves, thus resulting in retrograde blood flow. This interferes with the countercurrent heat exchanger mechanism, causing impaired sperm production.

There is also a seasonal effect on spermatogenesis, with sperm counts increasing in winter regardless of the temperature to which the scrotum is exposed.

Sperm production continues until the age of 80 or 90, although the production rate slows down after the age of 40.

Female Gametogenesis

Oogenesis

The female germ cell is called the oogonium, which develops into the primary oocyte and then into the secondary oocyte. At all stages of development, it is called by the general name ovum or egg (plural: ova). At birth the oogonium enters the prophase of meiosis I, forming the primary oocyte. However, immediately after it completes prophase, the meiosis I is arrested for several years. The remaining phases of meiosis I (metaphase, anaphase, and telophase) do not occur until puberty.

When meiosis I resumes at puberty, it is completed quickly and results in the formation of two daughter cells. One of the daughter cells, the secondary oocyte, receives most of the cytoplasm; the other, the first polar body, fragments and disappears. The secondary oocyte immediately goes into meiosis II, but the division stops again, this time at metaphase. It is at this stage that ovulation occurs. Meiosis II is completed only after a sperm penetrates the oocyte. When meiosis II resumes, the second polar body is cast off, and the fertilized ovum proceeds to form the embryo.

Folliculogenesis

At the time of birth, there are two million oogonia in the ovary, of which fewer than 300,000 ova are left by puberty; the others begin to develop, but without the support of cycling concentrations of hormones, they degenerate. Thereafter, once every 28 days, a group of ova that have been maturing for some time get recruited into more rapid development. Only one ovum will eventually be released; the rest of the developing follicles degenerate. A maturing primordial follicle grows successively into the primary, secondary, tertiary, and antral follicle (**Fig. 83.6**).

Primordial follicles are composed of an outer single layer of flat epithelial cells and a small immature oocyte arrested in the prophase of meiosis I. The epithelial cells and the oocyte are enveloped in a thin basal lamina. When the flat epithelial cells become cuboidal granulosa cells, the follicle is called a *primary follicle.*

Secondary follicles form when the granulosa cells inside the basal lamina divide mitotically to form a multilayered

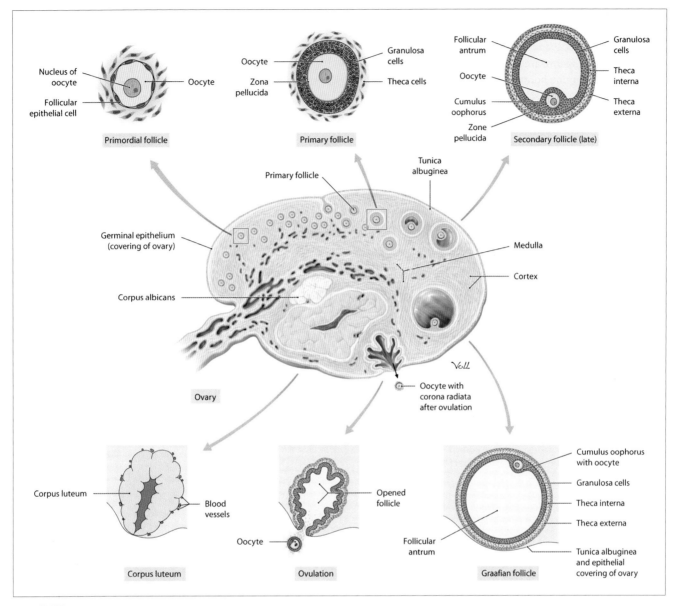

Fig. 83.6 Ovarian follicles. Note that the oocyte released from the ovary retains its coat of granulosa cells, called the cumulus oophorus or the corona radiata.

stratum granulosum. The oocyte enlarges and forms a coating of mucoid substance called the zona pellucida, which separates the granulosa cells from the oocyte.

Tertiary follicles are characterized by the formation of a fluid-filled cavity called the antrum. The stromal cells outside the basal lamina differentiate into two concentric layers of thecal cells called the theca interna and theca externa. One of the several tertiary follicles, called the dominant follicle, outgrows all the rest to form an antral (graafian) follicle.

It takes ~14 days for the primary follicle (~0.4 mm) to grow into a graafian follicle (~20–25 mm). Once every 28 days, one follicle, with the mature ovum in it, is released from the ovary (ovulation) into the abdominal cavity, where it enters the fallopian tube. The other follicles gradually regress through apoptosis and form the corpus albicans. Some of these events are discussed again in Chapter 90.

A primordial follicle can differentiate into the primary, secondary, and early tertiary follicle in the absence of FSH. It is only after reaching the early tertiary stage that its continued development depends on FSH and its own ability to secrete estrogen inside it. FSH receptors are located exclusively on the granulosa cells and LH receptors are located on the thecal cells. FSH regulates the growth and maturation of the follicle. LH regulates the function of the corpus luteum.

Summary

- Puberty (which occurs at 8–13 years of age for girls and 9–14 for boys) marks the development of reproductive fertility and the appearance of the secondary sex characteristics.

- Gametogenesis involves transforming primordial germ cells, which are diploid cells into germ cells that are haploid.

- Male gametes, sperm, are produced in the testes under the control of luteinizing hormone (LH) and follicle-stimulating hormone (FSH) (and testosterone) continuously from puberty.

- Female gametes, ova, are produced in the ovaries under the control of LH and FSH (and estrogen) starting at puberty and continuing through menopause.

Applying What You Know

83.1. What change in gonadotropin-releasing hormone (GnRH), luteinizing hormone (LH), or follicle-stimulating hormone (FSH) would result in Mr. Anderson's sperm count being decreased below normal? Explain.

83.2. There is reason to believe that Mrs. Anderson is ovulating normally. What is the state of the chromosomes in the ovulated egg that is released each cycle? Is it haploid, diploid, or something else?

The plasma levels of ovarian hormones are not constant, but show cyclical fluctuations. These fluctuations occur due to cyclic changes in the ovary (ovarian cycle). The hormones bring about cyclic changes in the uterine endometrium (uterine or menstrual cycle), the uterine cervix (cervical cycle), and the vagina (vaginal cycle). Cyclic changes also occur in the breast and in body temperature.

The onset of menstruation at puberty is called *menarche.* The occurrence of menstrual cycles marks the beginning of estrogen and progesterone secretion in substantial amounts. In early adolescence, the cycles are anovulatory, and the menses are irregular. The cessation of menses is called *menopause,* which typically occurs at about the age of 50 years and is associated with the cessation of estrogen and progesterone secretion.

The menstrual cycle is counted from the first day of menstruation (menstrual bleeding). A typical cycle has a length of 28 days, with ovulation occurring at about the middle of the cycle (**Fig. 84.1**). All the cycles, ovarian, uterine, cervical, and vaginal, can be divided into preovulatory and postovulatory periods. The length of the postovulatory period is fairly constant at ~14 days. When the length of the menstrual cycle is not exactly 28 days, the time of ovulation is estimated by subtracting 14 days from the duration of the menstrual cycle. Thus, in a 30-day cycle, ovulation occurs on the 16th day.

Preovulatory Period

Hormonal changes | The estrogen and progesterone levels are at their lowest at the beginning of the menstrual cycle (**Fig. 84.2**). There is progressive rise in the plasma estrogens until ovulation due to the secretion of estradiol by the granulosa cells of the growing ovarian follicle. The progesterone level remains very low and nearly unchanged during this period. The preovulatory changes in the uterus, cervix, and vagina are largely attributable to the rising estrogen levels. The preovulatory phase of the ovarian cycle is therefore referred to as the *estrogenic phase.*

The early growth of the ovarian follicle in the preovulatory period occurs under the combined influence of follicle-

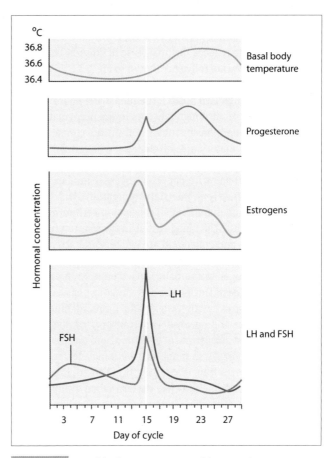

Fig. 84.2 Basal body temperature and hormonal concentrations through the menstrual cycle. Progesterone comes only from the corpus luteum. The increase in estrogen just prior to day 15 triggers the luteinizing hormone (LH) surge that brings about ovulation. FSH, follicle-stimulating hormone.

stimulating hormone (FSH) and luteinizing hormone (LH) on the granulosa and theca cells, respectively. However, FSH secretion gradually declines in the preovulatory period due to feedback inhibition at the anterior pituitary by the estrogens and inhibin secreted by the proliferating granulosa cells. The

	1	2	3	4	5	6	7	8	9	10	11	12	13	14	15	16	17	18	19	20	21	22	23	24	25	26	27	28
Ovary							Follicular phase								O	Luteal phase												
Uterus	Menstruation						Proliferative endometrium								Secretory endometrium													
Cervix							Watery mucus secretion								Thick mucus secretion													
Vagina							High glycogen content of epithelium								Low glycogen content of epithelium													

Fig. 84.1 Phases of the menstrual cycle as it affects the ovary, uterus, cervix, and vagina. Ovulation (O) occurs 14 days before the end of the cycle.

LH level rises slowly because there is not enough progesterone secretion to cause its feedback suppression.

Ovarian changes | The preovulatory period of the ovarian cycle is called the *follicular phase.* It is marked by follicular growth and secretion of estradiol by the developing follicles in response to FSH and LH from the pituitary. By the end of this phase, one follicle reaches the final stage of growth. The development of the ovarian follicle is shown in **Fig. 83.6**.

Uterine changes | During the preovulatory period, the uterus goes through two phases: the menstrual phase and the proliferative phase. Although it occurs in the preovulatory period, the *menstrual phase* is described in this chapter in the context of postovulatory uterine changes, where it will be better understood.

During the *proliferative phase,* estrogens stimulate mitosis of the stratum basale (endometrial proliferation), which regenerates the stratum functionale. The endometrium grows to ~4 mm in thickness. The blood vessels in the stratum functionale become long and coiled and are called spiral arteries. The uterine glands increase in length. The cells lining the glands accumulate glycogen but remain nonsecretory in this phase.

Cervical changes | During the preovulatory phase, estrogen makes the cervical mucus watery and more alkaline. These changes promote the survival and transport of sperm. The mucus is thinnest at the time of ovulation, and its elasticity, or *spinnbarkeit,* increases so much that by midcycle, a drop can be stretched into an 8 to 12 cm-long thin thread. In addition, it dries in an arborizing fern-like pattern when a thin layer is spread on a slide. The characteristic ferning pattern is due to crystallization of sodium chloride.

Vaginal changes | The vaginal epithelium cells mature under the effect of estrogen, resulting in the thickening and cornification of the vaginal lining. By evaluating the ratio of mature to immature cells microscopically in vaginal smears, this maturation can be indicated by what is known as the karyopyknotic index (KPI). KPI peak coincides with the estrogen peak near ovulation. Estrogen also increases the glycogen content of the epithelial cells, which are exfoliated throughout the menstrual cycle. The glycogen in the exfoliated cells is a rich substrate for bacterial flora, which breaks down glycogen into lactic acid and lowers the vaginal pH.

Breast changes | During menstruation, the decrease in estradiol and progesterone is associated with a decrease in the size of the mammary duct and acini. In the preovulatory phase, there is proliferation of mammary ducts under the influence of estrogens. A gradual increase of epithelial tissue occurs with each successive cycle.

Ovulation

Ovulation refers to the extrusion of the secondary oocyte from the graafian follicle into the peritoneal cavity. Ovulation is triggered by a sharp rise in the LH level, called the LH surge, which occurs 24 hours before ovulation. The LH surge occurs because when the plasma estrogen exceeds a critical concentration for long enough, it exerts a positive feedback (instead of the usual negative feedback) on the hypothalamic–hypophyseal axis, causing an increased release of gonadotropin-releasing hormone (GnRH) and a concomitant surge in pituitary LH secretion 24 hours later (**Fig. 84.3**). A lesser FSH surge also occurs simultaneously. The midcycle LH surge requires a plasma estradiol concentration of ~150 pg/mL for at least 36 hours, a condition that is normally achieved by day 13. The onset of the LH surge is a fairly precise indicator of ovulation.

General Model: Communication

The chemical (hormonal) information involved in driving the female reproductive cycle is among the most complex in the body, as it involves both negative feedback (common in the body) and positive feedback (uncommon).

Tests for ovulation | Progesterone is associated with a 0.5°C rise in *basal body temperature,* which occurs immediately following ovulation and which persists during most of the luteal phase. The basal body temperature dips during the follicular phase. This temperature increment is used clinically as a test for ovulation. The other test for ovulation is the *thinning of cervical mucus:* the persistence of spinnbarkeit and ferning of cervical mucus in the secretory phase indicates the absence of ovulation.

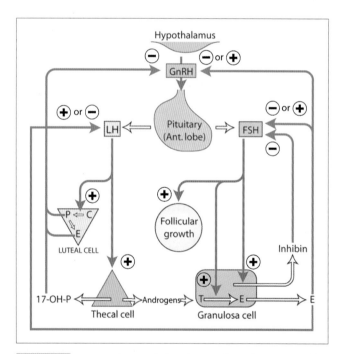

Fig. 84.3 Hormonal control of ovulation. Throughout most of the 28-day ovarian cycle, the effect of estrogen on the hypothalamic release of gonadotropin-releasing hormone (GnRH) is inhibitory (negative feedback). However, by day 13 (see **Fig. 84.2**), estrogen becomes high enough to prompt the hypothalamic cells to alter their function, so the effect of estrogen becomes stimulatory (positive feedback). Positive feedback is also present at the anterior pituitary. The result is a rapid increase in GnRH release and the luteinizing hormone (LH) and follicle-stimulating hormone (FSH) surge.

Postovulatory Period

Hormonal changes | The LH surge not only triggers ovulation, but also initiates the process of luteinization of the thecal and granulosa cells. FSH and LH stimulate the corpus luteum to secrete progesterone and estradiol. The plasma concentration of both progesterone and estradiol peak in the midluteal phase (day 21). Because progesterone is secreted in greater amounts (**Fig. 84.2**), the postovulatory phase is also called the *progestational phase.* FSH and LH levels continue to decline during the luteal phase due to negative feedback of estrogens and progesterone.

Ovarian changes | The ruptured follicle promptly fills up with blood, forming the corpus hemorrhagicum. Minor bleeding from the follicle into the abdominal cavity may cause peritoneal irritation and fleeting lower abdominal pain called *mittelschmerz.* This midcycle pain may be unilateral, indicating which of the two ovaries has ovulated. Thereafter, the clotted blood is replaced by yellowish, lipid-rich luteal cells (derived from the granulosa and thecal cells), forming the corpus luteum. Hence, the postovulatory phase of the ovarian cycle is called the *luteal phase.*

The oocyte that is released from the ovary is picked up by the fimbriated ends of the fallopian tube and is transported to the uterus. Fertilization occurs in the ampulla of the tube. *If fertilization does not occur,* the corpus luteum begins to degenerate by day 24 (luteolysis) and is eventually replaced by fibrous tissue, forming the corpus albicans. Luteolysis seems to be mediated by PGF_2 (a type of prostaglandin). *If fertilization occurs,* the functional life span of the corpus luteum is extended under the trophic influence of human chorionic gonadotropin (HCG) from the placenta, and it continues to secrete estradiol and progesterone until the third month of pregnancy, when the placenta takes over its endocrine function (the luteal–placental shift, see **Fig. 87.3**).

Uterine changes | The endometrium enters its secretory phase and is prepared for a possible implantation of the fertilized ovum. The endometrium (**Fig. 84.4**) thickens to ~5 mm, becomes hyperemic, and develops a scalloped "Swiss cheese" appearance. Progesterone halts endometrial mitosis and causes maturation of the endometrium. The glands elongate further and become tortuous. Their lumen becomes wider and is filled with mucus and a glycogen-rich secretion. The spiral arteries become longer, more coiled, and dilated. About 2 days before menstruation, the endometrium is infiltrated by neutrophils.

If there is luteolysis, there is a sudden drop in estrogen and progesterone levels, which cause arteriolar constriction, resulting in ischemia and necrosis of the stratum functionale, which is sloughed off. The stratum basale remains intact, and the total endometrial thickness reduces to ~2 mm. The vasospasm seems to be mediated by PGF_2. Bleeding starts when the arterioles relax. Because menstrual bleeding follows a sharp fall in the plasma concentration of ovarian hormones, it is also called *withdrawal bleeding.* Menstrual blood clots in the uterus but liquefies again in the vagina due to fibrinolysis. The average blood loss during menstruation is 40 mL (10–200 mL) over a period of 4 days.

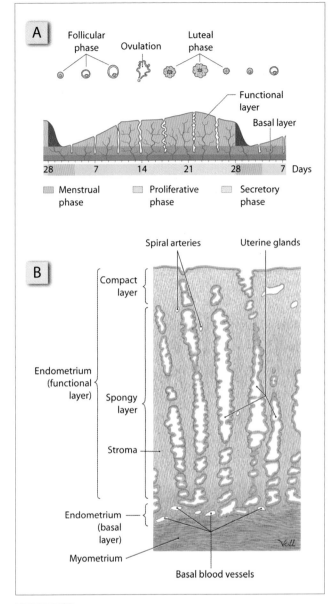

Fig. 84.4 (**A**) Ovarian and endometrial changes during the menstrual cycle. (**B**) Structure of the endometrium at the peak of the secretory phase.

Cervical changes | Progesterone makes the cervical mucus thick, tenacious, and cellular. It fails to form the fern pattern on drying, and the spinnbarkeit is no longer possible.

Vaginal changes | The glycogen content of the epithelial cells decreases during this phase. Consequently, less lactic acid is produced in the vagina by the bacterial flora. The rise in pH makes the vagina prone to infection by *Trichomonas vaginalis.* The epithelium becomes infiltrated by leukocytes.

Breast changes | In the luteal phase of the cycle, progesterone stimulates the proliferation of the terminal duct and alveoli, distention of the ducts, and hyperemia and edema of the interstitial tissue of the breast. All these changes, which cause a sense of breast fullness, regress during menstruation.

Summary

- The menstrual cycle, or ovarian cycle, is the result of the interaction of a large number of hormones whose concentrations change over a typically 28-day cycle.

- The cycle is driven by the increasing estrogen production by the dominant follicle.

- When estrogen levels are high enough and long enough, they cause the normally negative feedback of estrogen on the hypothalamus to become positive and generate the luteinizing hormone surge that produces ovulation.

Applying What You Know

84.1. Prior to her first marriage, Mrs. Anderson had been taking oral contraceptives. What might be the contents of such a pill, and how would it prevent ovulation?

Sperm Transport in the Male Tract

Sperm mature as they pass through the male ducts (**Figs. 85.1** and **85.2**). Transport of sperm through the male ducts does not require much sperm motility, as it is passively driven. There is an elevated pressure created by the secretion of fluid into elastic vessels as well as by the beating cilia. Spermatozoa show significant motility only after they are ejaculated.

General Models: Elasticity and Flow

Sperm transport through the male reproductive tract is a passive process in which several mechanisms create a pressure gradient, causing flow to occur. One mechanism generating an elevated pressure is the increase in the volume of fluid in the vessels making up the male reproductive tract; increasing the volume in an elastic structure results in increased pressure inside the structure.

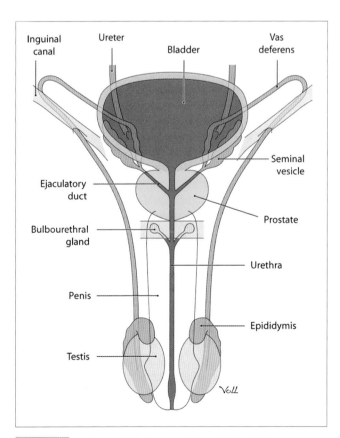

Fig. 85.1 Male reproductive tract. The epididymal duct continues into the vas deferens, which has thicker walls. Near its termination, the vas deferens joins the duct of the seminal vesicles to form the ejaculatory duct, which opens in the urethra.

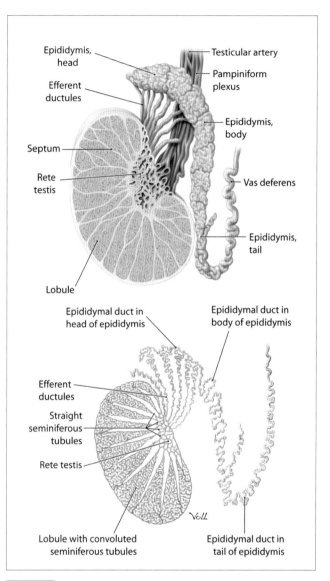

Fig. 85.2 Seminiferous tubules, rete testis, and epididymis. The seminiferous tubules in the testes drain into a plexus of epithelium-lined spaces called the rete testis. About a dozen efferent ducts from the rete testes drain into the epididymis. The epididymis is divided into the caput (head), the corpus (body), and the cauda (tail). It is made of over 6 m of coiled duct (the epididymal duct).

Sperm Passage through the Rete Testis

Sperm are concentrated as they pass through the rete testis. If the concentration does not occur, the sperm entering the epididymis become diluted in a large volume of fluid, and infertility results. The concentration occurs due to the reabsorption of sodium (Na^+) and water under the influence of estrogen. Spermatozoa leaving the rete testis are not fully motile and are therefore incapable of fertilizing the ovum.

Sperm Passage through the Epididymis

The sperm continue to mature and acquire motility during their 2- to 11-day passage through the epididymis. During this transit, the epididymis serves four major functions related to sperm: maturation, storage, decapacitation, and protection from immunologic damage.

Sperm maturation occurs in the proximal epididymis (caput and corpus epididymis) whereby sperm gain their ability to fertilize eggs. It involves (1) development of sperm motility with a higher velocity of forward progression and a straighter path; (2) development of zona-binding capacity due to development of zona pellucida 3 protein receptors on the sperm; (3) development of the ability to undergo acrosome reaction; (4) development of the potential to fuse with the egg; and (5) condensation of the sperm chromatin, which is later decondensed by the egg ooplasm.

Sperm storage | The storage capacity of the human epididymis is small and is exceeded after 2 weeks of abstinence. Continued abstinence results in sperm overflowing into the urine. Because these aged sperm still retain their viability, 2 weeks of abstinence is recommended for increasing the sperm output of oligozoospermic patients. For the same reason, sperm continue to be released in semen for a few weeks after vasectomy, often causing unwanted pregnancy unless additional contraceptive measures are taken.

During their storage in the epididymis, sperm come in contact with antioxidants, such as superoxide dismutase and glutathione peroxidase, which protect sperm from lipid peroxidation, and with acrosin inhibitor, which protects sperm from damage by leaking acrosomal enzymes.

Decapacitation of spermatozoa | Spermatozoa show motility only after they are ejaculated. The motility of the sperm, which is acquired in the head and body of the epididymis, is suppressed (decapacitated) again in the tail of the epididymis. The decapacitation keeps the sperm quiescent until they arrive at the right time and place for fertilization to be possible. Sperm motility is inhibited when the intracellular pH is acidic and stimulated when its intracellular pH is alkaline. Epididymal fluid contains lactates (and H^+ ions), which diffuse into the sperm (see **Fig. 85.3**), lowering the pH. Once outside the epididymis, the sperm finds itself in a Na^+-rich environment similar to plasma. The Na^+ is transported into the cell with bicarbonate ion (HCO_3^-), raising the intracellular pH and stimulating spermatic motility. This HCO_3^- cotransport with Na^+ cannot occur inside the epididymis because the epididymal

fluid has a low Na^+ and high potassium (K^+) concentration as compared with plasma.

Immune protection of spermatozoa | Immune tolerance to self develops in fetal life. As spermatozoa are only formed several years after the development of immune tolerance, sperm are considered "foreign" if they are encountered by the immune system. To prevent immunologic damage, sperm are separated within the epididymis from circulating immune cells. There are tight junctions in the epididymis that prevent paracellular transport. If the epididymal tubule is ruptured, as may occur after vasectomy, sperm antigens can encounter immune cells. Indeed, antisperm antibodies are present in the serum of men with epididymal occlusion.

Sperm Passage through the Urethra

During their passage through the urethra, the sperm come in contact with the secretions of seminal vesicles, prostate, and bulbourethral glands. The seminal plasma comes mostly from these accessory glands. During ejaculation, the accessory glands sequentially contribute their secretions to the seminal plasma. First, the bulbourethral glands secrete an alkaline solution with glycoproteins (the preejaculatory fluid) to neutralize the urinary tract acidity and lubricate the tract before ejaculation. Next, the epididymis and prostate contract together, discharging spermatozoa and prostatic secretions. Finally, the seminal vesicles contract and expel the spermatozoa to the exterior with their secretions.

Semen

Seminal fluid analysis is performed on samples obtained by masturbation after 24 to 36 hours of abstinence. Analysis should be performed within an hour. Normal semen is white or opalescent in color with a specific gravity of 1.028 and a pH of 7.35 to 7.50. The normal ejaculate volume is greater than 2 mL. Immediately after ejaculation, coagulation of the seminal fluid occurs, followed within 30 minutes by liquefaction.

Sperm | The normal sperm count is 40 to 100 million/mL, with fewer than 20% having abnormal morphology. For normal fertility, the sperm count should be at least 20 million/mL, and at least 60% of the sperm should be motile with normal morphology. However, many fertile men have lower counts, and many infertile men have higher counts.

Seminal plasma | The physiologic role of several constituents of seminal plasma is not known, but these constituents are estimated to assess the functioning of the accessory glands.

The *epididymis* contributes carnitine, glycerophosphocholine, and neutral α-glucosidase to the seminal fluid.

The *prostate* contributes ~20% to the volume of the semen. The prostatic fluid is slightly acidic (pH 6.5) due to the presence of citric acid. It contains substances important for sperm motility (notably albumin), fibrinolysin, acid phosphatase, and an antibacterial substance. It also contributes zinc and prostate-specific antigen to the seminal plasma.

The *seminal vesicle* contributes 70% to the volume of the semen. It contains fructose, citrate, ascorbic acid, prostaglandins, hyaluronidase, seminogelin, and fibrinolysin. The fructose is a source of energy for the spermatozoa. It is broken down into

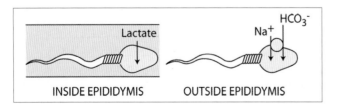

Fig. 85.3 In the epididymis, the entry of lactate (and its accompanying hydrogen ion) into the sperm lowers its pH. Once past the epididymis the cotransport of sodium (Na^+) and hydrogen carbonate ion (HCO_3^-) into the sperm increases its pH.

lactate through anaerobic glycolysis. Prostaglandins promote sperm transport by inducing tubal contractions. Hyaluronidase breaks down hyaluronic acid found in cervical mucus and thereby allows the sperm to pass easily through the cervix. Seminogelin causes coagulation of semen, and fibrinolysin dissolves the coagulum shortly after.

Insemination

Coitus allows the transfer of sperm from the male to the female reproductive tract. Successful coitus is the culmination of sexual arousal, which in both sexes has four stages: excitement, plateau, orgasm, and resolution.

During **sexual excitement,** parasympathetic activity is increased, resulting in vasocongestion in the genitalia. *In men,* there is dilatation of penile arteries and accumulation of blood in the corpora cavernosum and spongiosum, resulting in erection (penile tumescence). Vasoactive intestinal peptide and nitric oxide are important for penile erection. Increased blood flow to the testes causes an increase in testicular size. Contraction of the longitudinal muscles of the vas deferens lifts the testes closer to the body.

In women, vasocongestion of the vagina causes transudation of fluids from the vaginal epithelium, resulting in vaginal lubrication, which facilitates insertion of the penis without discomfort. Vasocongestion also occurs in the external genitalia and breast. There is a general increase in muscle tone, which results in nipple erection, sometimes in men too.

The **plateau phase** is characterized by the intensification of the changes seen during the phase of excitement. In *men,* blood pooling causes the glans to enlarge and become darker in color. Preejaculatory fluid from the bulbourethral glands trickles out of the penis. The fluid contains a few sperm and accounts for the poor safety rate of the withdrawal method of contraception.

In women, increased blood flow to the labia produces a deepening in the color of the labia minora and labia majora. The clitoris retracts. Swelling of the vaginal walls narrows the vaginal orifice. The uterus is elevated away from the vagina (tenting). There is increased size of the breast areola and reddening of the skin (sexual flush).

Orgasm is the climaxing of sexual excitement during intercourse. *In men,* it culminates in ejaculation, a forceful ejection of sperm from the urethra. Only sperm from the distal cauda epididymis enter the ejaculate. Ejaculation involves two processes: emission and expulsion of ejaculatory fluid. *Emission* is the entry of the ejaculatory fluid into the urethra. It is produced by rhythmic muscular contractions of the vas deferens, seminal vesicles, and prostate. *Expulsion* is the ejection of ejaculatory fluid out of the urethra. It is brought about by rhythmic muscular contractions of the urethra, aided by the contraction of bulbocavernous muscles. The sphincter vesicae contracts during ejaculation, preventing the ejaculatory fluid from entering the bladder.

In women, orgasm is characterized by rhythmic muscular contractions of the uterus and vagina. Unlike men, women are multiorgasmic: they are capable of experiencing more than one orgasm over a short period of time.

In the **resolution phase,** all the changes associated with sexual arousal revert to the prearousal state. *In men,* penile detumescence is caused by increased sympathetic nerve activity that constricts the penile arteries. Ejaculation is followed by a refractory period during which orgasm is not possible again. Women generally do not experience the refractory period.

Sperm Transport in the Female Tract

Sperm motility is essential for sperm migration out of the cervical mucus. It helps in sperm transport to the site of fertilization and is essential for penetrating the egg's investments. During intercourse, spermatozoa are deposited high up in the vagina. Soon after its deposition, the semen coagulates due to the presence of thrombin-like enzymes in the prostatic fluid and fibrinogen-like substrates (seminogelin) in the seminal vesicle fluid. The coagulum helps to retain the sperm in the vagina and protect them against the acidic vaginal pH. Within an hour of deposition, the coagulum is dissolved by the fibrinolysin present in the prostatic secretions, and the sperm migrate out of the coagulum.

During the secretory phase, the cervical mucus is watery and favors the passage of sperm through it. The same mucus, however, prevents the passage of sperm with abnormal head or subnormal flagellation and antibody-coated spermatozoa. This observation is put to diagnostic use in the in vitro cervical mucus contact test.

Sperm reach the uterine tubes within an hour of intercourse. Ejaculated spermatozoa have to reach the ampulla of the fallopian tube to fertilize the ovum (**Fig. 85.4**). The movement of spermatozoa is further assisted by contractions of the female tract, which is stimulated by prostaglandins present in the semen. The tubal fluid prevents capitation of spermatozoa until ovulation. After ovulation, the progesterone present in follicular fluid, which is released with ovulation, stimulates sperm capacitation.

Capacitation | Ejaculated sperm are ordinarily unable to fertilize the ovum in vitro. Sperm undergo capacitation: they gain the ability to fertilize eggs during their passage through the female tract. For capacitation to occur, the decapacitation factors acquired in the epididymis and seminal vesicle have to be removed. The follicular fluid entering the female tract during ovulation contains sterol-binding proteins that extract cholesterol from the sperm membranes. The decapacitation factors are lost with the cholesterol. Once a sperm cell is capacitated (**Fig. 85.5**), its tail shows hyperactivation, and its head acquires the capability to undergo the acrosome reaction.

Fertilization

Fertilization is the fusion of the haploid chromatin of the male and female gametes. The sperm usually meets the ovum in the ampulla of the fallopian tube. Fertilization occurs through the following steps.

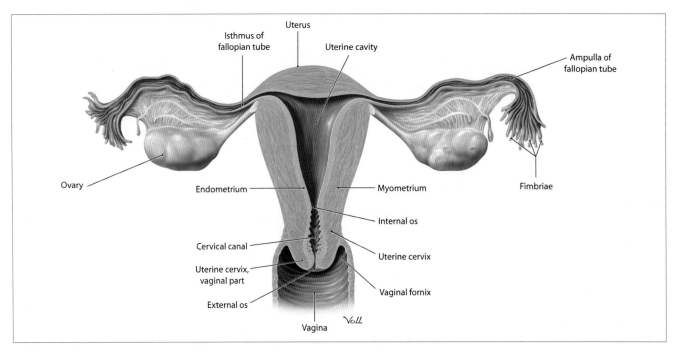

Fig. 85.4 Female reproductive tract. The uterus consists of the corpus (which includes the fundus) and the cervix, separated by a narrow isthmus. The cervical cavity communicates with the uterine cavity through the internal os and opens into the vagina through the external os. The upper part of the vaginal cavity extends around the cervix as the vaginal fornices. The fallopian tube consists of the infundibulum, ampulla, isthmus, and uterine part. The opening of the infundibulum into the peritoneal cavity is surrounded by fimbriae.

Penetration of Egg Coverings

The sperm has to pass through two layers of egg coatings before it can contact the oocyte directly. The outer coat is the cumulus oophorus (see **Fig. 83.6, lower right**), which consists

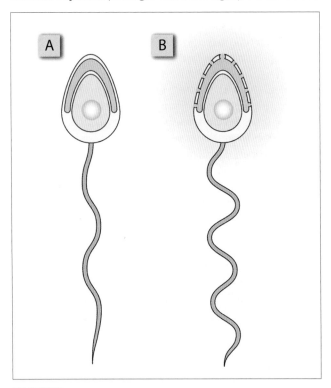

Fig. 85.5 Capacitation of spermatozoon. **(A)** Sperm before capacitation. **(B)** Capacitated sperm showing hyperflagellation and acrosomal reaction.

of granulosa cells embedded in a matrix composed mainly of hyaluronic acid. The inner coat is the zona pellucida (**Fig. 85.6A**), which is acellular and consists of a meshwork of glycoproteins.

The **penetration of the cumulus oophorus** is made possible by the hyaluronidase present on the sperm surface. Penetration is also aided by the hyperactivation of the sperm, which produces the required penetrative thrust by vigorous lashing of the sperm tail.

Penetration of the zona pellucida | The initial contact of the sperm with the zona pellucida (ZP) is a loose one. The contact becomes firmer by the binding of ZP3 (a zona pellucida glycoprotein) to a ZP3 receptor on the sperm. The interaction triggers the acrosomal reaction (**Fig. 85.5**) in which a protease called acrosin is released. Acrosin produces a penetration slit in the zona pellucida. Once inside the perivitelline space, the sperm fuses with the vitelline (egg) membrane. The binding occurs due to interaction of disintegrins (e.g., fertilin) present on the surface of acrosome-reacted sperm with integrins on the vitelline membrane. Thus, the acrosome reaction is important not only for the penetration of the zona pellucida, but also for the eventual fusion of the sperm cell with the egg membrane.

Activation of the Ovum

The fusion of the egg membrane with the sperm membrane depolarizes the membrane, stimulating the intracellular release of Ca^{2+} in the ovum. Certain sperm components called sperm-associated oocyte-activation factors (SAOAF) are required for the Ca^{2+} release. Insufficient SAOAF causes infertility and can be overcome by injection of SAOAF from other sperm.

Blocking of polyspermy | The rise in intracellular calcium promotes the exocytosis of cortical granules that are superficially situated in the unfertilized ovum. The cortical granules inhibit polyploidy by blocking a second sperm from entering the egg. The block occurs at two levels (**Fig. 85.6B**), the vitelline membrane and the zona pellucida. (1) When the cortical granules fuse with the vitelline membrane, large parts of the vitelline membrane are replaced by the membranes of the cortical granules for which sperm have no affinity. This constitutes the *vitelline block to polyspermy*. (2) The granules release glycosidases and proteases into the perivitelline space. Glycosidases alter the zona glycoprotein ZP3 so that it loses its affinity for the sperm receptors, while proteases degrade ZP3 so that it is unable to bind to acrosome-reacted spermatozoa. This constitutes the *zona block to polyspermy*.

Early Embryonic Development

At the time of ovulation, meiosis II is already in metaphase, and spindles form for separation of the second polar body. However, it is only after the entry of the sperm that the ovum extrudes the second polar body (**Fig. 85.7**). The chromosomes of the ovum assume the shape of a nucleus called the female pronucleus. At the same time, the nucleus of the spermatogonium transforms itself into the male pronucleus. The male and female pronuclei meet but do not fuse to form one nucleus.

Their nuclear membranes disappear, and their chromosomes become distinct. At this stage mitosis occurs, forming the two-cell stage embryo, with each cell having a distinct nucleus containing 46 chromosomes. The embryo is still surrounded by the zona pellucida.

By successive cleavages, the 16-celled *morula* (*morum = mulberry*) is formed (**Fig. 85.8**). The morula consists of an inner cell mass surrounded by an outer layer. Fluid from the uterine cavity enters the morula and partially separates the inner cell mass from the outer layer, which is now called the *trophoblast*. As the amount of fluid increases, the morula becomes cyst-like and is called a *blastocyst*.

Implantation

By the time the fertilized ovum reaches the uterus (**Fig. 85.9**), it is already a morula but is still surrounded by the zona pellucida, which prevents it from sticking to the walls of the uterine tube. The trophoblast tends to invade any tissue it comes in contact with. Once the zona pellucida disappears, the trophoblast sticks to the uterine endometrium. This is called implantation. The trophoblast invades the endometrium, and the blastocyst burrows deeper into the uterine mucosa until the whole of it is buried in the endometrium. This is called interstitial implantation to differentiate it from the central implantation, which occurs in some mammals where the blastocyst remains in the uterine cavity.

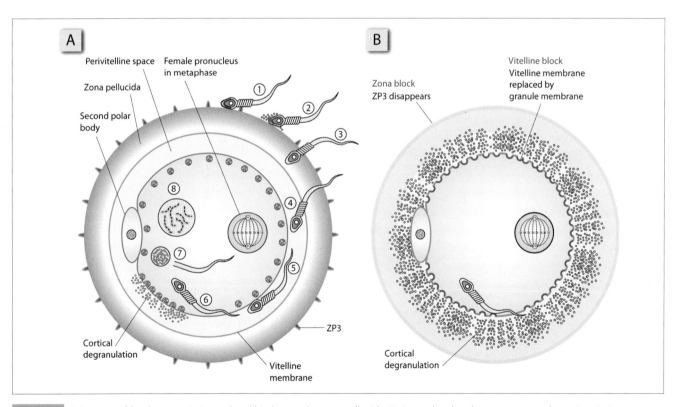

Fig. 85.6 **(A)** Stages of fertilization. 1. Sperm head binding to the zona pellucida. 2. Sperm head undergoes acrosomal reaction. 3. Sperm penetrates zona pellucida. 4. Sperm head enters perivitelline space. 5. Sperm head binds to oolemma. 6. Sperm in ooplasm. 7. Sperm tail disappears, and the nucleus decondenses. 8. Nucleus decondenses further to form the male pronucleus. **(B)** Zona and vitelline blocks to polyspermy. The zona block occurs due to the disappearance of ZP3, shown here in faded color. Vitelline block occurs due to extensive replacement of the vitelline membrane (*blue*) by the membrane of the cortical granules (*red*).

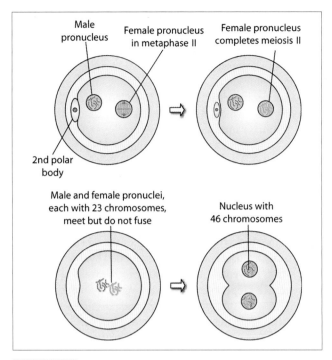

Fig. 85.7 Initial steps in the formation of the two-cell stage embryo.

Twenty Steps to Fertilization

1. Sperm is deposited high up in the vagina.
2. Semen first coagulates and then liquefies, allowing sperm to escape.
3. Healthy sperm pass through the cervical mucus barrier.
4. Sperm swim up to ampulla, aided by tubal contractions induced by prostaglandins in semen.
5. The tubal fluid inhibits sperm activation within ovulation.
6. Sterol-binding proteins present in the follicular fluid (released with ovulation) extract cholesterol from sperm, and decapacitation factors present in sperm are lost with cholesterol.
7. Capacitation causes hyperflagellation and the capacity to bind to the ovum.
8. Hyaluronidase present on sperm breaks down the matrix of cumulus oophorus.
9. Sperm penetrates cumulus oophorus through hyper-flagellation.
10. Sperm comes in contact with zona pellucida of ovum, and ZP3 present on zona pellucida binds to its receptors on the sperm surface.
11. The acrosomal reaction is triggered, and acrosin is released.
12. Acrosin produces a penetration slit in the zona pellucida.

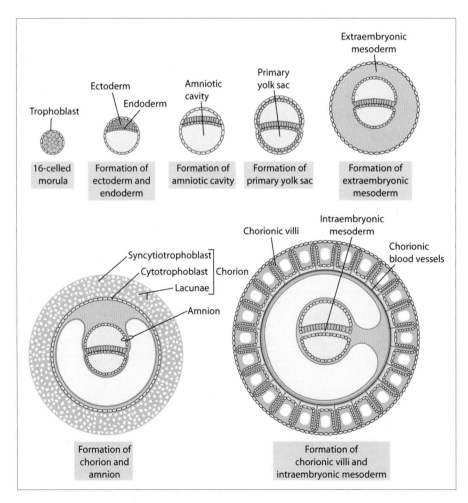

Fig. 85.8 Development of a morula (*top left*) into a blastocyst (*bottom right*).

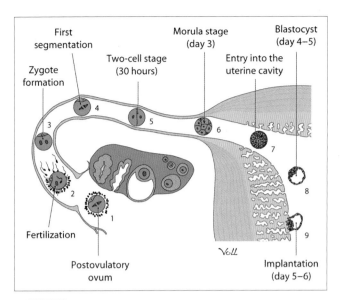

Fig. 85.9 Steps in the progression of the fertilized egg (2) to interstitial implantation in the wall of the uterus (9). The time span from fertilization to implantation of the blastocyst in the wall of the uterus is 5 to 6 days.

13. Sperm enters the perivitelline space, and disintegrins present on the sperm bind to integrins present on the vitelline membrane.
14. The sperm membrane fuses with the vitelline membrane.
15. Calcium is released from the intracellular reserves of the ovum.
16. Cortical granules of the ovum are exocytosed.
17. The vitelline membrane is replaced with membrane of cortical granules, resulting in the *vitelline block* to polyspermy.
18. ZP3 disappears from the zona pellucida under the influence of the cortical granules, resulting in the *zona block* to polyspermy.
19. The sperm tail disappears, and its nucleus decondenses to form the male pronucleus.
20. Mitosis results in the formation of the two-celled embryo.

Assisted Reproduction

In *intrauterine insemination* (IUI), sperm are placed directly in the uterus and are therefore not exposed to the acidic environment of the vagina. When the sperm count is very low, the sperm are placed directly in the uterine tube to avoid both the cervical and uterine passages, as in *gamete intrafallopian transfer* (GIFT). With *in vitro fertilization* (IVF), the sperm avoids all contact with the female genital tract. For IVF, sperm are obtained from the epididymis (microepididymal sperm aspiration), or from the testis (testicular sperm extraction). Sperm from more proximal regions of the tract are not very competent in producing in vitro fertilization. The sperm so obtained are introduced directly into the perivitelline space (*subzonal insemination,* or SUZI), bypassing the cumulus oophorus and zona pellucida. Hence, even immotile sperm can be made to fuse with the egg. Alternatively, the sperm is injected directly into the cytoplasm of the ovum, bypassing even the egg membrane. The procedure is called *intracytoplasmic sperm injection* (ICSI), and it allows even an immature germ cell to initiate pregnancy.

Contraception

Female Contraceptives
Barrier contraceptives like the diaphragm and cervical caps prevent sperm from meeting the ovum. The diaphragm is an elastic ring with a dome of rubber. These methods are associated with higher failure rates than the pill or the loop. Spermicidal cream is applied to the center of the diaphragm to increase its efficacy.

Intrauterine contraceptive devices (IUCDs) are inserted into the endometrial cavity to provide long-term contraception (up to several years). These devices are mostly made of plastic with either a serpentine shape (Lippe's loop) or a T configuration of polypropylene with helically shaped arms. Currently available IUCDs (the copper-T, copper-7, etc.) have greater efficacy due to added progesterone or copper. IUCDs act to prevent implantation and growth of the fertilized egg by causing a sterile inflammatory response of the endometrium. The sperm are phagocytosed by inflammatory cells in the endometrium.

Oral contraceptives contain estrogen, progesterone, or both. Estrogens induce feedback inhibition of follicle-stimulating hormone (FSH) secretion and inhibit development of the ovarian follicle, whereas progesterone inhibits the secretion of luteinizing hormone (LH) and hence prevents the LH surge from occurring. Ovulation is thus prevented. Progesterone makes the cervical secretion thick and viscid, blocking passage of sperm. Estrogens make the endometrium proliferative, preventing implantation. In practice, both hormones are combined, with progesterone inhibiting ovulation, and estrogen ensuring that the withdrawal bleeding is prompt and brief.

The *monophasic combined pill* is the most common type of oral contraceptive. The combined pill is taken for 21 days, starting from the 5th day of the menstrual cycle, followed by 7 days' gap during which withdrawal bleeding takes place. The *phased pill,* which may be biphasic or triphasic, uses different hormonal combinations during different phases of the menstrual cycle and is associated with a lower incidence of breakthrough bleeding. The *postcoital pill* ("morning after" pill) contains estrogen only, which is taken within 72 hours of coitus, and the *minipill* (progesterone only) is taken daily without interruption. These pills make the endometrium hyperproliferative or hypersecretory, respectively, and therefore unfit for implantation of the blastocyst. Moreover, the hypermotility of uterine tubes causes a rapid passage of ovum to uterus, expelling the conceptus, if any.

Long-acting injectables and implants are preferred as contraceptives by those who do not want to take oral pills daily. Examples include progestogens such as medroxyprogesterone acetate or norethindrone enanthate, which are administered intramuscularly once every 3 months. They act by inhibiting ovulation and thickening cervical secretions. Subdermal implants of levonorgestrel (a progestogen) provide effective contraception within 24 hours, and the effect lasts up to 5 to 6 years. These have been withdrawn from the market in some countries due to their adverse effects. Progesterone-containing intrauterine devices continuously release progesterone into the uterine cavity for 1 year. However, there is an increased risk of ectopic pregnancy with such devices.

Long-term hormonal contraceptives, mainly the estrogen component, have several adverse effects, such as weight gain, diabetes mellitus, impaired hepatic function, hypertension, increased incidence of thromboembolism, and increased risk of cervical, endometrial, and breast carcinoma. These side effects are not caused by nonsteroidal contraceptives, which act as estrogen antagonists and interfere with implantation of the fertilized ovum.

Tubectomy is a surgical method of sterilization involving excision of a small segment of the uterine tube.

Male Contraception

Coitus interruptus is withdrawal of the penis just before ejaculation during sexual intercourse. Full sexual pleasure is often not attained by this method. It has a high failure rate, partly because of failure of timely withdrawal and partly because of the presence of sperm in the preejaculatory emissions.

Mechanical devices like condoms are latex sheaths that are worn over the erect penis to prevent sperm from entering the female genital tract. Applying a spermicidal cream inside the condom increases the efficacy of the method. It is an inexpensive and reasonably reliable method of male contraception. It also provides significant protection against sexually transmitted diseases.

Thermal methods | Bathing the scrotum in hot (46°C) water for a few weeks reduces fertility for several months afterward. The suspensory briefs worn by men hold the testes close to the body, and because the testes are at body temperature, sperm counts gradually drop. The reliability of these methods is not established.

Vas-occlusive plugs are made of polyurethane or silicone rubber. They are injected in the liquid form into the vas deferens, where they harden in situ within 20 minutes, forming a barrier against sperm. The contraception is reversible, and fertility is restored after the plugs are removed.

Reversible inhibition of sperm under guidance (RISUG) uses styrene malic anhydride (SMA), a copolymer that is injected in combination with dimethyl sulfoxide into the vas deferens, where it coats the walls and partially blocks the lumen. RISUG is not a vas-occlusive plug because it only partially blocks the lumen of the vas deferens. It has other contraceptive effects. (1) The basic pH of the compound interferes with the acidic pH of sperm. (2) The positive electric charge associated with SMA causes the sperm membranes to rupture. SMA can be removed by flushing the vas deferens with an injected solvent and therefore allows multiple occlusions and reversals. It is a physiologically promising male contraceptive, but studies are needed to show high efficacy and reversibility along with high levels of safety and convenience.

Drugs causing azoospermia have not been found to be effective and reliable for male contraception. Azoospermic agents include testosterone, cyproterone, gossypol (a phenolic compound extract from the cotton plant), *Trypterigium wilfordii* (a vine used in traditional Chinese medicine), and nifedipine (an antihypertensive drug).

Vasectomy is a surgical, nonreversible (usually) method of sterilization involving excision of a small segment of the vas deferens.

Summary

- Sperm transport in the male reproductive tract is a passive process that is *not* dependent on the motility of the sperm.

- Insemination, whether natural as the result of intercourse or artificial, is required to allow the sperm and the ovum to meet and fuse.

- Sperm must undergo several transformations, some in the male reproductive tract, others occurring in the female tract, to be capable of fertilizing an ovum.

- Fertilization of the ovum by a sperm must be followed by implantation of the developing embryo in the wall of the uterus.

Applying What You Know

85.1. The morphology of Mr. Anderson's sperm seems to be normal. However, sperm must undergo several changes to be capable of fertilizing an ovum. What are these changes, and which are dependent on male functions and which on female processes?

85.2. Generate some possible (patho)physiologic mechanisms that might account for Mrs. Anderson's difficulty in becoming pregnant. Indicate whether each is a male or a female problem.

Normal Sexual Differentiation

The normal sexual differentiation in the embryo proceeds sequentially. The chromosomal (genotypic) sex determines the gonadal sex: it causes the indifferent gonad to develop into an ovary or a testis. The gonadal sex determines phenotypic sex—the internal and the external genitalia. The psychological sex is determined by both the gonadal sex (hormones) and phenotypic sex (appearance). The development of the brain is affected by androgens early in life. Early exposure of female human fetuses to androgens has masculinizing effects on behavior later during puberty.

General Model: Communications

Sexual differentiation is determined by the presence of XX or XY chromosomes and hormonal communications between cells.

Determination of Chromosomal Sex

The chromosomal sex is established at the moment of fertilization. The ovum contains 22 autosomal chromosomes + one sex chromosome (X). However, the spermatozoa are of two types: 50% of the spermatozoa have 22 autosomal chromosomes + an X chromosome; the remainder have 22 autosomal chromosomes + a Y chromosome. If the ovum is fertilized by an X-bearing sperm, the zygote has 44+XX chromosomes, and its chromosomal sex becomes female. On the other hand, if the sperm is Y-bearing, the zygote has 44+XY chromosomes, and its chromosomal sex becomes male. The human Y chromosome is smaller than the X chromosome. Hence, the sperm containing Y chromosome are lighter and swim faster up the female genital tract, reaching the ovum earlier than the X-bearing chromosomes. This may contribute to the fact that the global male birth rate is slightly higher than the female birth rate.

Barr body | Soon after cell division begins during embryonic development, one of the two X chromosomes in the female becomes functionally inactive. Even in abnormal individuals with more than two X chromosomes, only one remains active. The choice of which X chromosome remains active is random; hence, roughly half of the somatic cells contain an active X chromosome of paternal origin, and the rest contain an active X chromosome of maternal origin. In normal cells, the inactive X chromosome condenses and is present near the nuclear membrane as the Barr body or the sex chromatin. Thus, in an abnormal cell with three or more X chromosomes, there are two or more Barr bodies. The inactive X chromosome can also take up other forms. In up to 15% of the neutrophils, the inactive X chromosome forms a drumstick-like appendage projecting from the nucleus (**Fig. 86.1**).

If only one active X chromosome is necessary for normal feminine development, it is difficult to explain why chromosomal

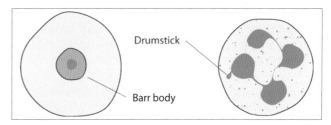

Fig. 86.1 Barr body and nuclear appendage.

disorders associated with a single X chromosome such as Turner syndrome (44+XO) should be associated with abnormalities. Hence, it is now believed that both of the X chromosomes are necessary for normal development and that the Barr body is reactivated just before oogenesis.

Differentiation of Gonadal Sex

Until the sixth week of intrauterine life, the fetal gonads are bipotential (undifferentiated): they have the rudiments of both male and female gonads (**Fig. 86.2**). The bipotential gonad consists of a medulla made of mesenchymal tissue and a cortical epithelium with primordial germ cells embedded in it. *In the genetic male,* the medulla of the bipotential gonad begins to differentiate into a testis, while the cortex regresses. *In the genetic female,* the cortex of the bipotential gonad differentiates into the ovary, while the medulla regresses. Testicular differentiation requires testis-determining factor (TDF), which is encoded by the SRY gene (sex-determining region of the Y chromosome) located near the tip of the short arm of the human Y chromosome. Under the influence of TDF, the Sertoli cells appear by the seventh week and start secreting müllerian inhibiting substance (MIS; see below). Leydig cells appear by the eighth week and start secreting testosterone. The embryonic ovary, in contrast, does not secrete any hormone.

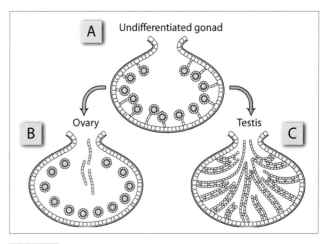

Fig. 86.2 **(A)** The undifferentiated (bipotential) gonad can differentiate into **(B)** an ovary with oogonia or **(C)** a testis with spermatogonia.

Differentiation of Internal Genitalia

The **male internal genitalia** are the rete testis, epididymis, vas deferens, and seminal vesicles. Until the seventh week of intrauterine life, the internal genitalia of the fetus have the rudiments of both male internal genitalia (the wolffian ducts) and the female internal genitalia (the müllerian ducts). A genetically male fetus with functional testes secretes testosterone and MIS. The testosterone (secreted from Leydig cells in the testes) stimulates the development of the wolffian ducts into male internal genitalia (**Fig. 86.3A**). MIS causes regression of the müllerian ducts by apoptosis. The action of both testosterone and MIS on internal genitalia is paracrine in nature and unilateral: if secreted from the left testis, they cause development of the left internal genitalia, and vice versa.

The **female internal genitalia** are the uterine tubes, uterus, and upper two-thirds of the vagina. In the absence of MIS, the müllerian ducts proliferate to form the uterine tubes, uterus, and upper two-thirds of the vagina. The development of the female external genitalia is independent of ovarian influence. By the eighth week, the müllerian ducts become committed to fully fledged development into female internal genitalia. In the absence of androgens, the wolffian ducts degenerate, and the external genitalia remain female (**Fig. 86.3B**).

Differentiation of External Genitalia

Until the eighth week of intrauterine life, the external genitalia of the fetus are bipotential; that is, they can develop along either male or female lines. Unlike the internal genitalia, which have distinct male and female rudiments, the external genitalia in both sexes develop from common rudiments, which are the urogenital sinus, the genital swellings, the genital folds, and the genital tubercle. In the absence of virilizing hormones, the fetal external genitalia develop along female lines. On the other hand, if the embryo has functional testes secreting testosterone, dihydrotestosterone (DHT) transforms the fetal external genitalia along male lines (**Fig. 86.4, Table 86.1**).

Aberrant Sexual Differentiation

Abnormalities of Chromosomal Sex

Abnormalities of chromosomal sex usually arise because of chromosomal nondisjunction during gametogenesis—a pair of chromosomes fails to separate, so that both go to one of the daughter cells during meiosis. The abnormal zygotes that can result from nondisjunction of one of the X chromosomes during oogenesis are shown in **Fig. 86.5**.

Klinefelter syndrome is also called seminiferous tubule dysgenesis. Its genotype is 47,XXY (i.e., 44+XXY), and it has an incidence of 1 in 500 males. It occurs in two forms: the classical form and the mosaic form. The *classical form* is due to meiotic nondisjunction, that is, chromosomal nondisjunction during gametogenesis. Meiotic nondisjunction is more common in the ovum than in the sperm. The *mosaic form* occurs due to mitotic nondisjunction, that is, chromosomal nondisjunction after zygote formation. It occurs due to anaphase lag. Mitotic nondisjunction can occur in a normal 46,XY or an

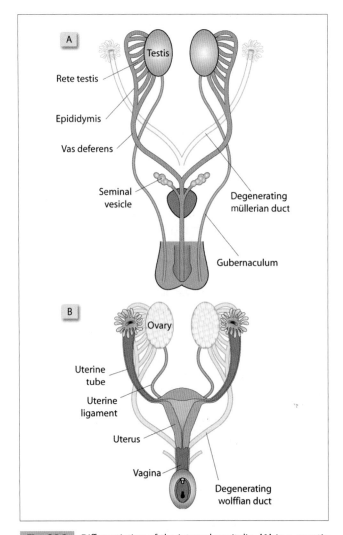

Fig. 86.3 Differentiation of the internal genitalia. **(A)** In a genetic male, the wolffian ducts differentiate into the male internal genitalia (rete testis, epididymis, vas deferens, seminal vesicles) under the effect of testosterone, while the müllerian duct regresses under the effect of müllerian inhibiting substance. **(B)** In a genetic female, the müllerian ducts develop into the female internal genitalia (uterine tubes, uterus, upper two-thirds of the vagina).

Table 86.1 Effect of Dihydrotestosterone (DHT) on the Differentiation of the External Genitalia

	In the Presence of DHT	In the Absence of DHT
Urogenital sinus	Develops into the prostate and prostatic urethra	Develops into the lower one-third of the vagina
Genital swellings	Fuse to form the scrotum	Develop into the labia majora
Genital folds	Elongate and fuse to form the shaft of the penis	Develop into the labia minora
Genital tubercle	Develops into the glans penis	Develops into the clitoris

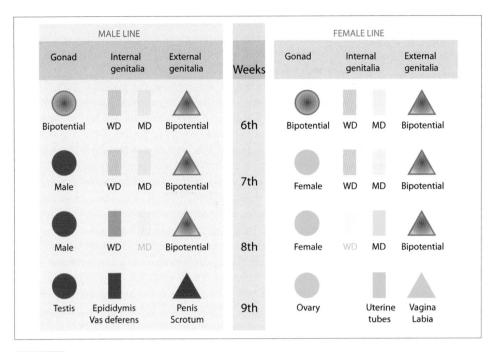

Fig. 86.4 Summary of sexual differentiation between the sixth and ninth week of intrauterine life. Red = male, blue = female. MD, müllerian duct; WD, wolffian duct.

abnormal 46,XXY zygote. The latter instance is called double nondisjunction.

Klinefelter syndrome is characterized by (1) normal male internal and external genitalia and psychosexual characteristics; (2) underdeveloped testes, hyalinization of tubules, azoospermia (no sperm present in seminal fluid), and infertility; (3) low levels of testosterone, with high levels of gonadotropins and estradiol; (4) tall build (due to increase in lower body segment) and obesity; (5) varicose veins, diabetes mellitus, thyroid abnormalities, and pulmonary diseases; and (6) mental deficiency.

Turner syndrome has an incidence of 1 in 3000 females. Fifty percent of them have the karyotype of 45,XO due to meiotic disjunction in either parent. Another 25% have the karyotype 46,XX/45,XO mosaicism due to mitotic disjunction. The remaining 25% have a structurally abnormal X chromosome with or without mosaicism.

Turner syndrome is characterized by (1) normal female internal and external genitalia and psychosexual characteristics; (2) bilateral streak gonads with infertility and primary amenorrhea and amastia; (3) characteristic facies with low posterior hairline, ptosis, epicanthus, low set ears, fish-like

Table 86.2 Phenotypic Characteristics in Different Types of Pseudohermaphroditism

	TST	MIS	DHT	Female Internal Genitalia	Male Internal Genitalia	External Genitalia
Female pseudohermaphroditism (Genetic XX)						
Exposure to TST in fetal life	+	–	+	Present, because MIS is absent	Absent, because exposure to TST usually occurs late	Male, because DHT is formed
Male pseudohermaphroditism (Genetic XY)						
Impaired testosterone secretion	–	+	–	Absent, because MIS secretion is unaffected	Absent, because TST is absent	Female, because DHT is absent
Persistent müllerian duct syndrome	+	–	+	Present, because MIS is absent	Present, because TST is present	Male, because DHT is present
5α-reductase deficiency	+	+	–	Absent, because MIS is present	Present, because TST secretion is normal	Female, because DHT is not formed
Receptor defect	+	+	+	Absent, because MIS is present	Absent, because TST is ineffective	Female, because DHT is ineffective

Abbreviations: DHT, dihydrotestosterone; MIS, müllerian-inhibiting substance; TST, testosterone.

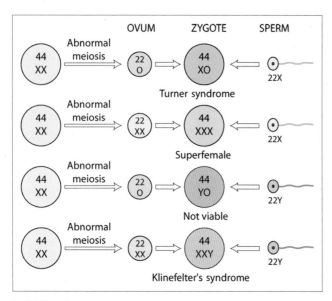

Fig. 86.5 Abnormalities of chromosomal sex. The XXX (superfemale) pattern is second in frequency only to the XXY pattern and is not associated with any obvious abnormalities. The YO zygote does not survive.

mouth, and micrognathia (small jaw); (4) short stature, webbed neck, shield-like chest, and cubitus valgus (a deformity of the elbows); and (5) coarctation of the aorta.

True hermaphrodites have both male and female gonads. Some of them have a testis on one side and an ovary on the other. Others have ovotestes, gonads containing both ovarian and testicular tissues. The internal genitalia correspond to the ipsilateral gonad. The external genitalia are ambiguous. Most hermaphrodites are brought up as males, but at puberty most of them become feminine, develop breasts, menstruate, and sometime even ovulate. Most of the true hermaphrodites have the genotype 46,XX. The rest have either 46,XY or mosaics. It is not clear why a normal genotype should be associated with true hermaphroditism. These XX genotypes probably have sufficient genetic material derived from the Y chromosome to induce growth of testicular tissue.

Abnormalities of Phenotypic Sex

A pseudohermaphrodite is an individual with the chromosomes and gonads of one sex and the genitalia of the other (**Table 86.2**).

A **female pseudohermaphrodite** is a genetic female with female gonads and internal genitalia, but male external genitalia. It occurs in genetic females exposed to high levels of androgens during the 8th to the 13th week of gestation. After the 13th week, the genitalia are fully formed, but exposure to androgens can cause hypertrophy of the clitoris. Female pseudohermaphroditism may be due to congenital virilizing adrenal hyperplasia, or it may be caused by androgens administered to the mother.

A **male pseudohermaphrodite** is a genetic male with male gonads, but female internal or external genitalia. It occurs due to deficiency of 17α-hydroxylase (causing impaired

testosterone secretion) or deficiency of 5α-reductase (causing reduced peripheral formation of dihydrotestosterone), or due to nonfunctional testosterone receptors (rendering androgens ineffective).

In the absence of testosterone, the wolffian duct fails to develop into the male internal genitalia. The female internal genitalia are not formed either, because the MIS secretion by the testes is usually unaffected and results in the regression of the müllerian duct. If MIS secretion is impaired but testosterone secretion is normal, it results in the persistent müllerian duct syndrome in which both the wolffian and müllerian ducts develop into male and female internal genitalia, respectively.

In the absence of dihydrotestosterone, the internal genitalia are male, and the external genitalia are female.

In *complete androgen resistance syndrome,* earlier called *testicular feminizing syndrome,* there is loss of function of the testosterone receptors due to mutation. The internal genitalia are therefore neither male (because testosterone is ineffective) nor female (because MIS is present). The external genitalia are female (because DHT is not formed), but the vagina ends blindly because there are no female internal genitalia. Individuals with this syndrome develop enlarged breasts at puberty and usually are considered normal women until they are diagnosed when they seek medical advice for absence of menarche.

Summary

- Chromosomal sex is determined by the presence (male) or absence (female) of a Y chromosome.

- Gonadal sex, whether a male or female reproductive tract develops, is determined by the presence (male) or absence (female) of testosterone and müllerian-inhibiting factor.

Applying What You Know

86.1. What factors determined whether Mrs. Anderson's child developed into a phenotypic female? Explain.

Placenta

After the implantation of the embryo, the endometrium is called the decidua because it is shed off at the end of pregnancy. The decidua resembles the secretory endometrium of the menstrual cycle. As the blastocyst grows, the trophoblast layer differentiates into two layers, the outer syncytiotrophoblast and the inner cytotrophoblast. The *syncytiotrophoblast* is a layer of cytoplasm containing multiple nuclei. It is formed by the fusion of several trophoblast cells. The *cytotrophoblast* layer ultimately differentiates into the chorionic villi. Fetal blood vessels grow into the chorionic villi (**Fig. 87.1**).

In the fully formed placenta, maternal blood circulates through the intervillous spaces; the fetal blood flows through the core of the chorionic villi. Hence, maternal and fetal blood do not mix together (**Fig. 87.2**). The placental membrane that separates the maternal and fetal circulation is made of four layers: syncytiotrophoblast, cytotrophoblast, connective tissue layer, and endothelium and basement membrane of the fetal blood vessels.

Placental Hormones

The syncytiotrophoblast of the placenta serves as an endocrine organ that secretes human chorionic gonadotropin, human chorionic somatomammotropin, human chorionic thyro-

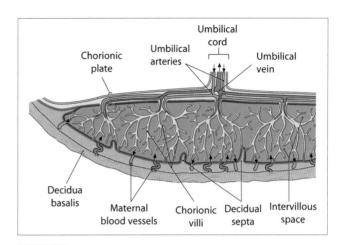

Fig. 87.2 Structure of a placenta showing the maternal and the fetal blood vessels.

tropin, relaxin, estrogens, and progestogens (**Fig. 87.3**). Both estrogens and progesterone are required for the initiation and maintenance of pregnancy. In the first 60 days of pregnancy, these hormones are produced mainly by the corpus luteum. Thereafter, the fetoplacental unit takes over the formation of estrogens and progestogens. This is known as the

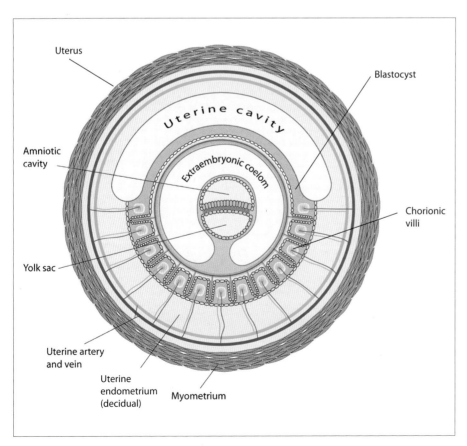

Fig. 87.1 A blastocyst in the wall of the uterus following implantation. Compare with **Fig. 85.8**.

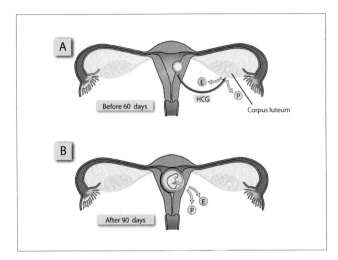

Fig. 87.3 Luteal-placental shift. **(A)** Estrogen and progesterone are produced by the corpus luteum during the first 60 days of pregnancy stimulated by human chorionic gonadotropin (HCG) from the corpus luteum. **(B)** By 90 days, these hormones are being produced by the placenta as the corpus luteum has degenerated. E, estrogens; P, progestogens.

luteal-placental shift. Hence, ovariectomy after 2 months does not interrupt pregnancy. The presence of placental hormones in maternal blood or urine indicates that the placenta is functioning normally.

Human chorionic gonadotropin (HCG) is a peptide hormone secreted by the syncytiotrophoblast soon after fertilization. It is detectable in maternal urine as early as 14 days after conception, which forms the basis for all pregnancy diagnostic tests. By the time a woman misses her period, her urinary HCG levels are high enough to be detected. HCG reaches a plasma peak between 60 and 90 days of gestation. Thereafter, the concentration falls to a low level and reduces to zero just before labor.

HCG has actions similar to those of luteinizing hormone (LH). It extends the life of the corpus luteum up to 60 days after conception, until the fetoplacental unit is able to synthesize its own estrogens and progesterone. (1) HCG stimulates the corpus luteum to secrete 17α-hydroxyprogesterone (see **Fig. 82.1**) and a smaller amount of progesterone. The blood level of 17α-hydroxyprogesterone is a reliable indicator of corpus luteal function because it is not produced by the placenta, which lacks 17α-hydroxylase. (2) In the male fetus, HCG stimulates the fetal testes to secrete testosterone, which is important for sexual differentiation. (3) HCG also stimulates the fetal adrenal cortex to secrete dehydroepiandrosterone sulfate (DHEAS), which is important for the placental synthesis of estriol.

Human chorionic somatomammotropin (HCS) structurally resembles pituitary growth hormone. Its concentration in serum rises steadily from the eighth week to term. Although less active than prolactin, it is produced in such large amounts that it may exert a lactogenic effect. It is also called human placental lactogen (HPL).

Human chorionic thyrotropin (HCT) is a placental hormone that resembles thyroid-stimulating hormone (TSH). Its concentration in serum follows a curve like that for HCG. The physiological role of HCT is unknown.

Relaxin is discussed in the next chapter.

Estrogens | All three types of estrogens, estrone, estradiol, and estriol, are produced in large quantities during pregnancy, and their concentration rises steadily throughout gestation, reaching their maximum at term (**Fig. 87.4**) and decreasing rapidly after parturition. Estriol, which is the weakest estrogen, is produced only during pregnancy. Its secretion not only indicates a healthy placenta, but also correlates well with the fetal growth. Falling estriol levels indicate impending fetal death.

Progesterone | The placenta secretes only progesterone, unlike the corpus luteum, which secretes both progesterone and 17α-hydroxyprogesterone (which has little biologic activity). Hence, after the luteal-placental shift, the 17α-hydroxyprogesterone level falls, but the progesterone level continues to rise until just before parturition (**Fig. 87.4**).

Fetoplacental Unit

The fetus, placenta, and mother are interdependent and constitute a functional unit called the fetoplacento-maternal unit or simply the fetoplacental unit. This interdependence is especially apparent in the placental synthesis of progesterone and estrogens and the fetal synthesis of cortisol, as explained below (**Fig. 87.5**).

General Model: Reservoir

To understand the origins of the estrogen, progesterone, and other hormones in the pregnant woman, it is important to keep in mind that we are dealing with a reservoir into which hormones flow from the woman's ovaries and from the fetoplacental unit.

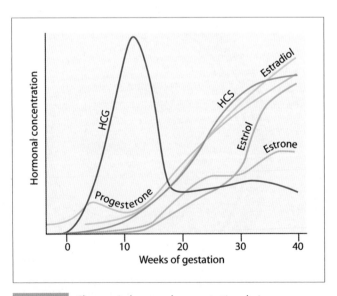

Fig. 87.4 Changes in hormonal concentration during pregnancy. Note the slight dip in progesterone secretion at about the 10th week of gestation. The dip coincides with the luteal-placental shift and occurs due to the decrease in the progesterone secretion by the corpus luteum. HCG, human chorionic gonadotropin; HCS, human chorionic somatomammotropin.

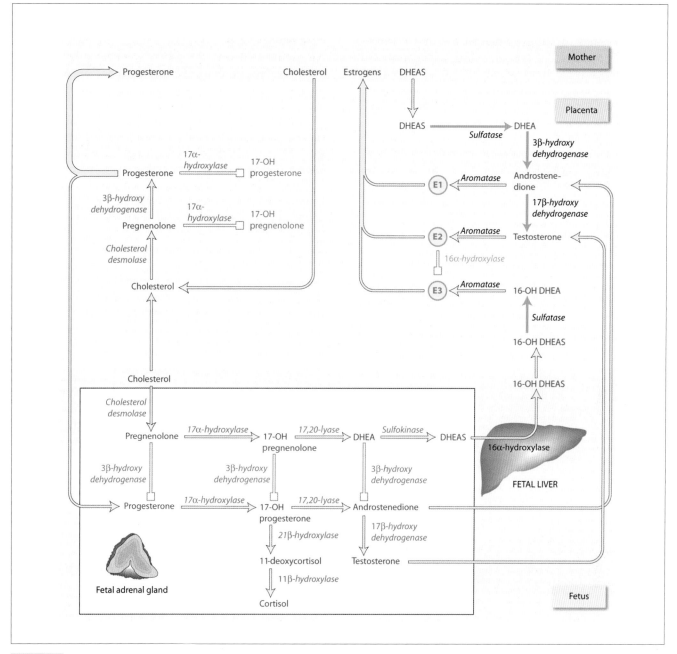

Fig. 87.5 Hormone synthesis in the fetoplacental unit. The mother provides much of the cholesterol required for steroid production by the placenta and dehydroepiandrosterone sulfate (DHEAS) needed to produce testosterone and estrogen. The mother receives large amounts of estrogen and progesterone from the fetoplacental unit. DHEA, dehydroepiandrosterone.

Placental synthesis of progesterone | The placenta synthesizes progesterone from cholesterol. Because it cannot synthesize its own cholesterol from acetate, it obtains the cholesterol from the maternal and fetal circulations. Ninety percent of the progesterone synthesized in the placenta diffuses back into the maternal circulation, resulting in the characteristic maternal changes in pregnancy. Ten percent of the progesterone synthesized in the placenta enters the fetal circulation, where it is converted to cortisol. Up to the 10th week of gestation, the fetus is dependent on placental progesterone for synthesizing corticosteroids because its own adrenal cortex is deficient in

3β-hydroxy dehydrogenase. After 10 weeks, the fetus is able to synthesize its own progesterone. It is also able to synthesize androstenedione and testosterone. These androgens diffuse into the placenta, where they are converted into estrogens.

Placental synthesis of estrone and estradiol | The placenta cannot synthesize estrone and estradiol from cholesterol because it lacks 17α-hydroxylase and 17,20-lyase. The placenta synthesizes estrone and estradiol from DHEAS, which it obtains from the maternal circulation. As with progestogens, 90% of the placental estrogens enter the maternal circulation, and the remainder enters the fetus.

Placental synthesis of estriol | The placenta cannot synthesize estriol from estrone because® it lacks 16α–hydroxylase. Hence, it obtains 16-hydroxy DHEA sulfate (16-OH DHEAS) from fetal circulation, removes the sulfate, and aromatizes it to estriol. Because the placental synthesis of estriol is entirely dependent on the 16-OH DHEAS produced by the fetal adrenal gland, the urinary excretion of estriol in the mother is an index of fetal health.

Fetal production of cortisol | The fetal adrenal cortex produces cortisol via the same pathways that operate in the adult adrenal glands (compare **Fig. 82.1** and **Fig. 87.5**). Cortisol is essential for the maturation of the fetal lungs (the production of surfactant) and the closure of the ductus arteriosus at birth.

Pregnancy Diagnostic Tests

All pregnancy diagnostic tests are based on the presence of HCG in urine, which can be detected as early as 14 days after conception, within a day or two of a missed period. The accuracy of these tests is ~99%.

In **biologic tests,** laboratory animals (frog, mouse, or rabbit) are injected with the patient's urine and observed for physiologic responses, such as ovulation or release of sperm. Although very sensitive, they have been abandoned, as they are cumbersome.

Immunologic tests are quick (give results in minutes), cheap, and accurate enough to replace biologic methods. The most commonly used immunologic test is the Gravindex test. The kit consists of Gravindex antigen (latex particles coated with HCG), Gravindex antibody (serum containing HCG antibodies), dark slide, sticks, and a pipette. If serum containing antibodies to HCG is allowed to react with HCG-coated red cells or latex particles, agglutination of the red cells or latex particles occurs. But if the serum is allowed to react with urine containing HCG prior to the reaction with red cells or latex particles, the agglutination of red cells or latex particles is inhibited because the antibodies are blocked by HCG from the urine (**Fig. 87.6**). Hence, inhibition of agglutination confirms pregnancy.

Maternal Changes in Pregnancy

Most of the physiologic changes associated with pregnancy are directly or indirectly related to the high concentrations of progesterone and estrogens in maternal blood, the dilatation of uterine blood vessels, and the elevation of the diaphragm. These are discussed below.

Effects of Progesterone and Estrogens
Amenorrhea is the first and best known change associated with pregnancy. It occurs because the high circulating levels of progesterone and estrogen prevent the normal cycling of the female reproductive system.

Breathing | Progesterone directly stimulates the respiratory center, resulting in a level of increased ventilation that is greater than that required to wash out the extra CO_2 produced by the fetus. Thus, maternal hyperventilation causes hypocapnia and respiratory alkalosis with bicarbonaturia.

Circulation | Estrogens increase uterine blood flow, helping to provide nourishment to the fetus through the placenta. Aldosterone, which is secreted in large amounts during pregnancy, causes fluid and electrolyte retention, resulting in hypervolemia, increase in renal blood flow, and increase in glomerular filtration rate (GFR). Water retention exceeds sodium retention, resulting in hyposmolarity of the extracellular fluid (ECF). Water retention also results in hemodilutional anemia, which is called the *physiologic anemia of pregnancy.* The resulting anemic hypoxia causes vasodilatation, reducing the peripheral resistance. The increased blood flow through the uterus (umbilicus) also contributes to the decreased peripheral resistance. Consequently, central venous pressure (CVP) is increased. The CVP also increases as a direct consequence of the increase in blood volume. The increase in CVP increases the cardiac output. Despite the increase in cardiac output, the mean blood pressure and even the systolic blood pressure remain normal because of

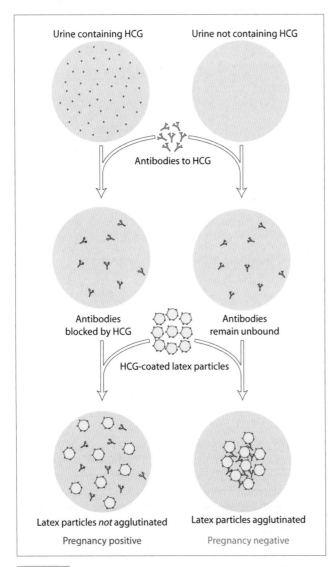

Urine containing HCG   Urine not containing HCG

Antibodies to HCG

Antibodies blocked by HCG   Antibodies remain unbound

HCG-coated latex particles

Latex particles *not* agglutinated   Latex particles agglutinated

Pregnancy positive   Pregnancy negative

Fig. 87.6 The immunologic basis of the Gravindex test. The detection of human chorionic gonadotropin (HCG) in the urine of a pregnant woman can occur as early as 14 days after conception.

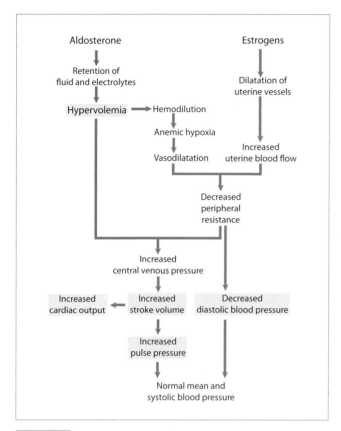

Fig. 87.7 Cardiovascular changes in pregnancy. The changes produced by estrogen and progesterone result in the increase in maternal cardiac output needed to perfuse the placenta and sustain the fetus.

the large fall in peripheral resistance. The peripheral resistance also decreases as a direct consequence of the increased uterine blood flow. These events are summarized in **Fig. 87.7**.

Plasma proteins | Estrogens stimulate liver enzymes to increase the synthesis of transport globulins that bind to thyroxine (TBG), corticosteroids and progestogens (transcortin), and estrogens (sex steroid-binding globulin). Despite the increase in transcortin, pregnant women are often in a state of *mild hyperadrenocorticism.* This is because the elevated placental progesterone competes with cortisol for binding sites on transcortin, thus increasing plasma-free cortisol. Estrogens also increase fibrinogen synthesis, resulting in *hypercoagulability of blood* and an increase of erythrocyte sedimentation rate (ESR). The hypercoagulability of blood is important in preventing excessive blood loss during placental separation. Increased synthesis of thyroxine-binding globulin results in increased binding of thyroxine and compensatory increase in thyroxine secretion. Estrogens also increase the hepatic synthesis of angiotensinogen, leading to increased angiotensin II synthesis and aldosterone secretion.

Glucose tolerance | Glucose tolerance is reduced in pregnant women due to the anti-insulin effects of progesterone, estrogen, and human chorionic somatomammotropin. A transient diabetes can be present during pregnancy, which is called *gestational diabetes.*

Gallbladder | Progesterone decreases the smooth muscle tone of the gallbladder and thereby predisposes to gallbladder stasis. Hence, gallstones are more common in women who have been pregnant several times.

Effects of Diaphragmatic Elevation
As the gravid uterus enlarges, the diaphragm is elevated. Elevation of the diaphragm affects the lung volumes and capacities of pregnant women (**Fig. 46.5**). It also rotates the apex of the heart upward and to the left, resulting in an outward shift of the apex beat, a left axis deviation in the electrocardiogram (ECG), and an increase in the cardiac shadow in the radiograph.

Summary

- The placenta provides the embryo/fetus with all of the materials it needs to grow and develop and removes the waste products it produces.

- The placenta is a source of hormones that are required to maintain the pregnancy.

- The maternal-placental-fetal unit is an endocrine "organ" that produces the hormones important to fetal development and changes in maternal physiology needed to sustain the pregnancy and bring about delivery at term.

Applying What You Know

87.1. During Mrs. Anderson's pregnancy, the placenta served as a barrier to exchange between her circulation and the circulation of her fetus. What substances are able to cross this barrier?

Hormones of Parturition and Lactation

Oxytocin

Oxytocin is a nonapeptide that is synthesized in the paraventricular and supraoptic nuclei of the hypothalamus and is stored in the posterior lobe of the pituitary gland. It causes (1) galactokinesis (see below) by stimulating the myoepithelial cells of the mammary gland and (2) stimulates uterine contractions. It plays a role in labor and is a useful therapeutic agent in the induction of labor. Along with estrogen, oxytocin is used therapeutically in arresting uterine bleeding.

Oxytocin secretion is stimulated by suckling and genital stimulation, as occurs during coitus and parturition. Oxytocin is also released in men during genital stimulation, but its role is not clear. Oxytocin secretion is inhibited by sympathetic discharge and circulating catecholamines; by pain and enkephalins; by emotional stress, especially fear; and by alcohol.

Relaxin

Relaxin is a polypeptide hormone secreted by the corpus luteum and placenta in women and by the prostate in men. During pregnancy, it relaxes the pubic symphysis and other pelvic joints and softens the cervix, facilitating parturition. In men, it probably has a role in sperm motility and sperm penetration of the ovum.

Prolactin

Prolactin is a polypeptide hormone secreted by the anterior pituitary acidophils. Its physiologic actions are (1) mammogenesis, lactogenesis, and galactopoiesis; and (2) suppression of gonadotrophin-releasing hormone (GnRH) secretion, which results in lactation amenorrhea.

Normally, the control of prolactin secretion is under constant inhibition by the prolactin-inhibiting factor (PIF) secreted in the hypothalamus. PIF is now known to be dopamine, which acts through D_2 receptors. Hence, prolactin secretion is disinhibited by dopamine antagonists such as metoclopramide. Prolactin secretion is stimulated by serotonin, which probably mediates the increase in prolactin secretion during sleep, and by vasoactive intestinal peptide (VIP), which mediates the suckling reflex. Prolactin secretion is also stimulated by estrogens and thyrotropin-releasing hormone (TRH).

Plasma prolactin levels start increasing by the eighth week of pregnancy and reach their peak 2 weeks before term (see **Fig. 87.4**). The increase is brought about by estrogens, which directly stimulate the pituitary lactotroph to synthesize and secrete more prolactin. After parturition, prolactin secretion falls, but the fall is gradual because prolactin secretion is stimulated during each session of suckling. Prolactin secretion is also stimulated by other factors of unknown physiologic significance; for example, it increases during sleep, exercise, and stress.

In **hyperprolactinemia,** galactorrhea occurs in only ~30% of cases. In women, the elevated prolactin causes infertility and amenorrhea; in men, it causes impotence and decreased libido. Treatment for prolactin hypersecretion includes administration of a dopamine agonist such as bromocriptine.

Parturition

Phases of Parturition

Parturition, the process of giving birth, encompasses three stages: (1) the preparation of the uterus for childbirth, (2) the actual process of childbirth, and (3) the recovery from childbirth. During parturition, the myometrium and the cervix undergo a series of events that are divided into four phases (**Fig. 88.1**).

Uterine phase 0 of parturition is the prelude to initiation of parturition and extends from before implantation until late

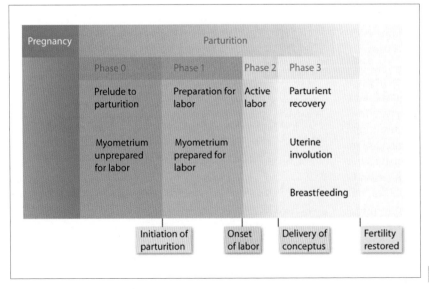

Fig. 88.1 Stages of parturition.

gestation. During this phase, the myometrium remains relaxed, and the cervix remains rigid and unyielding under the stimulation of progesterone. The conduction of action potentials by myometrial cells is slow, and myometrial contractility is low. There is increased degradation of endogenously produced *uterotonins* (humeral agents acting on the uterus), such as prostaglandins, oxytocin, and histamine by prostaglandin dehydrogenase, oxytocinase, and diamine oxidase, respectively.

Uterine phase 1 of parturition is the period of uterine preparation for labor. It is characterized by increased myometrial responsiveness to oxytocin and cervical ripening (softening). The *myometrial responsiveness* to oxytocin increases due to an increase in the number of oxytocin receptors in the myometrium. The number and size of gap junctions between the myometrial cells increase, resulting in faster conduction of action potentials between myometrial cells. *Cervical ripening* is mediated by the prostaglandins whose release is stimulated by estrogen. The cervix becomes soft and yielding due to the breakdown of collagen and an increase in hyaluronic acid, which has high water-retaining capacity.

General Model: Communications

The processes required to prepare the uterus for delivery involve several different examples of cell–cell communications. Some are examples of hormonal communication of information; others are examples of electrical interactions between adjacent cells.

Phase 2 of parturition is under the influence of oxytocin and prostaglandins (**Fig. 88.2**). It is the period of active labor, when uterine contractions bring about progressive cervical dilatation, fetal descent, and delivery of conceptus—the fetus, umbilical cord, and placenta (**Fig. 88.3**). It has further been divided into three stages. Stage I is the stage of cervical effacement and dilatation. The external opening of the cervix is normally closed. During labor, the cervical canal dilates and shortens, and the uterus, vagina, and cervix become one continuous canal in which the cervix is almost indistinguishable as a separate part. This is known as cervical effacement. Stage II is characterized by the expulsion of the fetus. Stage III is the stage of separation and expulsion of the placenta.

After the expulsion of the placenta, if the cord is not clamped until pulsations cease, an additional 100 mL of blood can be transferred into the neonate. However, clamping should not be delayed for more than 1 minute because too much blood (> 100 mL) will embarrass respiration and circulation. There is risk of blood loss to the placenta if the neonate is raised above the level of the uterus or if the cord is partially compressed, blocking venous return from the placenta, but not the arterial flow to the placenta.

Uterine phase 3 of parturition is the time of recovery of the mother. It involves uterine contraction and retraction to prevent postpartum hemorrhage, initiation of lactation and milk ejection to facilitate breastfeeding, involution of uterus,

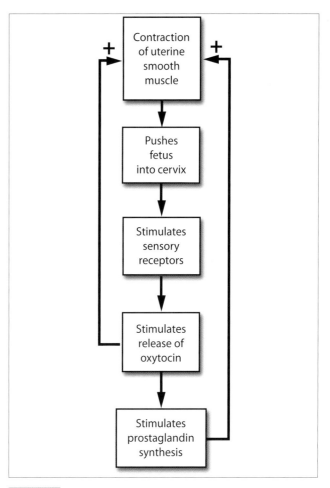

Fig. 88.2 The positive feedback mechanisms that drives parturition (labor and delivery of the fetus).

and restoration of fertility. Oxytocin and endothelin 1 are important regulators of phase 3 of parturition.

Initiation of Parturition

The stimuli that initiate parturition—that cause labor to begin—at the appropriate time for the fetus have not been definitively identified in humans.

Effects of high estrogen-to-progesterone (E:P) ratio | A high E:P ratio stimulates uterine contraction in the following manner. Progesterone relaxes uterine smooth muscles. On the other hand, estrogen causes increased secretion of oxytocin, increased synthesis of oxytocin receptors in the myometrium and decidua, increased synthesis of prostaglandins in the decidua, and increased synthesis of myometrial contractile protein. Prostaglandins increase the formation of gap junctions in the myometrium, enabling faster conduction of impulses.

Causes of high E:P ratio | The estrogen-to-progesterone ratio becomes high toward term due to a steep rise in plasma estrogen secretion and a slower rise in progesterone level (see **Fig. 87.4**). The rise in maternal estrogen level is triggered by a rise in fetal secretion of corticotropin-releasing hormone (CRH). The increase in CRH increases fetal adrenocorticotropic hormone (ACTH) secretion, which, in turn, increases the secretion of androgens from the fetal adrenal cortex. The

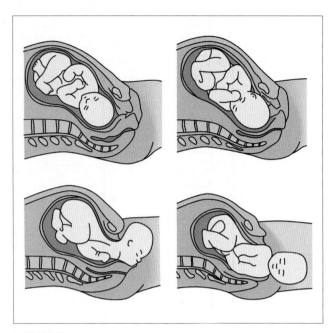

Fig. 88.3 Stages in the birth of the newborn (phase 2).

placenta converts these androgens to estrogens, which diffuse into maternal circulation (see **Fig. 87.5**). At the same time, the maternal progesterone level falls due to decreased contribution from fetal progesterone. Fetal production of progesterone decreases because the large amount of cortisol produced by the fetus inhibits the conversion of fetal pregnenolone to progesterone.

Parturition reflex | Once labor starts, uterine contractions dilate the cervix by pushing the fetal head into it. The dilatation sets up signals in afferent nerves that increase oxytocin secretion from the posterior pituitary. This is known as the *parturition reflex.* The oxytocin released contracts the myometrium further, increasing the intensity of labor pain, but culminating in the expulsion of the fetus.

Lactation

Phases of Lactation
Lactation is divided into four phases: mammogenesis, lactogenesis, galactokinesis, and galactopoiesis.

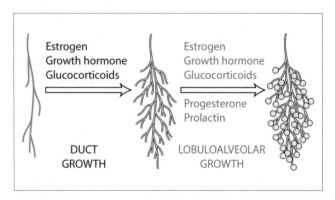

Fig. 88.4 Effect of hormones on development of the breast.

Mammogenesis is the preparation of the breasts. It involves both duct growth and lobuloalveolar growth. Duct growth is brought about by estrogens, growth hormone, and glucocorticoids. Lobuloalveolar growth requires, in addition to the hormones mentioned, progesterone and prolactin (**Fig. 88.4**).

Lactogenesis is the synthesis and secretion of milk from breast alveoli. Around midpregnancy, the alveoli become sufficiently differentiated to secrete small amounts of casein and lactose. After parturition, the breast secretes milk under the influence of prolactin, which stimulates the activity of the enzyme galactosyl transferase, leading to the synthesis of lactose. Growth hormone and thyroid hormone increase milk production.

Although the prolactin level is high during pregnancy, there is no milk secretion because estrogen and progesterone have a direct inhibitory action on lactogenesis. After parturition, there is a sharp fall in estrogen and progesterone levels. This removes the inhibitory effect on lactogenesis. Because the prolactin level is still high and mammogenesis is complete, lactogenesis occurs. Once lactation starts, it is not inhibited by administered progesterone because progesterone receptors are lost in lactating women. Limited secretion of milk, called *witch's milk,* also occurs from the breast of the newborn due to the influence of maternal prolactin.

Galactokinesis is also called milk ejection or milk letdown (**Fig. 88.5**). It is brought about by oxytocin, which stimulates the contraction of myoepithelial cells in the mammary alveoli and ducts. Oxytocin is released when the nipple is stimulated during suckling. Suckling stimulates the sensory nerve endings of the areola and the nipple. The impulses travel to the hypothalamus and cause reflex release of prolactin and oxytocin from the pituitary. Oxytocin secretion can also become conditioned so that the physical stimulation of the nipple no longer is required. Thus, lactating women can experience milk letdown in response to the sight, sound, and even thought of a baby. Such spontaneous milk release is associated with an increase in oxytocin secretion, but no increase in prolactin secretion.

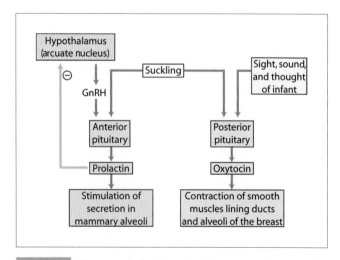

Fig. 88.5 The control of milk ejection by a neuroendocrine reflex mechanism. GnRH, gonadotrophin-releasing hormone.

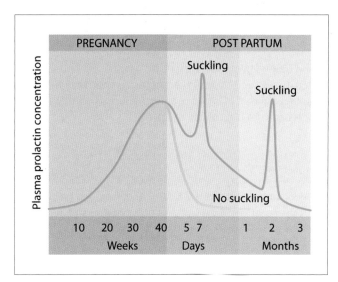

Fig. 88.6 Prolactin levels during pregnancy and suckling.

Galactopoiesis is the maintenance of lactation. Lactation is maintained by prolactin. After parturition, the estrogen and progesterone levels fall, and with them, the prolactin level also declines. However, there are periodic surges of prolactin that are associated with each episode of suckling (**Fig. 88.6**). These surges maintain lactation. In fact, lactation can continue indefinitely as long as suckling is continued, as in wet nurses who offer themselves for hire for suckling another's baby. The withdrawal of prolactin is associated with involution of the breast. The alveolar epithelium undergoes apoptosis and remodeling, and the gland reverts to its prepregnant state.

General Models: Communications and Energy

The ability of the mother to provide milk to nourish the newborn is dependent on a complex interplay of neural and chemical (hormonal) information. In addition, milk production by the mother requires the availability of energy and the necessary substrates for the synthesis of the components of milk. This is a definite challenge to the mother's physiology.

The high level of prolactin inhibits GnRH secretion, resulting in low levels of follicle-stimulating hormone (FSH) and luteinizing hormone (LH). Hence suckling, which stimulates prolactin secretion, is associated with anovulation and amenorrhea. Such amenorrhea is commonly called *lactation amenorrhea*.

Summary

- Parturition, delivery of the fetus at term, is possibly triggered by an increase of the ratio of estrogen to progesterone.

- Oxytocin stimulates contractions of the uterus, and its release is stimulated by the fetus pushing on the cervix.

- Lactation requires estrogen (to stimulate the development of the breasts for milk production), prolactin (to stimulate milk production), and oxytocin (to stimulate the ejection of milk).

Applying What You Know

88.1. Mrs. Anderson's labor was induced pharmacologically. What drugs might be used to accomplish this, and what mechanism(s) would initiate parturition?

Answers to Applying What You Know

Chapter 82

1 Mr. Anderson can only produce sperm if his testosterone level is high enough. What changes in the male reproductive endocrine system could lower his testosterone concentration?

Decreased gonadotrophin-releasing hormone (GnRH) from a primary problem in the hypothalamus would result in decreased luteinizing hormone (LH) and follicle-stimulating hormone (FSH) release from the pituitary. With reduced stimulation of the testes, circulating testosterone would be reduced.

If the primary problem were in the pituitary, there would also be decreased LH; therefore, FSH has exactly the same effect.

Two-thirds of the circulating testosterone is carried bound to albumin, with all but 2% of the remainder bound to another transport protein SHBP. A decrease in albumin could, at least in principle, reduce the size of the pool of testosterone being circulated and hence that is free in solution.

Finally, if the number of testosterone receptors on cells in the anterior pituitary were increased, the strength of the negative feedback of testosterone on LH secretion would increase; hence, LH levels would decrease, and testosterone would be decreased.

2 Mrs. Anderson apparently produces adequate quantities of estrogen and progesterone to maintain normal reproductive function. A decrease in the activity of which enzymes would result in a decrease in both estrogen and progesterone?

Androstenedione is the precursor for both testosterone and estradiol. The major precursor of androstenedione is dehydroepiandrosterone (DHEA). So, a reduction in the activity of 3β-hydroxy dehydrogenase, which converts DHEA into androstenedione, would cause reductions in both testosterone and estradiol.

Chapter 83

1 What change in gonadotropin-releasing hormone (GnRH), luteinizing hormone (LH), or follicle-stimulating hormone (FSH) would result in Mr. Anderson's sperm count being decreased below normal? Explain.

Spermatogenesis by the Sertoli cells requires adequate quantities of both FSH (which stimulates the Sertoli cells to produce sperm) and LH (which stimulates Leydig cells to make the testosterone required for spermatogenesis). Lack of either will hinder this process. Thus, if there were a primary problem in the hypothalamus, GnRH would be decreased; therefore, there would be decreased LH and FSH. A primary problem at the pituitary would have the same results. Whichever is the case, there would be an abnormally low sperm count.

2 There is reason to believe that Mrs. Anderson is ovulating normally. What is the state of the chromosomes in the ovulated egg that is released each cycle? Is it haploid, diploid, or something else?

At the time of ovulation, the oocyte has started, but not completed, the second stage of meiosis. As a result, the oocyte has a haploid number of chromosomes. Meiosis is only completed when the ovum is fertilized by sperm.

Chapter 84

1 Prior to her first marriage, Mrs. Anderson had been taking oral contraceptives. What might be the contents of such a pill and how would it prevent ovulation?

In principle, there are several sites in the female reproductive system where pharmacologic manipulation could either block ovulation or prevent conception. Inhibition of FSH and LH release by exogenous estrogen and progesterone, respectively, would prevent the LH surge; hence, no ovulation would take place. Blockade of the receptors for estrogen and/or progesterone at the thecal and granulosa cells would prevent the normal cycling of the system and prevent ovulation. Yet another avenue for blocking conception would be to prevent the changes to the cervix and/or the uterus that are needed if conception is to be successful.

The "pill" that is in widespread use today actually contains estrogen and progesterone in amounts that do both.

Chapter 85

1 The morphology of Mr. Anderson's sperm seems to be normal. However, sperm must undergo several changes to be capable of fertilizing an ovum. What are these changes, and which are dependent on male functions and which on female processes?

Sperm must undergo the processes of maturation, capitation, and activation. **Maturation** occurs in the epididymis and involves the acquisition of motility, the ability to bind to the zona pellucida of the ovum, the ability to undergo the acrosome reaction, the ability to fuse with the egg, and the condensation of sperm chromatin. **Capacitation** of sperm occurs in the female reproductive tract and involves the removal of the decapacitation factors that were added to the head of the sperm in the epididymis. Failure could occur because of "defects" in the sperm (a male problem) or because of abnormalities somewhere along the female tract. **Activation** of the sperm occurs when the sperm fuses with the ovum. Because this involves the sperm signaling the ovum to release calcium, a problem here could be due to either the sperm (male) or the ovum (female).

2 Generate some possible (patho)physiologic mechanisms that might account for Mrs. Anderson's difficulty in becoming pregnant. Indicate whether each is a male or a female problem.

The male must produce "good" sperm and "good" semen. The female must produce mucus in the cervix that is thin enough for sperm to penetrate it to enter the uterus. The fallopian tubes must be patent and their contractility normal to assist the movement of sperm toward the egg. The female must produce the decapitation factor, and the male's sperm must be capable of being decapitated. The sperm must be able to penetrate into the egg, the egg must be able to respond to prevent polyspermy, and the deoxyribonucleic acid (DNA) of the sperm and the egg must be able to combine. Obviously, there are a great many steps, some associated with the male and some with the female, that must occur for conception to occur.

Chapter 86

1 What factors determined whether Mrs. Anderson's child developed into a phenotypic female? Explain.

The development of a male reproductive tract requires the presence of testosterone (or dihydrotestosterone [DHT]) and müllerian inhibiting factor. In the absence of these two humoral agents (which would be the case in a zygote with XY chromosomes), a female reproductive tract develops.

Chapter 87

1 During Mrs. Anderson's pregnancy, the placenta served as a barrier to exchange between her circulation and the circulation of her fetus. What substances are able to cross this barrier?

The barrier to diffusion represented by the placenta must allow the transfer of oxygen (from mother to fetus) and carbon dioxide (from fetus to mother). Similarly, nutrients such as carbohydrates, fatty acids, and amino acids must be able to cross the placenta. In addition, there are a large number of hormones and chemical precursors of hormones that cross between mother and fetus.

On the other hand, some hormones do not appear to cross the placenta: some viruses and antibodies can cross, others cannot.

Chapter 88

1 Mrs. Anderson's labor was induced pharmacologically. What drugs might be used to accomplish this, and what mechanism(s) would initiate parturition?

Oxytocin is commonly used to induce labor. Oxytocin stimulates the contraction of uterine smooth muscle and stimulates the release of prostaglandins that also stimulate contractions. Thus, exogenous oxytocin can be expected to begin labor.

Section X Case Analysis:
Mrs. Anderson is having trouble getting pregnant.

Clinical Overview

Review of patient condition | Mr. and Mrs. Anderson, both 27 years old, are concerned because Mrs. Anderson has been unable to get pregnant over the past 2 years.

Etiology | Infertility can arise from many causes. In approximately one-third of the cases the problem is found to be with the female partner, in one-third of the cases the problem is with the male partner, and in the remaining one-third the problem arises from the couple or is simply not known.

For conception to occur, the man must produce an adequate number of sperm capable for fertilizing an egg, the woman must release a viable ovum each monthly cycle, and there must be no structural or functional barriers to the sperm reaching the ovum. Sources of infertility, then, encompass both male and/or female endocrine problems and anatomic problems.

Prevalence | Infertility, usually defined as being present if the couple does not conceive after 1 year of attempting to become pregnant, may affect more than 10% of couples.

Diagnosis | The diagnosis of the source of infertility obviously must consider both male and female problems. In this case, the wife's previous history of a successful pregnancy suggests that the problem is the husband's. Nevertheless, it is possible that since the wife's first pregnancy some problem has arisen. So, both male and female causes of infertility need to be explored.

Treatment | Obviously, no treatment can be planned until a diagnosis of the problem has been made.

Understanding the Physiology

For a man to produce sperm requires LH and FSH release from the anterior pituitary stimulating testosterone production from the Leydig cells and spermatogenesis from the Sertoli cells of the testes. An adequate number of sperm must be produced (Mr. Anderson's sperm count is low) and be present in the ejaculate for the probability of fertilization to be high enough. In addition, the sperm produced must be capable of maturation, capacitation, and activation, processes that occur in the male reproductive tract and the female tract. (The motility of Mr. Anderson's sperm is below normal.) In addition, the male reproductive tract must produce semen with appropriate concentrations of several substances that support sperm viability.

Anatomically, the most common problem that is encountered in studies of infertile men is the presence of a varicocele, abnormal veins within the spermatic cord, which results in an elevation of the temperature of the testes.

Females must regularly ovulate at the midpoint of their menstrual cycle. This requires appropriate release of GnRH from the hypothalamus, LH and FSH secretion from the anterior pituitary, and the production of estrogen by the ovaries. The ovum released must be capable of being fertilized. When released, the ovum must travel through the female reproductive tract and must meet the sperm that are moving from the vagina (where they have been deposited) to the fallopian tubes.

When the ovum is fertilized, it must then correctly implant itself in the wall of the uterus, which has been prepared for this by the hormonal changes that have occurred in the woman.

If any of these steps are defective, pregnancy will not result, and the couple will be infertile.

The accompanying flow chart (**Fig. X.1**) illustrates both the distribution of problems leading to infertility and the testing regime that is followed to diagnosis the problem.

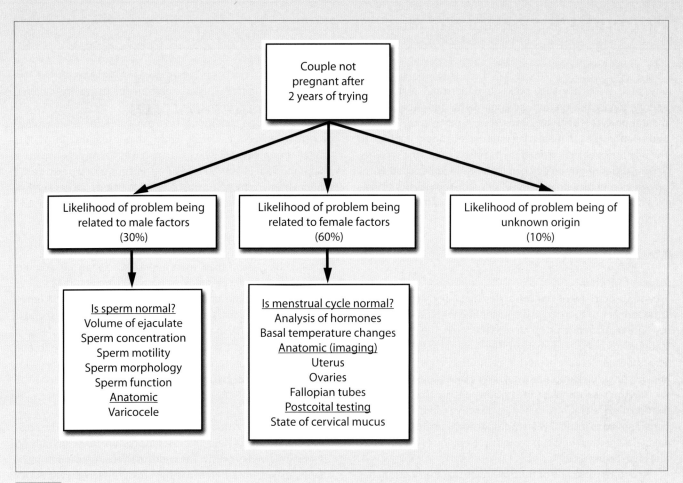

Fig. X.1 A flow chart illustrating the diagnostic procedures that can be used to determine the cause of infertility.

Appendix A   Principles of Physics in Physiology

Physics is a science that seeks to understand matter and energy, forces and motion, heat and light, and other fundamental processes that are observable in our world. The laws and relationships that have been uncovered apply not only to the inanimate objects around us, but also to all living systems. Several areas of physiology cannot be fully understood without an elementary knowledge of physics. Key physics principles that are important to our understanding of physiology are briefly discussed below.

Mechanics

Laws of Motion
Newton's first law of motion states that a body continues to be stationary or to move in a straight line with uniform velocity until it is acted upon by an external force. The law helps in defining force itself (see below). The law is also known as the *law of inertia.* Because of inertia, a stationary body cannot start moving on its own and a moving body cannot stop on its own.

Newton's second law of motion tells us that the acceleration or deceleration of a body is directly proportional to the force applied to it and inversely proportional to the mass of the body. The product of the mass and acceleration of a body gives the force acting on it.

Newton's third law of motion states that every action has an equal and opposite reaction.

Newton's three laws, first described in the 17th century, underlie our understanding of many physical phenomena and represent the foundation of much of physics.

Force
Force is anything that changes or tends to change the uniform motion of a body in a straight line. When you "push" or "pull" the sofa in your living room, you are applying a force to it, and the sofa will start to move; it will accelerate. There are many different kinds of forces that can affect the motion of objects, Friction, the result of interaction between an object and the surface on which it is found, acts like a force and alters the motion of objects in motion. Gravity (see below) is a force, and electrical and magnetic phenomena also act as forces. The chemical bonds holding molecules together are also forces.

Gravitational force, as applicable on earth, is a special kind of force that has two remarkable features: (1) It is always directed toward the center of the earth and thus defines the vertical. (2) It is directly proportional to the mass of the body. The acceleration produced by gravitational force is called *acceleration due to gravity.* A heavier body is pulled with a greater gravitational force (in accordance with Newton's law of gravitation). However, for a given force, a heavier body has less acceleration (in accordance with Newton's second law of motion). Therefore, the acceleration due to gravity does not vary with the mass of a body and remains absolutely constant at 9.8 m/sec/sec. In other words, all objects, regardless of their mass,

fall at the same rate. This acceleration due to gravity, denoted by g, is the weight of an object.

Under certain conditions (riding in a elevator or on a rollercoaster), we feel heavier or lighter than usual due to what is called the *apparent g,* which is denoted as Gz. Any change in Gz has important effects on cardiac output and blood pressure. Gz differs from g only when the body is subjected to other vertical accelerative forces in addition to the gravitational force.

Fluids

A solid object has a fixed mass and a fixed shape and volume. The atoms or molecules making up a solid are not free to move much because of intramolecular forces that are present. A liquid (fluid) has a fixed mass and a constant volume, but its shape is determined by the shape of its container. The molecules of a liquid have a much greater freedom to move relative to one another than is present in a solid. Water, which obviously includes body fluids, is the most common liquid found on earth.

Pressure
Pressure is the force per unit area exerted on a surface. The pressure of a column of fluid (hydrostatic pressure) depends only on its vertical height; neither the width of the column, nor its inclination makes any difference to the pressure exerted (**Fig. A.1A**). This concept is of importance in understanding the measurement of jugular venous pressure and the direct manometry of blood pressure. The dependence of fluid pressure on the height of the fluid column also explains why the venous pressure is higher in the dependent parts of the body (below the heart) and why the atmospheric pressure decreases at high altitudes. Its knowledge helps in estimating the pressure at different depths of the sea, which is important in deep-sea diving.

Fluid pressure is often expressed in terms of the vertical height of a fluid column because the pressure exerted by a fluid column is given by $h\rho g$, where h is the height of the fluid column, and ρ is the density of the fluid. The fluid of reference is usually mercury, but it can be water, saline, or even blood, whichever is convenient. The pressure exerted by 1 mm of mercury column, 1 mm Hg, is also called 1 torr. Because mercury is 13.6 times denser than water, 1 torr equals 13.6 mm of water pressure.

Even atmospheric pressure is commonly expressed in terms of the height of the mercury column that would counterbalance it. The pressure exerted by one atmosphere is 760 mm of mercury, or 760 torr. *Pressures recorded inside the body are usually referenced to atmospheric pressure.* Thus, a recorded mean blood pressure of 100 mm Hg is actually 100 mm Hg + 760 mm Hg in absolute terms. This method of specifying pressures in the body explains what it means when the measured pressure is said to be -7 mm Hg (or 763 mm Hg absolute pressure).

The mercury manometer (**Fig. A.1B**) is commonly used for measuring pressure. One limb of the manometer is connected to the system whose pressure is to be measured. The other limb of the manometer is left open to the atmosphere. The difference in the mercury column in the two limbs indicates the pressure of the system in excess of the atmospheric pressure.

Determinants of Flow

Fluid will flow (move) in a tube if there is a difference in pressure between the two ends of the tube. In a closed system, fluid flow will occur if there is a difference in pressure between two points in the system. The pressure difference is often referred to as a pressure gradient. Fluid flows from the region with high pressure to the region at low pressure. Of course, flow can only occur as long as the tube (or system) is patent (open along its entire length).

What determines the rate of flow (expressed as volume/unit time)? The larger the pressure gradient the greater the flow will be. However, in every system there is opposition to the occurrence of flow, commonly referred to as resistance. The greater the resistance (with the pressure gradient held constant), the smaller will be the flow. Thus, we can write an equation for flow:

$$Flow = \frac{P_1 - P_2}{R} \qquad (A.1)$$

This is a mathematical representation of the general model of flow.

The opposition to flow of a fluid, or resistance, is a property of the system, and it is described quantitatively by the Poiseuille equation:

$$R = \frac{8\eta L}{\pi r^4} \qquad (A.2)$$

where η is the viscosity of the fluid, L is the length of the vessel, and r is the radius of the vessel.

This tells us that as the length of the vessel increases it resistance to flow increases. Most significantly, it tells us that changes in the radius of a vessel will result in a very large change in resistance because r is raised to the 4th power.

Thus, when the flow rate, fluid viscosity, and tube radius remain constant, the pressure drop $(P_1 - P_2)$ along a tube is directly proportional to the length of the tube and inversely proportional to the tube radius, as illustrated in **Figs. A.2A** and **A.2B**.

Surface Tension

Surface tension is the property of a liquid surface, which causes it to behave like a stretched membrane. Because of surface

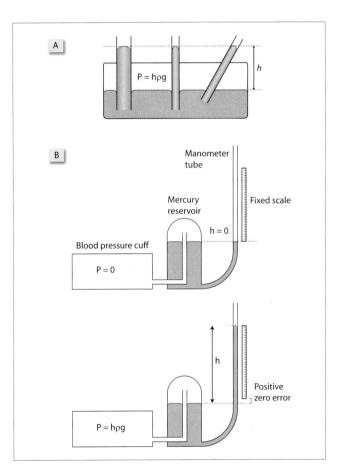

Fig. A.1 **(A)** Hydrostatic pressure in a column of fluid depends only on the vertical height of the fluid column. It is unaffected by the diameter of the column or the inclination of the tube. **(B)** A mercury manometer connected to a rubber cuff is used in sphygmomanometry. (*Above*) The cuff pressure is zero, and the mercury levels in the reservoir and manometer tube are equal. (*Below*) As the cuff pressure increases, the mercury level in the tube rises while the mercury level in the reservoir falls. The difference, h, in the mercury levels gives the cuff pressure.

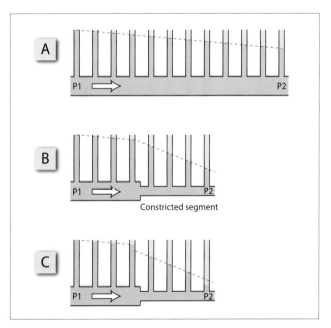

Fig. A.2 A horizontal tube is fitted with uniformly spaced manometers for measuring the pressure drop. **(A)** The pressure falls uniformly with length in accordance with the Poiseuille-Hagen formula; as length increases, the resistance increases, and pressure falls proportionately. **(B)** In a smaller tube, the resistance is increased, and pressure falls more steeply with distance (flow and flow velocity are low). **(C)** If flow velocity is higher, the pressure falls in the narrow segment in accordance with Bernoulli's principle.

tension, a drop of fluid tries to minimize its surface area. It therefore assumes a spherical shape because the surface-to-volume ratio is minimal for a sphere. The fact that a bubble does not collapse completely is due to the fact that the air inside it provides a distending pressure that exactly balances the collapsing pressure of the fluid shell.

The **law of Laplace** relates the tension, T, in the wall of a cylinder or a sphere, the transmural pressure, P, and the radius, R. For a cyliondrical structure such as a blood vessel, Laplace's law can be expressed as

$$T = P \times R \qquad (A.3)$$

For a sphere, the equation is

$$T = P \times R/2 \qquad (A.4)$$

Both equations A.3 and A.4 assume that the thickness of the wall, w, is small and can be ignored. However, if this is not the case, if the wall thickness is of the same order of magnitude as the radius, then the approximation does not hold. The Laplace equations then become

$$T = P \times R/w \qquad (A.5)$$

$$T = P \times R/2w \qquad (A.6)$$

The law of Laplace helps explain several interesting phenomena. (1) It explains how the thin-walled capillaries are able to withstand an internal distending pressure of 25 mm Hg, the normal capillary hydrostatic pressure. This is possible because capillaries have a very small radius, R. Thus, the tension, T, in their walls, the circumferential force acting to tear the wall, is small and does not exceed the mechanical strength of the wall. (2) The law of Laplace also explains why the dilated heart has to do more work. When the radius, R, increases, the wall tension, T, must go up, and it is T that determines the rate of oxygen consumption of the heart. (3) In accordance with the Laplace's law, the lower the functional residual capacity of the lungs, the more difficult it is to inflate it. (4) Because of Laplace's law, the greater the gastric filling, the lower is the pressure that causes gastric emptying. This is obviously beneficial to the process of digestion. (5) Laplace's law explains why reduction in detrusor muscle tension prevents the rise of intravesical pressure even as the bladder fills up to greater volume.

Viscosity

Viscosity is fluid friction. When fluid moves along a tube, it does so in the form of multiple layers, or laminae, that slip on one another, moving at different velocities due to friction between the layers and between the fluid and the wall of the tube. The lamina at the middle of the blood vessel moves fastest; the one closest to the vessel wall does not move at all. Thus, there is a velocity gradient of laminae, which is called the *shear rate*.

A Newtonian fluid is one in which the viscosity is independent of the shear rate. Blood is not a Newtonian fluid, although it is often possible to ignore this in analyzing many physiologic phenomena.

Just as friction affects the velocity of an object moving over a surface, viscosity affects the velocity of fluid flow. In a long, narrow tube of uniform radius, the relation of the flow rate (Q) with the pressure gradient ($P_1 - P_2$), that is, the pressure difference at the two ends of the tube, fluid viscosity (η), tube radius (R), and tube length (L), is given by the *Poiseuille-Hagen formula*.

$$Q = (P_1 - P_2) \times \frac{\pi}{8} \times \frac{1}{\eta} \times \frac{r^4}{L} \qquad (A.7)$$

This relationship is important in the understanding of hemodynamics. Because resistance varies inversely with the fourth power of the radius, even small changes in the vessel diameter cause large variations in blood flow through it, enabling effective regulation of blood flow through vascular beds. The relevance of the Poiseuille-Hagen formula is exemplified by the differences in the blood flow in the renal cortex and the renal medulla, where blood viscosity, capillary length, and capillary diameter all have a role in determining the distribution of flow that is present.

The same relationships that describe the flow of blood in the circulation also describe the flow of air in the airways of the lungs.

Turbulent versus Laminar Flow

At low velocities of flow (distance/unit time), a Newtonian fluid has a streamlined or laminar pattern of flow. There is little dissipation of energy in laminar flow, and such flow is quiet. However, at high velocities, the flow of fluid becomes turbulent and does not remain streamlined. The likelihood of turbulence being present is related to the diameter of the vessel and the viscosity of the blood. This likelihood is expressed by the *Reynolds number*.

$$Re = \frac{\rho DV}{\eta} \qquad (A.8)$$

where Re is the Reynolds number, ρ is the density of the fluid, D is the diameter of the tube (in cm), V is the velocity of the flow (in cm/sec), and η is the viscosity of the fluid (in poise). The higher the value of Re, the greater is the probability of turbulence. When $Re < 2000$, flow is usually not turbulent, whereas if $Re > 3000$, turbulence is usually present.

When flow is turbulent, there is dissipation of energy, and some of this lost energy is present as audible sound. Thus, turbulent flow of blood is responsible for cardiac murmurs (present when certain pathologies are present in the cardio-vascular system) and the Korotkoff sounds, which are used in measuring blood pressure with a sphygmomanometer.

Bernoulli's Principle

When fluid flow through a tube is constant, the total fluid energy—the sum of its kinetic energy and pressure energy—remains constant. This is known as *Bernoulli's principle*, and it helps us to understand several important hemodynamic phenomena. It explains, for example, why the fluid pressure is low in a blood vessel at places where its radius is less (**Fig. A.2C**); the flow velocity is increased here, and hence more of the total energy is present as kinetic energy, and less is present as pressure energy. It also explains the suction effect of venous blood flow on the thoracic duct terminating in the vein (see **Fig. 36.6**).

The fact that both the Poiseuille-Hagen formula and Bernoulli's principle describe the effect of tube diameter on fluid pressure need not be cause for confusion. The two formulas deal with different aspects of fluid energy. The Poiseuille-Hagen formula deals with the conversion of fluid pressure into heat and the resultant loss of fluid pressure as the fluid flows through a long tube of uniform diameter. It does not deal with the other forms of fluid energy like kinetic energy.

Work and Energy

Work is done when the point at which a force (F) is applied moves through a certain distance (D). Stated mathematically,

$$\text{Work done } (W) = F \times D \qquad (A.9)$$

Energy is the capacity for doing work and the unit of energy is the same as that of work, the joule. The energy that is associated with motion is called *kinetic energy* (KE) and is given by the formula

$$KE = \tfrac{1}{2}mv^2 \qquad (A.10)$$

where m is the mass of the body, and v is its velocity. The amount of kinetic energy that a body can gain by falling under the effect of gravity gives a measure of its potential energy (PE) and is given by the formula

$$PE = mgh \qquad (A.11)$$

where m is the mass of the body, g is acceleration due to gravity, and h is the height from which the body can fall.

When work is done by a body by expending its own energy, the work done is said to be positive. For example, a body that falls from a certain height expends its potential energy; therefore, the work done *by the body* is positive. Conversely, a body that is lifted against gravity gains in potential energy; therefore, the work done *on the body* is negative.

When a fluid (gas or liquid) is compressed by application of pressure, P, the fluid gains in energy, which is at least partly in the form of heat. The work done on the fluid is therefore negative and is given by

$$\text{Work done } (W) = -\Delta P \times \Delta V \qquad (A.12)$$

where ΔV is the small decrement in volume through which it has been compressed. Conversely, for expanding against an incumbent pressure, the fluid has to expend energy; therefore, it loses energy. The work done *by* the fluid is therefore positive and is given by

$$\text{Work done } (W) = +\Delta P \times \Delta V \qquad (A.13)$$

These concepts help us understand why the work done by the lungs or the heart is given by the area enclosed in its pressure–volume loop.

In the case of the lungs, the work done on the lungs is negative during inspiration because the lungs themselves do not expend any energy; rather, they are made to inflate by the inspiratory muscles. During inspiration, the lungs gain in elastic recoil energy. This recoil energy stored in the lungs is expended during expiration as the lungs deflate. Therefore, the work done by the lungs during expiration is positive. The work done on and by the lungs during inspiration and expiration are shown graphically in **Fig. A.3A**. When the work done during inspiration and expiration are added, we are left with a small amount of negative work done that is represented by the area enclosed within the *pressure–volume loop*. The negative work signifies that at the end of one breathing cycle, work has been done on the lungs *by* the respiratory muscles that have expended their energy. The lungs have not spent energy of their own; rather, they have gained some energy. This energy is the heat energy that has been generated by the frictional (viscous) forces inside the lungs.

In the same way, the area inside the ventricular pressure–volume loop of the cardiac cycle gives the positive work done *by* the ventricle in overcoming viscous resistance of blood flow (**Fig. A.3B**).

Heat and Temperature

The concepts of heat and temperature both refer to the motion of the atoms or molecules making up an object. *Temperature* is a measure of the average velocity of the moving particles and hence their average kinetic energy; the higher the temperature of the object the higher that average velocity. Thus, temperature is related to the thermal energy contained in an object by virtue of this constant movement of atoms and

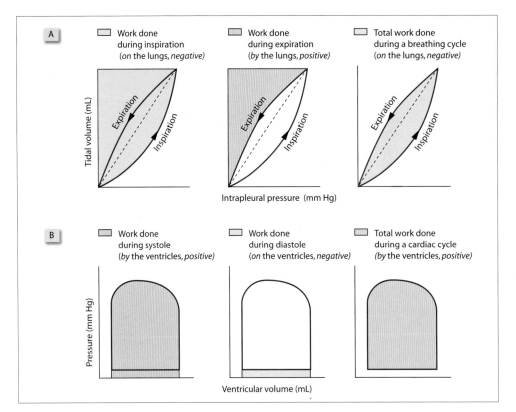

Fig. A.3 **(A)** Work done on the lung during breathing. **(B)** Work done by the ventricle during a cardiac cycle.

molecules. *Heat* is the thermal energy that is transferred from one system to another when there is a difference in temperature (a temperature gradient) between two locations or objects (**Fig. A.4**).

In nature, heat always flows from a higher temperature to a lower temperature. When the temperatures of two bodies are equal, no heat transfer occurs between them. When *conduction* occurs, the transfer of heat occurs through a medium whose molecules do not move about freely. Thus, when we hold an iron rod in fire, the iron atoms vibrate and transfer the heat from the fire to the hand through the rod. However, the iron

atoms do not move from their fixed places. When *convection* occurs, the molecules of the medium transfer heat by actually moving about, carrying the heat with them. A room radiator is an example of convective heating; the air above the radiator is heated and expands and cooler, denser air replaces it until it too is heated. No medium is required for heat transfer to occur by *radiation*. It is through radiation that heat from the sun travels through space and reaches us. Heat transfer occurs through all possible modes. If a medium is present and the molecules are free to move about, heat will travel through convection. If the molecules cannot move about, heat will tra-

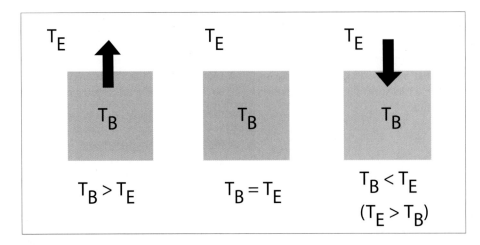

Figure A.4 When there is a difference in temperature between two objects, there will be a flow of heat from the hotter object to the colder object.

vel through conduction. Regardless of whether a medium is present or not, some heat will always travel through radiation.

Knowledge of the modes of heat transfer is relevant to the understanding of thermoregulation in the body and explains our behavioral responses to changes in environmental temperature. For example, it is through convection that the circulating blood maintains a fairly uniform temperature throughout the body. The body is cooled through the evaporation of sweat. We seek shade because it cuts off the direct radiation heat from the sun although we still feel the convective heat of hot air or the conductive heat of the ground we lie upon. We wear dark, coarse-textured clothes in winter because dark surfaces absorb radiated heat. We wear light-colored clothes in summer because they reflect back heat radiation. Thick woolen clothes that trap air in them reduce conductive and convective losses of body heat in winter. Convective currents are employed in the caloric stimulation test for testing vestibular functions.

Electricity

Electrical charge | Atoms are made of protons, neutrons, and electrons. A proton has a unit positive charge, an electron has a unit negative charge, and neutrons do not have any charge on them. A body containing equal numbers of protons and electrons is electrostatically neutral. When the number of electrons in a body exceeds the number of protons in it, the body develops a negative charge. Conversely, it develops a positive charge when the number of electrons is less than the number of protons in it. The SI (International System of Units) unit of charge is the *coulomb*, which equals the charge of 6.242×10^{18} electrons.

Current | The flow of charged particles is called an electric current. The SI unit of current is the *ampere*. A flow of 1 coulomb of charge every second is 1 ampere current.

Potential | The electrical potential of a body is the work done when a charge of +1 coulomb of charge approaches the body from infinity under the effect of the attractive or repulsive force that exists between the body and the charges. If the work done is 1 joule, the potential of the body is 1 *volt*, which is the SI unit of potential. Two charged bodies have 1-volt potential difference if 1 joule of work is done in moving a charge of +1 coulomb from one body to the other.

Resistance | The resistance of a conductor determines how much current it allows to pass through it when a potential difference is applied across it: for a given potential difference across a conductor, the current flowing through the conductor is inversely proportional to its resistance. This is known as the *Ohm's law*. If the current is 1 ampere when the potential difference is 1 volt, the resistance is said to be 1 ohm, which is the SI unit of resistance. Conductance is the reciprocal of resistance, and its SI unit is mho.

$$\text{Voltage} = \text{Current} \times \text{Resistance} \qquad (A.14)$$

An important derivation of Ohm's law is that when resistances ($R1, R2, R3 \ldots$) are added in series (**Fig. A.5A**), the total resistance (R) is given by

$$R_T = R_1 + R_2 + R_3 \ldots \qquad (A.15)$$

When R_1, R_2, and R_3 are connected in parallel (**Fig. A.5B**), the total resistance is given by the formula

$$1/R_T = 1/R_1 + 1/R_2 + 1/R_3 \qquad (A.16)$$

The resistance of a conductor varies directly with its length and inversely with its cross-sectional area. This principle is important in the understanding of nerve conduction and explains why nerve conduction velocity increases with axon diameter.

It is useful to note that the equation describing the flow of a fluid as a function of the pressure gradient that is present and the resistance to flow is analogous to the equation describing the flow of charges, electrical current. This is, of course, simply a restatement of the general model of flow.

Capacitance | The potential of a body is directly proportional to the amount of charge it contains. The greater the amount of charge a body contains, the greater is its potential. However, the extent to which the potential rises when a given amount of charge is imparted to it will differ for different bodies. A body that can hold a large amount of charge without much rise in its potential is said to have a high capacitance. Stated mathematically,

$$\text{Capacitance} = \frac{\text{Charge}}{\text{Potential}} \qquad (A.17)$$

Larger bodies have higher capacitance; therefore, the earth has a capacitance that can usually be regarded as infinite. Thus, the potential of earth (ground potential) remains unchanged no matter how much charge enters it. This stable ground potential is assumed to be zero and serves as a convenient reference for all electrical measurements. For the same reason, any

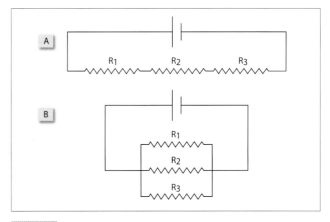

Fig. A.5 Resistances in series **(A)** sum ($R_T = R_1 + R_2 + R_3$); for resistances in parallel **(B)**, the total resistance is smaller than any single resistance ($1/R_T = 1/R_1 + 1/R_2 + 1/R_3$).

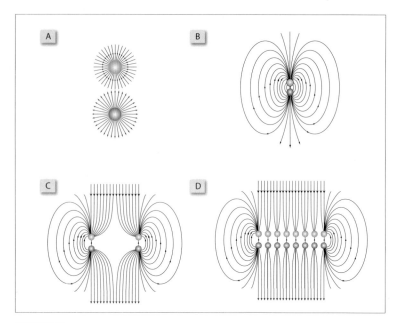

Fig. A.6 **(A)** The electric field of a positive charge (*red*) and a negative charge (*blue*). Each line is a vector representing the force and direction of the repulsive or attractive force exerted on a charge of +1 coulomb. **(B)** The lines of force around a dipole. **(C)** The lines of force when two dipoles are placed side by side. **(D)** When several dipoles are lined up, the current flowing along the long axis of the dipoles summate and are recorded by a distant electrode.

charged body, when grounded, loses all its charge to the earth, and its potential becomes zero.

A device that can store a large amount of charge is called a *capacitor*. A capacitor can hold a lot of charge, yet its potential remains low. On the other hand, a body with a low capacitance develops a high potential when it is charged. At high potentials, charge tends to "leak out"; hence, a body with low capacitance cannot hold much charge. A capacitor can be built by sandwiching a thin sheet of dielectric (nonconducting material) between two parallel metal plates. Such a capacitor is called a *parallel plate capacitor*. When a potential difference is applied to the plates, a large amount of charge gets stored in the plates. The nerve membrane behaves like a dielectric, and when both its surfaces are layered with ions of opposite charges, it acts like a parallel plate capacitor (see **Fig. 10.1**). Membrane capacitance is an important determinant of membrane excitability and conduction velocity of nerve membranes.

Electric Field of Dipoles

Electric field refers to the area of influence of an electric charge (or charges). The electric field of a single charged particle is depicted in **Fig. A.6A**. Each vector in the diagram represents the direction and force with which a positive charge of 1 coulomb moves (or tends to move) under the effect of the electric field. If an electric field is applied to a medium containing mobile charged particles, the charged particles start moving along the lines of the electric field, resulting in the flow of an electric current. This happens in body fluid where an electric field is set up by the heart.

A **dipole** is a pair of opposite charges lying close together. The electric field set up by a dipole is more complex. Each

dipole results in the flow of current between the opposite charges along multiple pathways as shown in **Fig. A.6B**. Although the conventional current flows from the positive to the negative charge, to a recording electrode placed at a distance, the current appears to flow along a vector directed from the negative to the positive charge.

Multiple dipoles located along a line result in a large resultant current. Each dipole generates a large field around it as shown in **Figs. A.6C and A.6D**. Only currents that travel straight along the axis of the dipole get added up and become strong enough to be picked up by a distant recording electrode. Knowledge of dipoles and their fields is essential to the understanding of electrocardiography and electroencephalography.

Appendix B Principles of Chemistry in Physiology

Chemistry is another physical science that is concerned with the structure and properties of matter and energy at the molecular level (atoms in combinations), and with the interactions, chemical reactions, that between them, Chemistry seeks to understand many phenomena that occur in the world around us. Chemistry describes and explains phenomena that we encounter when we seek to understand some of the phenomena in our bodies. Here we will review some important concepts from chemistry that help us to understand physiology.

Gases

Gases are a form of matter in which the constituent atoms or molecules move freely and randomly. The average distance between particles is large; hence, the density is low. Gases fill their container and are compressible. The laws that describe the behavior of gases have important applications in our understanding of the physiology of the respiratory system.

Universal Gas Law

The volume of a gas (V) is directly proportional to the absolute temperature (T) of the gas (Charles' law) and inversely proportional to the pressure (P) applied upon it (Boyle's law). The volume is also directly proportional to n, the number of moles of gas that are present (Avogadro's law). These three relationships can be combined to yield the ideal gas law. Stated mathematically:

$$PV = nRT \tag{B.1}$$

where R is the proportionality constant and is called the *universal gas constant*.

The variability in gas volume with temperature and pressure makes it imperative to express all gas volumes at standard temperature and pressure (STP). The standard temperature is 0°C (273 Kelvin), and the *standard pressure* is 1 atmosphere (760 mm Hg).

In physiology, gas volumes are often expressed at body temperature (37°C) and 1 atmosphere pressure (BTP = body temperature pressure).

Dalton's Law of Partial Pressure

When two or more gases are mixed, the total pressure exerted by the mixture is equal to the sum of the pressures exerted by the component gases when occupying the same volume.

Suppose 500 mL of oxygen (O_2) and 500 mL of nitrogen (N_2) in separate tanks (**Fig. B.1**) each have a temperature of 0°C and an initial pressure of 760 mm Hg. The valve separating the tanks is opened, and the gases are mixed. This creates a gas mixture with a volume of 1 L. What will be the final pressure exerted by the mixture? Because the final volume of the

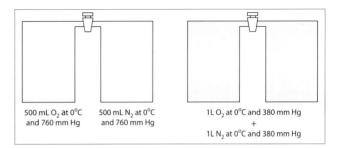

500 mL O_2 at 0°C and 760 mm Hg   500 mL N_2 at 0°C and 760 mm Hg   1L O_2 at 0°C and 380 mm Hg + 1L N_2 at 0°C and 380 mm Hg

Fig. B.1   An example of Dalton's law of partial pressures.

gaseous mixture is 1 L, each of the gases will come to occupy the available 1 L volume. In accordance with Boyle's law, the pressure of each gas will drop to 380 mm Hg. Finally, in accordance with Dalton's law of partial pressure, the pressure of the mixture will be 380 + 380 = 760 mm Hg.

In the above example, the pressure of 380 mm Hg is called the *partial pressure* of each of the constituent gases. It is calculated by the formula

$$P_{gas} = P_{total} \times \% \ of \ gas \ in \ mixture \tag{B.2}$$

For example, atmospheric air contains 21% O_2. Therefore, the partial pressure of oxygen in atmospheric air will be 760 × 21% = 160 mm Hg.

The partial pressure of a gas dissolved in a liquid is equal to the partial pressure of the gas in a gaseous mixture, which is in equilibrium with the liquid. In other words, there is no net flux of gas between the liquid and gas phases because the "concentration gradient" is zero.

The Partial Pressure of Water Vapor

When water vapor saturates a gas or a gas mixture, it exerts an additional pressure of 47 mm Hg at 37°C. This pressure is called the *saturated vapor pressure* or the *aqueous tension*. When air is saturated with water vapor, the concentration of all the other constituent gases decreases. However, the percentage composition of a gas mixture is always expressed, assuming that there is no moisture in it. For example, when we say that O_2 constitutes 21% of atmospheric air, we actually mean 21% of "dry" atmospheric air. If the air is saturated with water vapor, the saturated vapor pressure has to be deducted from the atmospheric pressure before calculating the partial pressure of constituent gases individually. For example, the partial pressure of O_2 (Po_2) in humidified atmospheric air (at 37°C) is (760 – 47) × 21% = 150 mm Hg.

In physiology, it is a common practice to record the volume of gases saturated with water vapor at body temperature and at atmospheric pressure. Volumes thus recorded are denoted as BTPS (S for saturated).

Solutions

A solution is a uniform mixture of two different substances, either solids in a liquid or a solid in another solid. We will be concerned only with solutions that are composed of substances (solutes) dissolved in water (the solvent). The cell is filled with an aqueous solution, and the space between cells is filled with a different aqueous solution.

Describing the Concentration of Solutions

When some substance is dissolved in water, the resulting solution has a concentration, which is simply the amount of substance per volume of solution:

$$Concentration = Amount/Volume \qquad (B.3)$$

We can specify the concentration in a variety of ways, but all relate to the idea of a "mole" of a substance. A mole (mol) is the name applied to 6.023×10^{23} atoms or molecules of a substance. The weight of one mole of atoms or molecules of any element or compound is exactly equal to the atomic or molecular weight of the element or compound expressed in grams (g). For example, the molecular weight of sodium chloride (NaCl) is 58.5 (Na = 23 and Cl = 35.5). Therefore, 6.023×10^{23} molecules (i.e., 1 mol) of NaCl weighs exactly 58.5 g. So, 1 mole of NaCl in 1 L of water gives a solution with a concentration of 1 mol/L (or 1000 mmol/L).

We can also specify a solution of ions by the number of charges that present per unit volume. If 1 mole of NaCl is dissolved in water, there will be 1 Equivalent (1000 mEq) of positive charges and 1 Equivalent of negative charges in solution. If the ion carries a charge of 2+ (like calcium), then there would be 2 Equivalents of positive charge in solution.

In physiology, all solutions are aqueous solutions, with water being the solvent.

Diffusion of Solutes

Simple diffusion | If there are two solutions of different solute concentrations separated by a membrane that is permeable to the solute, the solutes diffuse from higher to lower concentration. This is because the molecules in solution, due to their constant random motion, are more likely to be moving from a region of high concentration to a region of low concentration than vice versa. Thus, there is a net flux from high to low concentration until the concentration is the same everywhere. The greater the concentration of a substance in solution, the greater is the flux of solute that will occur. Hence, although solutes in both solutions are diffusing farther apart, there is a net flux of solutes from higher to lower concentration. The magnitude of the diffusing tendency (the flux, J) from one region to another is directly proportional to the cross-sectional area across which the diffusion takes place and the concentration gradient, which is the difference in concentration of the diffusing substance divided by the thickness of the boundary (*Fick's law of diffusion*). Thus,

$$J = -DA\frac{\Delta c}{\Delta x} \qquad (B.4)$$

where J is the net rate of diffusion, D is the diffusion coefficient, A is the area of the partition that separates the two solutions, and $\Delta c/\Delta x$ is the concentration gradient (i.e., the rate of change of concentration with distance). The minus sign is a sign convention that indicates the direction of diffusion. When solutes diffuse from higher to lower concentration, $\Delta c/\Delta x$ is negative, and therefore multiplying by $-DA$ gives a positive value.

Nernst potential | When two ionic solutions, A and B, of different concentrations (C_A and C_B) are separated by a permeable membrane, the ions tend to diffuse along their concentration gradient. Because ions are charged particles, their diffusion can be stopped by an appropriate electrical potential (E) applied across the membrane. The magnitude and polarity of the potential that must be applied to side A of the membrane for stopping the diffusion of ions (E_A) is given by the *Nernst equation:*

$$E_A = \frac{61}{z}\log\frac{[C_B]}{[C_A]} \qquad (B.5)$$

where z is the valence of the ion. This equation can also be written as

$$E_A = \frac{-61}{z}\log\frac{[C_A]}{[C_B]} \qquad (B.6)$$

In the example illustrated in **Fig. B.2**, with a concentration gradient of potassium (K^+) on side A (150 mEq/L) and side B (5 mEq/L), the Nernst equation gives a value of –90 millivolts (mV) across the membrane. This potential is called the *Nernst potential* for K^+ (E_K).

$$E_K = \frac{-61}{+1}\log\frac{150}{5}$$

It has *two* implications. (1) It means that –90 mV applied to side A will prevent any outward diffusion of the K^+. (2) It also means that if the K^+ concentrations are equal on both sides of the membrane, a potential difference of –90 mV applied to the membrane will result in the same ionic concentration ratio of 30 (i.e., 150 ÷ 5) across the membrane.

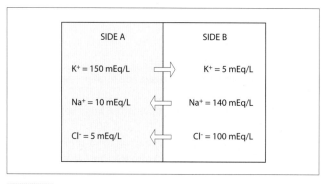

Fig. B.2 Ionic distribution in two compartments for illustrating the principles of Nernst potential.

Similarly, the diffusion of Na^+ will be prevented by a potential of +70 mV (E_{Na}) applied to side A, and the diffusion of Cl^- (E_{Cl}) will be prevented by applying a potential of –80 mV to side A because

$$E_{Na} = \frac{-61}{+1} \log \frac{10}{140}$$

$$E_{Cl} = \frac{-61}{-1} \log \frac{5}{100}$$

Thus, every ion distributed asymmetrically across the membrane has its own Nernst potential (E) that will prevent its diffusion. In other words, the Nernst potential of an ion gives the electrical equivalent of its diffusion energy.

Gibbs-Donnan equilibrium | If two compartments are separated by a semipermeable membrane, and one of the compartments contains diffusible ions (Na^+ and chloride [Cl^-]), the ions will soon distribute themselves equally across the two compartments (**Fig. B.3A**). If, however, one of the compartments (compartment A) contains impermeable ions, the typical equilibrium (with equal numbers of ions on both sides of the membrane) as observed in simple diffusion will not occur. Instead, a different type of equilibrium called the *Gibbs-Donnan equilibrium* (**Fig. B.3B**) will occur in which two conditions must be satisfied: (1) both the compartments must be electroneutral, and (2) the product of *diffusible* ions (anions and cations) must be equal in both compartments. The solution is shown in **Table B.1**.

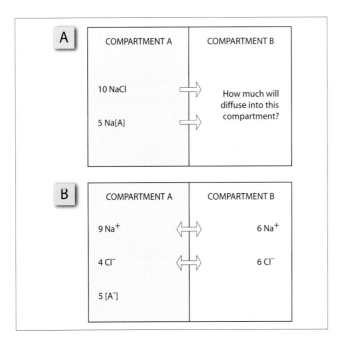

Fig. B.3 Ionic distribution in two compartments for illustrating the principles of Gibbs-Donnan equilibrium. *A* denotes an impermeable anion (negatively charged ion). **(A)** The initial state; sodium (Na^+) and chloride (Cl^-) will diffuse from compartment A to compartment B down their concentration gradients. **(B)** The equilibrium state: there is no net diffusion of Na^+ and Cl^- between the compartments. Note, however, that the concentrations of Na^+ and Cl^- are not equal in the two compartments.

Table B.1 Ionic Distribution at Gibbs–Donnan Equilibrium (See Fig. B.3)

	Inside	Outside
Total + charge	9 (Na^+)	6 (Na^+)
Total – charge	9 (4 Cl^- + 5 A$^-$)	6 (Cl^-)
Product of diffusible ions [Na^+] x [Cl^-]	36 (9 Na^+ × 4 Cl^-)	36 (6 Na^+ × 6 Cl^-)
Total number of ions	18 (9 + 4 + 5)	12 (6 + 6)

At equilibrium, compartment A will have a larger concentration of solutes (18) than compartment B (12). As a result, water will move from B to A due to osmosis and thereby decrease the solute concentration in compartment A. However, because the impermeable anion continues to be present in compartment A, the Gibbs-Donnan equilibrium is reestablished. As a result, compartment A would continue to have a higher solute concentration, no matter how much osmosis occurs.

All living cells contain impermeable proteins anions. This imposes the Gibbs-Donnan equilibrium, so that there are more ions inside the cell than outside it. As a result, water continuously moves into the cell by osmosis, which will inevitably rupture the cell. To survive, the cell must continuously pump out excess ions. It does so with the help of the ATP-driven Na^+-K^+ pump. When a cell dies, the pump stops, and the cell swells up; its microscopic appearance is known to pathologists as the "cloudy swelling."

Diffusion of Water

Osmosis is the movement of water across a semipermeable membrane that separates two solutions of different solute concentrations and restricts the movement of solutes across it. For osmosis to occur, it is not necessary for the membrane to be totally impermeable to the solute. A solute with limited permeability also produces osmosis, though to a lesser extent. The solute permeability is given by the *reflection coefficient* (s), which varies between 0 (freely permeable) and 1 (totally impermeable). The reflection coefficient is the probability of a solute molecule reflecting back from the membrane instead of passing through it. The reflection coefficient of a solute is not an absolute constant, but varies with the type of membrane. It will be zero for all solutes if the membrane has very large pores in it. Osmosis is proportional to the reflection coefficient as well as to the concentration gradient. Osmosis does not occur when the reflection coefficient is zero, that is when the membrane is freely permeable to the solute.

Osmotic pressure | The osmosis from a dilute to a concentrated solution can be prevented by increasing the hydrostatic pressure of the concentrated solution. The hydrostatic pressure necessary to prevent the osmosis is called the osmotic pressure of the solution (**Fig. B.4**).

Osmotic pressure, like freezing-point depression and boiling-point elevation, is a *colligative property*, that is it depends on the number rather than the type of particles in a solution. It is given by the *Van't Hoff relationship*:

$$\pi = RT \times \phi \, nC \qquad (B.7)$$

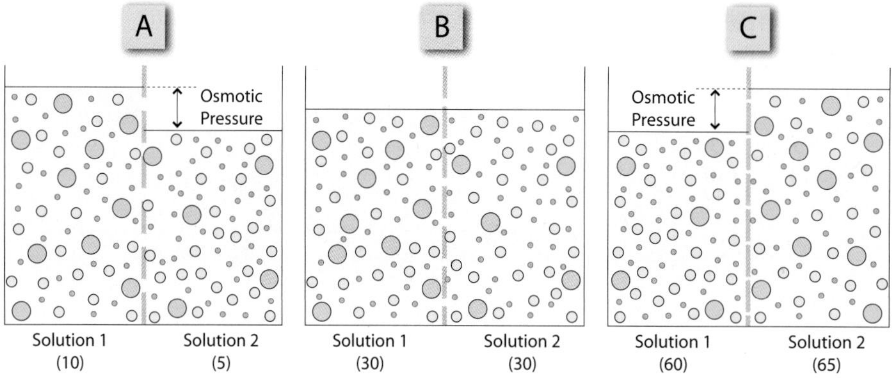

Fig. B.4 A membrane separates two solutions, 1 and 2, containing ions of three different sizes. Solution 1 contains 60 particles: 10 large, 20 medium-sized, and 30 small. Solution 2 contains 65 particles: 5 large, 25 medium-sized, and 35 small. The tonicity of the solutions depends on the membrane pore size. The figures below each solution indicate the number of osmotically active particles in it. **(A)** The pores allow only the medium and small particles to pass through, making solution 1 hypertonic. **(B)** The pores allow only the small particles to pass through, making the two solutions isotonic. **(C)** The pores are impermeable to particles of all sizes, making solution 2 hypertonic.

where π is the osmotic pressure, R is the universal gas constant, T is the absolute temperature, ϕ is the osmotic coefficient, n is the number of ions yielded by the dissociation of a solute molecule, C is the molar concentration (mol/L) of the solute.

The Van't Hoff equation shows that at a constant temperature, osmotic pressure is proportional to the number of particles in solution per unit volume of solution (given by $n \times C$ in the formula). The *osmotic coefficient* (ϕ) in the formula is not the same as the reflection coefficient. The osmotic coefficient does not depend on membrane characteristics: it is constant for a solute molecule and is assumed to be 1.0 in all approximate calculations.

Osmoles, osmolarity, and osmolality | One mole of osmotically active particles is called one *osmole* (osm). Thus, a molar solution of glucose contains 1 osmole, a molar solution of NaCl contains 2 osmoles (1 mol of Na^+ and 1 mol of Cl^-) while a molar solution of $CaCl_2$ contains 3 osmoles (1 mol of Ca^{2+} and 2 mol of Cl^-). The osmolar concentration of a solution expressed in osm/L is called *osmolarity*. When expressed as osmole per kilogram (osm/kg) of solution, it is called *osmolality*. Osmolarity is affected by temperature, which changes the volume of solution. Also, dissolution of solutes is associated with a slight rise in the volume of the solution. This increase is different for different solutes. Hence, when 1 mole of glucose is dissolved in 1 L of water, the osmolarity will be slightly less than 1 osm/L. Osmolality, however, is unaffected by temperature changes or the increased volume of the solution that accompanies dissolution. However, physiologic solutions are relatively dilute and the difference between the osmotic concentration expressed as osmolarity or osmolality is very small.

The measurement of osmolarity (nC) is based on the principle that the freezing point of a solution is depressed in proportion to the number of osmoles present in it. It is given by the formula:

$$nC = \Delta T_f / 1.86 \tag{B.8}$$

where ΔT_f is the reduction in the freezing temperature. The freezing point of normal human plasma averages -0.54°C, which corresponds to an osmolal concentration in plasma of 290 mOsm/L. This is equivalent to an osmotic pressure against pure water of 7.3 atmospheres.

Two solutions having identical osmolarity are called *isoosmolar*. They exert the same osmotic pressure and are therefore also called *isoosmotic*. If one of the two has greater osmolarity, it is said to be *hyperosmolar* or *hyperosmotic* in comparison to the other, which is called *hypoosmolar* or *hypoosmotic*. Except immediately after a sudden change in composition, all fluid compartments of the body are in osmotic equilibrium.

Tonicity | Given two solutions with different osmolarity separated by a membrane, it does not necessarily mean that there will be osmosis from the hypoosmolar to the hyperosmolar solution. Whether water movement occurs depends on the characteristics of the membrane and the particular solutes involved. This is made clear by the example illustrated in **Fig. B.4** in which the solutions have solutes of three different sizes: large, medium, and small.

The three solutes are present in different concentrations in the two solutions. Solution 1 contains 10, 20, and 30 particles, per unit volume of the large, medium, and small solutes, respectively. Solution 2 contains 5, 25, and 35 particles per unit volume. It is seen that the magnitude and direction of osmosis cannot be predicted without knowing the pore-size of the membrane. (A) If the pores exclude only the largest particles but allow the medium and small particles to pass through, solution 1 will be hypertonic with respect to solution 2 although the latter is hyperosmolar. This is because the number of osmotically active particles in solution 1 is 10 whereas solution 2 has only 5. (B) If the pores exclude the large and medium-sized particles but allow the small particles to pass through, the two solutions will become isotonic and no osmosis will occur. This is because the total number of osmotically active particles will be 30 in both solutions: 10 + 20 in solution 1 and 5 + 25 in solution 2. (C) If the pores do not permit any solute to pass through, solution 2 will be hypertonic with respect to solution 1: there will not be osmosis from compartment 1 to compartment 2. This is because the total number of osmotically active particles will be 60 in solution 1 and 65 in solution 2.

In real-life situations, the complexity of biologic membranes makes it impossible to predict accurately whether a solute particle will pass through it. Moreover, body fluids contain innumerable types of solutes, which is another reason why their tonicity cannot be predicted. The only way, therefore, of estimating the tonicity is to determine it experimentally. In clinical parlance, the word *tonicity* always refers to the tonicity of a solution with respect to an erythrocyte. In other words, it is the erythrocytic cell membrane across which the tonicity is tested. If the erythrocyte shrinks in a solution by losing water through osmosis, the solution is *hypertonic*. If the erythrocyte swells up in a solution by gaining water through osmosis, the solution is *hypotonic*. If the erythrocyte neither shrinks nor swells in the solution, the solution is called *isotonic*.

The fluid used in clinics for intravenous transfusion is both isotonic and isoosmolar to the plasma. A 0.9% saline solution is most often used for the purpose. The 0.9% NaCl solution is roughly isoosmolar (308 mOsm/ L) to the body fluids (290 mOsm/ L) as can be calculated easily.

Molecular weight of NaCl = 58.5

∴ 58.5 g NaCl contain 1 mol of NaCl molecules.

∴ A solution containing 58.5 g NaCl will contain 2 osm (1 osm of Na^+ and 1 osm of Cl^-)

∴ A solution containing 9 g NaCl contains $(2 \times 9)/58.5$ mol = 0.308 osm (or 308 mOsm)

∴ The osmolarity of a 9 g/L (0.9 g%) solution = 308 mOsm/L

A 5% glucose solution is also isotonic initially when infused intravenously, but as the glucose is metabolized, the solution gradually becomes hypotonic. An isoosmolar solution of urea will not be isotonic because urea rapidly diffuses into the erythrocytes.

Acids, Bases, and Buffers

Acids and Bases

Acids are substances that when dissolved in water and they dissociate, they increase the hydrogen (H^+) concentration in the water. Bases are substances that dissociate and can accept or combine with H^+ ions (thus removing them from solution). The concentration of H^+ ions in a solution is represented by the pH of the solution, where

$$pH = -\log_{10}[H^+] \qquad (B.9)$$

The pH inside cells is a powerful determinant of the activity of all enzymes; hence, it is critical that the body regulate pH so that it is maintained at a level that is compatible with normal physiologic function.

Buffers

The pH of a solution can be maintained at near constant levels with the help of buffers. Most body buffers comprise weak acids [HA] with their conjugate bases [NaA]. By the law of mass action:

$$k = \frac{[H^+][A^-]}{[HA]} \qquad (B.10)$$

where k is the dissociation constant.

$$[H]^+ = k \times \frac{[HA]}{[A^-]}$$

$$-\log[H^+] = -\log k - \log\frac{[HA]}{[A^-]}$$

$$pH = pk + \log\frac{[A^-]}{[HA]} \qquad (B.11)$$

The above equation is known as the *Henderson–Hasselbalch* equation.

The *buffering power* of the system is the number of moles of acid or base that must be added to 1 mole of the buffer to change its pH by 1 unit. The maximum buffering power of any buffer is 0.575. The buffering power of a buffer is maximal when the pH of the solution is identical with that of the pK value (**Fig. B.5**), that is when pH = pK, $[A^-]$ = [HA]. It also depends on the concentration of the buffer.

Chemical Equilibrium

All chemical reactions are potentially reversible, but they tend to proceed unidirectionally if one of the reactants or products is removed from the locale of the reaction. Consider the reaction shown below.

$$CO_2 + H_2O \xleftarrow{\underset{\text{anhydrase}}{\text{Carbonic}}} H_2CO_3 \leftrightarrow H^+ + HCO_3^-$$

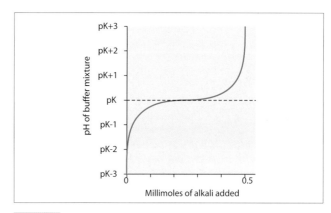

Fig. B.5 The titration curve of a buffer mixture with alkali. The buffering power is maximum at a pH that is equal to the pK.

The reaction will proceed in the forward direction (left to right) if at least one of the products is quickly removed, e.g., if the H^+ is buffered. On the other hand, if the carbon dioxide (CO_2) escapes from the reaction mixture, the reaction will proceed in the backward direction (right to left).

Chemical Constituents of Living Organisms

Water
The human body is 50 to 60% water, of which 60% is found inside the cells (intracellular water) and 40% is found between the cells (extracellular water).

Inorganic Solutes
Dissolved in the body's water are a very large number of solutes, some organic molecules (see below) and the others inorganic ions such a sodium (Na^+), potassium (K^+), chloride (Cl^-), bicarbonate (HCO_3^-), etc. The concentration of these inorganic solutes differs in intracellular and extracellular water and these differences are the result of biologic processes. In turn, these concentration differences drive important physiologic processes.

Organic Molecules
The molecules that make up living organisms all contain carbon atoms in some form. Although it was long believed that only living organisms could make certain compounds (one expression of the now discredited principle of vitalism), we now know that organic compounds behave like all other compounds found in nature.

Carbohydrates are molecules made up of carbon, oxygen, and hydrogen atoms (**Fig. B.6A**). They have the general formula (CH_2O)$_n$. Glucose, a simple sugar or monosaccharide, has the formula $C_6H_{12}O_6$ or (CH_2O)$_6$. Other simple sugars include fructose and galactose, which have the same formula but different structures. Monosaccharides can be combined into disaccharides (sucrose and lactose are examples) and into still larger molecules (polysaccharides). One particular important polysaccharide is glycogen.

Carbohydrates play many roles in living organisms. They make up an important component of the structure of the organism. Carbohydrates also play a key role in the storage, transportation, and generation of the energy used by the organism for all its work.

Fats (lipids) are also made up of carbon, hydrogen, and oxygen (**Fig. B.6B**). They are a diverse group of compounds that share several important properties. One such property is that they are not very soluble in water as they are nonpolar compounds. They are typically made up of a three-carbon molecule called glycerol and long-chain molecules called fatty acids. The number of fatty acids vary, with some lipids having only one fatty acid, whereas others are diglycerides or triglycerides (most common in the body).

Lipids have many, diverse roles in the body. One important category of hormones is lipids and all derive from cholesterol. Cell membranes are made of a variety of lipids (with imbedded proteins; see Chapter 2). Lipids are stored in adipose cells and represent the major storage form of energy to be used in powering the body.

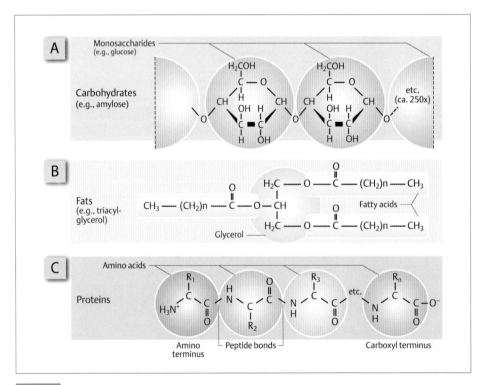

Fig. B.6 The major organic constituents of the body. **(A)** Carbohydrates, **(B)** fats, **(C)** proteins.

Proteins are molecules made up of a small number of components pieces, amino acids. Amino acids contain carbon, hydrogen, oxygen, nitrogen, and in some cases sulfur (**Fig. B.6C**). A protein is a molecule made up of a sequence of varying numbers of amino acids (proteins composed of only a small number of amino acids are sometimes referred to as peptides).

A protein is defined, in part, by this sequence of amino acids; this is referred to as the primary structure of a protein.

Hydrogen bonds between amino acids give rise to the secondary structure of a protein: the protein can "fold" into a sheet, or an α helix, or a random coil as result of the hydrogen bonds. The tertiary structure arises from interactions between parts of the protein molecule. For example, a helical protein may fold itself into a spherical structure. Finally, some proteins have a quaternary structure in which several polypeptides associate themselves in very specific ways. It is important

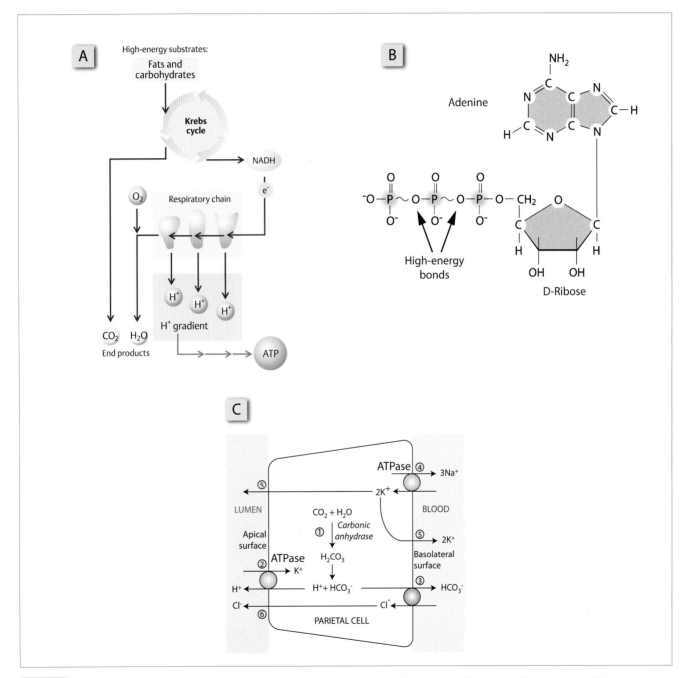

Fig. B.7 The storage of energy in high-energy phosphate bonds and the release of this energy in the body. **(A)** ATP is produced by several metabolic pathways, including the oxidation of fats and carbohydrates illustrated here. **(B)** Adenosine triphosphate (ATP) is a nucleotide containing two high-energy phosphate bonds. **(C)** One example of the use of ATP to do work in a cell. The hydrogen–potassium (H^+–K^+) exchanger and the sodium–potassium (Na^+–K^+) pump contain adenosine triphosphatase (ATPase), an enzyme that breaks one of the high-energy phosphate bonds, freeing energy to be used in moving solutes against their concentration gradients.

to remember that the structure of a protein plays an important role in determining its function. Conversely, proteins whose secondary, tertiary or quaternary structures are incorrectly formed either cannot carry out their normal function or they carry out functions with pathologic consequences.

Proteins serve many functions in the body. Proteins function as organic catalysts or enzymes, facilitating specific chemical reactions in the cell. Proteins are also an essential component of all cell membranes, serving as channels, transporters, and receptors. Finally, proteins make up the bulk of our muscles and the interaction between two proteins, actin and myosin, is what allows muscles to produce shortening or generate a force.

Nucleic acids (see **Fig. 3.1**) are complex molecules made up of nucleotides, complex molecules made up of a ring shaped base molecule, a sugar, and a phosphate. DNA (deoxyribonucleic acid) and RNA (ribonucleic acid) are large, information containing molecules with very special structures that are essential features of their function. DNA is found in the nucleus of cells and contains the genetic information describing that organism. RNA, which is derived from the organism's DNA, is found mainly in the cytoplasm and contains the information used to build proteins (enzymes). The smallest nucleotide, ATP (adenosine triphosphate) is used to store and transport energy to be used by every cell (see below).

Storage of Chemical Energy in Living Systems

The direct oxidation of fats and carbohydrates yields energy, but in a form that makes it difficult for a cell to capture and use; most of the energy released would be lost as heat (not usable by the cell and potentially damaging to it). Thus, the metabolism of glucose is performed in a stepwise process, with small amounts of energy being released at each step. This energy is used to create high-energy bonds in a compound call ATP, or adenosine triphosphate (**Fig. B.7A**). ATP is an RNA nucleotide made up of a ribose ring and an adenosine base (**Fig. B.7B**). Attached to the ribose are three phosphate groups. Energy is required to attach each phosphate; hence, ATP carries chemical energy that can be released and used to power all the processes of the cell (**Fig. B.7C**). Hydrolysis of the terminal phosphate yields ADP, adenosine diphosphate, an inorganic phosphate group, and energy that can be used to do the work of the cell.

Appendix C Abbreviations Used in Text

ACh	acetylcholine		ER	endoplasmic reticulum
AChE	acetylcholinesterase		ERV	expiratory reserve volume
AChR	acetylcholine receptor		FFA	free fatty acid
ACTH	adrenocorticotrophic hormone		FRC	functional residual capacity
ADH	antidiuretic hormone		FSH	follicle-stimulating hormone
ADP	adenosinediphosphate		FVC	forced vital capacity
ANS	autonomic nervous system		GABA	gamma-aminobutyric acid
ATP	adenosine triphosphate		gAMP	cyclic guanosine monophosphate
ATPase	adenosine triphosphatase		GFR	glomerular filtration rate
ATS	ascending thin segment		GH	growth hormone
AV	atrioventricular		GHRH	growth hormone-releasing hormone
AVP	arginine vasopressin		GIP	glucose-dependent insulinotropic peptide
BER	basic electrical rhythm			or gastric inhibitory peptide
BMR	basal metabolic rate		GLUT	glucose transporter
BUN	blood urea nitrogen		GnRH	gonadotropic-releasing hormone
cAMP	cyclic adenosine monophosphate		GRP	gastrin-releasing polypeptide
CBC	complete blood count		HCG	human chorionic gonadotropin
CBF	cerebral blood flow		HCS	human chorionic somatomammotropin
CCD	cortical collecting duct		HCT	human chorionic thyrotropin
CCK	cholecystokinin		HDL	high-density lipoprotein
CD	collecting duct		HPL	human placental lactogen
CNS	central nervous system		ICF	intracellular fluid
COMT	catechol-O-methyltransferase		IDDM	insulin-dependent diabetes mellitus
COPD	chronic obstructive pulmonary disease		IF	intrinsic factor
CRH	corticotrophin-releasing hormone		IGF	insulin-like growth factor
CTAL	cortical thick ascending limb		IMCD	inner medullary collecting duct
CVP	central venous pressure		INR	international normalized ratio (prothrom-
DAG	diacylglycerol			bin time)
DBP	diastolic blood pressure		IP3	inositol triphosphate
DCT	distal convoluted tubule		IPSP	inhibitory postsynaptic potential
DHEA	dehydroepiandrosterone		IRV	inspiratory reserve volume
DHEAS	dehydroepiandrosterone sulfate		JG	juxtaglomerular
DHT	dihydrotestosterone		LDL	low-density lipoprotein
DIT	diiodotyrosine		LES	lower esophageal sphincter
dL	deciliter (100 mL)		LH	luteinizing hormone
DL	diffusing capacity of lungs		MAO	monoamine oxidase
DNA	deoxyribonucleic acid		MBC	maximum breathing capacity
2,3-DPG	2,3-diphosphoglycerate		MCHC	mean corpuscular hemoglobin
DST	distal straight tubule			concentration
ECF	extracellular fluid		MCV	mean corpuscular volume
ECG	electrocardiogram		MEPP	miniature endplate potential
Em	membrane potential		MIS	müllerian inhibiting substance
EMG	electromyogram		MIT	monoiodotyrosine
EPP	endplate potential		mRNA	messenger ribonucleic acid
EPSP	excitatory postsynaptic potential		MSH	melanocyte-stimulating hormone

MTAL	medullary thick ascending limb
MVV	maximum voluntary ventilation
NIDDM	noninsulin-dependent diabetes mellitus
OMCD	outer medullary collecting duct
PAH	para-aminohippuric acid
PCT	proximal convoluted tubule
PEFR	peak expiratory flow rate
PG	prostaglandin
PIF	prolactin inhibitory factor
PK	protein kinase
POMC	pro-opiomelanocortin
PST	proximal straight tubule
PT	prothrombin time
PTH	parathyroid hormone
PTT	partial thromboplastin time
RBF	renal blood flow
RMP	resting membrane potential
RMV	respiratory minute volume
RNA	ribonucleic acid
RQ	respiratory quotient
RV	residual volume
SA	sinoatrial
SBP	systolic blood pressure
SGLT	sodium-dependent glucose transporters
SR	sacroplasmic reticulum
SRH	somatotropin-releasing hormone
SVC	slow vital capacity
T_3	triiodothyronine
T_4	thyroxine
TAL	thick ascending limb
TBA	thyroid-binding albumin
TBG	thyroid-binding globulin
TEPD	tubular electrical potential difference
TF/P	tubular fluid/plasma
TH	thyroid hormone (T_3 and T_4)
TLC	total lung capacity
TRH	thyrotropin-releasing hormone
TSH	thyroid-stimulating hormone
TXA	thromboxane A
VC	vital capacity
VIP	vasoactive intestinal polypeptide
VPRC	volume of packed red cells
V/Q	ventilation/perfusion
VT	tidal volume

Index

Note: Page numbers followed by *f* and *t* indicate figures and tables, respectively.

in exercise, 519
inhibition, 485
insulin and, 514–515, 514*f*
in red blood cells, 119–120, 119*f*
in starvation, 519, 519*f*
thyroid hormone and, 490
Glycoprotein(s), platelet, 145, 146, 147*f*
Glycosphingolipids, 9
Glycosuria, 398
renal, 403, 404*f*
GnRH. *See* Gonadotropin-releasing hormone
(GnRH)
Goblet cells
bronchial, 291, 292*f*
intestinal, 442
Goiter
cabbage, 490
definition, 490
euthyroid, 491
hypothyroid, 491
hypothyroid iodide, 490
Goitrin, 490
Goitrogens, 490
Goldman equation, 34, 36, 58
Golgi apparatus, 3, 3*f*, 4, 4*f*
cis (convex) side, 4
trans (concave) side, 4, 5
Golgi body, neuronal, 29*f*
Gonad(s), bipotential (undifferentiated),
555, 555*f*, 557*f*
Gonadal hormones, 476*t*
Gonadal sex, 555
differentiation, 555, 555*f*
Gonadotropin-independent precocity, 538
Gonadotropin-releasing hormone (GnRH),
476*t*, 481
actions (physiologic effects), 533, 544
as neurotransmitter, in autonomic
neurotransmission, 67*t*
and puberty, 537
secretion, 533
Gout, 5
G protein(s), 475, 477, 478*f*
inhibitory (G$_i$), 477, 479*f*
stimulatory (G$_s$), 477, 479*f*
Graded potential(s), 41, 41*t*
and action potentials, comparison, 41,
41*t*
Gram-negative bacteria, and disseminated
intravascular coagulation, 155
Granular casts, 398, 398*f*
Granular cells, renal. *See* Juxtaglomerular
cells
Granulocyte(s), 157–161
formation, 130, 131*f*, 132
segmented neutrophilic, 157*f*
Granuloma(s), 168, 169
Granulomere, platelet, 145
Granulosa cell(s), 534, 534*f*
Graves disease, 169*t*, 491–492
Gravindex test, 562, 562*f*
Gravitation, Newton's law of, 572

Gravitational force(s), 572
Gravity
acceleration due to, 572
and alveolar compliance, 316–317, 317*f*
and alveolar perfusion, 318
and alveolar ventilation, 316–317, 317*f*
and central venous pressure, 207
effect on circulation, 221–222, 221*f*
and intrapleural pressure, 317, 317*f*
and pulmonary circulation, 261–262,
262*f*
Gray-out, 222
Gray rami communicantes, 64, 64*f*
Growth, glucocorticoids and, 505
Growth hormone (GH), 476*t*, 484–485
actions (physiologic effects), 484–485
anabolic effects, 484
antiinsulin effects, 484–485
and carbohydrate metabolism, 484–485
deficiency, 485
disorders, 485
and fat metabolism, 484–485
hypersecretion, 485
hyposecretion, 485
insulin-like effects, 485
and insulin secretion, 514
lipolytic effects, 484–485
mechanism of action, 479–480, 479*f*
metabolic effects, 484–485
and protein metabolism, 484
renal effects, 484
secretion, 483, 483*f*, 484
cortisol and, 505
inhibition by somatostatin, 516
regulation, 484, 484*f*
stimuli for, 484
and skeletal growth, 484
Growth spurt, pubertal, 537, 537*f*
GRP. *See* Gastrin-releasing peptide (GRP)
GSR. *See* Galvanic skin resistance (GSR)
G-suit, 222
GTP. *See* Guanosine triphosphate (GTP)
GTT. *See* Glucose tolerance test (GTT)
Guanine (G), 17, 17*f*
Guanosine diphosphate (GDP), 475, 478*f*
Guanosine triphosphate (GTP), 475, 478*f*
in protein synthesis, 18–19
Guanylin, actions (physiologic effects), 450
Guanylyl cyclase, 475, 477, 477*t*, 478*f*
cytosolic, 477
membrane, 477
Gums (plant fiber), 424
Gz. *See* Apparent G

H

Haldane effect, 323–324, 324*f*
Halothane, adverse effects and side effects.
See Malignant hyperthermia
Hapten(s), 175
definition, 166
properties, 166

Haptocorrin, 138
Haptoglobin, 116, 128
Hartnup disease, 443
Hashimoto disease, 169*t*, 492
Haustra, 446
Haversian canals, 494, 495*f*
Hay fever, 169
Hb. *See* Hemoglobin
H-band, in muscle, 77, 77*f*, 82, 82*f*
HCG. *See* Human chorionic gonadotropin
(hCG)
hCS. *See* Human chorionic
somatomammotropin
HDL. *See* High-density lipoproteins (HDL)
Headache–post-lumbar puncture, 258
Heart. *See also* Cardiac
circulatory load on, 204–205
energy for, 251
hypereffective, 205
hypoeffective, 205
instantaneous electrical axis, 187
parasympathetic innervation, 234
pump function, 205
vascular factors and, 206–207
response to autonomic nerve impulses,
65*t*
response to circulating catecholamines,
65*t*
sympathetic innervation, 234
work done by, 219–220
Heart murmur(s), 199–200, 199*f*
in anemia, 121
Heart rate, 237
autonomic effects on, 103
effect on cardiac cycle, 199*t*, 200
response to Valsalva maneuver, 67
Heart sounds, 197*f*, 198–199
loud, 199
split, 199
Heat
definition, 576
flow, 576, 576*f*
muscle, 83–84
transfer, 576–577, 576*f*
by conduction, 576–577
by convection, 576–577
by radiation, 576–577
Heat exhaustion, 275
Heat loss
from body
nonevaporative, 273
scalp and, 272
insensible, 273
Heat stroke, 275
Heavy meromyosin (HMM), 77, 78*f*
Helicobacter pylori infection, 454
Helium-dilution (closed circuit) method, for
FRC estimation, 308, 309*f*
Hematinic factor(s), 134–140
definition, 134
Hematocrit (Hct), 119
Hematuria, 397

structure, 174, 175*f*
synthesis, 116
variable regions, 174
Immunologic memory, 166
Immunomodulation, 167–168
Immunosuppressant(s)
chemical, 168
physical, 168
Immunosuppression, therapeutic, 168
antibody-mediated, 168
antigen-induced, 168
nonspecific, 168
specific, 168
Immunotherapy
nonspecific, 167
specific, 167
Immunotoxin(s), 167
Implantation, 551, 553*f*
central, 551
interstitial, 551
Importins, 3
Incentive spirometry, 307
Incisura, 198, 199*f*
Indifferent electrode, 187
Infant respiratory distress syndrome, 304
Infection(s). *See also* Urinary tract
infection(s) (UTI)
susceptibility to, in nephrotic syndrome,
403
Inferior hypophysial artery, 482, 482*f*
Infertility, 547, 550, 557, 564
Inflammation
acute, hyperproteinemia in, 116
chronic, hypoproteinemia in, 116
corticosteroids for, 508–509
definition, 166
glucocorticoids and, 505
pathophysiology, 166
signs, 166
treatment, 508–509
Inhibin, 538
actions (physiologic effects), 533, 536,
536*f*
synthesis, 533*f*
Inhibitory postsynaptic potential (IPSP),
60–61, 61*f*
in autonomic neurotransmission, 67, 67*t*
and excitatory postsynaptic potential
comparison, 61*t*
summation, 61, 61*f*
Initial heat, of muscle, 84
Initial segment, 61, 61*f*
of axon, 29, 29*f*
Initial spike, 61, 61*f*
Initiation, of translation, 18–19, 18*f*
Inner membrane, mitochondrial, 4, 4*f*
Innervation ratio, of motor unit, 88
Innervation zone, of muscle, 88, 88*f*
Inorganic phosphate (P$_i$), in muscle
contraction, 81–82, 81*f*
Inositol triphosphate (IP$_3$), as second
messenger, 475, 477, 477*t*, 479*f*

Inotropic effects, 234
Insemination, 549
Inspiration
accessory muscles of, 294, 295
chest wall changes during, 294, 294*f*
muscles of, 294–295
Inspiratory capacity, 307*f*, 308
factors affecting, 310, 310*f*
Inspiratory off-switch neurons, 325–326,
326*f*
Inspiratory reserve volume, 307–308, 307*f*
Insulin, 476*t*
actions (physiologic effects), 13, 437,
480, 514–515
in absorptive state, 517, 517*f*, 518*f*
in postabsorptive state, 518
anticipatory secretion of, 452, 452*f*
antilipolytic actions, 514*f*, 515, 517, 518*f*
antinatriuretic effect, 515
and blood glucose levels, 514–515, 514*f*
and carbohydrate metabolism, 514–515,
517, 517*f*
deficiency, 520, 520*t*
and electrolyte balance, 515
and fat metabolism, 515, 517, 518*f*
formation, 513, 513*f*
hypokalemic action, 515
lipogenic actions, 514*f*, 515, 517, 518*f*
mechanism of action, 479–480, 479*f*
and membrane hyperpolarization, 515
metabolic effects, 514–515, 514*f*
and potassium balance, 515
and protein metabolism, 515, 517, 518*f*
secretion, 449
epinephrine and, 516
exercise and, 519
inhibition by pancreatic polypeptide,
516*f*, 517
inhibition by somatostatin, 516, 516*f*
regulation, 23, 481, 481*f*, 513–514
structure, 513*f*
therapy with, in diabetes, 522
Insulin-like growth factor(s), 476*t*, 514. *See
also* Somatomedin
cortisol and, 505
mechanism of action, 479–480, 479*f*
Insulin receptor(s), 479–480
Insulin resistance, 520, 520*t*
Integrator neurons, 326, 326*f*
Integrin(s), platelet, 145
Interatrial bundle(s), cardiac, 185, 185*f*
Interatrial pathway(s), cardiac, conduction
velocity, 186*t*
Intercalated cell(s), renal, 361*f*, 362
intercalated disks, 76
Intercellular junction(s), 7–8, 7*f*
Intercostal muscle(s)
external, 295, 295*f*
innervation, 327
internal, 295, 295*f*
Intercristal (intermembrane) space, 4, 4*f*
Interferon(s) (IFN), IFN-g, functions, 176

Interleukin(s) (IL), 131
IL-1, 176
IL-2, functions, 176
IL-4, 176
IL-5, 176
IL-6, 176
Interlobar artery(ies), renal, 357–358, 357*f*
Interlobar vein(s), renal, 358
Interlobular artery(ies), renal, 357–358,
357*f*
Interlobular vein(s), renal, 358
Intermediate filaments, 5, 6, 7, 79
Intermediolateral cells, 234, 239
Intermediomedial cells, 234, 239
Internal carotid artery(ies), 255, 255*f*
Internal genitalia, differentiation, 556, 556*f*,
557*f*
International standardized ratio (INR), 154
Internodal atrial pathways, 186
Internodal bundles, cardiac, 185, 185*f*
Interoreceptors, 54, 55*t*
Interpeduncular cistern, 257, 257*f*
Interstitial cells of Cajal (ICC), 429
Interstitial fluid, 114
Interstitial lung disease, 343, 343*f*
Interstitial oncotic pressure, increased, in
edema, 228–229
Interventricular septum, 196
cardiac, 185*f*
Intestinal blood flow, 267–268. *See also*
Mesenteric circulation
Intestinal brush border, digestive functions
of, 442
Intestinal obstruction, 454–455
Intestinal transit, disorders, 454–455
Intestinal villi
blood flow in, 267–268, 268*f*
countercurrent exchange in, 267–268,
268*f*
Intestine(s)
response to autonomic nerve impulses,
65*t*
response to circulating catecholamines,
65*t*
Intestinointestinal reflex, 442
Intracellular fluid (ICF), 114, 114*f*
osmolarity, 377, 377*f*
volume, 377, 377*f*
calculation, 114
measurement, indicators for, 114, 114*t*
Intracranial pressure, elevated, 259
and vomiting, 454
Intracranial temperature, 271
Intracytoplasmic sperm injection (ICSI), 553
Intraembryonic mesoderm, 552*f*, 559
Intraesophageal pressure, 301, 302*f*
Intrapleural pressure, 300, 301, 302*f*
changes during breathing, 302, 302*f*
gravity and, 317, 317*f*
Intrapulmonary pressure, 297–298, 301
changes during breathing, 302
forced, 301–302

Osteoid, 494
  mineralization, calcitriol and, 499
Osteomalacia, 422t, 495–496, 496f, 500
Osteon, 494, 495f
Osteonectin, 494
Osteopenia, in hyperparathyroidism, 500
Osteopetrosis, 496, 496f
Osteoporosis, 495
  cortisol-induced, 505
  disuse, 495
  involutional, 495
Osteosclerosis, 496
Ouabain, mechanism of action, 13
Outer membrane, mitochondrial, 4, 4f
Ovarian cycle, 543, 543f, 545, 545f
  estrogenic phase, 543–544
  follicular phase, 544, 545f
  luteal phase, 545, 545f
Ovarian hormones, 534–536
  effects on uterine smooth muscle, 101,
    535, 536
Ovary
  endocrine cells, 534
  fetal development, 555, 555f
  hormonal control of, 536, 536f
  hormones, 534–536
Ovulation, 541, 541f, 544
  hormonal control of, 544, 544f
  tests for, 544
  timing, in menstrual cycle, 543, 543f
Ovum (pl., ova), 540
  activation, 550
Oxaloacetate, in Krebs cycle, 467, 467f
Oxygen (O$_2$), 286
  arterial, partial pressure, regulation, 22t,
    330, 331f
  in arterial blood, 321t
  coefficient of utilization, 321, 322t
  consumption
    cardiac, 358
    renal, 358
  content, in arterial and venous blood,
    summary, 324f
  delivery to tissues, 321, 322t, 324f
  diffusion across respiratory membrane,
    318–319
  diffusion capacity for, measurement,
    319–320
  dissolved in plasma, 321, 321f
  hepatic supply, 269
  hyperbaric, 321, 333
  in intestinal villi, 268, 268f
  partial pressure, 321
    alveolar, 308, 316
    in arterial blood, 324f, 329
      regulation, 22t, 330, 331f
    in lungs, 324f
    in tissue, 324f
    in venous blood, 324f
  transport
    in blood, 321–322
    in tissue, 322–323

uptake from lung, 324f
in venous blood, 321t
Oxygen (O$_2$) dissociation curve
  of hemoglobin, 321–322, 323f
    acute versus chronic acidosis and, 322
    in exercise, 322
    shifts in, 322, 322f
    shift to right, at high altitude, 337t, 338
  of myoglobin, 322–323, 323f
Oxygen (O$_2$) therapy
  for hypoxia, 333
  for shock, 250
Oxygen (O$_2$) toxicity, 333
Oxyhemoglobin, 124–125, 321, 321f
Oxyntic cells. See Parietal cells
Oxytocin, 476t
  actions (physiologic effects), 564, 566,
    566f
  and milk letdown, 566, 566f
  and parturition, 565
  secretion, 484, 564
    regulation, 481, 481f
  synthesis, 564

P

PABA. See p-Aminobenzoic acid (PABA)
Pacemaker cells, gastrointestinal, 429
Pacemaker potentials
  in cardiac muscle, 103, 103f
    ionic basis, 103, 103f
  in smooth muscle, 100, 101f
    spikes in, 100, 101f
Paclitaxel, mechanism of action, 5
Pain, visceral, and vomiting, 454
Palpitation(s), in anemia, 121
PAM. See Pulmonary alveolar macrophages
Pancreas
  endocrine, 436
    functions, 513
  exocrine, 436
    deficiency, 455
  hormones, 476t
  response to autonomic nerve impulses,
    66t
  response to circulating catecholamines,
    66t
Pancreatic duct(s), 435f
Pancreatic function tests, 439–441
Pancreatic islet cells, 513, 513f
  α, 22t, 23, 513, 513f
  β, 513, 513f
  D cells, 513, 513f
  F cells, 513, 513f
  hypothalamic regulation of, 481, 481f
Pancreatic juice, 436–437
  analysis, 439–440
  constituents, 436
  enzymes in, activity, 437–439
  pH, 436
  secretion, 436
    cephalic phase, 436–437

intestinal phase, 436–437
  rate of, and ion concentration in, 436,
    437f
  regulation, 436–437
  volume, 436
Pancreatic polypeptide (PP)
  actions (physiologic effects), 517
  secretion, 513, 517
Pancreozymin, 449
Panhypopituitarism, 485
Pantothenic acid
  deficiency, 421t
  dietary sources, 421t
  functions, 421t
Papain, immunoglobulin splitting by, 174
Papilla, renal, 357
Papillary muscles, 196, 196f
Papilledema, 257, 259
Para-aminohippuric acid
  for measurement of renal blood flow, 223
  renal clearance
    as function of plasma concentration,
      393, 393f, 396f
    renal plasma flow and, 393–394
  renal handling of, 365, 365f, 367, 387
Parafollicular cells, thyroid, 487
Parallel elastic component (PEC), of muscle,
  91, 92f
Parasympathetic nervous system, 63–64,
  63f
  anatomy, 63f, 64
  functions, 64
  ganglia, 64
  postganglionic neurons, 64
  preganglionic neurons, 64
Parathyroid gland(s), 497, 497f
Parathyroid hormone (PTH), 476t, 494,
  497–498
  actions (physiologic effects), 388,
    497–498
  and calcitonin secretion, 498f
  and calcium balance (homeostasis), 388,
    497
  deficiency, 499
  excess, 500
  and phosphate balance (homeostasis),
    388, 497–498, 498f
  phosphaturic effect, 497
  secretion, in hypoparathyroidism,
    499–500, 500t
  and vitamin D synthesis, 499, 499f
Parathyroid hormone-related protein
  (PTHrP), 497
Paraventricular nucleus, 482f, 483–484
Parietal cells, 430, 431f
Paroxysmal supraventricular tachycardia,
  193, 194f
Partial pressure
  of carbon dioxide (CO$_2$)
    alveolar, 308, 316
    in arterial blood, 324f, 329
    regulation, 22t, 330, 331f

as osmotic diuretic, mechanism of action, 370
plasma. *See also* Blood urea nitrogen
  in chronic renal failure, 404
  factors affecting, 374
  as renal function indicator, 396
recycling, renal, 373*f*, 374, 386, 387*f*
renal handling of, 365–366, 386
transmembrane transport, 11
Urea clearance, 394
Urea cycle, 474, 474*f*
Urea-transport protein, 374, 386
Ureter(s)
  response to autonomic nerve impulses, 66*t*
  response to circulating catecholamines, 66*t*
Uric acid, renal handling of, 386–387, 387*f*
Uric acid crystals, in urine, 398
Uridine diphosphate (UDP) glucuronic acid, 126–127
Uridine diphosphoglucose, 470, 470*f*
Uridine triphosphate, 470, 470*f*
Urinary bladder
  accommodation, testing, 409
  capacity, testing, 409
  contractions, testing, 409
  motor innervation, 407, 407*t*
  mucous membrane epithelium, 406
  neuropathic, 408–409
  pain, 406*f*, 407
  parasympathetic innervation, 407, 407*t*
  response to autonomic nerve impulses, 66*t*
  response to circulating catecholamines, 66*t*
  sensations, testing, 409
  sensory innervation, 406–407, 406*f*
  smooth muscle, 406
  somatic motor innervation, 407, 407*t*
  sympathetic innervation, 407, 407*t*
  voluntary control of, 407, 408
   testing, 409
  wall, muscular coat, 406
Urinary sphincter(s), 406
  external, 406, 406*f*, 406*t*
  internal, 406, 406*f*, 406*t*
Urinary tract
  motor innervation, 407, 407*t*
  sensory innervation, 406–407, 406*f*
Urinary tract infection(s) (UTI), 397, 398
Urine
  alkaline, 397
  analysis, 397–398
  bilirubin in, 398
  casts
   cellular, 398, 398*f*
   noncellular, 398, 398*f*
  chemical analysis, 397–398
  chromatography, 396
  cloudy, 397, 397*t*
  color, 397, 397*t*
   in hemoglobinemia, 129

concentration, 357
crystals in, 398
formation, 354
heme pigments in, 398
ketones in, 398
microscopic examination, 398, 398*f*
nitrites in, 398
normal volume, 397
osmolarity, 397
  plasma osmolarity and, 376, 377*f*
  renal mechanisms determining, 372–374
output, factors affecting, 364, 364*f*, 366
physical examination, 397
proteins in, 397. *See also* Proteinuria
specific gravity, 396
  normal, 397
sugars in, 398
turbidity, 397, 397*t*
Urine anion gap, 402
Urobilin(s), 126*f*, 127, 448
Urobilinogen, 448
  excretion, 127
  formation, 126*f*, 127
Urobilinogen excretion, 398
Urodynamic studies, 409
Uroporphyrobilinogen-III, in hemoglobin synthesis, 124, 124*f*
Uterine cycle, 543, 543*f*, 545, 545*f*
  menstrual phase, 544
  proliferative phase, 544
Uterine tubes, fetal development, 556, 556*f*
Uterotonins, 565
Uterus. *See also* Endometrium; Myometrium
  fetal development, 556, 556*f*
  response to autonomic nerve impulses, 66*t*
  response to circulating catecholamines, 66*t*
  smooth muscle, ovarian hormones and, 101
Utrophin, 79

V

Vagina
  estrogens and, 535
  fetal development, 556, 556*f*
Vaginal cycle, 543, 543*f*, 544, 545
Vagus nerve, 64, 425
  and gastric secretion, 433
  and insulin secretion, 514
  and pancreatic secretion, 437
  and respiratory function, 290–291
Valsalva maneuver, 301
  blood pressure changes during, 241, 241*f*
  heart rate response to, 67
  and syncope, 257
Valsalva ratio, 67
Vanilloid receptor, 54
Vanillylmandelic acid (VMA), 511*f*, 514–515
Van't Hoff relationship, 581–582

Varicocele, 540
Vasa recta, 358
  countercurrent exchange in, 372, 374, 374*f*
Vascular disorders, 153, 154
  bleeding in, clinical features, 155*t*
  tests for, 153
Vascular function curve(s), 208*f*, 209, 209*f*
Vascular system, 214–215, 217*f*
  reservoir function, 214
Vas deferens, fetal development, 556, 556*f*
Vasectomy, 554
Vasoactive intestinal peptide (VIP), 232, 430, 449
  actions (physiologic effects), 442, 450, 450*f*
  excess, 456
  and respiratory function, 290–291
  and salivary secretion, 428
Vas-occlusive plugs, 554
Vasoconstriction
  cutaneous, 265, 272
  hypoxic, 263
Vasoconstrictor(s), 230
  circulating, 232–233
Vasodilatation
  cold, 265
  flow-induced, 230–231, 230*f*
  heat loss from, 273
  in immune response, 173
  poststenotic, 230–231, 230*f*
Vasodilator(s), 230
  circulating, 232
  for myocardial ischemia, 253
  sympathetic fiber, in muscle, 267, 267*f*
Vasomotor center, 234, 239
Vasooclusive crisis, in sickle cell anemia, 126
Vasopressin, 232
Vasovagal syncope, 256
VC. *See* Vital capacity
V$_D$. *See* Anatomic dead space
Vectorcardiography, 187
Vein(s), 215, 217*f*
  systemic
   response to autonomic nerve impulses, 65*t*
   response to circulating catecholamines, 65*t*
Venous pooling, 221, 241, 241*f*, 241*t*
Venous pumping, 207
Venous return, 207
Venous valves, 215, 217*f*, 218*f*
Ventilation, 286. *See also* Alveolar ventilation; Pulmonary ventilation
  assisted, 304–305, 305*f*
Ventilation–perfusion mismatch, in chronic obstructive pulmonary disease, 342
Ventilation–perfusion ratio, 316, 316*f*, 318, 318*f*
Ventilatory capacity, 313–314
Ventilatory support, 304–305, 305*f*